# European Manual of Medicine

**Series Editors**

W. Arnold, Munich, Bayern, Germany
U. Ganzer, Düsseldorf, Nordrhein-Westfalen, Germany

Presenting state-of-the-art procedures in all clinical medicine disciplines, the European Manual of Medicine book series aims to educate postgraduate students and residents in accordance with the U.E.M.S. charter on training medical specialists in the European Union. Each volume is a comprehensive reference devoted to a specific discipline, and the editors are internationally renowned specialists from different European Countries. The contents cover both diagnostic and therapeutic methods which are subdivided into essential procedures (those that are commonly employed in all European countries) and helpful procedures (which might be of further interest as well). The reader-friendly layout allows quick retrieval of information, and concise checklists and algorithms throughout each volume clearly present the pathway from patient complaint to diagnosis. This text book series is ideal for any practitioner in the European Union looking to gain a thorough understanding of the latest procedures in their field of interest. The European Union of Medical Specialists (U.E.M.S.) represents national associations of medical specialists in the European Union and its associated countries. Active at the European level since 1958, the UEMS promotes the free movement of European medical specialists while ensuring the highest quality of medical care for European citizens. More information can be found online at: www.uems.net

Antoinette am Zehnhoff-Dinnesen
Antonio Schindler · Patrick G. Zorowka
Editors

# Phoniatrics III

Acquired Motor Speech and Language
Disorders – Dysphagia – Phoniatrics
and COVID-19

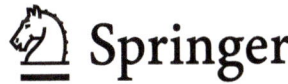

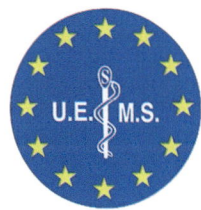

*Editors*
Antoinette am Zehnhoff-Dinnesen
Department of Phoniatrics and
Pedaudiology
University Hospital Münster
Münster, Germany

Patrick G. Zorowka
Department for Hearing, Voice and
Speech Disorders
Medical University Innsbruck
Innsbruck, Austria

Antonio Schindler
Luigi Sacco Hospital, Department of
Biomedical and Clinical Sciences
"L. Sacco", Phoniatrics
University of Milan
Milan, Italy

ISSN 2626-7845 ISSN 2626-7853 (electronic)
European Manual of Medicine
ISBN 978-3-031-48090-4 ISBN 978-3-031-48091-1 (eBook)
https://doi.org/10.1007/978-3-031-48091-1

This Springer imprint is published by the registered company Springer Nature Switzerland AG
The registered company address is: Gewerbestrasse 11, 6330 Cham, Switzerland

If disposing of this product, please recycle the paper.

# Foreword

The European Manual of Medicine (EMM) book series offers medical graduates and clinicians current state-of-the-art knowledge in accordance with the charter of the European Union of Medical Specialists (UEMS) in Brussels on training medical specialists in the European Union.

Like Volume "Phoniatrics I" (2020; ISBN 978-3-662-46780-0), which presents the topics Fundamentals, Voice Disorders, and Disorders of Language and Hearing Development, and Volume "Phoniatrics II," which covers the parts Dysglossia, Resonance Disorders, Velopharyngeal Insufficiency, Speech Fluency Disorders, Literacy Development Disorders, this volume "Phoniatrics III" offers phoniatric and ENT trainees, as well as members of related disciplines, a textbook/e-book of unique high quality.

"Phoniatrics III" includes the parts Acquired Motor Speech Disorders (Dysarthria, Dyspraxia), Acquired Language Disorders (Aphasia), Dysphagia, and Phoniatrics and COVID-19.

According to the principles of EMM, the established structure is used in addressing basics, special kinds of disorders, diagnosis/differential diagnosis, prevention, and rehabilitation/prognosis. Case studies, colour photos, tables, and supplementary audio and video samples, as well as detailed reference lists, provide a substantial amount of up-to-date information to the reader.

Antoinette am Zehnhoff-Dinnesen, as editor-in-chief (Münster, Germany), and the associated editors Antonio Schindler (Milan, Italy) and Patrick Zorowka (Innsbruck, Austria) have invited well-known, interdisciplinary experts from different countries to guarantee the excellent quality of this volume of the book series.

Special thanks go to Springer Nature, especially to Wilma McHugh, Daniela Heller, Timo Lange, Aruna Sharma, and Shanjini Rajasekaran for their precious help and assistance.

The signing series editors are extremely grateful for the work of all editors, but especially for the immense, untiring effort our friend and colleague, editor-in-chief, Antoinette am Zehnhoff-Dinnesen, has shown in creating this unique textbook.
Summer 2024

Munich, Germany                                                     Wolfgang Arnold
Lucerne, Switzerland
Düsseldorf, Germany                                                     Uwe Ganzer

# Preface

Volume III of the textbook *Phoniatrics* from the book series 'European Manual of Medicine', after Volume II with its 93 contributions, represents the final volume of a trilogy, providing the current basis for establishing high standards in patient care and improving training and education in phoniatrics. Although principally aimed at phoniatric and ENT trainees and specialised clinicians, it should also be of interest to medical students and physicians in specialties related to phoniatrics and to members of disciplines close to phoniatrics. This book provides guidance and internationally recognised standards in the current situation, where the extent and intensity of phoniatric training vary across different countries.

In addition to the complete textbook, individual e-chapters and e-books are also offered. To enhance understanding of the speciality, *Phoniatrics III* features, in 103 contributions, many colour photos, figures, tables, and case studies, often supplemented by audio and video samples. The aims of the book series are served by the majority of articles being written by more than one author, most of whom are from different countries. A total of 102 authors and co-authors contributed to this volume, representing 20 countries from four continents and 24 disciplines.

Whereas Volume I focused on the fundamentals of phoniatrics, voice disorders, and disorders of language and hearing development and Volume II highlighted dysglossia/resonance disorders/velopharyngeal insufficiency, speech fluency disorders, and literacy development disorders, Volume III illustrates acquired motor speech disorders (dysarthria, dyspraxia), acquired language disorders (aphasia), dysphagia, and phoniatrics and COVID-19. All these topics have been prepared according to the training programme and logbook *Medical Speech, Voice and Language Pathology, and Hearing and Swallowing Disorders* within the section Oto-Rhino-Laryngology of the European Union of Medical Specialists (UEMS) in Brussels.

We thank all authors and co-authors who invested their time and effort in this project, for their valuable contributions and crucial support.

Special thanks go to the external lectors who, in addition to the editors, provided in-depth research and analysis that significantly helped to achieve a high standard of knowledge transfer by their particular competence, proficiency, and expertise:

Enrico Alfonsi (Italy), Jacek Błeszyński (Poland), Jörg Bohlender (Switzerland), Francesca Bosco (Italy), Stefano Cappa (Italy), Melissa Catrini (Brazil), Sabine Crestani (France), Rémi Esclasson (France), Charles Ellis (USA), Daniele Farneti (Italy), Pascale Fichaux-Bourin (France), Simone Graf (Germany), Stefan Heim (Germany), Alexander Hemprich (Germany), Bibiána Hlebová (Slovakia), Irena Hočevar Boltežar (Slovenia), Michael Jungheim (Germany), Matti Lehtihalmes (Finland), Mari Markkanen-Leppänen (Finland), Rossella Muo (Italy), Tadeus Nawka (Germany), Karel Neubauer (Czech Republic), Lenka Neubauerova (Czech Republic), Arno Olthoff (Germany), Philippe Paquier (Belgium), Christina Pflug (Germany), Pirkko Rautakoski (Finland), Michel Rijntjes (Germany), Ilona Rubi-Fessen (Germany), John Rubin (United Kingdom), Uta Schick (Germany), Carola Schön (Germany), Heidrun Schröter-Morasch (Germany), André Smout (The Netherlands), Peter Sporns (Germany), Thomas Stamm (Germany), Miroslav Tedla (Slovakia), Rosemary Varley (United Kingdom), Darija Vranisek Bender (Croatia), Katarzyna Węsierska (Poland), Virginie Woisard (France), and Rachel Zeng (Germany).

The editors are much obliged and deeply grateful to the editors of the manual series, Wolfgang Arnold (Munich, Germany; Lucerne, Switzerland) and Uwe Ganzer (Düsseldorf, Germany), who initiated and decisively supported this important project.

Our special thanks go to Springer Nature, especially to Wilma McHugh, Daniela Heller, Timo Lange, Aruna Sharma, and Shanjini Rajasekaran for their substantial assistance and valuable advice.

The editors are deeply indebted to Dr. Trevor G. Cooper, lector for English language, for his excellent work and continued invaluable support as experienced scientist. His input decisively helped to complete this book.

We also thank Nicole Neptun for her work on some book parts, especially concerning the layout and the reference lists; Ross Parfitt for his diligent help in clarifying copyright questions; and Peter Matulat for his valuable support and advice in technical and IT matters.

To have a comprehensive textbook and e-book on phoniatrics in the English language is one keystone to provide an international basis of standards for improving training and education in this medical speciality. This activity supports the aim of the Union of the European Phoniatricians and the European Academy of Phoniatrics to establish a European Board Exam in Phoniatrics; we hope that *Phoniatrics III* will provide a comprehensive training tool for everyone interested in the field of communication disorders.

Summer 2024
Münster, Germany                                    Antoinette am Zehnhoff-Dinnesen
Milan, Italy                                                        Antonio Schindler
Innsbruck, Austria                                            Patrick G. Zorowka

# Contents

## Part V    Acquired Language Disorders (Aphasia)

## Part VI    Dysphagia

# About the Editors

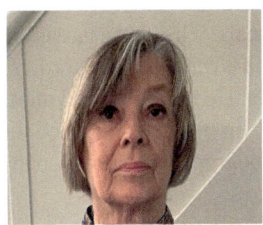

**Antoinette am Zehnhoff-Dinnesen** studied medical sciences in Düsseldorf and Bonn. In 1983, she became a medical specialist in ENT diseases, and in 1986, a medical specialist in phoniatrics and paedaudiology. In 1988, she gained her Habilitation from Düsseldorf University for her work on regulation of vocal amplitude and frequency during voice onset. In 1990, Dr. am Zehnhoff-Dinnesen was appointed Professor of Phoniatrics and Paedaudiology at the Medical Faculty of Philipps University in Marburg. The following year she became Professor at the Medical Faculty at the Westphalian Wilhelms University of Münster, where she was Head of the Clinic of Phoniatrics and Paedaudiology until her retirement in 2020. She is author or co-author of more than 160 original papers in German and English on various aspects of phoniatrics and paedaudiology and co-author of several books. Antoinette am Zehnhoff-Dinnesen is editor-in-chief of the book series European Manual of Medicine, Phoniatrics 1, 2 and 3. She has been both Secretary and President of the German Society of Phoniatrics and Paedaudiology, President of the Union of the European Phoniatricians (UEP), and has initiated and promoted the foundation of the European Academy of Phoniatrics as the founding director. She and her team have received several awards. Antoinette am Zehnhoff-Dinnesen is the honorary chairwoman of the Union of European Phoniatricians and an honorary member of the Polish Society of Otorhinolaryngologists and Head and Neck Surgeons, the Czech Society of Otorhinolaryngology and Head and Neck Surgery, the German Society of Phoniatrics and Paedaudiology, the European Academy of Phoniatrics, and the Confederation of German Hearing Screening Centres.

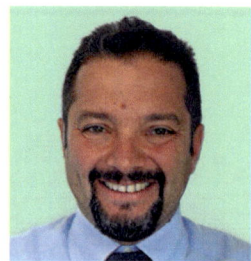

**Antonio Schindler** studied medicine at the University of Turin, Italy. He specialised in Phoniatrics in 2001 and in ENT in 2005. He is currently Head of the Phoniatric Unit at Sacco Hospital in Milan and Full Professor in Audiology at the University of Milan, where he Chairs the Bachelor degree in Speech and Language Pathology. He has chaired the Dysphagia Committee of the International Association of Logopaedics and Phoniatrics (IALP) and is General Secretary of the European Society for Swallowing Disorders. Dr. Schindler is an Associate Editor and reviewer for several international journals. His main areas of research include voice and swallowing disorders, child language, and aphasia. He has published more than 160 original articles in journals indexed in Scopus, in addition to monographs and book chapters in Italian and English.

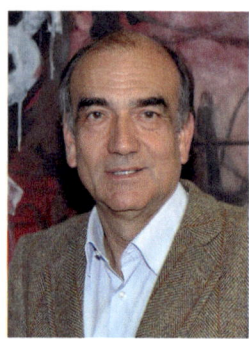

**Patrick G. Zorowka** received his doctorate from Martin Luther University Halle-Wittenberg in 1978. Between 1980 and 1985, he trained as an ENT specialist at the ENT department of the Martin Luther University Hospital Halle-Wittenberg. He also specialised in phoniatrics, paedaudiology, and allergology. After several years of clinical and managerial work at the ENT Department of the University Hospital of Cologne (1986–1988) and at the Department of Communication Disorders of the Johannes Gutenberg University of Mainz (1988–1996), he was appointed Professor of ENT and Phoniatrics-Audiology at the Department of Hearing, Speech and Voice Disorders of the Medical Faculty of Innsbruck in 1996. He was Director of the Department until his retirement in autumn 2022. Patrick Zorowka has been a board member and president of several scientific societies in the field of ENT, audiology, and phoniatrics. In recognition of his work, he has received several awards, e.g. the Annelie Frohn Award of the German Society for Phoniatrics and Paedaudiology and the Sponsorship Award of the Research Council of the German Society for Hearing Aid Acoustics, and has been an honorary member and corresponding member of several scientific societies. He has published more than 100 original articles and book contributions and is co-editor of professional journals.

# Abbreviations

| | |
|---|---|
| %SS | Percent stuttered syllables |
| 4S | Self-stigma of stuttering scale |
| AAC | Augmentative and alternative communication |
| AASP | Acute aphasia screening protocol |
| AAT | Aachen aphasia test |
| AAT-B | Aachen aphasia bedside test |
| ABaCo | Assessment battery for communication |
| ACA | Acquired childhood aphasia |
| ACE | Angiotensin-converting enzyme |
| ACE-III | Addenbrooke cognitive examination (third edition) |
| AChRAb | *Anti-acetylcholinesterase receptor antibodies* |
| ACL | Aphasia check list |
| AD | Ataxic dysarthria |
| aDBS | Adaptive deep brain stimulation |
| AF | Atrial fibrillation |
| A-FROM | Aphasia: Framework for outcome measurement |
| AIDS | Acquired immunodeficiency syndrome |
| AIDS | Assessment of Intelligibility of Dysarthric Speech |
| ALS | Amyotrophic lateral sclerosis |
| ALS-CBS | ALS cognitive behavioural screen |
| AMPAR | $\alpha$-Amino-hydroxy-5-methyl-4-isoxazolepropionic-acid receptor |
| AMSD | Acquired motor speech disorders |
| ANA | Anti-nuclear antibodies |
| ANCA | Anti-neutrophil circulating antibodies |
| AOS MFCC | AOS Mel-frequency cepstral coefficients |
| AOS/AoS | Apraxia of speech |
| AP | Antipsychotic |
| APACS | Assessment of pragmatic abilities and cognitive substrates |
| APM | Ambulatory Phonation Monitor |
| ASA | Acetylsalicylic acid |
| ASHA | American Speech–Language–Hearing Association |
| ASHA-FACS | ASHA-Functional assessment of communication skills |
| ASR | Automatic speech recognition |
| BADA | Batteria per l'Analisi dei Deficit Afasici |
| BAT | Bilingual aphasia test |
| BBS | Buried bumper syndrome |

| BDAE-3 | Boston diagnostic aphasia examination (third edition) |
| BEST-2 | Bedside evaluation screening test (second edition) |
| BMI | Body mass index |
| BNT | Boston naming test |
| BODS | Bogenhausener dysphagia-score |
| BOS | Background-orientated Schlieren |
| BTX | Botulinum toxin |
| BTX-A | Botulinum toxin type A |
| BZs | Benzodiazepines |
| CA | Conversation analysis |
| CA | Crossed aphasia |
| CADL | Communication activities of daily living |
| CANS | Central auditory nervous system |
| CAP | Community-acquired pneumonia |
| CAPD | Central auditory processing disorders |
| CAS | Childhood apraxia of speech |
| CAST | Computer-assisted speech therapy |
| CAT | Comprehensive aphasia test |
| CBS | Corticobasal syndrome |
| CCD | Charge-coupled device |
| CCN | Complex communication needs |
| CE | Cardio-embolic |
| CIAT | Constraint-induced aphasia therapy |
| CIDP | Chronic inflammatory demyelinating polyneuropathy |
| CILT | Constraint-induced language therapy |
| CIMT | Constraint-induced motor therapy |
| CIPNM | Critical illness polyneuromyopathy |
| CIT | Constraint-induced therapy |
| CL | Cleft lip |
| CMOS | Complementary metal-oxide semiconductor |
| CMS | Cerebellar mutism syndrome |
| CNS | Central nervous system |
| COPM | Canadian occupational performance measure |
| CP | Cerebral palsy |
| CPD | Cricopharyngeal dysfunction |
| CPG | Central pattern generators |
| CPM | Cricopharyngeal muscle |
| CPPs | Cepstral peak prominences |
| CPT | Communication partner training |
| CR | Clinical reasoning |
| CR | Computerised rehabilitation |
| CRDs | Complex repetitive discharges |
| CSE | Clinical swallowing examination |
| CSF | Cerebrospinal fluid |
| CSWS | Continuous spikes and waves during slow sleep |
| CT | Computed tomography |
|  | Chemotherapy |
|  | Cricothyroid muscle |

| | |
|---|---|
| CTGF | Connective tissue growth factor |
| CUSA | Cavitron ultrasonic surgical aspirator |
| CVA | Cerebral vascular accident |
| | Cerebrovascular disease and stroke |
| CVs | Consonant-vocal clusters |
| DHI | Dysphagia handicap index |
| DAB | Darley, Aronson, and Brown |
| DAF | Delayed auditory (aural) feedback |
| DAS | Developmental apraxia of speech |
| DBS | Deep brain stimulation |
| DDS | Dysphagia detection system |
| DF | Flaccid dysarthria |
| DHI | Deglutition handicap index |
| DIGEST | Dynamic imaging grade of swallowing toxicity |
| DISH | Diffuse idiopathic skeletal hyperostosis |
| DLD | Developmental language disorder |
| DM | Dermatomyositis |
| DM1 | Myotonic dystrophy type 1 |
| dmCPGs | Dorsomedial central pattern generators |
| DO-80 | Dénomination Orale d'images |
| DOZ | Double opposing Z-palatoplasty |
| DS | Down syndrome |
| DSP | Dynamic sphincter pharyngoplasty |
| DSS | Dysphagia severity scale |
| DTI | Diffusion tensor imaging |
| DWI | Diffusion-weighted sequences |
| DYMUS | Dysphagia in multiple sclerosis questionnaire |
| EAAT | Examination Aachen aphasia test |
| EBM | Evidence-based management |
| EBM | Evidence-based medicine |
| EBP | Evidence-based practice |
| ECAS | Edinburgh cognitive and behavioural ALS screen |
| ECD | Eruption control devices |
| ECO | European Cleft Organisation |
| ECOG | Eastern Cooperative Oncology Group |
| EDGC | European Dysphagia Group Questionnaire |
| EEG | Electroencephalography |
| EF | Executive functions |
| EGG | Electroglottography |
| EID | Elimination disorder |
| ELLM | Esame del linguaggio a letto del malato |
| EMA | Electromagnetic articulography |
| EMG | Electromyography |
| ENPA | Esame Neuropsicologico per l'Afasia |
| ENT | Ear, nose, and throat |
| EORTC | European Organisation for Research and Treatment of Cancer |
| EPG | Electropalatography |

| | |
|---|---|
| EPI | Echo planar imaging |
| ES | Equivalent score |
| ESPEN | European Society for Clinical Nutrition and Metabolism |
| ESSD | European Society for Swallowing Disorders |
| EYFP | Early years foundation profile |
| FAST | Frenchay aphasia screening test |
| FD | Flaccid dysarthria |
| FDA | Food and Drug Administration |
| FDA-2 | Frenchay Dysarthria Profile Assessment (second edition) |
| FDG-PET | Fluorodeoxyglucose-PET |
| FEES | Fibreoptic (flexible) endoscopic evaluation of swallowing |
| FEES(ST) | Fibreoptic evaluation of swallowing (with sensory testing) |
| FHS | Functional health status |
| FIM | Functional independence measure |
| FLAIR | Fluid-attenuated inversion recovery sequences |
| FM | Frequency modulated |
| FMPS | Frost Multidimensional Perfectionism Scale |
| fMRI | Functional magnetic resonance imaging |
| FOA | Fronto-orbital approach |
| FOIS | Functional Oral Intake Scale |
| FOTT | Facial oral tract therapy |
| FraDySc | Frankfurt dysphagia screening score |
| FS-IS | Feeding/swallowing impact survey |
| GABABR | γ-aminobutyric-acid receptor |
| GBS | Guillain-Barré syndrome |
| GER | Gastro-oesophageal reflux |
| GERD | Gastro-oesophageal reflux disease |
| GI | Gastro-intestinal |
| GPi/Gpi | Globus pallidus internus |
| GRN | Progranulin |
| GUSS | Gugging Swallowing Screen |
| Gy | Grey |
| HADS | Hospital Anxiety and Depression Scale |
| HD | Huntington disease |
| HD | High definition |
| HDTV | High-definition television |
| HeD | Hyperkinetic dysarthria |
| HME | Heat and moisture exchanger |
| HMs | Hidden Markov models |
| HNC | Head and neck cancer |
| HoD | Hypokinetic dysarthria |
| HRM | High-resolution manometry |
| HRQoL | Health-related quality of life |
| HU | Hounsfield units |
| IBM | Inclusion body myositis |
| ICF | International Classification of Function (Functioning, Disability and Health) |

| | |
|---|---|
| ICF-CY | International Classification of Functioning, Disability and Health–Children and youth version |
| ICT | Information and communication technology/ies |
| ICU(s) | Intensive care unit(s) |
| IDDSI | International Dysphagia Diet Standardisation Initiative |
| IFG | Inferior frontal gyrus (gyri) |
| IGF-I | Insulin-like growth factor-I |
| IMRT | Intensity-modulated radiation therapy |
| indels | Insertions and deletions |
| IOPI | Iowa oral performance instrument |
| I-PRO | Isometric progressive oropharyngeal |
| IQS | IQ screen |
| Jordan-3 | Jordan left-right reversal test (third edition) |
| K-CPT 2 | Connors kiddie continuous performance test |
| $L_{AFmax}$ | Maximum sound pressure level |
| LASCA | Lothian assessment for screening cognitions in aphasia |
| LAST | Language screening test (tool) |
| LCA | Lateral cricoarytenoid muscle |
| LCQ | La Trobe Communication Questionnaire |
| LD | Laryngeal dystonia |
| LD NOS | LD Not otherwise specified |
| LEMG | Laryngeal electromyography |
| LES | Lambert–Eaton syndrome |
| LHP | Laryngo-hyoidopexy |
| LOS | Lower oesophageal sphincter |
| LPAA | Life participation approach to aphasia |
| LPC | Laser-particle counter |
| LPC | Linear prediction coding |
| LPR | Laryngo-pharyngeal reflux |
| LSVT | Lee Silverman voice treatment |
| Lv | Logopenic/phonological variant |
| lv-PPA | Logopenic variant primary progressive aphasia |
| MAE | Multilingual aphasia examination |
| MAOIs | Monoamine oxidase inhibitors |
| MASA-C | Mann Assessment of Swallowing Ability-Cancer |
| MAST | Mississippi aphasia screening test |
| MBS | Modified barium swallow |
| MCST-A | Multimodal communication screening task for persons with aphasia |
| MD | Mixed dysarthria |
| MD | Multiple demand |
| MDADI | MD Anderson dysphagia inventory |
| MDT | Multidisciplinary team |
| MEBDT | Modified Evans blue dye test |
| MELAS | Myopathy, encephalopathy, lactic acidosis, and stroke |
| MFT | Myofunctional therapy |
| MG | Myasthenia gravis |
| mGluR5 | Metabotropic-glutamate-receptor 5 |

| MII | Multichannel intraluminal impedance |
| MIP | Munich intelligibility profile |
| MIT | Melodic intonation therapy |
| MLSE | Mini Linguistic State Examination |
| MMG | Mechanomyogram |
| MMOR | Modified multiple oral re-reading |
| MMS | Mini Mental State Examination |
| MNA | Mini Nutritional Assessment |
| MND | Motor neuron disease |
| MoCA | Montreal Cognitive Assessment |
| MOST | Madison Oral Strengthening Therapeutic |
| MPC | Measure of participation in conversation |
| MRI | Magnetic resonance imaging |
| MS | Multiple sclerosis |
| MS RES | MS Rapidly evolving severe |
| MS | Mean score |
| MSC | Measure of skill in supported conversation |
| MSD/MSDs | Motor speech disorder(s) |
| MT | Mapping therapy |
| MT-86 | Montreal-Toulouse aphasia battery |
| mtDNA | Mitochondrial DNA |
| MU | Motor unit |
| MUAPs | Motor unit action potentials |
| MUNOD | Medically unexplained oropharyngeal dysphagia |
| MVF | Multi-view videofluoroscopy |
| N/Afv | Non-fluent agrammatic variant |
| NBI | Narrow band imaging |
| NCV | Nerve conduction velocity |
| ND | Neurogenic dysphagia |
| NDD | National Dysphagia Diet |
| NDT | Neurodevelopmental therapy |
| NfV | Non-fluent variant |
| NGS | Nasogastric tube |
| NIBS | Non-invasive brain stimulation |
| NIDCD | National Institute on Deafness and other Communication Disorders |
| NIHSS | National Institutes of Health Stroke Scale/Score |
| NMES | Neuromuscular electrical stimulation |
| NPC | Nasopharyngeal carcinoma |
| NS | Nervous system |
| NTS | Nucleus tractus solitarii |
| NVC | Non-verbal communication |
| OC | Operant conditioning |
| OCD | Obsessive-compulsive disorders |
| OD | Oropharyngeal dysphagia |
| OFA | Orofacial apraxia |
| OMI | Oral motor intervention |

| OP | Operative therapy |
| OPMD | Oculopharyngeal muscular dystrophy |
| ORL | Otorhinolaryngology |
| ORLA | Oral reading for language in aphasia |
| OSA | Obstructive sleep apnoea |
| P/s | Particles/second |
| PABPN1 | poly(A)-binding-protein-nuclear 1 |
| PACE | Promoting aphasics communication effectiveness |
| PALPA | Psycholinguistic assessments of language processing in aphasia |
| PAP | Palatal augmentation prosthesis (prostheses) |
| PAS | Penetration/aspiration scale |
| PASAT | Paced auditory serial addition test |
| PC | Personal computer |
| PCA | Phonological components analysis |
| PCA | Posterior cricoarytenoid muscle |
| PCM | Pharyngeal constrictor muscles |
| pCMS | Paediatric cerebellar mutism syndrome |
| PD | Parkinson's disease |
| PECS | Picture exchange communication system |
| PEG | Percutaneous endoscopic gastrostomy |
| PEJ | Percutaneous endoscopic jejunostomy |
| PES | Pharyngo-oesophageal segment |
| PES | Pharyngeal electrical stimulation |
| PET | Positron emission tomography |
| PFS | Posterior fossa syndrome |
| PICA | Posterior inferior cerebellar artery |
| PIV | Particle image velocimetry |
| $P_M$ | Particle emission rate |
| PM | Polymyositis |
| PN | Parenteral nutrition |
| PNAM | Pre-surgical nasoalveolar moulding |
| PNF | Proprioceptive neuromuscular facilitation |
| PPA | Primary progressive aphasia |
| PPAOS | Primary progressive apraxia of speech |
| PPI | Proton pump inhibitors |
| PPN | Partial parenteral nutrition |
| PROMPT | Prompts for reconstructing oral muscular phonetic targets |
| PROMS | Patient-reported outcome measures |
| PSA | Post-stroke aphasia |
| PSI | Perception of stuttering inventory |
| PSNE | Phoneme-specific nasal emission |
| PSP | Progressive supranuclear palsy |
| PSW | Positive sharp waves |
| PWA/PwA | Person(s)/people with aphasia |
| pWM | Phonological working memory |
| PwMSD | People with motor speech disorders |
| QOL/QoL | Quality of Life |

| | |
|---|---|
| RAPIDS | Royal Adelaide Prognostic Index for Dysphagic Stroke |
| r-BANS | Repeatable battery for the assessment of neuropsychological status |
| RC | Reading comprehension |
| RCT | Radio-chemotherapy |
| RCT(s) | Randomised controlled trial(s) |
| REM | Rapid eye movement |
| RIG | Radiologically inserted gastrostomy |
| RSES | Rosenberg Self-Esteem Scale |
| rs-fMRI | Resting-state functional magnetic resonance imaging |
| RSs | Raw scores |
| RT | Radiotherapy |
| rTMS | Repetitive transcranial magnetic stimulation |
| SAND | Screening for aphasia in neurodegeneration |
| SARS-CoV-2 | Severe acute respiratory syndrome coronavirus 2 |
| SAS | Supervisory attentional system |
| SAT | Spinocerebellar ataxia type |
| SBMA | Spinobulbar muscular atrophy |
| SCA | Supported conversation for adults with aphasia |
| SD | Semantic dementia |
| SD | Spastic dysarthria |
| SD | Standard deviation |
| SF-6 | Short Form Health Survey |
| SFA | Semantic feature analysis |
| SGB | Supragastric belching |
| SiP | Swallowing intervention package |
| SIRFES | Simultaneous radiological and fibre(flexible)-endoscopic evaluation of swallowing |
| SIT | Sentence intelligibility test |
| SLD | Specific learning disorder(s) |
| SLDM | SLD in mathematics |
| SLI | Specific language impairment |
| SLP | Speech (and) language pathologist(s)/pathology |
| SLT(s) | Speech (and) language therapist(s)/therapy |
| SMA | Spinal muscular atrophy |
| SMART | Specific, measurable, achievable, relevant, and timed |
| SNVs | Single nucleotide variants |
| SP | Substance P |
| SPECT | Single-photon emission computed tomography |
| SPPARC | Supporting partners of people with aphasia in relationships and conversation |
| SPT | Sound production treatment |
| SSQ | Sydney Swallow Questionnaire |
| ST | Speech therapy |
| STM | Short-term memory |
| STN | Subthalamic nucleus |
| SV | Subject-verb |
| Sv | Semantic variant |

| | |
|---|---|
| SVD | Small-vessel disease |
| SWAL-QoL | Swallowing Quality-of-Life Questionnaire |
| TA | Thyroarytenoid/vocal muscles |
| TBI | Traumatic brain injury |
| TD | Typically developing |
| tDCS | Transcranial direct current stimulation |
| TDRS | Total dysphagia risk score |
| TGF-β | Transforming growth factor-beta |
| TLESR | Transient lower oesophageal sphincter relaxation |
| TMD | Texture-modified diet |
| TMF | Texture-modified food |
| TNA | Total nutrient admixture |
| TOLS | Trans-oral laser surgery |
| TOM | Therapy outcome measures |
| TPN | Total parenteral nutrition |
| TPTD | Tongue position tracking device |
| TR | Telerehabilitation |
| TTLS | Tracheo-tracheolaryngeal shunt |
| UAS | Ullevaal aphasia screening |
| UEP | Union of European Phoniatricians |
| UES | Upper oesophageal sphincter |
| UIS | UNESCO Institute for Statistics |
| UTBAS | Unhelpful beliefs about stuttering |
| VAS | Visual analogue scale |
| VFES | Videofluoroscopic examination of swallowing |
| VFS | Videofluoroscopy of swallowing |
| VFSS | Videofluoroscopic swallowing study/studies |
| VIM | Ventral (ventro) intermediate nucleus |
| vlCPGs | Ventrolateral central pattern generators |
| VOT | Voice onset time |
| VP | Velopharyngeal |
| VPS | Ventriculoperitoneal shunt |
| VR | Virtual reality |
| VT | Virtual therapist |
| VWS | Van der Woude syndrome |
| WAB-R | Western aphasia battery-revised |
| WAIS-IV | Wechsler Adult Intelligence Scale (fourth edition) |
| WCGH | Waldo County General Hospital |
| WE | Written expression |
| WGS | Whole-genome sequencing |
| WM | Working memory |
| WST | Water swallow test |
| XLP | Extended linear prediction |

# Part IV

# Acquired Motor Speech Disorders (Dysarthria, Dyspraxia)

Editors: Antonio Schindler, Antoinette am Zehnhoff-Dinnesen

Lectors: Enrico Alfonsi, Jacek Błeszyński, Stefano Cappa, Rémi Eclasson, Stefan Heim, Alexander Hemprich, Bibiána Hlebová, Rossella Muo, Karel Neubauer, Arno Olthoff, Philippe Paquier, Uta Schick, Thomas Stamm, Rachel Zeng

# Basics of Acquired Motor Speech Disorders (Dysarthria, Dyspraxia)

# 16

Daniele Farneti, Claudio Luzzatti, Arno Olthoff, Antonio Schindler, and Rachel Zeng

## 16.1 Definition of Acquired Motor Speech Disorders

Claudio Luzzatti and Antonio Schindler

The speech motor system includes several neural circuits involved in the planning, programming and execution of speech movements. Speech planning is the highest level in hierarchy and reflects the speech goal to be achieved; speech programming, however, is at a lower level and reflects the procedures necessary to accomplish the plans. Execution, finally, reflects the activity of the pyramidal, extra-pyramidal and neuromuscular systems.

*Acquired motor speech disorders* (AMSD) is a wide group of speech disorders due to impairment of the motor planning, motor programming and neuromuscular control (execution) of speech; AMSD share the following characteristics: they are not developmental in origin, they do not involve the language domains (phonology, lexicon, syntax and semantics) and the speech structures (lungs, larynx, pharynx, mouth) are preserved (Duffy 1994). Other neurological disorders affecting speech, but not included within AMSD, are acquired neurogenic stuttering, palilalia (compul-

**Supplementary Information** The online version contains supplementary material available at https://doi.org/10.1007/978-3-031-48091-1_1.

D. Farneti (✉)
Audiology Phoniatric Service, ENT Department, "Infermi" Hospital Rimini, Rimini, Italy
e-mail: daniele.farneti@auslromagna.it

C. Luzzatti
Department of Psychology, University of Milan Bicocca, Milan, Italy
e-mail: claudio.luzzatti@unimib.it

A. Olthoff
Department of Otorhinolaryngology, Phoniatrics and Pedaudiology, University Medical Centre Göttingen, Göttingen, Germany
e-mail: olthoff@med.uni-goettingen.de

A. Schindler
Luigi Sacco Hospital, Department of Biomedical and Clinical Sciences "L. Sacco", Phoniatrics, University of Milan, Milan, Italy
e-mail: antonio.schindler@unimi.it

R. Zeng
Department of Neurology, University Medical Centre Göttingen, Göttingen, Germany
e-mail: rachel.zeng@med.uni-goettingen.de

sive repetition of utterances), echolalia (unsolicited repetition of another's utterances) and aprosodia associated with right hemisphere damage (Duffy 2005a). Two main groups of speech disorders are found within the frame of AMSD: dysarthria and apraxia of speech.

*Dysarthria* is due to an impairment of the central or peripheral nervous system responsible for the execution of speech; it includes a variety of speech disorders characterised by abnormalities in strength, speed, range, steadiness, tone and accuracy of respiratory, phonatory, resonatory, articulatory, prosodic movements. Weakness, spasticity, incoordination, involuntary movements, excessive, reduced or variable muscle tone of speech organs can be found (Darley et al. 1969b).

*Apraxia of speech* (AoS) is a disorder of speech motor planning/programming, usually caused by a unilateral left-hemisphere brain damage (Ziegler et al. 2012). Several terms have been employed in the past to denote this same impairment: *anarthria* (Marie 1906), *aphemia* (Schiff et al. 1983), *phonetic disintegration* (Lecours 1976), as well as *foreign accent syndrome* (Marie 1907; Miller et al. 2006; Moen 2006; Pick 1919). AoS often accompanies Broca's aphasia, but the impairment may also appear in isolation. The impairment does not depend on paresis of the tongue, lips and velar muscles (Buckingham 1991; Johns and Darley 1970; Luzzatti 2012): patients suffering from AoS are unable to control the motor planning/programming of articulatory movements of lips, tongue pharynx and larynx, giving the impression of struggling for the realisation of the desired phonetic strings. The major mechanism underlying AoS is a loss of the ability to plan and programme the activity of the single muscles interacting in the production of the speech sounds. Unlike what occurs in dysarthria, AoS only affects the motor control of oral movements that are involved in the realisation of speech sounds, usually without any damage to the elementary nonarticulatory motor skills of mouth, lips and tongue and of the pharynx and larynx regions (e.g. sucking, chewing and swallowing), and it may be impaired in isolation from higher motor control of this functional region (i.e. there may be double dissociation with respect to oral apraxia).

## 16.2 Epidemiology of Dysarthria and Apraxia

Arno Olthoff and Rachel Zeng

### 16.2.1 Introduction

Dysarthria and apraxia of speech are *acquired motor speech disorders* that can result from dysfunction of various parts of the central and peripheral nervous system.

*Dysarthria* is an impaired articulation caused by movement disorders of the oropharyngeal muscle system. Since prosody is part of articulation, disorders of laryngeal and respiratory function must also be considered. *Dysarthria* results from a motor dysfunction whose origin can arise from cortical, pyramidal, basal ganglia, cerebellar, bulbar or neuromuscular defects or diseases. *Apraxia* is the clinical appearance of an impaired planning and programming of movement sequences and is attributed to disorders of the left (dominant) frontal lobe; the incidence and prevalence of these speech disorders depend on the underlying primary diseases, which include vascular, infectious, malignant, traumatic, autoimmune-mediated and neurodegenerative diseases.

### 16.2.2 Epidemiology Related to Different Causes

**Cortical defects and disorders** are mainly caused by *cerebrovascular events*. 70–80% of cerebrovascular events are ischaemic, the remaining being due to intra-cerebral or subarachnoid haemorrhage. Related to the world population, the respective incidence is about 1–2:1000/year and the prevalence about 1:1000 (Phipps and Cronin 2020). The incidence of cerebrovascular events such as *stroke* is considerably augmented after the age of 65 and further dramatically increased after the age of 85.

Advanced cortical neurodegeneration such as *Alzheimer's disease* can also affect the sensorimotor cortex and speech in about 5% of patients, even as a preclinical sign (Albers et al. 2015).

Concerning this, dementia's worldwide incidence of 1–2:1000/year and its prevalence of 6:1000 are high (Gautam and Sharma 2020). The increase in prevalence in very old age ranges up to 50:100 (>95 years) (Hou et al. 2019).

Another dementia syndrome typically characterised by impaired speech production is *primary progressive aphasia* (PPA), which is associated with fronto-temporal cortical degeneration. The non-fluent variant of PPA especially can exhibit apraxic symptoms, causing halting speech and dysprosody. To be differentiated from the non-fluent variant of PPA is *primary progressive apraxia of speech* (PPAOS), which is suggested to be a neurodegenerative disorder distinct from PPA with its own pathophysiology (Josephs et al. 2012). The prevalence of PPAOS has been estimated to be approximately 4–5:100,000; the prevalence of non-fluent variant PPA has been estimated to be 0.5–4 per 100,000 (Botha and Josephs 2019). In both diseases, the age of onset varies around 60 and no predominance in either men or women is suggested.

Less frequent causes of speech impairment due to cortical disorders include post-traumatic (head injury), post-inflammatory (encephalitis) or tumour-related cortical lesions.

**Basal ganglia neurodegeneration** seen in *Morbus Parkinson* is the most frequent neurodegenerative movement disorder with an incidence of 10–20:100,000 per year and a prevalence of 100–250:100,000 with values increasing in ages over 60 and further increasing over 80 years (Balestrino and Schapira 2020). It frequently causes dystonia of the oropharyngeal muscles and consequently dysarthria and dysphagia. Additional diseases of basal ganglia that can cause dysarthria and apraxia of speech are *progressive supranuclear palsy* (PSP) and *corticobasal syndrome* (CBS). These disorders, sometimes described as "atypical Parkinsonism", show a lower prevalence of approximately 5–7:100,000 (Lamb et al. 2016).

**Cerebellar disorders** lead to ataxic movement disorders that can also affect articulation. The main reasons are cerebrovascular events and other causes of cerebellar dysfunction covering a vast range of sporadic and acquired disorders such as neurodegenerative diseases, tumours, multiple sclerosis and para-neoplastic syndromes. There are also hereditary cerebellar ataxias such as *spinocerebellar ataxia type 3* (SCA), which is the most common autosomal-dominant ataxia with a prevalence of 1–4:100,000 (Ruano et al. 2014).

**Multiple sclerosis (MS)** can result in dysarthria and dysphagia through immune-mediated, demyelinating damage to various parts of the central nervous system, e.g. cortical, bulbar, cerebellar. MS is the main cause of non-traumatic neurological disabilities in young adults. The prevalence is estimated at 1–10:100,000 (Browne et al. 2014).

**Motor neuron diseases** such as *amyotrophic lateral sclerosis* (ALS) affect the cortex and the corticospinal tract. ALS comprises 80–90% of motor neuron diseases. The incidence of ALS is about 2:100,000/year with a main onset between the ages of 40 and 65. The prevalence is around 5:100,000. Men are more often affected than women (Worms 2001; Yedavalli et al. 2018).

**Bulbar motor dysfunctions** mainly result from *cerebrovascular events* or *ALS*. About 30% of ALS-patients have initial bulbar deficits and such sequelae as dysarthria and dysphagia, while the majority will develop them during the progress of disease (Yunusova et al. 2019).

In this context, *ALS* can also be seen as a *neuromuscular disease* whose clinical aspect can hardly be differentiated from such a **neuropathy** as *chronic inflammatory demyelinating polyneuropathy* (CIDP), especially in rare cases of CIDP with bulbar involvement. In CIDP, cranial nerve dysfunction can appear in 5–20% of all cases. The incidence of CIDP is about 1–2:100,000/year and its prevalence about 5:100,000 (Allen 2020). People of all ages can contract CIDP (Hattori et al. 2001).

Acute neuropathy diseases such as the "pharyngeal-cervical-brachial form" of the *Guillain–Barré Syndrome* (GBS) can also impair bulbar motor function leading to serious dysphagia. The incidence of this is about 1:100,000/year with predominance in men. The risk of developing GBS has its first peak in late adolescence/young adulthood and a second peak in the elderly;

the risk increases with age (Govoni and Granieri 2001).

**Peripheral nerve lesions** of the articulatory tract are mainly iatrogenic and caused by surgical treatment such as tumour surgery, leading to hemiparesis of the tongue or the soft palate.

**Myopathies** such as myositis and dystrophies are hereditary or idiopathic. Owing to its specific pattern of muscle involvement, dysphagia is the more common oropharyngeal symptom in myopathies, but in cases of severe facial and oral muscle weakness articulation can be impaired too. This applies especially to hereditary myopathies such as myotonic dystrophy type 1 (Curschmann-Steinert), which has a prevalence of 1:10,000 (Siciliano et al. 2001), and some congenital myopathies that are rare disorders with an estimated prevalence of 2:100,000 (Bagnall et al. 2006; Witting et al. 2017).

**Myasthenia gravis** is an immune-mediated disorder of the post-synaptic neuromuscular junction with an incidence of 0.17–2: 100,000/year and a prevalence of up to 18:100,000. The incidence increases with age, with an additional peak of female patients at young age and a predominance of males at old age (Carr et al. 2010). The disease is characterised by fluctuating weakness, which can affect bulbar functions leading to dysarthria and dysarthrophonia.

### 16.2.3 Summary

Cortical lesions due to cerebrovascular events (*stroke*) or neurodegeneration (*Alzheimer's disease*, PPA) are the main causes of dysarthria and speech apraxia. In elderly populations, the prevalence of each hugely increases with ageing into high percentage ranges (1–50:100). Since oropharyngeal muscles (tongue, palate, pharynx and larynx) are bilaterally represented in the sensorimotor cortex, disorders of the central nervous system generally lead to motor weakness or deceleration but not to unilateral or bilateral paralyses. Bilateral bulbar paralyses can be observed in rare (1–5:100,000) motor neuron disease (ALS) or neuropathy (CIDP, GBS). MS (1–10:100,000) can show symptoms of both with a major overlap of patients at young and midlife ages. Depending on the degree and pattern of motor dysfunction, patients with dysarthria may also have impaired deglutition (*dysphagia*). It particularly affects patients with bulbar involvement and neuromuscular disorders and is often of prime importance during disease progression.

## 16.3 Classification of Dysarthria

Daniele Farneti

Since Froeschels (1943) first classified dysarthria, various attempts have been made over the following decades to develop a classification of the disorder that is able to satisfy physiopathological and clinical needs (Duffy and Kent 2001). In this respect, the most important contribution has come from Darley et al. (1969a, b), devising what still today is recognised as the reference classification of dysarthria, also known as the Mayo Clinic classification system (or simply the Mayo system).

An exhaustive classification is, however, difficult to draw up, because the term dysarthria refers to a considerable number of aspects, compared with what it defines. In addition to articulation in the narrow sense, it includes breathing, voice and resonance. In fact, the normal perceptive verbal findings depend on the optimal functioning of these basic systems although the highest levels of functional integration (intelligence and emotional state) can inevitably interfere with the performance baseline.

Even though it is difficult to dissociate these basic activities physiologically, because of their close neuro-anatomical relationship in both the cortical and associated pathways, it is plausible clinically to assume that a motor defect of a basal activity may present various degrees of dysfunction, according to individual differences, location, type and extent of the disease, etc. One of the great advantages of the DAB classification is that it is easy to use in clinical practice and it was decidedly even more so in the pre-imaging period. It is a detailed classification that allows an accurate description of the patient's speech skills, most of which coincide with the localisation of the disease (Simmons and Mayo 1997). For this reason, although DAB was not conceived as a diagnostic tool (Kent 1994), it is in fact useful in clinical practice, not only for diagnostic purposes but also for therapeutic ones (Duffy 1994; Strand and Yorkston 1994).

Unfortunately, DAB is a classification based solely on perceptual parameters, as has for some time been documented by several authors, who have compared the poor correspondence between the findings of expert clinicians and the less expert: only 56% in the work of Zyski and Weisiger (1987). To know in advance the pathology or the location (by imaging) of the patient's lesion, permits a better description of the language model listened to, a better application of DAB and, for example, a better definition of a treatment plan. Following the work of Zyski and Weisiger (1987) and Fonville et al. (2008) reported poor accuracy in using the DAB classification when applied by neurologists and neurology trainees, and Van der Graaf et al. (2009) also came to the same conclusion for neurologists, residents in neurology and speech therapists. In these studies, the rate of correct classification ranged from about 35–40%.

A reasonable conclusion deduced from these studies is that in drawing up a classification the perceptual parameter should be accompanied by other objective parameters (Kim et al. 2011). Thus, in 2003, Guerra and Lovely reported encouraging data regarding the use of a classification that uses a combination of acoustic and perceptual data (Guerra and Lovely 2003), and Liss et al. (2009) reported how the consideration of rhythm metrics allows distinguishing between dysarthric speech and that of normal controls, and also among different subtypes of dysarthria, when the subtypes are chosen as highly repre-sentative of their classical description (Kim et al. 2011).

Unfortunately, to date a classification that uses more parameters and that has become as wide-spread as the DAB is not available in the litera-ture. Darley et al. (1969a, b) in their original papers listed the following types of dysarthria: flaccid, spastic, hypokinetic, hyperkinetic, ataxic and mixed.

## 16.4 Aetiology and Pathogenesis of Dysarthria

Daniele Farneti and Rachel Zeng

### 16.4.1 Aetiology

Articulation, breathing, voice and resonance, as the basic systems of speech, can be variously involved in dysarthria, with a huge variety of symptomatic manifestations detectable in the clinical setting (Duffy and Kent 2001). A speech disorder that is due to an alteration of the plan-ning and programming of motor sequences in the presence of normal muscle activity is termed apraxia of speech (AOS) and is a separate cate-gory from dysarthria (McNeil et al. 2009). The complexity mentioned above is inherent in the regulation of the motor system, which is devoted to this specific human expression (Dum and Strick 1992). More generally, the motor system is composed of multiple structures with a well-defined hierarchy: primary and associated corti-cal and sub-cortical structures, such as the basal ganglia, thalamus and cerebellum. The descend-ing pathways (Kuypers 1981) of the pyramidal and extra-pyramidal system, up to the neuromus-cular junctions, provide privileged connections between the structures of the motor system, alongside a dense network of reciprocal connec-tions, which ensures an extremely reverberant exchange of information.

This network supports and guarantees the con-trol of plasticity, precision, speed, range of motion and strength of the motor act, by means of conscious and unconscious activities. The complexity of the motor gesture is, however, influenced by sensory afferents and connections with the limbic system. This pattern of organisation ensures the vast range of our body movements, from basic movements of the limbs to the finest movements of the fingers or tongue and other articulators, during a verbal articulatory gesture. In an extreme synthesis, we can remind ourselves how the motor pathways that support speech production—the cortico-bulbar part of the pyramidal system—begin in the motor cortical areas (4 and 6), in the primary somato-sensory cortex (areas 1, 2, 3) and in the posterior parietal areas (areas 5, 7); descend into the corona radiata to cross the knee of the internal capsule; and terminate, directly or through inter-neurons, to the motor neurons of the cranial nerves (Martin 2003).

The cranial nerve nuclei involved in phono-articulation are the V, VII, IX, X, XI, XII and the phrenic nucleus, receiving both direct and cross afferents. The terminations of the cranial and phrenic nerves innervate the muscles of the pneumo-phono-articulation effectors (Martin 2003). In such a complex and composite system, one or more lesions can variously alter and compromise movements. The close anatomical relationship existing between the different structures mentioned above explains the close correlation with motor impairment and clinical symptomatology.

As already mentioned, breath, voice and resonance are basic systems that underlie spoken language. Their mutual and concurrent involvement is essential for adequate speech production. The sequence of events involving these basal activities can be summarised briefly. The pulmonary bellows provide the necessary energy for vocal fold vibration. The subglottal pressure needed to generate this overcomes the resistance of the vocal folds, of which the mucosal lining (fibro-elastic) is put into cyclical movement (the glottal cycle) (Farneti 2012).

This movement is the basis of phonation. The air being expired passes through the cavities of the vocal tract and is then conveyed into the oral or nasal cavity by the dynamics of the soft palate. This passage modifies the energy content of the sound produced by the larynx with a modification of its harmonic and formant architecture, which is closely tied to the movements of mobile (lips, tongue, veil) and fixed (teeth, alveolar and hard palate) articulators.

So, inconstant or altered respiratory dynamics, as made possible by an alteration in the dynamics of the respiratory muscles (diaphragm and inter-costal muscles), causes an expiratory airflow that is inadequate for phonation (hypophonic voice-reduced loudness or breathy voice) or articulation. Similarly, altered dynamics of the laryngeal musculature may affect the ability to adjust pitch and loudness of voice, necessary to express supra-segmental tracts, extremely important in verbal production, altering accent, intonation and prosody of speech (Murdoch et al. 1997).

An inadequate muscular activity, or muscle weakness, conditions a lack of glottal competence leading to a breathy and harsh voice quality. Under the opposite conditions, an overly muscular activity induces a strong vocal fold hyper-adduction with a strained or strangled voice quality.

Altered soft palate dynamics, with slow or weak movements, conditions an incomplete separation of the oral and nasal cavity during phonation, with nasalisation of phonemes usually lacking this feature.

Finally, an inappropriate timing, strength and speed of movement of the articulators are, separately or jointly, due to a reciprocal altered contact or approach, conditioning articulation errors, such as distortion of consonants or vowels, inappropriate silences and irregular articulatory breakdown (Freed 2012).

### 16.4.2 Pathogenesis

Starting with the DAB classification (Darley et al. 1969a, b), the following characteristics of impaired speech can be cited.

**Flaccid dysarthria (DF)** is due to an alteration in nerve transmission along the peripheral motor pathways and lower motor neurons that innervate the muscles involved in respiration, phonation, resonance and articulation (Singh and

Kent 2000). The main problems of the articulators are represented by muscle weakness and hypotonia. Patients with this type of articulation have a slow-laboured articulation, hypernasality and a hoarse-breathy phonation, although the characteristics of speech in flaccid dysarthria vary according to the nerves and muscles affected.

Among the main causes of FD may be mentioned: (1) Physical trauma responsible for 31% of DF observed in the Mayo Clinic in over 20 years (Duffy 2005b), mainly surgical trauma or vehicle accidents; (2) Brainstem stroke or cerebral-vascular accidents involving the cranial nerve nuclei, especially the IX, X and XI nerves anatomically adjacent in the trunk; (3) Myasthenia gravis, an autoimmune-mediated disorder of the neuromuscular junction, which alters the ability of muscles to maintain sustained performance leading to rapid fatigability; (4) Guillain–Barré Syndrome, where an inflammatory demyelination of peripheral nerves leads to severe muscle weakness or even complete paralysis; (5) Muscular dystrophy due to a progressive muscle degeneration; (6) Progressive bulbar palsy that can affect the upper and lower motor neurons; (7) Tumours of the trunk or along the course of the cranial nerves or the phrenic nerves, the latter of which innervates the diaphragm, the main muscle of respiration.

**Spastic dysarthria (SD)** occurred in 7.6% of dysarthria cases observed in the Mayo Clinic over 20 years (Duffy 2005b). It is due to a bilateral lesion in the central nervous system, more specifically the upper motor neurons (Murdoch et al. 1997; Nicolosi et al. 2006), which involves a combination of the pyramidal and extra-pyramidal system. The involvement of the two systems combines the clinical manifestations of SD: weakness, slow movement and spasticity (increased muscle tone). Some non-speech events are characteristic of SD: pseudo-bulbar effects, such as uncontrollable crying or laughing and drooling, and abnormal peripheral reflexes. Any disorder that bilaterally affects the pyramidal and extra-pyramidal pathways can determine SD: (1) Cerebral-vascular accidents involving the two hemispheres, likely at different times. In the case of an isolated episode, SD appears at a brainstem

location that involves the two systems of both sides; (2) Amyotrophic lateral sclerosis (ALS) affects the upper and lower motor neurons. When damage of the upper motor neuron is predominant, SD, hyperactive gag reflexes and jaw reflexes are more evident. In other cases, SD in ALS is mixed, spastic and flaccid; (3) Traumatic brain injury (TBI) can involve, in a manner variously extended or diffuse, the CNS and the PNS. Bilateral lesions can cause SD or mixed dysarthria: spastic or flaccid-ataxic spastic; (4) Multiple sclerosis can affect different areas of the CNS, producing an SD or mixed dysarthria; (5) Cerebral anoxia due to widespread neural damage of both sides of CNS; (6) Tumours of the brainstem; (7) Infections of the CNS or PNS of viral or bacterial aetiology.

**Ataxic dysarthria (AD)** is due to a lesion of the cerebellum or its connections (Cannito and Marquardt 2009). The cerebellum is mainly involved in circuits regulating timing, force, range and direction of muscular contraction during both planned and ongoing speech movements. Because of these properties, a lesion of the cerebellum causes important speech alterations.

In AD articulation is primarily compromised (Darley et al. 1969a, b) by imprecise consonant production, distorted vowel and irregular articulatory breakdown (Duffy 2005b). Prosodic alteration is also characteristic: equal or excess stress, prolonged phonemes and prolonged intervals between phonemes and mono-pitch and mono-loudness (Darley et al. 1969a, b). Other perceptive correlations can be harsh vocal quality, voice tremor or hypernasality.

Several pathological conditions cause AD. The following can be cited: (1) Degenerative diseases: Friedreich's ataxia, olivoponto-cerebellar degeneration, autosomal-dominant cerebellar ataxia of late onset, idiopathic sporadic late-onset cerebellar ataxia; (2) Stroke; (3) traumatic brain injury (TBI); (4) Tumours; (5) Toxic conditions: lead and mercury poisoning, alcohol, amides, drugs such as phenytoin or anti-seizure medication; (6) Infectious diseases of the CNS.

**Hypokinetic dysarthria (HoD)** is due to a disorder that affects the basal ganglia or the connections that they realise in the extra-pyramidal system (Singh and Kent 2000). This condition occurs primarily in Parkinsonism. The main symptoms of Parkinsonism (resting tremor, rigidity and bradykinesis) lead to hypokinetic speech, with mainly prosodic and articulation alterations (Darley et al. 1969a, b): in the former case, monopitch, reduced loudness, inappropriate silences, increased rate of speech and short rushes of speech can be cited; in the latter, imprecise articulation of consonants is due to a reduced range of movement of the articulators, involving stop consonants, fricatives and affricates, realising an articulatory undershoot (Duffy 2005b). Dysfluencies can also be heard: repeated phonemes or a word-phrase (palilalia). A harsh or breathy voice is frequent in HoD, whereas hypernasality is uncommon and usually mild.

The main causes of HoD are: (1) Idiopathic Parkinson's disease; (2) Neuroleptic-induced Parkinsonism: the second cause of Parkinsonism. It depends on the drugs (haloperidol, chlorpromazine, trifluoperazine, prochlorperazine) and the dosage levels; (3) TBI: involving the basal ganglia selectively or in the context of a more complex event; (4) Toxic metal poisoning: as in the long-term effect of manganese; (5) Postencephalitic Parkinsonism: mainly viral infection; (6) Stroke involving the basal ganglia in a multiple stroke condition.

**Hyperkinetic dysarthria (HeD)** is associated with damage involving the basal ganglia (Zraich and La Pointe 1997), mainly the striatum and its connections with the cortical motor areas (basal ganglia control circuits). Involuntary movements of body parts, such as chorea, myoclonus, tics, dystonia, essential tremor, are possible in this pathological condition. The speech in HeD depends on the severity of the pathology. It is characterised by alteration of prosody (prolonged intervals, variable rate of speech, mono-pitch, mono-loudness), articulation (imprecise consonant production, distorted vowels, prolonged phonemes), phonation (harsh vocal quality, excessive loudness variations, strained-strangled voice quality).

The main causes of HeD are: (1) Choreas: Sydenham's chorea, an autoimmune disorder which affects children from 5 to 15 years; Huntington's disease, a genetic neurodegenerative disorder that commonly develops between 30 and 50 years; (2) A rare manifestation after cerebral-vascular accidents involving basal ganglia and thalamus in a multiple, bilateral stroke condition; (3) Tardive dyskinesia: due to long-term taking of neuroleptics; (4) Anoxia, carbon monoxide poisoning.

**Mixed dysarthria (MD)** is characterised by a combination of pure dysarthrias (Singh and Kent 2000). It is more common than one might imagine: 27% of dysarthrias seen at the Mayo Clinic in 11 years (Duffy 2005b). MD is due to damage that involves two or more parts of the motor system. At the same time, a patient can present perceptive signs of two or more types of dysarthric speech with a predominance of one type in relation to the extent of the pathological event. So, for example, hypernasality (flaccid dysarthria) can coexist with strangled voice (spastic dysarthria) and consonant distortion (flaccid and spastic dysarthria). Brainstem lesions more frequently cause MD because of the proximity in this area of upper and lower motor neurons, or of TBI with involvement of the cerebellum and different cranial nerves. Among the more frequent conditions causing MD (some of which have already been mentioned) are: multiple sclerosis, multisystem atrophy (a collection of neurodegenerative conditions characterised by Parkinsonian movement disorders, cerebellar ataxia and autonomic nervous system dysfunction), amyotrophic lateral sclerosis, Wilson's disease (a rare hereditary disease due to an abnormal metabolism of dietary copper) and Friedreich's ataxia.

**Apraxia of speech (AoS)** As mentioned previously, AoS is a speech articulation disorder due to an alteration in the planning of motor sequences that characterise articulated voice, in the presence of normal muscle activity (McNeil et al. 2009). The absence of movement, as expressed by the term, is extremely unusual. Generally movements of the articulators are possible.

Apraxia can affect the execution of simple movements (ideomotor apraxia) or the combination and coordination of consecutive movements (ideatory apraxia). Ideatory apraxia also implies an impairment in the conception of an object or gesture. Apraxic syndromes of the oropharyngeal muscle system can be further differentiated in orofacial apraxia (OFA), also termed buccofacial apraxia, and apraxia of speech (AOS). OFA, a sub-category of ideomotor apraxia, is characterised by impairment in the non-verbal functions of cranial nerves, leading to an inability to blink, to open the mouth or to swallow voluntarily or on command, while reflex movements are well-preserved (Bakar et al. 1998). AOS refers to an impaired coordination of muscle movements affecting articulation; patients with AOS cannot sequence oral movements finalised to speech (Freed 2012). OFA and AOS are both attributed to disorders of the left (dominant) frontal lobe. More specifically, it is suggested that OFA is associated with the left middle frontal and premotor cortices, while AOS is linked to the left posterior inferior frontal gyrus and insula (Rohrer et al. 2010). Owing to the proximity of these areas, AOS and OFA can coexist in clinical cases of diffuse damage to the left frontal lobe. Additionally, AOS can be associated with aphasia if the lesion is close to the area of Broca.

Perceptually, AoS is characterised by errors of articulation and alteration of prosody. Less involved is respiration and seldom resonance and phonation. Articulation is mainly involved with errors in consonant clusters, consonants with distant points of articulation or those that involve articulators other than the lips or the tongue against the alveolar ridge. Non-sense, multisyllabic or unusual words are more distorted than common words or automatic speech. Fricatives and affricates are more often in error than other consonants, and substitutions are more frequent than distortion, omission or repetition. In AoS, prosodic errors are represented by slowness of connecting speech, reduction of normal variations of pitch and loudness, errors in stress placement, silent pauses at the initiation of a word and between syllables or words.

# References

Albers MW, Gilmore GC, Kaye J et al (2015) At the interface of sensory and motor dysfunctions and Alzheimer's disease. Alzheimers Dement 11(1):70–98

Allen JA (2020) The misdiagnosis of CIDP: a review. Neurol Ther 9(1):43–54

Bagnall AK, Al-Muhaizea MA, Manzur AY (2006) Feeding and speech difficulties in typical congenital nemaline myopathy. Adv Speech Lang Pathol 8(1):7–16

Bakar M, Kirshner S, Niaz F (1998) The opercular-subopercular syndrome: four cases with review of the literature. Behav Neurol 11(2):97–103

Balestrino R, Schapira AHV (2020) Parkinson disease. Eur J Neurol 27(1):27–42

Botha H, Josephs KA (2019) Primary progressive aphasias and apraxia of speech. Continuum 25(1):101–127

Browne P, Chandraratna D, Angood C et al (2014) Atlas of multiple sclerosis 2013: a growing global problem with widespread inequity. Neurology 83(11):1022–1024

Buckingham HW (1991) Explanations for the concept of apraxia of speech. In: Taylor-Sarno M (ed) Acquired aphasia, 3rd edn. Academic, New York, pp 269–307

Cannito MP, Marquardt TP (2009) Apraxia of speech: definition, differentiation, and treatment. In: McNeil MR (ed) Clinical management of sensorimotor speech disorders, 2nd edn. Thieme, New York

Carr AS, Cardwell CR, McCarron PO et al (2010) A systematic review of population based epidemiological studies in Myasthenia Gravis. BMC Neurol 10:46. https://doi.org/10.1186/1471-2377-10-46

Darley FL, Aronson AE, Brown JR (1969a) Clusters of deviant speech dimensions in the dysarthrias. J Speech Hear Res 12(3):462–496

Darley FL, Aronson AE, Brown JR (1969b) Differential diagnostic patterns of dysarthria. J Speech Lang Hear Res 12(2):246–269

Duffy JR (1994) Emerging and future issues in motor speech disorders. Am J Speech Lang Pathol 3(3):36–39

Duffy JR (2005a) Motor speech disorders, 2nd edn. Mosby, St. Louis

Duffy JR (2005b) Motor speech disorders. Substrates, differential diagnosis, and management, 3rd edn. Mosby, St. Louis

Dum RP, Strick PL (1992) Medial wall motor areas and skeletomotor control. Curr Opin Neurobiol 2(6):836–839

Farneti D (2012) Voice and dysphagia. In: Ekberg O (ed) Dysphagia: diagnosis and treatment. Springer, Berlin

Fonville S, van der Worp HB, Maat P et al (2008) Accuracy and inter-observer variation in the classification of dysarthria from speech recordings. J Neurol 255(10):1545–1548

Freed DB (2012) Motor speech disorders. Diagnosis and treatment, 2nd edn. Delmar-Cengage Learning, New York

Froeschels E (1943) A contribution to the pathology and therapy of dysarthria due to certain cerebral lesions. J Speech Disord 8(4):301–321

Gautam R, Sharma M (2020) Prevalence and diagnosis of neurological disorders using different deep learning techniques: a meta-analysis. J Med Syst 44(2):49. https://doi.org/10.1007/s10916-019-1519-7

Govoni V, Granieri E (2001) Epidemiology of the Guillain-Barré syndrome. Curr Opin Neurol 14(5):605–613

Guerra EC, Lovely DF (2003) Suboptimal classifier for dysarthria assessment: lecture notes in computer science. In: Sanfeliu A, Ruiz-Shulcloper J (eds) Progress in pattern recognition, speech and image analysis. Springer, Berlin

Hattori N, Misu K, Koike H et al (2001) Age of onset influences clinical features of chronic inflammatory demyelinating polyneuropathy. J Neurol Sci 184(1):57–63

Hou Y, Dan X, Babbar M et al (2019) Ageing as a risk factor for neurodegenerative disease. Nat Rev Neurol 15(10):565–581

Johns DF, Darley FL (1970) Phonemic variability in apraxia of speech. J Speech Hear Res 13(3):556–583

Josephs KA, Duffy JR, Strand EA et al (2012) Characterizing a neurodegenerative syndrome: primary progressive apraxia of speech. Brain 135(5):1522–1536

Kent RD (1994) The clinical science of motor speech disorders: a personal assessment. In: Till JA, Yorkston KM, Beukelman DR (eds) Motor speech disorders: advances in assessment and treatment. Brookes, Baltimore

Kent RD, Duffy JR, Slama A et al. (2001) Clinicoanatomic studies in dysarthria: review, critique, and directions for research. J Speech Lang Hear Res 44(3):535–51. https://doi.org/10.1044/1092-4388(2001/042). PMID: 11407559.

Kim Y, Kent RD, Weismerb G (2011) An acoustic study of the relationships among neurologic disease, dysarthria type, and severity of dysarthria. J Speech Lang Hear Res 54(2):417–429

Kuypers HGJM (1981) Anatomy of the descending pathways. In: Brooks VB (ed) Handbook of physiology, section 1: the nervous system. volume II: motor control, part 1. American Physiological Society, Bethesda

Lamb R, Rohrer JD, Lees AJ et al (2016) Progressive supranuclear palsy and corticobasal degeneration: pathophysiology and treatment options. Curr Treat Options Neurol 18(9):42. https://doi.org/10.1007/s11940-016-0422-5

Lecours AR (1976) The "pure form" of the phonetic disintegration syndrome (pure anarthria); anatomo-clinical report of a historical case. Brain Lang 3(1):88–113

Liss JM, White L, Mattys SL et al (2009) Quantifying speech rhythm abnormalities in the dysarthrias. J Speech Lang Hear Res 52(5):1334–1352

Luzzatti C (2012) La rieducazione dei deficit fonologici e dell'articolazione. In: Mazzucchi A (ed) La Riabilitazione Neuropsicologica: premesse teoriche e Applicazioni Cliniche, 3rd edn. Elsevier, Milano, pp 25–47

Marie P (1906) Révision de la question de l'aphasie: la troisième circonvolution frontale gauche ne joue aucun rôle spécial dans la fonction du langage. La Sem Méd 26:241–247

Marie P (1907) Présentation de malades atteints d'anarthrie par lésion de l'hémisphère gauche du cerveau

Martin JH (2003) Neuroanatomy texts and atlas, 4th edn. McGraw-Hill, New York

McNeil MR, Robin DA, Schmidt RA (2009) Apraxia of speech: definition, differentiation, and treatment. In: McNeil MR (ed) Clinical management of sensorimotor speech disorders, 2nd edn. Thieme, New York

Miller N, Lowit A, O'Sullivan H (2006) What makes acquired foreign accent syndrome foreign? J Neurolinguistics 19(5):385–409

Moen I (2006) Analysis of a case of the foreign accent syndrome in terms of the framework of gestural phonology. J Neurolinguistics 19:410–423

Murdoch BE, Thompson RC, Theodoros DG (1997) Spastic dysarthria. In: McNeil MR (ed) Clinical management of sensorimotor speech disorders, 1st edn. Thieme, New York

Nicolosi L, Harryman E, Kresheck J (2006) Terminology of communication disorders: speech-language-hearing, 4th edn. Williams and Wilkins, Baltimore

Phipps MS, Cronin CA (2020) Management of acute ischemic stroke. BMJ 368:16983. https://doi.org/10.1136/bmj.16983

Pick A (1919) Über Änderungen des Sprachcharakters als Begleiterscheinung aphasischer Störungen. Z Gesamte Neurol Psych 45:230–241

Rohrer JD, Rossor MN, Warren JD (2010) Apraxia in progressive nonfluent aphasia. J Neurol 257(4):569–574

Ruano L, Melo C, Silva MC et al (2014) The global epidemiology of hereditary ataxia and spastic paraplegia: a systematic review of prevalence studies. Neuroepidemiology 42(3):174–183

Schiff HB, Alexander MP, Naeser MA et al (1983) Aphemia: clinical-anatomic correlations. Arch Neurol 40:720–727

Siciliano G, Manca M, Gennarelli M et al (2001) Epidemiology of myotonic dystrophy in Italy: re-appraisal after genetic diagnosis. Clin Genet 59(5):344–349

Simmons KC, Mayo R (1997) The use of the Mayo Clinic system for differential diagnosis of dysarthria. J Commun Disord 30(2):117–132

Singh S, Kent RD (2000) Singular's illustrated dictionary of speech-language pathology. Delmar-Cengage Learning, New York

Strand EA, Yorkston KM (1994) Description and classification of individuals with dysarthria: a 10-year review. In: Till JA, Yorkston KM, Beukelman DR (eds) Motor speech disorders: advances in assessment and treatment. Brookes, Baltimore

Van der Graaf M, Kuiper T, Zwinderman A et al (2009) Clinical identification of dysarthria types among neurologists, residents in neurology, and speech therapists. Eur Neurol 61(5):295–300

Witting N, Werlauff U, Duno M (2017) Phenotypes, genotypes, and prevalence of congenital myopathies older than 5 years in Denmark. Neurol Genet 3(2):e140. https://doi.org/10.1212/NXG.0000000000000140

Worms PM (2001) The epidemiology of motor neuron diseases: a review of recent studies. J Neurol Sci 191(1-2):3–9

Yedavalli VS, Patil A, Shah P (2018) Amyotrophic lateral sclerosis and its mimics/variants: a comprehensive review. J Clin Imaging Sci 8:53. https://doi.org/10.4103/jcis.JCIS_40_18

Yunusova Y, Plowman EK, Green JR et al (2019) Clinical measures of bulbar dysfunction in ALS. Front Neurol 10:106. https://doi.org/10.3389/fneur.2019.00106

Ziegler W, Aichert I, Staiger A (2012) Apraxia of speech: concepts and controversies. J Speech Lang Hear Res 55:S1485–S1501

Zraich RI, La Pointe LL (1997) Hyperkinetic dysarthria. In: McNeil MR (ed) Clinical management of sensorimotor speech disorders, 1st edn. Thieme, New York

Zyski BJ, Weisiger BE (1987) Identification of dysarthria types based on perceptual analysis. J Commun Disord 20(5):367–378

# Special Kinds of Dysarthria

# 17

Guilia Biondi, Karel Neubauer,
and Philippe Paquier

## 17.1 Dysarthria in Children

Giulia Biondi and Karel Neubauer

### 17.1.1 Introduction

Dysarthria in children is caused, as in adults, by damage to those parts of the central or peripheral nervous system that control speech muscles, resulting in deficits of both speech (phonation, resonance, articulation) and non-speech movements (respiration, swallowing, etc.). Owing to a reduced range of motion, strength, speed, as well as coordination of articulatory muscles, children with dysarthria may exhibit voice alterations, hypernasality, vowel distortions, imprecise consonants and breathing rate control problems.

G. Biondi (✉)
Policlinico G. Rodolico - Department of Otorhinolaryngology, University of Catania, Catania, Italy

K. Neubauer
Clinic of Phoniatrics of University Hospital Prague, Charles University Faculty of Medicine, Prague, Czech Republic
e-mail: Karel.Neubauer@lf1.cuni.cz

P. Paquier
Clinical Neurolinguistics & Aphasiology, Brussels Center for Language Studies, Vrije Universiteit Brussels, Brussels, Belgium
e-mail: philippe.paquier@vub.be

Dysarthria is viewed as a disorder at the execution level of speech production, whereas disturbed planning or programming levels lead to different, and in some way more specific, disorders (developmental apraxia of speech—DAS—and possibly stuttering). The underlying disease can be congenital or acquired but, in any case, it can occur before or during the course of speech development, therefore interacting with the emerging language and speech processing system (Caruso and Strand 1999).

From this point of view, it is important to consider the:

- Biomechanical and neural maturation of speech development
- Interaction between language development and motor skill acquisition
- Increasing automaticity in motor processing

Furthermore, in most cases damage of the neural structures in the immature brain of children is often multiple, possibly associated with sensory functions, and consequently the subdivision established and accepted for adults (flaccid, spastic, dyskinetic, ataxic) is rarely applicable, while forms of mixed type, in which symptomatic clusters of either type may prevail, are more common (van Mourik et al. 1997). Conversely, some children may exhibit dysarthric characteristics of speech without any documented lesions of the nervous structures. During this time, children are developing other higher functions, and comorbidity is common, not only with other language functions but also with notable aspects of cognitive, psychological and relational functions.

In the medical literature, there are no reliable data on the prevalence and incidence of childhood dysarthria. A rough picture can be drawn from studies on cerebral palsy, which to some extent can parallel cases of dysarthria. In the USA, prevalence is estimated from 2.3 to 3.6 of every 1000 individuals, whereas the incidence of dysarthria among children is estimated to be 1–2 per 1000. From the same studies emerges a marked preponderance of the spastic type of the motor disorder (Yeargin-Allsopp et al. 2008).

When examining individual cases, it is important to consider age of onset, cause, natural course, site and severity of lesion, speech components involved and perceptual characteristics. Moreover, especially for subjects of school age, social/pragmatic aspects of communication can have a very high importance, even greater than that of the motor disorder itself (ASHA 2015).

With regard to the characteristics of the speech, the most typical features are the following: weak vocal quality (lack of respiratory support), marked difficulties with strength and accuracy of articulatory movements, distortion of vowels, weak articulatory contacts, imprecise or weakly targeted consonants, hypo- or hypernasality, rapid or slow speaking rate, generally weak, mushy, garbled, imprecise speech.

One bright point in childhood is the greater ability of the subject to recover from or compensate for the speech disturbance. This ability, more evident in the case of acquired neural damage, is attributable to neuroplasticity and a greater aptitude of the growing brain for the activation of other areas in partial replacement of those injured.

## 17.1.2 Terminology

Dysarthria is called a speech disorder owing to the organic damage to the nervous system. Dysarthria includes a number of types or syndromes of speech disorder that are caused by difficulties in muscle control of speech mechanisms and that are classified as motor speech disorders (MSDs) (Yorkston et al. 2010; Riesthal 2016; Duffy 2020). In dysarthria, they are affected to varying degrees in the basic modalities of motor speech—respiration, phonation, resonance and articulation.

Congenital or developmental dysarthria (childhood dysarthria) (Milloy 1991; Yorkston et al. 2010; McLeod and Baker 2017; Duffy 2020) arises from a congenital lesion of the nervous system, most commonly in cerebral palsy (CP) syndrome.

> Because children with cerebral palsy often have damage to both hemispheres and, in part, the brainstem damage, we find disorders of speech in them, that do not occur in adulthood. (Pfeiffer 1996, p. 156)

The frequency and clinical picture of individual types of developmental dysarthria is specific for this type of disability, and the care of children with developmental dysarthria is always a long-term process associated with stimulating the psychomotor development of such affected children (Neubauer 2016).

## 17.1.3 Aetiology and Prevalence

The most common cause of developmental dysarthria is cerebral palsy (CP) syndrome, the frequency of this syndrome long having been significant in the population. Kraus (2005) presents the results of a Swedish study of 2/1000 live births and reports that low-birth weight babies (up to 2500 g) account for 50% of CP cases. McLeod and Baker (2017) state "cerebral palsy is evident in approximately 2 per 1000 births, with approximately 35% of these children having speech difficulty" (p. 563). Less frequent but significant causes of developmental dysarthria are brain injuries in children (Allison et al. 2017) and manifestations of neurological syndromes and diseases, especially congenital disorders, degenerative neurological diseases and infectious diseases of the child's brain in the earliest period of life (Pennington 2012; Duffy 2020).

## 17.1.4 Symptomatology

The term developmental dysarthria includes disorders originating at the beginning of the body's development owing to organic damage to the child's central nervous system (CNS). The division of individual types of developmental dysarthria is based on the identification of manifestations of individual neurological syndromes present in the early trauma of the nervous system, especially CP syndrome. Current knowledge about the development of motor pathology in children with CP accepts the dynamic development of the symptoms of the disorder during the CNS maturation process. Developmental dysarthria syndrome is also a dynamic developmental process, during which non-constant and permanent disorders of speech development depend on the child's CNS maturation, his current general physical condition and the related state of motor speech functions—breathing, voice formation, articulation and motor skills of the active parts of the orofacial area (especially the tongue, velum closure and lip closure).

### Differential Types of Developmental Dysarthria

These include (Milloy 1991; Neubauer 1998, 2016; McLeod and Baker 2017):

**Bulbar type of developmental dysarthria (hypotonic dysarthria):** This is caused by damage to the motor nuclei of the elongated spinal cord and cranial nerves innervating the speech organs. It arises suddenly after accidents or surgical operations in this area rather than developmentally. Disorder of the type of mild paralysis with peripheral motor neuron involvement can be unilateral (e.g. facial nerve palsy n.VII. Facialis) or bilateral. In the case of bilateral failure, swallowing and chewing are often impaired. Speech is also more markedly impaired owing to disorders of the implementation of articulatory movements due to impaired innervation of the speech organs by cranial nerves.

**Spastic type of developmental dysarthria (pyramidal dysarthria):** This arises from a failure of the central motor neuron (pyramidal tract) and is part of the spastic form of CP. Speech is impaired in the area of targeted respiratory control and velopharyngeal occlusion. Disorders of speech rhythm and lip and tongue movement are present. Speech is convulsive and hard, with increased nasal resonance, as the movements are affected by spasticity; they are coarse, cumbersome and hypertonic with frequent slow and incomplete contractions, such as the pharyngeal closure.

**Athetoid, hyperkinetic/hypokinetic type of developmental dysarthria (extrapyramidal developmental dysarthria):** The cause is a disorder of the striatum or other nuclei of the subcortical areas, accompanying the dyskinetic forms of CP. Articulation can be quite indistinct owing to unsustained, involuntary (athetoid) movements of the tongue, some sounds are strongly uttered, others sound faint and indistinct. In hyperkinetic manifestations, speech is incomprehensible owing to involuntary movements of the speech organs, disrupting the articulation and strongly disrupting breathing with chest, the formation and stability of the voice. Hypertonic manifestations with reduced speech motility, common in adults with Parkinson's disease, are a rarer developmental syndrome, uncommon in children.

**Atactic type of developmental dysarthria (cerebellar dysarthria):** This accompanies damage to the cerebellum and its pathways. It can accompany CP and is a common consequence of cerebellar tumour, as tumours in this area of the brain are relatively common in children. Speech is explosively formed, with a distorted type of expression, emphasising the individual voices (vowels and consonants as well) of the word. Adiadochokinesis, clumsiness of the tongue, numerous stops in speech and manifestations of clinging, staying in individual articulatory positions are all important components of the pathology of speech in this type of developmental dysarthria.

**Mixed type of developmental dysarthria:** This includes a combination of manifestations of the above types of developmental dysarthria. It arises rather individually in more extensive lesions or degenerative CNS diseases.

## 17.1.5 Assessment

Clinical speech therapy assessment most often follows the results of neurological examination and is guided by an effort to define the disorders of speech communication present, their severity and impact on the communication skills of the individual. Its main goal is to identify the share of individual speech motor modalities in the stigmatisation of speech, in reducing or losing its intelligibility for the social environment. The subsequently created individual therapy plan is focused on the coordinated stimulation of all speech motor modalities, but with the predominance of stimulation of the area in which the development or renewal of the function for changing the state of speech communication is essential.

A comprehensive assessment of the condition, abilities and deficits of a child with a severe CNS disorder includes medical, physiotherapeutic, psychological and speech therapy diagnostics. The determination of a neurological diagnosis by a child neurologist and the performance of a psychological diagnosis of the child's mental and cognitive abilities provide essential information for the diagnosis of somatic and communication disorders, which should result in the establishment of an individual rehabilitation plan. The results of the evaluation of the somatic development of the child by a rehabilitation doctor and a physiotherapist are the basis for the development of the rehabilitation of the child's movement functions. Speech therapy diagnostics evaluates the manifestations of speech communication disorders and determines the plan of therapeutic activities with the child. For the overall evalua-

tion of the child's abilities, it is necessary to include the development of skills in the field of school teaching, in cooperation with the relevant special pedagogue of the counselling school facility.

**Objectives of clinical speech therapy examination are to:**
- Evaluate the achieved ontogenesis of the child's speech and communication skills
- Assess the differential cause of speech communication disorders
- Determine the type of developmental dysarthria and the severity of the impairment of communication with the environment
- Determine an individual plan of speech therapy care from each of the above areas

**Comprehensive diagnostics focuses on:**
- Possible visual and hearing impairments that could affect the condition and development of speech communication
- Breathing, voice production and presence of salivation
- Developing skills in eating and swallowing
- Comprehension of speech, content of speech and ability of phonemic differentiation
- Development of expressive speech skills—articulation, resonance and individual language skills: grammar (morphology and syntax), vocabulary
- Examination of the motility of the speech organs and the orofacial area
- Graphomotor skills and motor practice, pathological interactions of body and speech organs
- Development of school skills according to the age of the child

**The clinical examination of a child with developmental dysarthria is based on the use of:**
- Guidelines and scales for evaluating the ontogenesis of the child's speech and communication
- Specialised scales for assessing the abilities of children with dysarthria
- Aids for evaluating performance in each of the above areas

Evaluation of the child's development is achieved by using clinical diagnostic guidelines and assessment of available medical, psychological and physiotherapeutic diagnostics. The area of motor speech modalities (respiration, phonation, articulation, resonance) and prosody of a child's speech is assessed qualitatively by a clinical speech therapist, by listening, observation and processing of speech or video-recording. A pragmatically important area is the evaluation of the difference between the individual tasks of the examination and the spontaneous speech of the child (Neubauer 2011).

For the English-speaking language environment, McLeod and Baker (2017) state the use of some assessments that are specifically designed for children with dysarthria:

- Communication function classification system (Hidecker et al. 2011)
- Quick assessment for dysarthria (Tanner and Culbertson 1999, p. 281)

When diagnosing developmental dysarthria, especially in children with CP, it is necessary not to forget about the connection between the somatic state of the child and his ability of speech communication and not to conclude his evaluation on the basis of a single exposure. A procedure involving the examination of a child several times in a row, observation in a group of peers and in interaction with the family is a necessity. Manifestations of dysarthria, intelligibility of speech and the ability to perform assigned tasks can vary diametrically according to the mental state of the child, his current physical condition and body position, fatigue or unusual environment, situation and tasks (Neubauer 2011, 2018).

## 17.1.6  Therapy and the Intervention Process

The following areas should be taken into account when implementing speech therapy care for children with developmental dysarthria:

- Efforts to coordinate work with somatic rehabilitation
- Efforts to induce a relaxed stable position and relaxation in the therapy of speech skills
- An effort to minimise the interplay of the body and speech organs, not to cause the movement of speech organs at the cost of causing significantly increased spasticity of the body or an increase in involuntary uncontrollable movements (Neubauer 2002, 2011, 2016, 2018)

The clinical speech therapist should be acquainted with the basic principles of mobility development in children with CP, with their applications for the field of speech therapy intervention, and with the state of rehabilitation treatment of individual children with CP. The possibility of coordinating physiotherapeutic and speech therapy interventions is always a promising option for developing the effectiveness of care for the benefit of the child.

Care for children with severe congenital or early acquired CNS deficits should be started at an early stage, focusing on the development of vital functions and motor organs of speech organs. Owing to the frequent pathological development of orofacial motor skills, the issue of eating disorders in these children is closely connected with the area of verbal communication development. If an adequate position of the body and orofacial area is not provided when feeding the child, the development of adequate speech momentum will also be difficult in the development of vocal and speech communication.

The connection of speech therapy care with physiotherapy is significantly present in the rehabilitation procedures used:

- Bobath concept (Raine et al. 2009): Application of the so-called oral therapy to stimulate food intake and swallowing, development of orofacial motor skills; speech therapy using an inhibitory position determined by a physiotherapist. Neubauer (2002, 2011, 2018) describes the use of the concept and the principle of cooperation with a speech therapist in a team approach.

- Reflex locomotion therapy (Vojta 1993; Vojta and Peters 2018): The use of spasticity release or attenuation of involuntary movements in the period of time after the end of physiotherapy exercises; the possibility of increasing the stimulation of orofacial motor skills and breathing by using the trigger points in this area (e.g. the submandibular zone) during reflex rotation exercises (Neubauer 2002, 2011, 2018).
- Proprioceptive neuromuscular facilitation (PNF, Kabat's methodology, Adler et al. 2008): In the stimulation of speech momentum, involvement of exercises against resistance, use of isometric and isotonic methods of stimulation of orofacial momentum (Neubauer 2002, 2011, 2018).
- Orofacial regulatory therapy (Castillo–Morales concept): It is a directly specialised reflex methodology for the orofacial area, focusing on the activity of facial muscles, swallowing and speech. It uses tension, pressure and vibration in the facial and orofacial area and intensifies existing methods in this area (Morales 2006).
- Myofunctional therapy: An effective methodology for working with manifestations of muscle and functional imbalance in the orofacial area (Kittel 1999, 2001). Owing to its focus and types of exercise programme, it is intended for an intact population with developmental deficits rather than for the area of neurogenic disorders, but it also has its application in less severe manifestations of developmental dysarthria.

### 17.1.6.1 Stimulation of Spontaneous Motor Speech Skills

This involves establishing and maintaining eye contact as a basic precondition for the development of imitation and understanding of instructions and communication situations:

- Development of imitation of motor activities as a prerequisite for the development of imitation of articulatory movements.

- Use of massage of the orofacial area, frequent use of circular massage of the face and tongue, preferably in conjunction with interjectional content sounds—e.g. in a circular massage of the corner of the mouth to "u", stimulation of honking with a toy, etc.—the effort is to create a motor sensation associated with sound and content accompaniment.
- Transition from passive massage to active imitation of articulatory movements with visual, auditory and tactile feedback.
- An effort to stimulate phonological differentiation, differentiating sound-like words, linking these procedures with the development of impressive vocabulary with the use of manipulation with toys and visual aids.
- Consistent connection of audio and verbal expressions with language content at a motivational level, accessible to the child's current cognitive abilities.
- The use of all forms of motivation of the child for active communication, including the use of computer programs with auditory and visual feedback. The MENTIO voice program (Petržílková 2020) in the Czech language environment, program Sona-Speech II of KayPENTAX—acoustic analysis system for behavioural therapy (Jacobson 2016) in the English language environment are examples of complex PC programs, containing similar and more specific parameters than the older SpeechViewer program from IBM. They can be used for work with prosody and intonation of speech and allow a wide range of work with suprasegmental components of speech, sound, length, height, intensity and other parameters.

### 17.1.6.2 Development of Motoric of the Facial Area and Articulatory Abilities

This involves:

- A respect for the development of spontaneous speech skills, directing it towards improving the intelligibility of the child's speech and the development of multi-word sentences.
- The acceptance and development of spontaneous compensation mechanisms. Especially in

the case of more severe manifestations of dysarthria, it is necessary to accept alternative mechanisms of sound formation and these mechanisms must be directed to a satisfactory differentiation from other sounds.

- The use of preparatory breathing, phonation and motor exercises of speech organs. However, the contribution of these exercises to increasing the intelligibility of spontaneous speech needs to be realistically perceived. It mainly has a supporting function with the possibility of use in exercises, with speech production and reading.
- Equipping the articulation of individual sounds. It should be guided by realistic goals, to serve to improve speech intelligibility, not strictly by seeking intact articulation, especially in severe manifestations of dysarthria.
- The use of rhythmisation (Kábele 1988; Neubauer 2002, 2011, 2018), which plays a very important role in the development of speech intelligibility in children with dysarthria, as it supports the dynamics of speech movement in a global way within the framework of verbal and sentence expression, and creates space for increasing the precision of speech movements. The possibility of connecting the rhythmic movement of the hand and speech organs, the use of aids such as a buzzer or metronome. However, the use of rhythmic speech or reading must be evaluated individually in order to avoid provocation of the pathological movements of the speech organs and pathological movements of the body with orofacial movements.

### 17.1.6.3  The Process of Creating Individual Language Skills

At an inner and expressive level in a child with developmental dysarthria, the basic principles of communication development should be emphasised:

- Manifestations of communication disorders, in this case disorders of the development of motor speech skills, should not block the development of the child's inner language skills, the development of his visual and auditory perception or cognitive processes. A child with developmental dysarthria should complete an educational school programme at the level of their mental abilities and have adequate social contact with the environment and peers
- The effort to create an active stimulating communication environment in a family or institutional facility is not possible without the involvement of close persons and a wide team of facility staff. It includes the most frequent active communication situation, experiencing a sense of dialogue even at the lowest level of expression, using parallel speech procedures to comment on the activities of the child and surrounding persons, the use of corrective feedback for the development of sentence express and grammar
- Maximising the child's communication potential by the use of augmentative and alternative communication, if the severity of the disorder requires it (Neubauerová and Neubauer 2018)

### 17.1.7  Prognosis

The prognosis is frequently connected with the development of nervous system involvement, which was the cause of the onset and development of MSDs. Congenital of developmental dysarthria is a disorder that occurs with a wide range of causes, can vary in severity and can also develop in a prognostic variety. In the case of favourable healing of nerve tissue and restoration of functions after trauma, development is possible up to the area of mild residual difficulties in speech and practical disappearance of speech communication disorders. It can be documented in some people who have suffered from stroke or head injuries, children and adults.

In the case of developmentally more severe dysarthria, based mainly on CP but also in persistent organic causes, we can talk about functional improvement in terms of increasing self-control of motor skills, improving speech intelligibility and improving performance with regard to length and quality of speech. The complex prognostic picture also includes the successful introduction of compensation strategies—communication in writing, manual code, technical communication aid, PC with specialised software.

## 17.2 Cerebellar Mutism Syndrome in Children

Philippe F. Paquier

### 17.2.1 Introduction

Although transient and total, cerebellar-induced speechlessness has been exceptionally associated with non-tumoural aetiologies (Mariën et al. 2010); it is usually a tragic complication of paediatric posterior fossa surgery. Its incidence in children who have undergone posterior fossa tumour resection is estimated to be from 7% to 50% (Mariën et al. 2010). Even if it has occasionally been reported in adults (Mariën et al. 2010), the condition nevertheless is typically considered a paediatric syndrome, called the paediatric Cerebellar Mutism Syndrome (pCMS) (Gudrunardottir et al. 2016b).

The core features of pCMS are (De Smet et al. 2007):

1. Mutism occurs after resection of a cerebellar mass lesion.
2. There is generally a delayed onset of speech loss after an interval of a few hours up to 11 days after normal speech post-surgery.
3. Mutism is transient and usually lasts from 1 day to 6 months, but exceptions up to 2½ years of postoperative speechlessness have been documented.
4. Mutism is followed by a severe disorder of motor speech production, i.e. dysarthria—which usually recovers in 1–7 months, but in some instances a residual dysarthria has also been recorded >7 years after surgery.
5. There are frequent associations with other neurological disturbances, such as long tract signs, language impairments, cognitive abnormalities, behavioural and affective deficits.

The speechlessness is regarded as the hallmark symptom of the broader cerebellar mutism syndrome (CMS), previously also frequently termed the posterior fossa syndrome (PFS) (Schmahmann 2020). CMS covers a wider spectrum of postoperative, often frontal-like neuro-behavioural deficits that may include mood lability and irritability; apathy; unconcern; lack of bowel and bladder control without apparent gastroenterological, urological or pharmacological reasons; compulsive pre-sleep behaviour; autistic-like behaviour; decreased initiation of a wide range of voluntary activities including disrupted language dynamics, impaired voluntary eye opening (eye-lid apraxia), inhibited mastication and swallowing in the absence of neurological dysphagia (Catsman-Berrevoets and Aarsen 2010; Mariën et al. 2019). However, speechlessness is not always the core symptom of (p)CMS, as these patients may not present with true mutism but rather with severe verbal adynamia or very inhibited verbal output (De Smet et al. 2007).

The age-related discrepancy in frequency of occurrence of CMS in children and adults is often explained by (1) the higher incidence of posterior fossa tumours in children (Dolecek et al. 2012; Massimino et al. 2016) and (2) anatomical and functional postnatal maturational factors, the incomplete myelination of the descending cortico-ponto-cerebellar and ascending dentato-thalamo-cortical pathways, rendering children more vulnerable to the impact of a cerebellar lesion (Ildan et al. 2002). In addition, Pols et al. (2017) recently suggested surgery-related reasons for this age-dependent difference, in that compared with adults, children have a smaller intravascular volume, thus being less protected against hypovolaemia. This means that even a proportionately small quantity of intra-operative blood loss can result in a disturbance in oxygen delivery susceptible to induce local ischaemia at the surgical site and its immediate vicinity, including the deep cerebellar nuclei bilaterally.

## 17.2.2 Clinical Presentation

Typically, mutism in children with cerebellar tumours develops after a short period of relatively normal postoperative functioning. This "symptom-free" interval might be explained by the fading postoperative effects of intra-operative osmotherapy, administered to minimise cerebral oedema during the surgical intervention, along with the concomitant delayed onset of postoperative swelling and oedema. During the mute phase, high-pitched crying and whining may be observed, along with various concomitant neurological symptoms indicating cerebellar or brainstem damage (Küper and Timmann 2013). In addition, a wide spectrum of behavioural and affective disturbances may manifest, such as autistic behaviour, avoidance of social and physical contact with parents and caregivers, cortical blindness, compulsive pre-sleep behaviour, aggressiveness, forced crying and laughing with motor perseverations and severe apathy (Catsman-Berrevoets and Aarsen 2010).

After the alleviation of the postoperative mutism, the presence of dysarthria appears to be the rule. In a critical review of the literature, De Smet et al. (2007) found that 165 of 167 reliable cases (98.8%) unquestionably exhibited dysarthria after remission of mutism. In the two remaining children, these authors assumed that dysarthric symptoms were masked by a combination of overwhelming behavioural disturbances and lack of spontaneous verbal production.

Once speech resumes after the mute phase, motor speech deficits often do not display the typical ataxic speech symptoms found in adult patients with various types of cerebellar damage (Darley et al. 1975). Van Mourik et al. (1998) found a slow speech rate, rather than scanning of speech, to be the most prominent speech feature in a group of children who had undergone cerebellar tumour surgery. In two children with pCMS and persistent dysarthria at follow-up after cerebellar astrocytoma surgery, Aarsen et al. (2004) noted that the two more distinctive features of ataxic dysarthria—i.e. irregular articulatory breakdown and excess and equal stress—were absent. These observations were endorsed by a critical analysis by De Smet et al. (2007), which confirmed that prominent symptoms of ataxic dysarthria—i.e. irregular articulatory breakdown and scanning speech—are not necessarily the hallmark of dysarthria post-mutism. In a series of 40 children with pCMS, Catsman-Berrevoets and Aarsen (2010) described ataxic speech characteristics in only five children. In a long-term follow-up study of 24 children and adolescents—of whom 12 exhibited pCMS—who had undergone cerebellar tumour surgery, De Smet et al. (2012) observed typical ataxic speech symptoms in less than 25% of the patients. These authors suggested that the absence of ataxic speech features after cerebellar tumour surgery in children might be related to the underlying pathophysiology. Restricting the population under study to a more homogeneous aetiological group that requires surgery (e.g. by excluding heredoataxias and cerebrovascular diseases) might explain why non-ataxic speech characteristics are found to be more prominent in pCMS. Indeed, because of the close vicinity of the cerebellum and brainstem, the effects of the surgical intervention (e.g. postoperative spasm of the vessels supplying the cerebellum and the brainstem, causing ischaemia or oedema in brainstem structures) might be responsible for the occurrence of paretic rather than ataxic postoperative speech symptoms.

Besides motor speech deficits, a variety of concomitant non-motor language disturbances may manifest after remission of mutism, such as word-finding difficulties, agrammatism, disrupted language dynamics, comprehension deficits, reading and writing disorders (De Smet et al. 2013).

## 17.2.3 Recovery

Early optimistic assertions that dysarthria in pCMS recovers quickly and completely (Van Dongen et al. 1994) have been tempered by more recent follow-up studies documenting incomplete recovery of motor speech production in many patients (De Smet et al. 2007). For instance, Steinbok et al. (2003) reported seven patients with postoperative cerebellar mutism, of whom only one recovered normal speech; two other children displayed a residual dysarthria more than 7 years after surgery; in three children, motor speech production more than 3 years after surgery was said to be slow; another child was still mute 2½ years after surgery. In another long-term follow-up, auditory-perceptual motor speech analysis in 24 children who had undergone cerebellar tumour surgery, De Smet et al. (2012) found that all 12 children with pCMS exhibited dysarthria in the immediate post-mutism phase, and 11 of them (91.7%) had persistent motor speech deficits up to 12 years after surgery. These authors confirmed the findings of Huber et al. (2006) of persistent motor speech defects in a long-term follow-up of more than 5 years and endorsed their view that pCMS may be a poor prognostic factor for the presence of long-term dysarthria in children treated for cerebellar tumours.

## 17.2.4 Risk Factors

Several risk factors for the development of pCMS have been proposed. Catsman-Berrevoets et al. (1999) previously found an interaction between type and size of the lesion, i.e. pCMS is most likely to occur when the tumour resection concerns a large size medullo-blastoma with a diameter exceeding 5 cm (see also Pols et al. 2017). However, as pCMS may also be associated with smaller medullo-blastomas, as well as with other types of tumour or even with other aetiologies (Riva 1998; Fujisawa et al. 2005; Baillieux et al. 2007), additional risk factors were also suggested to play a role in its pathogenesis: midline tumour location (vermis or fourth ventricle) (Catsman-Berrevoets et al. 1999; Reed-Berendt et al. 2014); brainstem infiltration or compression (Robertson et al. 2006; Pols et al. 2017); post-surgical oedema of the pontine tegmentum (Van Dongen et al. 1994); lesions to the deep nuclei of the cerebellum (Puget et al. 2009; Albazron et al. 2019); and bilateral injury to the proximal dentato-thalamo-cortical pathways (Morris et al. 2009; Avula 2020), often associated with bilateral hypertrophic olivary degeneration of the inferior olivary nucleus resulting from disruption of the Guillain-Mollaret triangle (Patay et al. 2014; Avula et al. 2016). Postoperative meningitis and pre- or postoperative hydrocephalus were initially assumed to be of significance (Humphreys 1989; Ferrante et al. 1990), but more recent studies could not confirm this assumption (Gudrunardottir et al. 2011; Pols et al. 2017).

Surgical techniques are also considered to entail risk factors: presence and length of vermian incision (although with ambivalent evidence) (Kellogg and Piatt 1997; Avula et al. 2015; Cobourn et al. 2020; Schaller-Paule et al. 2021); extent of surgical resection (total resection seems to increase the risk of pCMS and does not necessarily improve the survival rate) (Catsman-Berrevoets and Patay 2018; Dhaenens et al. 2020); the use of Cavitron ultrasonic surgical aspirator (CUSA) with risk of causing thermal injury to the proximal efferent cerebellar pathway structures (Avula et al. 2015; Cobourn et al. 2020).

Interestingly, Pols et al. (2017) found that a 0.5 °C increase in mean body temperature in the first 4 days after surgery was an independent and highly significant predictor for pCMS, amplifying the odds ratio for its development almost five-fold. The authors explained this significant risk factor for pCMS as resulting from changing neuronal metabolic rates, which decrease under anaesthesia and increase again once anaesthesia wears off. Pols et al. (2017) postulated that a higher mean body temperature in the first days post-surgery might amplify metabolic stress to such a degree that the oxygen demands in the vicinity of the site of surgery are insufficiently met, especially when the circum-ambient brain tissues are in an already critical metabolic state. Pols et al. (2017) argued that their findings were consonant with data collected in stroke patients, in whom hyperthermia is linked to fairly large infarction volumes and poorer outcome.

As to the presence of pre-operative speech and language impairments (e.g. dysarthria, apraxia of speech, decreased mean length of utterance, anomia, reduced phonological verbal fluency, verbal adynamia), Di Rocco et al. (2011) and Bianchi et al. (2020) found that they were a strong risk factor for pCMS. Paquier et al. (2020) concluded that: "Referral to a speech/language pathologist for a comprehensive and systematic assessment of speech and language in children with cerebellar tumour is vital in order to facilitate the early detection and management of pCMS, with a view to reduce negative long-term consequences". Inserting data about pre-operative speech and language functioning into pre-operative pCMS prediction models (Liu et al. 2018) might well improve their accuracy and specificity (Dhaenens et al. 2020).

impact of a cerebellar lesion on a distant but anatomically and functionally connected supratentorial region (Mariën et al. 2019). In this respect, cerebellar damage is assumed to induce a decrease or loss of transmission of excitatory impulses from the deep cerebellar nuclei via the ascending cerebello-thalamo-cortical pathways to supratentorial brain areas (Mariën et al. 2010; Miller et al. 2010), thus resulting in the functional suppression of supratentorial cortical regions critically involved in neuro-cognition (and thus, language). Consistent with this assumption are the suggestions of Morris et al. (2009) that functional disruption of the white matter bundles containing efferent axons within the superior cerebellar peduncles might be a crucial underlying pathophysiological determinant of pCMS.

## 17.2.5 Pathophysiology

Despite the growing interest in pCMS, its exact pathophysiology remains unknown. A number of hypotheses have been put forward, supported by varying levels of evidence (for reviews, see Catsman-Berrevoets and Patay 2018; Mariën et al. 2019; Avula 2020): (1) postoperative vasospasm of the arteries supplying the cerebellum and the brainstem, leading to ischaemia and oedema in brainstem structures; (2) transient dysfunction of the A9 and A10 mesencephalic dopaminergic cell groups and ascending activating reticular system; (3) transient dysregulation of neurotransmitter release originating from the tumour resection and the alleviation of long-lasting compression of the brainstem by the tumour; (4) bilateral (surgical) damage to the dentate and interpositus nuclei or to the afferent or efferent pathways passing through these nuclei; (5) thermal injury causing damage to brain parenchyma and in particular to the proximal efferent cerebellar pathway structures (Purkinje cells of the cerebellum are thought to be selectively unprotected against heat injury); and (5) crossed cerebello-cerebral diaschisis reflecting the metabolic or blood perfusion

## 17.2.6 Treatment

As yet, there is no established treatment for the speech and language impairments in pCMS (Paquier et al. 2020). Attempts have been undertaken to reverse mutism in its acute stage by pharmacological intervention. Corticosteroids, fluoxetine, thyrotropin-releasing hormone, bromocriptine, midazolam and zolpidem have all been used with conflicting results (for reviews, see Lassaletta et al. 2015; Catsman-Berrevoets and Patay 2018; Mariën et al. 2019).

Drugs targeting acute and long-term pCMS-associated symptoms may result in symptom relief and improved quality of life (Molinari et al. 2020). Anecdotally, mostly single-case studies report rather ambivalent evidence of pharmacological effectiveness in cerebellar-related neuropsychiatric symptoms in children. Carbamazepine has been used for severe dysphoria and irritability (Turkel et al. 2004) and aripiprazole for agitation (Yap et al. 2012). Low doses of atypical antipsychotics and benzodiazepines may be useful in the postoperative course to favour engagement in speech/language, physical and occupational rehabilitation (Molinari et al. 2020).

### 17.2.7 Rehabilitation

Several authors agree on the need for individualised rehabilitation programmes combining speech/language, physical and occupational therapies to help restore communication and motor functioning (Morgan et al. 2011; Walker et al. 2014; Catsman-Berrevoets and Patay 2018). Consequently, rehabilitation strategies aiming at minimising the sequelae of a cerebellar injury are actually under scrutiny (Lassaletta et al. 2015; Hartley et al. 2019). However, to date few systematic rehabilitation trials focusing on diminishing or eradicating the long-term consequences of pCMS have been completed (Lassaletta et al. 2015; Catsman-Berrevoets and Patay 2018; Molinari et al. 2020). Cognitive rehabilitation needs to address several interrelated aspects of neurocognitive functioning that may be impaired to varying degrees, such as executive functions, memory, intentional and attentional processes, visuo-spatial and visuo-perceptual skills and non-verbal communication (Walker et al. 2014; Lassaletta et al. 2015). Moreover, as stressed by Walker et al. (2014), it is nonsensical to uncouple cognitive rehabilitation from behavioural and emotional problems or from the familial and environmental context, which have been proven to be much predictive of recovery from acquired brain damage. Outlining specific nursing strategies for the patients and their families is also of utmost importance (Parent and Scott 2011). These encompass managing acute symptoms and assisting the family through a period of intense anguish; coordinating the different actors' efforts (physicians, (neuro) psychologists, speech/language therapists, neuro-linguists, physiotherapists, occupational therapists); and supplying information to educational services and community representatives (Gudrunardottir et al. 2016a).

As recent evidence tends to show that the dentato-thalamo-cortical pathways are susceptible to neuroplasticity (Molinari et al. 2020), non-invasive (cerebellar) stimulation techniques such as transcranial direct current stimulation (tDCS) or transcranial magnetic stimulation (TMS) may be propitious in intensifying recovery by modulating the connectivity between the cerebellum and supratentorial brain areas (Grimaldi et al. 2014).

Currently, the range of postoperative challenges for children with pCMS necessitates an integrated approach to rehabilitation. Timely intervention with a long-term plan for the management and close scrutiny of speech and language is essential, as children remain vulnerable throughout development. As a group, children treated for brain tumours often face poor long-term quality of life outcomes owing to speech and language disorders, which comprise school failure and loss of friendships resulting in detrimental repercussions for healthy development and socialisation (Vanclooster et al. 2019, 2020; Paquier et al. 2020). As emphasised by Paquier et al. (2020), "Routine clinical management should be central to the rehabilitation of children with pCMS, with a systematic integrated approach to the management, assessment and treatment of speech and language disorders, and follow-up and early intervention. It is therefore recommended that rehabilitation of speech and language in children with pCMS involves multiphase implementation of evidence-based guidelines and recommendations that identify and highlight risk factors, specific deficits, and knowledge about progression over time".

### 17.2.8 Conclusion

Cerebellar-induced speechlessness is a well-known and deleterious complication of posterior fossa surgery that affects children far more often than adults. It is transient in nature, and mutism typically turns into dysarthria once speech resumes after the mute phase. Cerebellar-induced speechlessness is a symptom embedded in a constellation of associated devastating neurolinguistic, neurocognitive and neurobehavioural disturbances, termed the (paediatric) cerebellar mutism syndrome (CMS). Identifying risk factors/predictors for pCMS is crucial and may comprise a complete baseline assessment of speech and language. The complex and extensive symptomatology of pCMS highlights the importance of multidisciplinary management. The life-changing, chronic and pervasive impact of pCMS underscores the importance of rehabilitation and effective and early intervention (Paquier et al. 2020). Cognitive rehabilitation including speech and language therapy should be customised to suit the individual needs of the children. Given the large spectrum of cognitive, emotional, behavioural and social deficits in children who have had pCMS, a thorough longitudinal follow-up is important to mould an appropriate and personalised long-term rehabilitation programme that also improves their quality of life (Lassaletta et al. 2015; Catsman-Berrevoets and Patay 2018; Paquier et al. 2020). In addition to cognitive rehabilitation, the long-term emotional and behavioural sequelae of pCMS might well need to be addressed with tailored pharmacological interventions focusing on the children's individual specific clinical presentation (Molinari et al. 2020).

Current knowledge indicates that brainstem involvement and bilateral injury to the dentato-thalamo-cortical pathways are high risk factors for pCMS. Recent insights into the possible pathophysiological mechanisms support the notion that crossed cerebello-cerebral diaschisis disrupts the functional integrity of supratentorial cortical regions crucially involved in speech, language and other neurocognitive and neurobehavioural functions. Alternative techniques such as tDCS and TMS, in combination with cognitive interventions, seem to be propitious strategies to enhance recovery and neuroplasticity by acting on the cerebello-cerebral connectivity (Grimaldi et al. 2014), and may also bring about new opportunities in children with pCMS (Paquier et al. 2020). Given the paucity of controlled data on the therapeutic options, there is a need for systematic prospective trials evaluating the effects of different neurosurgical approaches, pharmacological interventions and neuro-rehabilitation strategies. Achieving a balance between optimal survival and minimal long-term sequelae will ultimately result in improved quality of life outcomes.

**Acknowledgments** This contribution incorporates research carried out by the Posterior Fossa Society (www.posteriorfossasociety.org) Working Group focusing on rehabilitation approaches and protocols (intervention and management) of pCMS.

# References

Aarsen FK, Van Dongen HR, Paquier PF et al (2004) Long-term sequelae in children after cerebellar astrocytoma surgery. Neurology 62:1311–1316

Adler S, Beckers D, Buck M (2008) PNF in practice. Springer, Berlin

Albazron FM, Bruss J, Jones RM et al (2019) Pediatric postoperative cerebellar cognitive affective syndrome follows outflow pathway lesions. Neurology 93:e1561–e1571

Allison A, Byorn L, Turkstra S (2017) Traumatic brain injury in children and adolescent. In: Johnson A, Jacobson B (eds) Medical speech language pathology. Thieme Medical Publisher Inc., New York, pp 103–118

ASHA (2015) Social communication disorder. http://www.asha.org/Practice-Portal/Clinical-Topics/Social-Communication-Disorders-in-School-Age-Children/. Accessed 18 Jun 2020

Avula S (2020) Radiology of post-operative paediatric cerebellar mutism syndrome. Childs Nerv Syst 36:1187–1195

Avula S, Mallucci C, Kumar R et al (2015) Posterior fossa syndrome following brain tumour resection: review of pathophysiology and a new hypothesis on its pathogenesis. Childs Nerv Syst 31:1859–1867

Avula S, Spiteri M, Kumar R et al (2016) Post-operative pediatric cerebellar mutism syndrome and its association with hypertrophic olivary degeneration. Quant Imaging Med Surg 6:535–544

Baillieux H, Weyns F, Paquier P et al (2007) Posterior fossa syndrome after a vermian stroke: a new case and review of the literature. Pediatr Neurosurg 43:386–395

Bianchi F, Chieffo DPR, Frassanito P et al (2020) Cerebellar mutism: the predictive role of preoperative language evaluation. Childs Nerv Syst 36:1153–1157

Caruso AJ, Strand EA (1999) Clinical management of motor speech disorders in children. Thieme, New York

Catsman-Berrevoets CE, Aarsen FK (2010) The spectrum of neurobehavioral deficits in the Posterior Fossa Syndrome in children after cerebellar tumor surgery. Cortex 46:933–946

Catsman-Berrevoets CE, Patay Z (2018) Cerebellar mutism syndrome. In: Manto M, Huisman TAGM (eds) Handbook of clinical neurology, vol. 155 (3rd series). The cerebellum: disorders and treatment. Elsevier, Amsterdam, pp 273–288

Catsman-Berrevoets CE, Van Dongen HR, Mulder PGH et al (1999) Tumor type and size are high risk factors for the syndrome of "cerebellar" mutism and subsequent dysarthria. J Neurol Neurosurg Psychiatry 67:755–757

Cobourn K, Marayati F, Tsering D et al (2020) Cerebellar mutism syndrome: current approaches to minimize risk for CMS. Childs Nerv Syst 36:1171–1179

Darley FL, Aronson AE, Brown JE (1975) Motor speech disorders. WB Saunders, Philadelphia

De Smet HJ, Baillieux H, Catsman-Berrevoets CE et al (2007) Postoperative motor speech production in children with the syndrome of 'cerebellar' mutism and subsequent dysarthria: a critical review of the literature. Eur J Pediatr Neurol 11:193–207

De Smet HJ, Catsman-Berrevoets CE, Aarsen F et al (2012) Auditory-perceptual speech analysis in children with cerebellar tumors: a long-term follow-up. Eur J Pediatr Neurol 16:434–442

De Smet HJ, Paquier PF, Verhoeven J et al (2013) The cerebellum: its role in language and related cognitive and affective functions. Brain Lang 127:334–342

Dhaenens BAE, Van Veelen MLC, Catsman-Berrevoets CE (2020) Preoperative prediction of postoperative cerebellar mutism syndrome. Validation of existing MRI models and proposal of the new Rotterdam pCMS prediction model. Childs Nerv Syst 36(7):1471–1480. https://doi.org/10.1007/s00381-020-04535-4

Di Rocco C, Chieffo D, Frassanito P et al (2011) Heralding cerebellar mutism: evidence for pre-surgical language impairment as primary risk factor in posterior fossa surgery. Cerebellum 10:551–562

Dolecek TA, Propp JM, Stroup NE et al (2012) CBTRUS Statistical report: primary brain and central nervous system tumors diagnosed in the United States in 2005–2009. Neuro Oncol 14:1–49

Duffy J (2020) Motor speech disorders. Substrates, differential diagnosis, and management. Elsevier, St. Louis, MO

Ferrante L, Mastronardi L, Acqui M et al (1990) Mutism after posterior fossa surgery in children. Report of three cases. J Neurosurg 72:959–963

Fujisawa H, Yonaha H, Okumoto K et al (2005) Mutism after evacuation of acute subdural hematoma of the posterior fossa. Childs Nerv Syst 21:234–236

Grimaldi G, Argyropoulos GP, Boehringer A et al (2014) Non-invasive cerebellar stimulation—a consensus paper. Cerebellum 13:121–138

Gudrunardottir T, Sehested A, Juhler M et al (2011) Cerebellar mutism: review of the literature. Childs Nerv Syst 27:355–363

Gudrunardottir T, De Smet HJ, Bartha-Doering L et al (2016a) Posterior fossa syndrome (PFS) and cerebellar mutism. In: Mariën P, Manto M (eds) The linguistic cerebellum. Elsevier & Academic Press, Amsterdam, pp 257–314

Gudrunardottir T, Morgan AT, Lux AL et al (2016b) Consensus paper on post-operative pediatric cerebellar mutism syndrome: the Iceland Delphi results. Child's Nerv Syst 32:1195–1203

Hartley H, Pizer B, Lane S et al (2019) Incidence and prognostic factors of ataxia in children with posterior fossa tumors. Neurooncol Pract 6:185–193

Hidecker M, Paneth N, Rosenbaum P et al (2011) Developing and validating the Communication Function Classification System for individuals with cerebral palsy. Dev Med Child Neurol 53(8):704–710

Huber JF, Bradley K, Spiegler BJ et al (2006) Long-term effects of transient cerebellar mutism after cerebellar astrocytoma or medulloblastoma resection in childhood. Childs Nerv Syst 22:132–138

Humphreys RP (1989) Mutism after posterior fossa tumor surgery. In: Marlin AE (ed) Concepts in pediatric neurosurgery. Karger, Basel, pp 57–64

Ildan F, Tuna M, Erman T et al (2002) The evaluation and comparison of cerebellar mutism in children and adults after posterior fossa surgery: report of two adult cases and review of the literature. Acta Neurochir 144:463–473

Jacobson B (2016) Assessment and treatment of voice disorders. In: Johnson A, Jacobson B (eds) Medical speech language pathology. Thieme Medical Publisher Inc., New York, pp 162–181

Kábele F (1988) Rozvíjení hybnosti a řeči dětí s dětskou mozkovou obrnou (Motility and speech development in children with cerebral palsy). Univerzita Karlova, Prague

Kellogg JX, Piatt JH (1997) Resection of fourth ventricle tumors without splitting the vermis: the cerebellomedullary fissure approach. Pediat Neurosurg 27:28–33

Kittel A (1999) Myofunkční terapie (Myofunctional therapy). Grada Publishing, Prague

Kittel A (2001) Myofunktionelle Therapie (Myofunctional therapy). Schulz-Kirchner Verlag GmbH, Idstein

Kraus J (ed) (2005) Dětská mozková obrna (Cerebral palsy). Grada Publishing, Prague

Küper M, Timmann D (2013) Cerebellar mutism. Brain Lang 127:327–333

Lassaletta A, Bouffet E, Mabbott D et al (2015) Functional and neuropsychological late outcomes in posterior fossa tumors in children. Childs Nerv Syst 31:1877–1890

Liu JF, Dineen RA, Avula S et al (2018) Development of a pre-operative scoring system for predicting risk of post-operative paediatric cerebellar mutism syndrome. Br J Neurosurg 32:18–27

Mariën P, De Smet HJ, Paquier P et al (2010) Cerebellocerebral diaschisis and postsurgical posterior fossa syndrome in pediatric patients. Am J Neuroradiol 31:e82. https://doi.org/10.3174/ajnr.A2198

Mariën P, Keulen S, Van Dun K et al (2019) Cerebellar mutism syndrome in children and adults. In: Manto M, Gruol DL, Schmahmann JD et al (eds) Handbook of the cerebellum and cerebellar disorders. Springer, Cham, pp 1–23

Massimino M, Biassoni V, Gandola L et al (2016) Childhood medulloblastoma. Crit Rev Oncol Hematol 105:35–51

McLeod S, Baker E (2017) Children's speech. An evidence-based approach to assessment and intervention. Pearson, Boston

Miller NG, Reddick WE, Kocak M et al (2010) Cerebellocerebral diaschisis is the likely mechanism of postsurgical posterior fossa syndrome in pediatric patients with midline cerebellar tumors. Am J Neuroradiol 31:288–294

Milloy N (1991) Breakdown in speech. Chapman & Hall, London

Molinari E, Pizer B, Catsman-Berrevoets C et al (2020) Posterior Fossa Society Consensus Meeting 2018: a synopsis. Childs Nerv Syst 36:1145–1151

Morales RC (2006) Orofaciální regulační terapie (Orofacial regulatory therapy). Portál, Prague

Morgan AT, Liégeois F, Liederkerke C et al (2011) Role of cerebellum in fine speech control in childhood: persistent dysarthria after surgical treatment for posterior fossa tumour. Brain Lang 117:69–76

Morris EB, Phillips NS, Laningham FH et al (2009) Proximal dentatothalamocortical tract involvement in posterior fossa syndrome. Brain 132:3087–3095

Neubauer K (1998) Poruchy řečové komunikace—diagnostika a terapie (Speech communication disorders—diagnosis and therapy). In: Preiss M (ed) Klinická neuropsychologie (Clinical neuropsychology). Geada Publishing, Prague

Neubauer K (2002) Terapie dysartrie (Dysarthria therapy). In: Lechta V (ed) Terapia narušenej komunikačnej schopnosti (Therapy of impaired communication skills). Osveta, Martin, pp 201–238

Neubauer K (2011) Terapie dysartrie (Dysarthria therapy). In: Lechta V (ed) Terapie narušené komunikační schopnosti (Therapy of impaired communication skills). Portál, Prague, pp 283–334

Neubauer K (2016) Speech-language therapy and neurogenic disorders of communication. Nakladatelství P, Mervart & Univerita Hradec Králové, Červený Kostelec

Neubauer K (2018) Dysartrie a řečová dyspraxie (Dysarthria and speech dyspraxia). In: Neubauer K (ed) Kompendium klinické logopedie (Compendium of clinical speech therapy). Portál, Prague, pp 416–441

Neubauerová L, Neubauer K (2018) Augmentativní a alternativní komunikace a klinická logopedická praxe (Augmentative and alternative communication and clinical speech therapy practice). In: Neubauer K (ed) Kompendium klinické logopedie (Compendium of clinical speech therapy). Portál, Prague, pp 697–713

Paquier PF, Walsh KS, Docking KM et al (2020) Postoperative cerebellar mutism syndrome: rehabilitation issues. Childs Nerv Syst 36:1215–1222

Parent E, Scott L (2011) Pediatric posterior fossa syndrome (PFS): nursing strategies in the postoperative period. Can J Neurosci Nurs 33:24–41

Patay Z, Enterkin J, Harreld JH et al (2014) MR imaging evaluation of inferior olivary nuclei: comparison of postoperative subjects with and without posterior fossa syndrome. Am J Neuroradiol 35:797–802

Pennington I (2012) Speech and communication in cerebral palsy. East J Med 17(4):171–177

Petržílková M (2020) Logopedický software a výukové počítačové programy (Speech therapy software and educational computer programs). www.mentio.cz/. Accessed 19 Dec 2020

Pfeiffer J (1996) Léčebná rehabilitace dětí sporuchou centrálního motoneuronu (Therapeutic rehabilitation of children with central motoneuron disorder). In: Trojan S, Druga P, Pfeiffer J et al (eds) Fyziologie a léčebná rehabilitace motoriky člověka (Physiology and therapeutic rehabilitation of human motor skills). Grada Publishing, Prague, pp 109–171

Pols SY, Van Veelen ML, Aarsen FK et al (2017) Risk factors for development of postoperative cerebellar mutism syndrome in children after medulloblastoma surgery. J Neurosurg Pediatr 20:35–41

Puget S, Boddaert N, Viguier D et al (2009) Injuries to inferior vermis and dentate nuclei predict poor neurological and neuropsychological outcome in children with malignant posterior fossa tumors. Cancer 115:1338–1347

Raine S, Meadows L, Lynch-Ellerington M (2009) Bobath concept: theory and clinical practice in neurological rehabilitation. Wiley-Blackwell, Chichester

Reed-Berendt R, Phillips B, Picton S et al (2014) Cause and outcome of cerebellar mutism: evidence from a systematic review. Child Nerv Syst 30:375–385

Riesthal M (2016) Assessment and treatment of neurogenic speech disorders. In: Johnson A, Jacobson B (eds) Medical speech language pathology. Thieme Medical Publisher Inc., New York, pp 119–134

Riva D (1998) The cerebellar contribution to language and sequential functions: evidence from a child with cerebellitis. Cortex 24:279–287

Robertson PL, Muraszko KM, Holmes EJ et al (2006) Incidence and severity of postoperative cerebellar mutism syndrome in children with medulloblastoma: a prospective study by the Children's Oncology Group. J Neurosurg 105:444–451

Schaller-Paule MA, Baumgarten P, Seifert V et al (2021) A paravermal trans-cerebellar approach to the posterior fossa tumor causes hypertrophic olivary degeneration by dentatenucleus injury. Cancers 13:258. https://doi.org/10.3390/cancers13020258

Schmahmann JD (2020) Pediatric post-operative cerebellar mutism syndrome, cerebellar cognitive affective syndrome, and posterior fossa syndrome: historical review and proposed resolution to guide future study. Childs Nerv Syst 36:1205–1214

Steinbok P, Cochrane DD, Perrin R et al (2003) Mutism after posterior fossa tumor resection in children: incomplete recovery on long-term follow-up. Pediatr Neurosurg 39:179–183

Tanner D, Culbertson W (1999) Quick assessment for dysarthria. Academic Communication Associates, Oceanside, CA

Turkel SB, Shu CL, Nelson MD et al (2004) Case series: acute mood symptoms associated with posterior fossa lesions in children. J Neuropsychiatry Clin Neurosci 16:443–445

van Dongen HR, Catsman-Berrevoets CE, Van Mourik M (1994) The syndrome of 'cerebellar' mutism and subsequent dysarthria. Neurology 44:2040–2046

van Mourik M, Catsman-Berrevoets CE, Paquier PF et al (1997) Acquired childhood dysarthria: review of its clinical presentation. Pediatr Neurol 17(4):299–307

van Mourik M, Catsman-Berrevoets CE, Yousef-Bak E et al (1998) Dysarthria in children with cerebellar or brainstem tumors. Pediatr Neurol 18:411–414

Vanclooster S, Bilsen J, Peremans L et al (2019) Attending school after treatment for a brain tumor: experiences of children and key figures. J Health Psychol 24:1436–1447

Vanclooster S, Van Hoeck K, Peremans L et al (2020) Reintegration into school of childhood brain tumor survivors: a qualitative study using the International Classification of Functioning, Disability and Health—

Children and Youth framework. Disabil Rehabil 43(18):2610–2620

Vojta V (1993) Mozkové hybné poruchyv kojeneckém věku (Cerebral movement disorders in infancy). Grada-Avicenum, Prague

Vojta V, Peters A (2018) Das Vojta-Prinzip: Muskelspiele in Reflexfortbewegung und motorischer Ontogenese (The Vojta principle: muscle play in reflex continuous movement and motor ontogenesis). Springer, Berlin

Walker D, Thomas SA, Talbot EJ et al (2014) Cerebellar mutism: the rehabilitation challenge in pediatric neuro-oncology: case studies. J Pediatr Rehabil Med 7:333–340

Yap JL, Wachtel LE, Ahn ES et al (2012) Treatment of cerebellar cognitive affective syndrome with aripiprazole. J Pediatr Rehabil Med 5:233–238

Yeargin-Allsopp M, Van Naarden Braun K, Doernberg NS et al (2008) Prevalence of cerebral palsy in 8-year-old children in three areas of the United States in 2002: a multisite collaboration. Pediatrics 121(3): 547–554

Yorkston K, Beukelman D, Strand E et al (eds) (2010) Management of motor speech disorders in children and adults. Pro-Ed, Austin

# Diagnosis and Differential Diagnosis of Acquired Motor Speech Disorders (Dysarthria, Dyspraxia)

# 18

Edoardo Nicoló Aiello, Enrico Alfonsi,
Mathieu Balaguer, Salvatore Biondi,
Stefano Cappa, Giuseppe Cosentino,
Mauro Fresia, Gregor Kasprian,
Ben A. M. Maassen, Donato Mecca, Rossella Muò,
Karel Neubauer, Gustavo Noffs, Danilo Patrocinio,
Cristina Polimeno, Timothy Pommée,
Paolo Prunetti, Vincenzo Sallustio,
Antonio Schindler, Massimiliano Todisco,
Iolanda Trittola, Adam P. Vogel, Virginie Woisard,
and Stefano Zago

Karel Neubauer and Salvatore Biondi shared first authorship.
Timothy Pommée, Mathieu Balaguer, and Virginie Woisard
shared first authorship.
Mathieu Balaguer, Timothy Pommée, and Virginie Woisard
shared first authorship.
Danilo Patrocinio passed away before the time of
publication.

E. N. Aiello
Department of Neurology and Laboratory
Neuroscience, Istituto Auxologico Italiano IRCCS,
Milan, Italy
e-mail: e.aiello@auxologico.it

E. Alfonsi (✉) · M. Fresia · M. Todisco
C. Mondino National Neurological Institute,
Clinical Neurophysiology Unit,
IRCCS Mondino Foundation, Pavia, Italy
e-mail: enrico.alfons@mondino.it;
mauro.fresia@mondino.it;
Massimiliano.Todisco@mondini.it

M. Balaguer
IRIT, Université de Toulouse, CNRS,
Toulouse INP, UT3, Toulouse, France
e-mail: mathieu.balaguer@irit.fr

S. Biondi
Policlinico G. Rodolico Department of
Otorhinolaryngology, Università di Catania,
Catania, Italy
e-mail: salvatore.biondi@tin.it

S. Cappa
Institute for Advanced Studies,
University of Pavia, Pavia, Italy
e-mail: stefano.cappa@isspavia.it

G. Cosentino
Department of Brain and Behavioral Sciences,
IRCCS Fondazione Mondinooi, University of Pavia,
Pavia, Italy
e-mail: giuseppe.cosentino@unipv.it

G. Kasprian
Department of Biomedical Imaging and Image-Guided
Therapy, Medical University of Vienna, Vienna, Austria
e-mail: gregor.kasprian@meduniwien.ac.at

D. Mecca · D. Patrocinio (Deceased) · C. Polimeno ·
V. Sallustio · I. Trittola
ASL Lecce, Rehabilitation Department, Phoniatric
and Communicative Disorders Rehabilitative Center,
Lecce, Italy
e-mail: meccado@libero.it;
cristina.polimeno@asl.lecce.it;
vincenzo.sallustio@asl.lecce.it;
antonellatrittola@libero.it

A. am Zehnhoff-Dinnesen et al. (eds.), *Phoniatrics III*, European Manual of Medicine,
https://doi.org/10.1007/978-3-031-48091-1_3

## 18.1 Evaluation of Verbal Communication: Phonetic, Phonological, Prosodic, Pragmatic Levels

Karel Neubauer and Salvatore Biondi

### 18.1.1 The Basis of Evaluation of Verbal Communication

The evaluation of verbal communication is a demanding multi-level process, which reflects the fact that verbal communication itself is a multi-level complex event, and which can be evaluated from many significantly different perspectives. In the field of evaluating the verbal expression of people who may suffer from a speech communication disorder, it is often preferred, especially in phoniatric and clinical speech therapy, to divide the phonetic, phonological, prosodic and pragmatic levels of the evaluated verbal expression. The use of this approach, i.e., the use of a linguistic point of view in diagnostics (Dlouhá et al. 2017), is a valid way of evaluating the verbal communication of a patient suspected of manifesting a speech disorder, which is a challenging task for any speech pathologist, owing to the complex nature of the verbal function. In children, the effort is even greater because the disorder occurs in a period of life in which the maturation processes and acquisitions are in full development. A complete evaluation cannot be limited to the expressive aspect, in particular to the production of the word, but must necessarily consider the receptive aspect, the cognitive abilities and the psychological background. The assessment procedures differ in the level of detail, distinguishing themselves in informal approaches, screening and specific tests (Wannberg et al. 2016).

The traditional division of approach into the fields of phonetics (especially the so-called articulatory phonetics: Ladefoged and Johnson 2014; Skarnitzl et al. 2016; Dlouhá et al. 2017), phonology, prosody and pragmatics is widely used.

R. Muò
Recupero e Rieducazione Funzionale, ASL Città di Torino, Turin, Italy
e-mail: rossella.muo@unito.it

K. Neubauer
Charles University Faculty of Medicine,
Clinic of Phoniatrics of University Hospital Prague,
Prague, Czech Republic
e-mail: Karel.Neubauer@lf1.cuni.cz

G. Noffs · A. P. Vogel
Centre for Neuroscience and Speech, The University of Melbourne, Parkville, VIC, Australia
e-mail: gustavo.noffs@unimelb.edu.au;
vogela@unimelb.edu.au

B. A. M. Maassen
Department Neurosciences/BCN,
Center for Language and Cognition,
University of Groningen Medical Center,
Groningen, The Netherlands
e-mail: b.a.m.maassen@rug.nl

T. Pommée
École d'orthophonie et d'audiologie,
Université de Montréal, Montreal, Canada
e-mail: timothy.pommee@umontreal.ca

P. Prunetti
C. Mondino National Neurological Institute, Pavia, Italy
e-mail: paolo.prunetti@mondino.it

A. Schindler
Luigi Sacco Hospital, Department of Biomedical and Clinical Sciences "L. Sacco", Phoniatrics,
University of Milan, Milan, Italy
e-mail: antonio.schindler@unimi.it

V. Woisard
Voice and Deglutition Unit in Larrey Hospital and Onco-Rehabilitation Unit in Oncopole Hospital, Larrey Hospital and Oncopole Hospital, Toulouse, France
e-mail: woisard.virginie@iuct-incopole.fr

S. Zago
Neurology Unit, IRCCS Fondazione Ca' Granda Ospedale Maggiore Policlinico, Milan, Italy
e-mail: stefano.zago@unimi.it

Contemporary, pragmatically orientated linguistics, especially phonetics, strives for a high level of interdisciplinarity and knowledge development, as well as a new approach to connecting psychological, neurophysiological and sociological knowledge with the field of speech communication (Landgraf 2015; Ladefoged and Johnson 2014):

> The interdisciplinarity promoted in current scientific practice does not favour phonology isolated from production and perceptual facts. (Skarnitzl et al. 2016, p. 11)

Therefore, the concept of contemporary phonetics may be preferred in the future, including not only segmental but also supra-segmental levels of speech communication, in conjunction with psycho-phonetic and socio-phonetic aspects of practical interpersonal communication (Skarnitzl and Volín 2018).

The traditional concept of phonetic, phonological, prosodic and pragmatic levels of evaluation of speech communication are:

- **The phonetic level**, which considers the articulatory production of speech sounds by the vocal tract, i.e., the ability to produce single phonemes and phonemic sequences (V, C, CV, VC, VCV…), depending on the parameters of movement such as range of motion, strength, speed, coordination, ability to vary muscular tension (Emerick and Hatten 1979; Hayden and Square-Storer 1999)
- **The phonological level**, concerned with the abstract characterisation of systems of sounds (i.e., phonemes) and their use to process spoken and written language. The broad category of phonological processing includes phonological awareness, phonological working memory and phonological retrieval (Wagner and Torgesen 1987; Dodd et al. 2006)
- **The prosodic level**, which refers to intonation, stress patterns, loudness variations and pausing, representing the melody of speech. It is also referred to as the "supra-segmental" or "para-linguistic" channel of communication (Sidtis and Van Lancker Sidtis 2003), in contrast to linguistic entities, which are discrete, unitary and combinatorial prosody expressed mainly by varying pitch, loudness and duration of segmental elements, representing the speaker's ability to blend sounds and words, to stress syllables and words, and to modify pitch appropriately. Gerken and McGregor (1998) define prosody as both a phonological and acoustic phenomenon. In dysarthric patients articulatory effort, phonetic errors, durational features (phone, syllable, word and phrase length), as well as voice production disorders of pitch and loudness, interfere with prosody (Peppé and McCann 2003)
- **The pragmatic level** (Russell and Grizzle 2008), which deals with how the context in which the verbal communication takes place contributes to meaning; in other words, the ability to use language in social interactions between speaker and listener(s) appropriately and effectively (Prutting and Kirchner 1987). Shriberg et al. (2001) categorise three subdomains of pragmatics of communicative acts:
  - **Verbal Aspects**: Speech acts (pair analysis, variety of speech acts); topics (selection, introduction, maintenance, change); turn-taking (initiation, response, repair/revision, pause time, interruption/overlap, feedback to speakers, adjacency, contingency, quantity/conciseness); lexical selection/use across speech acts (specificity/accuracy, cohesion, stylistic variations, the varying of communicative style)
  - **Paralinguistic Aspects**: Intelligibility and prosodics (intelligibility, vocal intensity, vocal quality, prosody, fluency) (Kent et al. 1989)
  - **Non-verbal Aspects**: Kinesics and proxemics (physical proximity, physical contacts, body posture, foot/leg and hand/arm movements, gestures, facial expression, eye gaze) (Kiernan and Reid 1987)

### 18.1.2 Informal and Formal Approaches to the Evaluation of Verbal Communication in Motor Speech Disorders

Informal approaches are achieved by observing both spontaneous and elicited verbalisations. Screenings use standard coded forms but are not particularly detailed. Both the informal approaches and the screenings aim to trace an overall profile of an essentially qualitative nature and are above all aimed at identifying any special needs of an educational or rehabilitative nature. The assessments logically follow informal approaches or screening, and include tests intended to gain a profile of the patient as completely as possible, including anatomical and functional aspects, even those not directly related to speech, such as respiration and feeding. Although the articulatory disorder is the most striking feature of dysarthria, a thorough evaluation has to extend observations to all levels of verbal communication.

Many protocols have been proposed for evaluating children with motor speech disorders. Watson and Pennington (2015) have listed and commented on those most frequently used in children, noting that Frenchay (Enderby and Palmer 2007) is the most used. On the other hand, in children standardised tests for adults are often applied, although incompletely, and limited to the aspects most relevant to the individual case.

In the field of motor speech disorders, standardised forms of evaluation are guided primarily by the effort to evaluate as accurately as possible the impact of the disorder on the intelligibility of the person's speech.

> The standardized Assessment of Intelligibility in Dysarthric Speakers (AIDS) has been a widely used measure of intelligibility, speaking rate, and communicative efficiency in people with dysarthria. (Duffy 2020, p. 79)

Other standardised forms in this area—the Sentence Intelligibility Test (SIT), Frenchay Dysarthria Profile Assessment (FDA-2) and Munich Intelligibility Profile (MVP)—are also predominant in the field of motor speech disorder

assessment of the intelligibility of speech (Brookshire and McNeil 2015; Riesthal 2016; Duffy 2020).

Their counterparts for achieving a comprehensive humanistic-orientated diagnosis of the difficulties of people with motor speech disorders are the rating scales of functional communication, communication effectiveness and psychosocial impact of acquired disorders, especially dysarthria and speech dyspraxia.

> For management decision-making and outcomes to be maximally effective, the influence of impaired speech on self-concept and day-to-day living should be understood. (Duffy 2020, p. 81)

For these reasons, the use of assessment materials such as the Visual Analogue Self-Esteem Scale (VASES, Brumfitt and Sheeran 1999) can be accepted as a highly valid approach, overcoming language barriers and loss of speech-intelligible communication in severe speech disorders (Neubauer 2018b).

The complex text by Togher (2018) emphasises the importance of the pragmatic level of evaluation of speech communication in the field of neurogenic communication disorders. It covers the methods of evaluating the pragmatic component of communication and discourse of speech, the possibility of their evaluation by such files as the La Trobe Communication Questionnaire (LCQ), currently the most commonly used tool performed by clinical speech therapists for evaluating discourse and pragmatics in adults with traumatic CNS. LCQ is used as a sensitive measure in the detection of positive communication results in the training programme of communication partners of people with neurogenic communication disorders, as it is with the reported Communicative Activities of Daily Living-2, presented in connection with the evaluation of the response to Promoting Aphasic Communicative Effectiveness (PACE) treatment.

> As the goal of speech pathology intervention is to improve the communication of people with ABI (acquired brain injury) in everyday contexts, the fields of discourse and pragmatics provide clinicians with the necessary tools to assess and treat people in the very contexts where they may be having difficulty. (Togher 2018, p. 130)

## 18.2 Evaluation of Non-verbal Communication

Cristina Polimeno, Danilo Patrocinio,
Vincenzo Sallustio, Donato Mecca,
Iolanda Trittola and Rossella Muò

### 18.2.1 Introduction

Non-verbal communication (NVC) is a general term used to refer to communication modes other than language that people may use to convey a message. Researchers generally agree that specific aspects to be observed under the domain of NVC include proxemics, body language (posture and positioning), gestures, facial expressions, eye contact and gaze (gaze shifts) (Prutting and Kirchner 1987). Paralinguistic aspects, such as intelligibility, voice quality, voice prosody and fluency (Prutting and Kirchner 1987), have sometimes been classified under either the NVC or the verbal communication pragmatic domains, as well as a separate domain. For example, according to Watzlawick's classic perspective the term NVC

> must comprise posture [and proxemics], gesture, facial expression, voice inflection, the sequence, rhythm, and cadence of the words themselves, and any other nonverbal expression of which the organism is capable, as well as the communicational clues unfailingly present in any context in which an interaction takes place. (Watzlawick et al. 1967–2011)

Whichever the classification, for people who have motor speech disorders (PwMSD), both NVC and paralinguistic aspects play a crucial role that need to be discussed.

### 18.2.2 Non-verbal Communication

According to the main classifications of MSD (ASHA 2022), for the purposes of this section, it is important to distinguish PwMSD due diseases that affect the motor system of the whole body, such as progressive neurodegenerative diseases, from PwMSD due to diseases that affect speech production only. In fact, while for the first group NVC is generally affected, at least from the moderate–severe stage of the disease, for the second group NVC may play a key role as an alternative and augmentative method of communication, as it can accompany, strengthen or replace verbal communication when it is lacking or not adequate (Rautakoski 2011). For example, the use of supplementation strategies in conjunction with natural speech (for example the use of gestures) has been reported as a useful strategy to enhance the intelligibility of dysarthric speech (Hanson et al. 2013). Moreover the speaker's use of body movements, especially hand gestures, is a significant aspect of NVC that contributes contextualising information, thus improving message comprehension (Garcia and Cannito 1996).

Facial expression is another fundamental component of NVC. The face is provided with considerable expressive and communicative potential; it consists of several elements that act with a high degree of coherence to express emotions and states of mind, manifest interpersonal attitudes, produce relevant signals of interaction and establish shifts and timing of conversation. The relationship between emotions and mimics is so close that facial expressions of emotion can be almost universally associated with specific emotions (Ekman and Friesen 1971). Facial expressions are almost always impaired in PwMSD, for example, as a consequence of cranial nerve disfunction, contributing to a reduced communication competence and limited emotion expression.

The lack of proficiency in NVC threatens the correct identification of the talker's intents, and a satisfactory sharing of meaning with the interlocutors, beyond the literal signification of the verbal utterance, and yields a poorly efficient communication.

When assessing PwMSD, the evaluation of other NVC aspects is infrequent. In the literature, the dated Prutting and Kirchner's "pragmatic" protocol is the only one dealing with this topic, albeit partially and broadly (Prutting and Kirchner 1987). It is a 30-item evaluation protocol divided into three main areas: verbal aspects, paralinguistic aspects and nonverbal aspects. For each item an external communication expert judges, using a

Likert scale, the patient's communicative acts as appropriate, inappropriate or not observed. More specifically, the non-verbal aspects considered in the protocol are kinesics and proxemics: physical proximity, physical contacts, body posture, foot/leg and hand/arm movements, gestures, facial expression and eye gaze.

### 18.2.3 Paralinguistic Aspects

Paralinguistic aspects include vocal characteristics such as pitch, supra-segmental features and rhythm. Words take on different meanings depending on the way they are pronounced and the inflections of the voice. Key factors are tone (determining the pitch profile of the voice), intensity (characterising the volume and emphatic accent of the voice), timing (determining the succession of speech and pauses), prosodic profile (based on the type of utterance: interrogative, exclamation, etc.) and emotional factors.

Paralinguistic aspects are generally one of the key impairment for PwMSD. An alteration in facial motility and in supra-segmental speech traits can cause extreme suffering in PwMSD: they feel themselves limited or deprived of the natural and spontaneous ability to express their emotions. Therefore, these subjects often experience psychological discomfort and depression, as it emerges from the analysis of the self-assessment questionnaire of dysarthria (Yorkston et al. 1994), reporting the subjective evaluation of speech characteristics and speech difficulties in social situations, as well as the compensation strategies adopted and the reactions of the interlocutors, or from other Quality of Life (QOL) self-assessment tools later developed (Piacentini et al. 2011, 2014).

The most common and well-known perceptual and instrumental protocols explore the speech and motor-speech abilities in patients affected with MSD, and usually include the evaluation of paralinguistic NVC aspects such as: speech rate, utterance and pause durations, rate-rhythm, correlation of prosody with intonation (fundamental frequency and its variations during speech production), stress patterning and naturalness. These aspects are exhaustively discussed in the relative book sections. Conversely, the evaluation of other NVC aspects is infrequent.

### 18.2.4 Complexity of Motor Speech Disorders

As the literature is lacking other more complex and validated tools, only an accurate evaluation performed by an expert clinician will be able to highlight, according to the ICF framework, the limitations and restrictions due to NVC impairment in patients affected by MSD. The phoniatrician needs to rely on verbal and non-verbal assessment systems that are flexible, linked to immediate contexts and cultural variables by definition, and that in physiological conditions tend to semantic and pragmatic tuning as a prerequisite for stability and sharing of meaning, and for communicative efficiency.

In addition, the ICF framework it is a suitable tool for highlighting the presence of other biological bonds that also occur for PwMSD. Indeed, impairment or alteration in the movements of body, head, arms and especially legs, facial expression muscles, oculomotor muscles and other structures involved in touching and rejecting, may in many ways compromise the functions attributed to the NVC and the achievement of semantic and pragmatic tuning. Since they condition the rehabilitation project and its outcome, the phoniatrician needs to detect especially the:

- Gestural lexicon depletion (emblems, deictic, illustrative, regulatory, adaptive gestures) that usually supports, regulates or replaces verbal communication
- Emotional lexicon depletion, mainly for paralinguistic aspects and facial expressions (inability to express basic emotions through facial expressions, audience effect disappearance, loss of social meaning of the smile, etc.); the presence of unmotivated non-verbal facial and vocal expressions (e.g., laughing or crying in supranuclear progressive palsy)
- Reduction in eye movements considered mainly as non-verbal communicative exchange regulator taking into account intercultural differences

- Reduced ability in space management in terms of interlocutor distance and orientation, postures, etc.)
- Reduction in initiative in physical contact with the interlocutor as relationship, power relation and cultural ritual regulator (i.e., salutation rituals), taking into account differences in cultural heritage (Arabic and Latin cultures rather than Northern, Japanese or Indian cultures)

Therefore, the "communicative state" of a patient with MSD appears to be a very complex issue. If a communicative and ecological perspective is used, the patient might actually disclose relational and social limitations and restrictions far beyond those traditionally evaluated by using a solely linguistic or motor-speech assessment. This aspect is well known by whoever has experienced a more prolonged open conversation with these patients.

## 18.3 Speech Motor Examination Protocol and Interventions for the Management of Dysarthria

Karel Neubauer

### 18.3.1 Introduction

The Speech Motor Examination Protocol is part of the motor speech test, which includes several components important for accurately describing signs and symptoms and making an appropriate diagnosis of speech. It includes acquiring a detailed history, examining the mechanism of speech during non-speech tasks, and assessing sound-perceptual speech characteristics and intelligibility. The majority of these components may be completed in most clinical settings, including acute care, inpatient rehabilitation, outpatient clinic and home health care settings (Riesthal 2016). A comprehensive assessment of a person with an acquired speech communication disorder includes, in accordance with the focus of speech-language therapy (SLT) and phoniatric diagnostics, the following items:

1. Design of case history (background questionnaire or interview or both)

   (a) Personal information and description of the problem
   (b) Medical history and previous services received
   (c) Occupational and social history

2. Speech diagnostic evaluation files

   (a) Speech Motor Examination Protocol and Oral Motor Examination Protocol (see Sect. 18.4)
   (b) Assessment scale due differentiation: dysarthria-apraxia of speech
   (c) Assessment of intelligibility of dysarthric speech (Brookshire and McNeil 2015)

3. Language screening and hearing screening (if appropriate)
4. Analysis of assessment data and Speech-Language Diagnosis
5. Recommendations and goals of the treatment plan (Shipley and McAfee 2016)

The Protocol for Motor Speech Evaluation respects the focus of speech disorder diagnostics, and its coexistence with neurological, ENT and neuropsychological diagnostics. It focuses on the evaluation of motor speech modalities and the influence of their dysfunction on the intelligibility and stigmatisation of speech. It mainly involves the auditory-perceptual method, which is considered the gold standard of assessment, because determining the presence or absence of a speech disorder is based on whether or not it is perceived by the listener (Riesthal 2016).

The form of Speech Motor Examination Protocol used is based on the adaptation of evaluation scales by Brookshire and McNeil (2015), Neubauer (2007) and Robertson and Fay (1993).

### 18.3.2 Speech Motor Examination Protocol

The following degrees and items have to be considered:

1. **Spontaneous Speech and Intelligibility**

   (a) Degrees: intact/mild disorders/moderate disorders/severe disorders/loss of function
   (b) Items:
      *Phoneme errors:* none/consistent/inconsistent/undetectable
      *Syllable/word errors*: none/consistent/inconsistent/undetectable
      *Intervals of fluent, error-free speech*: none/some/many/undetectable
      *Attempts to correct errors*: never/sometimes/often/undetectable
      *Successful error correction:* never/sometimes/often/undetectable
      *Difference*: spontaneous speech better/repetition better/no difference/undetectable
      *Stigmatisation of speech and overall effect on listener*: no problem/noticeable within normal range/slightly disturbing/strongly disturbing/blocking

2. **Articulation**

   (a) Degrees: intact/mild disorders/moderate disorders/severe disorders/loss of function
   (b) Items:
      *Irregular articulatory imprecision*: never/sometimes/often/constantly/undetectable
      *Imprecise consonants*: never/sometimes/often/constantly/undetectable
      *Distorted vowels*: never/sometimes/often/constantly/undetectable
      *Prolonged phonemes*: never/sometimes/often/constantly/undetectable
      *Repeated phonemes*: never/sometimes/often/constantly/undetectable
      *Weakened plosive consonants*: none/mild/moderate/severe/undetectable

3. **Resonance Factor and Prosody**

   (a) Degrees: intact/mild disorders/moderate disorders/severe disorders/loss of function
   (b) Items:
      *Non-intact nasal emission:* none/mild/moderate/severe/undetectable
      *Nasality in speech:* normal/somewhat hypernasal/very hyponasal/undetectable/somewhat hyponasal/very hyponasal
      *Rate of speech:* normal/somewhat slow/very slow/undetectable/somewhat fast/very fast
      *Variability of rate:* normal/less than normal/variable/very variable/undetectable
      *Excessive pauses:* none/within words/between words/between phrases/undetectable
      *Stress in speech:* normal/reduced/excessive/uncontrolled changes/undetectable
      *Abnormality:* none/short rushes of speech/intermittent fast rate/other abnormalities

4. **Phonation in Speech**
   (a) Degrees: intact/mild disorders/moderate disorders/severe disorders/loss of function
   (b) Items:
      *Loudness of voice:* normal/somewhat loud/very loud/undetectable/somewhat soft/very soft
      *Uncontrolled changes in loudness:* never/sometimes/often/constantly/undetectable
      *Diminishing loudness with sustained phonation:* none/moderate/severe/undetectable
      *Tremor in voice:* normal/soft/moderate/severe/undetectable
      *Harsh voice (raspy, rough):* none/mild/moderate/severe/undetectable

*Hoarse voice (wet, gurgly):* none/mild/moderate/severe/undetectable
*Breathy voice:* none/mild/moderate/severe/undetectable
*Other abnormalities of voice:*

5. **Respiration in Speech**

(a) Degrees: intact/mild disorders/moderate disorders/severe disorders/loss of function
(b) Items:
*Discoordination of breathing and speech:* never/sometimes/often/constantly/undetectable
*Problems with forced inspiration/expiration:* never/sometimes/often/constantly/undetectable
*Audible inhalation/exhalation:* never/sometimes/often/constantly/undetectable
*Speech length for one breath:* normal/somewhat short/very short/variable/undetectable

### 18.3.3 Analysis and Conclusions for Diagnosis: Interventions for the Management of Dysarthria

Evaluation of the presence of a neurogenic motor speech disorder is linked to the development of therapeutic intervention and management of the speech disorder. Its tasks are:

- To establish contact with a person with a speech communication disorder, create a sense of mutual trust and hope in the outcome of speech communication disorder therapy
- To carry out examinations according to the possibilities and general condition of the patient; in the case of a severe post-acute stage, at least by orientation and a screening examination; if the patient's condition allows, to perform a comprehensive examination
- On the basis of the examination, to contribute to the diagnosis of the type and extent of the deficit and to define the severity of the speech disorder

- To establish a plan of therapeutic intervention, an individual plan of clinical speech therapy
- If necessary, to initiate the work of other experts, such as an eye examination physician in determining the current possibility of adjusting the eye defect to support the resumption of reading and writing; possible assignment of hearing prosthetics, if the condition is complicated by a hearing impairment, etc.
- To establish contact with a physiotherapist to coordinate rehabilitation in the field of somatic disorders and speech communication, hand movements and graphomotoric skills, reading and writing
- To motivate family and nursing staff to work together (Neubauer 2018a)

In the field of management of people with acquired dysarthria, it is appropriate to summarise the basic principles outlined by therapeutic intervention programmes that have remained valid to this day (Darley et al. 1975; Rosenbek and LaPointe 1978; Robertson and Fay 1993; Yorkston et al. 1999; Freed 2000; Duffy 2013; Riesthal 2016) and that include:

- Compensation—the patient's learning to maximise the use of his remaining potential
- Purposeful activity—the patient's learning to do "on purpose" what he had been doing automatically before
- Monitoring—the patient's learning to monitor, check and criticise his own performance
- An early start—the patient's beginning at a very early stage to monitor, practise and compensate before succumbing to inefficient speech habits that are hard to eradicate
- Motivation—the therapist's encouraging the patient to "embark on and persist in a programme of therapy"

The above principles permeate the process of therapy for people with acquired dysarthria, are not limited to a particular aetiology, type or severity of dysarthria, and are followed by specific goals for therapy, carried out by daily systematic practice with specially selected and organised procedures in daily practice. The most common targets are:

- Helping the patient to become productive
- Modification of posture, muscle tone and strength
- Modification of respiration
- Modification of phonation
- Modification of resonance
- Modification of articulation
- Modification of supra-segmentals and prosody
- Providing alternative modes of communication

> …one does not treat a specific type of dysarthria (e.g., Flaccid, Spastic, Hypokinetic, etc.) or a specific type of neurological disease (e.g., Parkinson's Disease, Multiple Sclerosis, Pseudobulbar Palsy). The focus of therapy arises from, firstly, carefully analysing the affected parameters; secondly, grouping these in a logical manner (e.g., respiration and phonation; or facial musculature, diadochokinesis and articulation); and thirdly, bearing in mind the underlying pathology and associated physical and psychological factors. (Robertson and Fay 1993, p. 4)

## 18.4    Oral Motor Examination Protocol

Karel Neubauer

### 18.4.1 Introduction

Evaluation of oral motor skills is commonly included in the evaluation of motor speech disorders. This is because it improves assessment by focusing on the isolated movements of the lips, tongue, jaw and velopharyngeal structures, which cannot be achieved during speech tasks. The performance of the examined person in non-speech motor activities does not provide information that directly correlates with the performance in the modalities of motor speech. It is a complementary assessment that develops a complete picture of the patient's speech disorder (Duffy 2013; Riesthal 2016). Examination of the oral mechanism involves observing the patient's face, mouth, tongue and palate during a variety of tasks under various

conditions, including rest, during suspected postural problems, during movement. In each state, the purpose is to assess movement in these domains:

- Strength—the ability of a muscle to contract for a long time without excessive fatigue
- Symmetry—the appearance of both sides of the face at rest and during movement
- Range—the distance that the oral structure can move during the task
- Tone—continuous and passive partial contraction of the muscles of the oral structures
- Steadiness—the degree to which the oral structure exhibits aberrant movement (e.g., tremor) at rest or during movement
- Speed—the speed at which the oral structure is able to move
- Accuracy—successful execution of the motor movement (Duffy 2013; Riesthal 2016; Shipley and McAfee 2016)

The form of Sample Protocol of Oral Motor Examination used is based on the adaptation of evaluation scales by Riesthal (2016), Neubauer (2007), Robertson and Fay (1993).

### 18.4.2 Sample Protocol of Oral Motor Examination

Rating includes G (good—no noticeable deficit) or D (deficit) with possible comment

1. **Face and Lips at Rest and During Sustained Posture**
   (a) Strength/Symmetry/Range/Tone/Steadiness/Speed/Accuracy
   (b) G–D/G–D/G–D/G–D/G–D/G–D/G–D
2. **Face and Lips During Movement**
   (a) (Smile, pucker, open, close tight, puff up cheeks, hold against resistance)
   (b) Strength/Symmetry/Range/Tone/Steadiness/Speed/Accuracy
   (c) G–D/G–D/G–D/G–D/G–D/G–D/G–D
3. **Jaw During Rest and During Sustained Posture**
   (a) Strength/Symmetry/Range/Tone/Steadiness/Speed/Accuracy
   (b) G–D/G–D/G–D/G–D/G–D/G–D/G–D

4. **Jaw During Movement**
   (a) (Open wide and closing the mouth)
   (b) Strength/Symmetry/Range/Tone/ Steadiness/Speed/Accuracy
   (c) G–D/G–D/G–D/G–D/G–D/G–D/G–D

5. **Tongue During Rest and During Sustained Posture**
   (a) Strength/Symmetry/Range/Tone/ Steadiness/Speed /Accuracy
   (b) G–D/G–D/G–D/G–D/G–D/G–D/G–D

6. **Tongue During Movement**
   (a) (Stick straight out, move to left, right, left and right quickly, elevation, retraction, protrusion and lateral movement against resistance)
   (b) Strength/Symmetry/Range/Tone/ Steadiness/Speed/Accuracy
   (c) G–D/G–D/G–D/G–D/G–D/G–D/G–D

7. **Velopharynx at Rest**
   (a) Strength/Symmetry/Range/Tone/ Steadiness/Speed /Accuracy
   (b) G–D/G–D/G–D/G–D/G–D/G–D/G–D

8. **Velopharynx During Movement**
   (a) (Say "ah", elicit gag reflex by touching anterior faucial arches, posterior facial arches, or base of tongue)
   (b) Strength/Symmetry/Range/Tone/ Steadiness/Speed/Accuracy
   (c) G–D/G–D/G–D/G–D/G–D/G–D/G–D

### 18.4.3 Analysis and Conclusions for Diagnosis

Assessment tasks that may be included in a comprehensive examination of the oral mechanisms (Duffy 2013; Brookshire and McNeil 2015; Riesthal 2016; Neubauer 2018a) include observing:

- Symmetry, abnormal involuntary movement of eyes or lips, tremor-like movement of lips, fasciculations around the mouth or chin
- The position at rest and during sustained postures; the presence of abnormal involuntary movements, the same subsequently during movement
- The movement of jaw upon mouth opening, ability to maintain closed mouth against examiner's effort to open mouth, ability to

maintain open mouth against examiner's effort to close mouth
- All domains during sustained anterior protrusion of the tongue past the lips and lateral protrusion into the cheeks, with and without resistance
- All domains during rapid side-to-side movement of the tongue
- Symmetry, abnormal involuntary movement of palate during wide-open mouth position and for symmetry of movement during sustained phonation ("ah")

## 18.5 Objective Motor Speech Assessment

Gustavo Noffs, Ben A. M. Maassen, and Adam P. Vogel

### 18.5.1 Introduction

Speaking is one of the more complex motor activities humans perform. A series of time-aligned movements of respiratory muscles, the larynx and supraglottal articulators result in a speech sound (phoneme, syllable or word). A pre-planned sequence of sounds conveys meaning that can be understood by the listener. The complexity of our speech production system necessitates evaluation of a wide range of features, including isolated speech movement up to conversation level prosodic measures. These measures can become clinically meaningful when speech impairment is considered in the context of neurological and motor processes involved in speech production.

### 18.5.2 The Process-Orientated Approach to Speech Assessment

From a traditional, pathology-driven perspective, speech production may be divided into four main sequential stages: conceptualisation, formulation, motor preparation (or *programming*) and execution. Dysfunction during the formulation stage results in expressive aphasias, which are characterised by a varying combination of symptoms, including the inability to follow simple grammatical rules, a drastic reduction in fluency, restricted vocabulary and severe compromise of object-naming, among others (Damasio 1992). Aphasias (although not covered in this section) are generally classified as solely language dysfunctions and thus not included in motor speech disorders. Issues in the "programming" phase can result in apraxia of speech, which is characterised by non-systematic errors including speech hesitation, phonetic groping, intrusive vocalisation ("ben" for "pen"), preservatory substitutions ("pep" for "pet") and transposition of phonetic structures ("Arifca" for "Africa") (Ogar et al. 2005). People with apraxia of speech tend to produce better speech quality for phonetically easier (plosives, vowels) than for more difficult phonemes (fricatives) (Galluzzi et al. 2015). Lastly, the term dysarthria describes a group of disorders of motor speech execution. Speech errors in dysarthria are generally consistent across instances of similar phonetic properties (e.g., frequent voicing during voiceless consonants) and may include a wide range of speech features (e.g., vocal tremor, hoarseness, excessive nasalisation, slow speech rate, phonetic inaccuracy, poor loudness control, monotony) (Enderby 2013). Aphasias and apraxia arise from structural or functional neurological impairments, whereas dysarthria can result from impairment of neurological, muscular or osteoarticular structures.

Thus, the separate classification of expressive speech disorders in aphasia, apraxia and dysarthria is justified by their direct link to aetiological or topographical disease diagnosis. Knowledge of the underlying aetiology (e.g., spinocerebellar ataxia) will direct the investigation to phenotypical speech features (e.g., reduced speech agility), which translate into specific speech elicitation tasks (in this case, sequential motion rate—repeating "pa-ta" as quickly and clearly as possible for a few seconds) (Vogel et al. 2020). A comprehensive characterisation of speech dysfunction is similarly useful to assist in disease diagnosis when that aetiology is unknown (Enderby 2013).

Nonetheless, the processes involved in speech production are not disjunct, nor are language and speech motor execution (Guenther and Vladusich 2012; Kröger et al. 2020; Redford 2019; Ziegler et al. 2012). The interdependence between speech processes is reflected in the clinical presentations. While apraxia of speech, for instance, is traditionally classified separately from other motor speech deficits and from language, it is not necessarily independent of either (Molloy and Jagoe 2019; Ziegler et al. 2012), which is highlighted by the great difficulty that people with apraxia have in acquiring new language, while at the same time producing better speech quality for phonetically easier phonemes (bilabial in contrast to fricatives) (Ogar et al. 2005). Exploring the interplay between language and speech execution during examination, as well as between speech and other neurological functions, may assist in differential diagnosis or in detecting mild and subclinical impairments as discussed below.

Furthermore, aphasia, apraxia and dysarthria coexist (in different combination pairs) or appear at different disease stages in some conditions such as multiple sclerosis, progressive supranuclear Palsy and Parkinson's disease (Josephs et al. 2005; Noffs et al. 2018; Schalling et al. 2017). Conversely, an individual speech symptom (e.g., an increase in speech pauses) may arise through different mechanisms from those in aphasia (because of naming difficulties), apraxia of speech (hesitation) and dysarthria (poor respiratory support) (Terband et al. 2019).

Considering any set of speech features of interest, the interplay between the stages of speech production, and the eventual co-occurrence of dysfunctions, objective and meaningful measurement of speech should consider several factors: tasks required for eliciting speech features of interest, the complexity of tasks and their relationship to cognitive performance; the context where testing occurs, and the types of analysis adopted for making decisions about performance.

### 18.5.3 Stimuli and Tasks for Eliciting Meaningful Speech Samples

Speech assessment protocols cannot be administered without considering the role of cognition and linguistic features in the battery. Batteries of protocols should purposefully include a spectrum of tasks that fit along a continuum of complexity (Vogel et al. 2014) from tasks that are predominantly motoric (e.g., sustained vowel) to more cognitive-linguistically complex tasks (e.g., describing a picture scene or producing an unscripted monologue), see Fig. 18.1.

The motoric and linguistic complexity of a speech task can have an impact on the performance of a speaker. In short, individuals with a purely motor disorder will present with speech deficits across all tasks to a comparable degree. Individuals with a linguistic deficit will also present speech deficits (e.g., excessive speech pauses) but which increase with the degree of linguistic load. Contrasting speech metrics across tasks, as well as between speech metrics, allows an understanding of the contribution of language and speech to the observed deficit. This is of particular interest in diseases that affect both language and speech (e.g., Parkinson's, Huntington's, Multiple Sclerosis) (Chan et al. 2019; Magee et al. 2019; Noffs et al. 2018).

Next, we briefly discuss key characteristics of the structure, demand and context of speech tasks that influence the output and suggest a template protocol for eliciting speech (Table 18.1).

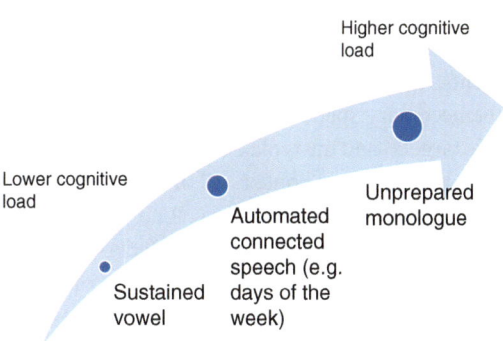

**Fig. 18.1** Common speech tasks across the cognitive load spectrum. Vogel © 2024

**Table 18.1** Basic speech tasks template. Based on Vogel et al. (2017a, 2020)

| Task | Characteristics | Demand type and utility |
|---|---|---|
| Sustained vowel (>4 s) Vowel glide/glissando | Very simple task (linguistically, phonetically and cognitively) | Typical performance to test phonatory instability and voice quality; maximum performance (with respective instruction) for measuring range/peak of loudness, frequency and respiratory support |
| Sequential and alternating speech motion (syllable alternation and repetition tasks) | Short task, cognitively and linguistically very simple but with moderate phonetic load | Maximum performance task, as typical performance meaningless. Measures articulatory agility and diadochokinesis |
| Reciting overlearned content (e.g., days of the week, months of the year, sequential counting) | Short and cognitively very simple, linguistically simple and phonetically variable | Usually, typical performance used as reference of low-demand motor speech performance. Detects moderate and severe impairment of respiratory support, syllable stress and intelligibility (phonetic accuracy) |
| Reading phonetically balanced passage/paragraph or set of words/sentences | Linguistically guided (although often unfamiliar) and phonetically diverse task | Typical performance, reference for measuring phonetic competency and prosody attributes |
| Semantically structured self-generated speech (picture description) | Linguistically challenging, phonetically variable. Relatively long task (may take minutes) | Usually typical performance demand, or light version of maximum performance. Reference task for assessing language attributes |
| Unstructured cued self-generated speech (telling personal story) | Cognitively moderate, linguistically and phonetically variable. Moderate to long task | Typical performance task. Used as proxy of real-world language abilities, prosody and phonetic preference. Cognitive load may help uncovering otherwise compensated deficits |

### 18.5.3.1 Speech Task Structure

Tasks with contrasting *phonetic structure* assist in identifying apraxia (greater difficulty with affricate and fricatives) (Ogar et al. 2005) and are useful for gauging the type and degree of dysarthria, particularly early progressive deficits once mild dysarthria is evident only in phonetically complex utterances (Kuruvilla-Dugdale et al. 2018, 2020). Phonetic complexity here refers to the required articulatory refinement and precision to produce an utterance. It includes the difficulty level of isolated phonetic targets, e.g., fricatives vs bilabial plosives, as well as the range of phonemic movements, the sequential difficulty level (related to the necessary speed of transition between phonemic targets) and the typical prosodic requirements of that utterance in context, all of which are linked to the severity of dysarthria (Lee et al. 2018; Rosen et al. 2008). To assess the effect of phonetic structure on speech, we suggest the use of a phonetically balanced structured task (usually in the form of reading a passage), and multiple short or long unstructured tasks, which allow for observing phonetic avoidance.

Varying the level of *linguistic complexity* may be desirable, as apraxia of speech and certain types of aphasia produce speech deficits that are proportional to the grammatical complexity of the task (Gorno-Tempini et al. 2011). While different speech tasks can be ranked according to linguistic complexity, the same task (i.e., the same text) does not challenge two individuals to the same degree, since language skills vary considerably between people. Thus, to "map" each person's status accurately, it is necessary to assess speech elicited by tasks at various linguistic levels.

Task *length* is critical in assessing motor breakdowns, decays, respiratory support and long-term variations. For example, a long and continuous phonation (in the form of a sustained vowel or voiced-only connected speech) is best for triggering the unintentional glottal adduction characteristic of spasmodic dysphonia, rather than the intermittent phonation common to most connected speech (Edgar et al. 2001; Roy et al. 2007). Furthermore, certain measures require a minimum task duration for analysis of the more stable segments, away from the loud speech onset (Tjaden and Watling 2003) or to derive long-term

metrics (e.g., long-term phonatory instability—related to vocal tremor) (Hartelius et al. 1997). Moderately long tasks involving naturalistic speech might additionally better reflect real-world speech difficulties. Caution must be exercised in applying lengthy tasks or protocols, particularly in fatigue-prone participants (e.g., Multiple Sclerosis, Myasthenia Gravis). We suggest a minimum of 4 s of uninterrupted performance for a sustained vowel, alternating and sequential motion rate tasks, and a minimum of 30 seconds for monologues or self-generated speech tasks.

Despite being separate abstract concepts, these task characteristics often vary together. For instance, word length, phonetic complexity and word-level linguistic complexity (i.e., a high probability word, common) are all intercorrelated (Gordon 2002; Haley and Jacks 2014; Kalimeri et al. 2015). Thus, speech tasks will also generally explore such characteristics in combination (i.e., from simple, overlearned and short utterances to linguistically complex, longer sentences with a wide phonetic structure).

### 18.5.3.2 Requirement Load of Speech Tasks

Reserve and compensation play significant roles in neurological output performance (Cabeza et al. 2018; Palmer et al. 2009). Measurement obtained from a *typical performance* (i.e., usual performance) likely reflect the balance between skill/impairment and compensatory mechanisms, particularly compensatory selection in neurologically impaired persons (i.e., alternative recruitment of unaffected structures/functions). For that purpose, speech tasks generally do not require additional instructions or might occasionally add "at a comfortable pace/level" to the task explanation. Conversely, requiring *maximum performance* (e.g., "as fast as you can") assists in exhausting the functional reserve and the compensatory upregulation, which is ample and proportionate in young, healthy subjects but limited in older or neurologically impaired persons (Cabeza et al. 2018). When reserve is depleted and upregulation fails, the resulting performance either plateaus below the expected or breaks down—often via neglect of articulatory accuracy. In addition to direct, overt elicitation through task instructions as commented on above, maximum performance may also be indirectly studied through the selection of speech targets that implicitly require high performance (e.g., words that require the fastest reshaping of the oral tract for their production, i.e., phonetic structure targets) (Rosen et al. 2008). We suggest opting for typical performance demand to assess appropriateness-related characteristics (e.g., phonetic precision, stress pattern, frequency and loudness steadiness) or when the examinee reports a complaint that occurs during typical use of their speech/voice. We suggest requesting maximum performance to investigate latent impairment, to estimate reserve/compensation capabilities or to determine working range (e.g., frequency, loudness, nasality).

*Cognitive and emotional load* influence speech performance (Huttunen et al. 2011; MacPherson et al. 2017). Manipulation of cognitive load in electing tasks of speech production, like that in maximum performance, may reduce the availability of compensatory mechanisms and expose otherwise covert speech deficits. Some cognitive loading occurs in self-generated long speech (i.e., monologues, via absence of a content-stimulating counter-speaker and absence of speech turns, characteristic of dialogues) and can be increased by requesting memory performance (recounting a story), and interpretation and synthesis of presented content. We do not recommend manipulation of emotional load in speech tasks for clinical assessments, for safeguard of examinees.

*Dual tasking* reduces speech performance of non-impaired individuals (Dromey and Bates 2005) but is disproportionally detrimental to people with Parkinson's Disease, often leading to a complete speech breakdown (Ho et al. 2002). The reduction in performance works both ways where the non-speech task performance is also affected. Speech production has largely been used as a secondary task to study the performance of other functions (e.g., gait, balance) and may produce a greater competitive demand than do silent concurrent tasks (e.g., auditory attention tasks, hand motor tasks) (Dromey and Bates 2005). The effect of a concurrent task on speech has not been well established for most conditions, making it gener-

ally unsuitable for clinical assessments but rather of ongoing interest in research.

Lastly, elicitation of speech varies in *the networks and systems involved*. Common examples include reading tasks, which rely on visual acuity (and literacy), and non-word imitation tasks, which rely completely on the auditory system for their performance. Long tasks such as monologues may also be affected by pronounced impairment of attention, short-term memory and consciousness fluctuation. The examiner must actively enquire and at times formally test the subject's competence in those functions that integrate the speech production performance loop.

### 18.5.3.3 Testing Context

*Practice and familiarity* with eliciting tasks affect speech various output characteristics (Gorno-Tempini et al. 2011; Kawachi 2002; Pen and Quinn 1997; Vogel et al. 2011). People with logopenic aphasia, for example, have more difficulty repeating (or even understanding) unfamiliar sentences (i.e., low probability sentences). Nonetheless, unfamiliarity affects all individuals, including neurotypical people, by causing a reduced speech rate and an increase in pauses. In general, the effect of familiarity is more evident for cognitively complex tasks such as reading a novel text aloud or describing a picture. Therefore, it might be desirable to control or account for the subject's level of familiarity with speech tasks. Running a training trial before the target testing trial is a simple strategy to mitigate unfamiliarity. Another approach is to contrast results arising from different levels of familiarity, once characteristics of the practice effect per se are known, i.e., the slope of change in performance between two or more consecutive trials, may be informative of cognitive and motor dysfunctions (Agostino et al. 2004; Schaefer and Duff 2017). The relationship between practice effect slope and impairment remains unexplored within speech production and is thus suitable only for experimental research.

Transient biological states will also influence speech performance, notably the circadian cycle (Vogel et al. 2010), hydration (Alves et al. 2019) and recreational drug use/intoxication (Shamei and Bird 2019; Sigmund and Zelinka 2011). The state of therapeutic drug effects (i.e., on vs. off) must also be considered, particularly those targeting the motor system, such as L-dopa (Pinho et al. 2018) and psychotropics (Mundt et al. 2012). Episodic states associated with ambient conditions will be discussed under Testing Environment. Except in experimental settings, we suggest testing people during commercial hours, well-hydrated and under the full effect of their therapeutic drugs when relevant. As with any measurement, consistency in testing conditions assists in optimising the reliability of results, particularly for longitudinal care and research.

### 18.5.4 Objective Analyses of Speech

Objective assessments of speech offer increased reliability (no inter- and intra-rater disagreements), reduced cost (no need for training of examiners or time-consuming perceptual analysis), facilitates scalability and remote examination. In research, objective measurements can also permit the use of more powerful statistical approaches and integration of multiple domains (e.g., scores from speech and other neurological dysfunctions). In this subsection, we will consider a few objective methods of measuring speech or speech-related phenomena, with a focus on acoustic analysis.

#### 18.5.4.1 Acoustic Analysis of Speech and Voice

Acoustic analysis of speech is an objective method for describing speech output. The sound produced by the speaker is mathematically decomposed for the calculation of various individual metrics (e.g., sound intensity) which describe discrete acoustic phenomena (e.g., the size of variation in air pressure during a determined short time-window). Thus a multi-parameter approach increases the meaningfulness of acoustic assessment given the nature of motor-speech production. Analyses often focus on measures related to speech quality, timing and control. There is a variety of voice quality measurements ranging from those mostly determined by constitutional characteristics (e.g., fundamental frequency largely determined by age and sex)

(Maturo et al. 2012) to metrics that mostly reflect an interplay between local structural status (e.g., laryngeal dehydration, nasal obstruction) and neurological control (e.g., vocal fold paralysis) (Delgado-Vargas et al. 2021; Vogel et al. 2017b; Wormald et al. 2008), including metrics such as cepstral peak prominence, jitter, shimmer and harmonics-to-noise ratio. Examples of acoustic measures of timing include inter-word intervals, percentage of silence within a sample, speech rate (see Vogel et al. (2012) for their application). At a more fine-grained, segmental level, acoustic analyses can be applied to measure, for instance, deviant voice onset time or disrupted co-articulatory transitions in apraxia (Terband et al. 2019). Acoustic measures of control gauge the accuracy of speech in reaching or sustaining (often implicit) targets, such as producing a steady, non-tremulous voice. Neurological function arguably determines most of the variation in control measurements. Examples include long-term instability of frequency and intensity in sustained vowels in Multiple Sclerosis (Hartelius et al. 1997) and reduced variability of fundamental frequency in connected speech in Parkinson's disease (Rektorova et al. 2016; Rusz et al. 2011).

To execute acoustic analyses, examiners dispose of many software options including open-source scripts and more user-friendly, commercially developed packages. They differ in accuracy and algorithms deployed to describe the signal (Burris et al. 2014; Tsanas et al. 2014), usability and cost (Vogel and Morgan 2009), with some high-quality free options (de Jong and Wempe 2009), e.g., *Praat* available at www.fon.hum.uva.nl/praat/. Nonetheless, the reliability of the resulting metrics will depend on the quality of the recorded speech signal. Next, we discuss two key determinants of the quality speech sound acquisition: testing environment and hardware.

- **Testing environment**: Testing conditions should either mimic that of the usual site of performance (e.g., classroom for workplace-related tests in teachers) or most commonly control for additional speech and voice stressors.
  **Non-acoustic factors**: Air or airborne particles often affect speech and voice. Ambient air that is very hot, very cold or dry will dehydrate the

speaker's airway, which reduces phonatory periodicity (Hemler et al. 1997; Zou et al. 2019) and likely increases the number of pauses and the rate of fatigue. Dusty or mouldy rooms, and poorly maintained airflow systems disperse common airborne triggers of respiratory allergic flares, inducing nasal blockage, coughing, sneezing and shortness of breath, possibly causing various speech and voice changes.

**Acoustic factors**: Background noise and room reverberation have major effects on speech assessment. Noise induces vocalising vertebrates (including humans) to increase their loudness involuntarily, which is known as the Lombard Effect (Luo et al. 2018). Room reverberation has the opposite effect, causing speakers to reduce their vocal loudness (Astolfi et al. 2019). Beyond just intensity, changes in vocal loudness are accompanied by multiple behavioural and resonance shifts, including changes in articulators speed and range (Kearney et al. 2017), in vocal noise (Brockmann-Bauser et al. 2019) and in the power ratio between harmonics (Nordenberg and Sundberg 2004).

In addition, noise and room reverberation have direct negative impacts on sound recording. Both decrease the general signal-to-noise ratio, distorting speech acoustic metrics that reflect or rely on periodicity or sound intensity contrasts, such as harmonics-to-noise ratio, cepstral peak prominence and intensity-based speech-silence ratios (Deliyski et al. 2005; Vogel and Maruff 2008). Reverberance has an additional frequency-selective effect on the recorded signal, depending on the distance between microphone and reflective surface in front of the speaker. If the length of the return travel (from the microphone to the reflective surface and back to the microphone) equals the wavelength of a periodic sound, the peak of the returning wave will coincide with the peak of the outgoing wave, summing up their amplitude at the microphone-point. Conversely if peak and valley meet, attenuation occurs. A reflective surface (e.g., a concrete wall) 43 cm from the microphone, for example, will dampen the amplitude of a periodic sound of wavelength 1.72 m (approximately 200 Hz) and boost the amplitude of 86 cm waves (400 Hz). Such selective frequency attenuation by near reflective surfaces is readily observable in experimental results (Bottalico et al. 2016) even when it is not the object of investigation—it is easy to imagine how it would affect sensitive speech acoustic metrics. Lastly, nearby electrical currents cause distortion or add noise to the recorded signal (Vogel and Morgan 2009).

- *From physics we know that electrical currents and moving magnetic fields cause electrical induction, i.e., an electrical current in a "distant" conducting material. This is relevant since sound is converted into an electric signal for its recording. The degree of induction depends on proximity, angle (between cables) and current magnitude in the source of interference. In most settings, simply making sure power cables are apart from recording equipment is sufficient. In hospital settings (or other facilities where high electrical currents are common), high gauge electric cables are sometimes present in common rooms' walls/floor/ceiling, carrying high electric current to (usually) nearby equipment (e.g., medical imaging—MRI and CT scans).*

- **Recording equipment and set-up**: *Speech can be recorded by using a variety of hardware options. Briefly, when considering whether recording hardware is suitable for the purpose, an examiner should consider why they are using the equipment, how portable it needs to be, its costs and whether the equipment should be calibrated and those undertaking subsequent analysis of recordings require further training [see Vogel and Morgan 2009 and Vogel and Reece 2021 for overviews of hardware and software].*

Microphones vary in self-generated noise (Peus 2004), electrical insulation and filtering of background noise. The polar pattern of microphones (directionality) also affects the amount of background noise captured (Vogel and Morgan 2009). Relative noise interferes with various acoustic measurements related to variation and periodicity (Deliyski et al. 2005; Vogel and Maruff 2008) (e.g., perturbations, standard deviation, harmonics-to-noise ratio, cepstral peak prominence); see (Švec and Granqvist 2010) for more on microphones.

The same applies for the positioning of microphones where proximity to sound source results in a greater signal magnitude and consequently smaller relative noise. Increasing the distance between sound source and microphone makes the signal more susceptible to non-free-field influences (e.g., reflection and refraction of sound in out-of-lab environments (Eargl 2003), which inflates measurements related to noise and perturbation or distortion (Titze and Winholtz 1993). A parallel between noise and dysarthria has been observed for intelligibility as assessed by a listener's transcription accuracy (Borrie et al. 2017). The angle of placement in relation to the sound source can also influence measurements, but to a smaller degree (Titze and Winholtz 1993) while the relation between the microphone and body parts can cause frequency-dependent distortions (Feigin et al. 1990).

Additionally, microphone sensitivity varies across frequencies. The distribution of sensitivity along the frequency spectrum is referred to as frequency response, which may influence the recorded signal in a predicable manner and thus be prone to a mathematical correction when necessary (Parsa et al. 2001). Frequency responsiveness further varies in relation to distance to sound source, depending on the polar pattern of microphones. A noticeable boost in low frequencies is observed for cardioid microphones (e.g., the Reference and the Directional) when that distance is shortened, known as proximity effect (Clifford and Reiss 2011). Frequency sensitivity influences spectral centroid and tilt measures and may affect metrics of relative harmonics/noise (e.g., cepstral peak prominence, harmonics-to-noise ratio).

- **Suggested Standard Practice** Except where otherwise required, e.g., for experiments on behavioural (e.g., the Lombard effect) or signal acquisition manipulation, speech assessments/recordings should be conducted in a room, that is:

  - Quiet (background noise <35 dB)
  - Non-reverberant; reverberant rooms are spacious (>4 × 4 m, high ceiling), with flat and solid reflective surfaces (e.g., solid walls, hard floor), lacking sound absorption (e.g., little or no furnishing)
  - With the speaker positioned away from walls in their 180° frontal plane (>1.8 m)
  - With power cables and power devices placed away from recording equipment (including from microphone cables). It is a good habit to listen to and inspect visually a short pilot recording sample with the equipment in final position, before the target recording/assessment session—electrical interference produces a low pitch buzz at 50 or 60 Hz (depending on the country)

- Additionally, related to hardware and set up, we recommend:

  - The use of a high-quality cardioid microphone where possible, head-mounted, positioned at about 5 cm from the mouth at a 45° angle. Alternatively, a lapel-attached or other at proximity to the speaker (but not directly in front of their mouth)

If deemed necessary, a strict control of environment biases requires the consistent use a sound-isolated, anechoic and electrically insulated room (or, at least, an electrically isolated room).

### 18.5.4.2 Electrophysiological and Kinematic Assessment of Motor Speech

Articulatory movement can be quantified by 3D imaging methods (such as ultrasound, X-ray, MRI) and anatomical site tracking (such as electropalatography, electromagnetic articulography). The utility of instrumental assessments can be determined, in part, by their relative connection to the speech behaviour they are attempting to describe, but also the time demand, cost and expertise required to administer and interpret the tests. The value of kinematic and physiological tools for describing speech lies in the information they can provide on the underlying mechanisms influencing output.

Motor control of speech can be explored by physiological protocols such as electromyography

(EMG) of the larynx (e.g., cricothyroid) or tongue (e.g., genioglossus) (Hardcastle 2006; Kubin et al. 2015). EMG uses wire electrodes embedded within target muscles or on the skin surface to record electrical activity of muscles. These sensors provide information on muscle activation (e.g., site, intensity and duration of activation) during speech. EMG may provide some insight into the underlying mechanisms driving disordered speech in some neuromuscular conditions. Its full utility as a diagnostic or therapeutic tool in clinical practice remains to be determined.

Electropalatography (EPG) is a sensor-based tool designed to measure tongue-to-palate contact by using sensors embedded in a palatal plate worn by the speaker (Lee 2021). Temporal and spatial data on tongue placement can be derived from isolated and connected speech (Hardcastle 1972). These parameters can in turn increase our understanding of speech-related timing and articulation (Folker et al. 2010) and even be used as a biofeedback tools for patients (Morgan et al. 2007). Similar to EPG, electromagnetic articulography (EMA) aims to provide data on placement, stability and consistency of speech motor behaviour. Unlike EPG, EMA provides information in 3D space. Older EMA systems required subjects to wear a helmet with transmitter coils attached to specific speech relevant anatomical sites (Folker et al. 2011). More recent EMA systems still utilise sensors but use low field-strength electromagnetic fields to measure kinematic outcomes (van Lieshout 2021).

### 18.5.4.3 Dynamic Imaging Methodologies

Dynamic imaging modalities such as ultrasound and magnetic resonance imaging (MRI) can provide visual data on articulatory movements associated with speech. Ultrasound uses high frequency sound waves to produce images and can be used to explore tongue movement and shape during speech. MRI can be used to visualise the vocal tract with the aim of obtaining images of dynamic articulation during speech. During use, an ultrasound probe is placed under the chin in either mid-sagittal or coronal view to derive an image of the tongue surface. Quantification of the tongue shape and corresponding movements can be challenging in both modalities. An assessors' ability to differentiate anatomical landmarks and accurately measure their speed and movement is partly determined by their expertise and experience, as well as the quality of images provided by the methods. In ultrasound and MRI, images produced during assessment can assist in treatment, both acting as visual biofeedback devices. Evidence supporting ultrasound or MRI as therapy tools is growing; however, studies remain small and underpowered, with no randomised controlled trials evaluating their efficacy (Sugden et al. 2019).

## 18.6 Clinical Examination of Motor Speech Disorders

Timothy Pommée, Mathieu Balaguer, and Virginie Woisard

### 18.6.1 Introduction

The goal of clinical assessment is to obtain clinical data to provide a diagnosis and to guide the management of the patient. It includes three different but dependent approaches: (1) an anatomical and sensorimotor examination of the vocal apparatus structures involved in speech production, (2) an assessment of speech by the examiner and (3) an assessment of the speech and communication impairment and of its functional impact by the patient or their peers.

The speech assessment is aimed at evaluating several dimensions of the speech disorder, which can be mapped to the three levels described in the ICF classification (World Health Organization 2001; Dykstra et al. 2007): *body structure and functions* (structural deficits/modifications and their stable or evolving nature, regarding respiration, phonation and articulation); *activities* (limitations on the patient's communication) and *participation* (interactions with the environment and psychosocial impact).

At the end of the assessment, data are synthesised to answer the following questions (Auzou 2007):

- What is the severity of the speech disorder?
- What are the main perceptual abnormalities allowing its description and their exchange with various therapists?
- What perception does the patient have of their complaint and what is it?
- What are the sensorimotor deficits associated with the speech disorder?

### 18.6.2 Anatomical and Sensorimotor Examination of the Structures Involved in Speech Production

The vocal apparatus is examined to assess the sensitivity, strength, speed, symmetry, accuracy, range of movement, steadiness and coordination of the anatomical structures involved in speech production. Some structures can be accessed directly by the eyes and the fingers of the examiner: chest, neck, jaw, face, cheeks, lips, tongue and palate. Others need instrumental assessment or are evaluated indirectly, such as the larynx. A fibrescopic evaluation is usually included in the clinical assessment for the phoniatrician. In any case the observation must be performed with the patient at rest, during static postures, during non-speech movements but also during speech. The aim is to assess the anatomy and functional capacities of each structure and their ability to be coordinated for speaking. The reader may refer to Sect. 18.4 for a more comprehensive description of the sensorimotor assessment.

### 18.6.3 Speech Assessment by the Therapist

#### 18.6.3.1 Tools and Levels of Granularity

For each of the different dimensions, various speech assessment methods are used (Rumbach et al. 2019). Clinicians can use visual analogue scales, Likert scales or direct magnitude estimation (Kent et al. 1989) to assess different concepts, both global (e.g., disorder severity, naturalness, speech clarity) or more specific (e.g., prosody, voice quality, speech rate). This assessment can be done at different levels of granularity, according to the aim of the evaluation: on isolated phonemes, syllables, (pseudo-)words, predictable or unpredictable sentences, reading passages or conversations (e.g., during the case history).

To obtain a quantitative measure that is more specific than an overall perceptual rating, the speech assessment usually includes orthographic stimuli transcriptions (usually of words or sentences) (Hustad 2006, 2008), but also assessment of the word/sentence comprehensibility by the use of closed sets of items (Kent et al. 1989; Hustad 2006) and assessment of narrative comprehensibility by questioning (Hustad 2008).

#### 18.6.3.2 Global and Specific Concepts to Assess

At the "activities" level, two aspects can be distinguished. The *functional aspect* of the patient's communication skills addresses the clinician's and the patient's primary goal. A *more analytical assessment* of speech intelligibility at the sub-lexical level provides a reliable outcome measure and gives the clinician more detailed insight of the speech parameters to focus on in therapy.

**Intelligibility** can be defined as the accuracy with which the acoustic signal is decoded by the listener in terms of "low-level" units (phonemes/phonemic groups/syllables) (Woisard et al. 2013; Ghio et al. 2018; Hustad 2008; Yorkston et al. 1996). To assess this acoustic-phonetic decoding, perceptual methods include the transcription and percentage of correct stimuli scores from repetition or reading aloud of isolated phonemes, syllables, pseudo-words or words in unpredictable sentences, or the use of minimal word pairs (i.e., any speech material that does not involve compensation processes). It can be supplemented by instrumental methods (see Sect. 18.7).

**Comprehensibility** can be defined as

the ability of the listener to interpret the meaning of the oral message produced by a speaker without regard to phonetic or lexical accuracy or correctness. (Woisard et al. 2013)

Comprehensibility is therefore a more *functional concept*, complementary to intelligibility in the "activities" level of the speech assessment. It takes into account many factors in the communication context (semantic, syntactic and discursive context, situational clues, gestures…) (Ghio et al. 2018; Hustad 2008; Yorkston et al. 1996), which can help the listener to compensate for a possible degradation of the speech signal (Ghio et al. 2018). Note that therapy goals aiming to reduce the speech deficits at a more analytical level (i.e., targeting intelligibility), along with compensatory approaches, will subsequently contribute to improving the patient's comprehensibility and functional communication (Yorkston et al. 1996; Palmer and Enderby 2007; Duffy 2013).

**The overall severity** of the speech disorder, last but not least, includes, in addition to comprehensibility (and thus intelligibility), such factors as voice quality, prosody, etc. While the concepts of intelligibility, comprehensibility and severity are interlinked (see Fig. 18.2), the choice of which one to assess depends, among other things, on the pathological context (Hustad 2008; Sussman and Tjaden 2012).

Finally, besides intelligibility, comprehensibility and severity, other dimensions can be rated, such as the naturalness or the clarity of the patient's speech or the perceived listener effort, but also more *specific parameters* such as speech rate, voice quality, prosody, nasality, etc. The same measurement tools and evaluation processes used for the global concepts will be applied to these parameters.

### 18.6.3.3  Limits of Perceptual Assessment

A first limit concerns the lack of consensus definitions of the concepts that are assessed. Indeed, definitions vary depending on the user's background and aims. What exactly is rated depends on the medium (e.g., pseudo-words vs. sentences) (Wannberg et al. 2016), on the tool (e.g., Likert scale vs. transcription) and on the instructions to the listening jury.

Furthermore, a high inter- and intra-rater variability of auditory-perceptual ratings has frequently been reported in the literature (Kearns and Simmons 1988; Kent 1996), depending on the assessed dimension and more importantly in

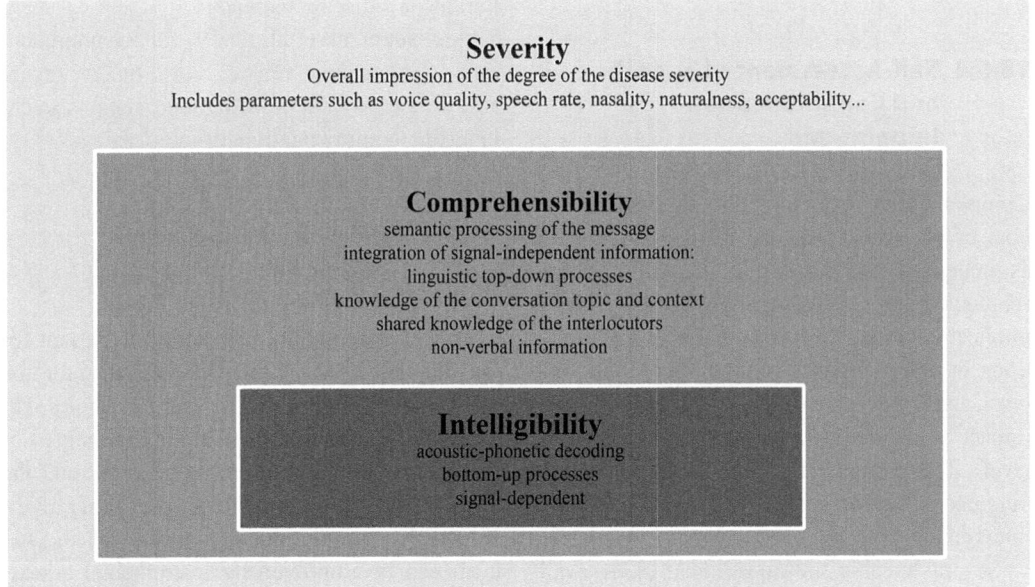

**Fig. 18.2**  Interrelations between speech concepts (Pommée et al. 2021a). With kind permission of John Wiley & Sons, Inc., Hoboken, New Jersey

the mid-range of the rating continua (Bunton et al. 2007). Each rater has their own expertise in the assessment of speech in various pathological contexts, whereby their internal referents are constructed (Kuruvilla-Dugdale et al. 2019). Inter-rater agreement was found to be higher for overall speech dimensions (e.g., naturalness, severity) than for specific speech dimensions (e.g., nasality) (Wannberg et al. 2016). Inter-rater variability is also influenced by poor definitions of the criteria to be assessed (Kent 1996). Intra-rater variability can be explained by continuously evolving internal referents and increasing familiarity (Hustad and Cahill 2003), but also and foremost by the cognitive availability at the time of each assessment (e.g., attention, tiredness…) and by the assessment context (Fex 1992).

While the auditory-perceptual assessment remains the gold standard in current clinical practice, its reliability is reduced by its subjective nature. To reduce the variability, databases of pathological speech recordings might help to induce more homogeneous internal anchors. Another solution is to resort to instrumental assessment methods to complement the perceptual assessment (see Sect. 18.7).

### 18.6.4 Self-Assessment of Speech and Communication Impairment

Complementary to the therapist's evaluations, the goal of the self-assessment by the patient is to estimate the functional impact on communication (perceived speech disorder or discomfort, communication effectiveness and perceived limitations in daily activities) at the "activities" ICF level, and the psychosocial consequences and the impact on the quality of life at the "participation" level. These elements have implications for outcome measurement and for planning intervention.

Several specific self-questionnaires are available. Although including elements assessing the

psychosocial impact, they mainly address items in functional dimensions: some target voice disorders (e.g., Voice Handicap Index: Jacobson et al. 1997; Voice Activity and Participation Profile: Ma and Yiu 2001), some are more speech-related (e.g., Speech Handicap Index: Rinkel et al. 2008; Phonation Handicap Index: Balaguer et al. 2020a; Fichaux-Bourin et al. 2009), some target communication (e.g., Communicative Participation Item Bank: Baylor et al. 2013; ASHA Quality of Communication Life: Paul et al. 2004), others are impairment-related (e.g., Living with Dysarthria self-report questionnaire: Hartelius et al. 2008; Dysarthria Impact Profile: Walshe et al. 2009).

Furthermore, the therapist can also provide more global questionnaires to assess the patient's self-reported quality of life. Again, several forms exist, such as the MOS SF-36 (Ware and Sherbourne 1992) and the QOL-DyS (Piacentini et al. 2011). Other questionnaires are dedicated to specific pathologies: the EORTC QLQ-C30 (Aaronson et al. 1993) and the FACT-G (Cella et al. 1993) for cancer patients; the Neuro-QoL (Cella et al. 2012) for neurological disorders; the ALSSQOL-R (Felgoise et al. 2011) for ALS patients; the PDQ-39 (Jenkinson et al. 1997) for Parkinson's disease patients.

See Neumann et al. (2019) for a comprehensive systematic review of quality-of-life assessment in adults with neurogenic speech-language-communication difficulties.

### 18.6.5 Synthesis of the Clinical Assessment

The synthesis of these data may be relevant for the diagnosis but is mainly necessary for the management of the disorder. Care strategies will depend on an interaction between the analysis of the speech disorder, the patient history and the available therapeutic methods (see Table 18.2). Knowledge of the pathophysiological mechanism can be improved by instrumental assessment (see Sect. 18.7).

**Table 18.2** Synthesis of assessment levels, tasks and outcome measures in motor speech disorders from Pommée et al. (2021b) reprinted by permission of Taylor & Francis Group, Abingdon, Oxon, UK

| ICF-levels | Dimensions of analysis | Tasks | Outcome measures |
|---|---|---|---|
| Global | Contextual information | Guided conversation with the patient and other stakeholders (peers, caregivers, health professionals…) | Patient history (medical diagnosis and history, associated deficits, age, living/working context, communication partners, main complaints, needs and priorities, communicational facilitators and barriers…) |
| Body structures and functions | Sensitivity and motricity | Verbal and non-verbal oro-facial motricity and sensitivity tasks<br>Respiration at rest and during speech<br>Posture | Strength, speed, amplitude, accuracy and coordination of movements of the tongue, lips, jaw, cheeks, velum, face<br>*Aerodynamic measures*[a]<br>Pneumophonic coordination |
|  | Phonation | Sustained vowels and running speech samples | *Objective voice quality measure, sound pressure levels and pitch, maximum phonation time*[a]<br>Subjective rating of overall voice quality and voice qualities (e.g., GRBAS-I, CAPE-V) |
| Activities | Articulation | Phoneme/syllable repetition<br>Diadochokinesis (pataka)<br>Simple vs. complex multisyllabic word repetition<br>Automatic speech | Phoneme inventory<br>Motor planning and programming vs. execution |
|  | Intelligibility | Repetition or reading of:<br>– Pseudo-words<br>– Minimal word pairs to test specific phonetic contrasts (e.g., TPI in French)<br>– Semantically unpredictable sentences | Percent-correct stimuli from transcription (phonemes/syllables/pseudo-words, words)<br>N.B. Ideally transcription by a colleague to avoid familiarity with the stimuli and with the patient's speech; large sets of pseudo-words to avoid recognition, with similarities/minimal pairs |
|  | Comprehensibility | Sentence comprehension tasks (e.g., sentence verification task, picture selection; ideally stimuli unknown to the listener)<br>Text reading<br>(Semi-)spontaneous speech | Ratings of speech comprehensibility, severity, naturalness, nasality (see Darley et al. 1969a, b for more rating criteria)<br>Deterioration over time/fatigability |
|  | Supra-segmental | Specific prosody-related tasks<br>Syntax/chunking (e.g., profiling elements of prosody in speech-communication, PEPS-C; Peppé and McCann 2003) | Intonation and intentions: use of declarative/interrogative/exclamatory/imperative sentences<br>Expression of emotions<br>Focus/contrastive stress expression<br>Syntactic chunking<br>Speech rate |
| Participation | Speech-related questionnaires | Speech handicap index, phonation handicap index, dysarthria impact profile or other specific questionnaires (e.g., Functional Assessment of Cancer Therapy Head and Neck) | Overall impact and specific dimensions |
|  | Overall quality-of-life questionnaires | Self-reported questionnaires (e.g., EORTC QLQ-C30, ALSSQOL-SF, PDQ-39, QOL-DyS, Neuro-QoL, MOS SF-36) | Overall quality of life and specific dimensions |

[a] These measures are exclusively instrumental (see Sect. 18.7)

## 18.7 Instrumental Examination of Motor Speech Disorders

Mathieu Balaguer, Timothy Pommée, and Virginie Woisard

### 18.7.1 Introduction

With regard to clinical examination, speech-related instrumentation extends the examiners' perception and makes their assessment objective, by providing valid and reliable speech measures. Moreover, the use of instrumental tools is relevant for comparing patients' results with reference values and allows follow-up measures with reference to a baseline. Instrumental methods can be described under two main headings: physiological methods and imaging techniques on the one hand, and acoustic measures, on the other.

### 18.7.2 Physiological Methods and Imaging Techniques

Physiological methods are crucial for identifying the links between pathological physiology and acoustic and perceptual attributes of dysarthria. An increasing number of methods are used (Murdoch 2011) and are more or less simple to operate. The choice of these methods depends on the targeted level of analysis: respiration, phonation, articulation.

**Anatomical and functional imaging**: Imaging techniques provide a visualisation of the anatomical structures involved in real-time speech and voice production. Videolaryngostroboscopy is an invasive examination that allows the visualisation of the glottis (Cohen et al. 2014). At the oral and pharyngeal levels, much of the early understanding about the behaviour of the articulators has come from X-ray studies, using videoradioscopy of speech. However, these techniques expose the patient to a high level of ionising radiation. Magnetic resonance imaging can overcome this issue but is currently limited by a slow rate of image acquisition (maximum 12 images/s for an acceptable loss of spatial definition, which might

be too low to represent accurately the precise movements involved in speech production) and by the noise of the device, preventing any good synchronisation with the speech signal. Furthermore, the patient needs to be in a supine position, which limits the ecological aspect of the speech and voice production. Lastly, ultrasonography could also be interesting for investigating the coarticulation effects during speech production, as well as to obtain articulatory measures (Barberena et al. 2014). While this technique is not commonly used and remains examiner-dependent, it can be implemented as a visual feedback during therapy (Bacsfalvi et al. 2007).

**Aerodynamic methods**: Aerodynamic methods describe the movement of the air in the respiratory and the upper aero-digestive tract. These methods provide information on phonatory, pneumophonic and articulatory functioning by measuring oral and nasal pressure or airflow and subglottal pressure (Teston 2007). These methods particularly give clues to understanding the efficiency of the phonatory breath, the pneumophonic coordination, the estimated subglottal pressure, the phonation quotient (the ratio of the vital capacity to the maximum phonation time), the velopharyngeal dynamics and the precision and coordination of labial and lingual movements. The combination with synchronised acoustic measurements allows the assessment of glottal efficacy and some specific linguistic phenomena, such as nasalisation or spirantisation (i.e., the noise generated during a stop consonant) (Ackermann et al. 1995). Finally, they can also be used to provide feedback for the patient during therapy.

**Electrophysiological techniques**: *Electromyography* (EMG) measures the electrical activity of the muscles during the contraction and relaxation phases of the muscles analysed (Kimaid et al. 2015). The electrodes can be placed, for example, on the thoracic and the cervico-scapular area to quantify the activity of the respiratory muscles. More specifically at the laryngeal level, *electroglottography* (EGG) determines the impedance between two electrodes placed on the neck on either side of the larynx. It allows a good representation of the vocal fold oscillation cycle because of its insensitivity to vocal tract effects and the absence of any aerodynamic noise (Herbst 2020).

**Kinematic measures**: Transduction devices provide data on the articulators' velocity, acceleration and trajectories in a two-dimensional mid-sagittal space, with optoelectronic or electromagnetic movement analysis systems (Goozée et al. 2000). A set of three to five coils creates a modulated magnetic field around the head of the patient. Receiving coils (sensors) are placed on different oral points (tongue, jaw, lips, velum), and can be located in the artificial magnetic field. Kinematic parameters are usually investigated on a sequence of syllables produced by the patient (Ackermann et al. 1995). This technique is an important research tool (Walsh and Smith 2012) and its clinical application is developing (Kaburagi et al. 2005; Berry et al. 2017).

**Palatography**: This technique dynamically records the points of contact between the tongue and the palate during speech, and thus allows assessment of the articulation between these structures. *Direct palatography* is an old technique requiring use of a paste composed of a black vegetal mixture applied on the surface of the tongue. A picture of the palate is taken just after the person has pronounced a specific phoneme (Ladefoged 1957). The main limitation of this technique is the ability to analyse only one articulation. *Electropalatography* (EPG) records the location and timing of tongue contacts with the hard palate during continuous speech, by using an artificial palate with electrodes placed in the patient's mouth (Barberena et al. 2017). Studies have demonstrated the value of using EPG to assess, diagnose and treat motor speech disorders (Murdoch 2011; Barberena et al. 2017). However, the necessity of manufacturing a customised palate for each patient limits the use of this technique to a single assessment.

## 18.7.3 Acoustic Measures

State-of-the-art instrumentation for acoustic methods has become easily accessible with efficient free software such as Praat (Boersma 2001)

and Wavesurfer (Beskow and Sjölander 2000). These programmes allow quantification and visual display of frequency-, intensity- and time-domain components of the speech signal (Barsties and Maryn 2013). Acoustic measures have the advantage of providing objective quantitative data to complement auditory-perceptual ratings and investigate signal components that cannot be heard, without requiring invasive methods. In a clinical context they allow targeting of specific phonemes, sound categories or speech parameters (e.g., to increase lip tension in plosives) when planning therapy. Furthermore, the visual representation of the speech signal can also be a source of visual feedback during therapy sessions. Even if acoustic analysis can be useful to supplement perceptual analysis, multi-parametric analysis is necessary to reflect the multidimensional nature of speech and take into account the lack of a strong link with auditory perception (Kreiman and Gerratt 1998). Acoustic measures should be used to supplement auditory-perceptual ratings, not replace them. Indeed, speech is highly variable (even more so in pathological speech), so how representative a speech sample at a given point in time is, can be questionable. Also, "norms" cannot be established, there being no potential answer to the question of the normality of speech: acoustic measures should rather be used to compare a patient or a patient group with their own baseline values.

Nonetheless, while the knowledge of their limits leads to caution in their interpretation, acoustic measures are valuable instruments and can be divided into three categories: those related to the laryngeal source (voicing), to the resonators (articulation of speech sounds) and to global speech parameters by using automatic speech recognition.

**Laryngeal source**: Phonation and voice quality measures can be informative in the assessment of motor speech disorders, because the voicing source contributes not only to phonetic contrasts at the phoneme level (e.g., voiced vs. unvoiced consonants), but also to supra-segmental aspects such as prosody. The most investigated are measures of instability, both of the fundamental frequency (e.g., jitter, i.e., short-term cycle-to-cycle variability, or standard deviation of F0) and of the sound pressure level (e.g., shimmer or standard deviation), as well as measures of additive noise in the voice signal (e.g., harmonics-to-noise ratio). Several authors have discussed the reliability of these perturbation measures, notably in severely disordered voices resulting in highly aperiodic acoustic signals. Measures in the cepstral domain, such as the smoothed cepstral peak prominence (CPPs) have shown promising results in severe voice disorders (Heman-Ackah et al. 2003). Furthermore, cepstral measures, along with long-term average spectrum measures (e.g., spectral tilt or slope), can be used on continuous speech samples (Lowell et al. 2011).

**Articulation of speech sounds**: Segmental acoustic measures are used to investigate speech intelligibility at the phoneme and syllable levels (see definition of intelligibility in Sect. 18.6), i.e., to assess vowel, glide and consonant articulation (Kent 1992; Miller 2013).

To date, vowels are investigated more than consonants (Balaguer et al. 2020b), mainly because they are by definition voiced, composed of periodic waveforms and can be sustained (in contrast to plosive consonants, for example), which makes them more convenient to analyse (see an example in Fig. 18.3).

The most commonly used vowel measures are based on steady-state formant values, such as the vowel space area (Fletcher et al. 2017), the articulatory-acoustic vowel space (Whitfield and Goberman 2017) and the formant centralisation ratio (Skodda et al. 2013). Dynamic vowel measures are also used to investigate formant shifts in phoneme transitions and to take into account coarticulation effects, e.g., the vector length (Ferguson and Quené 2014) or the formant movement ratio between static and dynamic vowels (Neel 2008).

Glide measures are by definition dynamic, as these phonemes transition from one state to another, e.g., second formant slope, reflecting vocal tract shape change rates (Martel-Sauvageau and Tjaden 2017).

For consonants, steady-state consonant measures include spectral moment measures (Jongman et al. 2000), spectral peak measures (Katz et al. 1991) and upper boundary frequency (Hohoff et al. 2003). Examples of dynamic measures are the spectral slope (Peeters 2004), the first formant offset frequency (Flege et al. 1992) and the locus equation based on the transition of the second formant (Martel-Sauvageau and Tjaden 2017).

In addition to spectral measures (i.e., in the frequency domain), those from the time domain are also used to investigate phonemes. The most common is the Voice Onset Time (VOT), which quantifies the time between the release (burst) of a stop consonant and the start of voicing. It studies the coordination between articulatory structures (constrictors) and phonatory structures (Morris 1989). Other time-domain measures include phoneme and burst duration measures (Kent and Kim 2003) and formant transition times. Examples of intensity-domain measures are phoneme intensities and the consonant/vowel intensity ratio.

**Overarching**: Supra-segmental acoustic measures can also be used to assess objectively specific parameters of speech, such as prosody (Van Santen et al. 2009). For example, the evolution of the fundamental frequency and of the intensity over time can be measured during utterances by using different speech modalities (assertion, question or order). Intensity, pauses and rate measures can also be used to assess the emphasis on a part of the utterance (focus/contrastive stress) as well as syntactic chunking. Other tools are used to measure speech or articulation rate automatically (De Jong and Wempe 2009)—the latter excluding pause intervals of the speech production—or to analyse rhythm patterns in pathological speech (e.g., envelope modulation spectra) (Liss et al. 2010).

**Global measures: automatic speech analysis**: The recent development of automatic speech recognition (ASR) allows a more global analysis of patients' speech performance. Different ASR system architectures exist (Keshet 2018), the

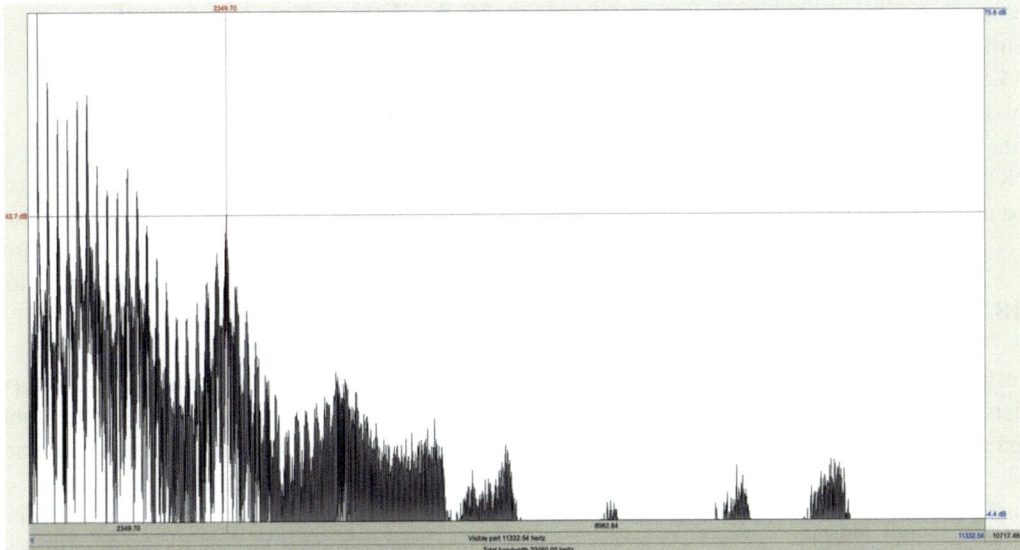

**Fig. 18.3** Example of a spectrum illustrating the frequency components of a sustained vowel/a/in Praat (frequencies on the x-axis and their sound pressure level on the y-axis), on which various measurements can be made, such as formant measures, spectral slope, harmonics-to-noise ratio, etc. Recorded by the authors and presented with permission from Paul Boersma (Boersma and Weenink 2021)

most commonly used at present being based on HMMs (Hidden Markov Models). After preprocessing of the signal to eliminate noise, spectral (LPC: Linear Prediction Coding) or cepstral (MFCC: Mel-Frequency Cepstral Coefficients) parameters are extracted over windows of 0–30 ms from the signal. These parameters are then compared by a decoder with (1) an acoustic model previously trained on numerous recordings, which represents statistically each phone of a language, and with (2) a pronunciation dictionary including the possible pronunciations of the words in a given language. Finally, (3) a language model is used to obtain an output of words corresponding to the best probability of phoneme and word chaining for a given language. The most recent systems are now fully integrated with algorithms that manage the acoustic and language models and the pronunciation dictionary at the same time. These ASR systems can be used to obtain statistics such as phonetic or lexical inventories. Highly developed and commonly used on healthy speech, few are yet really adapted to the recognition of pathological speech, mainly

because of a lack of data to train the models. However, various projects are emerging to address this issue (Google's Euphonia Project; C2SI, Woisard et al. 2020).

**Recording conditions**: A recording of the patient's speech is of high importance for the speech assessment. In order to obtain reliable acoustic data, the recording conditions have to be controlled. While for research purposes the recording context and parameters have to be kept constant throughout the experiments, for clinical purposes the parameters should at least be kept constant for each patient.

High quality microphones have become increasingly affordable. A head-mounted microphone is preferred, to allow for a consistent microphone-mouth distance and to maximise the signal-to-noise ratio (Švec and Granqvist 2010). The recording should be made in a quiet room, without noise sources such as fans, air-conditioners, computer hum, buzzing neon lights, etc., but also smartphones and other connected accessories such as smart watches, which can induce interference noise. Microphone foam covers avoid turbulence on plosives, fricatives or airflow noise. A minimum sampling rate of 44.1 kHz with a minimum amplitude resolution of 16-bit is recommended. The preferred audio file format is a ".wav" file (no compression; do NOT use. mp3), and the recordings should also be monophonic (Patel et al. 2018).

### 18.7.4 Conclusion

Instrumental assessment of motor speech disorders can supplement the clinician's perceptual assessment and provide additional reliable data in all stages of the clinical management, including:

- Increasing the accuracy of diagnosis through more reliable and more precise identification of abnormal functions that require modification
- Providing quantitative data for outcome measurement and documentation of therapeutic efficacy
- Expanding therapy modalities through the use of instrumentation for biofeedback (Baken and Orlikoff 2000)
- Using artificial intelligence, for instance to decrease the time-consuming processes of the speech assessment

Despite their advantages, instrumental methods are not yet widely used in motor speech disorders (except for research purposes). One reason may be a lack of widely accepted standards and normative data for speech tasks, measurement methods and specific parameters for instrumental measurements. Furthermore, instrumental measures are not yet sufficiently correlated with the patient's self-rated speech-induced impairment or quality of life (Lazarus et al. 2013). These tools and analyses have to be developed further to improve their accuracy and relevance. The subsequent diffusion and facilitation of access to instrumental techniques will provide clinical feedback to research and enhance the management of motor speech disorders.

## 18.8 Estimation of General Cognitive State

Stefano Zago and Edoardo Nicolò Aiello

Neuropsychological testing is the preferred method for identifying the presence, features, and severity of a cognitive impairment in neurological patients (World Health Organization 1993; American Psychiatric Association 2013; Cipolotti and Warrington 1995).

Cognitive domains (e.g., language, memory, attention) or subdomains (e.g., syntactic comprehension, verbal short-term memory) are not natural objects. They represent a grouping of mental faculties rooted in the brain that may thus be impaired by lesions or dysfunctions to particular structures of the central nervous system—this suggesting the existence of functionally distinct neurocognitive circuits. These unobservable cognitive constructs can be tested indirectly by measuring behaviour by objective neuropsychological tests. For example, in the Token Test, auditory comprehension is measured by means of counting the number of correct commands of increasing length and complexity that are decoded and executed by the patient through the manipulation of a deck of coloured tokens of different size and shape (De Renzi and Vignolo 1962). It has to be noted that neuropsychological tests may present with multiple sensory, motor, perceptual and cognitive demands—hence 'pure' domain-specific tests being the exception rather than the rule. Neuropsychologists have access to a number of tests that examine a variety of both instrumental (e.g., memory) and non-instrumental (e.g., attention) skills and abilities for the purpose of diagnosis, rehabilitation or baseline cognitive functioning assessment. In general, a 'test' should be a standardised measurement device—i.e., characterised by a specific procedure for administration and scoring. In addition, a test is 'normed', meaning there is some prescribed method for relating the test scores to a representative normal population sample, or in some cases to specific neurological aetiology (e.g., closed head injury, viral infections, Alzheimer's disease, aphasia).

There are many tests available for neuropsychologists to evaluate cognitive functions, either for global functioning or individual domains (Lezak et al. 2012). Some brief in-clinic and bedside tools such as the Mini Mental State Examination (MMSE) (Folstein et al. 1975, 2010), the Addenbrooke Cognitive Examination-III (ACE-III) (Hsieh et al. 2013) or the Montreal Cognitive Assessment (MoCA) (Nasreddine et al. 2005) are useful for a preliminary picture of global cognitive efficiency. With respect to language disorders, the Mini-Linguistic State Examination (MLSE) (Patel et al. 2020) has been developed for use in the assessment, clinical classification, and monitoring of progressive aphasic syndromes.

On the other hand, some fixed batteries such as the Wechsler Adult Intelligence Scale–IV (WAIS-IV) (Wechsler 2008) or the Repeatable Battery for the Assessment of Neuropsychological Status (r-BANS) (Randolph et al. 1998) examine multiple ability domains in a repeatable format and provide a general relative quotient on intellective and cognitive functioning. However, the more common approach today is to estimate a general cognitive state by using a flexible test battery, which involves testing a variety of cognitive domains or subdomains (Barr 2001).

The role of the clinical neuropsychologist as a 'test user' has been noted to include the responsibility of selecting, overseeing and scoring the test, measuring the pattern of severity of cognitive impairment and interpreting scores within a clinical and theoretical framework (Harvey 2012). The neuropsychologist has to check numerous systematic variables that undermine the validity of the neuropsychological exam, such as correct administration of the tests, age and education level (Arnett 2013). In addition, psychometric analysis should be supported through clinical-behavioural observation. The neuropsychologist is also trained to evaluate the patient's motivational and emotional states.

A specific issue arises owing to the presence of language difficulties, as many standardised

neuropsychological measures are verbally mediated (i.e., presented with verbal instructions and requiring verbal responses). Although assessment batteries designed for aphasia are still developing, at present there are only a few neuropsychological tests aimed at assessing global cognitive functioning of patients with language syndromes. A rare example is the Lothian Assessment for Screening of Cognition in Aphasia (LASCA) (Faiz 2016), a non-verbal assessment for screening cognition in post-stroke aphasic patients. Five cognitive domains are assessed: orientation, attention, memory, visual, and executive functioning. Another battery inspired by this principle is the Aphasia Check List (ACL) (Kalbe et al. 2005), which includes measures of cognitive abilities that rely on non-verbal tasks.

To conclude, estimation of a general cognitive state includes at least three types of knowledge: (1) knowledge of the faceted and interactive anatomo-functional organisation of the cognitive architecture; (2) knowledge of various cognitive profiles that can be determined in neurological and psychiatric fields and in psychological disorders; (3) up-to-date knowledge of the main neuropsychological tests.

## 18.9 Standard Neurological Examination

Stefano Cappa

A comprehensive neurological evaluation is required in any patient presenting with the onset of a motor speech disorder, in order to allow the differential diagnosis between aphasia, apraxia of speech and dysarthria.

An **assessment of language abilities** is necessary in order to evaluate the presence of a language disorder *(aphasia),* of which the motor speech disorder can be one component. This can be done clinically by following the guidelines of a brief standardised language examination (for example, the Aachener Aphasia Bedside Test of Biniek et al. 1992; the Aphasia Rapid Test of

Azuar et al. 2013). These screening test can be supplemented if required by a full language examination, such as the Aachen Aphasie Test (Huber et al. 1983), available in multiple languages. The difficult distinction between phonetic (motor) and phonological (linguistic) error is a crucial aspect of the differential diagnosis between apraxia of speech and aphasia (McNeil et al. 2017). Current neurobiological models of speech production are blurring the rigid distinction between abstract word form representations and their phonetic counterparts, and support an integrative view, which can account for this difficulty (Ziegler et al. 2012)

A **clinical speech examination** is based on careful listening while the patient speaks spontaneously, or is repeating sounds, words and sentences. This step is crucial for the differential diagnosis between *dysarthria and apraxia* of speech (AOS) (Ogar et al. 2005; Cappa and Gorno-Tempini 2009). The distinction is based on the classical definition of apraxia, i.e., a disorder in the execution of voluntary actions despite preserved muscle strength. AOS is a selective motor planning/programming disorder that results in defective coordination of the sequential articulatory movements involved in speech production (Wertz et al. 1984). Dysarthria, on the other hand, is a motor execution disorder, which can be due to impairment in the strength, coordination or tone of the muscles involved in speech production. The differential diagnosis between AOS and dysarthria is critically based on the qualitative analysis of errors. In AOS, the errors are highly inconsistent, more numerous in automatic than in volitional speech, and increase with phonemic sequences (multisyllabic words, in particular those including consonant clusters). Additional features are the initiation difficulty, the omissions, anticipation, perseveration and transpositions of syllables, and the abnormal prosody (Dabul 2000). These errors are considered to reflect defective timing and coordination of the articulators, due to dysfunction of motor control regions in the cerebral cortex. The precise cortical localisation of these control areas is controversial. The current neurobiological view of the speech production system includes several frontal, temporal and parietal areas, as well as subcortical structures (Sörös et al. 2006; Hickok 2012). The anterior part of the left insular cortex is often involved (Dronkers 1996), as well as the posterior part of the left inferior frontal gyrus (Hillis et al. 2004). In addition, the involvement of Broca's area is associated with persistent AOS (Trupe et al. 2013). A recently described white matter pathway, the frontal aslant tract, connecting the inferior frontal gyrus with SMA and pre-SMA, is also involved in programming speech production (Catani et al. 2012; Dick et al. 2013).

The features of *non-apraxic dysarthria* are more heterogeneous than in the case of AOS, as they reflect the mechanisms that are responsible for motor dysfunction (Duffy 1995; Kent et al. 2001). Phonation is also typically involved. Spastic dysarthria, often due to upper motor neuron involvement, is characterised by strained voice quality, low pitch, imprecise consonants, slow rate, hypernasality and hoarseness. Flaccid dysarthria, due to disorders affecting the peripheral nerves, the neuromuscular junction or the muscles, is associated with reduced loudness, hypernasality, monopitch and monoloudness. Symptoms that are considered typical of Parkinsonian dysarthria are monopitch, reduced stress, monoloudness, inappropriate silences and rapid speech rate. In the case of hyperkinetic basal ganglia disorders, the voice is often harsh, there may be vocal stoppages and hypernasality. Cerebellar, or ataxic, dysarthia is characterised by slow, slurred speech, with marked stress on each syllable and "explosive" phonation.

It must be stressed that dysarthria can often be mixed, and the Interpretation of the underlying mechanism is based on careful history-taking and on a complete clinical neurological examination, which is always required to detect:

• Symptoms and signs of pyramidal or extrapyramidal involvement. The assessment of tone, power, tendon reflexes, and the presence or absence of pathological reflexes is crucial for the assessment of spastic and Parkinsonian dysarthria, and is conducted following the standard procedures described, for example, as in (Campbell and DeJong 2005)

- Signs of cerebellar involvement, which are assessed based on the evaluation of muscle tone, coordination, standing and gait
- Signs of lower motor neuron involvement, which can be detected by the examination of facial and palatal movements and the gag reflex, and of trophism or movements of the tongue
- Signs of neuromuscular junction/muscle disorders, which can be detected by a careful muscle examination, including an assessment of possible worsening with sustained activity (suggesting the possibility of Myasthenia Gravis)

## 18.10 Laboratory Examinations (i.e., Serology, Immunology)

Stefano Cappa

The diagnostic work-up of a patient affected by a motor speech disorder should follow, as in any area of neurology, the formulation of a topographic diagnosis, with the differential diagnosis among the possible neurological diseases as a second step (Clarke et al. 2016). This crucial principle of clinical neurology should not be neglected, even in the present age of technological medicine, as the best guide to the appropriate and cost-effective use of health resources.

This basic concept needs to be underlined in contemporary clinical practice. Structural brain imaging, based on computed tomography and magnetic resonance imaging, and less extensively on functional imaging and positron emission tomography, are now frequently used in the case of suspected central nervous system involvement. Excessive reliance on brain imaging investigations should not lead to neglect of other potential causes of motor speech disorders, including peripheral nervous system and neuromuscular pathologies.

Laboratory screening tests of blood and urine are required in the suspicion of neurological manifestation of systemic disorders or when the hypothesis is of brain infection. Isolated dysarthria can be an infrequent manifestation of metabolic disorders, which can be diagnosed from clinical history and appropriate standard laboratory examinations. Screening for intoxication (aluminium, bismuth, toluene and many drugs) should be performed only in unexplained cases with an appropriate exposure history.

Genetic testing of DNA from white cells in the blood is useful for the diagnosis of Huntington's disease and other genetic disorders affecting cortical and subcortical structures involved in speech production, such as the group of spinocerebellar ataxias and hereditary spastic paraplegias, and lysosomal storage disorders. In any case, it should be conducted within appropriate medical genetics setting, following practice recommendations.

Immunological tests for anti-acetylcholine receptor antibodies are useful for the diagnosis of myasthenia gravis (MG), which can present as dysarthria, typically increasing in severity with continuing speech production (a manifestation of fatigability, in particular of the velar muscles).

Cerebrospinal fluid analysis is required in the case of suspected infection or multiple sclerosis. A spinal tap is now frequently considered as a biomarker for neurodegenerative disorders and can be useful for a differential diagnosis between Alzheimer's disease and the fronto-temporal dementia spectrum (Rivero-Santana et al. 2017). Neurofilament assay in the CSF can be helpful for the differential diagnosis of motor neuron disorders (Oeckl et al. 2016).

A biopsy of muscle or nerve is used to diagnose neuromuscular disorders. Dysarthria is frequently observed in polymyositis and is a prominent symptom of the (rare) oculopharyngeal form of genetic muscular dystrophy. Mitochondrial disorders in addition require neuroimaging and neurophysiological studies.

Electromyography (EMG) is used to diagnose nerve and muscle dysfunction and spinal cord disease. An EMG is usually done in conjunction with a nerve conduction velocity (NCV) test. The exam is crucial for the diagnosis of motor neuron disease, a frequent cause of bulbar or pseudobulbar dysarthria. In the case of suspected MG, single-fibre EMG may provide additional diagnostic information.

## 18.11 CT/MRI of the Brain and Other Neuroradiological Imaging

Gregor Kasprian, Antonio Schindler, and Silvia Rosa

### 18.11.1 Introduction

The diagnostic work-up of patients with a neurological disease leading to dysarthria usually includes the application of brain imaging techniques, which generally provide sufficient contrast to differentiate normal brain anatomy from pathological changes. As normal radiography of the skull does not directly resolve details on the human brain, multiplanar cross-sectional imaging techniques are used to diagnose structural abnormalities of the human brain radiologically. These techniques nowadays comprise computed tomography (CT) and magnetic resonance imaging (MRI). Furthermore, they can be combined with nuclear medicine techniques such as positron emission tomography (PET) or single-photon emission tomography (SPECT) in the form of PET-CT or PET-MRI.

### 18.11.2 Computed Tomography of the Brain

The technique of computed tomography was introduced in the early 1970s and is nowadays the workhorse for rapid head imaging (Ambrose and Hounsfield 1973). CT scanning uses a series of X-rays of the head taken from many different directions. Technically there are one (single source) or multiple (dual source) X-ray beam-emitting tubes rotating around the head of the patient. The X-rays or photons are detected originally by a single ring of electronic detectors. Increasing the number of detector rings for photon detection around the patient ("multi-detector row CT"—usually up to 64, but sometimes even 256 rows) has allowed an incredible increase in scanning speed, and generated submillimetre "image slices" of the human head and body. The most recent developments in CT technology use two rotating X-ray tubes (called "dual source" CT technology), which cover more imaged tissue within an even smaller amount of time. If the two tubes are operated at different voltages and the detectors can absorb different energy spectra, a more specific characterisation of the imaged tissue is possible (for further details see Kaza et al. 2012). For instance, this now allows the differentiation of extravascular iodine contrast agent and haemorrhage (which both appear "hyperdense" or bright on CT images—Fig. 18.4). These technical improvements have additionally provided better and more robust image quality with fewer movement artefacts than possible before. The typical effective radiation dose of a head CT nowadays lies in the range of 1.6 mSv, which approximately equals the amount received in 7 months of naturally occurring background radiation (Jaffe et al. 2010).

The combination of X-ray tubes and detectors alone does not automatically produce an image. CT scanning uses a computer programme that performs a numerical integral calculation on the measured X-ray series to estimate how much of the X-ray beam is absorbed in a small volume of the brain. Thereby digital data are produced and typically presented as grey-scale images of cross-sections of the head. The collected image is always in 3D and thus allows a reconstruction of the scanned object in three dimensions.

In approximation, the denser a material is, the brighter "whiter" a volume of it will appear on the scan, just as in the more familiar "flat" X-rays, where dense bone appears white. If an iodine-based contrast agent is administered intravenously, vessels can also be visualised non-invasively—an examination called "CT angiography" (Fig. 18.5). If CT angiography examinations are ordered, the side effects of iodine-based contrast agents need to be taken into account. The most feared adverse

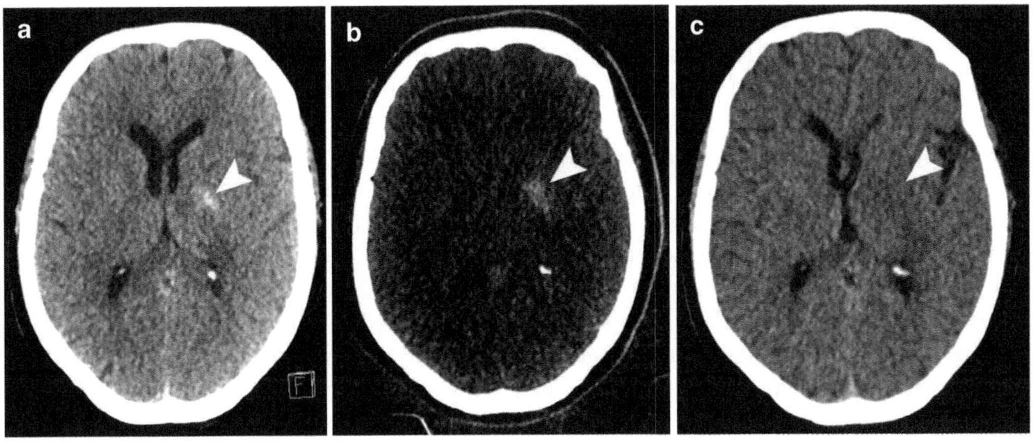

**Fig. 18.4** Dual Energy CT image of a patient who underwent thrombectomy after an ischaemic stroke of the left middle cerebral artery perforators. The arrowhead indicates a hyperdense lesion in the left basal ganglia (**a**), suggestive of haemorrhagic transformation of the ischaemic area. By using Dual Energy CT technology, the hyperdense change can be further differentiated with the iodine image (**b**) and the virtual non-contrast image (**c**). The brightness seen on the iodine image (**b**) indicates the presence of contrast agent in this area, which is not visible on the virtual non-contrast image (**c**). This helps the radiologist to differentiate between contrast agent leakage into ischaemia (as in this case) and haemorrhage. Kasprian © 2021

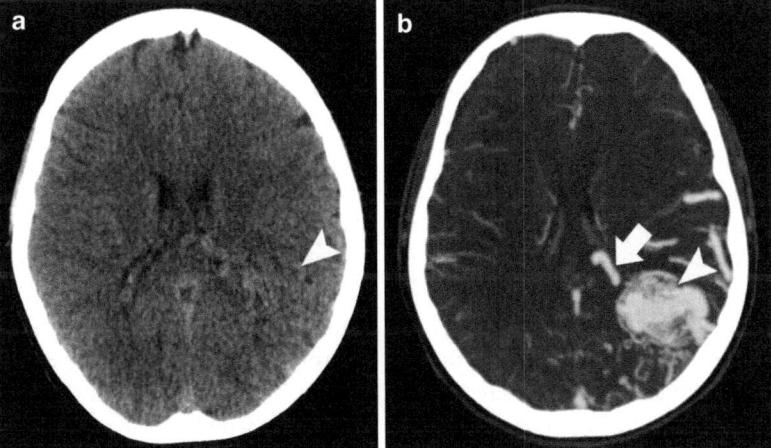

**Fig. 18.5** Non-contrast head CT (**a**) of a patient with recurrent therapy-resistant seizures (ictal aphasia) shows very subtle hyperdense structures in the left parietal lobe (arrowhead). CT Angiography with iodine-based intravenously administered contrast agent (**b**) allows the visualisation of the large arterio-venous malformation in the left parietal lobe. The arrow indicates a large draining vein. The arrowhead in (**b**) indicates the nidus of the vascular malformation. Kasprian © 2021

reaction is anaphylactic shock, nowadays occurring in 0.01–0.04% of i.v. iodinated contrast agent administrations with 1–3 deaths per 100,000–1,000,000 administrations (Kim et al. 2014; Wysowski and Nourjah 2006). The second-most common associated condition is contrast-induced nephropathy. In patients with pre-existing renal disease (multiple myeloma, renal transplant, nephrotic syndrome), intake of potentially nephrotoxic medication or application of other conditions with the potential to affect negatively renal function (diabetes mellitus, congestive heart failure, hypertonia, cirrhosis), iodinated contrast agent should be used with caution.

### 18.11.3  Strengths and Weaknesses of CT in the Diagnoses of Neurological Disease

The practical strengths of CT specifically lie in its rather wide availability and fast results. As the CT suite can be accessed without taking specific safety precautions, it grants fast patient logistics and a quick imaging procedure, mostly completed within 15 min. As a rule of thumb, CT is the imaging modality of choice in an acute setting. Patients with an acute onset of aphasia, are thus most likely to receive head CT imaging, as in most hospitals CT scanners are easily available for acute patients, whereas the logistics of MR scanners are usually more difficult.

The most common indication for acute head CT imaging is the exclusion or diagnostic proof of an intracranial haemorrhage. This presents itself bright/"white" on a non-contrast head CT. Despite contrast agents not having been used, extravascular blood appears bright on non-contrast-enhanced CT, as blood contains haemoglobin-bound iron, which absorbs radiation. Owing to these characteristics, head CT is the "reference standard" for the detection of an acute intracranial haemorrhage (Wintermark et al. 2013).

A major benefit of CT is the indirect ability to quantify the "radiodensity"—corresponding to its attenuation coefficient—of local tissue, in "Hounsfield" units (HU). These are comparable in all CT scanners (which is substantially different from MRI quantifications, which are known to differ a lot between scanners). As a rule of thumb, certain tissue characteristics present with distinct changes on non-contrast head CT: "hypodense" (dark) regions indicate the presence of a local increase of water, commonly in the form of oedema. Distilled water shows a HU of 0 (in every CT scanner in the world). If a lesion contains primarily fat it appears very dark on CT and has negative radiodensity, from $-120$ to $-90$ HU. If a lesion contains clotted blood, it usually appears bright on CT with values around $+50$ to $+75$ HU. Tumours usually contain many proliferating cells, leading to a higher local cell density, resulting in an increase in brightness ("hyperdensity") on non-contrast head CT. Calcifications are strongly hyperdense with values over $+300$ HU and are frequently encountered in "physiological" locations, such as the pineal gland, but also commonly occur in cavernoma (small hyperdense lesions, mostly without surrounding oedema) or calcified brain tumours.

Compared with MRI, the most eminent weakness of head CT is its relative insensitivity to acute physiological tissue changes and reduced capacity to resolve tissue contrasts, which are not resolvable by photon attenuation alone (for instance, the difference between cortex and white matter of the brain, particularly in regions such as the brainstem). This weakness is particularly relevant if early changes during ischaemic stroke need to be detected. The early signs of cerebral ischaemia on head CT are loss of grey-white differentiation, sulcal effacement and a hyperdense clot in the proximal vessels—as seen in the patient presenting with acute aphasia in Fig. 18.6 (Wintermark et al. 2013). However, these signs are frequently invisible during the early acute stage of cerebral ischaemia (within the first 3 h, Fig. 18.6b). Moreover, their identification is highly dependent on the experience of the assessing radiologist. Furthermore, some brain regions, such as the brainstem, are generally poorly contrasted by CT. It is not uncommon that patients with acute and severe neurological symptoms present with normal head CT findings for these reasons. Another weakness (which is also associated with MRI) is the occurrence of artefacts. Metals cause "streak" artefacts, which often interfere with the contrast of the surrounding tissue, leading to the inability to extract meaningful diagnostic information from the region surrounding the metal implant. In head CT, this is of particular relevance if patients with aneurysm clips or coils, or patients with dental implants, are imaged. Although to a lesser degree than MRI, CT is sensitive to patient motion, resulting in image series that do not cover the entire target regions and producing incorrect, negative results.

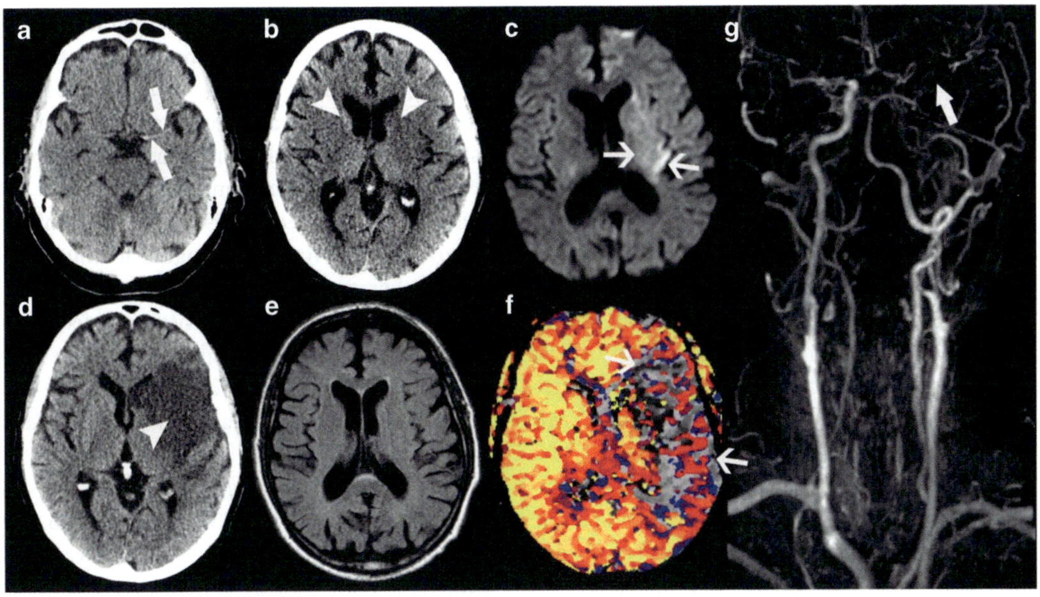

**Fig. 18.6** Evolution of an acute ischaemic stroke due to large vessel occlusion on non-contrast head CT (**a**, **b**, **d**) and MRI (**c**, **e**, **f**, **g**): 1 h after symptom onset (aphasia) an increased brightness of the left middle cerebral artery is noted on non-contrast CT (**a**, arrows)—the hyperdense media sign. At the same time point, extremely subtle CT findings are present in the middle cerebral artery territory, with a subtle loss of density in the region of the left caudate nucleus (left arrowhead compared with normal right arrowhead). About 1.5 h after the onset of symptoms contrast-enhanced MR angiography (**g**) depicts an occlusion of the left internal carotid artery and middle cerebral artery (arrow). Highly ischaemia-sensitive diffusion-weighted sequences (DWI) (**c**) shows diffusion restriction in the core area of the infarction (arrows, **c**), whereas no changes are seen in Fluid Attenuated Inversion Recovery Sequences (FLAIR) (**e**). Contrast-enhanced MR perfusion imaging allows the depiction of the tissue at risk (greyish colour code) in the middle cerebral artery territory (**f**, MR Perfusion tool; Dr. Christian Nasel, Univ. Clinics Tulln). Owing to contra-indications against thrombectomy, the ischaemia progressed and demarcated at late (12 h after clinical onset) non-contrast head CT (**d**). Note that the final extent of ischaemic tissue (**d**) corresponds to the amount of tissue at risk as predicted by MR perfusion (Fig. 18.6). Kasprian © 2021

## 18.11.4 Magnetic Resonance Imaging (MRI) of the Brain

The technique of MRI evolved during the early 1980s and was soon established as a major diagnostic neuroimaging technology. In addition to providing structural images of the human brain, MRI nowadays also provides insights into human brain function.

The technique of magnetic resultant imaging is based on the magnetic properties of protons/water molecules. A strong static magnetic field ranging from originally 0.5 Tesla (T) to the nowadays clinically used 1.5 T and 3 T (to experimentally used 7 T to 11 T) is combined with an electromagnetic impulse. The resulting electromagnetic wave emitted back by the patient is measured by coils that are positioned close to the patient. As water comprises 70–90% of most tissues, the characterisation of the distinct electromagnetic properties of water enables the differentiation of certain tissue types owing to their water content and distribution. Tissues with low water content (such as bone), usually provide low MR signals, whereas water-rich structures—such as the human brain and especially the brain of a neonate—provide a large MR signal. Certain techniques even allow the visualisation of water motion within a tissue, providing impressive visualisation of the architecture of the human brain white matter.

Gradients are used to locate the MR signals coming from the imaged tissue. Gradients are slight spatial variations in the magnetic field strength across the patient. Coils are used to receive the signals coming from the patient. Most neuroradiological MR examinations use a head coil with a certain number of channels. To put it simply, the more channels are built into a coil, the more images per time period can be collected. For spine imaging, cervical, thoracic and lumbar coil arrays are used. In addition to aspects of field strength, the quality of gradients and coils is crucial for the technical capabilities of a MR scanner.

Nowadays, MRI of the brain is the most commonly performed MR technology examination. For characterising different tissue types, and elaborating the characteristics of brain pathology, different sequences are used. A sequence is a combination of high-frequency impulses and gradients, which are deployed in a predefined spatio-temporal pattern, resulting in a characteristic appearance of certain tissues. A variety of technical parameters of each sequence can be modified by the operator before examining a patient, leading to different possibilities and options to optimise the detection and characterisation of brain pathologies (for further details see McRobbie et al. 2006).

In the following section the more commonly used neuro-MR sequences and their resulting contrast of the human brain grey and white matter are described.

**T1-weighted sequences**: These images provide excellent contrast between fluid-rich tissues and fat-containing tissues. On T1-weighted images the anatomy of the adult human brain is visualised as depicted in an anatomy textbook: the grey matter of the human brain is dark, the white matter appears bright. All grey matter nuclei, as well as the basal ganglia, are thus visualised rather greyish/dark, and all white matter tracts and structures—such as the corpus callosum—appear bright/white. Fluids and water such as the cerebrospinal fluid (CSF) do not result in a strong MR signal on T1-weighted sequences, and appear very dark/black (Fig. 18.7).

**T2-weighted sequences**: These cause an inverted contrast compared with T1 (and thus are not brain "anatomy"-like). Thus T2-weighted sequences depict grey matter structures as rather bright, and white matter structures as rather dark. Fluids such as water or CSF appear very bright on T2-weighted sequences. Consequently, oedema or fluid collections will result in a hyperintense or bright signal on T2-weighted sequences (Figs. 18.7 and 18.10).

**Fluid attenuated inversion recovery sequences**: FLAIR sequences are commonly used in head MRI and constitute the workhorse of most neuro-MR examinations. FLAIR uses the possibility of suppressing the signal of CSF combined with a T2-weighted sequence, resulting in a basic T2-weighted contrast, however, the CSF is visualised very dark (rather than on conventional T2-weighting, where CSF is typically

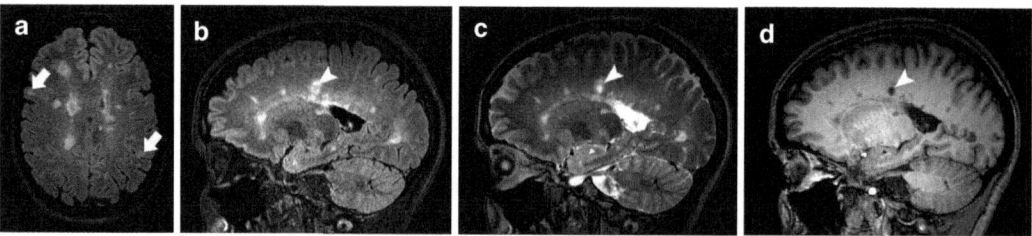

**Fig. 18.7** Patient suffering from relapsing-remitting Multiple Sclerosis (MS). FLAIR 3D sequence with axial (**a**) and sagittal (**b**) reconstructions. Sagittal T2-weighted 3D sequence (**c**) and T1-weighted sequence (**d**). The arrowhead marks a periventricular demyelinating lesion, which appears T2-weighted bright and T1-weighted hypointense (**d**). Marked T1 hypointensity indicates a long-standing lesion. The arrows (**a**) point to a juxtacortical MS lesion. Both demyelinating lesions are considered "characteristic" according to the MS diagnostic criteria (Filippi et al. 2016). Kasprian © 2021

**Fig. 18.8** MRI of a patient with post-stroke apraxia of speech. The arrowhead on FLAIR (**a**, **c**) and T1-weighted (**d**) images indicates the large post-ischaemic left hemispheric area (in neuroradiology all axial images are assessed as if the physician were looking from below) involving the inferior frontal gyrus in combination with the precentral gyrus (motor) in its lateral aspect. The arrow indicates the more acute ischaemic area in the right precentral gyrus region. DWI (apparent diffusion coefficient image) shows cytotoxic oedema confirming that the ischaemia was a recent event (dark areas in **b**). Kasprian © 2021

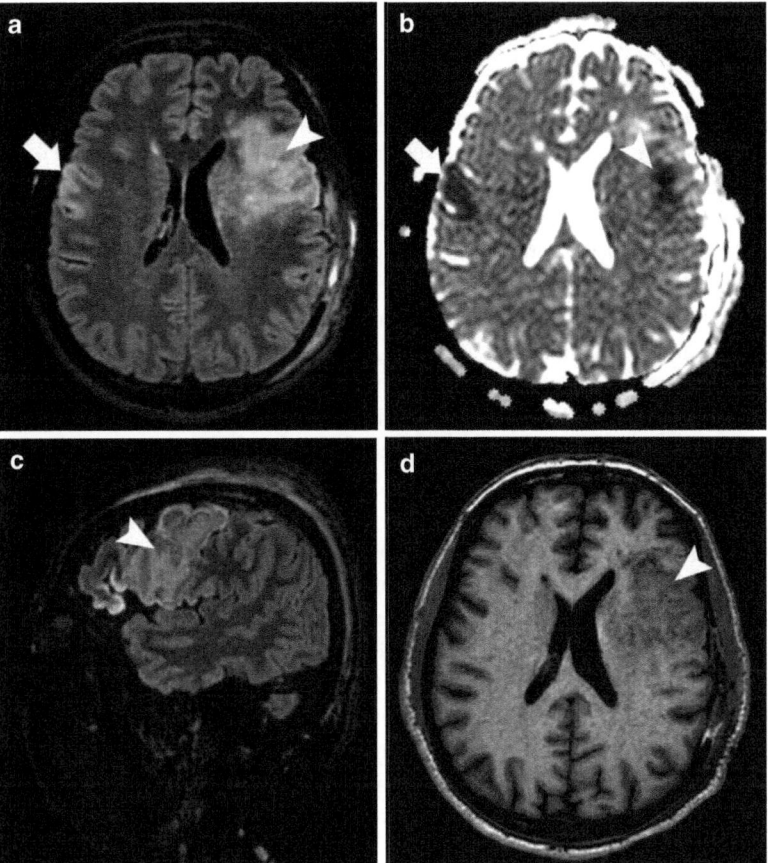

bright). This property enhances the contrast between brain pathologies, which mostly appear hyperintense on T2 and FLAIR, and the surrounding brain tissue. As normal brain tissue is darker than brain lesions or pathologies (Figs. 18.7, 18.8, and 18.10), the conspicuousness of brain tissue abnormalities is elevated. This helps radiologists identify lesions and pathologies relatively easily.

**Diffusion-weighted sequences (DWI)**: DWI is a technique that is sensitive to water and proton motion. By using different radiofrequency impulses at different time points, DWI enables the measurement of protons within the visualised tissue in a certain time period. This is particularly practical in imaging acute ischaemic stroke, as early changes on a cellular level, leading to intracellular oedema and cell swelling, can be sensitively picked up by DWI (Figs. 18.6 and 18.8). If cells swell during the early stages of ischaemia

owing to loss of osmotic regulation, DWI detects the local changes due to locally increasingly restricted proton motion. As of now, DWI is the most sensitive MRI imaging technique for visualising early ischaemia-related tissue damage (Figs. 18.6 and 18.8).

**Diffusion tensor imaging (DTI) and tractography**: Since DWI assesses microstructural changes in the brain parenchyma, the technique allows the characterisation of the microstructure of the human brain. The DWI technique of DTI provides DWI data covering a variety of directions in space, allowing geometrical covering and description of three-dimensional structures such as fibre tracts (tractography). A variety of mathematical approaches can be used, when postprocessing raw DTI data (for technical details see Jones 2012), resulting in the in vivo reconstruction and dissection of the three-dimensional fibre architecture of the human brain (Catani et al.

2002). For assessing the aphasic patient, knowledge about the involvement of structural language networks can provide information about the extent and nature of an individual pathology (Fig. 18.10). According to the recently evolved model of cortical language processing proposed by Hickok and Poeppel (2007), the neural architecture of phonemic processing is mainly related to two "streams" of neural activity. The ventral stream is represented by the inferior fronto-occipital and uncinate fascicles (Fig. 18.9), while the structural pathway of the dorsal stream is the arcuate and parts of the superior longitudinal fascicle (Fig. 18.9). With appropriate technical and neuroanatomical expertise, local deviations and alterations of language-related pathways (Fridriksson et al. 2018) can be depicted non-invasively. Intactness and microstructure of these pathways, moreover, correlate well with diverse aspects of language function (Catani et al. 2007).

**Functional MRI (fMRI)**: A special mode of sequence acquisition—"echo planar imaging" or EPI—is particularly sensitive to the magnetic effects of iron. Thus this method is capable of non-invasively detecting the level of oxygenation of blood haemoglobin. Owing to cerebral autoregulation of local brain blood supply, brain areas that are more active during certain functional processes tend to show an increase in blood supply and perfusion (neuronal activation

and blood flow are "coupled"). The increase of oxygenated blood in a specific area of the human brain correlates with its local functional activity at the neuronal level and can be measured indirectly by MRI. This measurement is frequently corrupted by noise from various sources and hence statistical procedures are used to extract the underlying signal. The resulting brain activation can be presented graphically by colour-coding the strength of activation across the brain or the specific region studied (Kent 1998).

By using fMRI it is possible to visualise brain regions that are active during certain cognitive tasks. Thus the characteristic areas associated with language comprehension and production can be non-invasively identified (Fig. 18.11). By using more advanced post-processing techniques on fMRI data, it is now possible to describe large parts of language-related brain activations as "language networks". These show lesion-specific alterations with different brain pathologies (tumours, malformations, epileptogenic lesions) leading to different patterns of language network changes (Foesleitner et al. 2020a). Network changes related to elective neurosurgical procedures can also be better understood by visualising the extensive alterations in these patients (Foesleitner et al. 2020b). This opens new ways of assessing clinically subtle aphasia and clinical understanding of the severity of language deficits at the individual level.

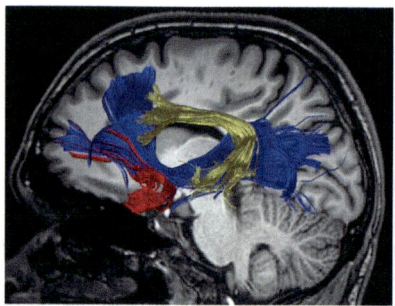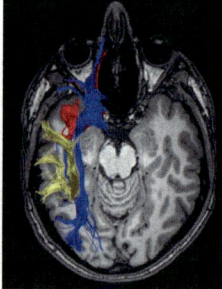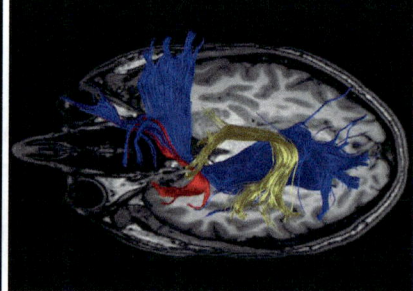

**Fig. 18.9** Diffusion tensor imaging (DTI)-based white matter pathway reconstructions of language-related pathways following the dual stream model of language processing: structural depiction of the ventral and dorsal stream in phonological processing. The ventral stream from the lateral and posterior temporal lobe follows the inferior fronto-occipital fascicle (blue) and the uncinate fascicle (red). The dorsal stream mainly follows the arcuate fascicle (yellow) connecting the inferior frontal gyrus to the supramarginal and superior and middle temporal gyri. Kasprian © 2021

## 18.11.5 Structural Pathology of the Brain

Computed tomography (CT) and magnetic resonance imaging (MRI) allow assessment of the site and size of focal, multifocal and diffuse brain damage. Depending on the setting (acute or chronic) and patient presentation, both CT and MRI are instrumental examinations in the neurological diagnostic process. From a phoniatrician's point of view, CT and MRI bring two key pieces of information: the impaired domain of the speech motor system (cortico-bulbar system, extrapyramidal system, cerebellar system, brainstem) and the presence of damage in the nonmotor system (diffuse cortical or subcortical damage, multifocal lesions, language areas lesions) (Figs. 18.7, 18.8, 18.9, 18.10, and 18.11).

Knowledge of the domain of the motor system is necessary for the classification of dysarthria subtypes, as perceptual assessment alone might be misleading (Fig. 18.7). Information on the nonmotor brain structures is equally important, as it allows the suspicion of potential impairment in linguistic or cognitive functions, both important in rehabilitation (Figs. 18.9 and 18.11). Communication approaches and augmentative alternative approaches (AAC) assume that verbal or cognitive skills for communication are preserved.

Overall, the neuroradiological assessment of potential brain abnormalities requires detailed knowledge about the underlying neuroanatomical functional architecture to be able to assess patients with dysarthria or aphasia appropriately.

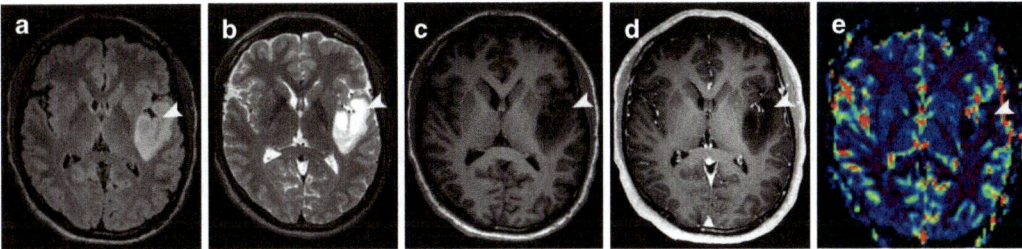

**Fig. 18.10** Axial series of FLAIR (**a**), T2-weighted (**b**), T1-weighted (**c**), T1-weighted with gadolinium-based contrast agent (**d**), perfusion-weighted/cerebral blood volume map (**e**) MRI in a patient with a low-grade glioma of the left superior temporal gyrus and insular region. The lesion (arrowhead) is FLAIR and T2-weighted hyperintense/bright and T1-weighted hypointense. As a rather characteristic of low-grade glioma, there is no clear contrast agent uptake (**d**). MR perfusion map indicates no significant hypervascularisation of the tumour also consistent with its low tumour grade. Kasprian © 2021

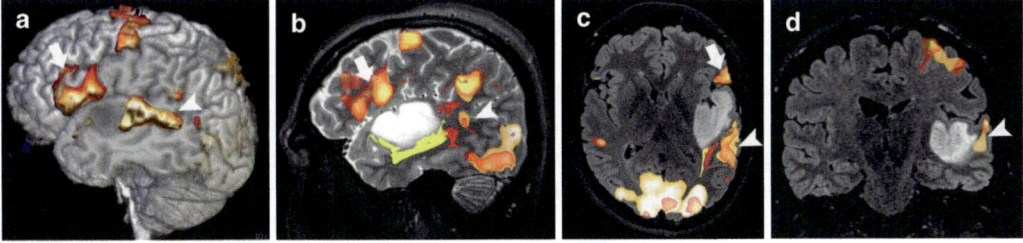

**Fig. 18.11** Functional language fMRI with a verb generation and a sentence completion task in the same patient as shown in Fig. 18.10. The orange and yellow areas mark those regions linked to increased blood flow due to neural activity. The Broca area in the left inferior frontal region (arrow) and the Wernicke regions in the left posterior temporal lobe (arrowhead) are significantly correlated with overt language comprehension and production tasks. The glioma shows a very close association with language activation and the language-associated pathways (inferior longitudinal fascicle in yellow and arcuate fascicle in red). Kasprian © 2021

## 18.12 Differential Diagnosis in Respect of Various Neurological Diseases

Stefano Cappa

The neural network subserving speech production includes multiple structures (Sörös et al. 2006):

- Cortical motor areas (SMA, cingulate, primary motor cortex, premotor cortex, anterior insula)
- Thalamus, basal ganglia, red nucleus
- Vermal and paravermal cerebellum
- Brain stem nuclei
- Neuromuscular junctions
- Articulatory muscles

Any disorder involving these structures can result in a motor speech disorder. It must be underlined that often the mechanisms of dysfunction are multiple (for example, in motor neuron disease dysarthria can be due to combined upper and lower motor neuron dysfunction; spinocerebellar degeneration can produce a combination of paretic and ataxic dysarthria, etc.).

**Apraxia of speech (AOS)** is the typical manifestation of a motor speech disorder due to cortical damage. The clinical features allowing a differentiation from dysarthria are discussed in Sect. 18.9. The differential diagnosis among the possible responsible neurological diseases is crucially based on the clinical presentation and on the associated clinical features. Sudden onset AOS is usually a manifestation of acute vascular damage (usually cardioembolic ischemic stroke) involving premotor and motor cortical areas of the left hemisphere (Graff-Radford et al. 2014). Extension to Broca's area and insular cortex is associated with the presence of aphasic manifestations (Itabashi et al. 2016).

A slowly progressive presentation of AOS suggests a diagnosis of neurodegenerative disease. The motor speech disorder is often the first manifestation of the *non-fluent agrammatic variant of primary progressive aphasia* (Gorno-Tempini et al. 2011), which is characterised by

the subsequent appearance of agrammatism in connected speech (simplification of grammatical forms, omissions, errors), word finding impairment and reading and writing disorder (Grossman 2012). The progression reflects the extension of the underlying pathology (often a tauopathy belonging to the front-temporal spectrum) from the left inferior frontal gyrus, pars opercularis, towards the supplementary motor area (SMA), insula, striatum, inferior parietal regions and underlying white matter, i.e., the regions structurally and functionally connected with the inferior frontal gyrus (Mandelli et al. 2016). In a minority of cases, AOS remains an isolated disorder, progressing in severity towards a complete speech loss, but associated with preserved language function (Josephs et al. 2012). Two subgroups can be identified, characterised, respectively, by prominent phonetic impairment (sound distortions) or by dysprosodic features (slow, segmented speech) (Utianski et al. 2018). The former subtype had imaging evidence of bilateral involvement of the supplementary motor area (SMA), of the precentral gyrus, and of the cerebellar crus, while the prosodic subtype had more focal atrophy of the SMA and of the right superior cerebellar peduncle.

**Dysarthria** due to neurological disease is seldom an isolated manifestation and is usually associated with other neurological signs and symptoms. Isolated speech and swallowing disorders can also be due to non-neurological diseases, such as cancers of the oral cavity, a possibility never to be neglected.

The sudden onset of motor speech impairment raises in the first place the diagnostic hypothesis of a cerebrovascular disorder. The differential diagnosis between AOS and dysarthria after an acute stroke is not always easy and is often based on the presence of additional signs, such as in the case of the *dysarthria-clumsy hand syndrome*, originally described by Charles Miller-Fisher, a stroke syndrome suggesting a capsular lacunar stroke (Arboix et al. 2004). Dysarthria is frequently observed in supratentorial (internal capsule) as well as brainstem (pontine) and cerebellar stroke. A left-sided hemispheric asymmetry has been reported (Urban et al. 2006).

The neurological sequels of *traumatic brain injury* often include dysarthria, with spastic or (more often) mixed features. A special case that should be kept in mind is the complete anarthria associated with quadriplegia present in the *locked-in syndrome*. Consciousness is preserved in this complete deafferentation syndrome, and communication is possible with eye movements and a variety of artificial interfaces (Vansteensel and Jarosiewicz 2020).

Simple partial seizures affecting the motor and premotor areas as well as the insular cortex can produce *ictal dysarthria.*

Dysarthria is a frequent feature of movement disorders. The most frequent condition affecting the basal ganglia is *Parkinson's disease*, which is typically associated with a hypokinetic form of dysarthria (monopitch, reduced loudness, accelerated rate, hypernasal quality). *Multiple system atrophy* is associated with hypokinetic (often high-pitched) or cerebellar dysarthria. *Progressive supranuclear palsy dysarthria* is usually low-pitched (with groaning in the advanced stage). Slurred speech is the most common early neurological manifestation of *Wilson's disease*. Choreic syndromes, including *Huntington's disease*, are also associated with hyperkinetic dysarthria, which reflects the presence of involuntary movements, resulting in high pitch and variable speech rate.

The cerebellum can be affected by many different pathologies that are associated with ataxic dysarthria. In addition to stroke, trauma and tumours, several neurodegenerative conditions affecting the cerebellum, such as the wide spectrum of *autosomal dominant cerebellar ataxias*, show prominent motor speech disorders.

The association of dysarthria, dysphonia and dysphagia with other signs and symptoms of upper and lower motor neuron dysfunction (weakness, atrophy and fasciculations) points to the diagnosis of the bulbar form of *motor neuron disease (MND)*. This is an important cause of slow onset, progressive motor speech impairment, usually with mixed features, which can be diagnosed on the basis of the typical EMG and clinical findings. Pure bulbar dysarthria is present in the *syndrome of spinal muscular atrophy*.

Other less frequent causes of bulbar involvement associate with dysarthria following the involvement of the IX, XII cranial nerve nuclei in *syringobulbia*, *cranial polyneuritis* and *brainstem tumours*.

Dysarthria is frequently observed in *multiple sclerosis*. The features are often mixed, reflecting the possible involvement of subcortical and cerebellar white matter. The differential diagnosis is usually not difficult, considering the overall clinical picture, and is supported by the appropriate examinations (MRI, cerebrospinal fluid analysis, evoked responses). Other rare demyelinating diseases (such as *Krabbe disease* and *metachromatic leukodystrophy*) can be diagnosed by metabolic and genetic examinations.

Motor speech disorders due to involvement of the neuromuscular junction and of the muscles of articulation can be observed in many diseases. The paretic dysarthria of *myasthenia gravis* (MG) is characterised by fatiguability and tends to increase in severity with prolonged articulation. The diagnosis is supported by its typical EMG findings and by the presence of IgG anti-acetylcholine receptor antibodies (AChRAb) in 75% of patients with MG. Another unusual muscular cause of dysarthria is *polymyositis*, which is diagnosed by the presence of inflammatory changes in a muscle biopsy. A rare form of late-onset, autosomal dominant muscular dystrophy affecting facial muscles (*oculopharyngeal dystrophy*) is due to an abnormal trinucleotide repeat expansion in the poly(A)-binding-protein-nuclear 1 (PABPN1) gene.

*Mitochondrial diseases* can be an unusual cause of dysarthria and dysphagia, which are however due to concomitant bulbar/pseudobulbar involvement rather than to muscle disease. Among the rare causes are also *lysosomal storage disorders* (*GM-2 gangliosidosis, Niemann-Pick type C*).

Speech disturbances may follow a number of *intoxications*, including to aluminium, toluene, alcohol, MPTP, hallucinogens and lithium. Many *drugs* (in particular antiepileptics) can be associated with dysarthria. Physical causes, such as *radiation damage*, *heat stroke* and *hypothermia*, can also be infrequently responsible for articulation impairment. Finally, systemic metabolic derangements, such as *hyperglycaemia* and *dialysis encephalopathy*, can present with speech disorders.

## 18.13    Clinical Neurophysiology in the Diagnosis and Treatment of Vocal Fold Motor Disorders

Enrico Alfonsi, Massimiliano Todisco, Mauro Fresia, Paolo Prunetti, and Giuseppe Cosentino

### 18.13.1    Electromyography (EMG): General Aspects

EMG is an electrophysiological technique commonly used for the diagnosis of neuromuscular disorders, i.e., diseases involving the peripheral nervous system, the neuromuscular junction or the striated muscles (Preston and Shapiro 2013). Over time, this investigation has also been extended to the study of exteroceptive and proprioceptive reflexes at the spinal and brainstem levels, as well to the study of voluntary and involuntary movements by means of an electro-kynesiographic approach. Therefore, EMG techniques can also be useful in the diagnostic framing of spasticity and different movement disorders, including myoclonus, tremor and dystonia.

#### 18.13.1.1    Resting Activity

The first part of the EMG examination consists of the evaluation of the activity of muscles at rest. In this case, some physiological activities can be observed. First, we normally record an "insertional activity", which is induced by the insertion of the needle-electrode into the muscle. In physiological conditions, this activity is characterised by a short-lasting EMG burst (less than 300 ms). Then neuromuscular activity can be recorded when the needle-electrode is inserted in the area of the neuromuscular junctions. This activity is represented by a background noise of the EMG trace, subcontinuous and very low in amplitude (30–60 µV) that is due to the spontaneous release of acetylcholine from the presynaptic terminal, which in turn activates the post-synaptic receptors located on the muscle fibre membranes. If the needle-electrode mechanically stimulates a nerve terminal, then a biphasic potential can be also recorded, characterised by an initial negative phase and a subsequent positive phase. This potential is called the "endplate potential" or "endplate spike", and has amplitudes ranging from 100 to 1000 µV with an irregular and high discharge rate. The endplate potentials appear for a few seconds and then abruptly cease.

In different pathological conditions, various kinds of abnormal electrical activity can be recorded in muscles at rest. First we have *muscle denervation*, a condition in which two kinds of potential due to activation of single muscle fibres can be recorded: (a) fibrillation potentials, i.e., biphasic and short-lasting potentials with an initial positive phase followed by a negative phase, with amplitude ranging from 100 to 1000 µV, and regular discharge frequency; (b) positive sharp waves (PSWs), i.e., potentials characterised by a positive phase that begins with a steep front with slow returns to the isoelectric. The PSWs have the same significance as fibrillation potentials but a different shape owing to the different position of the needle-electrode with respect to the denervated muscle fibres.

Another electromyographic sign of muscle denervation is represented by discharge of potentials with variable shape called "*complex repetitive discharges*" (CRDs). CRDs are expressions of the spontaneous electrical activity of a muscle area with extensive denervation. In this case, a closed circuit develops starting from the action potential of a denervated muscle fibre that is transmitted to adjacent fibres. Such kind of transmission is defined as "ephaptic" and characterised by the passage of the action potential from a muscle fibre to the contiguous ones without a chemical mediator but by diffusion of the electric field. This phenomenon can be observed in different excitable tissues and occurs both in physiological and pathological conditions (Preston and Shapiro 2013; Belenkov 1970). During a CRD, the diffusion of the electrical activity from the membrane of a denervated muscle fibre to nearby denervated fibres causes a discharge of high-frequency potentials that can last several seconds and stop abruptly when the muscle fibre membranes reach a condition of absolute refractoriness.

The *fasciculation* is a resting activity expression of the spontaneous discharge of a motor unit (MU). As fasciculations, *myokymias* are also expressions of MU activity, that in this case presents in the form of rhythmic activation. The term myokymia comes from the Greek mŷs—"muscle" + kŷmos—"wave" and refers to a localised quivering of a muscle. Fasciculations and myokymias can represent both physiological and pathological events. Fasciculations and myokymias can be observed in conditions of hypothermia (muscle cooling); after intense muscle activity (fatigue fasciculations); due to nicotinic stimulation of the neuromuscular plaque as in smokers (nicotine has an excitatory effect on the neuromuscular endplates); and as a side effect of anticholinesterase drugs. However, there are diseases in which the fasciculations are expression of an early damage of the motor neuron. This occurs in amyotrophic lateral sclerosis and, in general, in all diseases with damage of the lower motor neuron, such as spinal amyotrophy, chronic axonal motor neuropathy and chronic motor radiculopathy. Myokymias can be commonly observed in the orbicularis oculi muscle, resulting in small, visible contractions of part of the eyelid, typically the lower eyelid.

The *neuromyotonic discharge* is another resting activity caused by hyper-excitability of the motor axon membrane. This discharge is characterised by a very high frequency (up to 200 Hz) and lasts some seconds, featuring a progressive reduction in amplitude until the disappearance. Neuromyotonic discharges originate from the motor nerve terminal and are a consequence of an abnormal activity of voltage-gated K$^+$-channels of the motor axonal membrane.

Another type of high frequency potential, called *myotonic discharges*, can be observed upon insertion of the needle-electrode or its displacement within the muscle. These EMG discharges originate from the membrane of the muscle fibres and also show a high frequency (20–80 Hz) with a progressive decrease of amplitude and frequency. Myotonic discharges present a very characteristic sound from the EMG system amplifier, recalling that of a "dive bomber" and can be caused by different disorders of ionic channels of the muscle fibre membrane. These discharges are typically observed in patients with muscle diseases known as myotonic syndromes (i.e., myotonic dystrophies, congenital paramyotonia, different types of congenital and acquired myotonias). Clinically, the myotonic phenomenon appears as an impaired muscle relaxation after contraction. The repetition of muscle contraction in some myotonic syndromes, such as myotonic dystrophies, induces a progressive amelioration of this symptom until it disappears ("warming up" phenomenon). Conversely, in other forms of myotonia, such as paramyotonia congenita, the repetition of muscle activity tends to worsen the myotonia phenomenon progressively (i.e., the so-called paradoxical myotonia).

*Cramps* represent another type of resting activity. These are characterised by a prolonged discharge of all or most of the motor units of the muscle. The cramp can appear in normal subjects as an effect of metabolic conditions affecting the muscle, such as acidosis secondary to fatigue. Sometimes, the cramp can be expression of pathological conditions such as early neurogenic damage, as it can be observed in the initial stage of amyotrophic lateral sclerosis, or in chronic radiculopathy due to spondyloarthrosis or pathologies of the intervertebral discs.

In normal subjects, the muscles with sphincteric activity, such as the anal sphincter, the urethral sphincter or the upper oesophageal sphincter (especially in the striated portion represented by the cricopharyngeal muscle), may present "decelerating bursts" at rest resembling those of the complex repetitive discharges. However, this activity shows a discharge with progressive deceleration in frequency that recalls the sound emitted by a whale. The origin of these discharges is not yet known. However, it has been hypothesised that they are an expression of a physiological condition and are induced by the mechanical irritation of the nerve plexuses within the striated sphincters induced by the needle-electrode.

### 18.13.1.2 Voluntary Activity

EMG evaluation of muscle activity at rest is followed by the study of voluntary muscle activity. In this case, different parameters of the *motor unit action potentials* (MUAPs) are assessed. Motor units (MUs) represent the final common path of movement and are constituted by the lower motor neuron, its motor axon, and the muscle fibres innervated by the branches of the same motor axon. Each striated muscle contains fibres that are part of a high number of MUs. During a voluntary movement, MUs are recruited according to physiological modalities in relation to the type and the intensity of the activity made. There are two main modalities of MU recruitment: spatial recruitment, corresponding to the number of MUs recruited in the unit of time, and temporal recruitment, which refers to the number of times a given MU is activated in the unit of time (i.e., discharge frequency of the MU).

The number of muscle fibres in a MU is variable and depends on functional properties of the muscle. Generally, the muscles richest in "fast-twitch" fibres have a higher number of MUs, each of which contains relatively few muscle fibres (i.e., MUs with a high density of innervation). This occurs because these muscles allow the performance of very precise and accurate movements, being capable of expressing minimal variation in the force of contraction. Among these muscles we recognise the extrinsic eye muscles, muscles of the hand and laryngeal muscles. The muscles richest in "slow-twitch" fibres are those normally involved in postural activities, such as the soleus muscle, the quadriceps femoris and the axial muscles. These muscles comprise a small number of MUs, each of which contains a large number of muscle fibres.

During the routine EMG assessment the voluntary muscle activity is first analysed, by asking the patient to perform a slight voluntary contraction. In this way, single MUAPs can be easily detected and analysed. Amplitude, duration and morphology of the MUAP can be examined. MUAP waveform can be defined as simple, irregular or polyphasic. The latter term is used when the MUAP has more than three phases, i.e., its components cross the isoelectric line more than three times. MUAP duration represents the most reliable parameter when assessing pathophysiological changes of the MUAPs.

After single MUAP analysis, the spatial recruitment of MUAPs is examined by inviting the subject to perform a maximal contraction of the muscle under examination. In motor nerve axonopathy, EMG findings are defined as neurogenic and can be characterised by: (a) fibrillations, PSWs, CRDs and eventually fasciculations at rest; (b) higher amplitude, increased duration and increased percentage of polyphasic MUAPs; and (c) reduced spatial recruitment of MUAPs, even when performing a maximal effort.

In pathological conditions characterised by primary damage of muscle fibres (myopathies), fibrillations, PSWs and CRDs can be also observed at rest, as above. However, a high number of MUAPs show low amplitude and duration, and present with a polyphasic waveform. Moreover, we can observe an increased spatial recruitment of MUAPs, with an EMG interference pattern even when a slight muscle contraction is developed.

### 18.13.2 Laryngeal Electromyography (LEMG)

LEMG is an electrophysiological method used in the assessment of patients with vocal fold disorders. This is a niche technique used by clinical neurophysiologists, or even otolaryngologists and phoniatricians, with specific expertise in electromyographic techniques (Heman-Ackah et al. 2007).

Clinical application of LEMG is currently limited. This electrophysiological technique can be of great value for diagnosis of several neurological disorders affecting vocal fold motion, such as neurogenic damage, tremor and dystonia. In addition, LEMG has a relevant impact on treatment, since it allows precise guidance of the inoculation of botulinum toxin into vocal fold muscles. LEMG therefore represents a useful

**Fig. 18.12** Types of needle-electrodes for laryngeal EMG

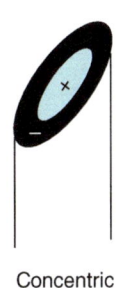
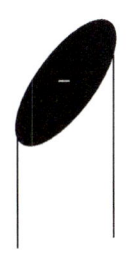
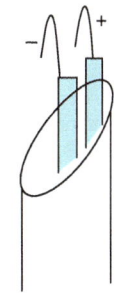

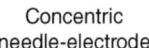
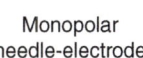

|  |  |  |
|---|---|---|
| Concentric needle-electrode | Monopolar needle-electrode | Bipolar hooked-wire needle-electrode |

approach to deepen our understanding of physiological and pathophysiological mechanisms underlying laryngeal motility (Kimaid et al. 2015; Ludlow 2015).

EMG recordings of laryngeal muscles rely on different types of needle-electrode (Fig. 18.12):

(a) The *concentric needle-electrode* is mainly used for the study of spontaneous muscle activity, parameters of MUAPs, and spatial recruitment of MUAPs of laryngeal muscles
(b) The *monopolar needle-electrode*, consisting of a needle-cannula, is usually employed to guide the correct inoculation of botulinum toxin into hyperactive laryngeal muscles; monopolar needle-electrodes can also be applied for direct stimulation of branches of the recurrent and superior laryngeal nerves in nerve conduction studies or in assessing laryngeal reflexes
(c) The *bipolar hooked-wire needle-electrode* can be used for electro-kinesiographic studies for evaluation of laryngeal movements

The activity of intrinsic muscles of the larynx is complex and yields rotational movements of the arytenoid cartilages, anterior–posterior displacement of the cricoarytenoid structures, and variations of vocal fold tension. Vocal fold movements are indeed able to develop vibratory frequencies greater than 100 Hz. Among laryngeal intrinsic muscles, the posterior cricoarytenoid muscle is solely responsible for vocal fold abduction. All remaining muscles lead to vocal fold adduction; in particular, the cricothyroid muscle

is solely a vocal fold tensor muscle, the lateral cricoaritenoid muscle and the interaritenoid muscle are solely vocal fold adductor muscles, the thyroarytenoideus muscle and the vocal muscle are responsible for both tension and adduction of vocal fold.

LEMG is performed with the patient lying supine and holding the neck hyper-extended, so that the larynx is closer to the skin, facilitating the identification of landmarks for insertion of the needle-electrode. This latter procedure causes a pricking sensation, similar to that reported after an intramuscular injection. Therefore, before this investigation, a topical application of anaesthetic sprays or creams can be advisable. A persistent local anaesthesia is not recommended, as it can easily alter the electrical activity of nerves and muscles. For LEMG recordings, a ground electrode is placed over a body site far from the neck, to facilitate the filtering of other contaminating electrical signals, such as heartbeat and breathing.

The muscles most commonly examined in LEMG and related recording procedures are detailed as follows (Figs. 18.13 and 18.14):

(a) The **cricothyroid muscle** is evaluated as a vocal fold tensor muscle. Among muscles examined in LEMG, the cricothyroid muscle is the only one innervated by the motor branch of the superior laryngeal nerve, since other muscles are innervated by the recurrent laryngeal nerve. The cricothyroid muscle is reached by inserting the needle-electrode in the upper border of the cricoid arch,

**Fig. 18.13** Vocal fold muscles commonly explored in laryngeal EMG. Reprinted from Alexandra Sieroslawska, Muscles of the Larynx (2022) https://www.kenhub.com/en/library/anatomy/muscles-of-the-larynx. With permission by KenHub GmbH Leipzig

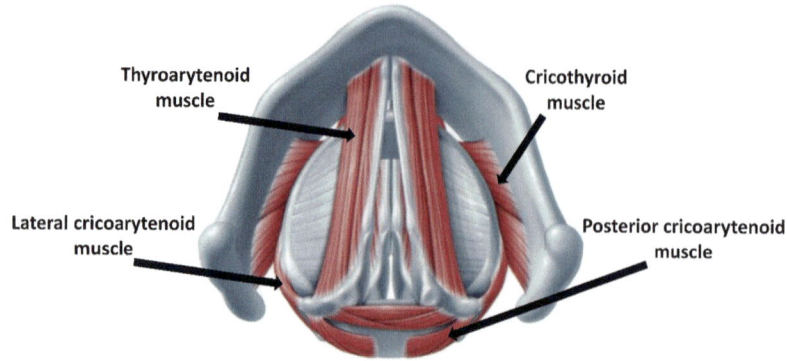

Thyroarytenoid muscle

Cricothyroid muscle

Lateral cricoarytenoid muscle

Posterior cricoarytenoid muscle

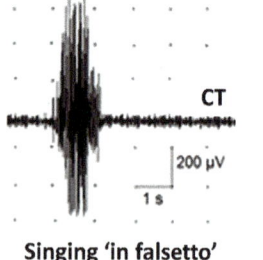

CT

200 µV

1 s

Singing 'in falsetto'

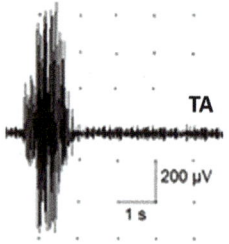

TA

200 µV

1 s

'eeeee'

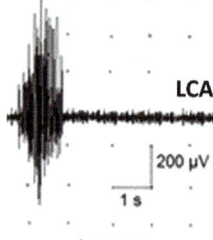

LCA

200 µV

1 s

'eeeee'

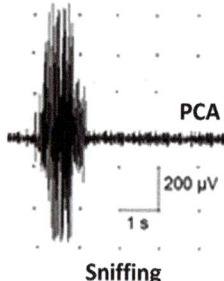

PCA

200 µV

1 s

Sniffing

**Fig. 18.14** Physiological activation of vocal fold muscles. *CT* cricothyroid muscle, *TA* thyroarytenoid/vocal muscles, *LCA* lateral cricoarytenoid muscle, *PCA* posterior cricoarytenoid muscle

approximately 1.5 cm from the midline, perpendicularly to the skin, at a depth of about 1 cm in relation to the thickness of the subcutaneous tissue. The correct position of the needle-electrode is verified by asking the patient to sing "in falsetto".

(b) The **thyroarytenoid** and **vocal muscles** are examined as vocal fold tensor and adductor muscles. These muscles are adjacent to the vocal folds and constitute a muscular complex whose medial portion is represented by the vocal muscle. These muscles are reached by inserting the needle-electrode just above the edge of the cricoid arch, at the midline, through the cricothyroid membrane, at an angle of approximately 45° upward and 30° laterally, to a depth of 1–2 cm. A proper recording is ascertained by asking the patient to say a prolonged "eeeee" or to perform a Valsalva manoeuvre.

(c) The **lateral cricoarytenoid muscle** is evaluated as solely a vocal fold adductor muscle. The approach to reach the muscle may

vary; one of the most commonly used methods involves inserting the needle-electrode through the cricothyroid membrane just above the cricoid cartilage at the midline, as with the TA muscle, but with a more lateral tilt of approximately 45° and a smaller upward angle of about 10°, deeper than the TA muscle. The lateral cricoarytenoid muscle is recruited by asking the patient to say a prolonged "eeeee".

(d) The **posterior cricoarytenoid muscle** is the only vocal fold abductor muscle, as mentioned above. Two techniques can be used for EMG recordings of this muscle. In the first case, the needle-electrode is inserted just laterally to the palpable lateral edge of the cricoid cartilage, perpendicular to the sagittal plane, and with a slight posterior tilt (approximately 15°) in the axial plane, to a depth of 1-3 cm. This technique is prone to mistakes, because the EMG activity of neighbouring muscles with different functions can be improperly recorded.

In particular, it is possible to confuse the EMG activity of the posterior cricoarytenoid muscle with that of the cricopharyngeal muscle, which is the main component of the upper oesophageal sphincter. The second technique is performed using a longer needle-electrode (of about 5 cm) inserted above the edge of the cricoid arch at the midline, with a 45° orientation in the axial plane and an upward angle of 20°–30°. The needle-electrode pierces the cricothyroid membrane and reaches the posterior wall of the laryngeal vestibule where this muscle is positioned. This second approach can be more traumatic for the patient than the first one and risks causing reflex spasms of the vocal folds. The posterior cricoarytenoid muscle can be activated by deep inhalations, such as sniffing, or even by asking the patient to say such sounds as "pi-pi-pi".

Normative parameters of MUAPs obtained from muscles commonly examined in LEMG by using concentric needle-electrode are given in Table 18.3

Intrinsic laryngeal muscles show high density of innervation and their MUAPs are very small. These properties influence the type and modality of activation of the muscles, which show a prominent capacity of modulating the spatial recruitment of their MUAPs (Ludlow 2015; Saran et al. 2021).

It is possible to study motor conduction of the recurrent laryngeal nerve (Fig. 18.15). In this regard, a monopolar needle-electrode stimulates the nerve along its course, close to the trachea, while the compound muscle action potential of thyroarytenoid, lateral cricoarytenoid or posterior cricoarytenoid muscles can be recorded by means of a needle-electrode. Normal values of the distal motor latency range between 1.3 and 3 ms for both anterior and posterior motor branches of the recurrent laryngeal nerve (Kimaid et al. 2015; Ludlow 2015).

**Table 18.3** Laryngeal EMG: normative values resulting from semi-automatic analysis of motor unit action potentials

| Muscles | Amplitude (μV) | Duration (ms) |
| --- | --- | --- |
| TA | 487 ± 394 (range: 100–1100) | 4.0 ± 2.1 (range: 3.2–6.3) |
| PCA | 441 ± 390 (range: 105–980) | 4.2 ± 2.7 (range: 3.0–6.3) |
| CT | 500 ± 482 (range: 103–1112) | 4.6 ± 2.6 (range: 3.4–7.4) |
| LCA | 504 ± 495 (range: 103–1045) | 4.4 ± 2.5 (range: 3.3–7.3) |

Mean values ± SD of 20 MUAPs obtained by concentric needle-electrode for each vocal fold muscle in 40 healthy subjects (aged between 18 and 80 years)
CT cricothyroid muscle, TA thyroarytenoid/vocal muscles, LCA lateral cricoarytenoid muscle, PCA posterior cricoarytenoid muscle

**Fig. 18.15** Motor conduction technique of the recurrent laryngeal nerve. Distance between stimulation site and lower border of the cricoid cartilage should be around 3 cm

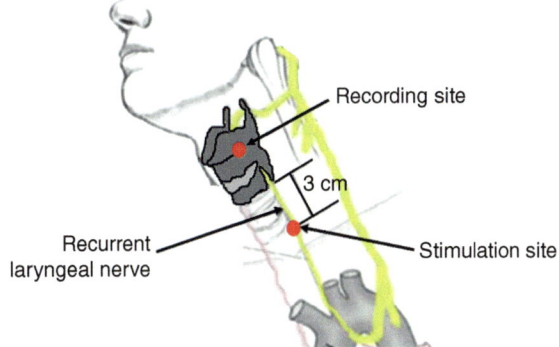

### 18.13.2.1 LEMG in Laryngeal Nerve Palsy

Lesions of the recurrent laryngeal nerve can originate from iatrogenic injuries or reflect various systemic or local diseases (Titche 1976; Sulica 2013). The iatrogenic origin of laryngeal nerve palsy is the most frequent and is mostly related to thyroid or carotid surgery. Laryngeal nerve lesions may also stem from extensive removal of oesophageal, pulmonary or mediastinal neoplasms (e.g., thymomas) or from cardiac surgery for aortic arch aneurysms. Non-iatrogenic causes are linked to several neuromuscular pathologies, such as idiopathic lesions of the recurrent laryngeal nerve, similar to idiopathic paralysis of the facial nerve and therefore of direct or immune-mediated viral origin. This origin is quite frequent among the non-iatrogenic causes of laryngeal nerve palsy. However, non-iatrogenic neuropathies of the recurrent laryngeal nerve can also be derived from more extensive neurodegenerative disorders, such as motor neuron disease or cranial polyradiculoneuritis; of note, in both conditions, the nerve lesion is often bilateral. The unilateral lesion of the recurrent laryngeal can be related to infiltrative lesions of neoplasms, such as malignancies of the thyroid, oesophagus, larynx, mediastinum (e.g., thymomas or lymphomas), or can originate from metastatic localisations in the neck or mediastinum. Compression of the recurrent laryngeal nerve from aneurysmal dilation of the aortic arch or from granulomatous inflammatory diseases (e.g., tuberculosis or sarcoidosis) are less common causes of laryngeal neuropathy (Titche 1976; Sulica 2013).

In the case of a selective injury involving the motor fibres of the superior laryngeal nerve, the EMG study of the cricothyroid muscle shows neurogenic abnormalities, whereas normal EMG findings are observed in the thyrarytenoid, lateral cricoarytenoid and posterior cricoarytenoid muscles, which are innervated by the recurrent laryngeal nerves as aforementioned (Kimaid et al. 2015; Ludlow 2015).

LEMG can also be used to identify an underestimated phenomenon that can largely influence reinnervation after recurrent laryngeal neuropathies, the so-called aberrant reinnervation (Crumley 1989). This is attributable to an incorrect regeneration of the axons, which reach muscles with an antagonistic function through regrowth on "false pathways", instead of reinnervating the original muscles. This phenomenon is represented by an atypical reinnervation of axons primitively belonging to the posterior branch of the recurrent laryngeal nerve and originally innervating the posterior cricoarytenoid muscle; these axons instead reach antagonist muscles, such as the lateral cricoarytenoid or the thyroarytenoid muscles. In case of vocal emission of aspirated sounds or simple inspirations, abduction of vocal folds does not occur, but the sound of the voice is strangled and there is often an inspiratory tirage. In addition, LEMG shows co-contraction between adductor and abductor muscles of vocal folds (Fig. 18.16). Sometimes a laryngospasm can also develop as result of this aberrant reinnervation, with consequent risk of prolonged apnoea and choking (Crumley 1989; Woo and Mangaro 2004). This phenomenon is substantially identical to the process which occurs in anomalous reinnervation of other nerve trunks, such as in peripheral facial paralysis or in reinnervations secondary to brachial plexus injury. Simultaneous needle-electrode recordings of antagonist muscles, such as abductor and adductor muscles of vocal fold, show paradoxical activation of the thyroarytenoid or lateral cricoarytenoid muscles or both during the inspiratory phase, being in co-contraction with the antagonist posterior cricoarytenoid muscle during both quiet and forced breathing. The injection of low doses of botulinum toxin at the level of the adductor muscles can result in a significant benefit for several months (Lekue et al. 2015).

LEMG is also valuable in discriminating between vocal fold palsy due to peripheral laryngeal neuropathies, and mechanical dysfunction of the cricoarytenoid joints due to sublussation or arthropathy. The latter phenomenon can develop when intubation is performed improperly or in rheumatoid arthritis involving cricoarytenoid joints (Ellis and Pallister 1975; Evman and Selcuk 2020; Pradhan et al. 2016; Woldorf et al. 1971). In these cases, LEMG does not show

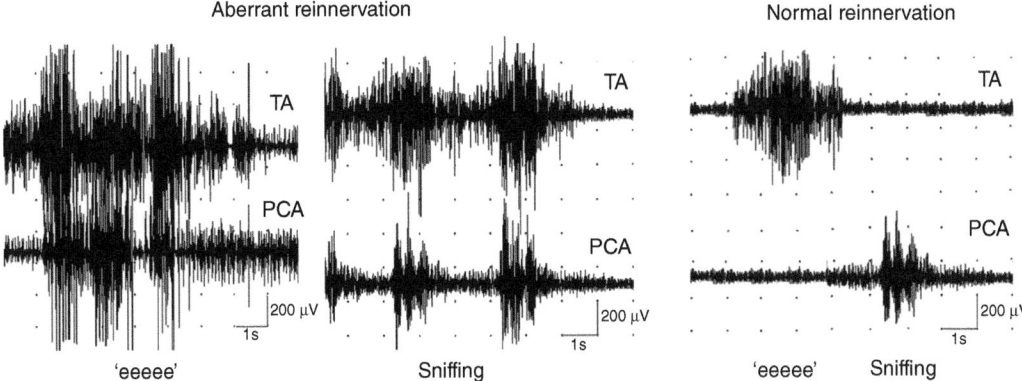

**Fig. 18.16** Examples of aberrant or normal vocal fold reinnervation after neurogenic lesion. *TA* thyroarytenoid/vocal muscles, *PCA* posterior cricoarytenoid muscle

neurogenic abnormalities of vocal fold muscles (Kimaid et al. 2015; Ludlow 2015).

### 18.13.2.2 LEMG in Disorders of Neuromuscular Transmission of Voice

In disorders of neuromuscular transmission such as myasthenia gravis, myasthenic syndromes and botulism, laryngeal muscles can be involved (Osserman and Genkins 1971; Mao et al. 2001). In particular, myasthenia gravis is an autoimmune disease due to failure in neuromuscular transmission related to dysfunction of post-synaptic receptors of acetylcholine in striated muscles. As result of involvement of laryngeal muscles, progressive dysphonia, and sometimes breathing deficits due to progressive vocal fold paralysis, can occur, which represent symptoms of myasthenia gravis in around 60% of cases. Dysphonia can even be the first symptom of myasthenia gravis in 6% of cases (Liu et al. 2007; Renard et al. 2015).

As a diagnostic technique, repetitive nerve stimulation can be performed with a monopolar needle-electrode for stimulation of the recurrent laryngeal nerve on the lateral edge of the trachea, and a coaxial needle-electrode in the laryngeal muscles for recording of the compound muscle action potential (Xu et al. 2009). However, according to our experience, this procedure has important technical limitations, given the poor stability deriving from the use of the

needle-electrode for signal recording. Furthermore, unlike recordings performed by means of surface electrodes, recordings through needle-electrodes are always only a partial expression of the electrical response from the examined muscle.

Single-fibre jitter represents the measurement of variation of the inter-potential interval between a couple of action potentials of muscle fibres belonging to the same motor unit. This investigation is able to evaluate alterations of the neuromuscular transmission (Preston and Shapiro 2013). Thus, this electrophysiological method can also be applied in laryngeal muscles when local deficits of neuromuscular transmission are suspected (Schweizer et al. 1999).

### 18.13.2.3 LEMG in Vocal Fold Motion Abnormalities due to Central Nervous System Disorders

Several alterations of vocal fold motility, which mainly include dystonic disorders of the larynx, can be derived from a primary focal disease, such as "spasmodic dysphonia", or can be part of a broader spectrum of complex neurological disorders, such as Parkinson's disease, multiple system atrophy or Wilson's disease.

As recently established by a Consensus Conference on this topic, the term "*laryngeal dystonia*" (LD) has been suggested to reflect better the clinical features of this disorder (Simonyan et al. 2021). Accordingly, LD will be used throughout this text instead of the term "spasmodic dysphonia". LD is a rare disease, having a prevalence of 1/100,000 (Nutt et al. 1988). However, this disorder is probably underestimated, given that a proper diagnosis is challenging when it relies on medical staff not specialised in neurological diseases involving speech. LD affects women in 80% of cases according to Adler et al. (1997), and often develops in middle-aged people, usually without clear prodromal or warning symptoms. Before the onset of speech abnormalities, LD patients may report previous upper respiratory tract infections (Schweinfurth et al. 2002). In some cases, "life events" (e.g., high emotional stress, recent bereavement, etc.) can precede the appearance of vocal disturbances. The chronic disease course of LD is generally characterised by an early worsening over a few months and a subsequent stabilisation, without further progression (Brin et al. 1998).

The differential diagnosis of LD, and of other vocal fold disorders, as a rule of thumb requires first the exclusion of organic diseases that may resemble or even be superimposed on various forms of LD. With this aim, a correct diagnosis of LD needs a "multidisciplinary team", which includes several specialists, namely otolaryngologist, speech therapist and neurologist. Vocal fold polyp and carcinoma, paralysis of the recurrent laryngeal nerve, and presbyphonia are the most frequent organic disorders mimicking LD. Of note, although very rare, presbyphonia is diagnosed after accurate clinical and instrumental investigations. Presbyphonic patients' voices are often comparable to those of subjects with mixed LD. However, features of vocalisation are essentially linked to anatomical and structural changes of laryngeal structures in presbyphonia, characterised by loss of vocal fold elasticity and reduction of glottal excursion during vocalisation. In such a situation, botulinum toxin treatment is ineffective, if not even harmful.

On the other hand, among central nervous system disorders causing speech impairment, spastic dysarthria has also to be taken into account. In this latter condition, vocal dysfunction is due to alterations of cortical-nuclear pathways and brainstem centres at the level of the pons or medulla oblongata, which control laryngeal muscles involved in sound emission. This disorder is responsible for a posterior rhinolalia, featured by a monotone voice and a slowing in word articulation. Of relevance, spastic dysarthria can mimic the adductor type of LD, especially when spastic hypertonia leading to dysarthria prevails on the adductor vocal fold muscles. LEMG of spastic dysarthria shows a tonic hyperactivity of the adductor and tensor vocal fold muscles, with limited phasic modulation during the emission of phonemes. This condition can occur in rare neurological diseases, such as primary lateral sclerosis (a variant of amyotrophic lateral sclerosis) and in particular chronic brain vascular diseases causing the so-called pseudobulbar syndrome. More frequently, involvement of the first motor neuron observed in spastic dysarthria is associated with variable degrees of damage of the second motor neuron (e.g., in amyotrophic lateral sclerosis); in this case, the vocal disturbance is clearly different and causes further phonatory and swallowing disturbances, also showing tongue hypomotility, sialorrhea and dysphagia. In any event, however, botulinum toxin treatment is ineffective or can even worsen the clinical picture.

LD involves the muscles responsible for vocal fold motion. In particular, LD patients present with involuntary spasms in different laryngeal muscles only during the emission of words, never during spontaneous breathing or emotional vocal expressions, such as laughing, crying, screaming. In LD, dysfunction of vocal fold motility usually occurs when emitting specific vowels or diphthongs or sounds. According to the clinical characteristics, various forms of LD have been distinguished: (a) adductor LD, (b) abductor LD, (c) mixed LD, (d) respiratory LD, (e) singer's LD:

(a) **Adductor LD** is due to a spasm of the tensor and adductor vocal fold muscles, mainly the thyroarytenoid, vocal and lateral cricoarytenoid muscles. This subtype is the most common form of LD, accounting for 80–85% of cases. In this form, the voice is hoarse, tense, with sudden bursts of intensity that cannot be modulated by the patient. Words such as "let us live", "heroic" or "flower bed" accentuate these alterations and can be employed as clinical tests to assess patients with suspicious adductor LD. This form usually undergoes a significant improvement after botulinum toxin injection

(b) **Abductor LD** is linked to hyperactivity of the posterior cricoarytenoid muscles, the only abductor vocal fold muscle. It is featured by a blown ("vented") voice. During utterance of a sentence, the vocal intensity is clearly less than optimal. This form of LD is much rarer than the adductor subtype and accounts for 15% of cases. Such words as "pail", "sissi" or "esso" emphasise the vocal disturbance. In general, the therapeutic response to botulinum toxin inoculation is worse than that found in adductor LD

(c) **Mixed LD** is even rarer and occurs in 0.5–1% of cases. In this LD subtype, both the adductor/tensor muscles and the abductor muscles of vocal folds are involved. Diagnosis of the mixed form is important in predicting the response to botulinum toxin treatment, which is often poor or absent

(d) **Respiratory LD** represents an extremely rare type of LD and is also known as abductor-respiratory laryngeal dysphonia. It is characterised by an apparently normal voice interspersed with a deep inhalation, which appears as suffocation to the listener and is caused by an exaggerated vocal fold abduction. A good response to botulinum toxin injection is reported

(e) **Singer's LD** is a particular form that is only detectable during singing and mainly affects professional or semi-professional singers (Chitkara et al. 2006). For this reason, singer's LD, which is not uncommon among singers, can be considered a professional dystonia. It is associated with a forced vocal fold adduction, presenting with strained and hoarse voice, vocal fatigue and loss of "vibrato sound". However, some patients also have spasms during vocal fold abduction, thus the vocal timbre appears vented with abrupt and sudden breath-ing pauses, and occasionally with compensatory vocal fold hyper-adduction during singing. Other subjects have the above-mentioned vocal dysfunction even during speaking, in conjunction with the presentation of their singing performance.

**Stridor** is a sharp noise, mainly during inspiration, caused by a mechanical vibration of vocal folds at a very high frequency (above 100 Hz). This laryngeal disorder is considered a "red flag" supporting the diagnosis of multiple system atrophy. This phenomenon originates from different pathophysiological mechanisms, such as neurogenic paralysis of abductor vocal fold muscles (Bannister et al. 1981) or dystonia of adductor vocal fold muscles (Vetrugno et al. 2007; Merlo et al. 2002), and is often associated with severe respiratory dysfunction and sudden death (Cortelli et al. 2019). This disturbance prevails during sleep, although in the advanced stages of the disease it can also be observed during daytime, variably affecting treatment and prognosis of these patients (Cortelli et al. 2019). Inoculation of low doses of botulinum toxin into hypertonic adductor vocal fold muscles has been shown to improve stridor transiently in patients with multiple system atrophy featuring laryngeal dystonic abnormalities without EMG evidence of neurogenic alterations (Merlo et al. 2002). In patients with multiple system atrophy, vocal fold abnormalities, detected at diurnal LEMG investigation, have been found to be correlated with the severity of nocturnal breathing alterations (Cortelli et al. 2019). In particular, an increasing severity of sleep-disordered breathing has been observed in several vocal fold patterns, from hypertonic adduction of vocal folds to paradoxical adductor activation during inspiration with or without neurogenic damage of abductor vocal fold muscles (Cortelli et al. 2019). Vocal fold patterns have also been associated with different pathophysiological mechanisms underlying stridor in multiple system atrophy phenotypes (Alfonsi et al. 2016). Indeed, the dystonic pattern has been shown to prevail in patients with the Parkinsonian subtype and stridor, while the mixed dystonic and neurogenic pattern has been related to stridor in subjects with the cerebellar phenotype (Todisco et al. 2020).

### 18.13.3 EMG-Guided Botulinum Toxin Type A (BTX-A) Injection for Treatment of Laryngeal Dystonia and Other Motility Disorders of the Vocal Folds

Although BTX-A is generally effective for treatment of LD, low or no therapeutic effectiveness has been reported in patients with essential vocal tremor or other types of motility disorders of the vocal folds (Blitzer et al. 1988; Blitzer and Brin 1991). It is noteworthy that vocal tremor is a frequent feature of LD (i.e., the so-called primary dystonic tremor), often involving the adductor muscles. Indeed, in about one third of patients, LD is also accompanied by a tremor component. In patients with dystonic tremor of the vocal folds, the EMG pattern is typically characterised by co-contraction of agonist and antagonist muscles (i.e., abductor and adductor muscles) at a frequency of about 5 Hz. EMG dischargers compatible with muscle spasms can be also observed in the form either of contraction of single laryngeal muscles or of co-contraction of adductor and abductor muscles, the tensor muscles of the vocal folds being frequently involved. Despite the above, the clinician should keep in mind that in many cases vocal tremor is not dystonic but associated with limb tremor. This is quite frequent in patients with essential tremor, who present with vocal tremor in about 20% or 30% of cases. Even when isolated, vocal tremor can represent an essential tremor variant. Such patients present with a characteristic "bleating" voice, and the EMG evaluation shows a rhythmic tremor activity at frequency ranging from 3–12 Hz, with alternating activation of agonist and antagonist muscles. A vocal tremor can be also present in patients with different Parkinsonian syndromes, such as Parkinson's disease, multisystem atrophy and progressive supranuclear palsy.

### 18.13.4 Approach to Treatment of LD with BTX-A by LEMG Guide

The treatment with BTX-A injection into the laryngeal muscles represents the "gold standard" therapy for LD (Blitzer et al. 1988; Dressler 2010). However, other treatments can be associated with BTX-A treatment or carried out as the first option, including drugs taken by mouth or voice rehabilitation or both. The latter can lead to clinical improvement in some patients with mild LD, even when applied as single treatment. Among the alternative pharmacological treatments are anticholinergics in the first place, such as trihexyphenidyl and benzotropine mesylate, which may occasionally induce some clinical benefit, even though this is often unsatisfactory and transient. Other drugs have been used with poor efficacy, such as non-selective beta-blockers (e.g., propranolol), some types of benzodiazepines (e.g., diazepam, clonazepam, etc.), and centrally acting muscle relaxants such as baclofen (Ludlow 2009).

The use an electromyographic guide capable of accurately identifying the laryngeal muscles to be infiltrated is highly recommended, if not mandatory, when performing the treatment with BTX-A. Therefore, this treatment should be always carried out by well-trained experts such as neurologists, neurophysiopathologists, phonologists or otolaryngologists with specific expertise in electromyographic recording of the pharyngo-laryngeal muscles. For BTX-A injection we should use very thin monopolar needle electrodes (i.e., 0.2–0.4 mm diameter) with an inner cannula face on which the syringe containing BTX can be inserted. Before injection of BTX-A, electromyography of the activity of the main adductor, abductor and tensor muscles of the vocal folds should be studied to ascertain the presence of a dystonic activity, which is indicated by prolonged EMG bursts (tonic spasms lasting longer than 400 ms) and reduced or absent phasic modulation (i.e., EMG activity peaks) during physiological activities such as vocalisations, in adduction, abduction and tension of the vocal folds, or in quiet and forced breathing (e.g., "sniffing", which requires activation of the abductor muscles). In this way the muscles to be treated can be correctly identified. It should be emphasised that even when treatment is effective, the patient's voice never turns to normal after BTX-A treatment, especially in older patients (Paniello et al. 2008, 2009; Cannito et al. 2008). This is because mechanisms of action of BTX-A in LD are much more complex than we believe and not the simple expression of the improvement of laryngeal muscles spasm. There may be a retrograde transport of BTX-A to the motor neurons of the injected laryngeal muscles (Moreno-López et al. 1997; Antonucci et al. 2008). Thus in turn, the physiological modulatory effects of the brainstem interneurons on the laryngeal motor neurons could be affected at the level of the CNS.

Central effects should also be taken into account to explain the reduction in muscle spasm following unilateral BTX injection in the untreated contralateral homologous muscles (Bielamowicz and Ludlow 2000). Changes in the sensory feedback from laryngeal structures due to inhibitory effects of BTX on the sensory afferents might also play a role, possible resulting in less mucous compression and reduced subglottal pressure in the trachea in the hyperadduction of the vocal folds during vocal emission. Regarding BTX-A doses to be used for treatment of LD, there are no standards, as treatment should be adapted to the type and severity of LD. Moreover, the choice of the BTX-A dose to be used in individual patients should take into account whether treatment is performed for the first time or it has been already performed.

Generally, at the first injection it is preferable to inject into single muscles lower BTX-A doses among those potentially effective. This will allow assessment of the efficacy and duration of treatment with minimal risk of side effects. Larger doses of BTX-A can be used in subsequent treatment sessions to achieve the optimal compromise between the treatment effectiveness and duration, and side effects. There are also no univocal rules to follow regarding the choice of injecting laryngeal muscles on one or both sides. Bilateral injection is more commonly performed in adductor type LD, whilst in the abductor forms it is generally preferable to treat only one side. This is in order to avoid potential dangerous respiratory dysfunction due to excessive reduction of the ventilatory space of the laryngeal vestibule. In selected cases, however, we could opt for using a higher BTX-A dose on one side, and a much lower dose contralaterally.

As a general criterion, when BTX-A injection is made bilaterally for treatment of adductor LD, a dose ranging from 1.0 to 2.5 U of Incobotulinumtoxin A or Onabotulinumtoxin A should be used to treat single muscles, using a concentration of 5 U/0.1 ml or 10 U/0.1 ml. For Abobotulintoxin A, equivalent doses range from 3.0 to 8.0 U with a concentration of 20 U/0.1 ml or 40 U/0.1 ml. Instead, when BTX-A is unilaterally injected, the recommended dose for Incobotulinumtoxin A and Onabotulinumtoxin A ranges from 2.5 U at first injection to 10 U when treatment is repeated over time. Corresponding doses of Abobotulinumtoxin A range from 8.0 to 30 U.

In patients with abductor LD, we normally choose to inject the posterior cricoarytenoid muscle (CAP) unilaterally. In these cases, doses ranging from 1.0 to 2.5 U of Incobotulinumtoxin A or Onabotulinumtoxin A (with a concentration of 5 U/0.1 ml or 10 U/0.1 ml) and from 3.0 to 8.0 units of Abobotulinumtoxin A (with a concentration of 20 U/0.1 ml or 40 U/0.1 ml) should be used. Only in selected cases (e.g., patients with severe abductor LD or who did not respond to repeated unilateral inoculation of an increasing amount of BTX-A) we might choose to inject the CAP on both sides, using a medium BTX-A dose on one side and a lower dose (i.e., from 0.5 to 1.0 U of Incobotulinumtoxin A or Onabotulinumtoxin A, or from 1.0 to 3.0 U of Abobotulinumtoxin A) on the opposite side. CAP should be injected bilaterally only in patients who did not present significant side effects after unilateral injection. A further increase in the BTX dose over time is generally not advisable in abductor type LD owing to the risk of major respiratory side effects.

The use of a different concentration would influence diffusion of the drug into the nearby tissues, which in turn could be responsible for possible side effects. Thus theoretically the use of a lower concentration could be preferable to reduce such a risk. In clinical practice, however, if we use too low a concentration, it may become difficult to inject precisely a small amount of drug such as that used for treatment of LD. Thus we believe that concentrations of 5 U/0.1 ml for Incobotulinumtoxin A or Onabotulinumtoxin A and 20 U/0.1 ml for Abobotulinumtoxin A are to be preferred.

In all cases, it is recommended to re-evaluate the patient clinically 3–6 weeks after BTX-A injection, both to assess the efficacy of treatment and the presence of possible side effects related to the treatment. Moreover, in the case of poor or absent therapeutic effect at first follow-up, and in the absence of side effects, the possibility of re-injecting BTX-A could be considered. With re-treatment we aim to enhance the effect of the first treatment of BTX-A injections of the same treated muscles, or we can choose to inject some other laryngeal muscles not previously treated. Ineffectiveness or major side effects of the BTX-A injection in LD could be consequences of either incorrect selection of the muscles to treat or choice of the BTX-A dose. In 17% of treated patients a swallowing disorder may occur after treatment, which is mild in most cases and generally has a short duration ranging from 1 week to 1 month. Mild bleeding or transient small haematomas in the injected vocal fold have been very rarely reported. These side effects can occur more frequently in patients being treated with anti-platelet agents or especially anticoagulants. A temporary suspension of anticoagulant therapy prior to treatment should be carefully considered, weighing the potential risks and benefits for each individual patient. However, major bleeding with serious clinical consequences related to the injection of BTX-A for treatment of LD has not been described so far. The frequency and type of side effects also depend on the type of LD being treated. In the adductor type, transient changes in voice and swallowing may occur that generally last from 1 to 6 weeks. Indeed, the patient could present a "blown" voice and some difficulty in ingesting liquids, with the risk of small inhalations into the airways. In patients treated for an abductor type LD, owing to the inoculation of the CAP muscle (even on one single side) there could appear some transient respiratory disturbance following strenuous physical activities, due to reduction of the laryngeal vestibule space.

When the BTX-A treatment fails to improve LD, last-resort surgical treatments could be considered, including selective lesion of the recurrent laryngeal nerve, laryngoplasty (Isshiki et al. 2000; Chan et al. 2004), myectomy (Koufman et al. 2006), myoplasty (Shaw et al. 2003) and denervation-reinnervation treatment strategy (Berke et al. 1999; Isshiki 1980). Currently, these treatments are available only in a very few ultra-specialised centres around the world. Deep brain stimulation (DBS) could represent another possible therapeutic option, considering its effectiveness for treatment of generalised dystonia when targeting the internal globus pallidus (Coubes et al. 2004). Future studies, however, are needed to investigate the use of DBS in patients with severe LD who cannot adequately be treated by BTX-A injection. In this regard, caution should be used considering that DBS may be of little use in the treatment of voice and speech deficits (Deuschl et al. 2006).

## 18.13.5 Conclusion

The LEMG represents a valuable tool in the clinical practice both for diagnosis purposes and for clinical quantification of vocal fold deficits. Indeed, thanks to LEMG we can obtain a great amount of information both when voice disturbances are due to a peripheral nerve injury (i.e., damage to the vagus nerve or its branches, the recurrent or superior laryngeal nerves) and when the motility disorders of the vocal folds are due to involvement of the CNS. This neurophysiological technique is also fundamental when we carry out treatment with BTX-A injection of the laryngeal muscles in patients with voice disorders such as LD and some kinds of vocal tremor.

## 18.14  Interpretation of Results of (Neuro-)Psychological Examinations

Stefano Zago and Edoardo Nicolò Aiello

Neuropsychological assessment has to be approached both qualitatively and quantitatively. Individuals' psychometric outcomes are indeed complemented with signs detected during both test execution (e.g., phonemic conduites d'approche during a confrontation naming task) and clinical interviews (e.g., uncriticised incorrect verb inflections), as well as with referred symptoms (e.g., tip-of-the-tongue phenomena in spontaneous speech) (Hannay and Lezak 2004). Qualitative clinical features also happen to be susceptible to a form of scoring (e.g., perseverance during a constructional-praxis task)—thus possibly becoming quantifiable (Somerville et al. 2000). However, although still inherently probabilistic, an accurate interpretation of potential qualitative markers of cognitive/behavioural dysfunctions is more dependent on practitioners' applied (e.g., clinical) background than it is on their methodological expertise (Monti et al. 2008; Kolakowsky-Hayner and Caplan 2011). By contrast, when it comes to drawing clinical judgements from test scores, care should be paid to the adopted statistical frameworks.

Practitioners have first to bear in mind fundamental psychometric properties that tests have to possess in order for them to be applicable—and thus test scores to be interpretable (Barr 2001). A test has to be valid—i.e., to measure what it is intended to (systematic error variability will be lower than the portion reflecting the target construct)—and reliable—i.e., to yield similar results on different administrations, other predictors remaining constant (random error variability will be lower than systematic components) (Willmes 2010). Epidemiological statistics have also to be addressed, such as sensitivity—i.e., the ability of a test to label a pathological performance as impaired—and specificity—i.e., labelling a normal performance as unimpaired (Rohling et al. 2017; Trevethan 2017). For instance, one would not uncritically regard a defective score on the Paced Auditory Serial Addition Test (PASAT) (Gronwall 1977) per se as supportive of a relevant attentive/executive deficit in an individual with suspected logopenic aphasia (Gorno-Tempini et al. 2011). Indeed, highly demanding and thus sensitive tests (e.g., the PASAT) may be inadequate as screeners or as the sole means through which a clinical inference is made (Brooks et al. 2011). Moreover, caution should be exerted when interpreting scores whose systematic error variability is possibly high—e.g., both linguistic (i.e., phonological) and extra-linguistic (e.g., short-term memory) components may underlie the performance on the PASAT (Strub and Gardner 1974).

Given that a test is psychometrically satisfactory, raw scores (RSs) yielded by its administration have to be quantitatively attributed a clinical, qualitative judgement (Willmes 2010). Performance levels are defined according to a comparison of RSs against point/interval norms—often by converting them into a common metric (Capitani 1997). When standardising RSs, one should pay attention to both the nature of the data and the adequacy of norm-inferring methods. Those requiring distributional assumptions (e.g., z-transformations, which assume that data converge to a normal distribution) should be cautiously adopted (Crawford 2003), as these criteria are often not met by neuropsychological data (e.g., normality and homogeneous variance violations owing to ceiling/floor effects and high inter-individual variability) (Malek-Ahmadi et al. 2017). Non-parametric approaches to RSs standardisation have therefore been traditionally preferred (e.g., Equivalent Scores, ESs) (Capitani and Laiacona 1997, 2017)—this being relevant for practitioners not falling into errors when interpreting results (e.g., underestimation of cognitive deficits severity) (Scherr et al. 2016). It has to be noted that not all standardisation procedures provide checks for inferential errors (Willmes 2010). For instance, the cut-off computed within the ESs method corresponds to the outer one-sided non-parametric lower tolerance limit, i.e., the highest observation in the "worst" 5% of a healthy sample that yields a ≥95% probability that at most 5% of the population performs below it (Capitani and Laiacona 2017). This allows practitioners to keep the error risk at 5% when judging a performance as defective (ibidem): the same precaution, however, is not considered when adopting as cut-off, e.g., either a percentile or a z-score (Crawford 2003; Willmes 2010; Capitani and Laiacona 2017). The representativeness of the normative sample from which norms are derived has also to be accounted when judging their quality (Willmes 2010).

Therefore, when it comes to fruition of both novel tests and updated norms—the latter being needed owing to socio-demographic changes (Siciliano et al. 2019), practitioners should always take into consideration methodological-statistical correctness of works (Bush 2010).

When interpreting RSs and standardising them, one should also bear in mind the statistical unit under investigation (Hambleton and Jones 1993). Although global test scores are often regarded as the only outcome (e.g., Classical Test Theory), single-item level approaches (e.g., Item Response Theory) are gaining ground (Martins et al. 2020). This last assertion happens to be true especially in the aphasiological field, where adaptive testing techniques happen to be intuitively applicable (e.g., a clinician administering only "difficult" items of a naming task to a patient clinically diagnosed with mild anomic aphasia after suffering a traumatic brain injury) (Edmonds and Donovan 2012).

A final remark has to be made on intervening constructs possibly bringing error variability into test scores—such as individual features (e.g., age, educational attainment, sex), psychological functioning (e.g., state of anxiety, personality traits) or environmental variables (e.g., background noises during the examination) (Kessels and Brands 2009). For example, regression-based norm-inferring methods (e.g., ESs) allow accounting for the influence of systematic variables such as age and education, by adjusting RSs via ad hoc equations—i.e., by computing Ass (Willmes 2010; Capitani and Laiacona 2017). Less trivial would be to control quantitatively for stochastic confounding factors (e.g., situational mood fluctuations)—which should nonetheless be qualitatively kept in mind by

practitioners when interpreting results of neuro-psychological examinations (Kessels and Brands 2009; Kolakowsky-Hayner and Caplan 2011).

## 18.15 Interpretation of Results of Logopaedic/SLP Examination

Iolanda Trittola, Danilo Patrocinio, Vincenzo Sallustio, Donato Mecca, and Cristina Polimeno

Patients suffering from motor speech disorders (MSD), when referred to phoniatricians and speech language pathologists (SLPs) for rehabilitation, usually have already received an aetiological and site-of-lesion diagnosis. Although specific evaluation purposes might vary with the intervention phase, the overall focus of the assessment is to "outline the profile of disabilities as well as the relational, communicative and linguistic potential of the patient in the various contexts of daily life": how he or she communicates, what obstacles, frustrations and expectations exist, what spontaneous compensations have been found, the willingness and elasticity to accept suggestions, the ability to adapt to the interlocutor in order to avoid continuing to adopt ineffective communicative behaviours (Rampone and Miletto 2010; Marini and Carlomagno 2004). Accordingly, the speech language rehabilitation specialists should operate with the aim of evaluating the following critical points (Duffy 2019; ASHA 2005, 2016), namely, the:

- Presence of dysarthria
- Presence of apraxia
- Type, level or severity of the verbal and non-verbal communicative impairment
- Presence of communicative associated disorders
- Prognosis of illness
- Treatment aims and the criteria for taking charge of the patients
- Perspective of patient and family
- Criteria for treatment suspension
- Suitable outcome measures.

The data available for phoniatricians and SLP will derive from (Duffy 2019; Pattee et al. 2019; RCP 2016; ASHA 2004) the:

- Evaluation of the phonetic, phonological, prosodic and pragmatic aspects of the verbal communication both for oral and written expression (academic skills)
- Evaluation of the non-verbal communication
- Speech motor-orientated protocols
- Oral motor-orientated protocols
- Health (and neurological) examination
- Psychological evaluation
- Instrumental examinations (e.g., endoscopic, acoustical, electrophysiological, imaging)
- Laboratory tests
- Evaluation of the emotional and relational aspects
- Patient and family counselling.

The previous statements suggest some considerations.

First, the collected data will be best used if linked to the International Classification of Functioning, Disability and Health (ICF) framework (World Health Organization 2014), because it strongly supports the rehabilitation specialists in comprehending and estimating both the patient's impairment and his activity limitations and restrictions in participation. Considering the residual and possibly recoverable abilities, and evaluating the environmental, contextual and personal factors that can act as barriers or facilitators on a case-by-case basis, the ICF framework may also provide guidance about type, duration and prognosis of the rehabilitative intervention. It is not always possible to interpret the patient's communicative limitations and his social restrictions solely due to his or her disability; it is also necessary to verify the communicative behaviour of the members of his or her family nucleus and caregivers, at home or through video analysis: the interlocutors' behaviour can be either a barrier or facilitator for relationships and socialising. Since dysarthria is a communication disorder, its complete or partial remedy should not be an exclusive task of the patient, but should involve all the interlocutors,

especially if they are healthy and in a condition to pursue more easily any adaptation useful for functional communication. The behaviour of the patient's family members and caregivers gives us the opportunity to interpret better what emerges from the narration or from the administration of evaluation tests; suggesting, if necessary, that phoniatricians and SLPs should take charge of the entire family/caregivers unit and thus conditioning the type, duration and prognosis of the treatment (ASHA 2004). For example, in anarthric subjects using an eye-controlled communicator, not only does the patient have to adapt to "talk" slowly by pointing his or her eyes at a screen, but the family members and caregivers (Baxter et al. 2012) also have to learn to listen and manage the sometimes very long silences associated with using that device.

Second, since three crucial tasks (respiratory, phono-articulatory and feeding functions) exploit the same anatomical structures, dysarthria is almost always associated with dysphagia and dysphonia to varying degrees. Therefore, the phoniatric and speech language assessment and its interpretation are quite complex; above all, the relationships and influences among disorders and symptoms have to be well defined, considering the underlying neurological disease (Duffy 2019; Pattee et al. 2019).

Third, although many technological procedures have been proposed, the most powerful tool for carrying out a functional communication-orientated evaluation is, to date, the expert ear (of the phoniatrician/SLP); it is the only tool able to perform from the first consultation a contextual, multiple and simultaneous assessment of the verbal and non-verbal communication components.

Fourth, the communication-orientated evaluation has to be able to identify the main factors impairing the verbal utterance intelligibility in patients affected by MSD, with the aim of addressing the treatment (e.g., prosody, speed or naturalness handling) to gain intelligibility.

Fifth, the focus on intelligence, memory and executing functions is a central topic because it influences the disorder prognosis, its evolution and sometimes the ability to assess the treatment (RCP 2016).

Sixth, the focus on the integrity of the sensorial afferents (auditory, tactile, kinaesthetic, pressure and taste sensors) both at the peripheral level and in their central processing (above all at the cerebellar and basal-subcortical circuit levels) is often neglected, but its role is crucial; it is important in understanding how the patient "senses" and rates his own motion, the (acoustic) result of those movements, and how the patient is able to detect and perceive any modification.

Seventh, it is essential to know the patient's feeling of his own disability. An MSD sufferer lives a non-easily solvable bereavement owing to the progressive loss of his speech intelligibility and to the non-verbal incompetence that prevents him from communicating his own emotions. In this regard, and considering that a health system also has in its mission the humanisation of the services and the increase in the satisfaction of the patient and of the operators, counselling is to be considered as the "humanising" tool par excellence (Patrocinio and Trittola 2005). SPL counselling in patients with MSD is a primary tool, whose essential aspects must be known and specific competence possessed. These counselling skills help the rehabilitative team to interpret the results of the SPL assessment, aiding in information, crisis support and problem-solving strategies. Counselling is useful in the decision-making process to take care of the patient according to the contexts (home care, outpatient care, day-hospital, hospitalisation, admission to a rehabilitation centre) as well as to modulate, measure and interpret the needs of the patient and the caregivers, respecting the times dictated by the emotions and feelings (denial, sense of guilt, anger, pain, frustration, etc.) evoked by the diagnosis.

Eighth, the phoniatrician and the SLP are components of a multidisciplinary team involving several professionals in the rehabilitative area (occupational and physical therapists, physiatrists, etc.) as well as in other disciplines (neurologists, respiratory disease specialists, etc.). This team has a physician as chief who is legally responsible for the individualised rehabilitation plan. If the predominant disorder is a communicative impairment, very often this professional is a phoniatrician. The responsible physician and the team will decide together on the rehabilitative approach and the timing, with a view to a highly personalised treatment on the basis of the results of the various evaluation steps and counselling conducted by the SLP. The accuracy of the decisions taken will be evaluated longitudinally over time, measuring the stability of the results achieved, the generalisation and maintenance of the new behaviour acquired, both in the motor-verbal area and in the cognitive, emotional and relational areas. The measures will derive from the repeated administration of the tests used for the assessment, or by referring to outcome scales, such as Therapy Outcomes Measures (TOM) (Enderby et al. 2013), bearing in mind that the final objective, for all the actors involved in the process of rehabilitation of MSDs, should be a functional communication that facilitates relationships, and pursuing the best possible quality of life for the patient and his or her family.

## 18.16 Cooperation with the Occupational Therapist: Interpretation of Results of Occupational Therapy

Karel Neubauer

The cooperation of a clinical speech therapist, phoniatrist and occupational therapist is an important part of the interdisciplinary team dedicated to the development of adequate care for people with neurogenic communication disorders, including those with acquired dysarthria or speech dyspraxia. This fact is repeatedly emphasised by the authors of current professional monographs devoted to the issue of comprehensive care in the field of acquired neurogenic communication disorders (Brookshire and McNeil 2015; Groher and Puntil-Sheltman 2016; Lopez 2016; Neubauer 2018a; Duffy 2020). The area largely corresponds to that of care for especially ageing and severely handicapped people (Kalvach and Švestková 2004; Lopez 2016).

The goal of occupational therapy as a non-medical field is to achieve the maximum possible self-sufficiency and independence of people with disabilities (physical, mental, sensory, cognitive) in the home, work and social environment. For this goal, contributing to the improvement of patients' quality of life, occupational therapy uses forms of functional and cognitive training, re-education of functional abilities and orientates these procedures primarily to the activities of everyday life in their entirety. It develops the functional potential of people in the field of skills, replacement activities, compensatory aids and also adjustments of the home environment to suit the patient's abilities.

An essential part of the occupational therapist's professional responsibility is to help the patient resume daily activities such as self-care, housekeeping, cooking, cleaning and more. The focus of the occupational therapist's activities in restoring momentum, coordination and muscle strength is focused on restoring these daily activities and the possibility of re-developing leisure activities and hobbies. The work activities used, the use of work tools and the creation of products are aimed at the process of restoring the abilities of everyday life, restoring work and professional skills, if the patient is able to do so.

In the field of cognition and communication, there is a direct connection with the fields of diagnostics and therapy of communication disorders. Sensory-motor and visuo-spatial disorders, which occupational therapists address in assessment and stimulation programmes, are related to the areas of visual perception, reading, writing and numerical performance; in order to influence these areas comprehensively for the benefit of the patient, mutual cooperation is frequent and important.

For mutual understanding in the field of interpretation of diagnostic and therapeutic conclusions, an understanding is needed at the level of terminological distinction of the content of the following: impairment-disability-handicap, in terms of the International Classification of Functioning, Disability and Health (ICF, World Health Organization 2001), as this differentiation is declared as an important part of the occupational therapy programmes performed. For example, a patient after a stroke suffering from half-body movement disorders and acquired dysarthria will have difficulty in both somatic abilities and speech. For comprehensive assistance, it will require (within a wider multidisciplinary team) the involvement of a clinical speech therapist and an occupational therapist. The non-intact system (impairment) here is motor skills and coordination of the body, and of the orofacial area. Disrupted activity (disability) here is self-sufficiency in motor activities—dressing, cooking, etc. on the other hand, it includes also intelligible oral speech. Handicap is present in the area of independence and mobility, and at the same time in communication with the social environment.

A widely used and well-known evaluation procedure based on the above approach is FIM (The Functional Independence Measure), which is not only part of a comprehensive multidisciplinary rehabilitation system in EU countries, but also the subject of a number of research and evaluation studies (Ravaud et al. 1999; Kalvach and Švestková 2004; Young et al. 2009). It also includes the area of communication assessment, focusing here on visual and auditory understanding and expression by verbal and non-verbal means. This is an expression of a functional evaluation set, focused on disability and the derived degree of handicap in communication.

# References

Aaronson NK, Ahmedzai S, Bergman B et al (1993) The European Organization for Research and Treatment of Cancer QLQ-C30: a quality-of-life instrument for use in international clinical trials in oncology. J Natl Cancer Inst 85(5):365–376

Ackermann H, Hertrich I, Scharf G (1995) Kinematic analysis of lower lip movements in ataxic dysarthria. J Speech Lang Hear Res 38(6):1252–1259

Adler CH, Edwards BW, Bansberg SF (1997) Female predominance in spasmodic dysphonia. J Neurol Neurosurg Psychiatry 63(5):688. https://doi.org/10.1136/jnnp.63.5.688

Agostino R, Currà A, Soldati G et al (2004) Prolonged practice is of scarce benefit in improving motor performance in Parkinson's disease. Mov Disord 19(11):1285–1293

Alfonsi E, Terzaghi M, Cosentino G et al (2016) Specific patterns of laryngeal electromyography during wakefulness are associated to sleep disordered breathing and nocturnal stridor in multiple system atrophy. Parkinsonism Relat Disord 31:104–109

Alves M, Krüger E, Pillay B et al (2019) The affect of hydration on voice quality in adults: a systematic review. J Voice 33(1):e113–e128

Ambrose J, Hounsfield G (1973) Computerized transverse axial tomography. Br J Radiol 46(542):148–149

American Psychiatric Association (2013) Diagnostic and statistical manual of mental disorders, 5th edn. American Psychiatric Association, Washington

Antonucci F, Rossi C, Gianfranceschi L et al (2008) Long-distance retrograde effects of botulinum neurotoxin A. J Neurosci 28:3689–3696

Arboix A, Bell Y, Garcia-Eroles L et al (2004) Clinical study of 35 patients with dysarthria-clumsy hand syndrome. J Neurol Neurosurg Psychiatry 75(2):231–234

Arnett PE (2013) Secondary influences on neuropsychological test performance. Oxford Academic Press, New York

ASHA (2004) Preferred practice patterns for the profession of speech-language pathology (preferred practice patterns). www.asha.org/policy/. Accessed 7 April 2021

ASHA (2005) Evidence-based practice in communication disorders (position statement). www.asha.org/policy. Accessed 7 April 2021

ASHA (2016) Scope of practice in speech-language pathology (scope of practice). www.asha.org/policy/. Accessed 7 April 2021

ASHA (2022) Dysarthria in adults. https://www.asha.org/practice-portal/clinical-topics/dysarthria-in-adults/#collapse_2. Accessed January 2022

Astolfi A, Castellana A, Puglisi GE et al (2019) Speech level parameters in very low and excessive reverberation measured with a contact-sensor-based device and a headworn microphone. J Acoust Soc Am 145(4):2540. https://doi.org/10.1121/1.5098942

Auzou P (2007) Les objectifs du bilan de la dysarthrie (the objectives of the dysarthria assessment). In: Auzou P, Rolland-Monnoury V, Pinto S et al (eds) Les dysarthries (dysarthria). Solal, Marseille, pp 189–195

Azuar C, Leger A, Arbizu C et al (2013) The aphasia rapid test: an NIHSS-like aphasia test. J Neurol 260(8):2110–2117

Bacsfalvi P, Bernhardt BM, Gick B (2007) Electropalatography and ultrasound in vowel remediation for adolescents with hearing impairment. Adv Speech Lang Pathol 9(1):36–45

Baken RJ, Orlikoff RF (2000) Clinical measurement of speech and voice, 2nd edn. Singular Publishing, San Diego

Balaguer M, Farinas J, Fichaux-Bourin P et al (2020a) Validation of the French versions of the speech handicap index and the phonation handicap index in patients treated for cancer of the oral cavity or oropharynx. Folia Phoniatr Logop 72(6):464–477

Balaguer M, Pommée T, Farinas J et al (2020b) Effects of oral and oropharyngeal cancer on speech intelligibility using acoustic analysis: systematic review. Head Neck 42(1):111–130

Bannister R, Gibson W, Michaels L et al (1981) Laryngeal abductor paralysis in multiple system atrophy. A report on three necropsied cases, with observations on the laryngeal muscles and the nuclei ambigui. Brain 104:351–368

Barberena LS, Brasil Brunah C, Michelon Melo R et al (2014) Ultrasound applicability in speech language pathology and audiology. Codas 26(6):520–530

Barberena LS, Portalete CR, Simoni SN et al (2017) Electropalatography and its correlation to the ultrasonography of the movement of speech analysis línguanas. Codas 29:2. https://doi.org/10.1590/2317-1782/20172016106

Barr WB (2001) Methodologic issues in neuropsychological testing. J Athl Train 36(3):297–302

Barsties B, Maryn Y (2013) Test-retest variability and internal consistency of the Acoustic Voice Quality Index. HNO 61(5):399–403

Baxter S, Enderby P, Evans P et al (2012) Barriers and facilitators to the use of high-technology augmentative and alternative communication devices: a systematic review and qualitative synthesis. Int J Lang Commun Disord 47(2):115–129

Baylor C, Yorkston K, Eadie T et al (2013) The Communicative Participation Item Bank (CPIB): item bank calibration and development of a disorder-generic short form. J Speech Lang Hear Res 56(4):1190–1208

Belenkov NY (1970) Ephaptic transmission of excitation as a factor in the synchronization of neuronal activity. In: Rusinov VS, Doty RW (eds) Electrophysiology of the central nervous system. Springer, Boston

Berke GS, Blackwell KE, Gerratt RR et al (1999) Selective laryngeal adductor denervation-reinnervation: a new surgical treatment for adductor spasmodic dysphonia. Ann Otol Rhinol Laryngol 108:227–231

Berry J, Kolb A, Schroeder J et al (2017) Jaw rotation in dysarthria measured with a single electromagnetic articulography sensor. Am J Speech Lang Pathol 26(2S):596–610

Beskow J, Sjölander K (2000) Wavesurfer - an open source speech tool. Proc Int Conf Spok Lang Process 4:464–467

Bielamowicz S, Ludlow CL (2000) Effects of botulinum toxin on pathophysiology in spasmodic dysphonia. Ann Otol Rhinol Laryngol 109:194–203

Biniek R, Huber W, Glindemann R et al (1992) The Aachen aphasia bedside test—criteria for validity of psychologic tests. Nervenarzt 63(8):473–479

Blitzer A, Brin MF (1991) Laryngeal dystonia: a series with botulinum toxin therapy. Ann Otol Rhinol Laryngol 100(2):85–89

Blitzer A, Brin MF, Fahn S et al (1988) Localized injections of botulinum toxin for the treatment of focal laryngeal dystonia (spastic dysphonia). Laryngoscope 98:193–197

Boersma P (2001) Praat, a system for doing phonetics by computer. Glot Int 5(9-10):341–345

Boersma P, Weenink D (2021) Praat, doing phonetics by computer. Computer program, version 6.1.40. https://www.fon.hum.uva.nl/praat/. Accessed 27 October 2021

Borrie SA, Baese-Berk M, Van Engen K et al (2017) A relationship between processing speech in noise and dysarthric speech. J Acoust Soc Am 141(6):4660. https://doi.org/10.1121/1.4986746

Bottalico P, Graetzer S, Hunter EJ (2016) Effects of speech style, room acoustics, and vocal fatigue on vocal effort. J Acoust Soc Am 139(5):2870. https://doi.org/10.1121/1.4950812

Brin MF, Blitzer A, Stewart C (1998) Laryngeal dystonia (spasmodic dysphonia): observations of 901 patients and treatment with botulinum toxin. Adv Neurol 78:237–252

Brockmann-Bauser M, Van Stan JH, Carvalho Sampaio M et al (2019) Effects of vocal intensity and fundamental frequency on cepstral peak prominence in patients with voice disorders and vocally healthy controls. J Voice 35(3):411–417

Brooks JBB, Giraud VO, Saleh YJ et al (2011) Paced auditory serial addition test (PASAT): a very difficult test even for individuals with high intellectual capability. Arq Neuropsiquiatr 69(3):482–484

Brookshire R, McNeil M (2015) Introduction to neurogenic communication disorders. Elsevier, St Louis

Brumfitt SM, Sheeran P (1999) Visual analogue self-esteem scale (VASES). Winslow Press, Oxon

Bunton K, Kent RD, Duffy JR et al (2007) Listener agreement for auditory-perceptual ratings of dysarthria. J Speech Lang Hear Res 50(6):1481–1495

Burris C, Vorperian HK, Fourakis M et al (2014) Quantitative and descriptive comparison of four acoustic analysis systems: vowel measurements. J Speech Lang Hear Res 57(1):26–45

Bush SS (2010) Determining whether or when to adopt new versions of psychological and neuropsychological tests: ethical and professional considerations. Clin Neuropsychol 24(1):7–16

Cabeza R, Albert M, Belleville S et al (2018) Maintenance, reserve and compensation: the cognitive neuroscience of healthy ageing. Nat Rev Neurosci 19(11):701–710

Campbell WW, DeJong RN (2005) DeJong's the neurologic examination. Lippincott Williams & Wilkins, Philadelphia

Cannito MP, Kahane JC, Chorna L (2008) Vocal aging and adductor spasmodic dysphonia: response to botulinum toxin injection. Clin Interv Aging 3:131–151

Capitani E (1997) Normative data and neuropsychological assessment. Common problems in clinical practice and research. Neuropsychol Rehabil 7(4):295–310

Capitani E, Laiacona M (1997) Composite neuropsychological batteries and demographic correction: standardization based on equivalent scores, with a review of published data. J Clin Exp Neuropsychol 19(6):795–809

Capitani E, Laiacona M (2017) Outer and inner tolerance limits: their usefulness for the construction of norms and the standardization of neuropsychological tests. Clin Neuropsychol 31(6-7):1219–1230

Cappa SF, Gorno-Tempini ML (2009) Clinical phenotypes of progressive aphasia. Future Neurol 4(2):153–160

Catani M, Howard RJ, Pajevic S et al (2002) Virtual in vivo interactive dissection of white matter fasciculi in the human brain. NeuroImage 17(1):77–94

Catani M, Allin MP, Husain M et al (2007) Symmetries in human brain language pathways correlate with verbal recall. Proc Natl Acad Sci USA 104(43):17163–17168

Catani M, Dell Aqua F, Vergani F et al (2012) Short frontal lobe connections of the human brain. Cortex 48:273–291

Cella DF, Tulsky DS, Gray G et al (1993) The functional assessment of cancer therapy scale: development and validation of the general measure. J Clin Oncol 11(3):570–579

Cella D, Lai J-S, Nowinski CJ et al (2012) Neuro-QOL: brief measures of health-related quality of life for clinical research in neurology. Neurology 78(23):1860–1867

Chan SW, Baxter M, Oates J et al (2004) Long-term results of type II thyroplasty for adductor spasmodic dysphonia. Laryngoscope 114:1604–1608

Chan JC, Stout JC, Vogel AP (2019) Speech in prodromal and symptomatic Huntington's disease as a model of measuring onset and progression in dominantly inherited neurodegenerative diseases. Neurosci Biobehav Rev 107:450–460

Chitkara A, Meyer T, Keidar A et al (2006) Singer's dystonia: first report of a variant of spasmodic dysphonia. Ann Otol Rhinol Laryngol 115:88–92

Cipolotti L, Warrington EK (1995) Neuropsychological assessment. J Neurol Neurosurg Psychiatry 58(6):655–664

Clarke C, Howard R, Rossor M et al (eds) (2016) Neurology: a queen square textbook, 2nd edn. Wiley, Somerset

Clifford A, Reiss J (2011) Proximity effect detection for directional microphones. Paper presented at the 131 Audio Engineering Society Convention. https://www.aes.org/e-lib/browse.cfm?elib=16001. Accessed 21 October 2021

Cohen SM, Thomas S, Roy N et al (2014) Frequency and factors associated with use of videolaryngostroboscopy in voice disorder assessment. Laryngoscope 124(9):2118–2124

Cortelli P, Calandra-Buonaura G, Benarroch EE et al (2019) Stridor in multiple system atrophy: consensus statement on diagnosis, prognosis, and treatment. Neurology 93:630–639

Coubes P, Cif L, El Fertit H et al (2004) Electrical stimulation of the globus pallidus internus in patients with primary generalized dystonia: long-term results. J Neurosurg 101:189–194

Crawford JR (2003) Psychometric foundations of neuro-psychological assessment. In: Goldstein LH, McNeil J (eds) Clinical neuropsychology: a practical guide to assessment and management for clinicians. Wiley, Chichester, pp 121–140

Crumley RL (1989) Laryngeal synkinesis: its signifi-cance to the laryngologist. Ann Otol Rhinol Laryngol 98:87–92

Dabul B (2000) Apraxia battery for adults: examiner's manual. Pro-ed, Austin

Damasio AR (1992) Aphasia. N Engl J Med 326(8):531–539

Darley FL, Aronson AE, Brown JR (1969a) Differential diagnostic patterns of dysarthria. J Speech Hear Res 12(2):246–269

Darley FL, Aronson AE, Brown JR (1969b) Clusters of deviant speech dimensions in the dysarthrias. J Speech Hear Res 12(3):462–496

Darley F, Aronson A, Brown J (1975) Motor speech disor-ders. Saunders, Philadelphia

de Jong NH, Wempe T (2009) Praat script to detect syl-lable nuclei and measure speech rate automatically. Behav Res Methods 41(2):385–390

De Renzi A, Vignolo LA (1962) Token test: a sensitive test to detect receptive disturbances in aphasics. Brain 85:665–678

Delgado-Vargas B, Acle-Cervera L, Sánz-López L et al (2021) Cepstral analysis in patients with a vocal fold motility impairment: advantages of the ceps-trum over time-based acoustic analysis. Eur Arch Otorrinolaringol 278(1):173–179

Deliyski DD, Shaw HS, Evans MK (2005) Adverse effects of environmental noise on acoustic voice quality mea-surements. J Voice 19(1):15–28

Deuschl G, Herzog J, Kleiner-Fisman G et al (2006) Deep brain stimulation: postoperative issues. Mov Disord 21(Suppl 14):S219–S237

Dick AS, Bernal B, Tremblay P (2013) The language con-nectome new pathways, new concepts. Neuroscientist 20(5):453–467

Dlouhá O, Krejčířová D, Nevšímalová S et al (2017) Poruchy vývoje řeči (speech disorders). Galén, Prague

Dodd B, Huo Z, Crosbie S et al (2006) Diagnostic evalu-ation of articulation and phonology (DEAP). Pearson, Harlow

Dressler D (2010) Botulinum toxin for treatment of dysto-nia. Eur J Neurol 17:88–96

Dromey C, Bates E (2005) Speech interactions with lin-guistic, cognitive, and visuomotor tasks. J Speech Lang Hear Res 48(2):295–305

Dronkers NF (1996) A new brain region for coordinating speech articulation. Nature 384(6605):159–161

Duffy JR (1995) Motor speech disorders. Substates, dif-ferential diagnosis and management. Mosby, St. Louis

Duffy JR (2013) Motor speech disorders: substrates, dif-ferential diagnosis, and management, 3rd edn. Mosby, St Louis

Duffy JR (2019) Motor speech disorders: substrates, differential diagnosis, and management, 4th edn. Elsevier, St. Louis

Duffy J (2020) Motor speech disorders. Substrates, differ-ential diagnosis, and management. Elsevier, St Louis

Dykstra AD, Hakel ME, Adams SG (2007) Application of the ICF in reduced speech intelligibility in dysarthria. Semin Speech Lang 28(4):301–311

Eargl JM (2003) Environmental effects and departures from ideal performance. In: Handbook of recording engineering. Springer, Boston, pp 65–73

Edgar JD, Sapienza CM, Bidus K et al (2001) Acoustic measures of symptoms in abductor spasmodic dyspho-nia. J Voice 15(3):362–372

Edmonds LA, Donovan NJ (2012) Item-level psychomet-rics and predictors of performance for Spanish/English bilingual speakers on an object and action naming bat-tery. J Speech Lang Hear Res 55(2):359–381

Ekman P, Friesen WV (1971) Constants across cultures in the face and emotion. J Pers Soc Psychol 17:124–129

Ellis P, Pallister W (1975) Recurrent laryngeal nerve palsy and endotracheal intubation. J Laryngol Otol 89:823–826

Emerick L, Hatten J (1979) Diagnosis and evaluation in speech pathology. Prentice Hall, Wallingford

Enderby P (2013) Disorders of communication: dysar-thria. Handb Clin Neurol 110:273–281

Enderby P, Palmer R (2007) Frenchay dysarthria assess-ment. Pro-Ed, Austin

Enderby P, John A, Petheram B (2013) Therapy outcome measures for rehabilitation professionals: speech and language therapy, physiotherapy, occupational ther-apy, 2nd edn. Wiley, Chichester

Evman MD, Selcuk AA (2020) Vocal cord paralysis as a complication of endotracheal intubation. J Craniofac Surg 31:e119–e120. https://doi.org/10.1097/SCS.0000000000005959

Faiz A (2016) Lothian assessment for screening cognition in aphasia (LASCA): a new nonverbal assessment of cognition. Procedia Soc Behav Sci 217:1052–1062

Feigin JA, Barlow NL, Stelmachowicz PG (1990) The effect of reference microphone placement on sound pressure levels at an ear level hearing aid microphone. Ear Hear 11(5):321–326

Felgoise SH, Walsh SM, Stephens HE et al (2011) The ALS specific quality of life-revised (ALSSQOL-R): user's guide. https://www.pennstatehealth.org/sites/default/files/Neurology/ALSSQOL-Manual.pdf. Accessed 19 January 2021

Ferguson SH, Quené H (2014) Acoustic correlates of vowel intelligibility in clear and conversational speech for young normal-hearing and elderly hearing-impaired listeners. J Acoust Soc Am 135(6):3570–3584

Fex S (1992) Perceptual evaluation. J Voice 6(2):155–158

Fichaux-Bourin P, Woisard V, Grand S et al (2009) Validation of a self assessment for speech disor-ders (phonation handicap index). Rev Laryngol Otol Rhinol 130(1):45–51

Filippi M, Rocca MA, Ciccarelli O et al (2016) MRI criteria for the diagnosis of multiple sclerosis: MAGNIMS consensus guidelines. Lancet Neurol 15(3):292–303

Flege JE, Munro MJ, Skelton L (1992) Production of the word-final English/t/–/d/ contrast by native speakers of English, Mandarin, and Spanish. J Acoust Soc Am 92(1):128–143

Fletcher AR, McAuliffe MJ, Lansford KL et al (2017) Assessing vowel centralization in dysarthria: a comparison of methods. J Speech Lang Hear Res 60(2):341–354

Foesleitner O, Nenning KH, Bartha-Doering L et al (2020a) Lesion-specific language network alterations in temporal lobe epilepsy. Am J Neuroradiol 41(1):147–154

Foesleitner O, Sigl B, Schmidbauer V et al (2020b) Language network reorganization before and after temporal lobe epilepsy surgery. J Neurosurg 134(6):1694–1170

Folker JE, Murdoch BE, Cahill LM et al (2010) Differentiating impairment levels in temporal versus spatial aspects of linguopalatal contacts in Friedreich's ataxia. Mot Control 14(4):490–508

Folker JE, Murdoch BE, Cahill LM et al (2011) Articulatory kinematics in the dysarthria associated with Friedreich's ataxia. Mot Control 15(3):376–389

Folstein MF, Folstein SE, McHugh PR (1975) "Mini-mental state": a practical method for grading the cognitive state of patients for the clinician. J Psychiatr Res 12(3):189–198

Folstein MF, Folstein SE, McHugh PR (2010) 5.2 Mini-mental state examination (MMSE). In: Manual of screeners for dementia. Springer, p 51

Freed D (2000) Motor speech disorders. In: Diagnosis and treatment. Singular Publishing Group, San Diego

Fridriksson J, den Ouden DB, Hillis AE et al (2018) Anatomy of aphasia revisited. Brain 141(3):848–862

Galluzzi C, Bureca I, Guariglia C et al (2015) Phonological simplifications, apraxia of speech and the interaction between phonological and phonetic processing. Neuropsychologia 71:64–83

Garcia JM, Cannito MP (1996) Influence of verbal and nonverbal contexts on the sentence intelligibility of a speaker with dysarthria. J Speech Hear Res 39:750–760

Gerken L, McGregor K (1998) An overview of prosody and its role in normal and disordered child language. Am J Speech Lang Pathol 7(2):38–48

Ghio A, Lalain M, Giusti L et al (2018) Une mesure d'intelligibilité par décodage acoustico-phonétique de pseudo-mots dans le cas de parole atypique (a measure of intelligibility by acoustico-phonetic decoding of pseudowords in the case of atypical speech). Proceedings of the XXXIIe Journées d'Études sur la Parole, Aix-en-Provence, France, pp 285–293

Goozée JV, Murdoch BE, Theodoros DG et al (2000) Kinematic analysis of tongue movements in dysarthria following traumatic brain injury using electromagnetic articulography. Brain Inj 14(2):153–174

Gordon JK (2002) Phonological neighborhood effects in aphasic speech errors: spontaneous and structured contexts. Brain Lang 82(2):113–145

Gorno-Tempini ML, Hillis AE, Weintraub S et al (2011) Classification of primary progressive aphasia and its variants. Neurology 76(11):1006–1014

Graff-Radford J, Jones DT, Strand EA et al (2014) The neuroanatomy of pure apraxia of speech in stroke. Brain Lang 129:43–46

Groher M, Puntil-Sheltman J (2016) Dysphagia unplugged. In: Groher M, Crary M (eds) Dysphagia. Clinical management in adults and children. Elsevier, St Louis, pp 1–18

Gronwall DMA (1977) Paced auditory serial-addition task: a measure of recovery from concussion. Percept Mot Ski 44(2):367–373

Grossman M (2012) The non-fluent/agrammatic variant of primary progressive aphasia. Lancet Neurol 11(6):545–555

Guenther FH, Vladusich T (2012) A neural theory of speech acquisition and production. J Neurolinguistics 25(5):408–422

Haley KL, Jacks A (2014) Single-word intelligibility testing in aphasia: Alternate forms reliability, phonetic complexity and word frequency. Aphasiology 28(3):320–337

Hambleton RK, Jones RW (1993) Comparison of classical test theory and item response theory and their applications to test development. Educ Meas Issues Pract 12(3):38–47

Hannay HJ, Lezak MD (2004) The neuropsychological examination: interpretation. In: Lezak MD et al (eds) Neuropsychological assessment, 4th edn. Oxford University Press, New York, pp 133–155

Hanson EK, Beukelman DR, Yorkstone KM (2013) Communication support through multimodal supplementation: a scoping review. Augment Altern Commun 29(4):310–321

Hardcastle WJ (1972) The use of electropalatography in phonetic research. Phonetica 25(4):197–215

Hardcastle WJ (2006) Electromyography. In: Hardcastle WJ, Hewlett N (eds) Coarticulation: theory, data and techniques. Cambridge University Press, Cambridge, pp 270–283

Hartelius L, Buder EH, Strand EA (1997) Long-term phonatory instability in individuals with multiple sclerosis. J Speech Lang Hear Res 40(5):1056–1072

Hartelius L, Elmberg M, Holm R et al (2008) Living with dysarthria: evaluation of a self-report questionnaire. Folia Phoniatr Logop 60(1):11–19

Harvey PD (2012) Clinical applications of neuropsychological assessment. Dialogues Clin Neurosci 14(1):91–99

Hayden D, Square-Storer P (1999) Verbal motor production assessment for children. Psychological Corporation, London

Heman-Ackah YD, Heuer RJ, Michael DD et al (2003) Cepstral peak prominence: a more reliable measure of dysphonia. Ann Otol Rhinol Laryngol 112(4):324–333

Heman-Ackah YD, Mandel S, Manon-Espaillat R et al (2007) Laryngeal electromyography. Otolaryngol Clin N Am 40:1003–1023

Hemler RJB, Wieneke GH, Dejonckere PH (1997) The effect of relative humidity of inhaled air onacoustic parameters of voice in normal subjects. J Voice 11(3):295–300

Herbst CT (2020) Electroglottography - an update. J Voice 34(4):503–526

Hickok G (2012) Computational neuroanatomy of speech production. Nat Rev Neurosci 13(2):135–145

Hickok G, Poeppel D (2007) The cortical organization of speech processing. Nat Rev Neurosci 8(5):393–402

Hillis AE, Work M, Barker PB et al (2004) Re-examining the brain regions crucial for orchestrating speech articulation. Brain 127(7):1479–1487

Ho AK, Iansek R, Bradshaw JL (2002) The effect of a concurrent task on Parkinsonian speech. J Clin Exp Neuropsychol 24(1):36–47

Hohoff A, Seifert E, Fillion D et al (2003) Speech performance in lingual orthodontic patients measured by sonagraphy and auditive analysis. Am J Orthod Dentofacial Orthop 123(2):146–152

Hsieh S, Schubert S, Hoon C et al (2013) Validation of the Addenbrooke's Cognitive Examination III in frontotemporal dementia and Alzheimer's disease. Dement Geriatr Cogn Disord 36(3-4):242–250

Huber W, Poeck K, Weniger D et al (1983) Der Aachener-Aphasie Test (AAT). Hogrefe, Göttingen

Hustad KC (2006) A closer look at transcription intelligibility for speakers with dysarthria: evaluation of scoring paradigms and linguistic errors made by listeners. Am J Speech Lang Pathol 15(3):268–277

Hustad KC (2008) The relationship between listener comprehension and intelligibility scores for speakers with dysarthria. J Speech Lang Hear Res 51(3):562–573

Hustad KC, Cahill MA (2003) Effects of presentation mode and repeated familiarization on intelligibility of dysarthric speech. Am J Speech Lang Pathol 12(2):198–208

Huttunen K, Keränen H, Väyrynen E et al (2011) Effect of cognitive load on speech prosody in aviation: evidence from military simulator flights. Appl Ergon 42(2):348–357

Isshiki N (1980) Recent advances in phonosurgery. Folia Phoniatr 32:119–154

Isshiki N, Tsuji DH, Yamamoto Y et al (2000) Midline lateralization thyroplasty for adductor spasmodic dysphonia. Ann Otol Rhinol Laryngol 109:187–193

Itabashi R, Nishio Y, Kataoka Y et al (2016) Damage to the left precentral gyrus is associated with apraxia of speech in acute stroke. Stroke 47(1):31–36

Jacobson B, Johnson A, Grywalski C et al (1997) The Voice Handicap Index (VHI): development and validation. Am J Speech Lang Pathol 6(3):66–70

Jaffe TA, Hoang JK, Yoshizumi TT et al (2010) Radiation dose for routine clinical adult brain CT: variability on different scanners at one institution. Am J Roentgenol 195(2):433–438

Jenkinson C, Fitzpatrick R, Peto V et al (1997) The Parkinson's disease questionnaire (PDQ-39): develop-

ment and validation of a Parkinson's disease summary index score. Age Ageing 26(5):353–357

Jones DK (2012) Diffusion MRI: theory, methods, and applications. Oxford University Press, Oxford

Jongman A, Wayland R, Wong S (2000) Acoustic characteristics of English fricatives. J Acoust Soc Am 108(3):1252–1263

Josephs KA, Boeve BF, Duffy JR et al (2005) Atypical progressive supranuclear palsy underlying progressive apraxia of speech and nonfluent aphasia. Neurocase 11(4):283–296

Josephs KA, Duffy JR, Strand et al (2012) Characterizing a neurodegenerative syndrome: primary progressive apraxia of speech. Brain 135(5):1522–1536

Kaburagi T, Wakamiya K, Honda M (2005) Three-dimensional electromagnetic articulography: a measurement principle. J Acoust Soc Am 118:428–443

Kalimeri M, Constantoudis V, Papadimitriou C et al (2015) Word-length entropies and correlations of natural language written texts. J Quant Linguist 22(2):101–118

Kalbe E, Reinhold N, Brand M et al (2005) A new test battery to assess aphasic disturbances and associated cognitive dysfunctions—German normative data on the aphasia check list. J Clin Exp Neuropsychol 27(7):779–794

Kalvach Z, Švestková O (2004) Geriatrická ergoterapie. In: Kalvach Z, Zadák Z, Jirák R et al (eds) Geriatrie a gerontologie. Grada Publishing, Prague

Katz WF, Kripke C, Tallal P (1991) Anticipatory coarticulation in the speech of adults and young children: acoustic, perceptual, and video data. J Speech Lang Hear Res 34(6):1222–1232

Kawachi K (2002) Practice effects on speech production planning: evidence from slips of the tongue in spontaneous vs. preplanned speech in Japanese. J Psycholinguist Res 31(4):363–390

Kaza RK, Platt JF, Cohan RH et al (2012) Dual-energy CT with single- and dual-source scanners: current applications in evaluating the genitourinary tract. Radiographics 32(2):353–369

Kearney E, Giles R, Haworth B et al (2017) Sentence-level movements in Parkinson's disease: loud, clear, and slow speech. J Speech Lang Hear Res 60(12):3426–3440

Kearns KP, Simmons NN (1988) Interobserver reliability and perceptual ratings: more than meets the ear. J Speech Hear Res 31(1):131–136

Kent RD (ed) (1992) Intelligibility in speech disorders. John Benjamins Publishing Company, Amsterdam

Kent RD (1996) Hearing and believing: some limits to the auditory-perceptual assessment of speech and voice disorders. Am J Speech Lang Pathol 5(3):7–23

Kent RD (1998) Neuroimaging studies of brain activation for language, with an emphasis on functional magnetic resonance imaging: a review. Folia Phoniatr Logop 50:291–304

Kent RD, Kim Y-J (2003) Toward an acoustic typology of motor speech disorders. Clin Linguist Phon 17(6):427–445

Kent RD, Weismer G, Kent JF et al (1989) Toward phonetic intelligibility testing in dysarthria. J Speech Hear Disord 54(4):482–499

Kent RD, Duffy JR, Slama A et al (2001) Clinicoanatomic studies in dysarthria: review, critique, and directions for research. J Speech Lang Hear Res 44(3):535–551

Keshet J (2018) Automatic speech recognition: a primer for speech-language pathology researchers. Int J Speech Lang Pathol 20(6):599–609

Kessels RP, Brands AM (2009) Neuropsychological assessment. In: Biessels G, Luchsinger J (eds) Diabetes and the brain. Contemporary diabetes. Humana Press, New York, pp 77–102

Kiernan C, Reid B (1987) Pre-verbal communication schedule (PVCS). https://www.worldcat.org/title/pre-verbal-communication-schedule-pvcs-manual/oclc/221071129. Accessed 19 October 2021

Kim M-H, Lee S-Y, Lee S-E et al (2014) Anaphylaxis to iodinated contrast media: clinical characteristics related with development of anaphylactic shock. PLoS One 9(6):e100154. https://doi.org/10.1371/journal.pone.0100154

Kimaid PAT, Crespo AN, Moreira AL et al (2015) Laryngeal electromyography techniques and clinical use. J Clin Neurophysiol 32(4):274–283

Kolakowsky-Hayner SA, Caplan B (2011) Qualitative neuropsychological assessment. In: Kreutzer JS et al (eds) Encyclopedia of clinical neuropsychology. Springer, New York, pp 2098–2099

Koufman JA, Rees CJ, Halum SL et al (2006) Treatment of adductor-type spasmodic dysphonia by surgical myectomy: a preliminary report. Ann Otol Rhinol Laryngol 115:97–102

Kreiman J, Gerratt BR (1998) Validity of rating scale measures of voice quality. J Acoust Soc Am 104:1598–1608

Kröger BJ, Stille CM, Blouw P et al (2020) Hierarchical sequencing and feedforward and feedback control mechanisms in speech production: a preliminary approach for modeling normal and disordered speech. Front Comput Neurosci 14:573554. https://doi.org/10.3389/fncom.2020.573554

Kubin L, Jordan AS, Nicholas CL et al (2015) Crossed motor innervation of the base of human tongue. J Neurophysiol 113(10):3499–3510

Kuruvilla-Dugdale M, Custer C, Heidrick L et al (2018) A phonetic complexity-based approach for intelligibility and articulatory precision testing: a preliminary study on talkers with amyotrophic lateral sclerosis. J Speech Lang Hear Res 61(9):2205–2214

Kuruvilla-Dugdale M, Threlkeld K, Salazar M et al (2019) A comparative study of auditory-perceptual speech measures for the early detection of mild speech impairments. Semin Speech Lang 40(5):394–406

Kuruvilla-Dugdale M, Salazar M, Zhang A et al (2020) Detection of articulatory deficits in Parkinson's disease: can systematic manipulations of phonetic complexity help? J Speech Lang Hear Res 63(7):2084–2098

Ladefoged P (1957) Use of palatography. J Speech Hear Disord 22(5):764–774

Ladefoged P, Johnson K (2014) A course in phonetics. Cengage Learning, Boston

Landgraf R (2015) Simulating complex speech-production environments. In: Niebuhr O, Skarnitzl R (eds) Tackling the complexity in speech. Charles University Prague, Prague

Lazarus CL, Husaini H, Anand SM et al (2013) Tongue strength as a predictor of functional outcomes and quality of life after tongue cancer surgery. Ann Otol Rhinol Laryngol 122(6):386–397

Lee A (2021) Electropalatography. In: Ball MJ (ed) Manual of clinical phonetics. Routledge, London

Lee J, Bell M, Simmons Z (2018) Articulatory kinematic characteristics across the dysarthria severity spectrum in individuals with amyotrophic lateral sclerosis. Am J Speech Lang Pathol 27(1):258–269

Lekue A, García-López I, Santiago S et al (2015) Diagnosis and management with botulinum toxin in 11 cases of laryngeal synkinesis. Eur Arch Otorrinolaringol 272:2397–2402

Lezak MD, Howieson DB, Bigler ED et al (2012) Neuropsychological assessment, 5th edn. Oxford University Press, New York

Liss JM, LeGendre S, Lotto AJ (2010) Discriminating dysarthria type from envelope modulation spectra. J Speech Lang Hear Res 53(5):1246–1255

Liu W, Xia Q, Men L et al (2007) Dysphonia as a primary manifestation in myasthenia gravis (MG): a retrospective review of 7 cases among 1520 MG patients. J Neurol Sci 260:16–22

Lopez R (2016) Caring for older adults. In: Johnson A, Jacobson B (eds) Medical speech-language pathology: a practitioner's guide. Thieme Medical Publisher, New York, pp 319–325

Lowell S, Colton R, Kelley R et al (2011) Spectral- and cepstral-based measures during continuous speech: capacity to distinguish dysphonia and consistency within a speaker. J Voice 25(5):e223–e232

Ludlow CL (2009) Treatment for spasmodic dysphonia: limitations of current approaches. Curr Opin Otolaryngol Head Neck Surg 17:160–165

Ludlow CL (2015) Laryngeal reflexes: physiology, technique, and clinical use. J Clin Neurophysiol 32:284–293

Luo J, Hage SR, Moss CF (2018) The Lombard effect: from acoustics to neural mechanisms. Trends Neurosci 41(12):938–949

Ma EP, Yiu EM (2001) Voice activity and participation profile: assessing the impact of voice disorders on daily activities. J Speech Lang Hear Res 44(3):511–524

MacPherson MK, Abur D, Stepp CE (2017) Acoustic measures of voice and physiologic measures of autonomic arousal during speech as a function of cognitive load. J Voice 31(4):e501–e509. https://doi.org/10.1016/j.jvoice.2016.10.021

Magee M, Copland D, Vogel AP (2019) Motor speech and non-motor language endophenotypes of Parkinson's disease. Expert Rev Neurother 19(12):1191–1200

Malek-Ahmadi M, Mufson EJ, Perez SE (2017) Statistical considerations for assessing cognition and neuropathology associations in preclinical Alzheimer's disease. Biostat Epidemiol 1(1):92–104

Mandelli ML, Vilaplana E, Brown JA et al (2016) Healthy brain connectivity predicts atrophy progression in non-fluent variant of primary progressive aphasia. Brain 139(10):2778–2791

Mao VH, Abaza M, Spiegel JR et al (2001) Laryngeal myasthenia gravis: report of 40 cases. J Voice 15:122–130

Marini A, Carlomagno S (2004) Speech analysis and speech pathology. In: Rehabilitation methodologies in speech therapy, vol 10. Springer, Milan

Martel-Sauvageau V, Tjaden K (2017) Vocalic transitions as markers of speech acoustic changes with STN-DBS in Parkinson's disease. J Commun Disord 70:1–11

Martins PS, Barbosa-Pereira D, Valgas-Costa M et al (2020) Item analysis of the Child Neuropsychological Assessment Test (TENI): classical test theory and item response theory. Appl Neuropsychol Child 1–11. https://doi.org/10.1080/21622965.2020.1846128

Maturo S, Hill C, Bunting G et al (2012) Establishment of a normative pediatric acoustic database. Arch Otolaryngol Head Neck Surg 138(10):956–961

McNeil MR, Ballard KJ, Duffy JR et al (2017) Apraxia of speech theory, assessment, differential diagnosis, and treatment: past, present, and future. In: van Lieshout P, Maassen B, Terband H (eds) Speech motor control in normal and disordered speech: future developments in theory and methodology. ASHA Press, Rockville, pp 195–221

McRobbie DW, Moore EA, Graves MJ et al (2006) MRI from picture to proton, 2nd edn. Cambridge University Press, Cambridge

Merlo IM, Occhini A, Pacchetti C et al (2002) Not paralysis but dystonia causes stridor in multiple system atrophy. Neurology 58:649–652

Miller N (2013) Measuring up to speech intelligibility. Int J Lang Commun Disord 48(6):601–612

Molloy J, Jagoe C (2019) Use of diverse diagnostic criteria for acquired apraxia of speech: a scoping review. Int J Lang Commun Disord 54(6):875–893

Monti A, Poletti B, Zago S (2008) 'Cogmarkers' for the diagnosis of dementia of Alzheimer's type. In: Galimberti D, Scarpani E (eds) Biomarkers for early diagnosis of Alzheimer's disease. Nova Science Publishers, New York, pp 11–28

Moreno-López B, Pastor AM, de la Cruz RR et al (1997) Dose-dependent, central effects of botulinum neurotoxin type A: a pilot study in the alert behaving cat. Neurology 48:456–464

Morgan AT, Liegeois F, Occomore L (2007) Electropalatography treatment for articulation impairment in children with dysarthria post-traumatic brain injury. Brain Inj 21(11):1183–1193

Morris RJ (1989) VOT and dysarthria: a descriptive study. J Commun Disord 22(1):23–33

Mundt JC, Vogel AP, Feltner DE et al (2012) Vocal acoustic biomarkers of depression severity and treatment response. Biol Psychiatry 72(7):580–587

Murdoch BE (2011) Physiological investigation of dysarthria: recent advances. Int J Speech Lang Pathol 13(1):28–35

Nasreddine ZS, Phillips NA, Bédirian V et al (2005) The Montreal Cognitive Assessment, MoCA: a brief screening tool for mild cognitive impairment. J Am Geriatr Soc 53(4):695–699

Neel AT (2008) Vowel space characteristics and vowel identification accuracy. J Speech Lang Hear Res 51(3):574–585

Neubauer K (2007) Diagnosis of ZNPŘK in adults. In: Neubauer K, Mikešová V, Obenberger J et al (eds) Neurogenic communication disorders in adults. Portál, Prague, pp 88–116

Neubauer K (2018a) Neurogenic disorders of communication and orofacial motor skills in adults. In: Neubauer K, Pospíšilová L, Škodová E et al (eds) Kompendium der klinischen Sprachtherapie. Portál, Prague, pp 223–252

Neubauer K (2018b) Dysarthria and speech dyspraxia. In: Neubauer K (ed) Compendium of clinical speech therapy. Portál, Prague, pp 416–441

Neumann S, Quinting J, Rosenkranz A et al (2019) Quality of life in adults with neurogenic speech-language-communication difficulties: a systematic review of existing measures. J Commun Disord 79:24–45

Noffs G, Perera T, Kolbe SC et al (2018) What speech can tell us: a systematic review of dysarthria characteristics in multiple sclerosis. Autoimmun Rev 17(12):1202–1209

Nordenberg M, Sundberg J (2004) Effect on LTAS of vocal loudness variation. Logoped Phoniatr Vocol 29(4):183–191

Nutt JG, Muenter MD, Aronson A et al (1988) Epidemiology of focal and generalized dystonia in Rochester, Minnesota. Mov Disord 3:188–194

Oeckl P, Jardel C, Salachas F et al (2016) Multicenter validation of CSF neurofilaments as diagnostic biomarkers for ALS. Amyotroph Lateral Scler Frontotemporal Degener 17(5-6):404–413

Ogar J, Slama H, Dronkers N et al (2005) Apraxia of speech: an overview. Neurocase 11(6):427–432

Osserman KE, Genkins G (1971) Studies in myasthenia gravis: review of a twenty-year experience in over 1200 patients. Mt Sinai J Med 38:497–537

Palmer R, Enderby P (2007) Methods of speech therapy treatment for stable dysarthria: a review. Adv Speech Lang Pathol 9(2):140–153

Palmer SJ, Ng B, Abugharbieh R et al (2009) Motor reserve and novel area recruitment: amplitude and spatial characteristics of compensation in Parkinson's disease. Eur J Neurosci 29(11):2187–2196

Paniello RC, Barlow J, Serna JS (2008) Longitudinal follow-up of adductor spasmodic dysphonia patients after botulinum toxin injection: quality of life results. Laryngoscope 118:564–568

Paniello RC, Edgar JD, Perlmutter JS (2009) Vocal exercise versus voice rest following botulinum toxin injections: a randomized crossover trial. Ann Otol Rhinol Laryngol 118:759–763

Parsa V, Jamieson DG, Pretty BR (2001) Effects of microphone type on acoustic measures of voice. J Voice 15(3):331–343

Patel N, Peterson KA, Ingram R et al (2020) The Mini Linguistic State Examination (MLSE): a brief but accurate assessment tool for classifying primary progressive aphasias. medRxiv. https://doi.org/10.1101/2 020.06.02.20119974. Accessed 4 Aug 2021

Patel RR, Awan SN, Barkmeier-Kraemer J et al (2018) Recommended protocols for instrumental assessment of voice: American Speech-Language-Hearing Association expert panel to develop a protocol for instrumental assessment of vocal function. Am J Speech Lang Pathol 27(3):887–905

Patrocinio D, Trittola I (2005) Counselling in phoniatrics and speech therapy. La Garangola, Padua

Pattee GL, Plowman EK, Focht Garand KL et al (2019) Provisional best practices guidelines for the evaluation of bulbar dysfunction in amyotrophic lateral sclerosis. Muscle Nerve 59(5):531–536

Paul D, Frattali C, Holland A et al (2004) Quality of communication life scale: manual. American Speech-Language Hearing Association, Rockville

Peeters G (2004) A large set of audio features for sound description (similarity and classification) in the CUIDADO project. IRCAM. https://hal.archives-ouvertes.fr/hal-01253651/document. Accessed 19 January 2021

Pen AE, Quinn R (1997) Task familiarity: effects on the test performance of Puerto Rican and African American children. Lang Speech Hear Serv Sch 28(4):323–332

Peppé S, McCann J (2003) Profiling elements of prosody in speech-communication (PEPS-C). http://www.peps-c.com/. Accessed 19 October 2021

Peus S (2004) Modern acoustic and electronic design of studio condenser microphones. Paper presented at the 116th Audio Engineering Society Convention in Berlin. Paper 6131. https://www.aes.org/e-lib/online/browse.cfm?elib=12692. Accessed 21 October 2021

Piacentini V, Zuin A, Cattaneo D et al (2011) Reliability and validity of an instrument to measure quality of life in the dysarthric speaker. Folia Phoniatr Logop 63(3):289–295

Piacentini V, Mauri I, Cattaneo D et al (2014) Relationship between quality of life and dysarthria in patients with multiple sclerosis. Arch Phys Med Rehabil 95(11):2047–2054

Pinho P, Monteiro L, de Paula Soares MF et al (2018) Impact of levodopa treatment in the voice pattern of Parkinson's disease patients: a systematic review and meta-analysis. Codas 30(5):e20170200. https://doi.org/10.1590/2317-1782/20182017200

Pommée T, Balaguer M, Mauclair J et al (2021a) Intelligibility and comprehensibility: a Delphi consensus study. Int J Lang Commun. https://doi.org/10.1111/1460-6984.12672

Pommée T, Balaguer M, Mauclair J et al (2021b) Assessment of adult speech disorders: current situation and needs in French-speaking clinical practice. Logoped Phoniatr Vocol. https://doi.org/10.1080/140 15439.2020.1870245

Pradhan P, Bhardwaj A, Venkatachalam VP (2016) Bilateral cricoarytenoid arthritis: a cause of recurrent upper airway obstruction in rheumatoid arthritis Malays. J Med Sci 23:89–91

Preston DC, Shapiro BE (2013) Electromyography and neuromuscular disorders: clinical-electrophysiologic correlations, 3rd edn. Saunders, St Louis

Prutting C, Kirchner D (1987) A clinical appraisal of the pragmatic aspects of language. J Speech Hear Disord 52(2):105–119

Rampone P, Miletto AM (2010) Role of the speech therapist. Acta Phon Lat 32:73–82

Randolph C, Tierney MC, Mohr E et al (1998) The Repeatable Battery for the Assessment of Neuropsychological Status (RBANS): preliminary clinical validity. J Clin Exp Neuropsychol 20(3):310–319

Rautakoski P (2011) Training total communication. Aphasiology 25:344–365

Ravaud JF, Delcey M, Yelnik A (1999) Construct validity of the functional independence measure (FIM): questioning the unidimensionality of the scale and the "value" of FIM scores. Scand J Rehabil Med 31(1):31–41

RCP (2016) National clinical guideline for stroke, 5th edn. Royal College of Physicians, London, p 151

Redford MA (2019) Speech production from a developmental perspective. J Speech Lang Hear Res 62(8s):2946–2962

Rektorova I, Mekyska J, Janousova E et al (2016) Speech prosody impairment predicts cognitive decline in Parkinson's disease. Parkinsonism Relat Disord 29:90–95

Renard D, Hedayat A, Gagnard C (2015) Isolated laryngeal myasthenia gravis for 26 years. Neuromuscul Disord 25:153–154

Riesthal M (2016) Assessment and management of neurogenic speech disorders. In: Johnson A, Jacobson B (eds) Medical speech-language pathology: a practitioner's guide. Thieme Medical Publisher, New York, pp 119–134

Rinkel RN, Verdonck-de Leeuw IM, van Reij EJ et al (2008) Speech Handicap Index in patients with oral and pharyngeal cancer: better understanding of patients' complaints. Head Neck 30(7):868–874

Rivero-Santana A, Ferreira D, Perestelo-Perez L et al (2017) Cerebrospinal fluid biomarkers for the differential diagnosis between Alzheimer's disease and frontotemporal lobar degeneration: systematic review, HSROC analysis, and confounding factors. J Alzheimers Dis 55(2):625–644

Robertson S, Fay T (1993) Working with dysarthrics. In: A practical guide to therapy for dysarthria. Winslow Press, Oxon

Rohling ML, Axelrod BN, Langhinrichsen-Rohling J (2017) Fundamental forensic statistics: statistics every forensic neuropsychologist must know. In: Bush SS et al (eds) APA handbook of forensic neuropsychology. American Psychiatric Association Publishing, Washington, pp 3–22

Rosen KM, Goozée JV, Murdoch BE (2008) Examining the effects of multiple sclerosis on speech production: Does phonetic structure matter? J Commun Disord 41(1):49–69

Rosenbek J, LaPointe L (1978) The dysarthrias: description, diagnosis, and treatment. In: Johns D (ed) Clinical management of neurogenic communication disorders. Little, Brown & Co., Boston

Roy N, Mauszycki SC, Merrill RM et al (2007) Toward improved differential diagnosis of adductor spasmodic dysphonia and muscle tension dysphonia. Folia Phoniatr Logop 59(2):83–90

Rumbach AF, Finch E, Stevenson G (2019) What are the usual assessment practices in adult non-progressive dysarthria rehabilitation? A survey of Australian dysarthria practice patterns. J Commun Disord 79:46–57

Russell R, Grizzle K (2008) Assessing child and adolescent pragmatic language competencies: toward evidence-based assessments. Clin Child Fam Psychol Rev 11(1-2):59–73

Rusz J, Cmejla R, Ruzickova H et al (2011) Quantitative acoustic measurements for characterization of speech and voice disorders in early untreated Parkinson's disease. J Acoust Soc Am 129(1):350–367

Saran M, Georgakopoulos B, Bordoni B (2021) Anatomy, head and neck, larynx vocal folds. In: StatPearls. StatPearls Publishing, Treasure Island

Schaefer SY, Duff K (2017) Within-session and one-week practice effects on a motor task in amnestic mild cognitive impairment. J Clin Exp Neuropsychol 39(5):473–484

Scherr M, Kunz A, Doll A et al (2016) Ignoring floor and ceiling effects may underestimate the effect of carotid artery stenting on cognitive performance. J Neurointerv Surg 8(7):747–751

Schalling E, Johansson K, Hartelius L (2017) Speech and communication changes reported people with Parkinson's disease. Folia Phoniatr Logop 69(3):131–141

Schweinfurth JM, Billante M, Courey MS (2002) Risk factors and demographics in patients with spasmodic dysphonia. Laryngoscope 112:220–223

Schweizer V, Woodson GE, Bertorini TE (1999) Single-fiber electromyography of the laryngeal muscles. Muscle Nerve 22:111–114

Shamei A, Bird S (2019) An acoustic analysis of cannabis-intoxicated speech. Can Acoust 47(3):108–109

Shaw GY, Sechtem PR, Rideout B (2003) Posterior cricoarytenoid myoplasty with medialization thyroplasty in the management of refractory abductor spasmodic dysphonia. Ann Otol Rhinol Laryngol 112:303–306

Shipley K, McAfee J (2016) Assessment procedures common to most communicative disorders. Assessment in speech-language pathology: a resource manual, 5th edn. Cengage Learning, Boston, pp 145–148

Shriberg L, Paul R, McSweeny J et al (2001) Speech and prosody characteristics of adolescents and adults with high functioning autism and Asperger syndrome. J Speech Lang Hear Res 44(5):1097–1115

Siciliano M, Chiorri C, Battini V et al (2019) Regression-based normative data and equivalent scores for Trail Making Test (TMT): an updated Italian normative study. Neurol Sci 40(3):469–477

Sidtis J, Van Lancker Sidtis D (2003) A neurobehavioral approach to dysprosody. Semin Speech Lang 24(2):93–105

Sieroslawska A (2022) Muscles of the larynx. Kenhub GmbH, Leipzig

Sigmund M, Zelinka P (2011) Analysis of voiced speech excitation due to alcohol intoxication. Info Tech Control 40(2):143–150

Simonyan K, Barkmeier-Kraemer J, Blitzer A et al (2021) NIH/NIDCD Workshop on research priorities in spasmodic dysphonia/laryngeal dystonia. Laryngeal dystonia: consensus on terminology, pathophysiology, and research priorities. Neurology 10:1212. https://doi.org/10.1212/WNL.0000000000011922

Skarnitzl R, Volín J (2018) Sound base of speech communication. In: Neubauer K (ed) Compendium of clinical speech therapy. Portál, Prague, pp 122–169

Skarnitzl R, Šturm P, Volín J (2016) Sound base of speech communication. Karolinum, Prague

Skodda S, Grönheit W, Mancinelli N et al (2013) Progression of voice and speech impairment in the course of Parkinson's disease: a longitudinal study. Parkinson's Dis 2013:389195. https://doi.org/10.1155/2013/389195

Somerville J, Tremont G, Stern RA (2000) The Boston Qualitative Scoring System as a measure of executive functioning in Rey–Osterrieth Complex Figure performance. J Clin Exp Neuropsychol 22(5):613–621

Sörös P, Sokoloff LG, Bose A et al (2006) Clustered functional MRI of overt speech production. NeuroImage 32(1):376–387

Strub RL, Gardner H (1974) The repetition defect in conduction aphasia: mnestic or linguistic? Brain Lang 1(3):241–255

Sugden E, Lloyd S, Lam J et al (2019) Systematic review of ultrasound visual biofeedback in intervention for speech sound disorders. Int J Lang Commun Disord 54(5):705–728

Sulica L (2013) Vocal fold paresis: an evolving clinical concept. Curr Otorhinolaryngol Rep 1:158–162

Sussman JE, Tjaden K (2012) Perceptual measures of speech from individuals with Parkinson's disease and multiple sclerosis: intelligibility and beyond. J Speech Lang Hear Res 55(4):1208–1219

Švec JG, Granqvist S (2010) Guidelines for selecting microphones for human voice production research. Am J Speech Lang Pathol 19(4):356–368

Terband H, Maassen B, Maas E (2019) A psycholinguistic framework for diagnosis and treatment planning of developmental speech disorders. Folia Phoniatr Logop 71(5-6):216–227

Teston B (2007) The instrumental study of gestures in the production of speech: Importance of aerophonometry. In: Auzou P, Monnoury-Rolland V, Pinto S et al (eds) Dysarthria. Solal, Marseille, pp 115–117

Trevethan R (2017) Sensitivity, specificity, and predictive values: foundations, pliabilities, and pitfalls in research and practice. Front Public Health 5:307. https://doi.org/10.3389/fpubh.2017.00307

Titche LL (1976) Causes of recurrent laryngeal nerve paralysis. Arch Otolaryngol 102:259–261

Titze IR, Winholtz WS (1993) Effect of microphone type and placement on voice perturbation measurements. J Speech Hear Res 36(6):1177–1190

Tjaden K, Watling E (2003) Characteristics of diadochokinesis in multiple sclerosis and Parkinson's disease. Folia Phoniatr Logop 55(5):241–259

Todisco M, Alfonsi E, Isaias IU et al (2020) Vocal fold electromyographic correlates of stridor in multiple system atrophy phenotypes. Parkinsonism Relat Disord 70:31–35

Togher L (2018) Pragmatics and discourse. In: LaPointe L, Stierwalt J (eds) Aphasia and related neurogenic language disorders. Thieme, New York, pp 124–134

Trupe LA, Varma DD, Gomez Y et al (2013) Chronic apraxia of speech and Broca's area. Stroke 44(3):740–744

Tsanas A, Zañartu M, Little MA et al (2014) Robust fundamental frequency estimation in sustained vowels: detailed algorithmic comparisons and information fusion with adaptive Kalman filtering. J Acoust Soc Am 135(5):2885–2901

Urban PP, Rolke R, Wicht S et al (2006) Left-hemispheric dominance for articulation: a prospective study on acute ischaemic dysarthria at different localizations. Brain 129(3):767–777

Utianski RL, Duffy JR, Clark HM et al (2018) Prosodic and phonetic subtypes of primary progressive apraxia of speech. Brain Lang 184:54–65

van Lieshout P (2021) Electromagnetic articulography. In: Ball MJ (ed) Manual of clinical phonetics. Routledge, London

Van Santen JPH, Prud'hommeaux ET, Black LM (2009) Automated assessment of prosody production. Speech Comm 51(11):1082–1097

Vansteensel MJ, Jarosiewicz B (2020) Brain-computer interfaces for communication. In: Ramsey NF, del Millán JR (eds) Handbook of clinical neurology, vol 168. Elsevier, Cambridge, pp 67–85

Vetrugno R, Liguori R, Cortelli P et al (2007) Sleep-related stridor due to dystonic vocal fold motion and neurogenic tachypnea/tachycardia in multiple system atrophy. Mov Disord 22:673–678

Vogel AP, Maruff P (2008) Comparison of voice acquisition methodologies in speech research. Behav Res Methods 40(4):982–987

Vogel AP, Morgan AT (2009) Factors affecting the quality of sound recording for speech and voice analysis. Int J Speech Lang Pathol 11(6):431–437

Vogel AP, Reece H (2021) Recording speech. In: Ball MJ (ed) Manual of clinical phonetics. Routledge, London

Vogel AP, Fletcher J, Maruff P (2010) Acoustic analysis of the effects of sustained wakefulness on speech. J Acoust Soc Am 128(6):3747–3756

Vogel AP, Fletcher J, Snyder PJ et al (2011) Reliability, stability, and sensitivity to change and impairment in acoustic measures of timing and frequency. J Voice 25(2):137–149

Vogel AP, Shirbin C, Churchyard AJ et al (2012) Speech acoustic markers of early stage and prodromal Huntington's disease: a marker of disease onset? Neuropsychologia 50(14):3273–3278

Vogel AP, Fletcher J, Maruff P (2014) The impact of task automaticity on speech in noise. Speech Comm 65:1–8

Vogel AP, Poole ML, Pemberton H et al (2017a) Motor speech signature of behavioral variant frontotemporal dementia: refining the phenotype. Neurology 89(8):837–844

Vogel AP, Wardrop MI, Folker JE et al (2017b) Voice in Friedreich ataxia. J Voice 31(2):243. https://doi.org/10.1016/j.jvoice.2016.04.015

Vogel AP, Magee M, Torres-Vega R et al (2020) Features of speech and swallowing dysfunction in pre-ataxic spinocerebellar ataxia type 2. Neurology 95(2):e194–e205. https://doi.org/10.1212/WNL.0000000000009776

Wagner R, Torgesen J (1987) The nature of phonological processing and its causal role in the acquisition of reading skills. Psychol Bull 101(2):192–212

Walsh B, Smith A (2012) Basic parameters of articulatory movements and acoustics in individuals with Parkinson's disease. Mov Disord 27(7):843–580

Walshe M, Peach RK, Miller N (2009) The dysarthria impact profile: validation of an instrument to measure psychosocial impact in dysarthria. Int J Lang Commun Disord 44(5):693–715

Wannberg P, Schalling E, Hartelius L (2016) Perceptual assessment of dysarthria: comparison of a general and a detailed assessment protocol. Logoped Phoniatr Vocol 41(4):159–167

Ware JE, Sherbourne CD (1992) The MOS 36-item short-form health survey (SF-36): I. Conceptual framework and item selection. Med Care 30(6):473–483

Watson RM, Pennington L (2015) Assessment and management of the communication difficulties of children with cerebral palsy: a UK survey of SLT practice. Int J Lang Commun Disord 50(2):241–259

Watzlawick P, Beavin JH, Jackson DD (1967–2011) Pragmatics of human communication. A study of interactional patterns, pathologies, and paradoxes. Norton, New York

Wechsler D (2008) Wechsler adult intelligence scale (WAIS-IV), 4th edn. NCS Pearson, San Antonio

Wertz RT, LaPointe LL, Rosenbek JC (1984) Apraxia of speech: the disorders and its management. Grune and Stratton, New York

Whitfield J, Goberman A (2017) Articulatory-acoustic vowel space: associations between acoustic and perceptual measures of clear speech. Int J Speech Lang Pathol 19(2):184–194

Willmes K (2010) The methodological and statistical foundations of neuropsychological assessment. In: Gurd J, Kischka U, Marshall J (eds) The handbook of clinical neuropsychology, 2nd edn. Oxford University Press, New York, pp 28–49

Wintermark M, Sanelli PC, Albers GW et al (2013) Imaging recommendations for acute stroke and transient ischemic attack patients: joint statement by the American Society of Neuroradiology, the American College of Radiology, and the Society of NeuroInterventional Surgery. Am J Neuroradiol 34(11):E117–E127

Woisard V, Espesser R, Ghio A et al (2013) From intelligibility to comprehensibility of speech, which measures in clinical practice? Rev Laryngol Otol Rhinol 134(1):27–33

Woisard V, Astésano C, Balaguer M et al (2020) C2SI corpus: a database of speech disorder productions to assess intelligibility and quality of life in head and neck cancers. Lang Resour Eval. https://doi.org/10.1007/s10579-020-09496-3

Woldorf NM, Pastore PN, Terz J (1971) Rheumatoid arthritis of the cricoarytenoid joint. Arch Otolaryngol 93:623–627

Woo P, Mangaro M (2004) Aberrant recurrent laryngeal nerve reinnervation as a cause of stridor and laryngospasm. Ann Otol Rhinol Laryngol 113:805–808

World Health Organization (1993) The ICD-10 classification of mental and behavioural disorders: diagnostic criteria for research. World Health Organization, Geneva

World Health Organization (2001) International classification of functioning, disability and health. https://www.who.int/standards/classifications/international--classification-of-functioning-disability-and-health. Accessed 7 November 2021

World Health Organization (2014) International classification of functioning, disability and health. www.who.int/classifications/icf/en/. Accessed 7 April 2021

Wormald RN, Moran RJ, Reilly RB et al (2008) Performance of an automated, remote system to detect vocal fold paralysis. Ann Otol Rhinol Laryngol 117(11):834–838

Wysowski DK, Nourjah P (2006) Deaths attributed to X-ray contrast media on U.S. death certificates. Am J Roentgenol 186(3):613–615

Xu W, Han D, Hou L et al (2009) Clinical and electrophysiological characteristics of larynx in myasthenia gravis. Ann Otol Rhinol Laryngol 118:656–661

Yorkston KM, Bombardier C, Hammen VL (1994) Dysarthria from the viewpoint of individuals with dysarthria. In: Till JA, Yorkston KM, Beukelman DR (eds) Motor speech disorders: advances in assessment and treatment. Brookes Publishing, Baltimore, pp 19–36

Yorkston KM, Strand EA, Kennedy MRT (1996) Comprehensibility of dysarthric speech. J Speech Lang Pathol 5(1):55–66

Yorkston K, Beukelman D, Strand R et al (1999) Management of motor speech disorders in children and adults. Pro-Ed, Austin

Young Y, Fan M, Hebel J et al (2009) Concurrent validity of administering the functional independence measure (FIM™) instrument by interview. Am J Phys Med Rehabil 88(9):766–770

Ziegler W, Aichert I, Staiger A (2012) Apraxia of speech: concepts and controversies. J Speech Lang Hear Res 55(5):S1485–S1501

Zou Z-F, Chen W, Li W et al (2019) Impact of vocal fold dehydration on vocal unction and its treatment. Curr Med Sci 39(2):310–316

# Prevention of Acquired Motor Speech Disorders (Dysarthria, Dyspraxia)

# 19

Giovanni Ruoppolo

## 19.1 Understanding the Importance of Early Diagnosis and Therapy of Speech and Swallowing Disorders due to Neurological Diseases

Giovanni Ruoppolo

Both dysphagia and dysarthria are highly prevalent among patients with neurological disorders. Early intervention in dysphagic patients is crucial to prevent the risk of aspiration, fluid depletion and malnutrition. Robust scientific evidence supports the relationship between swallowing deficits, excess morbidity and increased mortality rates (Martino et al. 2000). In particular oropharyngeal dysphagia is a common deficit after stroke, occurring in approximately 21–91% of patients. Of these subjects, 65% present this symptom within the first 5 days of hospitalisation, leading to a sixfold increase in risk for aspiration pneumonia and a threefold increase for mortality. In most stroke patients the mainstay of management is to keep them safe by means of a careful examination and management of swallowing while spontaneous recovery takes place (Singh and Hamdy 2006). In patients with trau-

matic brain injury, swallowing impairment also represents a significant problem, ranging from 25% to 93% (Lee et al. 2016).

In neurodegenerative diseases early intervention for swallowing disorders is also particularly important. The scientific literature has mainly focused on Parkinson disease (PD) and on amyotrophic lateral sclerosis (ALS). In PD more than 80% of patients develop dysphagia during the course of the disease (Suttrup and Warnecke 2016). Swallowing deficits are often significantly debilitating in the later stages of the disease, reducing the quality of life and contributing to dehydration, malnutrition and aspiration pneumonia, the leading cause of death of patients with PD. Behavioural therapies, the use of expiratory muscle strength training, compensatory manoeuvres and diet modifications can help patients to improve swallowing safety (Broadfoot et al. 2019; see Chap. 30). Early recognition of dysphagia in ALS is possible if there is periodic objective evaluation of swallowing in all the patients; this allows identification of those who need percutaneous endoscopic gastrostomy (PEG), giving them a higher probability of survival (Onesti et al. 2017).

In addition, in recent years research has continued to report the impact that dysphagia has on the quality of life (QoL) of neurological patients (see Sect. 28.8). In both PD and ALS, swallowing-related QoL scores worsen with disease progression. In the stroke population dysphagia also

G. Ruoppolo (✉)
Sapienza University, Rome, Italy

contributes to feelings of social isolation and altered relationships with family (Moloney and Walshe 2019).

The management of dysarthria, although not critical for survival, is also important because of the impact of the speech impairment on communication. Dysarthric subjects may experience isolation and restrictions on participation in family and working life. A significant correlation between the quality of life in dysarthric speakers and the severity of dysarthria has been reported (Brady et al. 2011; Piacentini et al. 2011). Unfortunately, many people with dysarthria are never referred for management because of ignorance about what can be done to help them (Duffy 2013). The decision to treat depends upon the degree of impairment, but activity limitation and participation restrictions must also be considered in addressing management issues and goals (Duffy 2013). For example, a mild articulatory imprecision might not reduce speech intelligibility but could restrict the work role of a professional; the same deficit might not limit the social interactions of a retired person. Obviously psychological and environmental factors must also be taken into account.

In the treatment of dysarthria it is generally agreed that early treatment is desirable; nonetheless, behavioural management should not begin until the patient is medically stable and medical management is complete or under way. In the field of motor speech disorders it is difficult to establish what constitutes an early treatment (Duffy 2013). Some evidence suggests that in stroke patients early treatment is most effective: motor learning mechanisms are operative during spontaneous stroke recovery and interact with rehabilitative training (Krakauer 2006). On the other hand it is possible that, both in stroke and in traumatic brain injury (TBI) subjects, a slight delay in treatment may permit structural and physiological changes that are important to prepare the patient for the positive changes that may occur with exercise (Kleim et al. 2003). In clinical reality, however, in acute care units there are few opportunities to submit the patient to speech rehabilitation, which usually begins after the patient is discharged and transferred to a rehabilitation hospital, and which is several days or weeks after acute injury. Dysarthria should be treated early, not only to achieve a better outcome and to counter activity limitation and participation restriction, but also to prevent the use by the subject of maladaptive compensatory strategies that further worsen the intelligibility of speech and result in a delay of the recovery. Moreover, if dysarthria persists, caregivers also tend to modify their verbal behaviour over time, with further frustration of the patient and of the family members.

With regard to neurodegenerative diseases, dysarthria is of particular importance in PD, owing to the high prevalence of this pathology. About 90% of individuals with PD develop an extra-pyramidal hypokinetic-hypertonic dysarthria characterised by reduced loudness, reduced pitch fluctuations and articulatory impairments. Early speech management, in particular the Lee Silverman Voice Treatment (Sapir et al. 2007), has shown improvements in speech functionality, at least in the short-term, reducing speech difficulties and improving the QoL of these patients (Broadfoot et al. 2019).

Any treatment for dysphagia or dysarthria should be based on the understanding of the underlying pathophysiological mechanism; for this reason a full phoniatric assessment must lead to the understanding of the specific anatomical or physiological deficit and should precede the prescription of rehabilitation (see Chap. 20). The pathophysiological assessment should be quantitative, as it represents the baseline for establishing goals and measuring changes over time. Medical diagnosis, usually performed by neurologists, is also of pivotal importance as it has prognostic implications.

## References

Brady MC, Clark AM, Dickson S et al (2011) The impact of stroke-related dysarthria on social participation and implications for rehabilitation. Disabil Rehabil 33:178–186

Broadfoot CK, Abur D, Hoffmeister JD et al (2019) Research-based updates in swallowing and communication dysfunction in Parkinson disease: implications for evaluation and management. Perspect ASHA Spec Interest Groups 4:825–841

Duffy JR (2013) Motor speech disorders. Substrates, differential diagnosis and management. Elsevier, St. Louis

Kleim JA, Jones TA, Schallert T (2003) Motor enrichment and the induction of plasticity before or after brain injury. Neurochem Res 28:1757–1769

Krakauer JW (2006) Motor learning: its relevance to stroke recovery and neurorehabilitation. Curr Opin Neurol 19:84–90

Lee WK, Yeom J, Lee WH et al (2016) Characteristics of dysphagia in severe traumatic brain injury patients: a comparison with stroke patients. Ann Rehabil Med 40:432–439

Martino R, Pron G, Diamant N (2000) Screening for oro-pharyngeal dysphagia in stroke: insufficient evidence for guidelines. Dysphagia 15:19–30

Moloney J, Walshe M (2019) Managing and supporting quality-of-life issues in dysphagia: a survey of clinical practice patterns and perspectives in the UK, Ireland and South Africa. Int J Lang Commun Disord 54:41–49

Onesti E, Schettino I, Gori MC et al (2017) Dysphagia in amyotrophic lateral sclerosis: impact on patient behavior, diet adaptation, and Riluzole management. Front Neurol 8:94. https://doi.org/10.3389/fneur.2017.00094

Piacentini V, Zuin A, Cattaneo D et al (2011) Reliability and validity of an instrument to measure quality of life in the dysarthric speaker. Folia Phoniatr Logop 63:289–295

Sapir S, Spielman JL, Ramig LO et al (2007) Effects of intensive voice treatment (the Lee Silverman Voice Treatment [LSVT]) on vowel articulation in dysarthric individuals with idiopathic Parkinson disease: acoustic and perceptual findings. J Speech Lang Hear Res 50:899–912

Singh S, Hamdy S (2006) Dysphagia in stroke patients. Postgrad Med J 82:383–391

Suttrup I, Warnecke T (2016) Dysphagia in Parkinson's disease. Dysphagia 31:24–32

# Rehabilitative Approaches and Prognosis for Acquired Motor Speech Disorders: Dysarthria and Dyspraxia

# 20

Tobias Bernasconi, Salvatore Biondi, Andrea Calvo, Adriano Chio, Ashley Craig, Philippe H. Dejonckere, Michelangelo Dini, Kurt Eggers, Roberta Ferrucci, Matteo Guidetti, Claudio Luzzatti, Anita McAllister, Donato Mecca, Karel Neubauer, Lenka Neubauerová, Danilo Patrocinio, Cristina Polimeno, Alberto Priori, Stefanie K. Sachse, Vincenzo Sallustio, Antonio Schindler, Iolanda Trittola, and Madeleine Wertsén

The original version of the chapter has been revised. A correction to this chapter can be found at https://doi.org/10.1007/978-3-031-48091-1_18

Danilo Patrocinio passed away before the time of publication.

**Supplementary Information** The online version contains supplementary material available at https://doi.org/10.1007/978-3-031-48091-1_5.

T. Bernasconi (✉)
Humanwissenschaftliche Fakultät, Department Heilpädagogik und Rehabilitation, University of Cologne, Köln, Germany
e-mail: tobias.bernasconi@uni-koeln.de

S. Biondi
Policlinico G. Rodolico - Department of Otorhinolaryngology, University of Catania, Catania, Italy
e-mail: salvatore.biondi@tin.it

A. Calvo · A. Chio
Department of Neuroscience 'Rita Levi Montalcini', University of Turin, Turin, Italy
e-mail: andrea.calvo@unito.it; adriano.chio@unito.it

A. Craig
University of Sydney, John Walsh Centre for Rehabilitation Research, Royal North Shore Hospital, St Leonards, NSW, Australia
e-mail: a.craig@sydney.edu.au

P. H. Dejonckere
Federal Agency for Occupational Risks, Brussels, Belgium

M. Dini
Foundation IRCCS Ca' Granda Ospedale Maggiore Policlinico, Milan, Italy
e-mail: angelica.desandi@policlinico.mi.it

K. Eggers
Thomas More University College, Thomas More Campus Sint-Andries, Antwerpen, Belgium
e-mail: kurt.eggers@thomasmore.be

R. Ferrucci
Policlinico, Fondazione IRCCS Ca' Granda Ospedale Maggiore, Milan, Italy
e-mail: roberta.ferrucci@unimi.it

## 20.1 Coordination of Rehabilitative Measures

Vincenzo Sallustio, Danilo Patrocinio, Donato Mecca, Cristina Polimeno and Iolanda Trittola

The planning of treatment and admission into a rehabilitation facility for patients suffering from motor speech disorders (MSD) are complex procedures (Duffy 2019). The rehabilitative team may consist of various professionals including phoniatricians, speech language pathologists, physiotherapists, psychomotricity therapists, occupational therapists, neurologists, neurosurgeons, pulmonologists, psychologists, neuropsychologists and physiatrists. The phoniatrician, as rehabilitator for training, is essential in this team, since the phoniatric evaluation assesses the type and severity of the MSD, which is the basis for establishing the rehabilitation plan. Although any member of the team is entitled to assume the responsibilities of coordinator and lead the team with regard to the customised rehabilitation plan development, in some countries, local legislation requires that the person in charge of the rehabilitation plan be a physician with specialised training in rehabilitation.

In any case, the approach of the rehabilitation team to dysarthria is "communicational", "ecological" and global; it proceeds according to both biological and humanistic guidelines and is managed according to efficiency criteria and evidence-based medicine (EBM) in the international classification of functioning, disability and health (ICF) framework (Sackett et al. 1996; Straus et al. 2011; WHA 2001).

The customised rehabilitative plan should take into account the:

- Patient's needs and preferences (or those of their relatives, if necessary).
- Patient's impairments, disabilities, limitations and restrictions.
- Patient's residual or recoverable abilities.
- Environmental, contextual and personal factors.

Furthermore, the criteria for the rehabilitative measure management and coordination should

M. Guidetti · A. Priori
Department of Health Sciences, "Aldo Ravelli"
Center for Neurotechnology and Experimental Brain
Therapeutics, University of Milan, Milan, Italy

Clinical Neurology Unit, Azienda Socio-Sanitaria
Territoriale Santi Paolo E Carlo, Milan, Italy
e-mail: matteo.guidetti@unimi.it;
alberto.priori@unimi.it

C. Luzzatti
Department of Psychology, University of Milan
Bicocca, Milan, Italy
e-mail: claudio.luzzatti@unimib.it

A. McAllister
CLINTEC Division of Speech and Language
Pathology, Karolinska Institutet, Stockholm, Sweden
e-mail: anita.mcallister@ki.se

D. Mecca · D. Patrocinio (Deceased) · C. Polimeno
V. Sallustio  I. Trittola
Phoniatric and Communicative Disorders
Rehabilitative Center, ASL Lecce, Rehabilitation
Department, Lecce, Italy
e-mail: meccado@libero.it;
cristina.polimeno@asl.lecce.it;
vincenzo.sallustio@asl.lecce.it;
antonellatrittola@libero.it

K. Neubauer
Clinic of Phoniatrics of University Hospital Prague,
Charles University Faculty of Medicine,
Prague 2, Czech Republic
e-mail: Karel.Neubauer@lf1.cuni.cz

L. Neubauerová
Institute of Social Work, Philosophical Faculty of the
University of Hradec Králové,
Hradec Kralova, Czech Republic
e-mail: lenka.neubauerova@uhk.cz

S. K. Sachse
FBZ-UK, University of Cologne, Cologne, Germany
e-mail: stefanie.sachse@uni-koeln.de

A. Schindler
Luigi Sacco Hospital, Department of Biomedical
and Clinical Sciences "L. Sacco", Phoniatrics,
University of Milan, Milan, Italy
e-mail: antonio.schindler@unimi.it

M. Wertsén
Clinic of Pedodontics and Special Dental Care,
Sahlgrenska University Hospital, Mölndal, Sweden
e-mail: madeleine.wertsen@vgregion.se

also consider the following factors (ASHA 2021), the:

- Age at onset of MSD development or acquisition.
- Medical (neurological) diagnosis, nature and site of lesion.
- Course of disease: congenital, improving stationary, progressive, fluctuating.
- Associated symptoms (dysphagia, respiratory disorders, cognitive or executive function impairments, upper/lower limb motor impairments, etc.)
- Speech and non-verbal communication impairment type and extent.
- Patient's psychological and behavioural profile.
- Health care system availability.
- Efficient caregiver availability at home.
- Patient's motivation (and that of their family).

The purposes to pursue, in agreement with the patient and their family, may be:

- To restore lost function and decrease the impairment (i.e., speech or surgical therapy in idiopathic unilateral vocal fold paralysis).
- Compensation: to promote the use of residual function and reduce the activity limitation (i.e., behavioural, prosthetic compensation, augmentative and alternative communication means).
- Reorganisation of work, social and relational activities suited to the feasible communication methods.
- Best quality of life possible for each patient.

The specific rehabilitation activities are driven by the current knowledge on neuroplasticity, procedural memory and motor learning. The rehabilitation team should discuss the possible types of intervention, their use in variable sequences and composition, as appropriate to the patient's clinical status, including:

- Pharmacological intervention.
- Surgical intervention (deep brain stimulation included).
- Prosthetic compensation (augmentative and alternative communication and computerised rehabilitation included).
- Behavioural compensation.
- Speech-language therapy.
- Counselling the patient and their family, seeking the best possible communicative conditions (control and modification of living environments, proxemics and orientation of the interlocutor, conversation shifts, conventional smart talk, etc.)
- Intervention on associated symptoms (i.e., dysphagia).

Some of these interventions, such as pharmacological and surgical, including botulinum toxin injection, must necessarily be decided under the responsibility of the physicians in the team.

The treatment of the motor speech disorder should be implemented in the general rehabilitation plan of the patients. As the underlying disease is neurological, the motor speech disorder in many cases is associated with movement disorders, language disorders, swallowing disorders, cognitive disorders, depending on the severity and stage of the disease and its aetiopathogenesis. It is therefore crucial for all components of the rehabilitation team to have a full awareness of all the needs of the patient and the plan to manage each of them.

## 20.2 Planning and Supervision of Speech Therapy Executed by Logopaedist/Speech and Language Pathologist (SLP)

Donato Mecca, Danilo Patrocinio, Vincenzo Sallustio, Cristina Polimeno and Iolanda Trittola

### 20.2.1 Introduction

Different approaches to the treatment of motor speech disorders (MSDs) have been reported, including pharmacological, surgical, prosthetic and rehabilitation (including brain stimulation techniques) (Jankovic and Tan 2020; Thies et al. 2021; Pinto et al. 2004; Wertheimer et al. 2014; Brabenec et al. 2021; Yorkston et al. 2001). The most adequate approach (or combination of different approaches) should be carefully defined in relation to the aetiopathology of the underlying disease and the specific characteristics of the MSD. Nevertheless, speech therapy (ST) is the most commonly used, documented and validated approach (Yorkston et al. 2010; Duffy 2019) and should be considered a specific primary component in the MSD rehabilitation process.

Beside the neurological diagnosis, a functional diagnosis should be included in order to plan a highly personalised approach for each patient, taking into consideration their specific aims. To draw a functional diagnosis, a proper physio-pathological interpretation of the impairment of both body functions and body structures, as well as activity limitations and participation restrictions, should be made. Baseline measures of all the previously mentioned domains should be assessed to allow the defining of expected changes, treatment effectiveness and possible suspension of treatment.

The primary purpose of rehabilitation in MSDs is to achieve the best possible outcome in terms of communicative participation. Two main approaches have been reported for ST for people with MSDs: a restorative and a compensatory approach. The first one focuses on the rehabilitation of motor speech impairment (WHA 2001); the second aims to provide tools and strategies to improve communication between the person with MSD, their family and their significant others (Lubinsky 1991).

The rehabilitation team for people with MSDs includes several professionals such as a phoniatrician, an SLP, a neurologist, a primary-care provider, a physiotherapist, a psychotherapist, a social worker and others. Within the rehabilitation team, the phoniatrician provides the functional diagnosis, based on both the clinical and instrumental examination and the SLP assessment results, agrees treatments goals with the SLP and the team members, defines follow-up timing and provides prognostic information. The follow-up assessments should be planned by taking into consideration several elements, such as aims and characteristics of the rehabilitation plan

(type of treatment, session rate and duration, setting) as well as the need for suspension of treatment and the actual needs and degree of motivation exhibited by the patient and caregivers. Each of these elements is shared, discussed and reviewed within the rehabilitation team. This multidisciplinary evaluation is intended not only to establish short- and long-term rehabilitation aims, but also to plan strategies, procedures and periodic follow-up. The rehabilitation team must supervise the motor speech impairment during the entire rehabilitation process in order to adopt changes in a timely manner when necessary.

Within the rehabilitation team it is appropriate to designate the role of the case manager from among the medical staff or other professionals such as social workers, SPLs, psychologists and technical health personnel. The function of the case manager is to facilitate and coordinate care for the patient and his or her family, working alongside the phoniatrician and the other rehabilitation team members to ensure not only the best possible outcome, but to promote the best possible quality of life (QOL).

## 20.2.2 Treatment Aims

Treatment aims should be carefully defined and shared with both the patients and their significant others. Being MSDs, in most cases consequences of degenerative disorders, a great effort should be spent on agreeing on realistic aims and avoiding non-realistic ones. For example, for people with severe dysarthria a non-realistic aim is to reach the recovery of completely unimpaired speech. Realistic aims are generally broader in scope and include, according to the severity of the MSD: promoting communication, including augmentative and alternative communication (AAC) tools for severe MSDs (Beukelman et al. 2007; Beukelman and Mirenda 2013), maximising the intelligibility for moderate MSDs, even at the expense of naturalness using techniques such as *pacing board* or *alphabet board* (Lang and Fishbein 1983), improving the communication effectiveness by acting on naturalness, accuracy and intelligibility for mild MSDs. No intervention or "preventive" intervention is generally needed for very mild MSD.

Depending on the severity of the MSD and the characteristics of the underlying disease (for example a degenerative disease), the ST should consider three different aims:

- to restore; that is, to make functional again the systems underlying verbal production altered by the symptoms,
- to carry out the function compromised by the symptoms through "compensation" strategies,
- to modify in a functional way the communicative behaviour of the patient by "adapting" to the current situation.

### 20.2.3 Beginning of Treatment

The treatment plan should start as early as possible. For MSDs due to acute events (i.e., stroke), this means to start the rehabilitation as soon as possible after the patient's clinical stabilisation, with the aim of an early restoration of an efficient communication; on the other hand, for chronic neurodegenerative diseases, an early start can help slow the effects on speech or prevent maladaptive compensation.

When planning treatment at this stage, the rehabilitation team should consider some elements that can be either facilitators or barriers according to individual case: the persistence of good linguistic and cognitive-decisional skills; the patient's and formal-informal carers' expectations; the patient's and formal-informal carers' compliance; the logistic organisation facilitating access to the outpatient clinic; previous speech therapies; the logistical support to conduct the training, also in telemedicine, both for rehabilitation purposes and supervision or periodic follow-ups.

### 20.2.4 Treatment Typology

Treatment type should consider the patient's needs and might be specific, global or step by step. *For current and future needs*, the immediate and future communicative needs should be considered. *For current needs* in acute care departments, the treatment should immediately facilitate communication by the use of AAC aids, even low-tech devices, and act specifically on speech as soon as possible. *For future needs*, the speech function decay in neurodegenerative chronic diseases should be predicted and a "preventive" intervention should be planned, acting on anatomical and functional subsystems, by preparing for the impairment progression and making the patient familiar with IT-based AAC systems. *Specific*: the rehabilitative action should be aimed at the subsystems responsible for the various symptom clusters (articulatory, respiratory, vocal, prosodic, resonance, etc.), according to the conscious learning model (declarative memory) or the motor learning model (procedural memory), with continuous or variable training. The rehabilitative action should also be aimed at the best available control of strength and muscle tone, direction, movement amplitude and pace, with regard to the neurological impairment typology (i.e., muscle strength has not to be enhanced in myasthenia); the treatment should elicit compensatory strategies. *Global*: the intervention of the rehabilitator is not directed exclusively to one of the subsystems affected, but involves all components of the subsystems involved in the verbal production, also using external and internal feedback; a typical example of such approach is the Lee Silvermann Voice Therapy (LSVT®) in Parkinson's Disease (McDonnell et al. 2018; Yuan et al. 2020). *Step by step*: by increasingly difficult tasks.

### 20.2.5 Session Rate and Treatment Duration

ST session rate, number and periodicity should be customised, keeping in mind many variables: impairment typology, disease progression, comorbidities, other contextual factors, patient's actual communicative abilities and needs, function recovery to be achieved, specific rehabilitative protocols (e.g., LSVT®). According to these variables, the rehabilitation team evaluates if a short and intensive treatment would be more effective than a prolonged one with sessions spaced over time or if drills would be more effective and better sustained by the patient. The number of sessions may change according to the function to be achieved, but it can never be decreased below a minimum; session rate can be reduced gradually over time (maintenance and generalisation period).

### 20.2.6 Setting

The setting may vary from acute care departments to outpatient department or to the patient's home, according to the adopted diagnostic therapeutic welfare and care pathway. Treatment may be delivered to single patients in a highly customised way, or in group sessions where, besides specific tasks for speech, it is possible to apply different strategies or test functional modality for the conversation. Other options include group therapy for maintenance and tele-rehabilitation (ASHA 2021). The setting should be activated in the hours most favourable for the patient (i.e., in the morning to avoid the motor fatigue accumulating during the day) or at the time of maximum effectiveness of the pharmacological therapy (i.e., in Parkinson Disease).

### 20.2.7 Treatment Suspension

It is advisable to discontinue the treatment when the planned aims are achieved or when the achieved modifications are in a steady state (plateau). In the planning of treatment suspension it is mandatory to use outcome measures (speech and quality of life measures).

### 20.2.8 Follow-Up

Follow-up represents a valuable way to verify the effectiveness of the treatment and the long-term stability of the achieved results, giving the option of recalibrating the rehabilitation plan according to the evolution of the communicative context. As well as during the planning phase, the emotional-relational and socio-cultural variables associated with patients' communication skills must also be taken into account during follow-up.

Follow-up might be periodic or scheduled at varying intervals according to the illness course and based on the outcome measures (ASHA-NOMS 2013; Hustad et al. 1998; Nogueira et al. 2019).

## 20.3 Rehabilitation of Dysarthria: Linguistic Principles

Karel Neubauer

### 20.3.1 Introduction

**Dysarthria** is a term for disorders of the motor execution of speech resulting from organic damage to the nervous system. It includes several types or syndromes of speech disorders that are caused by problems with the muscle control of speech mechanisms and classified as motor speech disorders (Motor Speech Disorders) (Love 1995; Freed 2000; Duffy 2005a; Brookshire 2007). In dysarthria, the basic modalities of the motor execution of speech—respiration, phonation, resonance and articulation—are affected to various extents.

**Acquired Dysarthria** (e.g., Brookshire 2007), which occurs during childhood, adulthood or with ageing, includes situations where the ongoing process of CNS maturation and the development of the speech skills of a child aged from newborn to 1–2 years is suddenly disrupted by trauma resulting from a brain injury, infection or an oncological disease of the nervous system. The above-mentioned causes—sudden trauma, disease or a tumour affecting the nervous system—frequently cause dysarthria even in the adult population, whereby in the case of ageing, elderly people in particular, they can cause specific problems for an already weakened organism (Neubauer 2016b, 2017b). The disorders that arise in this manner may improve spontaneously after their sudden onset and strong symptoms, but usually they require specialised logopaedic care and in some cases they may endure persistently.

**Anarthria** is used to describe the most severe disorders of motor speech modalities, where verbal communication with others is practically impossible; an inability to speak articulately due to the loss of, or undeveloped will for, the controlled movement of the speech organs, frequently also associated with the inability to form a voice–aphonia. Anarthria most often manifests itself in severe post-traumatic states after injuries and lesions to nervous tissue and is a symptom of some degenerative and progressive diseases of the nervous system, e.g., amyotrophic lateral sclerosis.

### 20.3.2 Differential Types of Acquired Dysarthria, and Related Syndromes

The syndrome of acquired dysarthria can be divided into a number of clinically distinguishable types. Dysarthria is present in a number of neurological syndromes; the normally used division of the types of dysarthria is also based on the interconnection of the results of neurological

**Table 20.1** Clinically distinguishable types of dysarthria, and the location of lesions in the nervous system (Love 1995; Freed 2000; Neubauer 2011)

| Type of dysarthria | Location of the lesion in the nervous system |
| --- | --- |
| Flaccid | Peripheral motor neuron |
| Spastic | Central motor neuron |
| Hypokinetic | Basal ganglia, and the nuclei of associated neural pathways |
| Hyperkinetic | Basal ganglia, and the nuclei of associated neural pathways |
| Ataxic | Cerebellum or its interconnection with neural pathways |
| Mixed For example: | |
| Mixed flaccid and spastic | Central and peripheral motor neuron, e.g. in amyotrophic lateral sclerosis |
| Mixed ataxic–spastic and flaccid | Cerebellum or the cerebellar neural pathways—Peripheral motor neuron and central motor neuron, e.g. in Wilson's disease |

diagnosis with clinically detectable examples of speech communication disorders (Freed 2000; Love 1995; Weismer and Kim 2010; Neubauer 2017b), see Table 20.1.

#### 20.3.2.1 Flaccid or Peripheral (Weak) Dysarthria

Present in impairments of the peripheral motor neuron, and usually a part of a neurological syndrome called bulbar paralysis, this is caused by damage to nuclei or to the course of the cranial nerves that innervate speech mechanisms. Neurologically, there are signs of peripheral paresis, with atrophy of the affected muscles and small muscle twitches–fasciculations.

The symptoms of dysarthria are especially pronounced in two-sided impairments of the cranial nerves, and its symptoms dominate in the form of a monotonous voice and slurred speech. This example of motor activity disorder is affected by lesions of certain cranial nerves that control the activities of facial muscles, performance of chewing and jaw movements, and the mobility of the soft palate or the tongue. A common symptom is disrupted breathing together with hypernasality, hoarseness and swallowing disorders. This type of dysarthria is present in infectious CNS diseases, myasthenia gravis and progressive bulbar paralysis.

#### 20.3.2.2 Spastic or Central Dysarthria

Caused by a disorder of the central motor neuron, and part of pseudobulbar paralysis, the impairment is localised in the area between the extended spinal cord and the white matter of the brain hemispheres. Neurologically, there are signs of central paresis with increased reflexes. The category of pseudobulbar paralysis also includes swallowing disorders, but there are no disorders of individual muscle movements; they are disorders involving overall mobility, and limitation and slowness of movement.

Speech is slow and laborious, words are stretched and longer speech is incomprehensible. Breathing is weakened; closures in articulated movements and palate-pharyngeal closures are slow and weakened.

The causes are mostly vascular conditions, CMP, strokes or multiple brain aneurysms.

### 20.3.2.3 Ataxic (Cerebellar) Dysarthria

Caused by damage to the cerebellum and the neural pathways associated with its activity, which neurologically form the so-called cerebellar syndrome, this includes badly targeted movements and poor co-ordination of muscle group activity, together with overall hypotonia.

Speech is irregular; syllables or words are forced out explosively (saccadic speech). Fluctuations appear in breathing, voice intensity and resonance. There are problems with speech rhythm and, in particular, the inaccurate pronunciation of consonants. A stickiness in the articulation position creates an impression of syllables being pronounced separately as words. This type of dysarthria is common in multiple sclerosis, in various cerebellar inflammations or tumours, or degenerative processes in this area.

### 20.3.2.4 Hypokinetic (Extra-Pyramidal) Dysarthria

Caused as part of the hypokinetic–hypertonic syndrome accompanying disorders of the activity of the basal ganglia, primarily in Parkinson's disease, here muscle activity is complicated by the rigidity and akinesia of the muscle groups. Often there are resting tremors and loss of motion automatisms.

Speech is monotonous; there may be an initial pause due to muscle stiffness followed by a rapid and inaccurate speech with palilalia—repetition of syllables or words. Breathing is insufficient and disrupted owing to disruption of the mobility of the respiratory muscles, and vocal expression is significantly weakened, eventually resulting in aphonia. Speech either slows down until it stops, or on the contrary increases in speed until it becomes an indistinct mumbling.

The most frequent cause is Parkinson's disease; sometimes cerebrovascular accident (CVA) or Parkinsonism caused by the effects of medicines.

### 20.3.2.5 Hyperkinetic (Extra-Pyramidal) Dysarthria

This is caused as part of the choreatic or athetoid syndrome and includes abnormal involuntary movements that disrupt normal motor activity, and to a various degree of severity, also speech skills. Overall muscle tone is decreased, and involuntary movement of muscle groups is increased.

Speech is loud, ranting and there is a noticeable lack of co-ordination with breathing movements. Speech mechanisms may be disrupted by sudden movements, or permanently disrupted by uncontrollable motion automatisms. The rate of speech fluctuates, and speech may be incomprehensible owing to the inability to control tongue and mouth movements, or the inability to control speech movements.

Causes are usually states occurring during the administration of drugs, in particular neuroleptics, to sensitive persons (so-called tardive dyskinesia), or degenerative CNS diseases.

### 20.3.2.6 Mixed Dysarthria

Neurological symptoms are signs of peripheral and central paresis; caused either by a combination of multiple CNS lesions, or in degenerative diseases, e.g., in amyotrophic lateral sclerosis.

Five types of mixed dysarthria are frequently cited in individual degenerative CNS diseases in adults (Table 20.1):

- Spastic-flaccid dysarthria–amyotrophic lateral sclerosis.
- Ataxic-spastic dysarthria–multiple sclerosis.
- Ataxic-spastic and flaccid dysarthria–olivopontocerebellar atrophy.
- Spastic-ataxic and hypokinetic dysarthria–Wilson's disease.
- Hypokinetic-spastic and ataxic dysarthria–progressive supranuclear paralysis.

Linguistic orientated diagnosis most often builds on the results of neurological examinations and is led by an effort to define the present speech communication disorders, their severity and their impact on the communication abilities of the affected person. The main

**Table 20.2** Frequently dominating motor speech modalities in individual types of dysarthria (Love 1995; Freed 2000; Neubauer 2011)

| Type of dysarthria | Dominating modality for therapy |
|---|---|
| Flaccid dysarthria | Orofacial motor activity |
| | Nasality—Velopharyngeal closure |
| Spastic dysarthria | Respiration |
| | Articulation |
| Hyperkinetic dysarthria | Respiration |
| | Articulation |
| Hypokinetic dysarthria | Phonation |
| | Resonance and prosody |
| Ataxic dysarthria | Articulation |
| | Prosody |

aim is to identify the contribution of individual speech motor modalities to the stigmatisation of speech, during the increase or loss of comprehensibility in a social environment. The subsequently formed individual therapy plan is aimed at the co-ordinated stimulation of all speech motor modalities, but with a predominance of stimulation of the area in which the renewal of the function for the change of the state of speech communication is fundamental (Table 20.2).

### 20.3.2.7 Dysarthria Caused by the Effects of Medicines

Long-term medication of neuroleptics with phenothiazine components (e.g., Haloperidol), which is effective in a number of psychiatric diseases, in particular schizophrenia, may negatively affect the activity of the extra-pyramidal nervous system, and cause uncontrollable rhythmic movements of the tongue, face, mouth and jaws in sensitive individuals. These symptoms then significantly disrupt speech production and comprehensibility, thus contributing to the social stigmatisation of the affected person. For these symptoms, which appear as extra-pyramidal hyperkinetic dysarthria, the term "tardive dyskinesia" has been introduced in the field of psychiatric care. It is probably the most prominent example of dysarthria caused by the effects of medicines.

Besides traditional medicative procedures used by psychiatrists to alleviate symptoms, at present the contribution of clinical speech therapy and timely logopaedic diagnosis is also recognised, especially in persistently enduring states. These persistent symptoms are not sufficiently controllable by treatment with medication; here we are dealing with persons for whom interruption of neuroleptic medication is not an option owing to the risk of a severe remission of the psychiatric disease—often these are chronic patients in psychiatric care, who have been using the medication for 10 years or more. Here, we recognise the need for periodic examination of these persons by an expert on speech communication disorders, the timely identification of orofacial dyskinesia and the commencement of speech therapy, which can prevent the development of severe speech abnormalities (Neubauer et al. 2007).

The above-mentioned issue is closely related to that of the effects of medicines in the area of speech, in particular speech motor modalities. Besides medicaments with a potentially positive effect on the motor activity of the speech organs, in this area there are very serious potential negative effects of medication on the speech communication of the medicated person. The best-known agent with a positive long-term effect on Parkinson's disease is levodopa (L-DOPA); other agents are used to increase muscular mobility (Baclofen etc.), but the interaction of these medicines does not exclude potential negative effects on speech motor activity. The most common risk-causing types of medicine, besides the above-mentioned neuroleptics, are sedatives and antidepressants, which may cause a reduction in salivation, problems with the motor activity of the speech organs, and cognitive difficulties in verbal memory and speech quality. A summary of the examples of the most risky agents are regularly listed overseas for the area of speech and language communication (Gravell and France 1991; Wheeler 1995); the broader issue of medication-induced communication and swallowing disorders is covered by authors (Remington and Fagan 2006) in a monograph, which also covers the area of speech fluency disorders and cognitive disorders.

### 20.3.2.8 Swallowing Disorders

Dysphagia—a swallowing disorder—is a common complication suffered by persons with dysarthria, because a lesion of the nervous system also affects the vital functions of the human orofacial tract: respiration and food intake. Some neurological syndromes, e.g., the bulbar syndrome in a two-sided lesion of the cranial nerves, also include speech function disorders (dysarthria, disorders of the mobility of the tongue and the mimic muscles) and vital functions (dysphagia, potential breathing and heart activity disorders). In dysphagia, the intake of food and liquids is made difficult or even impossible; in more serious cases the disorder may even be a life-threatening complication owing to the risk of aspiration (inhalation) of food, and in particular liquids, into the breathing mechanism.

A disorder of the vital functions of the orofacial tract, related to innervation disorders, is a common complication for persons suffering from acquired dysarthria. In particular, Parkinson's disease, multiple sclerosis, post-traumatic states and strokes are the most common listed causes of swallowing disorders. Dysphagia can occur in all types of acquired dysarthria, especially in a severe post-acute state after CNS trauma, or by contrast as an emerging symptom of a developed degenerative CNS disease. Severe swallowing disorders are regularly associated with examples of two-sided disorders of the peripheral motor neuron, resulting in a bulbar syndrome and symptoms of severe flaccid dysarthria. Severe two-sided lesions on the corticobulbar pathways may also result in the severe incidence of a pseudobulbar syndrome, mixed dysarthria and severe swallowing disorders.

Initiation of targeted therapy for the alleviation of swallowing disorders in more severe cases, where there is a risk of the aspiration of food into the airways, is possible only while co-operating with a team of health workers who will make a diagnosis (often with the help of instrumental methods) and approve the initiation of targeted therapy under the guidance of a doctor. The clinical speech therapist participates in the diagnosis together with the team of medical professionals and participates in the setting of the rehabilitation strategy. The diagnostic process enables clarification of the aetiology of the disorder, the designation of the types of swallowing disorder, and the subsequent targeting of compensation and therapeutic procedures in working with dysphagic patients. Most popular are compensation options involving change in the consistency of food and postural changes while eating, targeted according to the type and aetiology of the swallowing difficulties. The therapy also includes techniques aimed at changing muscle functions, which are based on speech therapy and rehabilitation exercises in the orofacial area (Murry and Carreau 1996; Tedla 2009).

### 20.3.2.9 Dysarthria and Speech Dyspraxia

Speech dyspraxia (speech apraxia) is classified as an individual motor disorder of speech communication (Kirshner 1995) on the boundary between dysarthria and motor aphasia and is a subject of both differential diagnosis and the creation of specialised therapeutic procedures.

At present, an opinion dominates that this disorder is apparently not caused exclusively by disruptions to the areas connected to the activity of the primary motor cortex, as in dysarthria (in speech apraxia, the muscles are not weakened, there is no disruption in muscle co-ordination or tone, and mobility is not restricted), but the programming of the speech itself is disrupted (instead, the localisation of the CNS disorder is connected to the secondary motor cortex and the pre-motor associative areas). From the perspective of disorders of the motor execution of the phonic sequences, emphasis is at present placed on the role of supra-syllabic (metric) mechanisms, which also play an important role in the induction of the symptoms of the disorder. A non-linear plan of the decoding and arrangement of the sounds of speech has an influence on the frequency and type of substitutions or elimination of the sounds and their perception (Ziegler et al. 2010).

The affected person makes varying errors while forming individual sounds, they incorrectly set the speech organs, and they link the arrangement of the sounds within a word to one another;

in the speech there is a presence of various phonemic disorders in the form of substitution, omission and perseverance of the articulation segments of the speech; in particular consonants. The problems escalate during the initiation of the speech, and minor instances are present in the prosody and cadence of the speech.

In addition, the clinical diagnosis of speech dyspraxia itself, and its clear differentiation from the symptoms of dysarthria and aphasia, are still a problem today; an opinion dominates regarding the common co-existence of the disorder with Broca's aphasia and certain types of dysarthria.

The dominant differential signs are a:

- Lack of language disorders, dysgrammatism.
- Lack of reading and writing disorders in relation to expressive aphasia.
- Variety of phonemic difficulties, as not found in dysarthria.

Speech dyspraxia may be further complicated by the presence of various forms of non-verbal dyspraxia, with which it should not be confused; oral dyspraxia or forms of ideomotor or ideatory dyspraxia are not directly connected with speech dyspraxia, because they express different forms of the deficit. The above-mentioned forms of dyspraxia are connected with the targeted imitation of motor activity (Králíček 2011); in speech dyspraxia the deficit is present in spontaneous speech.

### 20.3.2.10 Symptoms of Oral Dyspraxia

Oral dyspraxia is associated with disorders involving the repetition of demonstrated movements of the speech organs—movements of the tongue, the lower jaw and the orofacial muscles; the difficulties culminate in the execution of sequences of movements—in the imitation of two or more subsequent movements, in accordance with the demonstrated movement pattern.

The speech dyspraxia may also be complicated by the presence of various forms of non-verbal dyspraxia. The most common types are:

- Ideomotor (limbic) dyspraxia.
- Bucofacial (including oral) dyspraxia.
- Structural dyspraxia.

As mentioned in the preceding text—neither oral dyspraxia nor forms of ideomotor or ideatory dyspraxia are directly connected with speech dyspraxia, because they reflect different forms of the deficit. Non-verbal forms of dyspraxia are connected with the targeted imitation of motor activity; in speech dyspraxia the deficit is present in spontaneous speech.

Overseas, the diagnostic guidelines for this area are a part of specific tests for speech dyspraxia, which also include instructions and subtests for examining limbic and oral dyspraxia. Also used is the evaluation of the symptoms of oral dyspraxia as a co-existing factor in phatic disorders (e.g., the "Test of Oral and Limb Apraxia", Helm-Estabrooks and Albert 1991).

### 20.3.3 Clinical Assessment of Acquired Dysarthria

The area of clinical assessment of neurogenic motor disorders of speech communication dominates the continuity of the determination of the CNS lesion by the neurologist, the clinical evaluation of speech production and the subsequent clinical *Speech language therapy* (SLT) assessment of the symptoms of the speech communication disorders. On this is the subsequent therapeutic assistance procedure for persons handicapped in this manner most dependent.

The SLT diagnosis most often builds on the results of the medical examination and is based on the results of the clinical neurological examination during the determination of the type of dysarthria. It is led by the effort to define the speech communication disorders that are present, their severity and their impact on the communication abilities of the affected person. The main aim is to identify the speech motor modalities responsible for the stigmatisation of speech; for the reduction or loss of comprehensibility in a social environment.

To diagnose motor speech changes, examinations with diagnostic guidelines are used in clinical practice scales and examination forms for dysarthria. These are usually collections originally intended for children, referred to in the sections of text dealing with the diagnosis of developmental dysarthria. Their suitable adaptation and evaluation depend on the activity of an experienced clinical SLT who is able to evaluate the speech modalities on the basis of listening to, watching and processing magnetic tape or video recordings of the speech.

The most widely used diagnostic guideline in English-speaking countries is the "Dysarthria Profile"; an investigative scale used both in English-speaking countries and in the French adaptation since 1982. Its author is the British therapist Sandra Robertson. The scale includes entries related to the areas of:

- Respiration.
- Phonation.
- Facial muscle activity.
- Diadochokinesis (the accuracy of repeated movements).
- Reflex activity associated with swallowing, chewing and coughing.
- Articulation.
- Comprehensibility of reading and speech.
- Rate and prosody of speech.

The results are rated at five levels, from normal performance to the complete inability to perform the tests. The "Dysarthria Profile" is a type of therapeutic diagnostic aid aimed at setting a therapy plan and focusing on the most affected components of the motor speech profile. Furthermore, it enables the determination of the best-preserved abilities to compensate for the disorder (Robertson and Thompson 1986).

Another diagnostic method is Enderby's "Frenchay Dysarthria Assessment" from 1983, based on similar diagnostic principles as the "Dysarthria Profile". Its second, re-worked version from 2008 may be evaluated very positively, in particular owing to the higher involvement of linguistic criteria in the selection of diagnostic verbal materials, the development of model profiles for types of dysarthria and the obtaining of research standards for the control group of healthy persons (Enderby and Palmer 2008).

The diagnosis of neurogenic speech disorders is primarily a part of the co-operation between neurological medical clinical diagnosis and SLT clinical examinations. The SLT clinical assessment is based on the results of the neurological examinations and tries to define which speech communication disorders are present. Its main aim is to find the disorders responsible for the reduction or loss in speech comprehensibility.

In the diagnosis of motor speech changes, examinations with diagnostic guidelines are used in normal clinical practice scales and examination forms for dysarthria. Their evaluation depends on the activity of a qualified and experienced expert who is able to evaluate speech on the basis of listening to, watching and processing a recording or video recording of the speech. Usually this is a qualitative clinical examination, aimed at evaluating all the components of the speech profile—breathing, articulation, phonation, resonance, rate of speech and prosody.

### 20.3.3.1 Differential Diagnosis of Speech Dyspraxia

Since 1975, when verbal dyspraxia was classified as an independent motor disorder (Darley et al. 1975; Love 1995) on the boundary between dysarthria and motor aphasia, it has been the subject of both a differential diagnosis and the creation of specialised therapeutic procedures. Up to now, however, there have been differing opinions on the location of the CNS lesion in verbal dyspraxia.

The clinical diagnosis of verbal dyspraxia itself, with its clear differentiation from the symptoms of dysarthria and aphasia, remains a problem today. The most problematic phenomenon is the frequent co-existence of verbal dyspraxia with the symptoms of aphasia or dysarthria after CNS trauma.

In 1979, Barbara Dabul first published the specific test "Apraxia Battery for Adults", which includes a test for the examination of verbal dyspraxia and a subtest for the examination of limbic and oral dyspraxia. It is a three-degree scale showing mild–medium–severe disorders of the performance of tasks in spontaneous speech, word sequences and reading. In addition to this diagnostic material, there is also the similar "Comprehensive Apraxia Test" (Kirshner 1995). The evaluation of the symptoms of oral dyspraxia as a co-existing factor in phatic disorders is covered by the "Test of Oral and Limb Apraxia" (Helm-Estabrooks and Albert 1991).

Despite the persisting perception of this disorder as an unstable and ambiguous diagnostic unit, it is commonly part of complex processing in monographs and research programmes (Kirshner 1995; Brookshire 2007; Hedge and Davis 2010; Ziegler et al. 2010; Haynes and Pindzola 2012).

### 20.3.3.2 Assessment of Motor Speech Disorders with the Use of Acoustic Signal Analysis

The use of procedures for processing human speech that use frequency and spectral analysis of sound recordings in the diagnosis of motor speech disorders has long been a tempting and promising way of making the diagnostic process in this area objective. Speech analysis may be a form of increasing the objectivity and accuracy of the diagnosis of motor speech disorders, but owing to its absolute dependence on technical and IT facilities, it is currently implemented primarily within research projects, which have specialised time, technical and multi-disciplinary facilities available to them, which most clinical workplaces do not have at their disposal. The computer diagnostic recording programme MENTIO (Petržílková 2014), on the contrary, is an example of a diagnostic instrument aimed at using IT technology to capture, edit, describe and store sound recordings in SLT clinical practice. It also enables the use of the characteristics of spectral analysis, and the evaluation of frequency characteristics, in the course of diagnostic processing of recordings. The significance of this programme, which connects diagnostic values that are usable almost immediately (recording, description and storage) with the option of frequency analysis of the recording, may be invaluable for the future of SLT assessment in this area.

Other instrumental speech analysis procedures, such as electromagnetic articulography, electropalatography and ultrasonography of the oral cavity (Crystal 2010; Ferrand 2014) are at present mostly used in research programmes. They may, however, be utilised in the future as part of a suitable and easy-to-use evaluation programme for actual clinical motor speech disorder diagnosis. Their potential should, however, be targeted at the area of therapeutic assistance for these persons, and at the creation of instrumentally supported therapeutic intervention programmes.

### 20.3.4 Therapy of Impaired Central Motor Speech Functions

### 20.3.4.1 Use of Dysarthria and Speech Dyspraxia Therapy

A suddenly occurring disorder of the motor performance of speech, caused by trauma or a CNS disease is, in the adult population, connected primarily with CVA, head injuries and oncological or infectious brain tissue diseases. Speech disorders that arise in this manner may, after their sudden appearance and severe symptoms, spontaneously improve; more often however, they require specialised SLT care and in some cases they may permanently prevent the resumption of comprehensible speech; in persons handicapped in this way, a substitute communication system must be developed.

Parkinson's disease, multiple sclerosis and degenerative diseases of the CNS are very often accompanied by incurred and progressively worsening dysarthria. This group of affected persons was for a long time mostly neglected from a therapeutic perspective, although there is already very extensive information about the development of therapeutic programmes for persons with Parkinson's disease available (Ramig 1995). The therapy is led here by the effort to slow down or stop the development of dysarthria and choose an effective compensation strategy; the chances of improvement are affected primarily by the course of the developing disease and the induction of the patients' permanent activation.

### 20.3.4.2 Overview of the Methods and Tools of the Therapy

The methods and tools of SLT in adults with dysarthria may be summarised in these groups:

- The use of methods inducing muscle relaxation and body tone stabilisation in the area of speech organs.
- The modification of respiratory, phonatory, articulation and resonance exercises for the renewal and stabilisation of motor speech skills.
- Instrumental aids for the spectral display of the sound of speech and amplified feedback by sight and hearing, using delayed aural feedback and instruments based on the electromyogram.
- The use of non-verbal communication and communication aids in severe, persistently enduring, disorders of communication with the environment.
- Group procedures aimed at social group interaction, and at the transfer of skills from individual therapy to spontaneous speech.
- Rhythmic and intonation procedures inducing a speech stimulus, connected with mobility and the use of technical aids.

Speech dyspraxia in the area of therapeutic effectiveness requires specific procedures aimed at improving the pronunciation of individual sounds, and their initiation and verbal sequencing. This is why procedures used in articulation therapy in dysarthria are often modified for use in speech dyspraxia. Here the aim is to achieve the highest possible level of self-control during articulation, and the most fluent auto-correction of erroneous articulatory movements possible. With regard to the character of the disorder, the dominant procedures may be considered to be articulation exercises, rhythmic exercises and phonetic sound discrimination exercises (Neubauer et al. 2007; Neubauer 2018a).

### 20.3.4.3 The Use of Relaxation for Muscle Tension Stabilisation, and to Loosen Muscles

The stable and proportionate muscle tone of the entire body is a prerequisite for stable and optimal speech. Its inducement is therefore a highly sought-after effect of successful therapy. The relaxation exercises here are primarily tools for inducing self-control over the state of the muscle tone of the entire body, especially in the area of the speech organs. Both Jacobson's progressive relaxation training and autogenic training methods may be used. The first one of these works by using a targeted loosening of the muscle groups on the basis of experiencing a contrast between the maximum contraction and loosening. Autogenic training works more suggestively, by loosening the entire body and inducing feelings of adequate functioning of the internal organs and the body. The achievement of a suitable form of loosening and stabilisation of muscle tone, in particular the speech organs, is important and is a condition for the effectiveness of the therapy. For persons with severe full-body mobility disorders, it is individually necessary to use positioning aids for the limbs and to stabilise the upright sitting positions; supports or slings are also reported to have been used for the upper limbs in order to free the movements of the chest and the speech organs.

### 20.3.4.4 Orofacial Exercises for Restoring Mobility and Muscle Strength

Exercises for restoring the speech organs should be included continuously from the start of the therapy, or in a targeted manner according to the symptoms of apraxia in speech or the deterioration of repeated speech organ movements during speech. We should perform these exercises while inspecting them in the mirror several times a day, in order to induce the proper mobility and strength of the lips, tongue and mimic muscles. They include isotonic and isometric exercises against resistance, relaxation, and exercises focusing on the targeted movement of the speech organs.

Exercises aimed at improving the function of the palate-pharyngeal closure in hyperphonia can be very important. We use both the passive methods of stretching and massaging the soft palate and the active exercises of sucking, swallowing, also helping to stretch the palate with hand and body movements. Digital massages for inducing the gag reflex and overcoming velopharyngeal insufficiency are used mainly in the case of severe flaccid dysarthria.

### 20.3.4.5 Breathing and Phonation Exercises for Restoring Palate-Pharyngeal Closure Function

These are aimed at increasing the functional use of lung capacity and improving the strength and co-ordination of the respiratory muscles. Improvements achieved here have an impact on the improvement and stabilisation of speech phonation, articulation and prosody. We practise breathing deeply whilst ensuring that other body parts stay still, and we use phonation for vowels and rhythmic word sequences.

Exercises involving the initial sound of the voice, the optimal strength and pitch of the voice, and good co-ordination of breathing and phonation, utilise both the possibilities of strengthening speech by nasalisation and an expansion of the loosened resonance areas, and a practice of soft vocal expression according to the type of dysarthric difficulties. Of fundamental importance are the specific forms of breathing and phonation exercises for persons suffering from the hypokinetic form of acquired dysarthria as a result of Parkinson's disease (Neubauer 2011).

### 20.3.4.6 Articulation Exercises

These procedures are frequently connected to an effort to slow down the rate of speech while speaking and reading, and to accentuate and separate articulation movements while self-controlling them by listening to and inspecting them in a mirror. In the case of severe mobility disorder we sometimes use substitute articulation mechanisms. Most often, if the lips cannot close, a substitute closure is used for B-P-M sounds, which use a connection of the teeth to the lips, and if targeted movement of the tongue is not possible, we accept the formation of an acoustically distinguishable sound by moving the entire lower jaw and pressing the surface of the tongue against the palate.

Articulation tasks should have realistic goals and they should serve to improve speech comprehensibility, instead of focusing on intact articulation as in the case of children with only a problem in the development of articulation. It is necessary to use aids and probes to position the speech organs and stabilise body tone in the position in which the exercises are performed.

Besides using the positioning aids themselves—spatulas, probes and rubber pegs for positioning the angle of the jaw and the position of the tongue and lips—we often combine these procedures with the use of amplified or delayed aural feedback and the stimulation of speech organ movements.

### 20.3.4.7 Exercises for Word and Sentence Prosody, and Sentence Intonation

These mainly include the exercises of sentence intonation in different types of sentence, and communication with an adequate verbal accent. What has shown to be effective is the use of aids with graphically highlighted sections of sentences and words, and most of all the use of instrumental visual control methods with a programme that uses sound signal characteristics to illustrate movement sequences on a computer screen. By training the imitation of word and sequence patterns we stimulate speech that is distinguishable in intonation, and improvements in the prosody of longer words and sentences. The results of work with speech prosody in persons with dysarthria have been published by Bouglė et al. (1995) that uses the programme IBM Speech Viewer III. The MENTIO voice programme (Petržílková 2014) is currently available in Czech; it contains similar training parameters to those of the SpeechViewer programme, usable for work with prosody and speech intonation.

### 20.3.4.8 Rhythmic Movement Exercises

These have a wide range of compensation-motivation uses, with the possibility of rapidly influencing the comprehensibility of speech. They induce an articulation stimulus connected with the movement in every syllable or word. In this way they also help to set the pace of speech appropriate to the given motor and co-ordination abilities of the dysarthric person. By emphasising the first sound of a word, they improve the chances of treating rapid and confluent, slurred speech. Besides rhythmic exercises, shielded reading and graphic emphasis of syllables, words and sounds are also used.

### 20.3.4.9 Non-Verbal Communication and Communication Aids

These compensation procedures use, in enduring severe disorders, the ability to communicate by using writing, pictorial symbols or gestures. Their use depends on the motor and cognitive abilities of the dysarthric person. Alternative communication systems (such as pictograms and conceptual drawings) and systems of stimulating non-verbal communication (such as visual-action therapy and the use of gestures, sketches, etc.) are often adaptations of methods originally developed to treat phatic disorders (Helm-Estabrooks and Albert 1991). The use of a compensatory electronic and information and communication technology (ICT) aid with the option of recording and playing back sentence units, as well as voice amplifiers in the case of hypophony in Parkinson's disease sufferers, can be offered by workplaces for augmentative and alternative communication; these also include resources that gutturally and manually support the comprehensibility of "dysarthrics" speech (Feeley and Jones 2012a).

### 20.3.4.10 Group Therapy

Procedures aimed at social group interaction for the maximal imitation of an actual communication situation include, for example, PACE (Promoting Aphasics Communicative Effectiveness; Elman 2007); they also act as a usable transfer of methods from the area of aphasia, but here they serve to transfer skills from individual therapy to managed, thematic and spontaneous speech in a small group of persons with similar difficulties. In persons with acceptable speech comprehensibility, group interaction should be used under the leadership of a therapist who facilitates the spontaneous use of compensatory and newly renewed motor speech abilities in the widest possible range of social situations and activities, and in group support therapy.

### 20.3.4.11 Technical Aids and Instrumental Programmes

In dysarthria therapy, these aids are an important and increasingly used part of the procedures stimulating function renewal. They include standard clinical applications that use amplified aural feedback through headphones, often improving the quality of the dysarthric person's speech, just like using a telephone to solidify acquired communication skills. Another option is the utilisation of delayed auditory feedback (DAF) through headphones, which slows down the rate of speech and supports the formation of pauses between word units. Individually, an electronic metronome may also be used to induce rhythmic procedures, or a buzzer with sound and visual output may be used. Also of benefit is the use of video or sound recordings of exercises for the individual training of persons suffering from dysarthria. Clinical applications of the programme Speech Viewer III, in cases of persons with dysarthria, have resulted in improvements in the modulation of the basic voice frequency of persons who suffered from CNS injuries and Parkinson's disease (Bouglė et al. 1995; Le Dorze et al. 1992). Improvements in voice pitch and modulation in word expression and sentence intonation are presented in the form of 1–2 case studies in motivated persons. Despite the good results reported in case studies for persons with speech apraxia and acquired post-injury dysarthria, overseas we are still dealing with research rather than clinical therapeutic projects— just as with the use of other aids based on electrolaryngographs, electromyographical recordings and the use of a palate sensor and electropalatography (Love 1995; Neubauer 2011).

For the Czech and Slovak language area, the use of more complex sets of instruments was, until recently, restricted by their high cost. The use of "Speech Viewer", based on an IBM computer programme, which works with visual and aural feedback in the area of voice pitch and intensity, its voiced productions and use of sound articulation patterns, was associated with a high financial investment and minimal user support in case of problems with use in a language other than English (Neubauer et al. 2007). The original Czech MENTIO voice programme (Petržílková 2014), which contains similar training parameters to those of the SpeechViewer programme, usable for work with prosody and speech intonation, is available at minimal financial cost, owing to high support for the use of the programme in therapeutic intervention. It allows a broad spectrum of work with supra-segmental speech components, voicedness, length, pitch, intensity and other parameters.

### 20.3.5 Specific Procedures in the Area of Acquired Dysarthria

#### 20.3.5.1 Supporting the Renewal of Orofacial Mobility and co-Ordination in Adults

The therapeutic assistance for persons with most severe loss of speech organ mobility and the swallowing process is related to the renewal of movement co-ordination in the orofacial area. In the event that such severe disorders of the vital and vocal functions of the orofacial region persist, oral therapy and orofacial therapy procedures must be used.

Efforts to renew the mobility and movement co-ordination of the speech organs must be based on achieved desensitisation. The following principles must be observed:

- The person must be able to tolerate their mouth being touched without any defensive reactions; they must get used to this.
- In orofacial therapy procedures, the head must be positioned symmetrically to the body axis on the bed; a position where the top part of the body is supported should always be given preference.
- A transition to a sitting position, where the head is in a position symmetrically in the body axis, is a very important facilitative part of the therapy.
- Significant motor and tactile stimulation—circling and tapping on the lips, the tongue and the face, will support muscle mobility after desensitisation.
- Asymmetry in the position of the head, especially when it leans backwards, together with the opening of the mouth, makes swallowing and differentiation of speech organ mobility very difficult, or even impossible. A firm closure of the lips is an essential element of orofacial motor activity development.

At the beginning, speech organs are frequently massaged; circular massage of the speech organs is often used, most effectively when combined with emotive-verbal substantive sounds. For example, in the circular massage of the corner of the mouth into a "U". The aim is to encourage motor perception, coupled with a sound and content accompaniment. Subsequently, there is a transfer from passive massaging to the active imitation of articulation movements with visual, aural and tactile feedback. In addition to the facial muscle areas, the gums, the tongue surface and the centre of the hard palate are usually stimulated by circular massaging or repeated strokes, most commonly performed with the finger.

Stimulation is usually performed by:

- Circular massaging—in the speech organ area, small circles, 5–10 times per exercise.
- Tapping—fast, strong tapping.
- Tapping across the area of the other hand—put 1–2 fingers in place (usually the lip area) and tap firmly with the two fingers of the other hand to spread the stimulation across the entire area, for example, the upper lip.
- Stroking—especially across the lip area and when stimulating the inside of the mouth, 3–5 times per exercise; performing this using a finger is usually the most successful method, but if the person can tolerate it, a wooden spatula can be used; this is a more intense method.
- Vibration—most often used in connection with one of the above-mentioned movements.
- Using a small brush and, afterwards, ice sticks—initial stimulation with a small brush, and subsequent strokes with an ice stick, are performed in the mouth and facial area. The ice is also used to perform strokes across the tongue, and after inserting a piece of ice into the mouth and closing the lips, swallowing should occur.

The exercise should fundamentally be performed symmetrically on both sides of the face; a possible increase in the stimulation of half of the facial area will not be effective as a template with regard to the severity of the disability. When performing orofacial stimulation on adults with neurogenic motor deficits in the orofacial area to stimulate the renewal of mobility, a set of moderate exercises should be selected, individually, for each person according to their difficulties and in relation to the need to restore the ability to ingest food and to speak.

The suggested procedures can be highlighted as being fundamentally beneficial for:

- The stimulation of the oral cavity.
- The use of vibration to stimulate the oral cavity.
- The prolonged stretching of the face.
- Strengthening the function of the palato-pharyngeal closure, by blowing and sucking.
- Exercises for the improvement of tongue control while swallowing—mainly by sucking and swallowing whilst using a moistened gauze.

In terms of the dynamics of restoring orofacial mobility during favourable development, the given process must be respected as a renewal of already known functions on the terrain of a mature CNS. Acquired dysarthria in adults frequently presents differently from severe developmental dysarthria, and more locally differentiated from overall body mobility. This enables a significant proportion of people with this type of disability to make use of targeted renewal therapy aimed at speech organ mobility. According to author's clinical experience, isometric and isotonic forms of exercises perform an important function here. Isometric speech organ exercises are aimed at restoring muscle strength and the precise targeting of speech organ movements. A collection of mostly isometric procedures by authors from the Mayo Clinic in Rochester in the USA (Keith and Thomas 1989) contains 20 exercises, performed with a focus on restoring muscle strength and endurance in the speech organs.

### 20.3.5.2 Using Articulation and Rhythmic Procedures—Influencing the Comprehensibility and Dynamics of Speech

Owing to the nature of dysarthria as a CNS function disorder, articulation difficulties are usually caused by disorders of the mobility of the orofacial area, difficulties in the coordination of articulation movements and disorders of speech organ mobility dynamics. The articulation of individual sounds is secondarily affected or even prevented by these disorders, but the primary perceptional motor patterns of the articulation of individual sounds are potentially be preserved. For this reason, an intervention strategy aimed at influencing

speech rate and dynamics is more often effective than procedures targeted at the articulation of individual sounds (Neubauer et al. 2007; Neubauer 2011, 2017b, 2018a, b, c, d, e).

The basic aim of speech therapy here is to encourage sound articulation that is phonetically suitable and that does not prevent the comprehensibility of speech of a person with dysarthria. These efforts are a part of the orofacial motor activity stimulation procedures mentioned above, and they are usually supplemented with sound differentiation exercises.

The most common areas here are the differentiation:

- Of closing sounds in weakened mouth closure.
- Of voiced and unvoiced sounds in weakened exhalation dynamics and phonational insufficiency.
- Of the velar sounds K–G–CH in weakened velopharyngeal closure function.
- Between sibilants and sounds sounding like "D–T" or "Ď–Ť" in an adynamic shortened and weakened exhalation.

The procedures of differentiating between sounds are primarily based here on amplifying the differences between sounds during the use of aural, visual and tactile feedback. An amplification of the difference in the tactile perception of exhalation, in the perception of resonance in the area of the vocal cords whilst using a mirror, is a stable part of this articulation-differentiation exercise. For most people suffering from acquired dysarthria, however, a more fundamental problem is the transfer of individual articulation components into speech, where the rhythmic procedures play an important role.

Rhythmic procedures are a crucial area of global recovery procedures, and they have a wide range of compensation-motivation uses for the possibility of rapidly influencing the comprehensibility of speech in a variety of disorders. They induce a speech stimulus, connected with a movement (usually of the hand) with every syllable, or start of a word. In this way they also help to set a speech tempo appropriate to the given motor and co-ordination abilities of the persons suffering from dysarthria.

The motivational function of this approach arises from the need to pay adequate attention to the provision of motivation appropriate to the adult's age and mental abilities. The therapist should present procedures that aim to improve the comprehensibility of speech, and the use of rhythmic procedures is in our clinical experience a very versatile and effective way of helping persons with acquired dysarthria to renew their motor speech functions; it also contains considerable motivational potential, as long as the effectiveness of this procedure is demonstrated to the person with dysarthria at the outset of the SLT.

The most commonly listed aims of this therapeutic procedure, i.e., the inducement of control (especially self-control) of the rate of speech, and a reduction in excessive speech rate (Robertson and Thompson 1986; Freed 2000) should, in our clinical experience, be supplemented with the area of inducement of motorically stimulated articulation impulses and the restoration of speech organ mobility dynamics. Overcoming the phenomenon often known in clinical phoniatric diagnosis by the term "extinction of the articulation stimulus" is a fundamental goal of the intervention procedure, especially when dealing with the symptoms of more severe central dysarthria. When creating an individual SLT intervention plan, this form of therapy is most commonly used when dealing with the symptoms of ataxic dysarthria resulting from disorders of cerebellar functions, hypokinetic dysarthria resulting from Parkinson's disease, and central dysarthria resulting from strokes and brain injuries.

The above-mentioned goals will only be achieved with a sustained effort to use creative varieties of methods and technical aids that will enable an uncomplicated transition to the independent training of persons suffering from dysarthria. When using the therapeutic rhythmisation, we most commonly use simple technical aids such as a metronome or buzzer, the so-called shielded reading procedures (where the therapist collectively reads the beginnings of words or sets rhythmic sequences using their voice) and the graphical illustration of sounds, word parts and speech organ movements.

To induce quality self-control of speech rate (in ataxic or central dysarthria), the following variants are used:

- So-called tapping with a finger or a hand.
- Tapping when a buzzer sounds.
- Using a metronome for timing the repetition of word and sentence forms.
- The use of suitable reading material that enables an intensive and more long-term speech burden within the therapeutic session.

To slow down an excessive or unstable speech rate (hypokinetic dysarthria), the so-called deceleration aids have been proven to be effective:

- Charts with letters.
- Plastic tables with a series of boxes in which the finger may be placed gradually, word/syllable—for slowing and separating—during the utterance (pacing board, Duffy 2005a; Brookshire 2007).
- Adapted text with remote words, etc.

These aids extend the time period for the movement of the finger or hand during tapping, and they encourage the person with dysarthria to maintain a stable speech rhythm. Technical support means the use of:

- Delayed aural feedback for slowing the rate of speech (DAF).
- Amplified aural feedback through headphones within the scope of reading and spontaneous speech.

Amplified visual feedback by using a mirror, a video-camera or quality webcam is effective primarily when including newly-induced or renewed articulation movements in rhythmic exercises. During the intervention process, several methodical principles have been proven to be effective in the use of these methods and aids:

- We start with the rhythm of words after syllables; if there is a favourable response we can then make the transition to word rhythm, which enables more fluent speech with an emphasis only on the beginnings of individual words.
- A favourable response is the inducement and continuous improving the ability to use rhythm, from direct imitation to the independent mastering of parts of speech by a person with dysarthria.
- The arrangement of procedures, from reading to thematic monologue and dialogue, enables the linking of rhythm with the restoration of lexical and graphic abilities, and language ability stimulation.
- The dominant component is the effort to induce the spontaneous use of rhythm in speech, and to induce the self-control of own speech rather than just the mastering of a procedure in therapeutic sessions.
- The chosen form of tapping must be monitored, and possibly changed in the long term, e.g., from rhythm by using the finger to a leg movement, in order to reduce conspicuousness during spontaneous speech.

In adults with acquired dysarthria, sufficient attention must be paid to ensuring motivation appropriate to the adult's age and mental abilities. The therapist should present procedures aimed at improving speech comprehensibility, and they should clearly explain the importance of regular long-term therapy and supporting exercises; for example breathing exercises. The use of rhythm procedures is, in our clinical experience, a very versatile and effective way of helping persons suffering from acquired dysarthria to renew their motor speech abilities; it also contains considerable motivational potential, as long as the effectiveness of this procedure is demonstrated to the person with dysarthria at the outset of the SLT.

## 20.4 Rehabilitation of Apraxia of Speech

Claudio Luzzatti

### 20.4.1 Treatment of Apraxia of Speech (AoS)

Following the criteria outlined by Wambaugh et al. (2006), the training techniques employed for the treatment of AoS may be categorised in four main classes, on the basis of the major focus of the treatment:

- Techniques acting on the *voluntary control* of the articulatory kinematics.
- Techniques focused on *rhythm control.*
- Techniques focused on *intersystemic facilitation/reorganisation.*
- Techniques based on *augmentative* and *alternative* communication (AAC) procedures.

**The Techniques acting on the Voluntary Control of articulatory Kinematics** are based on the assumption that AoS depends on damage to the interface between phonological output and speech motor programming. These techniques aim at providing patients with phonetic information concerning the movements that are required to realise speech sounds, and bringing them to gain intentional control of the articulatory positions of vowels, and later on of consonant-vowel syllables, consonant clusters and multisyllabic strings.

The techniques grouped by Wambaugh and Martinez (2000) under this heading may be further divided into two major classes: (a) treatments inducing the activation of automatised elements by means of facilitation *(deblocking)* procedures (Basso 1977; Luria et al. 1969; Stevens 1989); (b) treatments aiming at breaking automatised schemata on which patients have lost intentional control owing to the AoS disorder, and at acquiring intentional control of speech production (Dabul and Bollier 1976; Rosenbek 1978). Despite their common goal, the two types of training procedure are based on opposite rehabilitation principles: in the first case, residual automatised articulatory patterns are facilitated and reinforced; in the second, inhibition of automatised elements and restoration of the impaired articulatory patterns on intentional basis are enhanced.

The rationale of the latter procedures is the remodelling of speech control (Luzzatti 2012a), based on proprioceptive, tactile and kinesthetic reinforcements, i.e., providing AoS patients with input information on the mutual position of the articulators, tension, temporal sequence, manner of articulation, and co-articulation [e.g., PROMPT—*Prompt of reconstructing oral muscular phonetic targets* (Square-Storer and Hayden 1989)]. Two major techniques are usually implemented in these methods: the use of drilling procedures and of sound pairs in minimal contrast (e.g., *Contrastive stress drill* (Wertz et al. 1984); SPT—*Sound Production Treatment* (Wambaugh et al. 1996)).

**The Techniques focused on Rhythm Control** assume that AoS depends on a primary deficit of a central mechanism that regulates rhythm in complex motor acts. However, such a hypothesis does not account for the frequent dissociation of AoS and ideo-motor apraxia (e.g., De Renzi et al. 1968), and the occasional dissociation of AoS and oral apraxia (e.g., De Renzi et al. 1966). The rationale of these techniques is the assumption that a treatment of rhythm control would restore proper temporal sequencing (e.g., Barlow et al. 2004), which would be specifically impaired in AoS, and in the remaining sorts of apraxic disorder.

**The Techniques focused on Intersystemic Facilitation/Reorganisation** assume that multisensory stimulation and activation of non-articulatory motor patterns reduce the severity of apraxic speech disorders.

**The Rationale of the Techniques based on AAC Procedures** is the assumption that AoS is resistant to any specific cognitive treatment. Therefore, functional recovery of the articulatory deficit depends only on non-articulatory communication skills (e.g., the use of the writing modality, mostly in association with electronic speech-generating devices).

## 20.4.2 Efficacy of the Apraxia of Speech Treatment

An analysis performed by West et al. (2005) for the *Cochrane Organization* aimed at confirming that individual treatments cause *significant* improvement (i.e., a degree of improvement that is significantly higher than that expected for spontaneous recovery) in patients with AoS

after focal vascular brain damage. None of the studies considered in the Cochrane review (1980–2004) actually corresponded to the criteria for a randomised clinical trial. A more recent analysis performed over the 1980–2007 period did not detect any further randomised case-control clinical trials (Luzzatti 2012b).

However, the analysis of studies employing a *single-case* or *multiple single-case methodology* could demonstrate the actual efficacy of individual treatment for AoS (Ballard et al. 2007; Basso et al. 2011; Dworkin et al. 1988; Knock et al. 2000; Mauszycki et al. 2024; Wambaugh 2009; Wambaugh and Nessler 2004; Wambaugh et al. 1996, 1998, 1999, 2017). The single-case analyses indicate that individual training of AoS by techniques acting on voluntary control of articulatory kinematics by means of contrastive stress drill (e.g., Wambaugh et al. 1996) improves the patients' speech performance even in chronic moderate-to-severe AoS cases. A relatively recent review (Ballard et al. 2015), updated to 2012, found 26 rehabilitation studies based on a single-case or multiple-single case methodology (meeting inclusion criteria): 24 of them tested efficacy of articulatory–kinematic (e.g., SPT) training procedures. Twenty-one of the studies satisfied criteria for an objective improvement of the post-treatment outcome. The efficacy seems to depend on treatment intensity with untreated material with the same phonetic characteristics of the material employed in the training phase and maintains its effect after treatment interruption. No clear evidence could be obtained in favour of either treatment that used sensory stimulation in the frame of an intersystemic facilitation/reorganisation training, or of techniques based on rhythm control, or on AAC procedures.

Nevertheless, since all studies reporting effective treatments were based on single case reports, no clear conclusion can be drawn about generalisability of such effects, since these studies usually do not specify either inclusion/exclusion criteria or the occurrence of drop-out cases. Furthermore, improvement after treatment is significant on experimental word and sentence lists, but no clear generalisation has been shown for the articulatory performance in ecological interactive speech conditions (connected speech).

## 20.5 Principles of Augmentative and Alternative Communication Interventions

Stefanie K. Sachse and Tobias Bernasconi

### 20.5.1 Introduction

Augmentative and alternative communication (AAC) is an intervention method for children, adolescents and adults whose

> natural speech is inadequate to meet all their communication goals.—Beukelman and Light (2020)

Some individuals with complex communication needs (CCN) might partly rely on speech and use AAC as additional (augmentative) means of communication, while others need AAC as an alternative to speech production. The overall purpose of AAC intervention is to enhance participation in education, employment, health care and family life (Light and McNaughton 2015). To achieve this goal, AAC intervention should provide short-term support for today's communication needs (intervention for today) as well as long-term support to prepare for future opportunities, needs etc. (intervention for tomorrow), and include not only the use of AAC modes, methods and strategies, but also a focus on natural speech and partner training (Beukelman and Light 2020; Braun 2020). The main focus of AAC interventions is on functionality of communication in the real world and in daily activities, thus it is essential continuously to assess the actual communication performance in real-life contexts (Light and McNaughton 2015; Sachse and Bernasconi 2020). The term used to describe the adequacy of communication in meeting the demands of daily interactions is communicative competence (Light 1989; Light and McNaughton 2014, 2015).

### 20.5.2 Communicative Competence

Communicative competence has been described as an interpersonal construct based on functionality of communication in real life contexts, and skills in four AAC-specific domains: linguistic competence, operational competence, social competence and strategic competence (Light 1989). Additionally, psychosocial factors such as motivation, attitude, confidence and resilience, as well as literacy skills, play an important role in successful communication in everyday interactions (Light and McNaughton 2014, 2015).

Light (1989) describes the four AAC-related areas as follows:

- **Linguistic competence** relates to the receptive and expressive language skills, as well as the linguistic code of the AAC system (such as symbols). Individuals need to learn their vocabulary and be able to combine words (syntactic skills) to express themselves.
- **Operational competence** describes both the technical skills to operate the communication devices (such as access methods and vocabulary retrieving; using such device features as volume control, deleting the last word, etc.), as well as the skills to use the system accordingly. That means that a child might have learned where the words "not" and "now" are on the device, but operational competence means that a child uses these words in different situations.
- **Social competence** relates to the pragmatic skills of knowing when to speak and when not, what to talk about, in what manner (Hymes 1972; Light 1989), as well as such socio-relational aspects of interaction as responsiveness to partners, the ability to put partners at ease (Light 1988). Examples are making eye-contact after the message button is pressed or nodding to express understanding or approval.
- **Strategic competence** describes the skill of AAC users "to make the best of what they do know and can do" (Light 1989), despite the limitations of the communication. This is a really important aspect that should get more attention within AAC intervention. It highlights the skill of individuals to decide upon the most efficient way to express themselves in a certain situation with the people present. It is the skill to know when to use, e.g., the signs and vocalisations that your sister under-

stands but not your teacher. It is self-evident that teachers and therapists do not insist on the use of the speech generating device (SGD) when they understand what an AAC user wants to express. The devices should expand the expressive skills in a meaningful way.

A balanced focus on these areas of the communicative competence model provides a helpful framework for AAC intervention planning for both aided and unaided AAC.

### 20.5.3 Unaided and Aided AAC

There is a wide range of AAC systems designed to meet the needs of individuals with CCN: unaided AAC does not require any external equipment or technology, and includes facial expressions, vocalisations, eye-blink-codes, gestures and signs. Aided AAC includes low-tech options such as communication boards and binders, as well as high-tech options such as speech-generating devices (dedicated AAC devices but also mobile technologies with AAC applications; Beukelman and Light 2020; for some examples see Reichmuth 2020).

Individual AAC users typically rely on multimodal communication systems (Braun 2020) because of the demands of different situations and the skills (or lack thereof) of different communication partners. In this sense, it is crucial to consider the advantages and disadvantages of the different communication modes (Table 20.3).

An example: Alex is an adolescent girl with cerebral palsy and dysarthria, using a high-tech eye gaze AAC-system (using both symbols and spelling with word-prediction) when talking to teachers, but with more familiar partners and in one-to-one situations she spells with the help of an alphabet board. Because she can't point to the letters, she uses a code with two head movements for one letter. Despite the time-consuming spelling technique, she is faster spelling with a partner than spelling with her device. Her strategic skills help her to choose the most efficient communication mode in a certain situation, and she chooses to spell often, because it's important to her to express herself in her own words.

Literacy skills expand the expressive skills of people with CCN tremendously and it's therefore critical to provide comprehensive literacy instruction as part of every AAC intervention.

**Table 20.3** Advantages and disadvantages of different AAC modes (Braun 2020; Beukelman and Light 2020; Erickson and Koppenhaver 2020)

| | Advantages | Disadvantages |
|---|---|---|
| Unaided AAC | Always present; often effective with familiar communication partners | Difficult or impossible to understand for non-familiar communication partners; (in absence of spelling skills:) difficult to communicate complex information; dependent on physical closeness and attention of the communication partner; can be difficult for participating in groups |
| Low-tech AAC | Communication and understanding possible with unfamiliar communication partner; easy to transport; rather simple to create and to adapt; effective with familiar communication partners | Symbols might seem somehow childish; depending on physical closeness and attention of the communication partner; depending on the co-construction skills of the communication partner; can be difficult to participate in groups |
| High-tech AAC | Possible to communicate with unfamiliar communication partners; possible to communicate despite physical distance; less dependent on the co-construction skills of the communication partner (compared with low-tech AAC); more independent possibilities to steer conversations; communication in groups | Long breaks within conversations; long time needed to learn to use the device; can break or be out of battery; dependent on somebody providing the device; in certain situations, difficult to use (i.e. bathroom); expensive; high pressure to use successfully |

"Until AAC users can spell, they depend on others to decide which words to provide them in aided AAC".—Erickson and Koppenhaver (2020)

Additionally, studies show that both intelligibility and comprehension of severely dysarthric speech are markedly improved when listeners are provided with alphabet and topic cues (Hustad and Beukelman 2001, 2002).

### 20.5.4 Overview of AAC Interventions

The complexity of AAC intervention results from the diverse needs of the heterogeneous group of individuals with CCN, with a wide range of therapy outcomes addressed, some directed at the impairment (body functions/structure) level of the International Classification of Functioning, Disability and Health (WHO ICF 2001/annual updates; McLeod and McCormack 2007) addressing comprehension or linguistic skills, and some directed at the activity/participation levels of the ICF, facilitating strategic skills and communicative effectiveness with a greater emphasis on real-life use (Murray et al. 2014).

> It's critical that interventionists focus on communication and do not become distracted too early by specific technological solutions [...]. A broad perspective on communication helps the interventionist's attention on the most essential elements first: building competence and independence—Dowden and Cook 2012

The model of communicative independence provides a helpful framework for the description of AAC intervention. The three types of communicators described are (Dowden 1999; Dowden and Cook 2012):

- **Emerging communicators** rely solely on non-symbolic modes of expression, such as facial expressions, body postures and vocalisations, and they are unable to communicate beyond "here and now". This group is rather dependent on familiar communication partners.
- **Context-dependent communicators** are not (yet) able to express anything they want, but they can use their AAC modes with certain familiar partners and express a certain number

of ideas. This group is dependent on context or on the support of the communication partner. Together with the familiar/skilled communication partners they can often use their AAC modes, strategies and expand their communication possibilities.

- **Independent communicators** have full communicative competence and can freely express their ideas, share their thoughts and feelings. They can communicate successfully with unfamiliar communication partners (Alex is an independent communicator).

These short descriptions of the different groups provide a first impression of the complexity of AAC intervention. It is not enough to provide a family with a set of manual signs or an adult with aphasia with a speech-generating device (Lüke and Vock 2019). Besides the decision on the communication modes, it is essential to describe the goals of the intervention in detail and to ask what advantage a certain intervention has for the person with CCN in terms of everyday life. Using the ICF can be helpful in finding meaningful everyday situations or activities to focus on (Bernasconi 2020). To be able (to learn) to communicate with different partners and in different settings it is important to combine different communication modes (Beukelman and Light 2020). Often, different intervention strategies are used (both in therapy and natural settings) and the intervention is directed to the individual and the communication partners (Squires et al. 2013). For these reasons, AAC intervention is best described as a complex intervention (de Silva et al. 2014; Squires et al. 2013; Zinkevich et al. 2019).

### 20.5.5 Studies and Reviews on AAC Intervention

An extensive review of meta-analyses and reviews on AAC intervention (Sachse in prep) reveals a very diverse description and focus of AAC-intervention research: it ranges from studies that focus solely on isolated skills such as requesting in a therapy setting (Alzrayer et al. 2014) or on the effect of AAC intervention on speech (Binger et al. 2008; Schlosser and Wendt 2008), to the different modes and strategies used (modelling and partner training, Biggs et al. 2018; Kent-Walsh et al. 2015) or barriers and facilitators to the use of high-tech AAC (Baxter et al. 2012), to reviews that focus on the needs of certain groups (autism spectrum disorder: Holyfield et al. 2017; treatment outcomes for children with childhood apraxia of speech: Murray et al. 2014) or younger children (Leonet et al. 2022). While the individual research is helpful in guiding practical decisions, we advocate a comprehensive understanding of AAC intervention, including at least the following components (Beukelman and Light 2020), descriptions of:

1. The indication or group according to the communicative independence model (Dowden 1999; Dowden and Cook 2012).
2. The communication modes used.
3. Intervention strategies (i.e., strategy instruction, prompting techniques, literacy as an integral part of intervention), description of partner training, description of strategies to ensure implementation (including modelling, environmental adaptation interventions, responsive social pragmatic intervention).
4. Meaningful outcomes addressed (regarding communicative competence, literacy skills, speech, quality of life or to decrease challenging behaviour; goals for today and for tomorrow) while taking the perspective of the children (Klang et al. 2016) and the social validity of the team into consideration (Logan et al. 2017).

## 20.5.6 Conclusion

The overall focus of AAC intervention should be on meaningful opportunities for communication and expanding participation in a variety of situations, and on such diverse communicative intents as expressing needs and wants, information transfer, social closeness and social etiquette or internal dialogue.

> The ultimate goal of AAC intervention is not to find a technological solution to communication problems but to enable individuals to efficiently and effectively engage in a variety of interactions and participate in activities of their choice—Beukelman and Light (2020)

## 20.6 Augmentative and Alternative Communication (AAC) Methods in Dysarthria/Apraxia

Lenka Neubauerová and Karel Neubauer

### 20.6.1 The Current Concept of AAC and the Field of Neurogenic Speech Communication Disorders

Augmentative and alternative communication (AAC) is in its current concept a multidisciplinary area that deals with the development of a constructive approach to communication of people who cannot effectively use common forms of interpersonal communication, especially speech communication, its written form and common forms of non-verbal communication modalities (gestures, intonation and sound dynamics, proxemics, etc.). AAC includes contributions from a number of disciplines, especially in the field of communication technologies, communication sciences, linguistics, rehabilitation, pedagogy and psychology. In many developed countries AAC intervention programmes and the use of AAC assistive technology are part of comprehensive rehabilitation care, intertwined with multi-departmental, especially medical programmes. These include the use of specific technologies with electronic aids and devices, as well as systems that are not primarily dependent on the use of these aids.

Knowledge in the field of AAC is focused on three main areas of interest:

- Processes of creating AAC programmes, use of communication systems and aids.
- AAC procedures developed to assist individuals with developmental communication disorders.
- AAC procedures developed to assist individuals with acquired communication disorders.

The common denominator for persons who benefit from the use of AAC procedures is always the severity, persistence or deterioration of the condition, which causes a serious difficulty or even impossibility of using common modalities of interpersonal communication. Frequently reported groups of such people are those with mental deficits, cerebral palsy (CP), pervasive developmental disorders, especially autism and sensory disabilities, and with multiple coexisting disabilities. These causes, associated with limited or minimal development of speech communication, lead to the employment of AAC procedures at an early or preschool age of the child, or at a later period, and may be part of a person's communication throughout his or her life. In the area of motor, neurogenically conditioned, disorders, it is mainly a group of children with severe manifestations of developmental dysarthria or anarthria, related to the development of the CP syndrome or other serious neurogenic diseases.

In the field of acquired disorders, the key areas are neurogenic emerging speech communication disorders—dysarthria, speech apraxia, aphasia—and the consequences of neurodegenerative diseases accompanied by dementia syndromes, such as Alzheimer's disease or vascular dementia. Loss of speech communication is also caused by conditions after traumatic CNS traumas and progressive neurological diseases—amyotrophic lateral sclerosis (ALS), progressive forms of multiple sclerosis (rapidly evolving severe relapsing remitting MS RES) (Johnson et al. 2012; Beukelman and Mirenda 2013; Neubauerová and Neubauer 2018).

## 20.6.2 AAC in Children with Developmental Dysarthria or Anarthria

One of the three more widespread areas of AAC use in children is for those who do not achieve the development of intelligible speech owing to severe neurogenic impairment of mobility and coordination, or severe manifestations of dysarthria to anarthria in CP, after CNS trauma or neurodegenerative diseases. Other areas are manifestations of the child's pervasive developmental disorder, especially autism, and the presence of a psychomotor delay in the child's development, which results in

permanent cognitive impairment (Clarke et al. 2012; Johnson et al. 2012).

In clinical practice, the coexistence of two or all of the above areas is very common, so it is a suitable starting point for detailed assessment of a person with communication disorders, their social environment and living conditions, especially in terms of obtaining a reasonable scope and focus of diagnostics before applying AAC procedures. Access to updated speech therapy, psychological and medical professional diagnostics can be considered a necessary precondition for a comprehensive evaluation of the possibilities of AAC intervention (Neubauerová and Neubauer 2018).

With the current stress mainly on augmentative communication, the importance of choosing a suitable method to support the development of the child's language skills, stimulate his ability to understand the content of communication and the development of his reading and writing is growing. Von Tetzchner and Matrinsen (2000) list three groups of children who use functional communication support with AAC, those:

- With an express disorder of language development (expressive language group).
- Using support for the development of language skills (supportive language group).
- Requiring an alternative communication code (alternative language group).

If we apply the above system to the reality of clinical speech therapy practice, it contributes appropriately to the diagnostic-therapeutic decision about the benefits of AAC and the choice of its form:

- The first group of children, owing to the serious difference between understanding and the possibility of their own speech production, will use a certain AAC system for effective communication with the environment in a long-term, frequent and lifelong way. This group is characterised by children with CP or severe dysarthria to anarthria, whose cognitive abilities allow the development of all language system components and understanding of the content of the language of people in the environment.

- The second group of children includes those for whom AAC is considered a temporary intervention that will support the development of comprehension of the language in the environment, and the development of their language skills of comprehension and expressive development for a relatively short time. AAC practices can help certain activities, such as developing a child's vocabulary. An example of this group are those with developmental dysphasia.
- The third group of children is characterised by a severe limitation in the development of both impressive language skills (understanding the content of the language message of those around them) and expressive speech skills. In children with severe cognitive deficits, mental deficits or severe developmental pervasive disorders, the use of AAC related to the state of their cognitive and educational abilities is appropriate, often with the perspective of life-long use across their daily programmes (Von Tetzchner and Matrinsen 2000; Neubauerová and Neubauer 2018).

Given the realistic perception of the diagnostic potential for prognosis of the child's communication and language skills, a pragmatic approach is appropriate to determine the relevant procedure and the extent of the involvement of AAC in the development of the therapeutic programme. Clarke et al. (2012) recommend respecting the following when evaluating this area:

- The child's physical condition, the presence of epilepsy or severe dietary problems.
- The child's personal interests and preferences, especially in building eye contact and attention.
- The child's cognitive development, involvement in the educational programme and the state of psychological diagnostics.
- The child's movement and coordination capabilities, which dictate the design of the programme and the necessary technical support.

**Table 20.4** Diagnostic evaluation of the development of understanding of symbols and signs and programme selection (Park 2002; Clarke et al. 2012; Neubauerová and Neubauer 2018)

| Level of understanding of symbols and signs | Decision to choose the AAC programme |
| --- | --- |
| Adequate level of physical age (at least 8–9 years of intact development) and developed reading ability and knowledge of spelling | Use of the written word as an augmentative system, involvement of grammar and spelling; use of the conversion of written speech into the voice speech output of the programme in ICT assistive technology or specialised software |
| Level 5 years. In the intact population, with a reduction in vocabulary volume | The user is often able to use (border area) a complex abstract symbolic system (Bliss system) |
| Level 3–4 years | Use of an abstract system of symbols with content reduction and support in the use or application of image communication symbols (pictograms, other iconic image systems) |
| Level 2 and a half to 3 years | Use of a mostly iconic system of visual communication; symbols in programme creation |
| Level 12–18 months of age | Use of iconic images and photographs in the form of a communication table or workbook |
| Level less than 12 months of age | Individual range of use of tactilely accessible three-dimensional symbols and objects in everyday repetitive activities |

- The child's temperament and personality, as well as the social environment.
- The family's attitude to the use of technology, involvement and possibilities of the school programme in their use.
- The child's age and development of his speech and language skills, the results of clinical speech therapy diagnostics.
- The degree of understanding of spoken expression and meaning of symbols in communication (see Table 20.4).

## 20.6.3 AAC in Adults with Acquired Dysarthria, Speech Apraxia and co-Existing Neurogenic Communication Disorders

AAC in the field of acquired disorders is seen primarily as a means of compensating for the difficulty or loss of speech communication in the environment. Such an attitude is in line with the statements of, for example, the American Speech-Language Hearing Association (ASHA) and other professional organisations in the field of Speech-Language Therapy (SLT). In clinical practice it is devoted to compensating for severe persistent communication disorders, driven by an effort temporarily or permanently to overcome the manifestations of disability in people with severe expressive communication disorders—that is, with severe disorders in motor speech, language system and written expression (ASHA 2005).

The above approach can be divided into three important segments of the use of AAC in the field of clinical speech therapy:

- By an individual in communication to develop understanding, to express his needs, if he cannot use speech at a given moment.
- Included directly in the therapeutic process simultaneously with specific methods of recovery therapy.
- A permanent means of support in the case of a persistent disorder that is a barrier to speech communication.

When AAC is used, especially in people with acquired neurogenic communication disorders, it is useful to define user groups according to the degree of support required within the communication process into two groups:

- The first group uses AAC as an expressive means of communication—i.e. people who understand spoken speech, but owing to their impaired expressive abilities, can only express themselves to a limited extent.
- The second group uses AAC to support speech production—i.e. people who express themselves verbally, but whose speech is incomprehensible without the use of a communication aid. This group also includes people who use AAC only to express themselves in a certain situation (Von Tetzchner and Matrinsen 2000; Neubauerová and Neubauer 2018).

These two approaches are relevant for people with aphasia (group 1) and with dysarthria or speech dyspraxia (group 2), and brings closer the noticeable tension between the concept of AAC as a compensatory means and that of a substitute for spoken speech. People without hearing loss especially, with a good understanding of speech communication (dysarthria-anarthria, speech apraxia), and those using extra-linguistic means of communication (voice modulation, voice dynamics), as well as those with expressive speech (severe mixed aphasia-global aphasia) are often not suitable candidates for visual system-only AAC, which replaces auditory-orientated communication. Beukelman and Mirenda (2013), Garrett and Lasker (2013), Feeley and Jones (2012b) and other authors associated with the field of SLT suggest the use of suitable AAC systems in people with aphasia or dysarthria with regard to the type and severity of the disorder. These people can effectively use:

- The compensatory function of AAC in combination with speech therapy, often with the use of a written form of verbal communication.
- Dual communication system with the use of vocal, voice communication and involvement of non-verbal communication AAC system.

## 20.6.4 Therapy in the Field of Clinical Speech and AAC

The clinical speech therapist should be able to perceive which AAC means can be used comprehensively for therapeutic assistance, not just using assistive technologies to provide "alternative speech" to non-speakers. It is appropriate to include in the diagnostic-therapeutic evaluation an understanding of the:

- Value and role of AAC and techniques for children and adults with severe speech and language deficits.
- Patient's needs as part of the overall system of so-called total communication.
- Design, methodology of use and appropriate involvement of differential types of AAC systems in these persons.
- Need to identify factors that are important in the assessment of the child or adult and his environment for the use of AAC resources.

The effective use of a file or system of graphic symbols is currently commonly linked to the use of PCs or portable types of computer, touch screen devices (smartphones, tablets) and output with digital or other speech technology or electronic communication aids producing speech recordings. These aids, especially for early and preschool children, should not prevail over non-electronic systems, such as cards with pictures, symbols, book aids etc. The use of both systems (high- or light-tech) should be in the right balance to support the child's development and motivation to communicate with the environment, not his dependence on a certain type of fun activity (Clarke et al. 2012). The development of the AAC system is intended to develop effective communication with the environment, and practical skills to communicate in everyday life. If the proposed way of using AAC resources is accepted by all persons with whom a person with communication disorders is in contact, the process of developing four main components of the ability to use AAC resources optimally will be adequately supported (Light et al. 1998; Beukelman and Mirenda 1992, 2013; Laudová 2003; Neubauerová 2013):

- Linguistic competence. Use of native language modalities (vocabulary and grammar) and mastery of codes (characters/symbols) required when using AAC.
- Operational competence. Motor and cognitive skills required to signal the message and to manage the technical skills required to operate the system.

- Social competence. Knowledge and skills included in the social rules of communication, e.g., adequate eye contact, maintaining a balance between self-expression and listening, the ability to start, hold and end a conversation and have knowledge of with whom, what, when and how to communicate.
- Strategic competence. Appropriate use of different communication strategies in different situations, flexibility in adjusting the communication style to suit the recipient, the ability to switch from one mode of communication to another (e.g., to use a communication table or computer according to immediate need or availability), the ability to "correct a conversation", i.e., to use a different way of expression if the other person does not understand.

For people with dysarthria, anarthria, speech apraxia and differential neurogenic communication disorders, communication systems with potential use in clinical practice include, in cases of problems with the use of written code The Picture Exchange Communication system— PECS, pictograms, the Makaton system, Bliss symbolism, character-to-speech and other character systems, are often associated with the compilation of a communication table used by individuals to communicate (Neubauerová et al. 2016). A communication log can be created from these tables, which, with diaries created according to the individual needs of their users, should contain a sufficiently large number of symbols that the individual has the widest possible communication. The list of terms is compiled with regard to the interests of the individual, and also his immediate surroundings contribute to his creation.

Words in the list that the individual can express differently are not included in the table. These are, for example, the terms "YES / NO / I DON'T KNOW", which can be represented through body language, most often associated with vocal intonation. However, if the individual is not able to do so, he should have these terms available in the communication diary in a special table intended for these terms and easily accessible. For example, through a last page that can be removed and placed next to all other communication tables. The selected symbol is indicated by pointing a finger or limb, directing the gaze, using a head pointer (a light source attached to the head), etc.

The ability to use eye movement and focus to communicate with a person who is physically paralysed and suffers from a loss of speech communication but has the ability to read, is a highly important AAC method for people with acquired anarthria. These conditions are present in advanced neurodegenerative diseases that do not affect human cognitive abilities (e.g., amyotrophic lateral sclerosis) or in persons after severe traumatic or other neurogenic traumas. The mass-produced device with a lightweight frame of transparent plastic, under the name The Frenchay E-trans Frame, has long been offered by the British company Speechmark Publishing, which demonstrates its importance and applicability. When using this communication system, both the user and the communication partner face each through in a window in the middle of the transparent frame and the edges of this frame are used to place letters, YES / NO answer symbols, etc. and coloured auxiliary points. In this position, eye movements are clearly identifiable with a side view, both horizontally and vertically. According to the agreed method of use, the user thus communicates to the communication partner the letter—part of the expression—and the entire expression with immediate confirmation by the communication partner's feedback. The e-trans system includes many advantages of using a low-tech type of tool that is independent of ICT technology. Here one can highlight the portability, minimum weight, the possibility of use, for example, in the bathroom in the bathtub, use at the bedside for people lying down, good possibility of use even in a state of increased fatigue, when the user is too tired for the demanding use of ICT technology (Neubauerová and Neubauer 2018).

The combination of technical aid and ICT technology with a computer system and specialised software is currently common, with the exception of simple electronic communicators, which play short verbal or multiword turns after activating the switch. These can be used only as a supplement to the communication system used;

on the other hand, ICT technologies enable a comprehensive solution of the communication system with the environment, which its user can manage in terms of motor, language and cognitive skills. Current specialised programmes offer support in development solutions mainly in the following parameters:

- Compilation, sorting, changes and extensions of communication tables from the AAC system used.
- Voice output producing intelligible digitised or ICT-generated speech.
- Conversion of voice or written input to output in the form of symbols or characters—manual playback—movement character, symbol presentation and its written output.
- Direct control of a computer programme by adjusting the touch input (keyboard, mouse, switch) or using a sensor (movement of the head, eyebrows, eyes, etc.) or an indicator (e.g., light from the pointer).
- Indirect control, most often by the so-called scanning, i.e., by selecting from the offered list of items by a switch and item cursor. Most often this is in the form of step, circular or linear scanning, which improves itself with a lower number of selected items. Multi-step scanning by sequentially selecting parts of an extensive vocabulary of items is a cognitively demanding operation that requires the user to have good judgement and motivation in the process of learning this skill, and it is a good choice for people with severe dysarthria, anarthria or with severe speech apraxia.

### 20.6.5 Prognosis and Use of AAC in Clinical Practice

Determination of prognostic factors by the use of AAC in people with dysarthria, anarthria, speech apraxia and coexisting disorders of speech communication is highly individual and variable, depending on the internal and external conditions of this process. In the case of stable motivation of participating persons, availability of a technical background and a prognostically positive or stable picture of the aetiology of the communication impairment of the affected person can be sufficient to establish an effective communication system with the environment. In the case of progressive disease, abrupt or creeping deterioration of cognitive or physical possibilities, the reality is to modify or change the original use of AAC resources in respect of the development of the disease.

The development of AAC for those who can benefit from its procedures may be hampered by clinical speech therapists who have a rather marginal interest in developing this form of communication and the involvement of AAC in the long-term therapeutic process management programme. Regarding the use of AAC, other experts, especially special educators, health professionals and social workers, often show little interest in deeper knowledge of speech communication disorders, understanding the difference between motor speech disorders, individual language system disorders and communication disorders resulting from the present cognitive deficit. These facts may lead to a limitation of mutual cooperation, unrealistic expectations in terms of the application of AAC and procedures of clinical speech therapy.

Respected published procedures in the application of the AAC system, especially in the provenance of experts from the USA and Australia (Beukelman and Mirenda 2013; Johnson et al. 2012) are mostly presented by speech therapy experts who focus on the area of AAC and show several inspiring characteristics, valid for this target group of people:

- The application of AAC procedures is developed differently for all groups of people with communication disorders, children, adults and seniors.
- The use of AAC procedures requires a high level of knowledge about the causes, manifestations and prognosis of communication disorders, including an understanding of the limits for the application of AAC.
- When applying technical (high-technology), computer and specialised support, the programme is guided by the interest of the person and the possibility of practical daily applica-

tion of AAC in communication with the environment, not by self-serving application of technology at the expense of direct interpersonal contact.

- The aim of the application of AAC is the application of all procedures leading to the goal—to improve the success of communication with the environment by any effective form of activity.

## 20.7 Cognitive Behavioural Therapy (CBT) and Transcranial Magnetic Stimulation (TMS)

### 20.7.1 Basic Knowledge of Psychological Treatment in Fluency Disorders

Kurt Eggers

#### 20.7.1.1 Introduction

In the Section on stuttering assessment (see Sect 8.1), we stated that although overt speech dysfluencies are the most characteristic symptom of stuttering, the diagnosis should not only focus on the overt symptoms, but also on a number of covert aspects such as underlying cognition and emotions associated with stuttering, and the impact that stuttering has on the client's day-to-day functioning. The same thing can be said for the treatment of stuttering.

Sheehan (1970) used the iceberg metaphor to describe stuttering, with only a small part of the iceberg above the waterline, i.e. the overt symptoms, and a much bigger part below referring to the covert aspects, including fear, shame, guilt, anxiety. Flattening the top of the iceberg will only cause the iceberg to rise again, so, just eliminating overt symptoms will cause relapse after a short time. Consequently, if treatment is only focused on the top of the iceberg by stuttering modification or fluency shaping techniques, one could argue that the whole stuttering problem is not effectively addressed (Guitar 2013). Therefore, addressing the covert aspects should form an integral part of any stuttering treatment, especially in people who have been stuttering for a long period of time and where covert aspects—most likely—will have developed further.

Several authors have described how the covert aspects are not only a consequence of the overt symptomatology but can also increase the overt stuttering severity (Conture 2001; Jones et al. 2020). Blood (1995) described that covert aspects, i.e. cognitive and affective reactions, are due to the subjective evaluations made by a person who stutters while experiencing speech interruptions. Van Riper (1982) stated how these covert aspects can be narrowed down to different types of fear/anxiety: fear for social punishment, for listener loss, for loss of self-control, for being stigmatised as a person who stutters. In stuttering, similar psychological mechanisms are involved, as can be seen in anxiety disorders. Individuals anticipate future danger, experience negative feelings and bodily symptoms, have low sense of self-efficacy to exercise control over their stressors, try to avoid fearful situations, and experience severe impairment in their daily functioning (Maniadaki 2017). This anxiety is caused and maintained by cognitive biases such as preferentially allocating attention towards the anticipation of stuttering (Lowe et al. 2016; McAllister et al. 2015).

There is a reasonable degree of consensus that children, adolescents and adults who stutter are at greater risk than population statistics would predict of experiencing and exhibiting behaviour that is characteristic of social anxiety, also referred to as social phobia (Craig et al. 2003; Craig and Tran 2014; Iverach et al. 2016; Smith et al. 2014). The co-existence of stuttering and anxiety has implications for assessment (see Sect. 8.1) and therapy, and has led to the development of a number of therapy programmes that incorporate strategies to manage or reduce anxiety associated with stuttering (e.g. Harley 2018; Kelman and Wheeler 2015; Menzies et al. 2019). Furthermore, it seems logical to conclude that psychological approaches that are typically being used to address anxiety in order to change dysfunctional beliefs and avoiding behaviour, such as cognitive-behavioural approaches, can also be applied for stuttering therapy (e.g. Boey 2010; Reddy et al. 2010).

So, in addition to direct therapy (working with the client on overt stuttering symptoms) and indirect therapy (working with the environment of children to create a fluency-enhancing environment), speech language therapists should also incorporate and apply psychology-based therapy components in their treatment of people who stutter, particularly in older children and adults. Such psychology-based therapies include cognitive behavioural therapy, personal construct therapy, narrative therapy, mindfulness, and acceptance and commitment therapy.

Finally, some might question if speech language therapists should be dealing with counselling aspects of people who stutter, or if working with emotions and cognitive change should be addressed by psychologists (Manning 2009). If clients are experiencing chronic life-adjustment problems, it is evident that referral to other professionals, such as counsellors and psychologists, is the most appropriate choice. Although communication disorders often result in serious problems on many levels, in most cases we are not working with people who have chronic life-adjustment problems. The vast majority of the people who stutter are ordinary people experiencing a normal reaction (i.e. emotions of stress and anxiety) to a very difficult communication problem (Luterman 2001). We agree with Manning's viewpoint that a comprehensive treatment should include client and family counselling, and that trying to achieve behavioural change in the absence of cognitive restructuring is a recipe for relapse. Hence, speech-language therapists specialised in working with stuttering must be trained in applying some of these psychology-based treatments.

## 20.7.1.2 Cognitive (Behavioural) Therapy

Cognitive behavioural therapy (CBT) is a form of psychological treatment, developed by Beck in the 50 s, that has been found to be effective for a range of problems including depression and anxiety disorders (Beck 2011). Numerous research studies suggest that CBT leads to significant improvement in the client's functioning and quality of life. CBT is based on the cognitive model, stating that the way in which individuals perceive a situation is more closely related to their reaction and interpretation of the situation than the situation itself. This can be helpful because it makes the world more predictable, but can also lead to errors. Beck stated that some people develop systematic, unhelpful biases in the way they interpret information, resulting in patterns of negative/unhelpful thinking. One of the core principles is that people can learn better ways of coping with these psychological adversities by efforts to change one's thinking patterns actively. This is done by identifying, evaluating and changing one's automatic thoughts, assumptions and core beliefs. Strategies to do so include (a) recognising one's distortions in thinking that are creating problems (e.g. catastrophising, mind reading, all-or-nothing thinking) and re-evaluating them in light of reality; (b) gaining a better understanding of the behaviour and motivation of others; (c) using problem-solving skills to cope with difficult situations; and (d) learning to develop a greater sense of confidence in one's own abilities.

The fact that people who stutter often feel anxious about specific (speaking) situations can be linked to negative/unhelpful thoughts or predictions of what is going to happen in these situations. These predictions can be about the stuttering itself ('I am sure I will stutter in that situation'), listener reactions ('People will start laughing') or how they will be perceived by others ('They will think I am incompetent'). Treatment gives clients insight into the link between their (automatic) thoughts, feelings and behavioural responses, focuses on problem-solving skills and aims to create more flexible thinking patterns.

CBT has been positively implemented in treatment for both individuals (e.g. Boey 2010; Blood 1995; Eggers 2020; Menzies et al. 2008) and groups (Fry et al. 2009) for stuttering, as well as in a stand-alone internet treatment for social anxiety in stuttering (Menzies et al. 2019). Different variants of this approach, such as Ellis's Rational emotive behaviour therapy (Ellis 2004), have also been successfully applied to the management of stuttering (Grossman 2020; Moleski and Tosi 1976).

### 20.7.1.3 Personal Construct Therapy

Personal construct therapy (PCT) was developed by Kelly (1955) and first applied to stuttering by Fransella (1970). Kelly considered each person as a scientist, engaged in a continuous process of hypothesising about one's environment and seeking evidence to test that understanding in terms of how it guides future events and behaviour (DiLollo et al. 2002; Manning 2010). The 'person-as-scientist' anticipates events, shapes behaviour accordingly, thus reducing uncertainty. The result of construing actions leads to the development of personal constructs. Kelly's idea of constructive alternativism states that all our present perceptions are open to question and reconsideration. Even the most obvious occurrences of everyday of life might appear totally transformed if we were inventive enough to construe them differently. Constructive alternativism states that there is always another way of construing events (Dalton 1983).

In stuttering therapy, PCT can be used to explore different ways one can talk (e.g. varying loudness, speed and pitch). Checking out the variety of ways or alternatives open to clients is part of the process of loosening constructs. In addition, when clients stutter, they can move beyond the feeling that there is only one way to speak, i.e. with a stutter. Loosening construing can lead to being able to make more choices, and ultimately to exercise better control in managing (stuttering) behaviour (Stewart and Birdsall 2001).

PCT has been implemented with people who stutter of different age ranges (Hayhow and Levy 1993; Shapiro 2011), offering a psychological framework to alter the clients' perception of himself with regard to his stuttering, and to the world in which he and his stuttering exists (Ward 2006). Both improvements in fluency, as well as decreases in anxiety have been reported (Botterill and Cook 1987).

### 20.7.1.4 Narrative Therapy

The application of PCT to stuttering has received widespread attention in Britain but much less in other countries, such as the United States. DiLollo et al. (2002) attribute this to the complexity of Kelly's (1955) theory, assessment that tends to be time-consuming, and the lack of collaboration between psychologists and speech-language therapists. An alternative treatment approach, adhering to the theoretical principles of a personal construct view, has gained considerable momentum is narrative therapy.

Narrative therapy (NT) has its origins in social constructionism, recognising that people construct their lives and identities socially and culturally, through language, discourse and communication (Ryan et al. 2015). NT was developed in the 80s (White 2000, 2007, White and Epston 1990) and is based on the idea that people understand their lives through their 'storying' of lived experience. NT begins with the narrative as told by the client; for people who stutter, this is often the stuttering-saturated narrative of how stuttering is central in the life of the client (Leahy et al. 2012). The process continues with externalising the problem through externalising conversations, assisting the client to separate the problem from oneself. In doing so, clients gain insight in and realise that the person is not the problem, but the problem is the problem. This implies that people who stutter make a shift from a 'stutterer'-perspective to a 'stuttering'-perspective. Through specific questioning techniques (e.g. outcome-, account-, possibility-, circulation- and re-description-questions), clients are invited to map the influence of the problem on their personal life and relationships and to 'rewrite and re-author their stories' to one that fits with their hopes, values and dreams.

NT can contribute to the long-term maintenance of more fluent speech (DiLollo et al. 2002), has been identified as a possible means of addressing the impact of stuttering on the person who stutters, and has been introduced as e.g. a core component of the Irish intervention programme 'Free to Stutter...Free to Speak' (Ryan et al. 2015).

### 20.7.1.5 Mindfulness- and Acceptance-Based Therapy

Mindfulness-based interventions (Kabat-Zinn 1996) and Acceptance and Commitment Therapy (ACT; Harris 2009) have been developed relatively recently and are sometimes labelled as 'third-wave behaviour therapies', which also include e.g. Dialectical Behaviour Therapy or Metacognitive Therapy. All of these therapies generally share an emphasis on acceptance and mindfulness (Merwin et al. 2019). Mindfulness and acceptance are closely related concepts. Mindfulness, described as intentionally focusing one's attention on the experiences occurring at the present moment in a non-judgmental and accepting way (Baer and Krietemeyer 2006), can be contrasted with states of mind in which attention is focused elsewhere, such as a preoccupation with memories or worries. Mindfulness results in decreased avoidance, increased emotional and attentional regulation, and acceptance. Acceptance can be described as willingness to experience a wide range of unwanted/unpleasant sensations, cognitions or emotional states without attempting to avoid, escape or terminate them.

Both professionals (e.g. Gregory 2003, Guitar 2013) and clients (e.g. Plexico et al. 2009a, b) have emphasised the importance of acceptance for the successful management of stuttering. Recent findings suggest that increased acceptance and less avoidance of stuttering are related to adaptive coping skills and increased quality of life among people who stutter (Plexico et al. 2009a, b). Mindfulness may be used as a valuable means for facilitating acceptance of stuttering-related behaviour, thoughts and feelings among people who stutter.

Different authors have described how these principles can be applied to the management of stuttering (e.g. Cheasman et al. 2015). Boyle (2011) concludes that the integration of mindfulness training and stuttering treatment appears practical and worthy of exploration and that mindfulness strategies adapted to stuttering may help in the management of cognitive, affective and behavioural challenges associated with stuttering.

### 20.7.1.6 Summary

The goal of this section was to provide doctors with an overview of the psychological approaches that are frequently being used by speech-language therapists in the overall management of stuttering, aimed at addressing its covert aspects, i.e. normal cognitive (irrational or dysfunctional thoughts and beliefs) and affective (social anxiety and avoidance behaviour) reactions to the experience of stuttering. These include approaches such as cognitive therapy, personal construct therapy, narrative therapy and mindfulness- and acceptance-based approaches. By no means did we have the intention to provide an all-encompassing overview of all treatments, and others used are e.g. solution-focused brief therapy and Dialectical therapy. They are applied by speech-language therapists in a counselling context, i.e. for the purpose of support or (re)education for behavioural problems not associated with mental illness (Crowe 1997). In case of chronic life-adjustment problems, referral to other professionals such as counsellors and psychologists, is evident.

### 20.7.2 Assistive Technology Used in the Treatment of Stuttering

Ashley Craig

### 20.7.2.1 Introduction

The treatment of stuttering has been dominated by behavioural, speech and psychological approaches, with the treatment modality largely dependent on the theoretical basis believed to cause the stuttering (Tran et al. 2011). For example, early theories assumed stuttering had a psychogenic basis, that is, the dysfluency was caused by underlying psychological deficits such as unconscious neurotic and psychosexual processes (Bloodstein and Bernstein Ratner 2008; Glauber, 1958). Others believed stuttering was caused by chronically high levels of anxiety, as argued by the approach-avoidance conflict or anticipatory-struggle theories, where stuttering was believed to occur owing to learned anxieties about speaking or from subconscious personality factors (Sheehan 1958). Treatments developed on the basis of these types of theory were principally psychotherapy-based (Bloodstein and Bernstein Ratner 2008). Psychologically based treatments alone have not proved to be effective in significantly reducing stuttering severity, though they may have some benefit for improving psychological reactions to the stuttering such as social anxiety (Bloodstein and Bernstein Ratner 2008; Menzies et al. 2008). In contrast, contemporary theories have argued that stuttering is a result of dysfunction in the speech sensory-motor control neural system with an inherited predisposition (Bloodstein and Bernstein Ratner 2008; Ludlow and Loucks 2003).

Notwithstanding the above, it is important to note that any elevated psychopathology associated with the disorder (such as elevated trait or social anxiety or depressive mood) is believed to be the result of negative reactions to the distress of living with the fluency disorder (Tran et al. 2011; Craig and Tran 2014). Consequently, more recent treatment approaches have targeted both speech/stuttering and psychological aspects of the disorder, with speech re-training and behavioural-contingent strategies, which have been found to be significantly effective in reducing stuttering and improving psychological states such as anxiety (Bothe et al. 2006; Craig and Tran 2006).

It has been recognised that clinicians have under-utilised technology in the treatment of stuttering (Packman and Meredith 2011). However, internet and world-wide web technology is now used by people who stutter, especially for access to educational resources concerning the nature and management of stuttering (Packman and Meredith 2011). Furthermore, technology used in the treatment of stuttering by speech pathologists, psychologists and others, has increased over the past 30–40 years or so, as described by Larry Molt (2019) in an excellent online resource. This section will summarise and briefly explore technology used in the treatment of stuttering, with special attention given to the efficacy of technology that utilises electromyography (EMG) feedback in combination with speech re-training and behaviour modification strategies to treat stuttering.

### 20.7.2.2 Overview of Technology Used in the Treatment of Stuttering

Molt (2019) provided a thorough breakdown of the types of technology used to help people who stutter to manage their disfluency. He classified types of technologies into the following:

- Devices that alter speech motor patterns. These include technology that alters a speech production pattern, such as a fork placed under the tongue, or the Idehara "Stutter-Cure" appliance, which consists of a palatal prosthesis similar to an orthodontic retainer, fitted into the mouth, against the hard palate (Van Riper 1973). The device includes a whistle, used to enhance continuous airflow when speaking, a factor known to reduce stuttering and increase fluency (Craig and Tran 2006). The person who stutters (PWS) is encouraged to maintain a whistling noise while speaking. There is little or no evidence of the efficacy of such devices, though if a PWS uses continuous airflow, fluency improves (Craig et al. 1996).
- Devices that provide feedback of physiological mechanisms. These for example include devices that provide feedback on respiratory, speech muscle and articulation timing. These types of technology have been used to help the PWS in identifying and altering speech production processes as part of therapy (Molt 2019). Physiological processes targeted include feedback on respiratory function, speech muscle EMG activity and feedback of phonatory/articulatory production and timing. An example of a respiratory device is called the "Breathing Monitor", included in the "Dr. Fluency" computerised stuttering treatment program (Friedman et al. 1999). The Breathing Monitor provides real-time feedback on respiratory flow, which can be used in training the PWS to regulate breathing; first without speech, followed by exercises involving breathing plus speech of graded complexity, beginning with single syllables and moving on to more complex speech, all the time maintaining appropriate air production. The CAFET (Computer Aided Fluency Establishment Trainer) device also provides feedback on the quality of voice onsets (Goebel 1994). Speech muscle feedback technology and its usefulness will be discussed in more detail below, given that a controlled trial has been conducted testing its efficacy (Craig et al. 1996).

- Devices that provide information on timing of speech, for example, in which the PWS is required to speak in time with a metronome. Metronome technology was widely used for the treatment of stuttering in the 1960s to 1980s, with wearable devices such as the Pacemaster. There is limited support for effectiveness (Berman and Brady 1973). A major problem was the unnatural sound of metronome speech produced, even if it improved fluency.
- Devices that alter speech feedback to the PWS. These include altered auditory feedback (AAF), including masked auditory feedback (MAF), delayed auditory feedback (DAF) and frequency-altered feedback (FAF), and combinations of these. MAF devices were popularised by the Edinburgh Masker (Dewar et al. 1979). The Edinburgh Masker uses a throat microphone (held by an elastic strap), a small control unit attached to a belt or carried in a pocket, and a headphone set. Masking is activated by vocalisation detected by the microphone, and masking stops when the PWS stops speaking. One problem for the Edinburgh Masker is the issue of having to wear a microphone around the neck, as well as when the PWS has non-vocalised or silent stuttering, as for example, in a stuttering block. Further, there is little or no evidence for the efficacy of MAF approaches. AAF devices are discussed in more detail directly below.

### 20.7.2.3 Altered Auditory Feedback

The use of AAF devices such as DAF in the treatment of stuttering has been prevalent since the mid-twentieth century (Bloodstein and Bernstein Ratner 2008; Ingham 1984; Packman and Meredith 2011). DAF became popular when evidence that delaying the feedback of a person's speech reduced stuttering frequency (Ingham 1984). DAF mostly slows speech rate, and research has found that the same effect can be achieved by asking the PWS to slow down their speech without DAF (Bloodstein and Bernstein Ratner 2008; Packman and Meredith 2011). FAF involves feedback of altered frequency of the speech of a PWS (Stuart et al. 2004; Casa Futura Technologies 2015). AAF devices have been widely used in the treatment of stuttering with commercial AAF products available (Bakker 2006; Bloodstein and Bernstein Ratner 2008) that employ masking, DAF and FAF. One example is the SpeechEasy device that employs DAF and AAF. The SpeechEasy device is believed to help reduce stuttering because the person using the device hears their voice slightly delayed and at a different pitch. Their voice is therefore perceived as the voice of someone else, and this effect helps to reduce stuttering frequency. This phenomenon is called choral speech, i.e. talking in unison, and this effect is well known to reduce stuttering and induce fluency (Kalinowski and Saltuklaroglu 2003). Evidence does exist for the efficacy of SpeechEasy in reducing stuttering, especially when reading but less so when speaking in a conversation (Foundas et al. 2013; Stuart et al. 2004). Another similar device is a small unobtrusive ear device called the SmallTalk, a device that also employs AAF, DAF and FAF and that comes with headphones and microphones (see Casa Futura Technologies (2015) for the website on their technology). The efficacy of AAF devices has been investigated with mixed findings (Foundas et al. 2013; Gallop and Runyan 2012; Packman and Meredith 2011; Pollard et al. 2009).

### 20.7.2.4 Electromyography Feedback

Electromyography (EMG) feedback (Craig and Cleary 1982; Craig et al. 1996) is designed to help the person who stutters to control speech muscle activity associated with their stuttering behaviour by teaching them (a) to reduce muscle activity/tension to low levels before speaking with a computer-based speech muscle activity biofeedback; (b) to lower overall levels of muscle tension in the face while speaking; (c) to learn to control speech muscle tension, called EMG mastery, in the absence of the computer biofeedback; (d) to help them raise their levels of confidence, increase their sense of control over their speech and stuttering, and raise their levels of self-

esteem. EMG biofeedback therapy attempts to train the PWS to become aware of and to control tension in their speech muscles.

EMG biofeedback utilises at least two EMG channels in a biomonitoring system (Craig et al. 1996), consisting of a computer feedback and electrodes attached to various speech muscles, providing immediate and sensitive feedback of muscle activity. Silver-silver chloride electrodes are attached to speech muscles on the PWS's face in muscles such as the zygomaticus, levator anguli oris, depressor anguli oris muscle sites and superior and inferior obicularis oris muscles. A grounding electrode is usually placed near the active biofeedback site. Figure 20.1 shows the process of treating the EMG activity signals so they can be understood by the PWS, allowing learning to occur. A typical biofeedback device comprises the EMG amplifier unit, recording and reference electrodes, electrode cables and a PC with a stereo microphone port. The PC screen displays the EMG waveforms, their power spectrum and a meter to measure muscle contraction levels by using various feedback forms such as audio/visual formats (see http://www.neuromotionphysio.com/about/our-equipment/ for a typical EMG feedback system setup).

Training begins on a specific muscle and then learning is transferred to other speech muscles, once control at the first site has been learnt. In a controlled trial (Craig et al. 1996), the PWS were taught to raise and lower their muscle tension without speaking by using visual or auditory biofeedback. When achieved, a hierarchy system was initiated, commencing with repeating simple one-syllable words and progressing to more complex, multi-syllabic words, then on to conversational speech. Fluency skills should be reinforced by behavioural modification strategies, such as reward, assignments and telephone calls. EMG signal-based games can also be played to maintain interest and reinforce EMG mastery. Follow-up should occur regularly (Craig et al. 1996).

Evidence suggests that EMG biofeedback is best delivered in a behavioural modification programme (Craig and Cleary 1982; Craig et al. 1996). Controlled trials (Craig et al. 1996; Hancock et al. 1998) have shown that EMG biofeedback can be effective in reducing stuttering

**Fig. 20.1** Showing raw electromyography activity in the upper trace, rectified EMG activity in the middle trace and smoothed activity in the bottom trace that is used in the biofeedback. The EMG signal is amplified, filtered and processed so that it can be sensibly displayed to the PWS by means of visual or auditory feedback. With kind permission of Brian Kaminski at Advancer Technologies

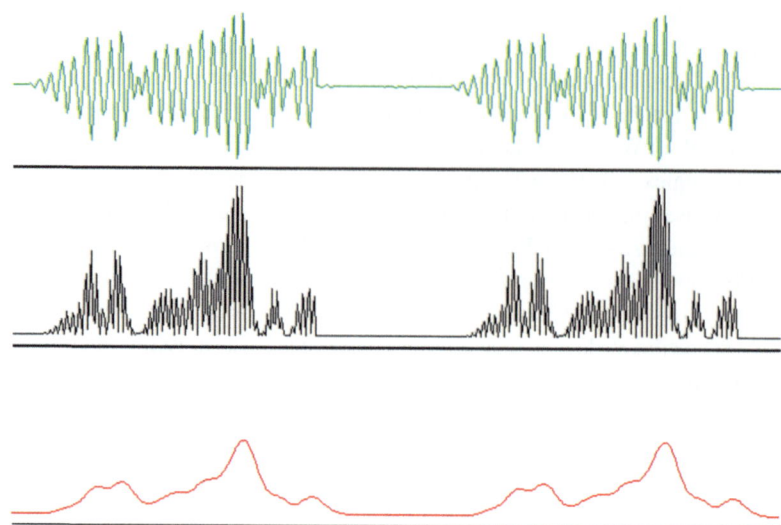

when in a combined therapeutic programme that includes airflow techniques, a regimen of achievable behavioural goals, assessment of behavioural outcomes, rewards, transfer and maintenance procedures, and that employs behavioural assignments to reinforce skills, and cognitive behavioural therapy techniques to address anxiety and social fears. A replication study also found benefits, but to a lesser extent than in the original trials (Block et al. 2004; Craig et al. 1996; Hancock et al. 1998); however, this study has been criticised because it did not utilise response-cost strategies (Bothe et al. 2006). EMG feedback is currently rarely used for the treatment of stuttering.

### 20.7.2.5 Conclusions and Implications

Technology is being used for the treatment of stuttering. While many stuttering people I know say that devices such as those discussed above are helpful and enhance their ability to communicate verbally, the efficacy of most devices has a long way to go before gold standard evidence is available for any device currently in use. It should be understood that technology is always a component of a therapy package, and it is best that the technology is not the sole component. It is also crucial that principles of treatment should be adhered to by clinicians to ensure that stuttering treatment effectiveness is optimised. These include (a) taking a

comprehensive diagnosis by using a behavioural approach (e.g. measuring stuttering frequency and speech rate) as well as psychological measures (e.g. social anxiety); (b) clinicians' conducting therapy in a professional, caring and accepting manner, working on developing a positive relationship with the PWS; (c) gaining the support of family and friends to assist the PWS in self-managing; (d) employing appropriate response cost methods, such as effective rewards and negative reinforcements, whatever the age of the PWS; (e) encouraging the PWS to learn relaxation strategies and to be sure they are engaging in frequent pleasant life events; (f) encouraging self-responsibility and self-management; (g) employing follow-up and anti-relapse strategies (Craig et al. 2011; Craig and Tran 2006).

## 20.8 Surgical Techniques for Dysarthria Treatment

Philippe H. DeJonckere

### 20.8.1 Background

Dysarthria has been defined as a neurological motor speech impairment causing the speech musculature to be slow, weak or imprecise

(Duffy 2013). There is a poor co-ordination of movements, involving breathing, voice production, resonance and oral articulation (Yorkston 1996). People with dysarthric speech typically sound less intelligible or slurred because of poor oral control of articulators, particularly the tongue. Speech can also sound underpowered and lacking expressiveness because of weak respiratory control and impaired vocal/velopharyngeal function.

Dysarthrias result from sensorimotor impairments of articulatory movements. In contrast to dysglossias, which often concern only specific areas of phonation and articulation, dysarthric speech consists of a global de-differentiation of speech motorics (Schröter-Morasch and Ziegler 2005a). Problems of impaired motor control are mainly caused by damage to primary cortical zones or to cortically originating or subcortical motor projection systems and disturb speech as well as swallowing. Problems of impaired motor programming (apraxia of speech) in general are caused by (left) cortical lesions involving motor association cortex or secondary cortical zones (Mosera et al. 2016).

Parkinson's disease, stroke, traumatic brain injury, amyotrophic lateral sclerosis and cerebral palsy represent important clinical diagnoses in which dysarthria is a frequent and debilitating symptom (Yorkston 1996). Dysarthria includes a wide severity range, from lapses in speech accuracy, or fatigue related to speech, until complete unintelligibility (Mitchell et al. 2017).

## 20.8.2  Surgical Approaches

In cases of Parkinson's disease, several surgical approaches have been proposed to manage the motor symptoms in general. Pinto et al. (2004) specifically reviewed the effects of these surgical procedures on dysarthria.

Functional neurosurgery procedures such as (stereotaxic) thalamotomy, pallidotomy and deep brain stimulation have actually been tried out to treat Parkinsonian symptoms. Some significant improvement after surgical treatment has been observed for motor impairment of limbs;

however, the effect on Parkinson's disease (PD) dysarthria is more commonly deleterious (word blocking, hypophonia, palilalia, dysfluency) than it is beneficial (Volkmann et al. 1998). Notwithstanding this, some positive changes in phonatory and articulatory measures in patients with PD who underwent unilateral posteroventral pallidotomy have also been reported (Schulz et al. 1999).

Pallidotomy for an overactive globus pallidus can reduce tremor and rigidity, but Mourao et al. (2005) have found that this treatment provides little improvement on the functional use of communication for Parkinson patients and can actually cause further speech deterioration if the procedure is done bilaterally.

Electrical stimulation of an overactive subthalamic nucleus has been shown to improve all the cardinal symptoms of Parkinson's disease. Some studies with this method have demonstrated that although loudness, pitch and motor movements may improve after stimulation, they do so at the price of decreased intelligibility (Dias et al. 2006; Pinto et al. 2004; Rousseaux et al. 2004; Cohen et al. 2009).

Because of the risk of deleterious effects on speech, several of these procedures have been abandoned for the treatment of Parkinson's disease (Moya-Galé and Levy 2019).

Summarising, the effect of most treatments for Parkinson's disease on dysarthria remains unsatisfactory. The pathophysiology of dysarthria is complex and, at least in part, different from that of general motor dysfunction (Pinto et al. 2004).

## 20.8.3  Velopharyngeal Inadequacy as a Component of Dysarthria

Velopharyngeal inadequacy (a generic term) is a common relevant component of dysarthria, as impaired motor control can include paresis of the soft palate and pharyngeal walls. When velopharyngeal inadequacy has a neurogenic aetiology, it is usually referred to as velopharyngeal incompetence (rather than insufficiency) (Trost-Cardamone 1989).

Velopharyngeal incompetence may be a contributing factor to the speech disorder in dysarthric patients, as it implies the presence of hypernasality, inappropriate nasal escape and decreased air pressure during speech (Rilo et al. 2013). However, in case of velopharyngeal incompetence secondary to neurological conditions, the speech symptomatology is dependent not only upon the extent of velopharyngeal incompetence and the type of neurological condition, but also on the involvement of remaining structures of the speech mechanism (Dworkin and Johns 1980). When hypernasality appears to be a significant component of dysarthric speech, a reduction of the nasal air escape, either by fitting an oral prosthesis or by velopharyngeal surgery, may improve intelligibility and nasal regurgitation.

Velopharyngeal insufficiency can be improved by plastic surgery of the velopharynx or pharynx. Velopharyngoplasty (a connection between the velum and dorsal pharyngeal wall in the shape of cranially or caudally pedunculated flaps) can be successful if residual contraction of the lateral and posterior muscles of the pharynx is still possible. However, these are affected by central lesions just as often as the velum itself. Because of shrinking of the flaps and formation of scar tissue the success of an operation often does not last. If the velum still has a residual but insufficient lifting function, attempts can be made to create velopharyngeal contact by augmenting the back wall of the pharynx with body tissue or artificial material.

As stated by Gart and Gosain (2014) in a review article, although many techniques are available for velopharyngeal inadequacy, there are no conclusive data to guide procedure choice, and newer surgical techniques continue to evolve. The most commonly used techniques for the surgical management of velopharyngeal insufficiency (in general) are:

- Furlow palatoplasty, or double opposing Z-palatoplasty (DOZ): this restores the velar levator musculature to a more physiological condition and simultaneously lengthens the velum. This technique may be used in cleft palate patients, in order to create a full velar muscle ring. This can better be done, however, in a complete muscle revision with straight line incisions in the velum avoiding a big Z-scar (Elsherbiny et al. 2018).
- Pharyngeal flap: a static structure that reduces the size of the velopharyneal port and relies on the lateral wall motion for closure.
- Dynamic sphincter pharyngoplasty (DSP): this augments the pharyngeal musculature to improve lateral wall motion.
- Posterior pharyngeal augmentation: injectable or implantable alloplastic and autologous materials, particularly fat, are used to augment the posterior pharyngeal wall in selected cases (Cantarella et al. 2012). Alloplastic materials have mostly been abandoned because of unforeseeable postoperative displacement and unwanted reactions, whereas fat injections under endoscopic control are successful; they may be repeated after shrinking.

A survey of speech outcomes of velopharyngeal surgery in general (Kummer et al. 2012) shows considerable variability in the methods for evaluating and reporting speech outcomes following surgery. Further, there are no large clinical trials that have tested whether these treatments are effective specifically in dysarthric patients.

In dysarthric patients, the same limitations apply as for prostheses, as possible improvement will be restricted to nasality (Pinto and Pegoraro-Krook 2003). A simple test that can be predictive for improvement of intelligibility is to fill the nasal cavities to some extent, e.g. with cotton wool.

All prosthetic and surgical measures require close cooperation between speech therapist, phoniatrician, dentist/maxillofacial surgeon and ENT specialist.

### 20.8.4 Hypophonia as a Component of Dysarthria

Furthermore, hypophonia and breathiness can also contribute to poor speech intelligibility in cases of peripheral paresis of the vocal fold caused by lesion of the nucleus of the vagal nerve with atrophic excavation of the vocal fold and loss of glottal closure (Schröter-Morasch and Ziegler 2005a, b). According to Dashtipour et al. (2018), hypophonia is one of the more pronounced symptoms of Parkinsonian speech. In cases of dysarthria surgical methods for voice improvement are to be used cautiously, but vocal fold augmentation procedures (collagen, hyaluronic acid, calcium hydroxylapatite, autologous fat…) (Berke et al. 1999; Sewall et al. 2006; Hamdan et al. 2018) and medialisation laryngoplasty can be indicated in selected cases (Jayaraman and Das 2024). They may reduce vocal fatigue and be a useful adjunct to voice therapy (Ramig et al. 2008; Levy et al. 2020). However, relevant clinical trials specifically dealing with dysarthric patients are lacking.

If spasticity appears to be a relevant component of dysarthria, the only medication of any significance is injection of botulinum toxin in cases of severe spasticity of the orofacial muscles or in cases of focal dystonia, in particular spasmodic dysphonia (Schröter-Morasch and Ziegler 2005a, b).

## 20.8.5 Conclusion

Dysarthrias result from sensorimotor impairments of articulatory movements. Dysarthric speech consists of a global de-differentiation of speech motorics. Velopharyngeal incompetence may be a contributing factor to the speech disorder in dysarthric patients, as it implies the presence of hypernasality, inappropriate nasal escape and decreased air pressure during speech. Furthermore, hypophonia and breathiness can also contribute to poor speech intelligibility in cases of peripheral paresis of the vocal fold caused by lesion of the nucleus of the vagal nerve with atrophic excavation of the vocal fold and loss of glottal closure. Techniques of velopharyngoplasty and of vocal fold augmentation can, in selected cases, have a positive effect on these specific and limited components of dysarthria, but relevant clinical trials specifically dealing with dysarthric patients are lacking.

Furthermore, the effect of most surgical treatments for Parkinson's disease on dysarthria remains unsatisfactory. Because of the risk for deleterious effect on speech, most of these procedures have been abandoned. Mitchell et al. (2017) produced a systematic Cochrane review about interventions for dysarthria and summarised that there is insufficient evidence to conclude whether any one treatment is better than any other or whether treatment is better than general support or no treatment.

## 20.9 Principles of Computer Rehabilitation of Dysarthria/Apraxia

Salvatore Biondi and Karel Neubauer

### 20.9.1 Introduction

Although the first applications of the personal computer (PC) in the field of verbal communication pathology concerned the diagnostic aspect, the new technologies did not take long to establish themselves in the field of rehabilitation. In this direction, the evolution has been rapid both for the enormous diffusion among the population of computers in their various forms, and for the technological advances of the equipment. The evolution concerned not only the computational power of machines but also the human–machine interaction, interconnectivity, portability and the miniaturisation of components. All this has given rise to a particular branch of rehabilitation, *computerised rehabilitation* (CR) which has achieved rapid success owing to its versatility, availability and diffusion. The rapid increase in resources and devices for electronic therapy is therefore transforming the therapeutic process (Theodoros 2012; Kim et al. 2024).

The computer, thanks to specific speech analysis and recognition algorithms, is able to produce audiovisual feedback and therefore improve the awareness and intentionality of a specific function and in particular of the quality and correctness of speech production. It can also propose models that act as targets and promote a progressive remodelling of the voice, speech and language. In this condition, the speech therapist's work is supported in activities that help the client find the most useful strategies to cancel or reduce types of deviant behaviour. However, the computer remains a tool and does not replace the rehabilitator who is the professional able to organise the treatment, as well as to provide important psychological and relational supports that the machine is not able to offer. The therapist maintains the task of elaborating the treatment planning on the basis of his or her training and experience (Popovici and Belciu 2012).

The use of this technical background in the field of communication disorders affects in principle the whole area, called Information and Communication Technologies (ICT), which can be developed and used for the benefit of people with these disorders. ICT resources in this area can be divided into:

- Desktop PC programmes that are run from storage media or directly from the memory disk of the computer—the use of speech therapy intervention programmes and specialised programmes for diagnosing the development, status and disorders of communication skills.
- Mobile technology—smartphones and tablets—the use of portable technology of this type with the iOS and Android operating systems and a touch screen. They already include a wide range of programmes from nontargeted, rather motivational and stimulation programmes to sophisticated applications of diagnostic and therapeutic programmes for mobile technology.
- Applications using the www network for sharing repositories, from which it is possible to draw materials for the intervention program. These are aids of the nature of an Internet portal or website, which contain illustrative therapeutic materials, sets of targeted exercises for a certain area of stimulation and comprehensive therapeutic programs.
- Communication and educational technologies that use the Internet for the implementation of video transmission in the programmes of therapeutic sessions and for communication between

persons with speech communication disorders and their family members, therapist, etc.

The sessions carried out with the help of the computer in the presence of the therapist achieve a condition referred to as *computer-assisted speech therapy* (CAST). A different situation is that in which the computer replaces the human intervention and itself acts as a *virtual therapist* (VT): in this case the machine interacts with the patient in the absence of the speech-language pathologist (SLP) and special software manages a series of practical exercises for the patients. The control of the patient and the gradual progression of the programme are carried out by the SLP with meetings at set intervals or even remotely (Phoebe Chen et al. 2016).

In both cases, the human–machine interaction with the patient requires the existence of robust speech recognition and speech verification algorithms with respect to the sources of variability of speech, even of deteriorated, as in the case of dysarthric speakers (Saz et al. 2009).

The rehabilitation activity draws on established and shared codified methodologies, among which prevail those that refer to classical or *operant conditioning* (OC) techniques and, more recently, to *motor learning* (ML) theories (Maas et al. 2008). Often, however, the therapist acts in an eclectic way, also drawing on contributions from different schools of thought (theory of mind, psychotherapy, counselling, etc.).

## 20.9.2 Instrumentation

From a historical point of view, after the first proposals around the 1980s, well-developed commercial programmes began to appear in the 1990s. We can mention Speech Viewer by IBM (IBM 1992) and Speech tools by Kay Elemetrics running on common commercial desktops or laptops. To overcome the limits of the sound cards of medium-low range computers Kay Elemetrics has marketed specific hardware equipment such as Visi Pitch and CSL Lab. with which it is also possible to carry out quantitative and reliable diagnostic investigations. Speech Viewer went out of production at the end of the 1990s, while

**Fig. 20.2** Therapy of verbal memory, attention and naming with connection of visual, sound and movement mode in a person with cognitive-communication disorder after CNS trauma. PC therapeutic programme MENTIO. Courtesy of Mentio®. Photo: Karel Neubauer

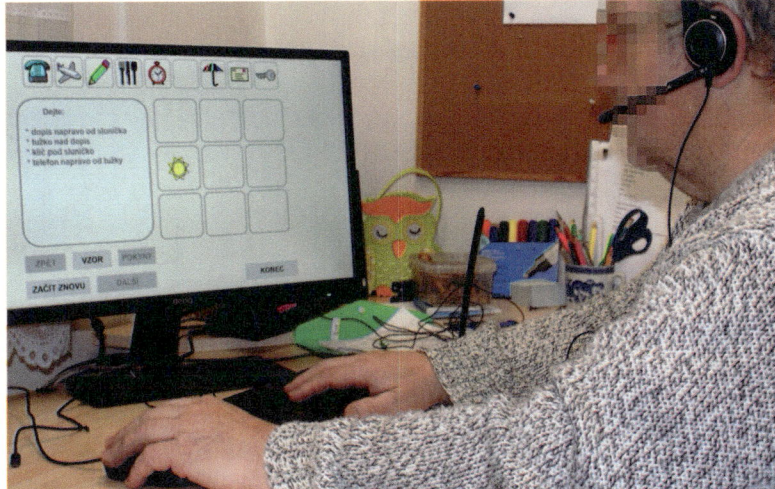

**Fig. 20.3** Global reading of words, assignment to illustrative material in a person with aphasia after a stroke. PC therapeutic programme MENTIO. Courtesy of Mentio®. Photo: Karel Neubauer

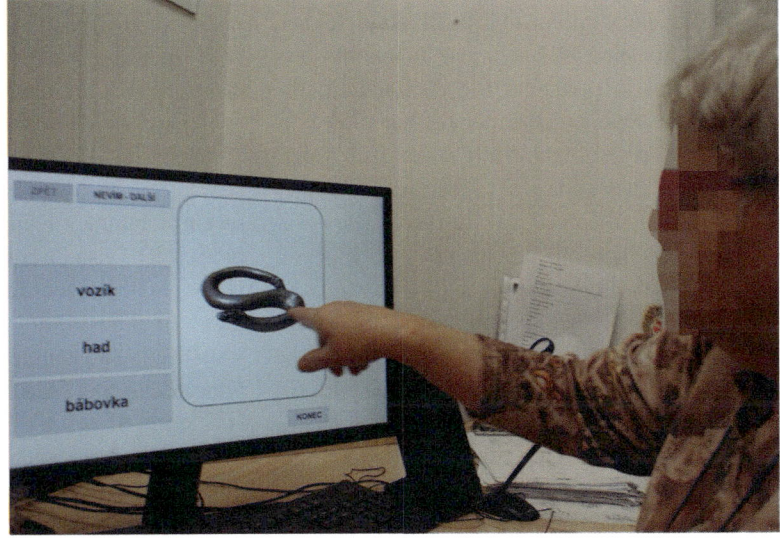

Pentax Medical took the place of Kay Elemetrics (Pentaxmedical 2021), expanding its range of products as can be found on its website. An example of a comprehensive set of diagnostic and therapeutic software is the set of MENTIO programmes used in the Czech and Slovak language environments. It enables the performance of SLP diagnostics by using multiple levels of recording and spectrographic analysis of voice expression and connection with therapeutic programmes for people with motor, linguistic and cognitive-communication disorders, especially aphasia and dysarthria (see Figs. 20.2, 20.3 and 20.4; Petržílková and Neubauer 2007; Petržílková 2020; Neubauer 2018c).

Over the next few years, more software programmes were gradually added (Eriksson et al. 2005). Most are designed for use on home computers for homework even with no need for great precision. More elaborate systems that use complex equipment such as Electropalatography,

Electroglottography, Electromagnetic articulography, Plethysmography, etc. (Murdoch et al. 1999; Katz and McNeil 2010; Giacchini et al. 2013) are not very common and reserved for highly specialised or research centres. More

**Fig. 20.4** Use of an internet repository for language therapy of a person with acquired dysarthria after a stroke. Linking loud reading, description of the thematic image and writing. Courtesy of © 2021 Zuzana Průchová. Photo: Karel Neubauer

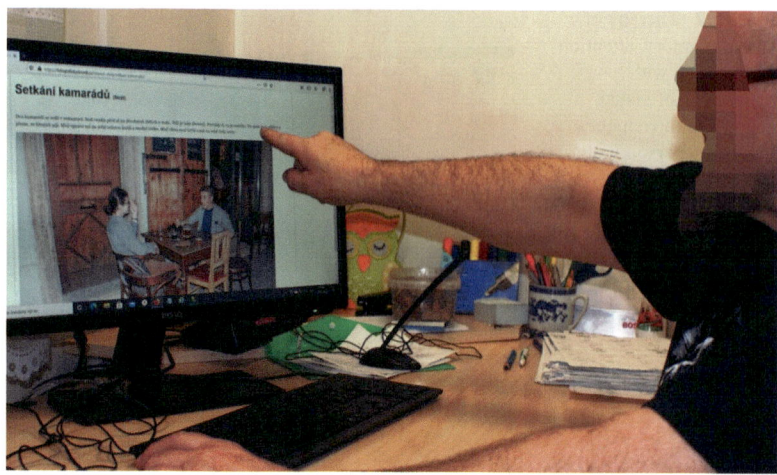

recently, tablets and smartphones have arrived on the market that combine in a small, powerful and compact machine all the main functions of a desktop and in particular the central unit, the monitor, the keyboard, the modem that allow portability and ease of use, while audiovisual interconnectivity has expanded. This last possibility had a very rapid spread, giving rise to teleworking, teleteaching, telemedicine which have become increasingly established. In the wake of this evolution, further specific applications have appeared dedicated to the rehabilitation of the voice and speech and language, opening a new era in telerehabilitation (TR) (Theodoros 2012). A quick internet search yields a truly rich sample of specific software possibilities.

Remote work with the patient meets these important needs:

- Makes up for the shortage of therapists.
- Reaches patients with mobility problems, in quarantine or isolation.
- Allows carrying out of home care sessions.
- Promotes family participation in the rehabilitation programme.

TR is on the way to becoming an integral part of language pathology treatment and imposes the need for SLP's to adapt to this new modality of health care. Remote activity combined with interconnectivity can allow *group sessions* by teleconference. The group sessions encourage the cooperation and competition among pupils and promote the pragmatic communication skills of patients (Tobolcea and Danubianu 2010), while from the point of view of results they are not inferior to individual treatment in person (Wales et al. 2017).

In addition to the visualisation of the acoustic characteristics of the patient's speech, the most recent computers equipped with cameras combine video visualisation of articulatory movements and their recording for subsequent reviews. This visual possibility in addition to the acoustic visualisation constitutes a formidable *augmented biofeedback* tool for self-control, error correction and self-verification of progress achieved. Visual feedback is also potentially able to activate the *mirror neuron system* that has been found active in all phases of the motor learning process (Buccino and Riggio 2006). The role of mirror neurons opens up interesting research prospects for the future.

From the point of view of the SLP, data recording and storage allow the analysis of the training sessions, the evaluation of the effectiveness of the applied methods, guaranteeing the gradual, ordered progression of the treatment correlating it to the improvements achieved (or any regressions).

Finally, technological advances do not stop, promising as of now new possibilities for the near future related to the introduction of machines equipped with *artificial intelligence* (Liss and Berisha 2020; Deka et al. 2024).

## 20.9.3 Principles of Treatment

The distinction of the therapeutic approach to speech motor disorders into three categories proposed by Duffy involves *behaviour-modifying methods*, *prosthetic intervention* and *medical procedures*. The use of computers is widely applied in the first of these categories (Schröter-Morasch and Ziegler 2005b). In the literature, no contribution sets specific general principles for computerised rehabilitation. This is certainly because the computer is not a method but rather a tool. However, from examination of the literature, shared criteria applicable in this sector of activity can be identified.

Keeping in mind that the goal of the treatment is to maximise communication, the objectives can be divided into restitution, compensation and adaptation of the verbal function, while the intervention procedures can be divided into *communication-oriented* and *speech-oriented* (Duffy 2005b).

In the most severe cases, those of anarthria patients, in which a functional use of the word is not possible, the goal is to adapt the condition of the subject to communication needs, and the treatment is almost exclusively communication orientated. In these cases the computer represents a useful tool in the management of *augmentative alternative communication*. PCs, tablets and smartphones have progressively replaced the low-tech tools used in the pre-digital era (symbols, icons, graphic characters, etc.). Patients with significant motor limitations that may prevent normal use of the machine require specially modified peripherals (e.g., mouse, joystick, stylus or button box). More recently speech synthesis programmes have made the computer speak. Alternative augmentative communication is now widely codified and applied according to specific methodologies (Ball et al. 2012).

Communication orientated interventions do not exclusively concern the most serious cases. Even in less serious cases of speech deterioration, the PC is able to intervene usefully in the improvement of non-verbal aspects such as leg and hand/arm movements, gestures, facial expression, eye gaze, vocalisations not articulated but with communicative value, and in short everything related to communicative pragmatics.

In cases where a recovery or an improvement in speech is foreseeable, the rehabilitation is *speech orientated*. In this direction, the contribution of the computer on phonation, articulation, resonance and prosody is extraordinarily effective. It is appropriate to examine the fundamental points. These distinctly concern: the man–machine interface, the machine, the caregiver, the method.

(a) The man-machine interface.
   - the machine,
     1. patient awareness of the parameters that we intend to modify (*purposeful activity* according to Darley et al. (1975), *baseline of operant conditioning, cognitive stage of Motor Learning*),
     2. patient's ability to interact with the instrument and exchange information with it.
   - the patient.
     1. attraction and interest,
     2. increased sense of independence,
     3. autonomy.
(b) The machine.
   - Input peripherals capable of being activated by the patient (adaptations may be necessary).
   - Ability to detect the parameters of the activities to be modified.
   - Ability to provide feedback according to a precise sensory modality.
   - Choice of feedback frequency (real time or deferred).
   - Demonstration on monitor of the activity and movements of the articulatory organs.
   - Visualisation of the acoustic characteristics of the voice.
   - Highlighting the structure of the word.
   - Rewarding graphic / playful representations (especially for children).
(c) SLP or trained family member.
   - Assessment of the disorder.
   - Determination of the objectives to be achieved.
   - Definition of the specific training for the activity to be modified.

- Promotion of the patient's awareness of the training.
- Grading of the ordered difficulty and progression of the exercises.
- Management of trial / error processes.
- Enrollment of other caregiver who can assist the patient.
- Assignment of the activities to be carried out in the absence of the therapist.
- Ability to manage more people in case of group activities or teleconference.

(d) Management of the treatment.

In the case of speech-orientated treatment, the ultimate goal is to change the motor behaviour that gives rise to the production of the word. The rehabilitation activities are currently managed according to principles that refer to operative conditioning or motor learning. The preliminary stages are corresponding for both methodologies:

- Baseline measures of the behaviour.
- Structure of practice.
- Successive approximation.
- Stimulus-response sequence.

The progression is diversified in its consequences: for OC the response is followed by reinforcement in the case of a correct response while for ML the response provides feedback that can be distinguished from internal to external (Ruscello and Vallino 2014). The speech-language treatment literature following ML recognises the performance distinctions in different terms by exploring acquisition (performance during practice), maintenance (retention) and generalisation (transfer) (Maas et al. 2008).

## 20.10 Deep Brain Stimulation

Alberto Priori, Matteo Guidetti,
Michelangelo Dini and Roberta Ferrucci

### 20.10.1 Introduction

Deep brain stimulation (DBS) is a surgical option that was approved by the Food and Drug Administration (FDA) as a treatment for essential tremor in 1997, advanced Parkinson's disease in 2002, primary segmental and generalised dystonia in 2003 and obsessive-compulsive disorders (OCD) in 2009. Furthermore, it has also been used in research studies for treatment of chronic pain and selected affective disorders (Boccard et al. 2015; Graat et al. 2017). DBS is not currently employed for treatment of motor speech disorders.

DBS involves implanting electrodes that are positioned within a specific brain nucleus. The electrodes produce electrical impulses that modify brain activity in a controlled and reversible way. Stimulation is controlled by a pacemaker-like device placed under the skin in the patient's upper chest. A wire connects this device to the intracranial electrodes (Amon and Alesch, 2017).

The target nucleus of DBS varies according to the type of symptoms to be addressed. For essential tremor, the target location for electrode placement is the ventro-intermediate nucleus (VIM) of the thalamus, while for dystonia and symptoms related to Parkinson's disease (rigidity, bradykinesia/akinesia and tremor) electrodes are implanted in the globus pallidus internus (GPi) and in the subthalamic nucleus (STN) (Kern and Kumar 2007). DBS surgery can be unilateral or bilateral. Unilateral or bilateral electrode placement depends on the presenting symptoms and whether symptom location is unilateral, bilateral or midline (Hemm and Wårdell 2010).

The effect of DBS on the physiology of brain cells and neurotransmitters is still uncertain and debated. While stimulation can suppress some neural elements (e.g., cell bodies), other neural elements (e.g., myelinated axons) can be activated and potentially entrained to the frequency of stimulation (Thevathasan and Gregory 2010). Moreover, the target nucleus itself may not be responsible for the clinical effects but rather its efferent or afferent projections (Gradinaru et al. 2009).

Frequency, voltage and pulse width of the electric signal sent from the neurostimulator device are variables that must be manipulated in order to obtain the best control of symptomatic behaviour and the fewest side effects. Of the latter, motor speech difficulties have been often reported (Herzog et al. 2003; Krack et al. 2003; Putzke et al. 2003; Rodriguez-Oroz et al. 2005; Romito et al. 2002). Indeed, while DBS is not specifically employed in the treatment of voice or speech difficulties, speech may be affected by DBS.

## 20.10.2 Applications in Essential Tremor

Essential tremor is a movement disorder characterised by postural and action tremor that may affect limbs, head, neck and other body regions. In 25–30% of patients this disease may affect voice (Silek and Dogan 2023). Pharmacological treatments for tremor are limited and results are often poor, or no benefit is reported. Several studies have demonstrated that DBS of the VIM of the thalamus significantly reduces tremor of the upper extremities, head, voice and trunk (Koller et al. 2001; Ondo et al. 1998; Sydow et al. 2003). Long-term studies ranging from 1–7 years have shown significant improvement in patients with voice tremor, ranging from 15 to 100% (Lyons and Pahwa 2008). The improvement was more pronounced with bilateral stimulation and decreased over time, probably because of disease progression (Lyons and Pahwa 2008). Among the most common adverse events of DBS in patients with essential tremor, dysarthria is reported in 17% of patients with unilateral implant and in 63% of patients with bilateral implants (Pahwa et al. 2006). Dysarthria, as other complications related to the stimulation, is generally mild and most often may be eliminated with stimulation parameter adjustments.

## 20.10.3 Applications in Parkinson's Disease

Parkinson's disease is a neurodegenerative disorder whose main clinical features are represented by progressive impairment of limb and speech motor control. DBS-STN should be considered only for patients responsive to L-dopa. When the motor fluctuations and the involuntary move-

ments of advanced stage Parkinson cannot be managed with adjustments of L-dopa or other anti-Parkinson medications, but the patient remains L-dopa responsive, DBS-STN may provide an alternative (Welter et al. 2002). Researchers examining the effect of DBS surgery on speech of patients with Parkinson's disease have employed a variety of experimental designs (e.g. assessment of speech before and after DBS-STN; comparison of speech "on" versus "off" stimulation; comparisons of effects of L-dopa versus DBS-STN; comparisons of effects of left versus right STN stimulation). Results of this research have often shown no improvement or deterioration of speech following surgery (Bejjani et al. 2000; Krause et al. 2004; Thobois et al. 2002). One study, which examined the effect of bilateral DBS-STN on speech in patients with idiopathic Parkinson's disease by using acoustic analysis, found that none of the acoustic parameters analysed worsened when the stimulator was turned on (D'Alatri et al. 2008). Moreover, although some acoustic parameters improved in the condition stimulation "on", either with or without medication, this did not reflect a functionally useful change in the patient's speech performance. Some beneficial effects of DBS-STN in Parkinsonian patients were demonstrated in a study that examined force measurement of the upper and lower lips and of the tongue before and after STN stimulation (Gentil et al. 1999). After surgery and with stimulators turned "on", measurements of maximum force and reaction time improved. These findings were replicated in another study that showed a reduction in speech pauses, as well and an increase in phonemic length during stimulation (Pinto et al. 2003). Another study showed a significant difference in speech between bilateral stimulation "on" and "off". As speech is a bilateral motor activity mainly controlled by the dominant hemisphere, a balanced tuning of bilateral ganglia circuits may allow avoidance of negative effects on speech (Santens et al. 2003). Finally, in patients with Parkinson's disease, DBS-STN does not appear to confer any protection against the decline of speech motor control that occurs in the long-term (Krack et al. 2003).

### 20.10.4 Applications in Primary Dystonia

Primary dystonia is a movement disorder that occurs in patients who have no signs of structural abnormality in the central nervous system. It is characterised by sustained muscle contractions that cause twisting and repetitive movements or abnormal postures (Pana and Saggu 2017). Dystonia may be classified on clinical examination according to its distribution: focal dystonia, affecting a single body part in isolation; segmental dystonia, affecting adjacent body parts or a segment of the body; hemi-dystonia, involving one side; generalised dystonia, affecting two or more body segments. Dystonia may be associated with tremor. DBS is indicated for primary dystonia treatment when motor dysfunction causes severe disability despite medication or botulinum toxin. The Gpi is the target nucleus (Kern and Kumar 2007). The response of dystonia to DBS is delayed; it can take months for beneficial effects to become apparent. Conversely, dystonia returns rapidly when stimulation stops (Thevathasan and Gregory 2010). Benefit of pallidal DBS in primary and segmental dystonia are generalised, without significant differences between limbs and axial muscles. However, the results of randomised trials have shown low improvement of speech and swallowing (Kupsch et al. 2006; Vidailhet et al. 2005). Moreover, speech abnormalities are the most common stimulation-related adverse events in patients with dystonia undergoing DBS therapy (Tagliati et al. 2011).

### 20.10.5 Technological Advances: Adaptive DBS

Currently, DBS technology is clinically applied using open-loop stimulation strategies, i.e., providing continuous stimulation. For many indications, however, uninterrupted delivery of energy to the brain may limit patients' therapeutic potential, besides increasing battery consumption. Moreover, constant stimulation of the STN in Parkinson's disease has been associated with speech impairments and increased risk of falls (Moreau et al. 2008; Xie et al. 2017). From the assumption that stimulation should be delivered only when needed, adaptive deep brain stimulation (aDBS) has the potential to remedy DBS disadvantages. It relies on a closed-loop model that allows automatic optimisation of the stimulation parameters (frequency, voltage and pulse width) according to actual symptoms' condition (Priori et al. 2013). Feedback variables representing the clinical state of the patient are indeed monitored to trigger the stimulus delivery (Priori et al. 2013; Basu et al. 2013; Wang et al. 2020; Mitchell and Starr 2020). Thus far, several technologies have been tested, and several papers have reported the clinical application of aDBS in human movement disorder patients (Arlotti et al. 2019; Little et al. 2013; Rosa et al. 2015). For example, bilateral aDBS over VIM and the nucleus Ventralis Oralis Posterior (VOP) significantly reduce tremor in essential tremor patients (Yamamoto et al. 2012) and in tremor-dominant Parkinson's disease patients (Malekmohammadi et al. 2016). aDBS has shown its clinical potential especially in Parkinson's disease patients. Indeed, aDBS-STN showed superior motor improvement by 20–30% compared with DBS after 10 min of stimulation (Little et al. 2013), and reduced levodopa-induced dyskinesia by almost 50% after 2 h (Rosa et al. 2015). Similar results were reached by bilateral aDBS implantations (Little et al. 2015, 2016), in patients with previous DBS implant (Velisar et al. 2019; Arlotti et al. 2019) and when patients were free to move in a real-world setting for long periods of stimulation time (Arlotti et al. 2018; Rosa et al. 2017). As DBS technology advances, a growing body of evidence is indicating the clinical potentials and benefits of aDBS, which will be disclosed in the future.

### 20.10.6 Conclusions and Future Prospects

In conclusion, current evidence indicates that DBS of the VIM of the thalamus in patients with essential tremor reduces voice tremors, with minimal side effects (dysarthria in particular) that are easily remedied by adjusting stimulation parameters. Conversely, opinions regarding the efficacy of DBS-STN for the improvement of speech in patients with Parkinson's Disease are mixed, with most studies reporting no effect, and others reporting minor improvements with limited functional relevance. In addition to mixed evidence regarding the short-term results, DBS-STN seems unable to protect against the long-term decline of speech motor control typically observed in these patients. Finally, DBS of the Gpi in patients with dystonia shows significantly less efficacy on speech abnormalities than that on other symptoms; moreover, speech impairment represents one of the more common adverse effects of DBS-Gpi in patients with dystonia.

The fundamental goal for future developments of DBS technology and application is to provide an increasingly safe, less invasive and more accurate methodology to treat an increasing number of pathologies (Krauss et al. 2021). In this sense, for example, the scientific community has been investigating the application of new types of electrodes to be implanted, smaller and better able to prevent temperature fluctuations (Aum and Tierney 2018) or the use of advanced neuroimaging techniques to improve the targeting of anatomical regions for implantation (Krauss et al. 2021). Increased neurophysiological knowledge will also allow better control of waveform shape in order to reach an optimised stimulation (Krauss et al. 2021). Furthermore, promising results have been gained by new technologies applied to DBS treatments, such as closed-loop strategies; their ability to deliver contingency-based and optimised stimulation, indeed, needs to be further explored in order to satisfy more accurately the clinical need of the patients.

## 20.11  Oral Motor Devices

Anita McAllister and Madeleine Wertsén

Several oral motor devices have been designed to train both children and adults to compensate for speech motor disorders and hypernasality. In this section we provide an overview of different intra-oral devices such as palatal plates and oral screens that aim to improve speech in different patient groups. The focus is on adults but reviews reporting intervention outcomes in children and teenagers are also included. Some compensatory and augmentative devices and their use are discussed, as well as prognoses and scientific support for interventions using different devices related to a disorder.

### 20.11.1  Introduction

Intra-oral treatment by different methods and devices to improve a speech disorder dates back at least 2000 years to the Greek Demosthenes. According to the historian Plutarch, he had "an inarticulate and stammering pronunciation" that he overcame by speaking with pebbles in his mouth (Murphy 2020). In modern medicine several more sophisticated, individually designed and commercially available intra-oral treatment devices have been developed. Treatment with intra-oral devices may also aim at establishing or reestablishing saliva control, swallowing and proper bolus transport. This is, however, beyond the focus of the present section.

Speech disorders affect several aspects of communication, participation and quality of life, in both children (Feeney et al. 2012) and adults (Neumann et al. 2019). Primarily two types of disorder are included in motor speech disorders (MSD), dysarthria and apraxia (see Chap. 16). In children, speech disorders can be classified according to the Speech Sound Disorder Classification System (Shriberg et al. 2010) including four categories: childhood apraxia of speech, dysarthria, co-occurring dysarthria and childhood apraxia of speech, and speech motor delay.

Speech disorders commonly occur owing to neurological diseases or lack of oral tissue. They may also be a result of cancer surgery or radiation therapy, and in children be due to craniofacial anomalies. A comorbidity of swallowing disorders and problems with mastication are common in patients with dysarthria and muscular weakness (Clark et al. 2003).

The aim of interventions for all motor speech disorders (MSD) is to establish or re-establish appropriate speech movements or, in some cases, to compensate for a paralysis or deviant anatomy.

In the research on motor learning a fundamental principle has been suggested to be the amount of practice (Maas et al. 2008; Schmidt et al. 2019). However, the necessary amount of practice and the active participation and motivation for the intervention can be difficult to achieve in patients with a comorbidity of cognitive or psychiatric disorders. The required amount of practice, and the distribution of trained tasks and feedback may also differ between different patient groups (Kwon et al. 2015; McAllister et al. 2018; Schmidt et al. 2019). In patients with very compromised oral motor function the intervention may instead focus on compensatory intervention methods such as palatal lifts, palatal augmentation prostheses (PAP) or obturators and compensatory strategies (see Sect. 20.11.2.1 below).

## 20.11.2 Different Oral Motor Devices

The first distinction regarding intra-oral devices is between the individually designed and those that are commercially available, not requiring an individual fitting. Treatment goals may also differ, with more active training devices aiming at improved function, and augmentative devices compensating for loss of function or tissue in the mouth or palate. Depending on the treatment goals and design of the device, it may be important to assess and follow the progression of treatment in a multi-professional team including both a speech and language pathologist (SLP) and a dentist.

### 20.11.2.1 Palatal Plates

Palatal plates are individually designed on a plaster model made from an impression of the upper jaw. The palatal plate is made of acrylic and provided with metal cubes, balls or wheels on bars, etc. that correspond to the intended training or articulatory target (Fig. 20.5a, b). The training is typically performed 10–30 min at least twice a day.

In a review evaluating outcomes for children and youth with motor speech disorders, the effects of interventions with palatal plates ad modum Castillo Morales for 56 children 4 to 9:6 years old with Down Syndrome (DS) were assessed (McAllister et al. 2018). Two of the studies included were Randomised Controlled Trials (RCT) (DS) (Carlstedt et al. 2001, 2003). Two studies reported longitudinal effects following 4 years of treatment (Carlstedt et al. 2003; Bäckman et al. 2007). All three studies reported positive effects on speech or specific orofacial functions related to speech, such as lip-rounding, tongue position or tongue mobility following the

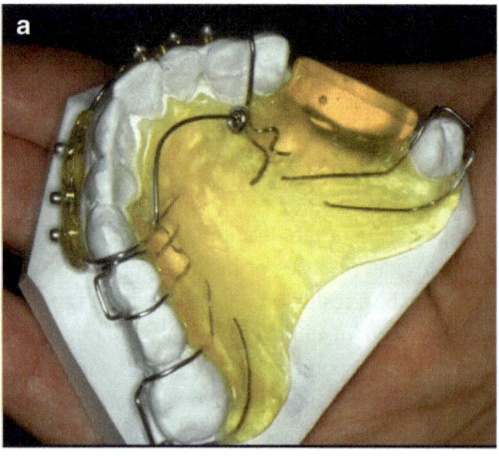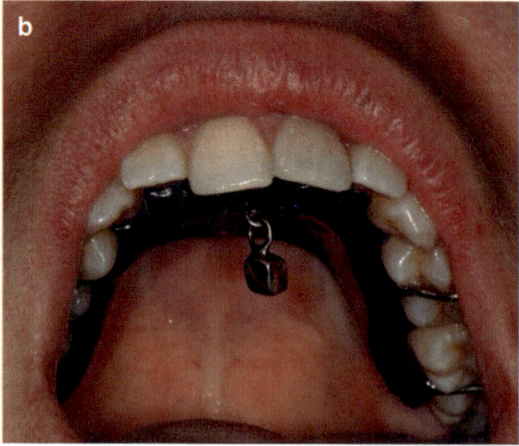

**Fig. 20.5** (a) The metal wheel is moved sideways to train lateralisation of the tongue. (Photo, Wertsén, Clinic of Orofacial Medicine, Mölndal). (b) A palatal plate with metal cube in situ (Photo, Wertsén, Clinic of Orofacial Medicine, Mölndal)

intervention. Similar results are reported in a systematic review by Javed and coworkers. They included eight clinical studies reporting on palatal plate intervention in a total of 241 children with DS (Javed et al. 2018). They report that

> most of the included studies suggest that palatal plate therapy in combination with physiotherapy/orofacial regulation therapy according to Castillo Morales/speech and language intervention seems effective in improving orofacial disorders in children with DS.—Javed et al. 2018

In adults, palatal plates are mainly used in relation to velopharyngeal impairments (Shifman et al. 2000) or swallowing disorders (Hägg and Larsson 2004). The clinical use of palatal plates to improve speech appears to be rare. Only a few studies reporting treatment effects following intervention with palatal plates have been found, and no reviews. Hägg and Larsson (2004) report results from a case series of seven patients with orofacial disorders and dysphagia following their first stroke. The intervention included manual orofacial regulation ad modum Castillo Morales and a palatal plate. A total of 31 variables was assessed, including head control, facial variables, lips, tongue, jaw and velum. The authors report pronounced improvements after a 5-week intervention on facial variables and muscles in the lips and tongue, and swallowing, judging by results from the Swallowing Capacity Test (Nathadwarawala et al. 1992). All patients also self-rated a decreased severity of their problems after treatment.

In another investigation of orofacial dysfunction and dysphagia following the first stroke, interventions with palatal plates or oral screens were compared (Hägg and Tibbling 2015). A total of 31 patients was included with 13 patients treated with a palatal plate and 18 with a standardised oral screen (Iqoro *screen*, IQS). Both interventions were carried out over a period of 3 months. The palatal plate group started treatment a median of 59 weeks after the stroke and the oral screen group after a median of 5 weeks. The authors reported significantly improved facial activity in both groups. However, owing to differences in the time elapsing after the stroke it is difficult to separate treatment effects from spontaneous recovery in the oral screen group. The palatal plate training also included tongue mobility parameters with a potential effect on speech, however no such outcomes were reported.

**Electropalatography (EPG)** (EPG) is a method of determining tongue-palate contact during speech (Morgan Barry 1989). Tongue-palate contact is important for speech clarity, but assessment of tongue movements during speech is difficult, since most speech sounds of the tongue are obscured by the lips or teeth. Thus, EPG has been used both to increase our understanding of different speech disorders and as an intervention method (McAuliffe and Ward 2006; Hardcastle et al. 1985). Using EPG with a home training device increases flexibility for the patient, who can consequently increase the number of repetitions of a target. Visual real-time feedback of tongue-palate contact is provided on a screen (Hardcastle et al. 1991). This biofeedback can be a way for the patient to adopt an external focus of attention of speech movements that may be beneficial for learning (Maas et al. 2008).

Recently, positive results were reported in a randomised controlled trial of children and adolescents with Down syndrome (DS) receiving 12 weeks of intervention with EPG or treatment as usual (Wood et al. 2019). Wood and coworkers found that those who had received EPG training and visual feedback were more likely to maintain and improve speech than those on the usual treatment. Positive results have also been reported for DS children in earlier studies by the same research group (Cleland et al. 2009).

Only a few studies report effects of EPG intervention in adults (McAuliffe and Ward 2006) and the number of participants is usually one or in single digits. Goldstein et al. (1994) reported positive results following an extensive intervention period of 1 year in a patient with dysarthria after a traumatic head injury. The intervention was divided into several steps and included both palatal-lift and EPG training. The EPG-palate was also modified to provide palatal lift. At the end of the intervention, improved articulation and overall intelligibility was reported (Goldstein et al. 1994). Kelly and coworkers report out-

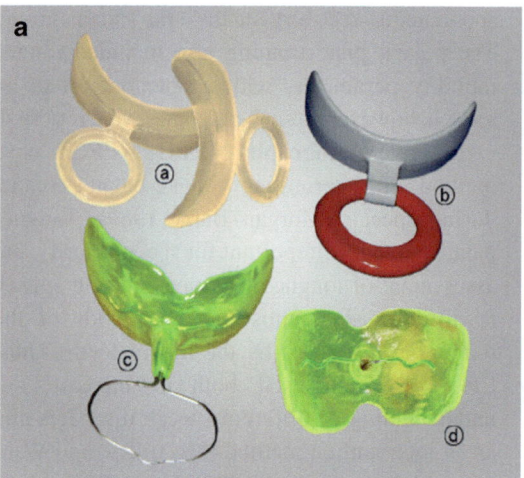
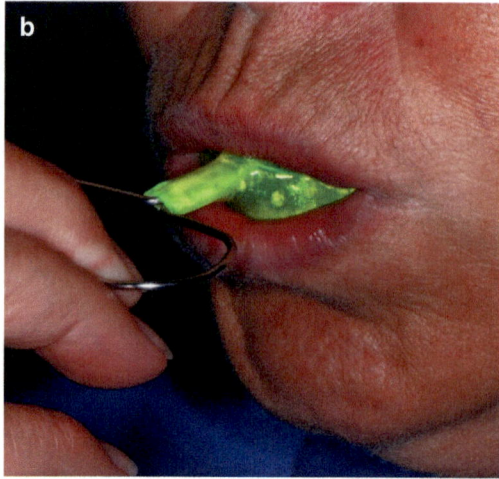

**Fig. 20.6** (**a**) (a) Soft screen Ulmer (b) Hard OS II (c) and (d) Custom made oral screen (Photo, Wertsén, Clinic of orofacial Medicine, Mölndal). (**b**) Custom-made oral screen in situ. Prefabricated (Photo, Wertsén, Clinic of orofacial Medicine, Mölndal)

comes from a three-year clinical trial with EPG both in therapy and assessment of 34 adults with acquired dysarthria (Kelly et al. 2000). In the study, EPG was compared with conventional speech and language therapy in a cross-over design where participants were treated with both methods but in a randomised order. All participants received 6 weeks of conventional speech therapy and 6 weeks of EPG-therapy, twice weekly. They reported positive results from both interventions and that EPG-therapy was significantly more effective in improving tongue/palate contact (Kelly et al. 2000). Patients who started with EPG and continued with speech therapy had better results than those who started with the speech intervention.

### 20.11.2.2 Oral Screens
Oral screens can be prefabricated or custom made. The prefabricated screens are either soft or hard and made of acrylic with a handle (Fig. 20.6a, b). The custom-made screens are produced in plaster from impressions of the upper and lower jaws. These screens are preferred in cases with severe malocclusion or loss of all or part of the mandible. The soft screens are usually intended for children but have, in some cases, also been used in adults (Baram et al. 2020). The oral

screen is placed in the space between the lips and the teeth. The patient grabs the handle and pulls the screen straight forward while sucking as hard as possible. The amount of exercise recommended varies between different therapists, but short sessions twice to three times daily is usually recommended (Hägg and Anniko 2008; Wertsén and Stenberg 2020).

Oral screen training in adults typically focuses on rehabilitation of lip and oral motor problems such as drooling, food retention, bite wounds and impaired transport of the bolus due to acquired neurological disease, trauma, infections or treatment of head and neck cancer. Studies have shown that training with an oral screen can improve orofacial and oral motor function and swallowing after stroke and facial palsy (Hägg and Anniko 2008; Hägg and Tibbling 2015; Hägglund et al. 2020; Wertsén and Stenberg 2020) and in patients with Parkinson's disease (Baram et al. 2020). In a randomised controlled trial, Hägglund and coworkers compared effects of 5 weeks intervention with orofacial sensory-vibration stimulation with an electric toothbrush to additional oral neuromuscular training with a prefabricated oral device (Muppy®) (Hägglund et al. 2020). Results showed significant improvement in both groups after training. At 12 months, the intervention group had improved further whereas the controls, using sensory-vibration stimulation, had deteriorated. Significant between-group differences in swallowing rate (*P* = 0.032) and lip force (*P* = 0.001) (Hägglund et al. 2020) were found. Sjögreen and coworkers investigated effects of treatment with an oral screen on speech production in eight teenagers with myotonic dystrophy type 1 (DM1). A majority demonstrated improved lip force but only four had a significant change. This increased lip strength also did not lead to improved labial or bi-labial articulation during speech (Sjögreen et al. 2010). In our own clinical experience, many patients report improved speech following the intervention. Although this has not been studied and reported in a systematic way, it seems reasonable that improved oral motor and lip function would lead to improved labial articulation during speech (Kent 2015).

A common way to measure the outcome of this training is to measure lip force (Hägg and Anniko 2008; Sjögreen et al. 2010; Wertsén and Stenberg 2017a, b, 2020). However, studies use different methods for measuring lip force and the result can differ depending on screen size and whether the examiner controls for the participant's sucking or clenching the jaws. These factors complicate comparisons across studies. The material of the oral screen may also affect results. One study showed that lip force values measured with a soft prefabricated oral screen in healthy adults were markedly unreliable (Wertsén and Stenberg 2017b). Despite these problems, the overall picture is that oral motor and lip dysfunction can improve after training with an oral screen.

### 20.11.2.3 Compensatory Devices

These devices are designed to compensate for loss of function or tissue. Commonly these appliances have been aimed at re-establishing closure of the nasal cavity and achieving improved position of the soft palate to enhance velopharyngeal closure.

**Palatal Lifts** A palatal lift is an appliance supporting the function of the velopharyngeal valve. It is preferably used where there is remaining soft palate tissue but without sensory function. Usually, a palatal plate is produced and extended over the soft palate, where the extension is built so that a cranial pressure against the velum is obtained (Fig. 20.7). Selley and coworkers constructed a palatal lift consisting of a stainless-steel wire, bent to a loop in a U-shape that was fixed to a palatal plate for 30 patients following their first stroke (Selley et al. 1995). The plate was anchored to the teeth in the upper jaw with clasps, with the loop extending onto the soft palate. The authors' clinical impression was that the appliance rapidly improved swallowing ability. In some patients the loop was removed after swallowing ability had improved, but the symptoms returned, and the patients requested a replacement of the loop, resulting in improved swallowing (Selley et al. 1995). Usually, the fitting and adjustment of a palatal lift requires several visits to a team with a dentist and a speech and language pathologist to achieve comfort and optimal speech.

Palatal insufficiency or palatal incompetence is associated with an inability to achieve velopharyngeal closure. The insufficiency results in deviant speech and resonance related to the inability. The treatment with a palatal lift has a rather long history starting around 1960 with early reports by Gibbons and Blumer (1958) and Lang and Kipfmueller (1969) (Kipfmueller and Lang 1972). The study by Kipfmueller and Lang included 18 patients with velopharyngeal incompetence or velopharyngeal insufficiency of different origins and showed that the palatal lift improved speech intelligibility by reducing

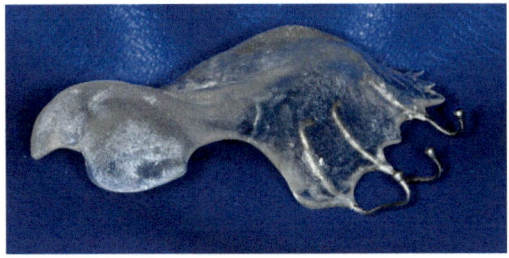

**Fig. 20.7** A custom-made palatal lift with extension to the soft palate. Ball clasps for retention. The final design and adjustments were made while using a fibre-endoscope. (Photo, Wertsén, Clinic of orofacial Medicine, Mölndal)

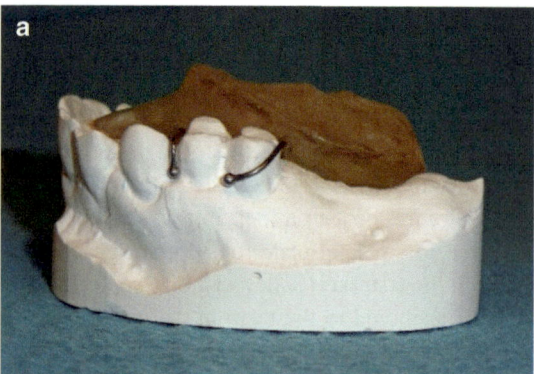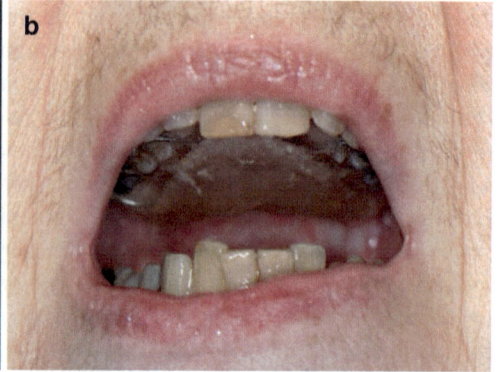

**Fig. 20.8** (**a**) A palatal augmentation prosthesis for severe tongue dysfunction (Photo, Wertsén, Clinic of orofacial Medicine, Mölndal). (**b**) Palatal augmentation prosthesis in situ (Photo, Wertsén, Clinic of orofacial Medicine, Mölndal

perceived consonant errors (Kipfmueller and Lang 1972). Alfwaress and coworkers investigated 30 patients (8–67 years) diagnosed with dysarthria after traumatic brain injury and stroke (Alfwaress et al. 2017). More than 90% of the patients had mixed dysarthria and hypernasality. The patients received a custom-made palatal lift prosthesis. Treatment results showed a decreased nasalance score and an increased sequential motion rate, sound pressure level and speech rate. In a case report Rilo and coworkers report a significant reduction in hypernasality by using a palatal lift in a 20-year-old patient with velopharyngeal incompetence due to brain injury (Rilo et al. 2013).

**Palatal Augmentation Prosthesis (PAP)** The PAP was developed to improve the patients´ ability to speak and swallow. It is an individually designed augmentation made with elastic imprint material on a palatal plate attached to the teeth by clasps. During the setting of the material the patient is asked to repeat words and sentences (Fig. 20.8a, b). The impression material is replaced with acrylic.

Cantor and coworkers first described a PAP in 1969 (Cantor et al. 1969). Several studies followed, which reported improved articulation (Davis et al. 1987; Wheeler et al. 1980; Aramany et al. 1982; Robbins et al. 1987; Logemann et al. 1989; Marunick et al. 2004; de Carvalho-Teles et al. 2008).

Oral surgery can also affect sensory function, with impaired sensory function and abnormal movement patterns. Speech intelligibility may be affected if tongue-palate contact is lacking or too weak. Löfhede and coworkers evaluated the production of velar speech sounds by listener assessment before and after intervention. The study showed significant improvement after PAP intervention in 12 of 19 patients (Löfhede et al. 2020).

### 20.11.3 Discussion

Several studies on intra-oral devices report improvements following intervention. This is related to the well-known risk of publishing bias where positive outcomes are reported more often than negative. In studies of effects of intra-oral devices, results are most often related to swallowing and sometimes also a general report on improved orofacial function (Sjögreen et al. 2018). One reason for the lack of reported results related to speech may be a lack of a speech language pathologist/therapist in the research team.

Another problem is that studies often are small, including a limited number of participants or only a single case. Methodological problems affecting the assessment of reported treatment effects have also been found. Consequently, the prognosis-related palatal plate intervention in adults with dysarthria and acquired apraxia of speech is difficult to predict.

Several studies with positive results after oral screen intervention have been reported. Included were stroke patients with dysphagia and orofacial dysfunction after stroke, patients with peripheral palsy (Hägg and Anniko 2008, Hägg and Tibbling 2015, Hägglund et al. 2020, Wertsén and Stenberg 2020) and patients with Parkinson's disease (Baram et al. 2020). Commercially available oral screens (Hägg and Anniko 2008; Hägg and Tibbling 2015; Baram et al. 2020; Hägglund et al. 2020) or individually designed screens (Wertsén and Stenberg 2020) were used. Baram et al. (2020) reported significantly improved jaw opening, chewing time and oral hygiene following a 2-month intervention, also including jaw exercises. A second assessment in those randomised to late intervention after 2-months showed no improvement (Baram et al. 2020). Hägglund et al. (2020) compared effects from sensory-vibration stimulation to a prefabricated oral screen in stroke patients with dysphagia. After therapy both groups had improved but at 12 months the effects of the oral screen intervention continued to improve whereas effects from sensory-vibration stimulation deteriorated (Hägglund et al. 2020). Wertsén and Stenberg (2020) found significant improvement in patients 7–14 months after stroke and 14–28 months after onset in patients with peripheral palsy. In the stroke-group, muscles around the mouth improved when pouting and smiling; in the peripheral palsy group little improvement could be seen when pouting and smiling but patients reported less or no drooling. In stroke patients, a period of spontaneous recovery occurs depending on studied function. Motor functions typically improve during the first 3 months following onset (Kwakkel and Kollen 2013), while cognition and language may continue to improve up until 12 months (Cassidy and Cramer 2017). In some studies, this overlap between spontaneous recovery and intervention makes it challenging to determine treatment effects.

Studies on treatment effects following EPG training also report promising results. The training can be intensive, with a high number of weekly sessions owing to home training devices. The visual feedback of palate-tongue contact patterns may also be beneficial for learning (Maas et al. 2008). If a combination of interventions methods is used, it may be important to consider the order of these interventions, since one study showed better effects when starting with EPG

followed by speech therapy (Kelly et al. 2000). It seems reasonable to assume that EPG, with the visual feedback, improves patient's awareness and understanding of tongue-palate contact for specific speech targets. This improved spatial and temporal control and understanding is also beneficial in speech therapy.

The intra-oral devices mentioned in this section all have potential to increase treatment intensity for the patient. An increased number of repetitions of a task may be one important factor related to improved function (Maas et al. 2008; Sjögreen et al. 2018). In EPG the visual feedback on tongue palate contact patterns may have several beneficial effects on patients learning.

In some cases, the indications for different devices could be expanded. For example, indications for PAP may also include patients with neurological disorders and impaired tongue mobility, since a lowering of the hard palate can improve a patient's ability to achieve tongue-palate contact. This could have beneficial effects on both speech and swallowing.

The technical development in the area is rapid, with several researchers and companies working on improved usability for the patient. In a recent master thesis, Pastore (2018) proposed a novel so-called Tongue Position Tracking Device (TPTD). This is a wireless device combining electro-palatography and glossometry that enables the investigator to determine tongue-hard palate contact patterns and also to measure the distance between the tongue and palate during continuous speech or other tongue movements. TPTD is connected to an application via Bluetooth. The application provides real-time visual feedback during training.

### 20.11.4 Conclusion

Despite several positive reports following treatment with different intra-oral devices, the result of this overview clearly shows that more intervention studies are needed. Both specific and more detailed reports, as well as reports on patient evaluations of the interventions, are needed. Complicating factors when assessing treatment outcomes are patient heterogeneity and recruitment, study design, the design of the intra oral device, intervention duration and reported outcomes. For oral screens reported outcomes indicate positive effects on swallowing.

## 20.12 General Principles on Drug Treatment

Adriano Chio and Andrea Calvo

Dysarthria is frequent in many neurological disorders, owing to the involvement of different nervous pathways, both peripheral and central. In a number of neurodegenerative disorders, it represents one of the main symptoms, and for this reason there is continual literature on clinical trials for the treatment of speech disorders. For example, there are several papers on speech pharmacotherapy in cerebellar ataxias, in particular Friedreich's ataxia, in motor neuron disease and in movement disorders. However, no evidence-based efficacy for any drug has been found for the treatment of dysarthria (Costantini et al. 2013; Vogel et al. 2014). The response to aetiological or symptomatic treatment, such as L-dopa in Parkinson's disease or steroids in multiple sclerosis, is the most effective approach in those disorders.

One example of dysarthria drug treatment is dysarthria management in Amyotrophic lateral sclerosis (ALS); in ALS bulbar functions are involved at onset in 30% of cases, but almost 70–80% of ALS patients develop signs and symptoms in this region. Bulbar clinical manifestations in ALS patients are characterised by dysarthria, which causes communication problems, more severe when upper limb movements are impaired (when writing is no longer possible); dysphagia, with consequent drooling, also affects dysarthria, as impairment in saliva management further impairs speech. The management of these symptoms is difficult (EFNS Task Force, Andersen et al. 2012). While no drug is available for speech improvement, drooling is treated with several off-label drugs that have an anticholinergic effect, in particular with tricyclic antidepressants, antispasmodics (e.g., scopolamine) or botulin toxin (Table 20.5).

**Table 20.5** Medications for sialorrhoea in amyotrophic lateral sclerosis

| Scopolamine | 1.5 mg bid or tid |
|---|---|
| Amitriptiline | 5–50 mg qd, bid or tid |
| Atropine | Drops 0.5–1% three or four times |
| Glycopirrolate | Nebulised or i.v. |
| Botulin toxin type A in salivary glands | 25–100 UI for each gland |
| Radiotherapy in salivary glands | No clear protocols |

Speech language pathologists (SLP) manage the bulbar symptoms of ALS patients through many care settings and are aware of the need to provide patient education to prevent complications related to dysphagia.

There is a consensus among SLPs that during clinical evaluation a screening for dysphagia in ALS patients is recommended, even in the absence of bulbar symptoms; unfortunately, there is still no consensus on the types of assessments. The need for objective instrumental evaluations to assess dysphagia is also accepted by most SLPs, but the timing and indication of these instrumental evaluations is not standardised. In collaboration with SLPs, neurologists can better direct dysphagia treatment within multidisciplinary models where clinicians can collaborate effectively through improved coordination of care. Further research is required to determine the best way to assess and handle dysphagia in patients with ALS (Epps et al. 2020).

Recent developments in neuroimaging, staging systems development, patient-reported outcome measures and the advent of novel instrumental speech and evaluation strategies for swallowing offer new insights into ALS bulbar dysfunction. However, in order for these approaches to be adopted into standard clinical practice and pharmacological studies, their measuring properties, diagnostic accuracy and longitudinal monitoring abilities have to be rigorously tested. The development of broad international collaborations and relentless biomarker testing efforts give rise to optimism for the development of validated bulbar evaluations, which in turn will lead to recommendations for best practice, allow for well-timed clinical interventions and promote precise stratification of patients in clinical trials (Yunusova et al. 2019).

A recent review highlighted that neurogenic dysphagia is not simply a symptom, but a multi-aetiological condition, depending on the underlying disorder, with various phenotypic patterns. Phenotypes of dysphagia, according to flexible endoscopic evaluation of swallowing (FEES) criteria, may promote differential diagnosis of unknown aetiology in patients with dysphagia (Warnecke et al. 2020).

## 20.13 Therapy of People with Dementia: The Role of Speech Language Pathology

Karel Neubauer

### 20.13.1 The Role of Speech Language Pathologists

The role of clinical speech language therapists (SLTs), phoniatricians and audiologists in helping people with dementia was summarised in an official statement published by ASHA (American Speech-Language-Hearing Association) for the first time in 1988 (Ripich 1992), to:

- Contribute to comprehensive diagnosis and care of patients with Alzheimer's and similar diseases by assessing the level of their communication skills.
- Contribute to uncovering the contribution of possible unrecognised and misinterpreted communication disorders to the diagnosis of dementia.
- Participate in the interdisciplinary development of treatment programmes designed to facilitate and maintain functional communication of these persons for as long as possible.
- Help those around them and their families understand their communication disorders, specific deficits and needs.

In the current view of the role and importance of clinical SLTs, in addition to the above, the approach to swallowing and eating disorders and the importance of clinical speech language therapy (SLT) in screening, diagnosis and therapy of cognitive-communication disorders in people with dementia are accentuated.

> Speech-language pathologists (SLPs) play a central role in the screening, assessment, diagnosis, and treatment of persons with dementia. The professional roles and activities in speech-language pathology include clinical/educational services (diagnosis, assessment, planning, and treatment); prevention and advocacy; and education, administration, and research—ASHA (2016)

The primary goal of therapy, including SLT, is a rehabilitation programme with realistic goals and usable methods of work that will build an alternative to hopelessness and resignation from a bleak life perspective. A comprehensive therapeutic assistance programme for people with dementia is implemented through the involvement of pharmacological, psychotherapeutic, rehabilitation and non-pharmacological approaches and methods, including a clinical speech therapist, and must be pursued to support the basic principles of dementia therapy (Neubauer 1999a, 2003; Holmerová et al. 2009), and involves:

- Urgently addressing issues of assistance and adaptation to the situation and introducing therapeutic measures to maintain and improve the current capabilities of the disabled person.
- Active exercise, training of physical and mental abilities and emphasising retained skills, not disorders.
- Promoting the active attitude of the treated person and the use of retained abilities in everyday life.
- Promoting proper treatment of existing and future symptoms and diseases by the attending physician, as good physical condition is a prerequisite for a stable mental condition.
- Proper supportive medication treatment by the attending physician to deal with sleep disorders, affectivity, restlessness, anxiety, etc. is a prerequisite for effective rehabilitation.

- Providing psychotherapeutic assistance to the patient and his or her family.
- Use of rehabilitation care, work therapy, SLT and cognitive training to help actively a person suffering from dementia.

The aims, methods and forms of the rehabilitation process for people with dementia are necessarily modified according to the results of medical and psychological diagnostics, determined on the basis thereof. For non-medicative therapeutic procedures, the most important is the diagnosis of dementia, the current stage of development of the dementia syndrome and the predicted development and prognosis of the disease.

The difference between the manifestations of dementias referred to as cortical or subcortical, possibly mixed, determines the dominant area and goals of therapy, but often its possibilities and prognosis too. In cortical dementia, the therapy focuses primarily on cognitive and phatic disorders; in contrast, subcortical dementia is less cognitive, memory is impaired, motoric and communication disorders are more dominant—dysarthria, dysphagia, dysphonia, etc. Some types of subcortical dementia therapeutically have more favourable options and prognosis than cortical forms of dementia.

The prognosis of the disease must necessarily correspond to the setting of realistic goals of the therapeutic process. Only in reversible forms of dementia can a great extent of the recovery of lost skills and abilities be expected. For other, especially benign static forms, maximising the conserved potential and inducing appropriate compensation strategies are paramount. In the progressive form of dementia, the main goal is to slow down the progressive loss, maintaining the highest possible level of independent life in the current stage of the disease. Progressive forms of dementia syndrome require repeated adaptation of forms and methods of therapy, always to achieve the maximum degree of loss compensation and quality of life. Because it is difficult to predict the dynamics of the development of dementia symptoms—even in the diagnosis of

progressive disease—the symptoms can only be stabilised in the long term. Therefore, it is not possible to proceed passively here or to deprive a person with dementia of an active therapeutic programme.

## 20.13.2 Therapy of Speech Communication Disorders

Therapy of communication disorders performed or managed by clinical SLTs must necessarily be intertwined with procedures for the rehabilitation of cognitive disorders into a single therapeutic programme. Depending on the type and stage of dementia, the programme monitors improvement, slowing down or compensating for disorders and deterioration of a person with dementia. Therefore, the application of all methods of cognitive rehabilitation procedures—such as validation therapy, group re-socialisation methods or reality orientation therapy—is a frequent part of therapy predominantly focused on working with communication disorders in people with dementia. Orientation and comprehensive specialisation education of clinical SLTs in specific and best practices to help people with dementia is a highly desirable extension of professional competence and preferred specialisation (Carozza 2016; Horner et al. 2016). Involvement of therapeutic intervention by clinical SLTs for people with dementia has been underestimated for a long time by those in the medical and psychological community. A similar situation in the past was in the area of swallowing disorders—dysphagia—and it can be expected that practical support of the implementation of professional health care in the area of cognitive-communication disorders in people with dementia will rise in the future.

The basic principle of therapy of speech communication disorders in people with dementia is to maximise the preserved communication potential in order to maintain meaningful communication of the patient with the environment for the longest possible time by any usable forms. This therapy supports:

- Maintaining communication competence.
- Maintaining adaptive and facilitating communication behaviour.
- Maintaining and creating opportunities for communicating with the environment.
- Improving the interaction between a person with dementia and caregivers.
- Maintaining respect for themselves and dignified communication behaviour.
- Reducing emotional stress during contact with the environment.
- Keeping behaviour and emotional experience at a socially acceptable level.

Individual and group forms of work respect the type and degree of the disorder in a person with dementia (Brookshire 2007; Neubauer 1999b, 2003, 2018a; Bourgeois 2011).

### 20.13.2.1 Therapy in the Early Stages of Development of Dementia Syndrome

Therapeutic assistance to persons in the early stages of dementia with preserved insight into their own communication, at least to the level that allows motivation for their own active cooperation with the therapist, and insight into the implementation of therapeutic assignments, involve the use of SLT components of speech. Techniques of SLT of phatic disorders, in conjunction with memory and cognitive training techniques, may be essential for patients with reversible or early-diagnosed symptoms of the onset of dementia syndrome. Methods of care must be adapted to the dominant cognitive and memory disorders and to a different picture of individual language skill disorders from that in most people with aphasia. They can build on mostly more intact expressive phonological and syntactic abilities, overcome dominant semantic disorders, word amnesia, speech initiation difficulties, and promote coherence and a clear goal of spoken expression.

The most commonly used are adaptive communication strategies, including the use of external aids, communication aids and clearly formulated informative messages about their problems, often in written form. The communication facilitation strategy seeks to maintain appropriate procedures for finding words in the form of semantic (content related) and phonemic (phonetic and rhythmic) help hints. Other approaches seek to promote cohesion in conversation by creating an outline for the topic. Group procedures can be based on the traditional concept of group sessions in clinical SLT. For people with dementia at an early stage of the disease, they can be used to practise adaptive and facilitation procedures, provide feedback from the therapist and other group members, create a coherent activating and emotionally stimulating environment, or provide direct demonstrations of family cooperation with the person suffering dementia or with staff of the institution.

### 20.13.2.2 Therapy in Advanced Stages of Development of Dementia Syndrome

At this stage of dementia, most people already experience disorders of all elements of language expression. Understanding of not only more complicated but also simple conversational conversions is limited. Initiation of dialogue is often not possible and the coherence of the utterance is seriously violated, even in short parts of speech.

The loss of insight into one's life situation and the practical cessation of the possibilities of recovering learning leads to the necessity of changing the dominance of therapeutic procedures in favour of indirect or counselling procedures of communication therapy. Individual activity is based on the possibility of maintaining stimulation of cognitive and memory functions in a non-directed dialogue in a motivationally positive atmosphere, in which the person with dementia is willing to cooperate during exercises and contact stimulation.

**Group Activities** seek to support the remaining communication opportunities of these people by using simple topics at multiple levels. If one level fails, no response or conversation is reached, so we go to a simpler or another topic. Intensive sound stimulation and creation of the opportunity to comment on the subject are used, even at the non-verbal communication level and with strong visual and tactile stimulation. Institutional environments can often hamper the ability to perform regular therapy and achieve a quiet, undisturbed therapeutic environment. Another important factor is the choice of members of a group at a similar cognitive and communication level. Group activities provide an ideal environment for demonstrating appropriate procedures to facilitate communication of carers with persons with the syndrome of dementia.

**Indirect or Counselling Communication Techniques** seek to change the environment in which a person suffering from dementia lives and to improve communication between the patient and their surroundings, using the ways in which caregivers communicate. If the patient is no longer able to adjust their behaviour, the manner of speaking and the behaviour of those around them can be changed. However, there is a clear need for long-term practical work under the guidance of an experienced therapist to incorporate these rules into the communication behaviour of the family or professionals around the person with dementia. Targeted adjustments in a personal or group environment that can stimulate communication and cognition can prevent the risk of deterioration. Uncovering the potential for improving the visual, auditory and tactile orientation and psychosocial environment stimulates opportunities and motivation to communicate, especially for institutionalised persons with communication disorders (Bayles 1995; Lubinski 1995).

### 20.13.2.3 Dysarthria and Dysphagia in Dementia Syndrome

Swallowing disorders and dysarthria are frequent manifestations, mainly in the area of subcortical and mixed dementia (Parkinson's disease, vascular dementia, etc.) or present as an additional complication, e.g., after CNS trauma in a person with dementia.

In milder manifestations of dementia, SLT can be performed to improve speech quality and intelligibility. In the case of more severe symptoms of dysarthria in persons with severe development of dementia syndrome, deterioration of respiratory capacity and the risk of severe incoordination of speech and breathing should be prevented through breathing and movement exercises.

In the case of swallowing difficulties, the composition of the diet and the position of body and head should be adjusted to the benefit of a person with dementia. If the level of cooperation of a person with dementia allows it, movement of muscles in the orofacial area is involved. The procedures are modified in the field of dysarthria and dysphagia therapy, with predominantly indirect compensatory strategies that are most useful in the often limited cooperation of people with dementia (Neubauer 2016a, 2017a, 2018e).

### 20.13.2.4 Interconnection of Cognitive and Communication Methods

Procedures for the treatment of cognitive abilities of people with dementia have been developed and are used by professionals from several areas: psychiatrists, psychologists, psychomotor therapists and occupational therapists, psychotherapists, clinical speech therapists, special educators, rehabilitation and social workers. They are aimed at stimulating not only the performance of cognitive processes, but also at managing the emotional, behavioural and social difficulties that this development brings.

Therapeutic approaches on the profession of clinical SLTs have been published by Brookshire (2007) and Carozza (2016), focusing on group therapy of people with dementia in the care of clinical SLT (Hopper 2007). The current approach in this area increasingly accentuates group activities for people with dementia, involving elements of drama therapy, music therapy, art therapy, and dance and movement therapy. For people with severe dementia, the preferred approach is also to involve a multisensory programme of activities based on the Marie Montenssori approach (Brookshire 2007, p 596). The above directions are related to the increasingly emphasised aspect of quality of life, preservation of activities, interests and social communication of people with dementia syndrome.

The degree to which the symptoms of dementia are found in the rehabilitated person is crucial for determining the appropriate approach and methods of cognitive therapy. In the early, mild stage of dementia, these are primarily procedures to support the maintenance of a person's social skills, adaptation of the environment, and intensive stimulation of cognitive abilities. In advanced, moderate and more severe stages of the disease, it is crucial to maintain adequate emotional experience and behaviour, to continue to stimulate cognitive functions adequately, and to use non-verbal communication options.

This implies that in the early stages of the disease, the social capacity of a person with dementia is improved by adjustments to the environment, reality orientation therapy, psychotherapy, resocialisation or remotivation procedures and reminiscence therapy. The current cognitive abilities of a person with dementia are stimulated by memory and sensory training, targeted cognitive stimulation and the use of external memory aids.

In particular, people in the late stages of dementia may be helped to maintain adequate social behaviour and emotional experience. Validation therapy, behavioural methods, together with primarily non-verbal techniques—music therapy, art therapy, ergotherapy—are mainly used. Movement and dance therapy (Ripich 1992; Neubauer 1999b; Carozza 2016) are of great importance for maintaining the physical condition and mobility of people with dementia.

A comprehensive approach to the problems of people with dementia cannot do without combining cognitive abilities therapies and communication therapy. For this reason, the above-mentioned procedures are often applied in individual and group speech therapy, most often in the form of memory, attention training and using external compensatory memory aids (Wilson 1982; Bourgeois 1990, 1992, 2007, 2011). This area is a widely recognised and highly validated part of therapeutic assistance for people with dementia syndrome.

Validation therapy, reminiscence therapy and music therapy (Benjamin 1995; Neubauer 1999b; Orange et al. 1995; Carozza 2016) are suitable for therapists with psychotherapeutic education and training, who are more focused on managing the emotional and social problems of people with dementia. For the creation of programmes involving memory and attention stimulation, and interconnection of speech and memory rehabilitation, in clinical practice the EBM (evidence-based management) approach has proven effective. This

involves the use of keeping daily diary records, reading them in an attempt to reproduce the feelings, writing the content of the record, and involvement of memory stimulation in the form of modified crosswords, word lotto, etc., with possible support of ICT (Information and Communications Technology) multimedia background and specialised programmes (Van Vliet 1996; Neubauer 1999a, 2018d; Brookshire 2007).

Horner et al. (2016) have published a meta-analysis of an extensive set of studies, aimed at finding and evaluating such approaches in therapeutic assistance to people with dementia, that can rely on the results of evaluation in an Evidence-Based Management (EBM). They highlight the following approaches (p 79):

- Educational programmes for people in helping professions.
- Cognitive stimulation programmes.
- ICT-supported cognitive stimulation programmes.
- Reality orientation therapy.
- Stimulating contact with the social environment.
- Reminiscence therapy.
- Prolonged responses on stimulus tasks.

The authors point out the presence of positive partial effects of these programmes on the cognitive and communication skills of people with dementia. They present a promising potential for the development of new and effective adaptation of best practice therapies for people suffering from dementia symptoms.

## 20.14 Prognosis of Neurogenic Speech Disorders

Karel Neubauer and Antonio Schindler

Neurogenic speech disorders that occur in adults result from several of the more common mechanisms of damage to the human nervous system (NS) (Brookshire and McNeil 2015; Neubauer 2018b; Duffy 2020):

- Cerebrovascular disease and stroke (CVA).
- Traumatic tissue damage to the NS.
- Tumours and infections of the NS.
- Degenerative diseases of the NS.

The origin and persistence of motor speech disorders are represented to a very large extent by these aetiologies. Enderby and Emerson (1995) report 280 people with acquired CVA-based dysarthria and brain tissue lesions, head injuries and degenerative neurological diseases, per 100,000 of the population. According to the authors, this is a more common neurogenic disorder of speech communication than aphasia (150 per 100,000) or acquired dysphonia (max. 89 per 100,000) inhabitants. Subsequent prognosis in people with dysarthria or speech dyspraxia is often associated with the development of the NS, when this is the cause of speech communication disorders. The primary organic disorder can be of varying degrees of severity, and can also, in particular depending on the condition of the NS of the affected person, develop a prognostic variety. In the case of favourable healing of nerve tissue and restoration of functions after trauma, development is possible up to the area of mild residual difficulties in speech, and practical disappearance of speech communication disorders. This can also be documented in some people who have suffered from CVA or head injury, in children and in adults. If the basis of the communication disorder is a neurodegenerative disease, it is necessary to take into account the long-term unfavourable development of manifestations, especially depending on the development of the symptomatology of the CNS disease of the affected person. The aim is to support the maintenance of quality communication with the environment for as long as possible and thus contribute to maintaining the quality of life of a person with dysarthria or speech dyspraxia.

With regard to the practical clinical situation and also the development of therapeutic assistance for a person with acquired motor speech disorder, prognosis is a key concept for both the patient and the clinician; in fact, while the patient is interested in whether and how much his speech will improve in order to organise his life, for the clinician the prognosis in one of the key elements in establishing the plan of treatment, its goal and its termination. Unfortunately, it is very unlikely that a patient with an acquired motor speech disorder will have his previous speech restored, but prognosis may enormously vary according to several factors.

Prognosis can be referred to either the underlying disease (e.g., Parkinson's) or the speech disorder (e.g., hypokinetic dysarthria); in some cases disease prognosis and speech prognosis will be related to each other, in others they will diverge: e.g., while Parkinson's disease will progress, hypokinetic dysarthria may improve owing to Lee Silverman Voice Therapy. For disease prognosis, different situations may be encountered:

- Progressive diseases such as neurodegenerative diseases, where neuromuscular control will either worsen slowly, as in Parkinson's disease, or rapidly, as in amyotrophic lateral sclerosis.
- Exacerbating-remitting diseases, such as multiple sclerosis, where motor and non-motor symptoms will worsen during exacerbating phases, while they will improve afterwards.
- Chronic diseases, such as stroke or traumatic brain injury, characterised by a sudden deterioration of neuromuscular control, followed by an improvement and finally reaching a plateau (the chronic phase).

Disease prognosis depends not only on the natural history of the disease, but also on the possible treatments: pharmacological (for Parkinson's disease, myasthenia gravis, multiple sclerosis) or surgical treatments (deep brain stimulation). The goal of speech treatment is strongly related to the disease prognosis: for progressive diseases, it might be important to reduce progression of speech symptoms and communication restrictions; for exacerbating-remitting diseases, the focus is on acceleration of symptoms removal; for chronic diseases it is pivotal to improve speech and guarantee communication.

Speech prognosis may be related to two main factors:

- Cognitive-linguistic impairment.
- Motor speech impairment.

In fact, impairment of cognitive or linguistic functions may severely affect the possibility of adopting communication or augmentative/alternative strategies, thus reducing treatment options. Motor speech impairment, on the other hand, can be improved by speech therapy, prosthetic or surgical treatments. Other factors that have an impact on speech prognosis are motivation, environmental needs, communications partners, availability of speech treatment, financial and family support and structure of the health care system. Although a number of accepted relationships can be mentioned—for example, between the characteristics of the lesion and impaired function in CNS trauma (extent and location of the lesion, presence and duration of severe impaired consciousness, etc.) and the level of healing of a person's cognitive and communication skills after a nerve tissue lesion (Coelho et al. 2016), these relationships lack clear validity. Some people show a surprising level of recovery, or conversely its stagnation, neither of which correlates with the above factors. Factors such as the internal motivation of the affected person, the capacity of his or her will and the influence of the social environment play a difficult but undoubtedly important role. The importance of a therapeutic relationship that contributes to the development of the social and motivating dimension of helping a person with a communication disorder is aptly characterised by Brookshire and McNeil (2015, p. 215):

> Education, counselling, and support may not affect a patient's scores on standardized tests, yet they are important to patients and families immediately after the onset of aphasia … delaying or eliminating counseling, education, and support during the first weeks after the patient becomes aphasic may have important and irreversible negative effects on the patient and the patient's family.

The above statement can undoubtedly be applied to people with severe motor speech disorders and emphasises the impact of comprehensive therapeutic assistance, including family, social and institutional environment, for activating and motivating people with neurogenic speech disorders.

# References

Alfwaress FSD, Bibars AR, Hamasha A et al (2017) Outcomes of palatal lift prosthesis on dysarthric speech. J Craniofac Surg 28(1):30–35

Alzrayer N, Banda DR, Koul RK (2014) Use of iPad/iPods with individuals with autism and other developmental disabilities: a meta-analysis of communication interventions. Rev J Autism Dev Disord 1:179–191

Amon,A., & Alesch, F. (2017). Systems for deep brain stimulation: review oftechnical features. *Journal of NeuralTransmission, 124*, 1083-1091.

Andersen PM, Abrahams S et al (2012) EFNS Task Force on Diagnosis and Management of Amyotrophic Lateral Sclerosis; EFNS guidelines on the clinical management of amyotrophic lateral sclerosis (MALS)—revised report of an EFNS task force. Eur J Neurol 19(3):360–375

Aramany MA, Downs JA, Beery OC et al (1982) Prosthodontic rehabilitation for glossectomy patients. J Prosthet Dent 48(1):78–81

Arlotti M, Marceglia S, Foffani G et al (2018) Eighthours adaptive deep brain stimulation in patients with Parkinson disease. Neurology 90(11):e971–e976. https://doi.org/10.1212/WNL.0000000000005121

Arlotti M, Palmisano C, Minafra B et al (2019) Monitoring subthalamic oscillations for 24 hours in a freely moving Parkinson's disease patient. Mov Disord 34(5):757–759

ASHA (American Speech-Language-Hearing Association) (2005) Roles and responsibilities of speech-language pathologists with respect to augmentative and alternative communication. Position statement. DOI:https://doi.org/10.1044/polici.PS2005-0013

ASHA (American Speech-Language-Hearing Association) (2016) Roles and responsibilities of speech-language pathologists. Available via https://www.asha.org/PRPSpecificTopic.aspx?folderid=8589935289&section=Roles_and_Responsibilities. Accessed 20 Feb 2020

ASHA (American Speech-Language-Hearing Association) (2021) Telepractice (Practice Portal). Available via www.asha.org/Practice-Portal/Professional-Issues/Telepractice/. Accessed 2nd April 2021

ASHA-NOMS (American Speech-Language-Hearing Association—National Outcomes Measurement System) (2013) Adults in Health Care. Functional Communication Measures (FCMs). Speech Language Pathology. American Speech-Language-Hearing Association. Available via www.asha.org/NOMS. Accessed 14 Nov 2021

ASHA (American Speech-Language-Hearing Association) (2021) Augmentative and Alternative Communication (Practice Portal). Available via www.asha.org/Practice-Portal/Professional-Issues/Augmentative-and-Alternative-Communication/. Accessed 17 Jan 2021

Aum DJ, Tierney TS (2018) Deep brain stimulation: foundations and future trends. Front Biosci (Landmark Ed) 23:162–182

Bäckman B, Grever-Sjölander AC, Bengtsson K et al (2007) Children with Down syndrome: oral development and morphology after use of palatal plates between 6 and 48 months of age. Int J Paediatr Dent 17(1):19–28

Baer RA, Krietemeyer J (2006) Overview of mindfulness- and acceptance-based treatment approaches. In: Baer RA (ed) Mindfulness-based treatment approaches: clinician's guide to evidence base and applications. Elsevier Academic Press, Amsterdam, pp 3–17

Bakker K (2006) Technical support for stuttering treatment. In: Bernstein Ratner N, Tetnowski J (eds) Current issues in stuttering research and practice. Lawrence Erlbaum Associates, Mahwah, pp 205–237

Ball L, Fager S, Friek Olsen M (2012) Augmentative and alternative communication for people with progressive neuromuscular disease. Phys Med Rehabil Clin N Am 23(3):689–699

Ballard KJ, Maas E, Robin DA (2007) Treating control of voicing in apraxia of speech with variable practice. Aphasiology 21(12):1195–1217

Ballard KJ, Wambaugh JL, Duffy JR et al (2015) Treatment for acquired apraxia of speech: a systematic review of intervention research between 2004 and 2012. Am J Speech Lang Pathol 24(2):316–337

Baram S, Karlsborg M, Bakke M (2020) Improvement of oral function and hygiene in Parkinson's disease: a randomised controlled clinical trial. J Oral Rehabil 47(3):370–376

Barlow SM, Finan DS, Park S-Y (2004) Central pattern generation and sensorimotor entrainment of respiratory and orofacial systems in humans. In: Maassen B, Hulstijn KR et al (eds) Speech motor control in normal and disordered speech. Oxford University Press, Oxford, pp 211–224

Basso A (1977) Il Paziente Afasico. Feltrinelli, Milan

Basso A, Cattaneo S, Girelli L et al (2011) Treatment efficacy of language and calculation disorders and speech apraxia: a review of the literature. Eur J Phys Rehabil Med 47(1):101-21. PMID: 21448123

Basu I, Graupe D, Tuninetti D et al (2013) Pathological tremor prediction using surface electromyogram and acceleration: potential use in 'ON–OFF' demand driven deep brain stimulator design. J Neural Eng 10(3):036019. https://doi.org/10.1088/1741-2560/10/3/036019

Baxter S, Enderby P, Evans P et al (2012) Barriers and facilitators to the use of high-technology augmentative and alternative communication devices: a systematic review and qualitative synthesis. Int J Lang Commun Disord 47:115–129

Bayles K (1995) Language in ageing and dementia. In: Kirshner H (ed) Handbook of neurological speech and language disorders. M Dekker Inc., New York, NY, pp 351–372

Beck JS (2011) Cognitive behavior therapy: basics and beyond, 2nd edn. The Guilford Press, New York

Bejjani BP, Gervais D, Arnulf I et al (2000) Axial Parkinsonian symptoms can be improved: the role of levodopa and bilateral subthalamic stimulation. J Neurol Neurosurg Psychiatry 68(5):595–600

Benjamin B (1995) Validation therapy. An intervention for disoriented patients with Alzheimer's disease. Top Lang Disord 15(2):66–74

Berke GS, Gerratt B, Kreiman J et al (1999) Treatment of Parkinson hypophonia with percutaneous collagen augmentation. Laryngoscope 109(8):1295–1299

Berman PA, Brady JP (1973) Miniaturized metronomes in the treatment of stuttering: a survey of clinician's experiences. J Behav Ther Exp Psychiatry 4(2):117–119

Bernasconi T (2020) ICF und UK: Chancen einer aktivitätsbezogenen Perspektive. In: Boenisch J, Sachse SK (eds) Kompendium Unterstützte Kommunikation. Kohlhammer, Stuttgart, pp 365–371

Beukelman DR, Light J (2020) Augmentative and alternative communication: supporting children and adults. Paul H Brookes Publishing Co. Inc., Baltimore, MD

Beukelman D, Mirenda P (eds) (1992) Augmentative and alternative communication. Management of severe communication disorders in children and adults. Paul H. Brookes Publishing Co. Inc., Baltimore, MD

Beukelman D, Mirenda P (eds) (2013) Augmentative and alternative communication. Supporting children and adults with complex communication needs. Paul H. Brookes Publishing Co. Inc., Baltimore, MD

Beukelman DR, Garrett KL, Yorkston KM (2007) Augmentative communication strategies for adults with acute or chronic medical conditions. Paul H Brookes Publishing Co. Inc., Baltimore, MD

Biggs EE, Carter EW, Gilson CB (2018) Systematic review of interventions involving aided AAC modeling for children with complex communication needs. Am J Intellect Dev Disabil 123:443–473

Binger C, Berens J, Kent-Walsh J et al (2008) The effects of aided AAC interventions on AAC use, speech, and symbolic gestures. Semin Speech Lang 29:101–111

Block S, Onslow M, Roberts R et al (2004) Control of stuttering with EMG feedback. Adv Speech Lang Pathol 6:100–106

Blood GW (1995) A behavioral-cognitive therapy program for adults who stutter: computers and counseling. J Commun Disord 28:165–180

Bloodstein O, Bernstein Ratner N (2008) A handbook on stuttering, 6th edn. Thomson Delmar, Clifton Park

Boccard, S. G., Pereira, E. A., & Aziz, T. Z. (2015). Deep brain stimulation for chronic pain. *Journal of ClinicalNeuroscience, 22*(10), 1537-1543.

Boey R (2010) Sociaal cognitieve gedragstherapie voor stotteren: adolescenten en volwassenen (Social cognitive behavioral therapy for stuttering: adolescents and adults). VVL, Belsele

Bothe AK, Davidow JH, Bramlett RE et al (2006) Stuttering treatment research 1970–2005: I. Systematic review incorporating trial quality assessment of behavioral, cognitive, and related approaches. Am J Speech Lang Pathol 15(4):321–341

Botterill W, Cook F (1987) Personal construct theory and the treatment of adolescent dysfluency. In: Rustin L, Purser H, Rowley D (eds) Progress in the treatment of fluency disorders. Taylor & Francis, London, pp 147–165

Bouglé F, Ryalls J, LeDorze G (1995) Improving fundamental frequency modulation in head trauma patients: a preliminary comparison of speech-language. Therapy conducted with and without IBM Speech Viewer. Folia Phoniatr Logop 47(1):24–32

Bourgeois M (1990) Enhancing conversation skills in patients with Alzheimer's disease using a prosthetic memory aid. J Appl Behav Anal 23(1):29–42

Bourgeois M (1992) Evaluating memory wallets in conversations with patients with dementia. J Speech Hear Res 35(6):1344–1357

Bourgeois M (2007) Memory books and other graphic cuing systems. Health Professionals Press, New York, NY

Bourgeois M (2011) Dementia. In: LaPointe L, Stierwalt JAG (eds) Aphasia and related neurogenic language disorders. Thieme Medical Publishers Inc., New York, NY, pp 223–232

Boyle MP (2011) Mindfulness training in stuttering therapy: a tutorial for speech-language pathologists. J Fluen Disord 36:122–129

Brabenec L, Klobusiakova P, Simkoa P et al (2021) Noninvasive brain stimulation for speech in Parkinson's disease: a randomized controlled trial. Brain Stimul 14(3):571–578

Braun U (2020) Entwicklung der Unterstützten Kommunikation in Deutschland—eine systematische Einführung (Development of Supported Communication in Germany—a systematic introduction). In: Boenisch J, Sachse SK (eds) Kompendium Unterstützte Kommunikation (compendium of supported communication). Kohlhammer, Stuttgart, pp 19–32

Brookshire R (2007) Introduction to neurogenic communication disorders. Mosby Elsevier, St. Louis, MO

Brookshire R, McNeil M (2015) Introduction to neurogenic communication disorders. Elsevier Mosby, St. Louis, MO

Buccino G, Riggio L (2006) The role of the mirror neuron system in motor learning. Kinesiology 38(1):1–13

Cantarella G, Mazzola RF, Mantovani M et al (2012) Fat injections for the treatment of velopharyngeal insufficiency. J Craniofac Surg 23:634–637

Cantor R, Curtis TA, Shipp T et al (1969) Maxillary speech prostheses for mandibular surgical defects. J Prosthet Dent 22(2):253–260

Carlstedt K, Henningsson G, McAllister A et al (2001) Long-term effects of palatal plate therapy on oral motor function in children with Down syndrome evaluated by video registration. Acta Odontol Scand 59(2):63–68

Carlstedt K, Henningsson G, Dahllöf G (2003) A four-year longitudinal study of palatal plate therapy in children with down syndrome: effects on oral motor function, articulation and communication preferences. Acta Odontol Scand 61(1):39–46

Carozza L (2016) Communication and aging. Plural Publishing Inc., San Diego, CA

Casa Futura Technologies (2015) Technology for treating stuttering and Parkinson's speech. http://casafuturatech.wpengine.com/smalltalk-anti-stuttering-device/. Accessed 1 Feb 2022

Cassidy JM, Cramer SC (2017) Spontaneous and therapeutic-induced mechanisms of functional recovery after stroke. Transl Stroke Res 8(1):33–46

Cheasman C, Simpson S, Everard R (2015) Acceptance and speech work: the challenge. Procedia Soc Behav Sci 193:72–81

Clark HM, Henson PA, Barber WD et al (2003) Relationships among subjective and objective measures of tongue strength and oral phase swallowing impairments. Am J Speech Lang Pathol 12(1):40–50

Clarke M, Price K, Jolleff N (2012) Augmentative and alternative communication. In: Kersner M, Wright J (eds) Speech and language therapy. The decision-making process when working with children. Routledge Taylor & Francis Group, London, pp 221–233

Cleland J, Timmins C, Wood SE et al (2009) Electropalatographic therapy for children and young people with Down's syndrome. Clin Linguist Phon 23(12):926–939

Coelho C, Youse K, Eagan E (2016) Assessment and management of traumatic brain injury. In: Johnson A, Jacobson B (eds) Medical speech language pathology. Thieme Medical Publisher Inc., New York, NY, pp 83–102

Cohen SM, Elackattu A, Noordzij JP et al (2009) Palliative treatment of dysphonia and dysarthria. Otolaryngol Clin N Am 42:107–121

Conture EG (2001) Stuttering: its nature, diagnosis and treatment. Allyn & Bacon, Boston

Costantini A, Giorgi R, D'Agostino S et al (2013) High-dose thiamine improves the symptoms of Friedreich's ataxia. BMJ Case Rep 22:2013

Craig AR, Cleary PJ (1982) Reduction of stuttering by young male stutterers using EMG feedback. Biofeedback Self Regul 7(3):241–255

Craig A, Tran Y (2006) Fear of speaking: chronic anxiety and stuttering. Adv Psychiatr Treat 12(1):63–68

Craig A, Tran Y (2014) Trait and social anxiety in adults with chronic stuttering: conclusions following meta-analysis. J Fluen Disord 40:35–43

Craig A, Hancock K, Chang E et al (1996) A controlled clinical trial for stuttering in persons aged 9 to 14 years. J Speech Hear Res 39(4):808–826

Craig A, Hancock K, Tran Y et al (2003) Anxiety levels in PWS: a randomized population study. J Speech Lang Hear Res 46:1197–1206

Craig A, Blumgart E, Tran Y (2011) Resilience and stuttering: factors that protect people from the adversity of chronic stuttering. J Speech Lang Hear Res 54(6):1485–1496

Crowe TA (1997) Counseling: definition, history, rationale. In: Crowe TA (ed) Applications of counseling in speech-language pathology and audiology. Williams & Wilkins, Baltimore, pp 3–39

Crystal D (2010) The Cambridge encyclopedia of language. University Press, Cambridge

D'Alatri L, Paludetti G, Contarino MF et al (2008) Effects of bilateral subthalamic nucleus stimulation and medication on Parkinsonian speech impairment. J Voice 22(3):365–372

Dabul B (1979) Apraxia battery for adults. ProEd, Austin, TX

Dabul B, Bollier B (1976) Therapeutic approaches to apraxia. J Speech Hear Disord 41(2):268–276

Dalton P (1983) Psychological approaches to the treatment of stuttering. In: Dalton P (ed) Approaches to the treatment of stuttering. Imprint Routledge, London, pp 106–135

Darley FL, Aronson AE, Brown JR (1975) Motor speech disorders. WB Saunders, Philadelphia, PA

Dashtipour K, Ali Tafreshi A, Lee J et al (2018) Speech disorders in Parkinson's disease: pathophysiology, medical management and surgical approaches. Neurodegener Dis Manag 8(5):337–348

Davis J, Lazarus C, Logemann JA et al (1987) Effect of a maxillary glossectomy prosthesis on articulation and swallowing. J Prosthet Dent 57(6):715–719

de Carvalho-Teles V, Sennes LU, Gielow I (2008) Speech evaluation after palatal augmentation in patients undergoing glossectomy. Arch Otolaryngol Head Neck Surg 134(10):1066–1070

Deka C, Shrivastava A, Abraham A, Nautiyal S, Chauhan P (2024) AI-based automated speech therapy tools for persons with speech sound disorder: a systematic literature review. Speech, Language and Hearing 1-22. 10.1080/2050571X.2024.2359274.

Dewar A, Dewar AD, Austin WTS et al (1979) The long-term use of an automatically triggered auditory feedback masking device in the treatment of stammering. Br J Disord Commun 14(3):219–229

De Renzi E, Pieczuro A, Vignolo LA (1966) Oral apraxia and aphasia. Cortex 2(1):50–73

De Renzi E, Pieczuro A, Vignolo LA (1968) Ideational apraxia, a quantitative study. Neuropsychologia 6(1):41–52

de Silva MJ, Breuer E, Lee L et al (2014) Theory of change: a theory-driven approach to enhance the Medical Research Council's framework for complex interventions. Trials 15:267. https://doi.org/10.1186/1745-6215-15-267

Dias AE, Barbosa ER, Coracini K et al (2006) Effects of repetitive transcranial magnetic stimulation on voice and speech in Parkinson's disease. Acta Neurol Scand 113(2):92–99

DiLollo A, Neimeyer RA, Manning WH (2002) A personal construct psychology view of relapse: indications for a narrative therapy component to stuttering treatment. J Fluen Disord 27(1):19–42

Dowden P (1999) Different strokes for different folks. Augment Commun News 12(1–2):7–8

Dowden P, Cook AM (2012) Improving communicative competence through alternative selection methods. In: Johnston SS, Reichle J, Feeley KM et al (eds) AAC strategies for individuals with moderate to severe disabilities. Brookes, Baltimore, MD, pp 81–118

Duffy JR (2005a) Motor speech disorders: substrates, differential diagnosis, and management. Elsevier/Mosby, St Louis, MO

Duffy JR (2005b) Motor speech disorders. Substrates, differential diagnosis, and treatment. Elsevier, St Louis MO

Duffy JR (2013) Motor speech disorders: substrates, differential diagnosis, and management, vol 1, 3rd edn. Elsevier Health Sciences, St Louis, MO

Duffy JR (2019) Motor speech disorders: substrates, differential diagnosis, and management, 4th edn. Elsevier, St. Louis, MO

Duffy J (2020) Motor speech disorders. Substrates, differential diagnosis, and management. Elsevier, St. Louis, MO

Dworkin JP, Johns DN (1980) Management of velopharyngeal incompetence in dysarthria: a historical review. Clin Otolaryngol 5:61–74

Dworkin JP, Abkarian GG, Johns DF (1988) Apraxia of speech: the effectiveness of a treatment regimen. J Speech Hear Disord 53(3):280–294

Eggers K (2020) Addressing cognitions and emotions in people who stutter using Beck's cognitive therapy. Two-day workshop presented at Dilgem Istanbul, Turkey

Ellis A (2004) Rational emotive behavior therapy: it works for me—it can work for you. Prometheus Books, Amherst

Elman R (2007) Group treatment of neurogenic communication disorders. The expert clinician's approach. Plural Publishing, San Diego, CA

Elsherbiny A, Amerson M, Sconyers L et al (2018) Time course of improvement after re-repair procedure for VPI management. J Plast Reconstr Aesthet Surg 71:895–899

Enderby P, Emerson J (1995) Does speech and language therapy work? A review of the literature. Whurr, London

Enderby P, Palmer R (2008) Frenchay dysarthria assessment 2. Pro-Ed, Austin, TX

Epps D, Kwan JY, Russell JW et al (2020) Evaluation and management of dysphagia in amyotrophic lateral sclerosis: a survey of speech-language pathologists' clinical practice. J Clin Neuromuscul Dis 21(3):135–143

Erickson KA, Koppenhaver D (2020) Comprehensive literacy for all: teaching students with significant disabilities to read and write. Paul H. Brookes Publishing Co., Baltimore, MD

Eriksson E, Bälter O, Engwall O et al (2005) Design recommendations for a computer-based speech training system based on end-user interviews. Proc Tenth Intl Conf Speech Computers 483–486 10th International Conference on Speech and Computer (SPECOM 2005), 17th–19th October 2005, Patras, Greece

Feeley K, Jones E (2012a) The use of augmentative strategies to enhance communication of verbal mode users. In: Johnson S, Reichle J, Feeley K et al (eds) AAC strategies for individuals with moderate to severe disabilities. Brookes Publishing, Baltimore, MD

Feeley M, Jones E (2012b) The use of augmentative strategies to enhance communication of verbal mode users. In: Johnson S, Reichle J, Feeley K et al (eds) AAC strategies for individuals with moderate to severe disabilities. Paul H. Brookes Publishing Co. Inc., Baltimore, MD, pp 347–363

Feeney R, Desha L, Zivana J et al (2012) Health-related quality-of-life of children with speech and language difficulties: a review of the literature. Int J Speech Lang Pathol 14(1):59–72

Ferrand C (2014) Speech science: an integrated approach to theory and clinical practice. Pearson Education Inc., Upper Saddle River, NJ

Foundas AL, Mock JR, Corey DM et al (2013) The SpeechEasy device in stuttering and nonstuttering adults: fluency effects while speaking and reading. Brain Lang 126(2):141–150

Fransella F (1970) Stuttering: not a symptom but a way of life. Br J Disord Commun 5:22–29

Freed D (2000) Motor speech disorders. Diagnosis and treatment. Singular Publishing Group, San Diego, CA

Friedman A, Fetterman E, Jolson Y (1999) Dr. fluency computerized stuttering treatment program User's guide (version 2.3). Speech Therapy Systems Ltd, Jerusalem

Fry J, Botterill W, Pring T (2009) The effect of an intensive group therapy program for young adults who stutter: a single subject study. Int Speech Lang Pathol 11:12–19

Gallop RF, Runyan CM (2012) Long-term effectiveness of the SpeechEasy fluency-enhancement device. J Fluen Disord 37(4):334–343

Garrett L, Lasker J (2013) Adults with severe apraxia and apraxia of speech. In: Beukelman D, Mirenda P (eds) Augmentative and alternative communication. Supporting children and adults with complex communication needs. Paul H. Brookes Publishing Co. Inc., Baltimore, MD, pp 405–445

Gart MS, Gosain AK (2014) Diagnosis and management of velopharyngeal insufficiency following cleft palate repair. J Cleft Lip Palate Craniofac Anomal 1:4–10

Gentil M, Tournier CL, Pollak P et al (1999) Effect of bilateral subthalamic nucleus stimulation and dopatherapy on oral control in Parkinson's disease. Eur Neurol 42(3):136–140

Giacchini V, Wiethan FM, Ceron MI et al (2013) The use of electroglottography, electromyography, spectrography and ultrasound in speech research—theoretical review. Rev CEFAC Epub. https://doi.org/10.1590/S1516-18462013005000049

Gibbons B, Blumer HH (1958) The palatal lift; a supportive-type speech aid. J Prosthet Dent 8(2):362–369

Glauber IP (1958) The psychoanalysis of stuttering. In: Eisenson J (ed) Stuttering; a symposium. Harper & Row, New York, pp 71–120

Goebel MD (1994) CAFET Program. Annandale Fluency Clinic, Annandale

Goldstein P, Ziegler W, Voge M et al (1994) Combined palatal-lift and EPG-feedback therapy in dysarthria: a case study. Clin Linguist Phon 8(3):201–218

Graat,I., Figee, M., & Denys, D. (2017). The application of deep brain stimulation in the treatment of psychiatric disorders. *International Review of Psychiatry, 29*(2), 178-190.

Gradinaru V, Mogri M, Thompson KR et al (2009) Optical deconstruction of parkinsonian neural circuitry. Science 324(5925):354–359

Gravell R, France J (1991) Speech and communication problems in psychiatry. Chapman Hall, London

Gregory HH (2003) Stuttering therapy: rational and procedures. Allyn & Bacon, Boston

Grossman HL (2020) Rational emotive behavior therapy for stuttering (REBT). Webinar presented for the Stuttering Foundation

Guitar B (2013) Stuttering: an integrated approach to its nature and treatment, 4th edn. Lippincott, Williams & Wilkins, Baltimore

Hägg M, Anniko M (2008) Lip muscle training in stroke patients with dysphagia. Acta Otolaryngol 128(9):1027–1033

Hägg M, Larsson B (2004) Effects of motor and sensory stimulation in stroke patients with long-lasting dysphagia. Dysphagia 19(4):219–230

Hägg M, Tibbling L (2015) Effect of oral IQoro R and palatal plate training in post-stroke, four-quadrant facial dysfunction and dysphagia: a comparison study. Acta Otolaryngol 135(9):962–968

Hägglund P, Hägg M, Levring Jäghagen E et al (2020) Oral neuromuscular training in patients with dysphagia after stroke: a prospective, randomized, open-label study with blinded evaluators. BMC Neurol 20:405. https://doi.org/10.1186/s12883-020-01980-1

Hamdan AL, Khalifee E, Tabet G (2018) Unilateral vocal fold paralysis in Parkinson disease: case report and review of the literature. J Voice 32(6):763–766

Hancock K, Craig A, Campbell K et al (1998) Two to six year controlled trial stuttering outcomes for children and adolescents. J Speech Lang Hear Res 41(6):1242–1252

Hardcastle WJ, Morgan Barry RA, Clark CJ (1985) Articulatory and voicing characteristics of adult dysarthric and verbal dyspraxic speakers: an instrumental study. Br J Disord Commun 20(3):249–270

Hardcastle WJ, Gibbon FE, Jones W (1991) Visual display of tongue-palate contact: electropalatography in the assessment and remediation of speech disorders. Int J Commun Disord 26(1):41–74

Harley J (2018) The role of attention in therapy for children and adolescents who stutter: cognitive behavioral therapy and mindfulness-based interventions. Am J Speech Lang Pathol 27(3S):1139–1151

Harris R (2009) ACT made simple. New Harbinger Publications, Oakland

Hayhow R, Levy C (1993) Working with stuttering: a personal construct approach. Winslow Press, Bicester

Haynes W, Pindzola R (2012) Diagnosis and evaluation in speech pathology. Pearson Education Inc., Upper Saddle River, NJ

Hedge M, Davis D (2010) Clinical methods and practicum in speech-language pathology. Delmar Cengage Learning, Clifton Park, NY

Helm-Estabrooks N, Albert M (1991) Manual of aphasia therapy. Pro Ed, Austin, TX

Hemm, S., &Wårdell, K. (2010). Stereotactic implantation of deep brain stimulationelectrodes: a review of technical systems, methods and emerging tools. *Medical & biological engineering &computing, 48*, 611-624.

Herzog J, Volkmann J, Krack P et al (2003) Two-year follow-up of subthalamic deep brain stimulation in Parkinson's disease. Mov Disord 18(11):1332–1337

Holmerová I, Jarolímová E, Suchá J (2009) Péče o pacienty s kognitivní poruchou (care for patients with cognitive impairment). EV public relations, Prague

Holyfield C, Drager KDR, Kremkow JMD et al (2017) Systematic review of AAC intervention research for adolescents and adults with autism spectrum disorder. Augment Altern Commun 33:201–212

Hopper T (2007) Group cognitive-communication treatment for people with dementia. In: Elman R (ed) Group treatment of neurogenic communication disorders. The expert clinician's approach. Plural Publishing, San Diego, CA

Horner J, Norman M, Ripich D (2016) Assessment and management of dementia. In: Johnson A, Jacobson B (eds) Medical speech language pathology. Thieme Medical Publisher Inc., New York, NY, pp 72–82

Hustad KC, Beukelman DR (2001) Effects of linguistic cues and stimulus cohesion on intelligibility of severely dysarthric speech. J Speech Lang Hear Res 44:497–510

Hustad KC, Beukelman DR (2002) Listener comprehension of severely dysarthric speech. J Speech Lang Hear Res 45:545–558

Hustad KC, Beukelman DR, Yorkston KM (1998) Functional outcome assessment in dysarthria. Semin Speech Lang 19:291–302

Hymes DH (1972) On communicative competence. In: Pride JB, Holmes J (eds) Sociolinguistics. Penguin, Harmondsworth, pp 269–293

IBM (1992) Announcement Letter Number 292–280 dated May 26, 1992. https://www-01.ibm.com/common/ssi/ShowDoc.wss?docURL=/common/ssi/rep_ca/0/897/ENUS292-280/index.html&lang=en&request_locale=en

Ingham R (1984) Stuttering and behavior therapy. College-Hill Press, San Diego

Iverach L, Jones M, McLellan LF et al (2016) Prevalence of anxiety disorders among children who stutter. J Fluen Disord 49:13–28

Jones R, Eggers K, Zengin-Bolatkale H (2020) Temperamental and emotional processes. In:

Zebrowski P, Anderson J, Conture E (eds) Stuttering: characteristics, assessment, and treatment, 4th edn. Thieme Medical Publishers, New York

Jankovic J, Tan EK (2020) Parkinson's disease: etiopathogenesis and treatment. J Neurol Neurosurg Psychiatry 91:795–808

Javed F, Akram Z, Barillas AP et al (2018) Outcome of orthodontic palatal plate therapy for orofacial dysfunction in children with Down syndrome: a systematic review. Orthod Craniofac Res 21(1):20–26

Jayaraman DK, Das JM (2023) Dysarthria. In: StatPearls [Internet]. Treasure Island (FL): StatPearls Publishing; 2024 Jan–. PMID: 37279355

Johnson S, Reichle J, Feeley M et al (2012) AAC strategies for individuals with moderate to severe disabilities. Paul H. Brookes Publishing Co. Inc., Baltimore, MD

Kabat-Zinn J (1996) Full catastrophe living. Piatkus, London

Kalinowski J, Saltuklaroglu T (2003) Choral speech: the amelioration of stuttering via imitation and the mirror neuronal system. Neurosci Biobehav Rev 27(4):339–347

Katz WF, McNeil MR (2010) Studies of articulatory feedback treatment for apraxia of speech based on electromagnetic articulography. Perspect Neurophysiol Neurogenic Speech Lang Disord 20(3):73–79

Keith R, Thomas J (1989) Speech practice manual for dysarthria, apraxia, and other disorders of articulation. BC Decker Inc., Philadelphia, PA

Kelly GA (1955) The psychology of personal constructs. Norton, New York

Kelly S, Main A, Manley G et al (2000) Electropalatography and the Linguagraph system. Med Eng Phys 22(1):47–58

Kelman E, Wheeler S (2015) Cognitive behaviour therapy with children who stutter. Procedia Soc Behav Sci 193:165–174

Kent RD (2015) Nonspeech oral movements and oral motor disorders: a narrative review. Am J Speech Lang Pathol 24(4):763–789

Kent-Walsh J, Murza KA, Malani MD et al (2015) Effects of communication partner instruction on the communication of individuals using AAC: a meta-analysis. Augment Altern Commun 31:271–284

Kern,D. S., & Kumar, R. (2007). Deep brain stimulation. *The Neurologist, 13*(5), 237-252.

Kim Y, Kim M, Kim J, Song T-J (2024) Efficacy and feasibility of a digital speech therapy for post-stroke dysarthria: protocol for a randomized controlled trial. Front. Neurol. 15:1305297. https://doi.org/10.3389/fneur.2024.1305297

Kipfmueller LJ, Lang BB (1972) Treating velopharyngeal inadequacies with a palatal lift prosthesis. J Prosthet Dent 27(1):63–72

Kirshner H (1995) Apraxia of speech. In: Kirshner H (ed) Handbook of neurological speech and language disorders. M Dekker Inc., New York, NY, pp 41–55

Klang N, Rowland C, Fried-Oken M et al (2016) The content of goals in individual educational programs for students with complex communication needs. Augment Altern Commun 32:41–48

Knock TR, Ballard KJ, Robin DA et al (2000) Influence of order of stimulus presentation on speech motor learning: a principled approach to treatment for apraxia of speech. Aphasiology 14(5):653–668

Koller WC, Lyons KE, Wilkinson SB et al (2001) Long-term safety and efficacy of unilateral deep brain stimulation of the thalamus in essential tremor. Mov Disord 16(3):464–468

Krack P, Batir A, Van Blercom N et al (2003) Five-year follow-up of bilateral stimulation of the subthalamic nucleus in advanced Parkinson's disease. N Engl J Med 349(20):1925–1934

Králíček P (2011) Úvod do speciální neurofyziologie (introduction to special neurophysiology). Galén, Prague

Krause M, Fogel W, Mayer P et al (2004) Chronic inhibition of the subthalamic nucleus in Parkinson's disease. J Neurol Sci 219(1–2):119–124

Krauss JK, Lipsman N, Aziz T et al (2021) Technology of deep brain stimulation: current status and future directions. Nat Rev Neurol 17(2):75–87

Kummer AW, Clark SL, Redle EE et al (2012) Current practice in assessing and reporting speech outcomes of cleft palate and velopharyngeal surgery: a survey of cleft palate/craniofacial professionals. Cleft Palate Craniofac J 49(2):146–152

Kupsch A, Benecke R, Müller J et al (2006) Pallidal deep-brain stimulation in primary generalized or segmental dystonia. N Engl J Med 355(19):1978–1990

Kwakkel G, Kollen BJ (2013) Predicting activities after stroke: what is clinically relevant? Int J Stroke 8(1):25–32

Kwon YH, Kwon JW, Lee MH (2015) Effectiveness of motor sequential learning according to practice schedules in healthy adults; distributed practice versus massed practice. J Phys Ther Sci 27(3):769–772

Lang AE, Fishbein V (1983) The "pacing board" in selected speech disorders of Parkinson's disease. J Neurol Neurosurg Psychiatry 46(8):789. https://doi.org/10.1136/jnnp.46.8.789

Lang BR, Kipfmueller LJ (1969) Treating velopharyngeal inadequacy with the palatal lift concept. Plast Reconstr Surg 43(5):467–477

Leahy MM, O'Dwyer M, Ryan F (2012) Witnessing stories: definitional ceremonies in narrative therapy with adults who stutter. J Fluen Disord 37:234–241

Leonet O, Orcasitas-Vicandi M, Langarika-Rocafort A, Mondragon NI, Etxebarrieta GR (2022) A Systematic Review of Augmentative and Alternative Communication Interventions for Children Aged From 0 to 6 Years. LANG SPEECH HEAR SERV SCH 53:894-920. https://doi.org/10.1044/2022_LSHSS-21-00191

Laudová L (2003) Augmentativní a alternativní komunikace (augmentative and alternative communication). In: Škodová E, Jedlička I (eds) Klinická logopedie (clinical speech therapy). Portál, Prague, pp 561–577

Le Dorze G, Dionne L, Ryalls J et al (1992) The effect of speech and language therapy for a case of dysarthria associated with Parkinson's disease. Eur J Disord Commun 27(4):313–324

Levy ES, Moya-Galeb G, Chang YHM et al (2020) The effects of intensive speech treatment on intelligibility in Parkinson's disease: a randomised controlled trial. EClinical Medicine 24. https://doi.org/10.1016/j.eclinm.2020.100429. Accessed 7 Nov 2021

Light J (1988) Interaction involving individuals using augmentative and alternative communication systems: state of the art and future directions. Augment Altern Commun 4:66–82

Light J (1989) Toward a definition of communicative competence for individuals using augmentative and alternative communication systems. Augment Altern Commun 5:137–144

Light J, McNaughton D (2014) Communicative competence for individuals who require augmentative and alternative communication: a new definition for a new era of communication? Augment Altern Commun 30:1–18

Light J, McNaughton D (2015) Designing AAC research and intervention to improve outcomes for individuals with complex communication needs. Augment Altern Commun 31:85–96

Light J, Roberts B, Dimarko R et al (1998) Augmentative and alternative communication to support receptive and expresive communication for people with autism. J Commun Disord 31:153–180

Liss J, Berisha V (2020) How will artificial intelligence reshape speech-language pathology services and practice in the future? Available via https://academy.pubs.asha.org/2020/08/how-will-artificial-intelligence-reshape-speech-language-pathology-services-and-practice-in-the-future/ Accessed 10 Nov 2021

Little S, Pogosyan A, Neal S et al (2013) Adaptive deep brain stimulation in advanced Parkinson disease. Ann Neurol 74(3):449–457

Little S, Beudel M, Zrinzo L et al (2015) Bilateral adaptive deep brain stimulation is effective in Parkinson's disease. J Neurol Neurosurg Psychiatry 87(7):717–721

Little S, Tripoliti E, Beudel M et al (2016) Adaptive deep brain stimulation for Parkinson's disease demonstrates reduced speech side effects compared to conventional stimulation in the acute setting. J Neurol Neurosurg Psychiatry 87(12):1388–1389

Löfhede H, Wertsén M, Havstam C (2020) Palatal augmentation prostheses in individuals treated for head and neck cancer: effects on speech and oral transport. Head Neck 42:1882–1892

Logan K, Iacono T, Trembath D (2017) A systematic review of research into aided AAC to increase social-communication functions in children with autism spectrum disorder. Augment Altern Commun 33:51–64

Logemann JA, Kahrilas PJ, Hurst P et al (1989) Effects of intraoral prosthetics on swallowing in patients with oral cancer. Dysphagia 4(2):118–120

Love R (1995) Motor speech disorders. In: Kirshner H (ed) Handbook of neurological speech and language disorders. M Dekker Inc., New York, NY, pp 23–39

Lowe R, Menzies R, Packman A et al (2016) Assessing attentional biases with stuttering. Int J Lang Commun Disord 51:84–94

Lubinski R (1995) Dementia and communication. Singular Publishing Group, San Diego, CA

Lubinsky R (1991) Dysarthria: a breakdown in interpersonal communication. Pro-Ed Inc., Austin, TX

Ludlow CL, Loucks T (2003) Stuttering: a dynamic motor control disorder. J Fluen Disord 28(4):273–295

Lüke C, Vock S (2019) Unterstützte Kommunikation bei Kindern und Erwachsenen (Assisted Communication in children and adults). Springer, Berlin, Heidelberg

Luria AR, Naydin VL, Tsvetkova LS et al (1969) Restoration of higher cortical function following local brain damage. In: Vinken PJ, Bruyn GW (eds) Handbook of clinical neurology, vol 3. Elsevier, Amsterdam, pp 368–433

Luterman DM (2001) Counseling persons with communication disorders and their families, 4th edn. Pro-Ed, Austin

Luzzatti C (2012a) La rieducazione dei deficit fonologici e dell'articolazione (Phonological and articulation deficits). In: Mazzucchi A (ed) La Riabilitazione Neuropsicologica: Premesse teoriche ed applicazioni cliniche (Neuropsychological Rehabilitation: theoretical premises and clinical applications), 3rd edn. Elsevier, Milan, pp 25–47

Luzzatti C (2012b) Rieducazione dell'aprassia dell'articolazione (Apraxia of speech). In: Cantagallo A, Cappa S, Vallar G et al (eds) La Riabilitazione Neuropsicologica—un'analisi basata sul metodo evidence-based medicine (neuropsychological rehabilitation—an analysis based on the evidence-based medicine method). Springer, Milan, pp 149–159

Lyons KE, Pahwa R (2008) Deep brain stimulation and tremor. Neurotherapeutics 5(2):331–338

Maas E, Robin DA, Austermann Hula SN et al (2008) Principles of motor learning in treatment of motor speech disorders. Am J Speech Lang Pathol 17(3):277–298

Malekmohammadi M, Herron J, Velisar A et al (2016) Kinematic adaptive deep brain stimulation for resting tremor in Parkinson's disease. Mov Disord 31(3):426–428

Maniadaki K (2017) Let's talk about stuttering in a journal of child psychology. J Child Psychol 1(1):1–2

Manning WH (2010) Clinical decision making in the diagnosis and treatment of fluency disorders, 3rd edn. Delmar, Clifton Park

Marunick M, Tselios N, Arbor A (2004) The efficacy of palatal augmentation prostheses for speech and swallowing in patients undergoing glossectomy: a review of the literature. J Prosthet Dent 91(1):67–74

Mauszycki SC, Bunker LD, Bailey DJ et al (2024) Speech Intelligibility Outcomes Associated With Treatment for Acquired Apraxia of Speech: Magnitude of Change and Stability of Measurement. Am J Speech Lang Pathol 13:1-15. doi: 10.1044/2024_AJSLP-24-00104. Epub ahead of print. PMID: 39270061

McAllister J, Kelman E, Millard S (2015) Anxiety and cognitive bias in children and young people who stutter. Procedia Soc Behav Sci 193:183–191

McAllister A, Brodén M, Gonzalez Lindh M et al (2018) Oral sensory-motor intervention for children and adolescents (3–18 years) with developmental or early acquired speech disorders—a review of the literature 2000–2017. Ann Otolaryngol Rhinol 5(5):1221. Available via https://www.jscimedcentral.com/Otolaryngology/otolaryngology-5-1221.pdf. Accessed 14 Sept 2021

McAuliffe MJ, Ward EC (2006) The use of electropalatography in the assessment and treatment of acquired motor speech disorders in adults: current knowledge and future directions. NeuroRehabilitation 21(3):189–203

McDonnell MN, Rischbieth B, Schammer TT et al (2018) Lee Silverman Voice Treatment (LSVT)-BIG to improve motor function in people with Parkinson's disease: a systematic review and meta-analysis. Clin Rehabil 32(5):607–618

McLeod S, McCormack J (2007) Application of the ICF and ICF-children and youth in children with speech impairment. Semin Speech Lang 28:254–264

Menzies RG, O'Brian S, Onslow M et al (2008) An experimental clinical trial of a cognitive-behavior therapy package for chronic stuttering. J Speech Lang Hear Res 51(6):1451–1464

Menzies RG, Packman A, Onslow M et al (2019) In-clinic and standalone internet cognitive behavior therapy treatment for social anxiety in stuttering: a randomized trial of iGlebe. J Speech Lang Hear Res 62(6):1614–1624

Merwin R, O'Rourke S, Ives L et al (2019) Chapter 16—Third-wave cognitive-behavioral therapies for the treatment of anxiety among children and adolescents. In: Compton SN, Villabø MA, Kristensen H (eds) Pediatric anxiety disorders. Academic Press, Cambridge, pp 335–357

Mitchell KT, Starr PA (2020) Smart neuromodulation in movement disorders. Handb Clin Neurol 168:153–161

Mitchell C, Bowen A, Tyson S et al (2017) Interventions for dysarthria due to stroke and other adult-acquired, non-progressive brain injury (review). Cochrane Database Syst Rev 2017(1):CD002088

Moleski R, Tosi DJ (1976) Comparative psychotherapy: rational-emotive therapy versus systematic desensitization in the treatment of stuttering. J Consult Clin Psychol 44:309–311

Molt L (2019) A brief historical review of assistive devices for treating stuttering. https://www.mnsu.edu/comdis/isad8/papers/molt8/molt8.html. Accessed 26 Aug 2019

Moreau C, Defebvre L, Destée A et al (2008) STN-DBS frequency effects on freezing of gait in advanced Parkinson disease. Neurology 71(2):80–84

Morgan Barry RA (1989) EPG from square one: an overview of electropalatography as an aid to therapy. Clin Linguist Phon 3(1):81–91

Mosera D, Basilakos A, Fillmore P et al (2016) Brain damage associated with apraxia of speech: evidence from case studies. Neurocase 22(4):346–356

Mourao LF, Aguiar PM, Ferraz FA et al (2005) Acoustic voice assessment in Parkinson's disease patients submitted to posteroventral pallidotomy. Arq Neuropsiquiatr 63(1):20–25

Moya-Galé G, Levy ES (2019) Parkinson's disease-associated dysarthria: prevalence, impact and management strategies. Res Rev Parkinsonism 9:9–16

Murdoch BE, Pitt G, Theodorus DG et al (1999) Real-time continuous visual biofeedback in the treatment of speech breathing disorders following childhood traumatic brain injury: report of one case. Pediatr Rehabil 3(1):5–20

Murphy JJ (2020) Demosthenes. Greek statesman and orator. In: Encyclopædia Britannica. Available via https://www.britannica.com/biography/Demosthenes--Greek-statesman-and-orator. Accessed 30 June 2020

Murray E, McCabe P, Ballard KJ (2014) A systematic review of treatment outcomes for children with childhood apraxia of speech. Am J Speech Lang Pathol 23:486–504

Murry T, Carreau R (1996) Clinical manual of swallowing disorders. Plural Publishing, San Diego, CA

Nathadwarawala KM, Nicklin J, Wiles CM (1992) A timed test of swallowing capacity for neurological patients. J Neurol Neurosurg Psychiatry 55:822–825

Neubauer K (1999a) Diagnostika kognitivních poruch u demencí, nefarmakologické postupy v rehabilitaci demencí (diagnosis of cognitive disorders in dementia, non-pharmacological procedures in dementia rehabilitation). In: Jirák R (ed) Demence (dementia). Maxdorf Prague, pp 19–32

Neubauer K (1999b) Psychoterapeutické přístupy v rehabilitaci kognitivních poruch u dospělých osob s demencí (psychotherapeutic approaches in the rehabilitation of cognitive disorders in adults with dementia). In: Jirák R (ed) Demence (dementia). Maxdorf Prague, pp 97–108

Neubauer K (2003) Syndrom demence a poruch komunikace (dementia syndrome and communication disorders). In: Škodová E, Jedlička I (eds) Klinická logopedie (clinical speech therapy). Portál, Prague, pp 180–206

Neubauer K (2011) Terapie dysartrie (dysarthria therapy). In: Lechta V et al (eds) Terapie narušené komunikační schopnosti (therapy impaired communication capabilities). Portal, Prague, pp 283–333

Neubauer K (2016a) Acquired dysphagia. In: Neubauer K (ed) Speech-language therapy and neurogenic disorders of communication. P-Mervard & University of Hradec Králové, Česvený Kostelec, pp 85–86

Neubauer K (2016b) Speech-language therapy and neurogenic disorders of communication. Pavel Mervart and University of Hradec Králové, Červený Kostelec

Neubauer K (2017a) Acquired neurogenic dysphagia in adults. In: Neubauer K (ed) Assessment and treatment of adult persons with acquired disorders of communication and neurogenic dysphagia. Internationale Stiftung Schulung, Kunst, Wien, pp 133–160

Neubauer K (2017b) Assessment and treatment of adult persons with acquired disorders of communication and neurogenic dysphagia. Internationale Stiftung Schulung, Wien

Neubauer K (ed) (2018a) Kompendium klinické logopedie (compendium of clinical speech therapy). Portal, Prague

Neubauer K (2018b) Neurogenní poruchy komunikace a orofaciální motoriky u dospělých osob (neurogenic communication and orofacial motor disorders in adults). In: Neubauer K (ed) Kompendium klinické logopedie (compendium of clinical speech therapy). Portál, Prague, pp 221–252

Neubauer K (2018c) Dysartrie a řečová dyspraxie (Dysarthria and speech dyspraxia). In: Neubauer K (ed) Kompendium klinické logopedie (compendium of clinical speech therapy). Portál, Prague, pp 416–441

Neubauer K (2018d) Syndrom demence a KKP (kognitivně-komunikační poruchy) dementia syndrome and KKP (cognitive-communication disorders). In: Neubauer K (ed) Kompendium klinické logopedie (compendium of clinical speech therapy). Portál, Prague, pp 479–498

Neubauer K (2018e) Dysfagie—poruchy polykání (dysphagia—swallowing disorders). In: Neubauer K (ed) Kompendium klinické logopedie (compendium of clinical speech therapy). Portál, Prague, pp 542–559

Neubauer K, Obenberger J, Mikešová V et al (2007) Neurogenní poruchy komunikace u dospělých. Portál, Prague

Neubauerová L (2013) Alternativní a augmentativní komunikace u cílových skupin oboru psychopedie. Alternative and augmentative communication in the target groups of the field of psychopedia. In: Dlouhá J (ed) Úvod do psychopedie. Introduction to psychopedia. Gaudeamus, Hradec Králové

Neubauerová L, Neubauer K (2018) Augmentativní a slternativní komunikace a klinická logopedická praxe (augmentative and alternative communication and clinical speech therapy practice). In: Neubauer K, Pospíšilová L, Škodová E et al (eds) Kompendium klinické logopedie (compendium of clinical speech therapy). Portál, Prague, pp 697–713

Neubauerová L, Černá M, Neubauer K (2016) Wykorzistanie komunikacji akternatywnej i wspomagajacej i przez osoby niepelnosprawne w Republice Czeskej (Using alternative and supportive communication by people with disabilities in The Czech Republic). In: Blesziński J, Kochan K, Skorek E (eds) Ekukacyjne oblicza komunikacji (the educational faces of communication). Uniwersytet Zielonogórski, Zielona Góra

Neumann S, Quinting J, Rosenkranz A et al (2019) Quality of life in adults with neurogenic speech-language communication difficulties: a systematic review of existing measures. J Commun Disord 79:24–45

Nogueira D, Reis E, Ferreira P et al (2019) Measuring quality of life in the speaker with dysarthria: reliability and validity of the European Portuguese version of the QoL-DyS. Folia Phoniatr Logop 71(4):176–190

Ondo W, Jankovic J, Schwartz K et al (1998) Unilateral thalamic deep brain stimulation for refractory essential tremor and Parkinson's disease tremor. Neurology 51(4):1063–1069

Orange J, MacLean M, Ryan J et al (1995) Application of the enhancement model for long-term care residents with Alzheimer's disease. Top Lang Disord 15(2):20–35

Packman A, Meredith G (2011) Technology and the evolution of clinical methods for stuttering. J Fluen Disord 36(2):75–85

Pahwa R, Lyons KE, Wilkinson SB et al (2006) Long-term evaluation of deep brain stimulation of the thalamus. J Neurosurg 104(4):506–512

Pana, A., & Saggu, B. M. (2017). Dystonia.

Park K (2002) Objects of reference in practice and theory. SENSE, London

Pastore G (2018) Tongue position tracking device (TPTD): a discreet wireless electropalatography and glossometry device. Unpublished master thesis in Bioengineering. Graduate College, University of Illinois, Chicago, IL

Pentaxmedical (2021) Available via: https://www.pentax-medical.com/pentax/en/94/16/Multi-Speech-Model--3700-Sona-Speech-II-Model-3650. Accessed 10 Nov 2021

Petržílková M (2014) Počítačové programy Mentio [online] (Mentio computer programs [online]). Mentio [cit. 10.3.2014]. Available http://www.mentio.cz/ Accessed 6 Nov 2021

Petržílková M (2020) Logopedický software a výukové počítačové programy (speech therapy software and computer tutorials) (online) Available www.mentio. cz/. Accessed 19 Dec 2020

Petržílková M, Neubauer K (2007) Terapie porušených centrálních motorických řečových funkcí (Therapy of impaired central motor speech functions). In: Neubauer K, Mikešová V, Obenberger J et al (eds) Neurogenní poruchy komunikace u dospělých (Neurogenic communication disorders in adults). Portál, Prague, pp 130–143

Phoebe Chen YP, Johnson C, Lalbakhsh P et al (2016) Systematic review of virtual speech therapists for speech disorders. Comput Speech Lang 37:98–12

Pinto J, Pegoraro-Krook MI (2003) Evaluation of palatal prosthesis for the treatment of velopharyngeal dysfunction. J Appl Oral Sci 11(3):192–197

Pinto S, Gentil M, Fraix V et al (2003) Bilateral subthalamic stimulation effects on oral force control in Parkinson's disease. J Neurol 250(2):179–187

Pinto S, Ozsancak C, Tripoliti E et al (2004) Treatments for dysarthria in Parkinson's disease. Lancet Neurol 3(9):547–556

Plexico LW, Manning WH, Levitt H (2009a) Coping responses by adults who stutter. Part I. Protecting the self and others. J Fluen Disord 34:87–107

Plexico LW, Manning WH, Levitt H (2009b) Coping responses by adults who stutter. Part II. Approaching the problem and achieving agency. J Fluen Disord 34:108–126

Pollard R, Ellis JB, Finan D et al (2009) Effects of the SpeechEasy on objective and perceived aspects of stuttering: a 6-month Phase 1 clinical trial in naturalistic environments. J Speech Lang Hear Res 52(2):516–533

Popovici DV, Belciu CB (2012) Professional challenges in computer-assisted speech therapy. Procedia Soc Behav Sci 33:518–522

Priori A, Foffani G, Rossi L et al (2013) Adaptive deep brain stimulation (aDBS) controlled by local field potential oscillations. Exp Neurol 245:77–86

Priori, A.,Maiorana, N., Dini, M., Guidetti, M., Marceglia, S., & Ferrucci, R. (2021).Adaptive deep brain stimulation (aDBS). In InternationalReview of Neurobiology (Vol. 159, pp. 111-127): Elsevier.

Putzke JD, Wharen RE, Wszolek ZK et al (2003) Thalamic deep brain stimulation for tremor-predominant Parkinson's disease. Parkinsonism Relat Dis 10(2):81–88

Ramig L (1995) Speech therapy for patients with Parkinson's disease. In: Koller WC, Paulson G (eds) Therapy of Parkinson's disease. Marcel Dekker Inc., New York, NY, pp 539–550

Ramig LO, Fox C, Sapir S (2008) Speech treatment for Parkinson's disease. Expert Rev Neurother 8(2):299–311

Reddy RP, Sharma MP, Shivashankar N (2010) Cognitive behavior therapy for stuttering: a case series. Indian J Psychol Med 32:49–53

Reichmuth K (2020) Principles of augmentative communication methods. In: am Zehnhoff-Dinnesen A, Wiskirska-Woznica B, Neumann K et al (eds) European manual of medicine: Phoniatrics 1. Springer, Berlin

Remington T, Fagan S (2006) Drug-induced communication and swallowing disorders. In: Johnson A, Jacobson B (eds) Medical speech-language pathology. A practitioner's guide. Thieme Medical Publishers Inc., New York, NY, pp 363–378

Rilo B, Fernández-Formoso N, da Silva L et al (2013) A simplified palatal lift prosthesis for neurogenic velopharyngeal incompetence. J Prosthodont 22(6):506–508

Ripich D (1992) Language and communication in dementia. In: Ripich D (ed) Handbook of geriatric communication disorders. ProEd, Austin, TX, pp 255–283

Robbins KT, Bowman JB, Jacob RF (1987) Postglossectomy deglutitory and articulatory rehabilitation with palatal augmentation prostheses. Arch Otolaryngol Head Neck Surg 113(11):1214–1218

Robertson S, Thompson F (1986) Working with dysarthrics. A practical guide to therapy for dysarthria. Winslow Press, Oxon

Rodriguez-Oroz MC, Obeso JA, Lang AE et al (2005) Bilateral deep brain stimulation in Parkinson's disease: a multicentre study with 4 years follow-up. Brain 128(10):2240–2249

Romito LM, Scerrati M, Contarino MF et al (2002) Long-term follow up of subthalamic nucleus stimulation in Parkinson's disease. Neurology 58(10):1546–1550

Rosa M, Arlotti M, Ardolino G et al (2015) Adaptive deep brain stimulation in a freely moving parkinsonian patient. Mov Disord 30(7):1003–1005

Rosa M, Arlotti M, Marceglia S et al (2017) Adaptive deep brain stimulation controls levodopa-induced side effects in Parkinsonian patients. Mov Disord 32(4):628–629

Rosenbek JC (1978) Treating apraxia of speech. In: Johns DF (ed) Clinical management of neurogenic communicative disorders. Little, Brown & Co, Boston, MA, pp 191–241

Rousseaux M, Krystkowiak P, Kozlowski O et al (2004) Effects of subthalamic nucleus stimulation on parkinsonian dysarthria and speech intelligibility. J Neurol 251(3):327–334

Ruscello D, Vallino L (2014) The application of motor learning concepts to the treatment of children with compensatory speech sound errors. Perspectives. ASHA 24(2):39–47

Ryan F, O'Dwyer M, Leahy MM (2015) Separating the problem and the person: insights from narrative therapy with people who stutter. Top Lang Disord 35:267–274

Sachse SK (in prep) Evidenzsynthese zur Wirksamkeit von UK-Interventionen (Compilation of evidence on the effectiveness of UK interventions)

Sachse SK, Bernasconi T (2020) Ziele formulieren und Maßnahmen beschreiben mit dem ABC-Modell (evidence synthesis on the effectiveness of UK interventions). In: Boenisch J, Sachse SK (eds) Kompendium Unterstützte Kommunikation (compendium of supported communication). Kohlhammer, Stuttgart, pp 203–216

Sackett D, Rosenberg W, Gray J et al (1996) Evidence based medicine: what it is and what it isn't: it's about integrating individual clinical expertise and the best external evidence. BMJ 312:71–72

Santens P, De Letter M, Van Borsel J et al (2003) Lateralized effects of subthalamic nucleus stimulation on different aspects of speech in Parkinson's disease. Brain Lang 87(2):253–258

Saz O, Yin SC, Lleida E et al (2009) Tools and technologies for computer-aided speech and language therapy. Speech Comm 51:948–967

Schlosser RW, Wendt O (2008) Effects of augmentative and alternative communication intervention on speech production in children with autism: a systematic review. Am J Speech Lang Pathol 17:212–230

Schmidt RA, Lee TD, Weinstein CJ et al (2019) Motor control and learning: a behavioral emphasis, 6th edn. Human Kinetics Publisher, Champaign, IL

Schröter-Morasch H, Ziegler W (2005a) Rehabilitation of impaired speech function (dysarthria, dysglossia). GMS Curr Top Otorhinolaryngol Head Neck Surg 4:Doc15. Published online 2005 Sep 28. PMCID: PMC3201013 PMID: 22073063

Schröter-Morasch H, Ziegler W (2005b) Sprachstörungen. Rekonstruktive Verfahren bei Sprachstörungen (Dysarthrie, Dysglossie). Reconstructive procedures in speech dysfunction (dysarthria, dysglossia). Laryngorhinootologie 84(Suppl 1):S213–S220

Schulz GM, Peterson T, Sapienza CM et al (1999) Voice and speech characteristics of persons with Parkinson's disease pre- and post-pallidotomy surgery: preliminary findings. J Speech Lang Hear Res 42:1176–1194

Selley WG, Roche MT, Pearce VR et al (1995) Dysphagia following strokes: clinical observations of swallowing rehabilitation employing palatal training appliances. Dysphagia 10(1):32–35

Sewall GK, Jiang J, Ford CN (2006) Clinical evaluation of Parkinson's-related dysphonia. Laryngoscope 116(10):1740–1744

Shapiro DA (2011) Stuttering intervention: a collaborative journey to fluency freedom, 2nd edn. Pro-Ed, Austin

Sheehan JB (1958) Conflict theory of stuttering. In: Eisenson J (ed) Stuttering; a symposium. Harper & Row, New York, pp 121–166

Sheehan JG (1970) Stuttering: research and therapy. Harper & Row, New York

Shifman A, Finkelstein Y, Nachmani A et al (2000) Speech-aid prostheses for neurogenic velopharyngeal incompetence. J Prosthet Dent 83(1):99–106

Shriberg LD, Fourakis M, Hall SD et al (2010) Extensions to the speech disorders classification system (SDCS). Clin Linguist Phon 24(10):795–824

Silek,H., & Dogan, M. (2023). Voice Analysis in Patients with Essential Tremor. *Journal of Voice*.

Sjögreen L, Tulinius M, Kiliaridis S et al (2010) The effect of lip strengthening exercises in children and adolescents with myotonic dystrophy type 1. Int J Pediatr Otorhinolaryngol 74:1126–1134

Sjögreen L, Gonzalez Lindh M, Brodén M et al (2018) Oral sensory-motor intervention for children and adolescents (3–18 years) with dysphagia or impaired saliva control secondary to congenital or early-acquired disabilities: a review of the literature, 2000 to 2016. Ann Otol Rhinol Laryngol 127(12):978–985

Smith KA, Iverach L, O'Brian S et al (2014) Anxiety of children and adolescents who stutter: a review. J Fluen Disord 40:22–34

Square-Storer P, Hayden D (1989) PROMPT treatment. In: Square-Storer P (ed) Acquired apraxia of speech in aphasic adults. Taylor and Francis, London, pp 165–186

Squires JE, Valentine JC, Grimshaw JM (2013) Systematic reviews of complex interventions: framing the review question. J Clin Epidemiol 66:1215–1222

Stevens ER (1989) Multiple input phoneme therapy; an approach to severe apraxia and expressive aphasia. In: Square-Storer P (ed) Acquired apraxia of speech in aphasic adults. Lawrence Erlbaum, Hillsdale, NJ, pp 220–238

Stewart T, Birdsall M (2001) A review of the contribution of personal construct psychology to stammering therapy. J Constr Psychol 14:215–225

Straus S, Glasziou P, Richardson W et al (2011) Evidence-based medicine: how to practice and teach it, 4th edn. Churchill Livingstone Elsevier, Edinburgh

Stuart A, Kalinowski J, Rastatter MP et al (2004) Investigations of the impact of altered auditory feedback in-the-ear devices on the speech of people who stutter: initial fitting and four-month follow-up. Int J Lang Commun Disord 39(1):93–113

Sydow O, Thobois S, Alesch F et al (2003) Multicentre European study of thalamic stimulation in essential tremor: a six year follow up. J Neurol Neurosurg Psychiatry 74(10):1387–1391

Tagliati M, Krack P, Volkmann J et al (2011) Long-term management of DBS in dystonia: response to stimulation, adverse events, battery changes, and special considerations. Mov Disord 26(Suppl 1):S54–S62

Tedla M (ed) (2009) Poruchy polykání (swallowing disorders). Tobiáš, Havlíčkův Brod

Theodoros D (2012) A new era in speech-language pathology practice: innovation and diversification. Int J Speech Lang Pathol 14(3):189–199

Thevathasan W, Gregory R (2010) Deep brain stimulation for movement disorders. Pract Neurol 10(1):16–26

Thies T, Mücke D, Dano R et al (2021) Levodopa-based changes on vocalic speech movements during prosodic prominence marking. Brain Sci 11:594–617

Thobois S, Mertens P, Guenot M (2002) Subthalamic nucleus stimulation in Parkinson's disease: clinical evaluation of 18 patients. J Neurol 249(5):529–534

Tobolcea I, Danubianu M (2010) Computer-based programs in speech therapy of dyslalia and dyslexia-dysgraphia. BRAIN Res Artif Intell Neurosci 1(2):52–63

Tran Y, Blumgart E, Craig A (2011) Subjective distress associated with chronic stuttering. J Fluen Disord 36(1):17–26

Trost-Cardamone JE (1989) Coming to terms with VPI. Cleft Palate J 26:68–70

Van Riper C (1973) The treatment of stuttering, 2nd edn. Prentice-Hall, Englewood Cliffs

Van Riper C (1982) The nature of stuttering, 2nd edn. Prentice Hall, Englewood Cliffs

Van Vliet L (1996) In: Logopaedica I (ed) Stratégia terapie při poruchách mnestických funkcí (strategic therapy for disorders of anamnestic functions). Liečreh, Bratislava, pp 12–16

Velisar A, Syrkin-Nikolau J, Blumenfeld Z et al (2019) Dual threshold neural closed loop deep brain stimulation in Parkinson disease patients. Brain Stimul 12(4):868–876

Vidailhet M, Vercueil L, Houeto JL et al (2005) Bilateral deep-brain stimulation of the globus pallidus in primary generalized dystonia. N Engl J Med 352(5):459–467

Vogel AP, Folker J, Poole ML (2014) Treatment for speech disorder in Friedreich ataxia and other hereditary ataxia syndromes. Cochrane Database Syst Rev 10:CD008953

Volkmann J, Sturm V, Weiss P et al (1998) Bilateral high-frequency stimulation of the internal globus pallidus in advanced Parkinson's disease. Ann Neurol 44:953–961

Von Tetzchner S, Matrinsen H (2000) Introduction to augmentative and alternative communication. Whurr, London

Wales D, Skinner L, Hayman M (2017) The efficacy of telehealth-delivered speech and language intervention for primary school-age children: a systematic review. Int J Telerehabil 9(1):55–70

Wambaugh JL (2009) Understanding and management of acquired apraxia of speech: contribution of the Department of Veterans Affairs. Aphasiology 23(9):1127–1145

Wambaugh JL, Martinez AL (2000) Effects of modified response elaboration training with apraxic and aphasic speakers. Aphasiology 14(5):603–617

Wambaugh JL, Nessler C (2004) Modification of sound production treatment for apraxia of speech: acquisition and generalization effects. Aphasiology 18(5):407–427

Wambaugh JL, Doyle PJ, Kalinyak MM et al (1996) A minimal contrast treatment for apraxia of speech. Clin Aphasiol 24:97–108

Wambaugh JL, West JE, Doyle PJ (1998) Treatment for apraxia of speech: effect of treating sound groups. Aphasiology 12(7):731–743

Wambaugh JL, Martinez AL, McNeil MR et al (1999) Sound production treatment for apraxia of speech: overgeneralization and maintenance effects. Aphasiology 13(9):821–837

Wambaugh JL, Duffy JR, McNeil MR et al (2006) Treatment guidelines for acquired apraxia of speech: treatment descriptions and recommendations. J Med Speech Lang Pathol 14(2):35–67

Wambaugh JL, Nessler C, Wright S et al (2017) Effects of blocked and random practice schedule on outcomes of sound production treatment for acquired apraxia of speech: results of a group investigation. J Speech Lang Hear Res 60(6S):1739–1751

Wang DD, Chen W, Starr PA et al (2020) Local field potentials and ECoG. In: Pouratian N, Sheth S (eds) Stereotactic and functional neurosurgery. Springer, Cham, pp 107–117

Ward D (2006) Stuttering and cluttering: frames for understanding and treatment. Psychology Press, Hove

Warnecke T, Labeit B, Schroeder J (2020) Neurogenic dysphagia: a systematic review and proposal of a classification system. Neurology. Publish Ahead of Print. https://doi.org/10.1212/WNL.0000000000011350

Weismer G, Kim Y (2010) Classification and taxonomy of motor speech disorders: what are the issues? In: Maasen B, Van Lieshout P (eds) Speech motor control. New development in basis and applied research. Oxford University Press, Oxford, pp 229–241

Welter, M., Houeto, J., Tezenas du Montcel, S., Mesnage, V., Bonnet, A., Pillon, B., … Cornu, P. (2002). Clinical predictive factors of subthalamic stimulation in Parkinson's disease. *Brain, 125*(3), 575-583.

Wertheimer J, Gottuso AJ, Nuno M et al (2014) The impact of STN deep brain stimulation on speech in individuals with Parkinson's disease: the patient's perspective. Parkinsonism Relat Disord 20(10):1065–1070

Wertsén M, Stenberg M (2017a) Measuring lip force by oral screens. Part 1: Importance of screen size and individual variability. Clin Exp Dent Res 3(3):87–92

Wertsén M, Stenberg M (2017b) Measuring lip force by oral screens part 2: the importance of screen design, instruction and suction. Clin Exp Dent Res 3(5):191–197

Wertsén M, Stenberg M (2020) Training lip force by oral screens. Part 3: outcome for patients with stroke and peripheral facial palsy. Clin Exp Dent Res 6(3):286–295

Wertz RT, La Pointe LL, Rosenbek JC (1984) Apraxia of speech in adults: the disorder and its management. Grune & Stratton, Orlando, FL

West C, Hesketh A, Vail A et al (2005) Interventions for apraxia of speech following stroke (Cochrane review). In: The Cochrane Library, issue 4. John Wiley & Sons, Chichester, pp 1–10

WHA (World Health Assembly) (2001) Resolution WHA 54.21. International classification of functioning, disability and health. Available via https://www.who.int/standards/classifications/international-classification-of-functioning-disability-and-health. Accessed 14 Nov 2021

Wheeler D (1995) Communication and swallowing problems in the frail older person. Top Geriatr Rehabil 11(2):11–25

Wheeler RL, Logemann JA, Rosen MS (1980) Maxillary reshaping prosthesis effectiveness in improving speech and swallowing of postsurgical oral cancer patients. J Prosthet Dent 43(3):313–319

White M (2000) Reflections on narrative practice. Dulwich Centre Publications, Adelaide

White M (2007) Maps of narrative practice. Norton, New York

White M, Epston D (1990) Narrative means to therapeutic ends. Norton, New York

Wilson B (1982) Memory therapy in practice. In: Wilson B, Moffat N (eds) Clinical management of memory problems. Aspen Public, London, pp 89–111

Wood S, Timmins C, Wishart J et al (2019) Use of electropalatography in the treatment of speech disorders in children with Down syndrome: a randomized controlled trial. Int J Lang Commun Disord 54(2):234–248

World Health Organization (2001) International Classification of Functioning, Disability and Health (ICF) Annual updates available via: https://www.who.int/standards/classifications/international--classification-of-functioning-disability-and-health. Accessed 7 Nov 2021

Xie T, Padmanaban M, Bloom L et al (2017) Effect of low versus high frequency stimulation on freezing of gait and other axial symptoms in Parkinson patients with bilateral STN DBS: a mini-review. Transl Neurodegener 6:13. https://doi.org/10.1186/s40035-017-0083-7

Yamamoto T, Katayama Y, Ushiba J et al (2012) On-demand control system for deep brain stimulation for treatment of intention tremor. Neuromodulation 16(3):230–235

Yorkston KM (1996) Treatment efficacy: Dysathria. J Speech Lang Hear Res 39(5):46–57

Yorkston KM, Spencer KA, Duffy JR et al (2001) Evidence-based practice guidelines for dysarthria: management of velopharyngeal function. J Med Speech Lang Pathol 9(4):257–273

Yorkston KM, Beukelman DR, Strand EA et al (2010) Management of motor speech disorders in children and adults, 3rd edn. Pro-Ed Inc., Austin, TX

Yuan F, Guo X, Wei X et al (2020) Lee Silverman Voice Treatment for dysarthria in patients with Parkinson's disease: a systematic review and meta-analysis. Eur J Neurol 27(10):1957–1970

Yunusova Y, Plowman EK, Green JR et al (2019) Clinical measures of Bulbar dysfunction in ALS. Front Neurol 10:106. https://doi.org/10.3389/fneur.2019.00106. eCollection 2019

Ziegler W, Staiger A, Aichert I (2010) Apraxia of speech: what the deconstruction of phonetic plans tells about the construction of articulate language. In: Maasen B, Van Lieshout P (eds) Speech motor control. New development in basis and applied research. Oxford University Press, Oxford, pp 3–21

Zinkevich A, Uthoff SAK, Boenisch J et al (2019) Complex intervention in augmentative and alternative communication (AAC) care in Germany: a study protocol of an evaluation study with a controlled mixed-methods design. BMJ Open 9:e029469. https://doi.org/10.1136/bmjopen-2019-029469

# Part V

# Acquired Language Disorders (Aphasia)

Editors: Antonio Schindler, Antoinette am Zehnhoff-Dinnesen

Lectors: Francesca Bosco, Stefano Cappa, Melissa Catrini, Charles Ellis, Matti Lehtihalmes, Karel Neubauer, Lenka Neubauerova, Philippe Paquier, Pirkko Rautakoski, Michel Rijntjes, Ilona Rubi-Fessen, Rosemary Varley, Katarzyna Węsierska

# Basics of Acquired Language Disorders: Aphasia

Stefano Cappa, Daniela Ginocchio,
Barbara Maciejewska, Francesco Mozzanica,
and Antonio Schindler

## 21.1 Definition of Aphasia

Barbara Maciejewska and Antonio Schindler

The term 'aphasia', derived from old Greek a-pha-tos (speechless), was first introduced by Armand Trousseau in 1964 to describe patients who had lost their ability to speak (Tesak and Code 2008). However, the first explicit reference to the role of the brain in language disturbances is found in the Hippocrates' Corpus, where Hippocrates referred to two different types of language disturbance: aphonos ('without voice') and anaudos ('without

Barbara Maciejewska and Antonio Schindler shared first authorship

S. Cappa (✉)
Institute for Advanced Studies, University of Pavia, Pavia, Italy
e-mail: stefano.cappa@iusspavia.it

D. Ginocchio · F. Mozzanica
San Giuseppe Hospital, Milan, Italy
e-mail: francesco.mozzanica@unimi.it

B. Maciejewska
Department and Clinic of Phoniatrics and Audiology, Poznan University of Medical Sciences, Poznan, Poland
e-mail: barbaramaciejewska@ump.edu.pl

A. Schindler
Luigi Sacco Hospital, Department of Biomedical and Clinical Sciences "L. Sacco", Phoniatrics, University of Milan, Milan, Italy
e-mail: antonio.schindler@unimi.it

hearing'), corresponding to the two major aphasia syndromes. Broca made a breakthrough with his case studies and identified the third frontal convolution as a centre for the control of articulated speech. Carl Wernicke distinguished seven variants in the language disturbances associated with brain pathology: cortical motor; cortical sensory; conduction; transcortical motor; subcortical motor; transcortical sensory; subcortical sensory (Tesak and Code 2008). Despite the validity of Broca's and Wernicke's original observations, the definition, as well as classification, of language disorders is considerably more complex (more information in Sect. 12.3).

Aphasia means speechlessness and is not a disease, but a symptom. It is a loss or impairment of language function as a consequence of brain damage. It could be said that aphasia is an impairment of the system of language communication formed after brain damage (Benson and Ardila 1996). Despite a clear basic definition and its acceptance among scientists, investigators and clinicians, the agreement between them is illusory. Several definitions of aphasia are given below, according to the clinical perspectives they come from.

It is important to know the differences and the consequences of different meanings and interpretations of the word '*language*'. '*Language*' is defined as a communication system, and as a result aphasia is treated as a linguistic problem. '*Language*' disorder means a problem with

A. am Zehnhoff-Dinnesen et al. (eds.), *Phoniatrics III*, European Manual of Medicine, https://doi.org/10.1007/978-3-031-48091-1_6

speech, so aphasia is evaluated by speech language pathologists. What is more, *'language'* is a cognitive function, leading to disorders in behaviour, thus aphasia is a branch of psychiatry as well as neuropsychology. *Language* and speech are functions of the brain, so that neuroscientists, such as neuroanatomists, neuropsychologists and neuropathologists, treat aphasia as a pathology of the nervous system. As language problems in aphasic patients are also a result of brain damage, aphasia belongs to the field of neurology. Thus:

- In *medicine/neurology*, aphasia is considered an acquired neurological disorder, leading to a language impairment due to damage in the brain areas responsible for language production or processing, resulting in abnormalities of speech production or understanding or both (Kirshner 2016a).
- In *neuropsychology*, aphasia means a loss or impairment of verbal communication that occurs as a consequence of brain dysfunction (Sinanović et al. 2011)
- From a *functional* viewpoint, aphasia is mainly communication impairment (Papathanasiou et al. 2013)
- The *linguistic* aspect of aphasia focuses on an impairment of language function as a system of communication after brain damage (Benson and Ardila 1996)
- In the *rehabilitation* world, following the principles underlying the International Classification of Functioning, Disability and Health (ICF) (Galletta and Barrett 2014), aphasia is defined as 'an acquired selective impairment of language modalities and functions resulting from a focal brain lesion in the language-dominant hemisphere that affects the person's communicative and social functioning, quality of life, and the quality of life of his/her relatives and caregivers' (Papathanasiou et al. 2013).
- From a *phoniatric* point of view, it is advisable to use the term aphasia selectively for acquired language impairment due to brain lesions in the language-dominant hemisphere affecting interpersonal communication.

Because language is one of the cortical functions and its many aspects originate in definite brain areas, the different language components (phonology, morphology, syntax, semantics) across different modalities (speaking, reading, writing, signing) in both expression and comprehension may be impaired in aphasia (Purves et al. 2018), resulting in problems with communications. The distinction between language and the related sensory and motor abilities on which it depends is crucial. So it is important to distinguish aphasia from other communication and speech disorders such as motor speech disorders, cognitive-communication disorders, hearing problems and dementia.

There is clinical evidence that the ability to move the muscles of the mouth, tongue, larynx and pharynx can be affected without abolishing the ability to use spoken language to communicate (even though a motor deficit may make communication difficult). Similarly, damage to the auditory pathways can impede the ability to hear without interfering with language functions (Purves et al. 2018). Aphasia diminishes or abolishes the ability to comprehend or to produce language while sparing the ability to perceive the relevant stimuli and to produce words. Damage to specific regions of the brain can affect essential language functions, destroying the ability to recognise or use the symbolic value of words, thus depriving adult aphasic patients of the linguistic understanding, grammatical organisation and intonation that distinguishes language from nonsense.

It is important to distinguish aphasia from related afflictions (Kirshner 2016b; McNeil 2008):

- Dysarthria: An acquired disorder of speech production due to problems with nerves innervating the speech articulators.
- Dysphonia: Difficulty or lack of voice production.
- Dysglossia: An acquired disorder of speech production due to abnormal anatomy of speech articulators jaw, lips, tongue, palate.

Other differential diagnoses to consider (Josephs et al. 2006; Kirshner 2016b; Christman et al. 2017) include:

- Apraxia of speech: An impairment in the motor planning and programming of the speech articulators, characterised by slow speaking rate, abnormal prosody and distorted sound substitutions, additions, repetitions and prolongations; sometimes accompanied by groping, and trial and error articulatory movements.
- Cognitive-communication disorder: Problems with communication that have an underlying cause in a cognitive deficit rather than a primary language or speech deficit.
- Altered mental status from encephalopathy or delirium.

Aphasia, dysarthria and apraxia can coexist, but often occur separately. Aphasia may involve other language symptoms, such as writing or reading problems, unlike dysarthria, anarthria and dysphonia. The latter can be distinguished by evaluation of language (tests of word and sentence comprehension, naming, repetition, spontaneous speech, reading and writing), as well as tests of articulation (tests assessing the strength, coordination, rate and range of movement of the muscles of speech articulation) and motor speech programming.

The basic elements of aphasia are that it is:

- An *acquired* language disorder (therefore all language impairments due to child deafness, congenital motor impairment or selective but developmental in origin are excluded).
- A *disorder of language, not only speech* (phonation, articulation), that may involve comprehension or expression or both, across different modalities; spoken language expression, spoken language comprehension, written expression, reading comprehension.
- Due to *brain damage.*

An aphasic patient remains a challenge of huge importance for phoniatricians. Attention is particularly directed to medical, linguistic, psy-

chological and cultural aspects of diagnosis, as well as to treatment and rehabilitation.

## 21.2 Epidemiology of Aphasia

Barbara Maciejewska

### 21.2.1 Definition of Aphasia

Language is a specific human feature. It provides humans with communication as well as allowing learning and the exchange of information. The loss or impairment of language is one of the more devastating cognitive impairments. The language problems lead to faulty communication and can also affect speaking, reading and writing. It is a life-changing condition and has a large impact on a patient's quality of life, health condition and daily interactions. As a result, it is a medical as well as social problem (Klippi et al. 2012; Efstratiadous et al. 2012). Aphasia is defined as an acquired language disorder caused by brain damage (Kirshner 2016a). It is a group of conditions that have overlapping signs and symptoms. A key feature of these conditions is impairment of language skills rather than speech only. It is an impairment of comprehension or formulation of language caused by damage to the cortical centre for language (Le and Lui 2023). As a result, aphasia should be distinguished from congenital and developmental language disorders (e.g. dysphasias) as well as from speech problems (such as dysarthria, dyspraxia, dysglossia). More information can be found in Sect. 21.1.

### 21.2.2 Incidence and Aetiologies of Aphasia

According to the National Institute on Deafness and Other Communication Disorders (NIDCD), in the USA there are 180,000 new aphasia cases a year, and 1 of every 272 Americans is affected with aphasia (Le and Lui 2023).

It can be caused by many different brain diseases, disorders and lesions to the language areas of the brain. Aphasia can be seen in focal brain damage such as penetrating brain injuries, brain tumours, head injuries and other mass lesions (Le and Lui 2023; Bobba et al. 2019; Kirshner 2016a). Traumatic brain injury frequently disrupts discourse and produces language impairments that are often part of a syndrome of general cognitive dysfunction. About one-third of severely head-injured persons have problems with communication as a result of aphasia (Grochmal-Bach et al. 2009). Focal encephalitis and infections (abscesses) also cause aphasia; e.g. the herpes simplex virus causes encephalitis, with a predilection for the orbital frontal lobes and temporal lobes (Kirshner 2016a; Chaudhuri and Kennedy 2002).

However, the condition is most commonly seen in patients after such cerebrovascular accidents as ischaemic and haemorrhagic strokes (Kirshner 2016a, b; Klippi et al. 2012; Mitchell et al. 2020; Khedr et al. 2020). Approximately one-third of stroke patients (21–38%) develop aphasia (Engelter et al. 2006; Klippi et al. 2012; Kauhanen et al. 2000). Atrial fibrillation (AF) especially represents a high-risk factor for ischaemic stroke with aphasia (Khedr et al. 2020). In Europe and USA, the reported annual incidence of the most common type of aphasia, post-stroke aphasia, is 43–60 per 100,000 inhabitants (Engelter et al. 2006; Berthier et al. 2011).

The incidence of post stroke-aphasia is age-dependent. Aphasic stroke patients are older than non-aphasic stroke patients; their mean age being 80 years versus 75 years according to Engelter's study (Engelter et al. 2006) and 65.2 vs 63.8 years in Wilson's research (Wilson et al. 2019) in the aphasia group and non-aphasia group, respectively. Patients who are younger than 65 years have a 15% chance of being affected, compared with those who are older than 85 years, who have a 43% chance of developing the condition (Engelter et al. 2006). The risk of aphasia increased in stroke patients by 1–7% for each year of age (Engelter et al. 2006).

Stroke-type (ischaemic or haemorrhagic) aphasia appears to have no connection with the frequency of communication impairment, but stroke severity does. Higher rates of aphasia are seen in patients with more severe stroke: only 1%

survive a severe stroke with communication intact (Mitchell et al. 2020).

Gender differences are observed in the severity of aphasia on admission, with women having more severe aphasia than men (Pedersena et al. 2004). However, sex was no longer a significant determinant of aphasia severity after a year, and the outcome for language function was predicted only by the initial severity of the aphasia and stroke, but not by age, sex or type of aphasia.

Patients suffering from post-stroke aphasia have greater morbidity and mortality than stroke patients without aphasia (Ellis et al. 2012).

Referring to the aetiologies of aphasia, epileptic aphasia is described. The main acquired epileptic aphasia is known as Landau-Kleffner syndrome. However, it generally affects children from 3 to 7 years of age. It is a rare neurological disorder characterised by severe and prolonged receptive language deterioration, with patients suffering from total loss of auditory/verbal comprehension and expression (Qiu et al. 2017). Aphasia as an exclusive symptom of epilepsy in adults is rare. Qiu et al. report a unique case of aphasic status epilepticus as the isolated symptom of epilepsy in an adult woman. Aphasia in adults with drug-resistant focal epilepsy can be observed in patients who undergo surgery with resection of language areas (Mnatsakanyan et al. 2018).

Speech and language impairments can be the most prominent presenting symptoms of a neurodegenerative disease. Aphasia can also result from primary progressive aphasia (PPA) (Tee and Gorno-Tempini 2019), which is a neurodegenerative disorder characterised by a primary dissolution of language. PPA can be classified into three subtypes on the basis of specific speech and language features: semantic dementia (SD), progressive non-fluent aphasia and logopenic progressive aphasia (lv-PPA) (Josephs et al. 2008; Matías-Guiu and García-Ramos 2013).

### 21.2.3 Frequency of Different Patterns of Aphasia

Common types described in studies of aphasia are as follows: global, Broca's, Wernicke's, transcortical motor, transcortical sensory, mixed transcortical, conduction, anomic, crossed, subcortical (Davis 2007; Bobba et al. 2019; Pedersena et al. 2004; Khedr et al. 2020). This is a common classification in the literature because its reliability and validity have been well described and because it allows results to be compared with those of other studies (for more see Sect. 21.1).

Because of the many types of aphasia, classification can be difficult. Each type of aphasia classification is an attempt to organise and group aphasic syndromes (Ardila 2010; Kirshner 2016a).

According to the literature the most frequent type is global aphasia—more than half of episodes (El-Tallawy et al. 2019; Khedr et al. 2020). The classic aphasia types such as Broca's or Wernicke's ones are also common. They affected one quarter of aphatic patients in Pedersen study (Pedersena et al. 2004). In Kherd's study, Broca's aphasia was observed in 27.7% and Wernicke's in 11.1% (Khedr et al. 2020); in El-Tallawy's study values were 8.4% and 2.8%, respectively (El-Tallawy et al. 2019). Subcortical aphasia is also common (15.9%) (El-Tallawy et al. 2019). Taking into consideration speech fluency, aphasia can be fluent (29%) and non-fluent (60%) (Engelter et al. 2006).

However, 'clear' types are rare. Aphasia has many manifestations, because the pathological processes can affect various language-related cortical brain areas at the same time. About 15% of patients are unclassifiable according to the main described types (Khedr et al. 2020). Moreover, numerous studies have reported the evolution of types of aphasia during recovery (Kauhanen et al. 2000; Pedersena et al. 2004).

Nevertheless, to characterise better the observed aphasia the patient suffers from, it is worth investigating various language abilities such as spontaneous speech, naming, comprehension, repetition, reading, writing-associated signs (apraxia, hemiparesis, hemianopia) (Kirshner 2016a).

## 21.2.4 Concomitant Speech Disorders

Not only aphasia (where language is affected) but also dysarthria (where speech production and intelligibility are affected) is a common conse-

quence of stroke. Post-stroke dysarthria is also often observed. It is worth mentioning that the most common presentation of communication impairment in patients after stroke is to have a combination of aphasia and dysarthria.

In some studies, 28% of stroke patients had both aphasia and dysarthria, 24% had dysarthria only, and 12% had aphasia only (Mitchell et al. 2020; Kirshner 2016a, b).

## 21.2.5 Perspectives

The role of phoniatricians is to identify communication impairment such as aphasia. It is crucial to prevent permanent disability, poor psychological well-being, health outcomes and social isolation in patients suffering from language problems. Rehabilitation of aphasic patients is a challenge. Aphasia recovery is a complex long-lasting and time-consuming process, which may involve neural changes (Crosson et al. 2019; Pulvermüller and Berthier 2008). It needs cooperation of the patient, phoniatrician, neurologist and speech language therapist, but it should be noted that even patients with global aphasia on admission might fully recover their language function (Pedersena et al. 2004; Crosson et al. 2019). This is because of neuroplasticity—the structural and physiological changes that occur at the synaptic, cellular and macro-structural levels in the brain (Mohr 2017; Crosson et al. 2019). Functional and structural neuroimaging in aphatic patients provide information that brain systems can change as a result of therapy (Crosson et al. 2019).

## 21.3 Classification of Aphasia and its Symptomatic Profile

Barbara Maciejewska and Antonio Schindler

## 21.3.1 Introduction

The neural organisation of language is complicated. Language is a complex behaviour and belongs to the higher cognitive functions. Thus it is not a product of a small, isolated, circumscribed region of the brain, but a consequence of cooperation of different areas linked together by a complicated neuronal network (Schoeman and Van der Merwe 2010). As a result, classifying the subtypes of language problem in aphasia is difficult (Kolb and Whishaw 2003). However, the analysis of language deficit in patients with aphasia and its classification is of primary importance for several reasons. First, classification requires knowing the main impairment and communication problem and the severity of aphasia. Second, this makes it easier to provide prognosis, to analyse the evolution of the disease and to decide on rehabilitation plans. Finally, the type of the aphasic patients' symptoms is a crucial procedure that favours and simplifies communication among the clinicians involved in patient treatment and follow-up (Wilson et al. 2009).

Aphasia is an acquired language disorder and a heterogeneous entity in severity, aetiology and symptoms; most aphasic patients present a constellation of symptoms that cannot be reliably classified in only one particular syndrome (Basso 2003; Cherney and Small 2009). Depending on the reasons for the disease, different classification criteria are used (Schindler and Miletto 2005; Grabias and Kurkowski 2012; Schoeman and Van der Merwe 2010). It is difficult to find universal agreement on the classification of aphasia types.

### 21.3.2 Aphasia Subtypes: Attempts at Classification

Over 20 aphasia classifications have been proposed since Broca's first report of a language disturbance associated with brain pathology (Ardila 2010). He described the variety of aphasia types 'alogia', 'verbal amnesia', 'aphemia' and 'mechanic alalia'. In 1874, C. Wernicke was the first to propose classification of aphasias on the basis of the anatomical correspondence of the various aspects of language impairment, with a posterior centre and an anterior centre connected by an anatomical pathway (the arcuate fasciculus), damage to which would give rise to sensory, motor and conduction aphasia, respectively

(Viader 2015; Nasios et al. 2019; Tremblay and Dick 2016; Hagoort 2013). This concept has been further elaborated to culminate in the well-known Lichtheims 'house' scheme.

The Wernicke–Lichtheim model of language representation and language network based on the Wernicke–Lichtheim–Geschwind model is common and well-known (see: Tremblay and Dick 2016; Nasios et al. 2019; Hagoort 2013; O'Sullivan et al. 2019). The model predicts only five patterns of aphasia: (1) Broca's aphasia; (2) Wernicke's aphasia; (3) conduction aphasia; (4) transcortical motor aphasia; (5) transcortical sensory aphasia (O'Sullivan et al. 2019; Tremblay and Dick 2016). The classical model focuses on cortical structures, excluding subcortical regions and relevant connections, based on an outdated brain anatomy (Nasios et al. 2019). However, it is perhaps still useful for understanding the types of aphasia and its classical syndromes (Table 21.1).

Probably, the oldest and most applied criterion to classify aphasia is to follow the so-called Wernicke–Lichtheim–Geschwind model. According to this, three main centres exist: acoustic, motor and concept, and a different subtype of aphasia arises depending on which of the centres or their

**Table 21.1** Clinical features and linguistic deficits, type of aphasia according to the Wernicke–Lichtheim–Geschwind model (according to: Tremblay and Dick 2016; Nasios et al. 2019; Hagoort 2013; O'Sullivan et al. 2019; Mesulam 2016)

| Damaged brain region | Main linguistic deficit | Type of aphasia |
|---|---|---|
| Motor centre | Production | Broca's aphasia |
| Acoustic centre | Comprehension | Wernicke's aphasia |
| Motor-acoustic tract | Repetition | Conduction aphasia |
| Acoustic-concept tract | Comprehension, preserved Repetition | Transcortical sensory aphasia |
| Motor-concept tract | Production, preserved repetition | Transcortical motor aphasia |
| Motor (M) + acoustic (A) + concept (C) Centre | Comprehension, production, repetition, naming | Global aphasia |

connections is damaged (Nasios et al. 2019). The two more influential aphasia classifications are the Boston Group classification (by Geschwind, Benson, Alexander, Goodglass, Kaplan and others) and Luria's aphasia system (Ardila 2010).

The Boston Group classification represents a development of Wernicke's ideas about brain centres of language. In this classification, aphasias can be fluent or non-fluent, as well as cortical, subcortical or transcortical (Ardila 2010).

Luria proposed seven aphasia subtypes relating to particular language-processing defects: motor efferent or kinetic, motor afferent or kinesthetic, acoustic-agnosic, acoustic-amnesic, amnesic, semantic and dynamic (Akhutina 2016). Other aphasia types, classified by characteristics of verbal expression include just two types: fluent and non-fluent (Clough and Gordon 2020; Le and Lui 2023). Fluent aphasias include Wernicke's, transcortical sensory, conduction and anomic; non-fluent aphasias include Broca's, transcortical motor and global.

Various points of view were integrated by Benson and Ardila, who created a classification based on two anatomical criteria: (1) pre-Rolandic aphasia (anterior, non-fluent) or post-Rolandic (posterior, fluent) and (2) peri-Sylvian aphasias (aphasias with pathology in the peri-Sylvian language area) or extra-Sylvian aphasia (due to damage beyond this area) (Ardila 2010).

Since the introduction of CT and MRI in the 1980s, new language deficits have been found (Duffy 2005). CT and MRI scans brought new concepts, e.g. 'subcortical aphasias', which are called 'dissident' because they do not fit the clinical profile of classical aphasic syndromes. The so-called thalamic and striato-capsular aphasias have been described. Thalamic aphasia is characterised by word-finding deficit, paraphasia (mainly semantic), neologisms, perseveration, circumlocution, reduced spontaneous speech output, while repetition and comprehension are relatively preserved. Striato-capsular lesions may present with an atypical constellation of language deficits and their description in terms of classical aphasia syndrome is not useful; possible charac-

teristics of striato-capsular lesion are deficits in generative language and naming.

Aphasia is a language disturbance, and consequently not only a neurological/anatomical background is important but neuropsychological as well as neurolinguistic perspectives are also required. Hence, new aphasia classifications are related to linguistic and cognitive neuropsychology (Viader 2015; Ardila 2010). The neuropsychological concept is Luria's neuropsychological theory of language and speech (Akhutina 2016). The target of the linguistic analysis is only the language disorder, regardless of any anatomical correlation (Viader 2015)

The linguist Roman Jakobson proposed that the major aphasic syndromes are related to the two basic linguistic operations of selecting (language as paradigm) and sequencing (language as syntagm). He stressed the importance of the paradigmatic/syntagmatic dichotomy, corresponding to selection and combination, respectively, of linguistic elements (phonemes/morphemes/words). Contrary to pure linguistics, cognitive neuropsychology aims at uncovering the brain areas that support specific speech processes (Viader 2015). Aphasia is seen as a disruption of cognitive processes underlying language tasks, such as sentence comprehension and word naming. Cognitive representations are distributed across regions of the brain and activation of these areas is needed to evoke semantic representations (Tippett et al. 2014).

A new classification of aphasic syndromes has been suggested by Ardila (2010), Buckingham (2010) and Marshall (2010) (Table 21.2), with there being two fundamental forms of aphasia: Primary and secondary. Primary (or 'central') aphasias are due to problems with language-processing mechanisms affecting the language system itself (phonology, lexicon, semantics, grammar) and are linked to impairments in the lexical/semantic and grammatical systems of language (Wernicke-type and Broca-type aphasias). Secondary (or 'peripheral') aphasias are the result of other problems, such as memory impairment, attention disorders or perceptual problems. Secondary aphasias impair some peripheral mechanisms required to produce language (con-

**Table 21.2** New classification of aphasias, according to Ardila (2010)

| Types of aphasia | Main problem | Subtypes of aphasia | Description |
|---|---|---|---|
| Primary (central) aphasias | Language system | Wernicke-type | Phoneme and word selection are deficient |
| | | Broca-type | Wrong sequencing of speech elements/grammar impaired |
| Secondary (peripheral) aphasias | Mechanisms of production | Conduction aphasia | Inability to reproduce aloud the auditory information that is heard |
| | | Supplementary motor area (SMA) aphasia | Impairment of initiation and maintaining voluntary speech |
| Dysexecutive aphasia | Language executive control | Extra-sylvian (transcortical) motor aphasia | The active use and executive control of the language is limited |

duction aphasia and aphasia of the supplementary motor area), or the executive control of the language (extra-Sylvian or transcortical motor aphasia). As a result, language is limited (Ardila 2010). Sometimes language is not impaired, but the patient cannot use it appropriately because of executive control impairments (dysexecutive aphasia).

To sum up: in primary central aphasias, language is disintegrated and thus impaired; in secondary peripheral aphasias, some mechanism required to produce the language is altered, so language is limited.

Despite its age, the concept of two main types of aphasia described by Broca in 1861 and Wernicke in 1874 is still present. Increasingly often it is said that there are only two major aphasic syndromes: Wernicke-type aphasia and Broca-type aphasia. Language is only disintegrated in Wernicke and Broca aphasia; in the other forms of aphasia, language is not disintegrated but limited (Ardila 2010; Marshall 2010). The localisation of the main brain damage and different perspectives of aphasia are briefly presented by Grabias and Kurkowski (2012). Namely, aphasia of Broca's area has been described from different perspectives: anatomically as anterior, physiologically as motor, psychologically as expressive, neuropsychologically as coding, linguistically as syntagmatic, neurolinguistically as combination and communicatively as non-fluent. Whereas aphasia of Wernicke's area has been characterised as posterior, sensory, perceptive, decoding, paradigmatic, selection and fluent.

Nowadays, syndromic classification has turned towards a more flexible and mostly descriptive conceptualisation, taking into account the difficulty in reliably classifying the aphasic patient population. For clinical practice, the best way is to describe the deficits and impairments of language in aphasic patients.

### 21.3.3 Classical Aphasia Subtypes: A Brief Summary (from Bartlett and Pashek 1994; Grabias and Kurkowski 2012; Mitchell et al. 2021; Tippett et al. 2014; Schoeman and Van der Merwe 2010; Viader 2015)

#### 21.3.3.1 Wernicke's Aphasia (Sensory, Receptive, Acoustic, Syntactic Aphasia)

This is usually due to a lesion in the posterior superior temporal lobe of the dominant hemisphere, although involvement of the parietal and occipital lobe is possible. The major difficulty in Wernicke's aphasia is putting together objects or ideas and the words that signify them. It leads to a severe deficit in auditory comprehension, with fluent but incoherent spontaneous speech. Speech tends to be paraphasic (including both semantic [e.g. chair instead of table] and phonemic [e.g. book instead of look] paraphasias), uncorrected but well-articulated sentences, often to the point of neologistic jargon, conveying little meaning. Thus, in Wernicke's aphasia, speech is fluent and well structured, but makes little or no sense because words and meanings are not correctly linked.

### 21.3.3.2 Transcortical Sensory Aphasia

The lesions responsible for transcortical sensory aphasia are not very precise, but involve large areas of the temporo-parietal-occipital region, often sparing at least partially the Wernicke's area.

In this type of aphasia repetition is preserved, but the patients present with severe comprehension deficit, while spontaneous speech is fluent with paraphasias (verbal rather than phonemic), frequently using information-poor words, such as place or thing, conveying little meaning. Patients have fluent and paraphasic speech and can repeat verbatim, but understand little of what they repeat or read.

### 21.3.3.3 Broca's Aphasia (Expressive, Efferent Motor, Verbal, Motor Aphasia)

Broca's aphasia is due to a lesion of the dominant hemisphere fronto-parietal cortex, but might also be limited to the frontal operculum, third frontal convolution or anterior insula. It is characterised by non-fluent and agrammatical spontaneous speech: the absence of small, function words leads to the label telegraphic speech, while the impoverishment of grammatical forms to the label agrammatical speech; phonemic paraphasias and perseverations, together with dysprosody (abnormal melody and rhythm of speech) complete the picture. Patients are unable to express themselves appropriately because the organisational aspects of language (its grammar) have been disrupted. Auditory comprehension is preserved for understanding most conversation, though it may be below normal limits at formal testing.

### 21.3.3.4 Transcortical Motor Aphasia

This is usually seen after lesions appear close to Broca's area (the inferior posterior frontal area or the superior parasagittal frontal area). The clinical picture is characterised by a reduction of spontaneous speech almost until muteness; speech is non-fluent, troubled by phonemic and global paraphasias and without connective words, while repetition, comprehension, naming and reading are preserved.

### 21.3.3.5 Mixed Transcortical Aphasia

This form combines both the motor and sensory elements common to the transcortical aphasias. Patients cannot write and have severe speaking and comprehension impairment, but with unaffected repetition.

### 21.3.3.6 Conduction Aphasia

This disorder arises from lesions to the pathways connecting the relevant temporal and frontal regions—the arcuate fasciculus in the subcortical white matter that links Broca's and Wernicke's areas. Spontaneous speech production is relatively normal, fluent and correct, although minor phonemic paraphasias may be introduced. The linguistic deficit includes impairment of repetition and anomia. Interruption of this pathway may lead to an inability to produce appropriate responses to heard communication, even though the communication is understood.

### 21.3.3.7 Anomic Aphasia (Nominal, Amnestic Aphasia)

The lesion is at the angular gyrus; the main feature is a difficulty with naming. Patients tend to produce fluent, well-articulated and grammatically correct speech. Language comprehension is intact, and repetition is normal. Patients have difficulties with word finding. Selected naming deficit may be an evolution of different subtype of aphasia (Broca's, Wernicke's, conduction aphasia), usually due to relatively small brain lesions, as well as in diffuse and multifocal brain damage, or in degenerative dementia.

### 21.3.3.8 Global Aphasia

This type of aphasia is caused by a wide lesion of the dominant fronto-temporo-parietal cortex, lesions vary in size and location but tend to follow the left middle cerebral artery distribution. This is the most severe form of aphasia. It leads to severe communication difficulties because of deficits in all language domains: comprehension, naming, repetition, reading, writing and reading are severely impaired. Patients can only produce a few recognisable words, speech is non-fluent and reduced to a few words with impairment of language and auditory comprehension. Patients are unable to read or write.

Despite its classic subtypes (Table 21.3), the language disorder aphasia seldom occurs as an isolated symptom, it is very rarely pure and usually mixed, so patients do not fit into any of the aphasia subtypes described above. Moreover aphasia, dysarthria, apraxia can coexist. Mitchell et al. (2021) showed that 64% of 88,974 stroke patients were communication-impaired, and 28% not only had aphasia but also dysarthria, 24% had dysarthria only and 12% had aphasia only (Mitchell et al. 2021).

### 21.3.4 Beyond the Classification: Other Forms of Aphasia

In addition to the syndromes above, there are many other possible combinations of deficits that do not exactly fit into any existing categories or classification systems. These are so-called exceptional aphasias and the main ones are presented below.

#### 21.3.4.1 Crossed Aphasia (CA)
This occurs when a person demonstrates language impairment secondary to right hemisphere lesion. Most aphasias in right-handed individuals are caused by left hemispheric injury; crossed aphasia following a right-hemispheric lesion is rarely observed. A right-handed person who develops aphasia following a right-hemispheric stroke exhibits crossed aphasia. The prevalence of CA in right-handed patients is reported to be from 0.4% to 3% of all aphasic syndromes (Kim et al. 2013).

#### 21.3.4.2 Subcortical Aphasia
This results from damage to subcortical regions of the brain (e.g. thalamus or basal ganglia), and symptoms can mirror those that arise from cortical lesions. Main symptoms depend on the location and size of the subcortical lesion.

#### 21.3.4.3 Primary Progressive Aphasia (PPA)
Despite its name, this is a type of dementia. It is characterised by a gradual loss of language function in the context of relatively well-preserved memory, visual processing and personality until the advanced stages (Mesulam 2001; Rogers 2004). The recognition that focal neurodegenerative disease can cause primary progressive aphasia allows investigation of language deficits caused by cerebral atrophy of regions of the brain not typically damaged by stroke (Tippett et al. 2014).

#### 21.3.4.4 Cerebellar Aphasia
The cerebellum does not appear in either the classical or modern models describing the neuroanatomy of language. However, neuro-scientific evidence has established the view that the cerebellum participates in a much wider range of functions than conventionally accepted (Marien et al. 2000; van Dun and Mariën 2016). Much research has implicated the cerebellum in cognitive and behavioural-affective functions, as well as language at a higher than the articulatory level. Scientists discuss the involvement of the cerebellum in a broad spectrum of non-motor language functions through a dense network of crossed and reciprocal cerebello-cerebral connections. Clinical

**Table 21.3** Aphasia types and criteria for classification (according to Kirshner 2016a, b)

| Aphasia type | Fluency | Auditory comprehension | Repetition | Naming |
|---|---|---|---|---|
| Broca's | Non-fluent | Relatively good | Impaired | Impaired |
| Global | Non-fluent | Impaired | Impaired | Impaired |
| Transcortical motor | Non-fluent | Relatively good | Good | Impaired |
| Wernicke's | Fluent | Impaired | Impaired | Impaired |
| Conduction | Fluent | Good | Impaired | Impaired |
| Anomic | Fluent | Good | Good | Impaired |
| Transcortical sensory | Fluent | Impaired | Good | Impaired |

evidence and imaging studies point to cerebellar involvement in motor speech production; verbal fluency and lexical/semantic retrieval; grammatical/syntactical processing; reading, writing, metalinguistic skills; and verbal working memory. These observations have led to the hypothesis of a cerebellar-induced aphasia (Nasios et al. 2019). However, the idea of a cerebellar-induced aphasia is still a matter of debate.

### 21.3.5 Key Points

- Aphasia is not pure, it seldom occurs as an isolated symptom.
- The best way to describe a particular aphasia is by describing the types of deficit, because types of aphasia overlap and no classification system is ideal.
- Often other motor impairments coexist, including bucco-facial apraxia (impairment of voluntary movement oral and facial muscles), apraxia of speech, dysarthria, ideomotor apraxia (impairment in miming tool use) and dysarthria.
- Evaluating the patient's ability to name, repeat, comprehend, read and write at the bedside; doing brain imaging; and considering neuropsychological testing are crucial to the diagnosis and description of aphasia.

## 21.4 Aetiology and Pathogenesis of Aphasia

Francesco Mozzanica and Daniela Ginocchio

Aphasia is a clinical syndrome due to brain disorders of multiple aetiology. Several regions of the brain are known to be responsible for language function, including Broca's and Wernicke's areas, and the transcortical and subcortical pathways which connect them (Hu et al. 2018; Sul et al. 2016). However, lesions in other areas can also affect large-scale language networks, resulting in aphasia (Sul et al. 2016; Cappa 2011; Crinion et al. 2013). According to the nature of speech fluency, aphasia can be classified as fluent (characterised by the ability to produce connected speech with sentence structure relatively intact, but lacking meaning) and non-fluent (characterised by halting and effortful speech production and grammar impairment). Typically, fluent aphasia is determined by damage posterior to the central sulcus in the language-dominant hemisphere, while non-fluent aphasia frequently results from damage in the front half of the language-dominant hemisphere, anterior to the central sulcus (Brookshire and McNeil 2014). In the majority of the cases, the damage has a vascular origin, i.e. acute stroke. Other causes include a brain tumour, traumatic brain injury, cerebral hypoxia, cerebral haemorrhage, cerebral infections and neurodegenerative disorders (Finch and Copland 2014). Most of the non-vascular neurological conditions that may cause aphasia are insidious, rather than abrupt, in onset (Al-Khindi et al. 2010; Fitzgerald et al. 2010). These insidious conditions make their presence known slowly over a period of time, sometimes with intermittent periods of stabilisation.

For brain tumours, aphasia is related to the pathological involvement of brain language areas, and in this case the language impairment typically develops gradually. Tumours affecting brain tissues may be either primary or secondary (metastatic tumours more frequently related to breast, lungs, pharynx and larynx carcinomas) and determine a swelling of the brain tissue that represents one of the major causes of observable symptoms. Localised symptoms commonly appear in the early stages, while a gradual intensification of symptoms and more generalised dysfunction typically occur as tumour grows, with consequent swelling of brain tissue and increase of intracranial pressure. The type and number of symptoms, as well as their rate of progression, are determined by the size, rate of growth and location of the tumour. For example, patients with gliomas, the most common benign brain tumour, develop aphasia in approximately 24% of cases (IJzerman-Korevaar et al. 2018). Usually symptom development may span several years because gliomas grow slowly. Conversely, glioblastoma multiforme, the most common primary malignant tumour, grows rapidly with symptoms typically developing during a period of few months (Brookshire and McNeil 2014).

Infections of the central nervous system may also determine aphasia. *Streptococcus pneumoniae*, *Neisseria meningitidis* and *Haemophilus influenzae* may induce acute bacterial meningitis, which is characterised by the abrupt onset of fever, headache and meningismus, and in survivors neurological sequelae including aphasia, ataxia, paresis, hearing loss and cognitive impairment (Davis 2018). As far as viral infections are concerned, they are more commonly related to a general infection (such as mumps) or as a consequence of insect transmission or animal bites (such as equine encephalitis). In these cases, the symptom development may be very rapid, followed by gradual improvement (as in viral meningitis) or very slow, without any improvement (as in acquired immunodeficiency syndrome, AIDS) (Brookshire and McNeil 2014).

Aphasia is frequent in acute and subacute stroke situations, affecting from 21 to 38% of patients surviving stroke (Hoffmann and Chen 2013). Factors that increase an individual's likelihood of experiencing stroke and aphasia are genetic factors, hypertension, diabetes, dyslipidaemia, cigarette smoking, obesity, atrial fibrillation, inactivity, sleep-disordered breathing, inflammation, infections, excessive consumption of alcohol and dietary intake high in fat and sodium (Meschia et al. 2016). In stroke patients, aphasia syndromes are predictive of lesion location, stroke pathophysiology and recovery (Croquelois and Bogousslavsky 2011). Most patients with aphasia undergo multimodality magnetic resonance imaging (MRI) or computed tomography (CT) in the course of their stroke workup. Consequently, the location of the damaged brain area is usually known (Hills et al. 2004). Nowadays, the detection of the mechanism that finally leads to language impairment is the most important factor for preventing a recurrence or worsening of an aphasia syndrome, since the natural course varies with the pathogenesis. Aphasia subtypes and pathogenesis, in fact, have some significant associations. In particular, anomic aphasia appears significantly associated with small-vessel disease (SVD), while global aphasia patients mostly have cardioembolic (CE) causes that lead to the occlusion of the middle cerebral artery before it branches. Wernicke's aphasia is frequently related to haemorrhage or CE that determines the occlusion of the posterior temporal and parietal branches of the middle cerebral artery (Hoffmann and Chen 2013). Broca's aphasia can be caused by SVD, haemorrhage, large vessel disease or CE that causes an occlusion of the anterior branches of the middle cerebral artery.

As far as the lesion location (which finally determines the characteristic of aphasia) is concerned, damage to the area of the inferior frontal gyrus is usually associated with mild and transient language impairment. In other cases, the infarct may be in the territory of the anterior branches of the middle cerebral artery with possible damage of the frontal operculum cortex (Brodmann's areas 44 and 45), the underlying white matter, the insula and the basal ganglia, as well as the inferior sector of the pre-central gyrus. In the acute stage of this condition, a small and circumscribed infarct of the frontal operculum can also produce a non-fluent language deficit with all the characteristics of Broca aphasia (Brookshire and McNeil 2014). In Wernicke's aphasia, the lesion is usually located in the posterior sector of the superior temporal gyrus (Brodmann's area 22) with extension in the middle and inferior temporal gyri (Brodmann's areas 37, 20 and 21) and into part of the inferior parietal lobule, destroying the lower sector of the supramarginal and the angular gyri (Brodmann's areas 40 and 39) (Brookshire and McNeil 2014). Conductive aphasia is caused by damage to the supra-synaptic cortex and underlying white matter, with damage to the arcuate fasciculus – the white matter pathway that connects the two main language centres, the posterior and anterior language areas: the Wernicke area and the Broca area (Catani and Mesulam 2008). Interestingly, tractography studies have demonstrated that in addition to the long direct segment connecting Wernicke's area with Broca's area, there is an indirect pathway consisting of two segments: the anterior one links Broca's territory with the inferior parietal lobule, while the posterior one links the inferior parietal lobule with Wernicke's territory (Catani and Mesulam 2008). Global aphasia is related to extensive damage to the frontal, parietal and temporal regions. Transcortical aphasia is caused by dominant-hemisphere brain damage that spares the central region (Wernicke's area, Broca's area and the arcuate fasciculus) but disconnects all or parts of the central region from the rest of the brain. Frequently, the damage may involve the angular gyrus (Brodmann's area 39) and the posterior sector of the middle temporal gyrus (Brodmann's area 37). On occasion, the lesions may extend into the lateral aspect of the occipital lobe (Brodmann's areas 18 and 19). Anomic aphasia is frequently related to lesions located exclusively in the left temporal pole (Brookshire and McNeil 2014).

Finally, primary progressive aphasia (PPA) comprises a heterogeneous group of neurodegenerative proteinopathies with diverse clinical profiles and underlying pathological substrates that share a propensity to target language networks of the human brain. There are three major variants of PPA: semantic, non-fluent/agrammatic and logopenic. In particular, the semantic variant is closely associated with TDP-43 pathology (a nuclear factor involved in regulating RNA metabolism), which determines dysfunction and atrophy of the semantic memory network, most severe in the antero-mesial temporal lobe and generally predominantly left-sided initially. The non-fluent/agrammatic variant is most often associated with primary tauopathies (characterised by abnormal metabolism of misfolded $\tau$ (tau) proteins and consecutive intracellular accumulation) that determine dysfunction and atrophy predominantly involving the left peri-Sylvian cortices centred on the inferior frontal gyrus and anterior insula. The logopenic variant is often associated with Alzheimer pathology and with dysfunction and atrophy usually involving left temporo-parietal cortices predominantly (Ruksenaite et al. 2021).

## 21.5 Neurological Diseases Causing Acquired Language Disorders

Stefano Cappa

Acquired language disorders can follow from any pathological process affecting the multiple cortical and subcortical structures involved in language function. One of the main contributions of functional neuroimaging in normal subjects engaged in language tasks has been the description of the manifold language networks, which extend beyond the classical 'language areas' of clinical neurology (Price 2012). This information is now integrated by large-scale studies of aphasic patients, taking advantage of new, advanced quantitative methods of lesion imaging (Seghier et al. 2016; Fridriksson et al. 2018). Current understanding of the neural mechanisms of language, supported by both clinical and imaging evidence, is based on the concept of multiple processing streams, subserving different aspects of language organisation. One of the more influential models (Hickok and Poeppel 2007) includes a dorsal and a ventral pathway (respectively, above and below the Sylvian fissure). The former connects, via the arcuate and superior longitudinal fasciculi, the inferior frontal gyrus (IFG) and premotor cortex to the posterior superior temporal lobe, including the planum temporale (area Spt) in the temporo-parietal junction of the Sylvian fissure. The ventral pathway involves several fibre tracts running through the extreme capsule (inferior longitudinal fasciculus, temporofrontal extreme capsule fasciculus and uncinate fasciculus) connecting the IFG with the superior temporal gyrus.

These two main pathways support different aspects of language comprehension (mapping auditory input, respectively, to meaning for the ventral pathway, and to articulation for the dorsal pathway). In the case of production, the dorsal pathway is considered to be necessary for repetition (providing auditory feedback during speech production) and for syntactic structure building (Friederici 2018). The language system is lateralised to the left hemisphere, but the right hemisphere contributes to several aspects of language processing. The ventral pathways in the Hickok and Poeppel (2007) model, responsible for accessing the mental lexicon from speech sounds, are bilaterally organised. The notion of a central role of the right hemispheric in prosodic processing has also been supported by recent studies (Friederici 2017). Additional contributions to language processing are provided by subcortical structures and the cerebellum (Mariën and Borgatti 2018).

Given the extent of the language network, it is not surprising that language disorders can be found in many neurological conditions, either as the primary clinical feature (aphasic syndromes) or as a component of the clinical presentation. In clinical practice, a crucial distinction is between (1) aphasias due to focal vascular lesions affecting the language-dominant hemisphere and (2) progressive aphasias due to neurodegeneration. Aphasic syndromes, however, can be observed in (3) many other common neurological conditions (in particular, closed head injury and tumours).

### 21.5.1 Vascular Aphasic Syndromes

The vascular aphasic syndromes have heterogeneous clinical presentations, which reflect the site and extent of cerebrovascular damage (infarction or haemorrhage). The traditional clinical classification is based on the fluency/non-fluency distinction for production (Goodglass and Kaplan 1983), on the presence or absence of auditory comprehension impairment and on the status of repetition (Abutalebi and Cappa 2008). The

Boston classification of aphasic syndromes (Benson 1979) reflects the location of damage in the language-dominant hemisphere but does not provide direct information about the brain mechanisms responsible for the different aspects of language function (Table 21.4). An in-depth analysis based on psycho-linguistic models of normal performance in specific language processes (such as word finding or sentence parsing) is the focus of the cognitive neuropsychological approach to aphasic disorders (Hillis 2002) and is required to draw inferences about the brain mechanisms responsible for specific aspects of language organisation, such as phonology, lexical semantics and morphosyntax (Friederici 2017).

### 21.5.2 Primary Progressive Aphasia Types (PPA)

Primary progressive aphasias are the consequence of neurodegenerative disorders affecting the language networks in a relatively selective way (at least in the early stages). The current classification reflects the most frequent location of brain involvement and is based on the assessment of production, comprehension and repetition abilities

**Table 21.4** Vascular aphasic syndromes (based on Abutalebi and Cappa 2008)

| Type | Production | Comprehension | Repetition |
|---|---|---|---|
| Broca | Non-fluent | + | − |
| Global | Non-fluent | − | − |
| Wernicke | Fluent | − | − |
| Conduction | Fluent | + | − |
| Transcortical motor | Non-fluent | + | + |
| Transcortical sensory | Fluent | − | + |
| Mixed transcortical | Non-fluent | − | + |
| Anomic | Fluent | + | + |

**Table 21.5** Primary progressive aphasias

| Type | Articulation | Naming | Single word comprehension | Repetition | Syntactic comprehension |
|---|---|---|---|---|---|
| Nfv | Impaired | Impaired Phonological/phonetic errors | Preserved | Impaired | Impaired |
| Sv | Normal | Impaired Semantic errors | Impaired | Preserved | Relatively preserved |
| Lpv | Slow, hesitant | Impaired Phonological errors | Preserved | Impaired | Impaired |

(Gorno-Tempini et al. 2011) (Table 21.5). There is a probabilistic relationship between the aphasic phenotype and the underlying pathological process (Spinelli et al. 2017). The non-fluent agrammatic variant (NfV) is often due to a tauopathy (Grossman 2012), the semantic variant (Sv) is usually associated with a TDP-43 pathology (Mackenzie et al. 2010) and the logopenic/phonological variant (Lv) predicts a diagnosis of atypical Alzheimer's disease (Mesulam et al. 2008). The syndromes belonging to the PPA spectrum are often familial, and about half of cases have a positive family history. Aphasia has been reported as an unusual presentation of sporadic prion disease (Johnson et al. 2013).

### 21.5.3 Language Disorders in Other Neurological Diseases

Acquired language disorders in the young age group are often a consequence of closed head injury. While classical aphasia can be observed in the case of focal damage to the language areas and their connections, the most frequent long-term clinical picture in survivors of severe head injury is an impairment of narrative abilities, due to defective organisation of discourse structure (Coelho et al. 2013).

Brain tumours affecting the language networks can also be associated with aphasia. While the clinical presentations may be similar to those of vascular aphasia, some features may be different. For example, gliomas involving the left premotor cortex and the arcuate fasciculus are more likely to cause aphasia than when infiltrating Broca's area (Bizzi et al. 2012). In general, the neoplastic compression or infiltration process is associated with slow progression and possible compensation by neighbouring structures, resulting in aphasic symptoms that are mild and aspecific (word-finding difficulties), also in the case of large space-occupying lesions (Cappa and Cipollotti 2008).

Aphasia can (infrequently) be observed in multiple sclerosis and in infectious disorders of the nervous system, especially herpes encephalitis. It has also been reported as a reversible side effect of drugs, such as Topiramate (Cappa et al. 2007) and Zonisamide.

## References

Abutalebi J, Cappa SF (2008) Language disorders. In: Cappa SF, Abutalebi J (eds) Cognitive neurology. A Clinical textbook. Oxford University Press, New York

Akhutina T (2016) Luria's classification of aphasias and its theoretical basis. Aphasiology 30(8):878–897

Al-Khindi T, Macdonald RL, Schweizer TA (2010) Cognitive and functional outcome after aneursysmal subarachnoid hemorrhage. Stroke 41(8):519–536

Ardila A (2010) A proposed reinterpretation and reclassification of aphasic syndromes. Aphasiology 24(3):363–394

Bartlett CL, Pashek GV (1994) Taxonomic theory and practical implications in aphasia classification. Aphasiology 8:103–126

Basso A (2003) Aphasia and its therapy. Oxford University Press, New York

Benson DF (1979) Aphasia, alexia and agraphia. Churchill Livingstone, New York

Benson DF, Ardila A (1996) Aphasia: a clinical perspective. Oxford University Press, New York

Berthier ML, Pulvermüller F, Dávila G et al (2011) Drug therapy of post-stroke aphasia: a review of current evidence. Neuropsychol Rev 21(3):302–317

Bizzi A, Nava S, Ferrè F et al (2012) Aphasia induced by gliomas growing in the ventrolateral frontal region: assessment with diffusion MR tractography, functional MR imaging and neuropsychology. Cortex 48(2):255–272

Bobba U, Munivenkatappa A, Agrawal A (2019) Speech and language dysfunctions in patients with cerebrocortical disorders admitted in a neurosurgical unit. Asian J Neurosurg 14(1):87–89

Brookshire RH, McNeil MR (2014) Introduction to neurogenic communication disorders, 8th edn. Mosby, St Louis

Buckingham HW (2010) Aristotle's functional association psychology. The syntagmatic and the paradigmatic axes in the neurolinguistics of Roman Jakobson and Alexander Luria: an anatomical and functional quagmire. Aphasiology 24(3):395–403

Cappa SF (2011) The neural basis of aphasia rehabilitation: evidence from neuroimaging and neurostimulation. Neuropsychol Rehabil 21(5):742–754

Cappa SF, Cipollotti L (2008) Cognitive and behavioural disorders associated with space occupying lesions. Cognitive neurology. A clinical textbook. Oxford University Press, New York, pp 161–182

Cappa SF, Orteli P, Garibotto V et al (2007) Reversible nonfluent aphasia and left frontal hypoperfusion during topiramate treatment. Epilepsy Behav 10(1):192–194

Catani M, Mesulam M (2008) The arcuate fasciculus and the disconnection theme in language and aphasia: history and current state. Cortex 44(8):953–961

Chaudhuri A, Kennedy PG (2002) Diagnosis and treatment of viral encephalitis. Postgrad Med J 78(924):575–583

Cherney LR, Small SL (2009) Aphasia, apraxia of speech, and dysarthria. In: Stein J et al (eds) Stroke recovery and rehabilitation. Demos Medical, New York, pp 155–182

Christman SS, Buckingham HW, Sneed KE (2017) Cognitive-communication disorder. In: Kreutzer J et al (eds) Encyclopedia of clinical neuropsychology. Springer, Cham

Clough S, Gordon JK (2020) Fluent or nonfluent? Part A. Underlying contributors to categorical classifications of fluency in aphasia. Aphasiology 34:515–539

Coelho C, Lê A, Mozeiko J et al (2013) Characterizing discourse deficits following penetrating head injury. Am J Speech Lang Pathol 22(2):S438–S448

Crinion J, Holland AL, Copland DA et al (2013) Neuroimaging in aphasia treatment research: quantifying brain lesions after stroke. NeuroImage 73:208–214

Croquelois A, Bogousslavsky J (2011) Stroke aphasia: 1500 consecutive cases. Cerebrovasc Dis 31(4):392–399

Crosson B, Rodriguez AD, Copland D et al (2019) Neuroplasticity and aphasia treatments: new approaches for an old problem. J Neurol Neurosurg Psychiatry 90(10):1147–1155

Davis GA (2007) Cognitive pragmatics of language disorders in adults. Semin Speech Lang 28(2):111–121

Davis LE (2018) Acute bacterial meningitis. Continuum (Minneap Minn) 24(5):1264–1283

Duffy JR (2005) Motor speech disorders. Substrates, differential diagnosis, and management, 3rd edn. Elsevier Mosby, St. Louis

Efstratiadous EA, Chelas EN, Ignatiou M et al (2012) Quality of life after stroke: evaluation of the Greek SAQOL-39g. Folia Phoniatr Logop 64(4):179–186

Ellis C, Simpson AN, Bonilha H et al (2012) The one-year attributable cost of poststroke aphasia. Stroke 43(5):1429–1431

El-Tallawy HN, Gad AHES, Ali AM et al (2019) Relative frequency and prognosis of vascular aphasia (follow-up at 3 months) in the Neurology Department of Assiut University Hospital. Egypt J Neurol Psychiatry Neurosurg 55:41. https://doi.org/10.1186/s41983-019-0086-7

Engelter ST, Gostynski M, Papa S et al (2006) Epidemiology of aphasia attributable to first ischemic stroke: incidence, severity, fluency, etiology, and thrombolysis. Stroke 37(6):1379–1384

Finch E, Copland DA (2014) Language outcomes following neurosurgery for brain tumours: a systematic review. NeuroRehabilitation 34(3):499–514

Fitzgerald A, Aditya H, Prior A et al (2010) Anoxic brain injury: clinical patterns and functional outcomes. A study of 93 cases. Brain Inj 24(11):1311–1323

Fridriksson J, den Ouden DB, Hillis AE et al (2018) Anatomy of aphasia revisited. Brain 141(3):848–862

Friederici AD (2017) Language in our brain. MIT Press, Cambridge, MA

Friederici AD (2018) The neural basis for human syntax: Broca's area and beyond. Curr Opin Behav Sci 21:88–92

Galletta EE, Barrett AM (2014) Impairment and functional interventions for aphasia: having it all. Curr Phys Med Rehabil Rep 2:114–120

Goodglass H, Kaplan E (1983) Assessment of aphasia and related disorders. Lea and Febiger, Philadelphia

Gorno-Tempini ML, Hillis AE, Weintraub S et al (2011) Classification of primary progressive aphasia and its variants. Neurology 76(11):1006–1014

Grabias S, Kurkowski M (2012) Speech therapy—theory of speech disorders. UMCS, Maria Curie-Sklodowska University, Lublin

Grochmal-Bach B, Pachalska M, Markiewicz K et al (2009) Rehabilitation of a patient with aphasia due to severe traumatic brain injury. Med Sci Monit 15(4):67–76

Grossman M (2012) The non-fluent/agrammatic variant of primary progressive aphasia. Lancet Neurol 11(6):545–555

Hagoort P (2013) MUC (memory, unification, control) and beyond. Front Psychol 4:416. https://doi.org/10.3389/fpsyg.2013.00416. Accessed 13 Aug 2021

Hickok G, Poeppel D (2007) The cortical organization of speech processing. Nat Rev Neurosci 8(5):393–402

Hillis AE (2002) The handbook of adult language disorders. Psychology Press, New York

Hills AE, Wityk RJ, Beauchamp NJ et al (2004) Perfusion-weighted MRI as a marker of response to treatment in acute and subacute stroke. Neuroradiology 46(1):31–39

Hoffmann M, Chen R (2013) The spectrum of aphasia subtypes and etiology in subacute stroke. J Stroke Cerebrovasc Dis 22(8):1385–1392

Hu XY, Zhang T, Rajah GB et al (2018) Effects of different frequencies of repetitive transcranial magnetic stimulation in stroke patients with non-fluent aphasia: a randomized, sham-controlled study. Neurol Res 40(6):459–465

IJzerman-Korevaar M, Snijders TJ, de Graeff A et al (2018) Prevalence of symptoms in glioma patients throughout the disease trajectory: a systematic review. J Neuro-Oncol 140(3):485–496

Johnson DY, Dunkelberger DL, Henry M et al (2013) Sporadic Jakob-Creutzfeldt disease presenting as primary progressive aphasia. JAMA Neurol 70(2):254–257

Josephs KA, Duffy JR, Strand EA et al (2006) Clinicopathological and imaging correlates of progressive aphasia and apraxia of speech. Brain 129(6):1385–1398

Josephs KA, Whitwell JL, Duffy JR et al (2008) Progressive aphasia secondary to Alzheimer disease vs FTLD pathology. Neurology 70(1):25–34

Kauhanen ML, Korpelainen JT, Hiltunen P et al (2000) Aphasia, depression, and non-verbal cognitive impairment in ischemic stroke. Cerebrovasc Dis 10:455–461

Khedr EM, Abbass MA, Soliman RK et al (2020) A hospital-based study of post-stroke aphasia: frequency, risk factors, and topographic representation. Egypt J Neurol Psychiatry Neurosurg 56:2. https://doi.org/10.1186/s41983-019-0128-1

Kim WJ, Yang EJ, Paik NJ (2013) Neural substrate responsible for crossed aphasia. J Korean Med Sci 28(10):1529–1533

Kirshner KS (2016a) Aphasia and aphasic syndromes. In: Daroff R et al (eds) Bradley's neurology in clinical practice, 7th edn. Elsevier, London, pp 123–144

Kirshner KS (2016b) Dysarthria and apraxia of speech. In: Daroff R et al (eds) Bradley's neurology in clinical practice, 7th edn. Elsevier, London, pp 145–147

Klippi A, Sellman J, Heikkinen P et al (2012) Current clinical practices in aphasia therapy in Finland: challenges in moving towards national best practice. Folia Phoniatr Logop 64(4):169–178

Kolb B, Whishaw IQ (2003) Fundamentals of human neuropsychology, 6th edn. Worth publishers, New York, p 502. 505, 511

Le H, Lui MY (2023) Aphasia. In: StatPearls [Internet]. Treasure Island (FL): StatPearls Publishing; 2024 Jan-. Available from: https://www.ncbi.nlm.nih.gov/books/NBK559315/

Mackenzie IR, Neumann M, Bigio H et al (2010) Nomenclature and nosology for neuropathologic subtypes of frontotemporal lobar degeneration: an update. Acta Neuropathol 119(1):1–4

Mariën P, Borgatti R (2018) Language and the cerebellum. In: Handbook of clinical neurology, vol 154. Elsevier, Philadelphia, pp 181–202

Marien P, Engelborghs S, Pickut B et al (2000) Aphasia following cerebellar damage: fact or fallacy? J Neurolinguist 13(2–3):145–171

Marshall J (2010) Classification of aphasia: are there benefits for practice? Aphasiology 24(3):408–412

Matías-Guiu JA, García-Ramos R (2013) Primary progressive aphasia: from syndrome to disease. Neurologia 28:366–374

McNeil MR (2008) Clinical managenents of sensorimotor speech disorders, 2nd edn. Thieme Medical Publisher Inc, New York

Meschia JF, Bushnell C, Boden-Albala B et al (2016) Guidelines for the primary prevention of stroke: a statement for healthcare professionals from the American Heart Association/American Stroke Association. Stroke 45(12):3754–3832

Mesulam M (2001) Primary progressive aphasia. Ann Neurol 49:425–432

Mesulam MM (2016) Aphasia, memory loss, and other focal cerebral disorders. In: Hauser S, Josephson SA (eds) Harrison's neurology in clinical medicine, 3rd edn. McGraw-Hill Education/Medical, New York, pp 142–156

Mesulam M, Wicklund A, Johnson N et al (2008) Alzheimer and frontotemporal pathology in sub-

sets of primary progressive aphasia. Ann Neurol 63(6):709–719

Mitchell C, Gittins M, Tyson S et al (2020) Prevalence of aphasia and dysarthria among inpatient stroke survivors: describing the population, therapy provision and outcomes on discharge. Aphasiology 32(Supp1):145–146

Mitchell C, Gittins M, Tyson S et al (2021) Prevalence of aphasia and dysarthria among inpatient stroke survivors: describing the population, therapy provision and outcomes on discharge. Aphasiology 35(7):950–960

Mnatsakanyan L, Vadera S, Ingalls CW et al (2018) Language recovery after epilepsy surgery of the Broca's area. Epilepsy Behav Case Rep 9:42–45

Mohr B (2017) Neuroplasticity and functional recovery after intensive language therapy in chronic post stroke aphasia: which factors are relevant? Front Hum Neurosci 11:332. https://doi.org/10.3389/fnhum.2017.00332

Nasios G, Dardiotis E, Messinis L (2019) From Broca and Wernicke to the neuromodulation era: insights of brain language networks for neurorehabilitation. Behav Neurol 9894571:1. https://doi.org/10.1155/2019/9894571

O'Sullivan M, Brownsett S, Copland D (2019) Language and language disorders: neuroscience to clinical practice. Pract Neurol 19(5):380–388

Papathanasiou I, Coppens P, Potagas C (2013) Aphasia and related neurogenic communication disorders. Jones and Barlett Learning, Burlington (MA)

Pedersena PM, Vinterb K, Olsenc TS (2004) Aphasia after stroke: type, severity and prognosis. Cerebrovasc Dis 17:35–43

Price CJ (2012) A review and synthesis of the first 20 years of PET and fMRI studies of heard speech, spoken language and reading. NeuroImage 62(2):816–847

Pulvermüller F, Berthier ML (2008) Aphasia therapy on a neuroscience basis. Aphasiology 22(6):563–599

Purves D, Augustine GJ, Fitzpatrick D et al (eds) (2018) Neuroscience, 6th edn. Oxford University Press, New York

Qiu JQ, Cui Y, Sun LC et al (2017) Aphasic status epilepticus as the sole symptom of epilepsy: a case report and literature review. Exp Ther Med 14(4):3501–3506

Rogers M (2004) Aphasia, primary progressive. In: Kent RD (ed) The MIT encyclopedia of communication disorders. MIT Press, Cambridge, MA, pp 245–249

Ruksenaite J, Volkmer A, Jiang J et al (2021) Primary progressive aphasia: toward a pathophysiological synthesis. Curr Neurol Neurosci Rep 21(3):7. https://doi.org/10.1007/s11910-021-01097-z

Schindler A, Miletto AM (2005) (eds) Il paziente afasico. Valutazione multifattoriale. Omega edn. Torino

Schoeman R, Van der Merwe G (2010) Aphasia, an acquired language disorder. SA Fam Prac 52(4):308–311

Seghier ML, Patel E, Prejawa S et al (2016) The PLORAS database: a data repository for predicting language outcome and recovery after stroke. NeuroImage 124(B):1208–1212

Sinanović O, Mrkonjić Z, Zukić S et al (2011) Post-stroke language disorders. Acta Clin Croat 50(1):79–94

Spinelli EG, Mandelli ML, Miller ZA et al (2017) Typical and atypical pathology in primary progressive aphasia variants. Ann Neurol 81(3):430–443

Sul B, Kim JS, Hong BJ et al (2016) The prognosis and recovery of aphasia related to stroke lesion. Ann Rehabil Med 40(5):786–793

Tee BL, Gorno-Tempini ML (2019) Primary progressive aphasia: a model for neurodegenerative disease. Curr Opin Neurol 32(2):255–265

Tesak J, Code C (2008) The older history of aphasia. In: Milestones in the history of aphasia: theories and protagonists. Psychology Press, New York, pp 3–17

Tippett DC, Niparko JK, Hillis AE (2014) Aphasia: current concepts in theory and practice. J Neurol Transl Neurosci 2(1):1042. PMID: 24904925; PMCID: PMC4041294

Tremblay P, Dick AS (2016) Broca and Wernicke are dead, or moving past the classic model of language neurobiology. Brain Lang 162:60–71

van Dun K, Mariën P (2016) Cerebellar-induced aphasia and related language disorders. In: Mariën P, Manto M (eds) The linguistic cerebellum. Academic Press Elsevier, London, pp 107–134

Viader F (2015) The classification of aphasias: a brief history. Rev Neuropsychol 1(1):5–14

Wilson MA, Martínez-Cuitiño M, Joanette Y (2009) An instrument to quickly and reliably classify aphasic patients' symptoms in syndromes based on cognitive assessments. Psychol Neurosci 2(2):157–162

Wilson SM, Eriksson DK, Brandt TH et al (2019) Patterns of recovery from aphasia in the first 2 weeks after stroke. J Speech Lang Hear Res 62(3):723–732

# Special Kinds of Aphasia

# 22

Philippe Paquier

## 22.1 Aphasia in Children

Philippe F. Paquier

### 22.1.1 Introduction

The term *aphasia* when used with reference to a paediatric population denotes three pathological conditions: congenital aphasia, developmental aphasia and acquired aphasia. *Aphasia* does not cover language impairments associated with predominant behavioural disorders (e.g., autism spectrum disorder, attention deficit hyperactivity disorder, psychosis), basic sensory deficits (e.g., deafness), syndromic and non-syndromic intellectual disability of genetic origin (e.g., Down syndrome, consanguinity with autosomal recessive non-syndromic intellectual disability), major environmental or language deprivation (e.g., child abuse and neglect, feral children).

### 22.1.2 Congenital Aphasia

Congenital aphasia refers to a language disorder that is a consequence of significant pre-, peri- or early post-natal damage to the brain structures responsible for language. Because of the early disruption of brain mechanisms crucial for language acquisition, children with congenital aphasia fail to develop normal linguistic functions (e.g., Pizzamiglio et al. 2004; Northam et al. 2018). However, the concept of congenital aphasia is a disputed one, as several studies have shown that infants with congenital unilateral brain injuries are capable—if they do not develop epilepsy—of attaining language abilities that are well within the normal range, that is, they are not clinically aphasic (Bates 1999). This resilience to early brain damage has been explained by a significant degree of post-lesional neuroplasticity (Aram 1999), of which an extreme example is represented by the transfer of language functions to the right hemisphere in the case of an early left hemisphere lesion (Hertz-Pannier 1999). Furthermore, Staudt et al. (2002) have shown in patients with early left brain injury that right hemisphere recruitment for language during an fMRI word generation task occurs in brain regions that are homotopic to the left hemisphere areas involved in language processing under normal circumstances. Such a pattern of right hemisphere language (re)organisation after early left brain lesion has been explained by the hypotheses of equi-potentiality and of progressive lateralisation (Basser 1962; Lenneberg 1967).

The hypothesis of equi-potentiality states that during the first 2 years of life, cerebral dominance for language is not well established, and that

P. Paquier (✉)
Clinical Neurolinguistics & Aphasiology, Brussels Center for Language Studies, Vrije Universiteit Brussels, Brussels, Belgium
e-mail: philippe.paquier@vub.be

© The Author(s), under exclusive license to Springer Nature Switzerland AG 2025
A. am Zehnhoff-Dinnesen et al. (eds.), *Phoniatrics III*, European Manual of Medicine,
https://doi.org/10.1007/978-3-031-48091-1_7

throughout that time the two hemispheres simultaneously play an equally active role in language processing. The hypothesis of progressive lateralisation claims that subsequently right hemisphere involvement in language processing progressively decreases with age, resulting in the gradual transfer of most language functions towards the left hemisphere until puberty, the age at which the process of language lateralisation is assumed to be completed. These hypotheses predict that the right hemisphere has full potential for assuming control of language in case of early left hemisphere injury.

Despite the dramatic capacity to shift language functions to the opposite hemisphere (François et al. 2016; Lidzba et al. 2017a), it nevertheless appears that the right hemisphere is not capable of fully accommodating language functions after early left hemisphere damage. Using fMRI, Beharelle et al. (2010) have indeed shown that left hemisphere regions remain critical for language in the face of early left focal brain injury, even when there is a right hemisphere takeover of language functions. Their findings are supportive of a strong ontogenetic predisposition of left brain regions for the maturation of linguistic functions. Their suggestion probably also accounts for the observation that in cases of early left hemispherectomy—the ultimate instance of unilateral brain damage—the sole right hemisphere does not appear to be sufficient to ensure full-blown linguistic proficiency (Danelli et al. 2013). Taken together, these and other observations (e.g., Aram 1999; Lidzba et al. 2017b) challenge the hypotheses of equi-potentiality and of progressive lateralisation by demonstrating that early left brain damage leads to subtle but clinically relevant linguistic sequelae and does not permit high level linguistic skills to develop normally.

### 22.1.3 Developmental Aphasia

Developmental aphasia, also termed *dysphasia*, *specific language impairment* (SLI) and *developmental language disorder* (DLD), is typically diagnosed when, for no obvious reason, a child fails to develop normal language skills despite adequate non-verbal intelligence, hearing acuity, neurological condition, psycho-emotional development and

environmental or language stimulation (Bishop and Adams 1992). Recent advances in the study of developmental language disorders, however, indicate that a definition of dysphasia that includes the notion of 'no known neurological deficits' (Weismer 2013) is no longer tenable. For instance, in a subgroup of children with dysphasia, the occurrence of sleep electro-encephalographic abnormalities (i.e. spike-and-wave activation in sleep, SWAS, formerly known as continuous spikes and waves during slow sleep, CSWS), which can also be observed in children with acquired epileptic aphasia (Landau-Kleffner syndrome), suggests the existence of a spectrum of nocturnal epileptiform activity and language impairment that ranges from dysphasia at one end to acquired epileptic aphasia at the most affected other (Billard et al. 2009; Overvliet et al. 2010). On the other hand, the discovery of cyto-architectonic brain abnormalities (e.g., cortical dysplasia, grey matter heterotopias) in children with dysphasia (Cohen et al. 1989; Preis et al. 1998), along with the demonstration of cerebral and cerebellar SPECT-perfusion defects (Oki et al. 1999; Tzourio et al. 1994) and of structural anomalies of the language connectome (Vydrova et al. 2015) in individuals with dysphasia, also points to a neuronal involvement in the cause of developmental language disorders. Finally, the last main strand of research by means of linkage studies and molecular genetic analyses has brought to the fore that in some instances of inherited developmental speech and language disorders, the language deficit is associated with functional and structural brain anomalies (Watkins et al. 1999, 2002). Collectively, these observations suggest that a clear distinction between dysphasia and congenital aphasia is no longer maintainable in all aspects.

### 22.1.4 Acquired Aphasia

Acquired childhood aphasia (ACA) pertains to a childhood language disorder caused by an identified, non-congenital brain injury that is sustained after onset of language acquisition, and that disrupts already developed language skills. Whereas in congenital aphasia and dysphasia the—identified or unknown—pathological process that hinders language acquisition is already present before language starts to emerge, in ACA, on the contrary, the pathological process that compromises language is sustained after a period of language development.

Since the first elaborated studies on ACA published in the nineteenth century, and for over more than 100 years, ACA has traditionally been considered a non-fluent aphasia irrespective of lesion location and characterised by rapid and dramatic recovery abilities (Paquier and Van Dongen 1998). In their landmark paper on childhood aphasia, however, Woods and Teuber (1978) presented several conclusions that were inconsistent with the classical teaching on ACA. Since then, ACA has been acknowledged to display an adult-like heterogeneity of aphasia syndromes, to exhibit adult-like anatomo-clinical correlations between aphasia syndrome and aphasiogenic lesion locations (Paquier and Van Dongen 1996), to be mainly related to left brain lesions—that is, crossed aphasia in dextral children is as rare as in adults (Mariën et al. 2004), and to be particularly prone to an incomplete recovery from aphasia that entails subtle but persistent language sequelae, future academic failure and incapacitating socio-professional problems (Martins 2004). Chilosi et al. (2008) introduced the term 'illusory recovery' to denote these deleterious repercussions present many years after onset of aphasia in spite of a spuriously good clinical recovery.

It appears that at least five—often interdependent—variables convey prognostic value as to the outcome of ACA: age at lesion onset, aphasia type, aetiology, lesion site, lesion size (see Paquier and Van Dongen (1996) for a critical discussion). Of these, the role of age at lesion onset has undoubtedly spawned the hottest debate, since the traditional claim that unilateral aphasiogenic lesions acquired before puberty do not leave any permanent language sequelae (cf. hypotheses of equi-potentiality and of progressive lateralisation). Martins (2004) could not confirm the prognostic value of age at onset but underscored the role of language-related and lesion-related variables in the recovery process. Chilosi et al. (2008) reconsidered the role of age at onset by proposing that long-term linguistic deficits might be the consequence of the absence of consolidated representations of complex linguistic knowledge in the young brain. In this respect, Rowan et al. (2007)

revealed degeneration of cortico-subcortical pathways in children who had sustained an arterial ischaemic stroke confined to the basal ganglia at a very young age. This process might well be responsible for the delayed appearance of linguistic difficulties at the age that written language is acquired (Gout et al. 2005), and might explain why younger children are more vulnerable to the effects of early subcortical strokes—hence, why prognosis is less favourable in preschool children than school-age children.

The relationship between age at lesion onset and outcome of ACA remains an abstruse question. Although left brain lesions sustained later in life are less likely to lead to an inter-hemispheric transfer of language skills than early lesions (Müller et al. 1999; Lidzba et al. 2017b), evidence for a right hemispheric takeover of language functions can nevertheless be suggested in some children who become aphasic at or after puberty (Elkana et al. 2011)—as documented in adults as well (e.g., Belin et al. 1996; Pillai 2010). However, increased right hemisphere involvement in language tasks, as shown by fMRI, does not seem to be a marker of successful or adequate recovery from aphasia. Elkana et al. (2011) found in children who sustained brain injury after language acquisition, that better recovery from aphasia was linked to more left than right lateralisation of fMRI activations in anterior and posterior language regions, as found in adults. In addition, in one child scanned twice, 3 years apart, these authors could establish that the improvement in her language skills over time was associated with a substantial reduction of right hemisphere fMRI activation rather than with a prominent increase in left hemisphere fMRI activation. Elkana et al. (2011) thus corroborated the findings in adults of Saur et al. (2006) and Pillai (2010) that effective language recovery is principally related to ipsilateral adaptive changes with only a subservient contribution from contralateral homotopic regions. Poorer recovery from aphasia appears to be correlated with greater right hemisphere than perilesional left hemisphere fMRI activation (Lidzba et al. 2017b), suggesting that increased right hemispheric recruitment might well be the reflection of maladaptive plasticity. In sum, these recent findings are clearly at variance with the traditional teaching on hemispheric equi-potentiality for language.

## 22.1.5 Conclusion

Children with developmental or acquired language disorders display a variety of linguistic deficits, which may range from the subtle but clinically relevant to the quite severe. The origin of the language impairment can be related to congenital brain damage (congenital aphasia) or brain injury acquired later in life (acquired aphasia), but a primary language acquisition failure of unknown origin can also account for a developmental language disorder (developmental aphasia or dysphasia). Recent advances in structural and functional brain imaging, modern electrophysiology and molecular genetics suggest an overlap between neuro-developmental language disorders and congenital aphasia. Traditional, quite optimistic views on the almost unlimited potential for neuroplastic accommodation of language functions in the case of focal and circumscribed paediatric brain damage, leading to well-flourished language skills given an early lesion, or to complete recovery from aphasia given injury acquired later in life, have been seriously tempered by contemporary knowledge. Apart from the nature of the lesion, it is clear that other lesion-related and language-related variables act on the recovery process. Further insights into the neurobiology of developmental and acquired childhood language disorders will unquestionably improve our diagnostic and therapeutic intervention strategies.

## References

Aram DM (1999) Neuroplasticity: evidence from unilateral brain lesions in children. In: Broman SH, Fletcher JM (eds) The changing nervous system: neurobehavioral consequences of early brain disorders. Oxford University Press, New York, pp 254–273

Basser LS (1962) Hemiplegia of early onset and the faculty of speech with special reference to the effects of hemispherectomy. Brain 85:427–460

Bates E (1999) Plasticity, localization, and language development. In: Broman SH, Fletcher JM (eds) The changing nervous system: neurobehavioral consequences of early brain disorders. Oxford University Press, New York, pp 214–253

Beharelle AR, Dick AS, Josse G et al (2010) Left hemisphere regions are critical for language in the face of early left focal brain injury. Brain 133(6):1707–1716

Belin P, Van Eeckhout P, Zilbovicius M et al (1996) Recovery from nonfluent aphasia after melodic intonation therapy: a PET study. Neurology 47(6):1504–1511

Billard C, Fluss J, Pinton F (2009) Specific language impairment versus Landau-Kleffner syndrome. Epilepsia 50(Suppl 7):21–24

Bishop DVM, Adams C (1992) Comprehension problems in children with specific language impairment: literal and inferential meaning. J Speech Hear Res 35(1):119–129

Chilosi AM, Cipriani P, Pecini C et al (2008) Acquired focal brain lesions in childhood: effects on development and reorganization of language. Brain Lang 106(3):211–225

Cohen M, Campbell R, Yaghmai F (1989) Neuropathological abnormalities in developmental dysphasia. Ann Neurol 25(6):567–570

Danelli L, Cossu G, Berlingeri M et al (2013) Is a lone right hemisphere enough? Neurolinguistic architecture in a case with a very early left hemispherectomy. Neurocase 19(3):209–231

Elkana O, Frost R, Kramer U et al (2011) Cerebral reorganization as a function of linguistic recovery in children: an fMRI study. Cortex 47(2):202–216

François C, Ripollés P, Bosch L et al (2016) Language learning and brain reorganization in a 3.5-year-old child with left perinatal stroke revealed using structural and functional connectivity. Cortex 77:95–118

Gout A, Seibel N, Rouvière C et al (2005) Aphasia owing to subcortical brain infarcts in childhood. J Child Neurol 20(12):1003–1008

Hertz-Pannier L (1999) Brain plasticity during development: physiological bases and fMRI approach. J Neuroradiol 26(Suppl 1):66–74

Lenneberg E (1967) Biological foundations of language. John Wiley, New York

Lidzba K, de Haan B, Wilke M et al (2017a) Lesion characteristics driving right-hemispheric language reorganization in congenital left-hemispheric brain damage. Brain Lang 173:1–9

Lidzba K, Küpper H, Kluger G et al (2017b) The time window for successful right-hemispheric language reorganization in children. Eur J Paediatr Neurol 21(5):715–721

Mariën P, Paquier P, Engelborghs S et al (2004) Crossed aphasia in children. In: Fabbro F (ed) Neurogenic language disorders in children. Elsevier, Amsterdam, pp 147–180

Martins IP (2004) Persistent acquired childhood aphasia. In: Fabbro F (ed) Neurogenic language disorders in children. Elsevier, Amsterdam, pp 231–251

Müller RA, Rothermel RD, Behen ME et al (1999) Language organization in patients with early and late left-hemisphere lesion: a PET study. Neuropsychologia 37(5):545–557

Northam GB, Adler S, Eschmann KCJ et al (2018) Developmental conduction aphasia after neonatal stroke. Ann Neurol 83(4):664–667

Oki J, Takahashi S, Miyamoto A et al (1999) Cerebellar hypoperfusion and developmental dysphasia in a male. Pediatr Neurol 21(4):745–748

Overvliet GM, Besseling RMH, Vles JSH et al (2010) Nocturnal epileptiform EEG discharges, nocturnal epileptic seizures, and language impairments in children: review of the literature. Epilepsy Behav 19(4):550–558

Paquier P, Van Dongen HR (1996) Review of research on the clinical presentation of acquired childhood aphasia. Acta Neurol Scand 93(6):428–436

Paquier P, Van Dongen HR (1998) Is acquired childhood aphasia atypical? In: Coppens P et al (eds) Aphasia in atypical populations. Lawrence Erlbaum Associates, Mahwah, pp 67–115

Pillai JJ (2010) Insights into adult postlesional language cortical plasticity provided by cerebral blood oxygen level–dependent functional MR imaging. Am J Neuroradiol 31(6):990–996

Pizzamiglio MR, Piccardi L, Nasti M et al (2004) Language disorder in a child with early left thalamic lesion. Neurocase 10(4):308–315

Preis S, Engelbrecht V, Huang Y et al (1998) Focal grey matter heterotopias in monozygotic twins with developmental language disorder. Eur J Pediatr 157:849–852

Rowan A, Vargha-Khadem F, Calamante F et al (2007) Cortical abnormalities and language function in young patients with basal ganglia stroke. NeuroImage 36(2):431–440

Saur D, Lange R, Baumgaertner A et al (2006) Dynamics of language reorganization after stroke. Brain 129(6):1371–1384

Staudt M, Lidzba K, Grodd W et al (2002) Right-hemispheric organization of language following early left-sided brain lesions: functional MRI topography. NeuroImage 16(4):954–967

Tzourio N, Heim A, Zilbovicius M et al (1994) Abnormal regional CBF response in left hemisphere of dysphasic children during a language task. Pediatr Neurol 10(1):20–26

Vydrova R, Komarek V, Sanda J et al (2015) Structural alterations of the language connectome in children with specific language impairment. Brain Lang 151:35–41

Watkins KE, Gadian DG, Vargha-Khadem F (1999) Functional and structural brain abnormalities associated with a genetic disorder of speech and language. Am J Hum Genet 65(5):1215–1221

Watkins KE, Vargha-Khadem F, Ashburner J et al (2002) MRI analysis of an inherited speech and language disorder: structural brain abnormalities. Brain 125(3):465–478

Weismer SE (2013) Developmental language disorders: challenges and implications of cross-group comparisons. Folia Phoniatr Logop 65(2):68–77

Woods BT, Teuber HL (1978) Changing patterns of childhood aphasia. Ann Neurol 3(3):273–280

# Special Kinds of Acquired Language Disorders: Aphasia

Edoardo Nicolò Aiello, Sue Berger, Stefano Cappa, Teresa Difonzo, Anne Escher, Lisa Gerhards, Kristina Jonas, Andrea Marini, Fanny Meneguzzi, Rossella Muò, Jana Quinting, and Stefano Zago

**Supplementary Information** The online version contains supplementary material available at https://doi.org/10.1007/978-3-031-48091-1_8.

E. N. Aiello (✉)
Department of Neurology and Laboratory Neuroscience, Istituto Auxologico Italiano IRCCS, Milan, Italy
e-mail: e.aiello@auxologico.it

S. Berger · A. Escher
Department of Occupational Therapy, Boston University, Boston, USA
e-mail: sueb@bu.edu; aaescher@bu.edu

S. Cappa
Institute for Advanced Studies, University of Pavia, Pavia, Italy
e-mail: stefano.cappa@isspavia.it

T. Difonzo · S. Zago
Neurology Unit, IRCCS Fondazione Ca' Granda Ospedale Maggiore Policlinico, Milan, Italy
e-mail: teresa.difonzo@policlinico.mi.it; stefano.zago@unimi.it

L. Gerhards · J. Quinting
Department of Special Education and Rehabilitation, University of Cologne, Cologne, Germany
e-mail: lisa.gerhards@uni-koeln.de; jana.quinting@uni-koeln.de

K. Jonas
Department of Special Educational Needs in Language and Communication, Paderborn University, Paderborn, Germany
e-mail: kristina.jonas@uni-paderborn.de

A. Marini · F. Meneguzzi
Department of Languages and Literatures, Communication, Education and Society, University of Udine, Udine, Italy
e-mail: andrea.marini@uniud.it

R. Muò
Recupero e Rieducazione Funzionale, ASL Città di Torino, Turin, Italy
e-mail: rossella.muo@unito.it

## 23.1 New Developments on Language Assessment in Aphasia: From Traditional Assessment to Multilevel Analyses of Narrative Discourse

Andrea Marini and Fanny Meneguzzi

### 23.1.1 Introduction

This section focuses on language assessment in people with aphasia (PWA) after stroke. Importantly, we limit the discussion to such patients and do not extend it to the assessment of language in patients with aphasia due to neurodegenerative processes (i.e., primary progressive aphasia), traumatic brain injury or other causes.

A large percentage of stroke patients experiences language difficulties (Rohde et al. 2018). This means that the potential presence of aphasia, its type and gravity must be adequately assessed to guide both diagnosis and rehabilitation. Growing evidence suggests that language processing is a complex cognitive function that is implemented in an extensive neural network (e.g., Indefrey 2011; Piervincenzi et al. 2016) and consists of a micro-linguistic and a macro-linguistic dimension (Glosser and Deser 1990; Marini et al. 2005). The former allows individuals to organise phonemes into morphological strings and words (i.e., lexical processing) and generate the syntactic context required by each word (i.e., morpho-syntactic processing) for the generation of well-formed sentences (i.e., syntactic processing). The macro-linguistic dimension, on the other hand, selects the contextually appropriate meaning of a word or a sentence within a given context (i.e., pragmatic processing) and allows speakers to integrate utterances in a coherent discourse (i.e., discourse processing). Importantly, this complex infrastructure relies on the multifaceted interaction between different cognitive systems (e.g., memory, attention, perception, motor control) and executive functions (such as inhibition, updating, planning, and monitoring) (Miyake et al. 2000; Diamond 2013).

This complexity suggests that an accurate language assessment is not a simple procedure but a dynamic process that requires well-trained expert clinicians (e.g., neuropsychologists, speech-language therapists) using tests with solid psychometric properties (e.g., test-retest reliability, internal consistency, sensitivity, specificity: Murray and Coppens 2013, Salter et al. 2006, Streiner and Norman 2000). In this section, a brief overview of some of the more common batteries of tests used for language assessment will be provided. It will also include a discussion of the usefulness of multilevel procedures of discourse analysis for both diagnosis and rehabilitation.

### 23.1.2 An Overview of Some of the Major Batteries of Tests for Language Assessment in People with Aphasia

Since the seminal descriptions by Paul Broca (1861) and Carl Wernicke (1874), language assessment has mainly focused on a limited range of micro-linguistic skills (e.g., phonological, morphological, semantic, and syntactic), while neglecting the macro-linguistic dimension. Nonetheless, over time both informal and formal procedures have been developed to gather relevant information about the patients' linguistic and cognitive skills in the broader context of their social context, spontaneous recovery, and psychological distress (e.g., Murray and Coppens 2013; Vogel et al. 2010). Obviously, such procedures vary depending on whether the patient is still in the acute/subacute (Kiran 2012) or chronic (Hillis 2005) phase after the stroke.

In the acute stage after the lesion, PWA show unstable clinical characteristics that significantly affect their attention. For this reason, the assessment in the acute phase must be performed in a reasonably short amount of time (ideally, not exceeding 30 minutes: Lapointe and Stierwalt 2018). A number of batteries of tests have been developed for bedside linguistic assessment. They include the Frenchay Aphasia Screening Test (FAST, Enderby and Crow 1996; Language:

Different languages; Administration time: 10 minutes), the Language Screening Tool (LAST, Flamand-Roze et al. 2011; Language: French, German; Administration time: 2 minutes), the ScreeLing (Doesborgh et al. 2003; Language: Dutch; Administration time: 30 minutes), the Mississippi Aphasia Screening Test (MAST; Nakase-Thompson et al. 2005; Languages: English, Czech, Spanish; Administration time: 5–10 minutes), the Acute Aphasia Screening Protocol (AASP, Crary et al. 1989; Language: English; Administration time: 10 minutes), the Ullevaal Aphasia Screening test (UAS, Thommessen et al. 1999; Language: Norwegian; Administration time: 5–15 minutes), the Esame del linguaggio a letto del malato (ELLM, Allibrio et al. 2009; Language: Italian; Administration time: 20–30 minutes), the Bedside Evaluation Screening Test-2 (BEST-2, Fitch-West et al. 1998; Language: English; Administration time: 20 minutes), and the Aachen Aphasia Bedside Test (AAT-B, Biniek et al. 1992; Language: German, Italian, Thai; Administration time: 15–40 minutes). These screening tests usually assess a restricted range of linguistic skills and functions. For this reason, for an accurate diagnosis of the type and gravity of aphasia, clinicians will need to administer more complete batteries of tests once the patient enters the chronic stage.

For the chronic phase several standardised batteries of tests are currently available in different languages. Such batteries usually focus on specific aspects of language processing and have been developed according to either neuropsychological or neuro-linguistic criteria. Those developed according to neuropsychological criteria allow clinicians to assess not only language but also those cognitive skills that underlie linguistic abilities. Among these are the Esame Neuropsicologico per l'Afasia (ENPA, Capasso and Miceli 2001; Language: Italian; Administration time: 120 minutes), the Batteria per l'Analisi dei Deficit Afasici (BADA, Miceli et al. 1994; Language: Italian; Administration time: 240 minutes), the Psycholinguistic Assessments of Language Processing in Aphasia (PALPA, Kay et al. 1996; Language: English; Administration time: not reported), and the Comprehensive Aphasia Test (CAT, Swinburn et al. 2004; Language: English; Administration time: 60–120 minutes).

The batteries of tests developed according to a neuro-linguistic approach focus on a thorough description of the levels of linguistic processing, allowing for a clear description of the type and gravity of aphasia. Here are some examples of such batteries: the Aachen Aphasia Test (AAT, Huber et al. 1984; Language: Different languages; Administration time: 90 minutes), the Esame del Linguaggio II (Ciurli et al. 1996; Language: Italian; Administration Time: not reported), the Western Aphasia Battery-Revised (WAB-R, Kertesz 2006; Language: English; Administration Time: >60 minutes), and the Boston Diagnostic Aphasia Evaluation, III edition (BDAE-3, Goodglass et al. 2000; Language: English; Administration time: 30 minutes till 6 hours).

Overall, employing naming, fluency, lexical, and grammatical comprehension tasks, as well as reading and writing tasks, such batteries of tests allow clinicians to perform a detailed assessment of the patient's oral and written linguistic skills. Of note, in some batteries (e.g., AAT) it is also possible to perform a qualitative analysis of the patient's discourse skills.

The patients' pragmatic skills can also be assessed by administering specific batteries of tests. For example, the Assessment of Pragmatic Abilities and Cognitive Substrates (APACS, Arcara and Bambini 2016) and the Assessment Battery for Communication (ABaCo, Angeleri et al. 2019). Furthermore, additional observations can be made by administering the Communicative Abilities of Daily Living test (CADL, Holland 1980), which assesses communication skills in simulated contexts, and the American Speech-Language and Hearing Association-Functional Assessment of Communication Skills test for adults (ASHA-FACS, Roth 2011), which indirectly assesses those pragmatic skills that are required for a functional communication in six major domains: social communication, primary needs, reading, writing, activities with manipulation of numbers, and the ability to plan daily life activities.

A further issue concerns language assessment in bilingual patients with aphasia (Marini et al. 2012). A systematic assessment of their languages is needed to have a clear picture of the patient's overall linguistic skills. To date, this issue is still quite unexplored. Nonetheless, the Bilingual Aphasia Test (BAT; Paradis and Libben 1987) offers a good compromise. This battery of language assessments is articulated in three major sections. Part A is basically a questionnaire that allows the clinician to have an idea of the patient's bilingual history (e.g., how many and which languages did she or he speak in different contexts and how did she or he acquire them [at what age, where, etc.]). Part B is formed by tasks assessing the patient's phonological, morphological, syntactic, semantic, and discourse skills. Importantly, this section has been adapted to approximately 70 languages. Therefore, it allows clinicians to compare the performance of a patient across his or her languages. Finally, Part C assesses the patient's translating skills in his or her languages.

### 23.1.3 On the Utility of Multilevel Analyses of Narrative Discourse in People with Aphasia

Over the past few years, increasing attention has been devoted to the issue of the validity and reliability of the currently available tests for language assessment in PWA (e.g., Rohde et al. 2018; Thomson et al. 2018; El Hachioui et al. 2017). Unfortunately, even though El Hachioui et al. (2017) commented on the validation studies for eight tests for acute stroke patients, reporting the sensitivity of such tests in differentiating between aphasic and non-aphasic stroke patients (e.g., FAST, LAST, UAS, MAST), Rohde et al. (2018) highlighted that none of the 56 tests included in their review reported diagnostic data in differentiating aphasic and non-aphasic stroke patients. This strongly limits their applicability and supports the need for the development of diagnostically robust tests for a reliable diagnosis of aphasia in stroke patients.

Recent reviews highlight that procedures of discourse analysis may provide a much clearer picture of the real linguistic and communicative skills of PWA (e.g., Bryant et al. 2016; Linnik et al. 2015; Armstrong 2000). Speech samples can be elicited in a number of ways: picture descriptions tasks (e.g., Nicholas and Brookshire 1993), story retelling tasks (Saffran et al. 1989), recounting personal events (e.g., Glosser and Deser 1990) or descriptions of procedures (e.g., Ulatowska et al. 1983). These speech samples can be taped, transcribed, and then analysed. The narrative analysis can focus on the structural characteristics of the elicited speech samples or on their functional features or both. The former focuses on the assessment of the levels of productivity of a patient, as well as his or her lexical, grammatical, and narrative skills. The functional analysis focuses on the patient's ability to identify, select, and produce appropriate pieces of information at the conceptual and lexical level. Marini et al. (2011) developed a multilevel procedure of discourse analysis that allows clinicians to perform both structural and functional analyses that proved highly sensitive in detecting the presence of language impairment in patients with brain injury. Indeed, such a procedure is much more informative than traditional standardised linguistic tests, as it helps clinicians to determine (1) the exact nature of the linguistic impairment, (2) the way specific micro-linguistic difficulties might affect macro-linguistic processing and vice versa, and (3) the putative efficacy of innovative rehabilitation protocols. Indeed, a number of investigations have clearly shown that approaches of this kind highlight the presence of subtle linguistic difficulties when traditional batteries of tests failed to detect significant linguistic difficulties, such as in non-aphasic individuals with mild traumatic brain injury (e.g., Galetto et al. 2013). Furthermore, recent evidence suggests that multilevel procedures of discourse analysis can even identify the subtle improvements induced by thrombolysis in persons with stroke aphasia in the hypercute phase (Andreetta et al. 2024). Furthermore, such analyses are effective in assessing linguistic recovery after rehabilitation. For example, Larfeuil and Le Dorze (1997) showed that the administration of traditional standardised aphasia tests failed to show any improvement in a group of PWA after 6 weeks of language stimulation. Nonetheless, the analysis of their narrative language elicited with a picture description task highlighted the presence of a significant improvement in their communicative effectiveness. Similar findings were also reported by Marini et al. (2007). In this case on the post-therapy assessment, traditional standardised aphasia tests showed minimal changes, even if the patients' levels of informativeness, as measured with a multilevel procedure for discourse analysis, improved significantly. Interestingly, such analyses also showed that in persons with anomic aphasia the lexical impairment might affect the macro-linguistic organisation of their speech samples (Andreetta et al. 2012) and that anodic stimulation over the left inferior frontal gyrus enhances the levels of lexical informativeness in chronic non-fluent PWA (Marangolo et al. 2013).

Acknowledgement: This contribution was supported by PRIN 2022 PNNR, n. P2022M9JCM, project title: Standardization of the Multilevel prOcedure for discOurse analysis and Training program for narrative production in healthy adults - SMOOTH Avv. pub. n. 1409 14/09/2022 - PRIN 2022 PNRR M4C2 Inv.1.1 Ministero dell'Università e della Ricerca (Financed by EU, NextGenerationEU) - CUP G53D23007250001.

## 23.2  Evaluation of Non-Verbal Communication with People with Aphasia

Rossella Muò

Non-verbal communication consists of a heterogeneous set of communication means, other than language, which people may use to convey a message. Within non-verbal means of communication the use of voice and prosody, facial expressions, eye contact and eye movement, drawing, gestures and body movements are generally included (Prutting and Kirchner 1987; van der Meulen et al. 2010). In some contexts, other elements such as posture or clothing are also included within the label of non-verbal communication. For our purposes, only those communication acts within the communication domain with at least a partial intentionality by those who convey it will be considered (Bara 1999), so that during an interaction each participant can purposely choose to exchange some information by using either verbal or non-verbal means or both. In clinical settings with people who have acquired communication and language disorders, non-verbal communication plays a key role as an alternative and augmentative method of communication, as it can accompany, strengthen, or replace verbal communication when it is lacking or not adequate (Rautakoski 2011). This is often the case for people with moderate to severe aphasia. When a person experiences abrupt inability (or reduced ability) to communicate through language, non-verbal communication means offer a crucial role in revealing the person's communicative competence and in conveying their communicative intention. For example, people with severe aphasia have been shown to use drawings, gestures, facial expression, gaze, pointing, pantomime and body language, as well as the prosody of their voice, to communicate. Moreover, several communication strategies have been reported, such as pointing out a message from word lists or graphic resources, or indicating numbers with their fingers. Non-verbal communication also contributes to supporting and regulating discourse, such as regulating taking turns, and to promoting interpersonal/social aspects of communication, for example, transmitting emotional content (Rautakoski 2011).

Several approaches and concepts can be found in fields close to that of non-verbal communication, for example, multimodal communication, augmentative and alternative communication, and functional communication. Although they share much in common, they are not completely overlapping concepts. In the speech-language pathology literature, multimodal typically refers to communication in any modality outside speech, regardless of how many modalities are used. Strictly speaking, the term multimodal refers to communication of the same message via more than one channel, either simultaneously or serially (Pierce et al. 2019). The label multimodal is also applied to a diverse range of interventions (see Pierce et al. 2019 for a review). Augmentative and Alternative Communication (AAC) includes all of the ways we share our ideas and feelings without talking, but the term also refers to a specific rehabilitation approach that helps people with severe communication disorders who cannot use spoken words, by providing both unaided systems (i.e., done with the body, such as gestures or facial expressions) and aided systems (i.e., either basic or high-tech devices) for communicating in their environment (ASHA 2020). In the field of AAC, people can either use multiple non-speech systems (multimodal communication) or a single system (unimodal) to communicate (van der Meulen et al. 2010; Pierce et al. 2019). Functional communication is defined as "the ability to receive or to convey a message, regardless of the mode, to communicate effectively and independently in a given natural environment" (Frattali et al. 2017). This means that in order to communicate in an effective and independent way in a specific environment, people with communication disorders can mix spoken words and one or more non-verbal communication means, to the best of their competence.

During the last decades a deep transformation of the aphasia concept has occurred, moving from a closely linguistic point of view to a broader communicative one and finally to a more extensive social and environmental framework. This transformation has also been reflected in changes in the way that communication and language disorders are assessed. Recent guidelines (Canadian Stroke Best Practice 2019) recommend broadening the focus of rehabilitation from the impairment level only (that is language and cognitive impairment) to a full set of domains related to the language impairment, including functional communication and level of communication activities, daily living participation, and well-being, as indicated by the International Classification of Functioning, Disability and Health (ICF) framework (World Health Organization 2001). Following this suggestion, the assessment of non-verbal aspects of communication should always be carefully considered, as it may contribute to the reaching of higher levels of communication functioning, especially when spoken words alone are no more an effective means of conveying messages.

Despite there being at present no tests or protocols specifically addressed to assess each non-verbal communication skill in persons with communication disorders or aphasia (for example, gestural skills are usually considered only in terms of presence/absence of apraxia), some useful tools can be found to reach the aim of expanding the assessment of non-verbal communication skills.

The importance of adding to the formal assessment procedure an informal assessment performed through clinical observations has been underlined (Thomson et al. 2018). The main aim of performing an informal assessment reflects the need to take into account all those aspects that may be difficult to highlight with standardised tests, such as the description of all the non-verbal strategies used during a conversation or the subjective difficulties encountered while using a newly suggested non-verbal communication strategy. Informal assessment is moreover fundamental for the inclusion of the opinion of the persons with aphasia and their significant others in the assessment procedure.

Assessment of "functional and pragmatic aspects of communication, including compensatory strategies" is recommended as per International guidelines (RCSLT 2005). Since non-verbal communication is usually considered a part of pragmatic competence, pragmatic protocols usually include items regarding this. Above all, the *Pragmatic Protocol* (Prutting and Kirchner 1987) includes the assessment of non-verbal aspects of kinesics and proxemics, such as physical proximity (i.e., the distance that the speaker and listener sit or stand from each other), physical contact (i.e., the number of times and placement of contacts between speaker and listener), body postures (such as leaning forwards, moving away from the partner or moving side to side), foot/leg and hand/arm movements (touching self or objects), gestures (to support, complement or replace verbal behaviour), facial expression (positive, negative or neutral), and eye gaze (at each other or reciprocal). Each of the aforementioned aspects is assessed as appropriate, if it facilitates the communicative interaction; neutral, neither helping nor detracting; or inappropriate, if it detracts from the communicative exchange and penalises the individual. Judgements should take into account the person with aphasia, his or her communication partner and the context where the conversation takes place.

Another useful tool that can be used to summarise the competence level in using non-verbal communication is the International Classification of Functioning, Disability and Health (ICF), where two specific activity and participation codes are provided: Communicating with/receiving non-verbal messages (d315) and Producing non-verbal messages (d335) (WHO 2001). For each code a qualifier can be added to rate both the performance (first qualifier) and the capacity without assistance (second qualifier). Scores ranging from 0 (i.e., no difficulty) to 4 (i.e., complete difficulty) can be assigned.

Since specific assessment tools for gestures are lacking, a deep informal evaluation, including gesture intentionality, gesture types and roles in producing and maintaining informativeness during conversation, is suggested in order to steer rehabilitation to increase communicative outcomes for people with aphasia. Types of gestures may include co-verbal production, used to accompany and strengthen linguistic productions (for detailed classification see, for example, Ekman and Friesen 1969), and intentional gestures, often used to replace spoken words and facilitate naming when there is a production deficit. Intentional gestures can support communicative exchange and partners' comprehension and they can include both simple and more complex gestures, such as deictic gestures (i.e., pointing), iconic gestures (i.e., reproduction of some physical characteristic of a given object or person), emblematic gestures (i.e., gestures with known and shared meaning within a given cultural group) and pantomime. A person's ability to draw or sketch should also be assessed informally in order to obtain useful information to define a complete communicative profile and to plan a rehabilitation programme, in particular with regard to compensatory and support strategies.

Several approaches underline the importance of a comprehensive assessment of communication skills, considering as a whole verbal, para-verbal and non-verbal skills (for example, total communication, life participation or functional communication approach) (Rautakoski 2011;

Brown et al. 2011; Frattali et al. 2017). The functional communication approach suggests considering the ability to communicate effectively and independently in a given environment. The American Speech-Language and Hearing Association—Functional Assessment of Communication Skills for Adults (ASHA-FACS) (Frattali et al. 1995) can be considered as a useful assessment tool to highlight if the overall communication abilities of a person with aphasia, including non-verbal communication, allow them to participate in an independent and qualitative adequate way in communication activities of daily living (i.e., social participation, communication of basic needs, reading, writing, and calculating, and daily planning).

Among the evaluation tools that are focused on the whole communication abilities of the person with aphasia, the *Scenario Test* (van der Meulen et al. 2010, cultural adaptation for UK in Hilari et al. 2018) was specifically designed to assess multimodal communication, by examining the ability to convey a message, verbally or non-verbally or both, in daily life scenarios. Although specifically addressed to plan and evaluate treatments based on the Augmentative and Alternative Communication strategies, it can be used to highlight the person's ability to use different communication means, including non-verbal communication, to convey daily life messages. Moreover, the Scenario Test examines communication in a dialogue between the person with aphasia and the examiner, who acts as a helpful communication partner.

The importance of the conversational partner, who acts as a conversational ramp to support the communication abilities of people with aphasia, has been underlined and recently reviewed (see for example Simmons-Mackie et al. 2016). The Kagan Scales *Measure of Skill in Supported Conversation (MSC)* and *Measure of Participation in Conversation (MPC)* (Kagan et al. 2004) can be considered useful tools both to rate the conversation partner's ability in providing support for the person with aphasia, as well as the level of participation in conversation by adults with aphasia. Within the Kagan Scales, non-verbal communication strategies are listed, which include gestures, writing, drawing and pictographic resources. The assessment is intended for exploring the conversation abilities of communication couples. On the one hand, the focus of the assessment is on the partner's ability both to use nonverbal communication to reveal the person with aphasia's competence, and to understand the conveyed message that can be produced through spoken words or non-verbal strategies or a mix of the two. On the other hand, the assessment explores the person with aphasia's ability to use nonverbal communication means to connect socially with the partner (interaction); to exchange information, opinions and feelings (transaction) and to understand the conversation partner's verbal and non-verbal messages. It has been highlighted that people with aphasia are often unsuccessful in using non-verbal communication strategies without the guidance and support of the conversation partner. The importance of communication partner training approaches to improve the couples' ability to strengthen their successful communication strategies and to avoid the less successful ones has been underlined and reviewed (Kagan 1998; Kagan et al. 2001; Nykänen et al. 2013; Simmons-Mackie et al. 2016).

In conclusion, the importance of considering non-verbal communication skills in the assessment of people with moderate or severe aphasia has been highlighted. Although an exhaustive list of all tools is beyond the aims of this presentation, some useful tools are described to help clinicians provide a better description of both non-verbal communication strategies used by their clients and their global communication effectiveness.

## 23.3 Estimation of General Cognitive State

Stefano Zago and Edoardo Nicolò Aiello

Neuropsychological testing is the preferred method for identifying the presence, features, and severity of a cognitive impairment in neurological patients (World Health Organization 1993; American Psychiatric Association 2013; Cipolotti and Warrington 1995).

Cognitive domains (e.g., language, memory, attention) or subdomains (e.g., syntactic comprehension, verbal short-term memory) are not natural objects. They represent a grouping of mental faculties rooted in the brain that may thus be impaired by lesions or dysfunctions to particular structures of the central nervous system—this suggesting the existence of functionally distinct neurocognitive circuits. These unobservable cognitive constructs can be tested indirectly by measuring behaviour by objective neuropsychological tests. For example, in the Token Test, auditory comprehension is measured by means of counting the number of correct commands of increasing length and complexity that are decoded and executed by the patient through the manipulation of a deck of coloured tokens of different size and shape (De Renzi and Vignolo 1962). It has to be noted that neuropsychological tests may present with multiple sensory, motor, perceptual and cognitive demands—hence 'pure' domain-specific tests being the exception rather than the rule. Neuropsychologists have access to a number of tests that examine a variety of both instrumental (e.g., memory) and non-instrumental (e.g., attention) skills and abilities for the purpose of diagnosis, rehabilitation or baseline cognitive functioning assessment. In general, a 'test' should be a standardised measurement device—i.e., characterised by a specific procedure for administration and scoring. In addition, a test is 'normed', meaning there is some prescribed method for relating the test scores to a representative normal population sample, or in some cases to specific neurological aetiology (e.g., closed head injury, viral infections, Alzheimer's disease, aphasia).

There are many tests available for neuropsychologists to evaluate cognitive functions, either for global functioning or individual domains (Lezak et al. 2012). Some brief in-clinic and bedside tools such as the Mini Mental State Examination (MMSE) (Folstein et al. 1975, 2010), the Addenbrooke Cognitive Examination-III (ACE-III) (Hsieh et al. 2013) or the Montreal Cognitive Assessment (MoCA) (Nasreddine et al. 2005) are useful for a preliminary picture of global cognitive efficiency. With respect to language disorders, the Mini-Linguistic State Examination (MLSE) (Patel et al. 2020) has been developed for use in the assessment, clinical classification, and monitoring of progressive aphasic syndromes.

On the other hand, some fixed batteries such as the Wechsler Adult Intelligence Scale–IV (WAIS-IV) (Wechsler 2008) or the Repeatable Battery for the Assessment of Neuropsychological Status (r-BANS) (Randolph et al. 1998) examine multiple ability domains in a repeatable format and provide a general relative quotient on intellective and cognitive functioning. However, the more common approach today is to estimate a general cognitive state by using a flexible test battery, which involves testing a variety of cognitive domains or subdomains (Barr 2001).

The role of the clinical neuropsychologist as a 'test user' has been noted to include the responsibility of selecting, overseeing and scoring the test, measuring the pattern of severity of cognitive impairment and interpreting scores within a clinical and theoretical framework (Harvey 2012). The neuropsychologist has to check numerous systematic variables that undermine the validity of the neuropsychological exam, such as correct administration of the tests, age and education level (Arnett 2013). In addition, psychometric analysis should be supported through clinical-behavioural observation. The neuropsychologist is also trained to evaluate the patient's motivational and emotional states.

A specific issue arises owing to the presence of language difficulties, as many standardised neuropsychological measures are verbally mediated (i.e., presented with verbal instructions and requiring verbal responses). Although assessment batteries designed for aphasia are still developing, at present there are only a few neuropsychological tests aimed at assessing global cognitive functioning of patients with language syndromes. A rare example is the Lothian Assessment for Screening of Cognition in Aphasia (LASCA) (Faiz 2016), a non-verbal assessment for screening cognition in post-stroke aphasic patients. Five cognitive domains are assessed: orientation, attention, memory, visual, and executive functioning. Another battery

inspired by this principle is the Aphasia Check List (ACL) (Kalbe et al. 2005), which includes measures of cognitive abilities that rely on non-verbal tasks.

To conclude, estimation of a general cognitive state includes at least three types of knowledge: (1) knowledge of the faceted and interactive anatomo-functional organisation of the cognitive architecture; (2) knowledge of various cognitive profiles that can be determined in neurological and psychiatric fields and in psychological disorders; (3) up-to-date knowledge of the main neuropsychological tests.

## 23.4 Standard Neurological Examination in Aphasia

Stefano Cappa

After the assessment of the level of consciousness, the crucial step in the neurological examination of an aphasic patient is the clinical language examination, to be subsequently supplemented by a standard aphasia test. This includes four simple steps:

**Language Production**
Listening to the patient speaking provides crucial information. Extended production can be elicited by an open conversation, or by requests to narrate an event or to describe a complex picture. A basic judgement to be applied to production is 'fluency'. The assessment of fluency is based on an evaluation of phrase length (i.e., the longest uninterrupted sequence of words produced by the patients), speech articulation, the presence of phonological and lexical errors (paraphasias), grammatical abilities, and prosody. From these parameters, an aphasic patient can usually be defined as fluent or non-fluent. Non-fluent patients produce short sentences or single words, usually have articulation disorders, may produce paraphasias and grammatical errors, and have an altered prosody. Conversely, fluent patients produce grammatically well-structured, longer sentences, with a variable number of phonological and lexical errors; their articulation is unim-

paired, and prosody sounds normal. The examination of production is completed by an assessment of the naming abilities, asking the subject to name objects or parts of objects present in the room.

## Language Comprehension

The ability to understand language produced by others can be assessed at the single word level, placing three or four items in front of the subject and asking the patient to point to the item named by the examiner. Sentence comprehension is assessed with verbal commands or with yes–no questions.

## Repetition

The ability to repeat syllables, words, and sentences indicates the status of phonological skills, and if preserved it suggests an integrity of the immediately perisylvian language areas (Broca, Wernicke, supramarginal gyrus) and of their connections.

## Written Language

A fast but comprehensive examination of written language includes reading aloud of word and sentences, understanding of written commands, dictation of words and sentences, and narrative writing.

This clinical examination allows a basic classification of the aphasic syndrome in the case of stroke-associated aphasia in the post-acute stage. The brief neurological examination of stroke patients in the acute stage is completed by the assessment of visual fields, facial movement, upper and lower limb power, tone and reflexes and somatosensory perception, and can be assisted by the use of standardised scales (Bushnell et al. 2001).

In the case of primary progressive aphasia (PPA), it is diagnostically very important to perform an in-depth examination of motor function. Several pathologies associated with PPA are characterised by motor symptoms. The corticobasal degeneration syndrome is frequently associated with the non-fluent/agrammatic variant (N/Afv) or with milder language dysfunction (Dodich et al. 2019), and features alien hand

symptoms as well as asymmetrical rigidity, myoclonus, and apraxia (Mathew et al. 2012). Progressive supranuclear palsy can also be associated with speech and language impairment (Catricalà et al. 2019), which is considered one of the core clinical features of cognitive dysfunction in the current diagnostic criteria (Höglinger et al. 2017). The crucial aspects of neurological examination are ocular motor dysfunction, postural instability, and akinesia. The presence of muscle weakness, wasting, and fasciculations is diagnostic of the association of motor neuron disorder with PPA (Tan et al. 2019).

Several screening tests are available for stroke aphasia (El Hachioui et al. 2017) and PPA (Battista et al. 2017).

## 23.5 Tests of Neuropsychological Functions

Stefano Zago and Teresa Difonzo

Neuropsychological assessment can help define cognitive deficits, clarify diagnoses, and develop optimal management plans for patients with cognitive deficits (Schroeder et al. 2019). The more common tests are available in paper-and-pencil format but there are also some computerised versions, and in the future there will always be more opportunities for collecting neuropsychological data with digital technology (Parsons and Duffield 2019).

The current neuropsychological test armamentarium includes those with different goals that can be classified according to how selectively they evaluate target cognitive functions. Screening tests (i.e., first-level tests) serve the aim of providing practitioners with a rapid estimate of global or specific functioning, whereas second-level, domain-specific/multi-domain, tests are administered in order to perform an in-depth analysis within a given function or a range of functions.

Today the neuropsychologist can choose a set of neuropsychometric tools suitable to the majority of patients with some flexibility—adding or subtracting tests on the basis of the observations made during the test administration or on the specific referral reason. In some cases, the need to have a quick and easy measure of global cognitive functioning leads the neuropsychologist to adopt brief cognitive screening tools, such as the Mini Mental State Examination (MMSE, Folstein et al. 1975, 2010), the Montreal Cognitive Assessment tool (MoCA, Nasreddine et al. 2005) or Addenbrooke's Cognitive examination-revised (Mioshi et al. 2006). Some screening tests can also be disease-specific—i.e., designed to assess those domains/functions that are typically found to be impaired in patients affected with a given condition. Examples are the Mini-Mental Parkinson, in which items evaluating executive function is included to capture better Parkinson's disease-related cognitive changes (Mahieux et al. 1995) and the ALS Cognitive Behavioural Screen (ALS-CBS) for fronto-temporal spectrum disorders (e.g., dysexecutive signs) in patients with amyotrophic lateral sclerosis (ALS)—given the biological link between ALS and fronto-temporal degenerations (Woolley et al. 2010). As a screening measure for evaluating the language domain, the Mini-Linguistic State Examination has been developed (Patel et al. 2020).

An in-depth neuropsychological evaluation requires the application of different cognitive tests by domain (e.g., language, memory, attention, practice, visuospatial abilities, executive functions) to build flexible neuropsychological batteries. Several publications have catalogued the broad range of neuropsychological tests used in practice today, including their values and limits (e.g., Schroeder et al. 2019; Fujii 2017; Lezak et al. 2012). Different standardised tests concerning aspects of language are available, such as naming (e.g., Boston Naming Test, Kaplan et al. 1983), comprehension (e.g., Token Test, De Renzi and Vignolo 1962), and verbal fluency (e.g., Letter Fluency), etc. For memory assessment, tests typically consist of memorising numbers (e.g., Digit Span forward and backwards, Wechsler 1939), words (e.g., Rey Auditory Verbal Learning Test, Rey 1941), pictures (e.g., Free and Cued Selective Reminding Test, Buschke 1984) or short stories that have to be recalled after a delay or recognised among distracters.

Regarding the attention domain, timed tasks that require the participant to detect numbers (e.g., Attentional Matrices, Spinnler and Tognoni 1987) or symbols (e.g., Multiple Features Target Cancellation, Gainotti et al. 2001) as quickly as possible are usually administered. Practice is generally assessed with drawing tasks (free drawings or copying; e.g., Rey-Osterrieth complex figure, Rey 1941) or by tasks requiring the patient to imitate gestures (e.g., make the sign of the cross) or perform actions on verbal command (e.g., prepare a letter for mailing). Visual perception is in most cases assessed with visual tasks in which pictures of common and uncommon objects have to be recognised, which can also be presented from unusual views or by overlapping outlines to assess agnosia (the inability to recognise objects or scenes). Finally, the 'executive domain' regards higher-order cognitive processes, such as planning, response inhibition, attentional set-shifting. Executive functions are then examined by tasks that require planning (e.g., Tower of London, Shallice 1982), inhibitory control (e.g., Stroop Color and Word Test, Stroop 1935; Hayling Sentence Completion Test, Burgess and Shallice 1997), set-shifting (e.g., Wisconsin Card Sorting Test, Berg 1948), decision-making (e.g., Iowa Gambling Task, Bechara et al. 1994), etc.

Numerous test batteries for aphasia diagnosis, which constitutes the first step towards a well-founded language therapy, have been developed. The more popular and widely translated are the Multilingual Aphasia Examination (MAE, Jones and Benton 1995), the Western Aphasia Battery (WAB-R, Kertesz 2006) and the Examination Aachen Aphasia Test (EAAT, Miller et al. 2000). More recently, some neuropsychological batteries have also been proposed for specific neurological diseases. One example of this is the Edinburgh Cognitive and Behavioural ALS Screen (ECAS), specifically designed for ALS. It includes a range of tests sensitive to cognitive impairment in ALS (i.e., language, fluency, and executive functions) and an assessment of ALS non-specific functions (i.e., memory and visuospatial) (Niven et al. 2015). Another example is the Screening for Aphasia in NeuroDegeneration battery (SAND) specifically tailored to primary progressive aphasia patients and to describe language impairment in relation to this disease phenotype and cognitive status (Catricalà et al. 2017).

## 23.6 Laboratory Examinations (i.e., Serology, Immunology) in Aphasia

Stefano Cappa

The standard indications for laboratory examinations aimed at the assessment of risk factors and of possible contributing systemic disorders in cerebrovascular disease apply to all patients with aphasia due to ischaemic or haemorrhagic stroke (Brainin and Heiss 2019). A special case is the suspicion of vasculitis, which requires a complete inflammatory panel, including anti-neutrophil circulating antibodies (ANCA) and anti-nuclear antibodies (ANA). Aphasia can be one manifestation of autoimmune encephalitis, which can be diagnosed with assays of serum or cerebrospinal fluid (CSF) antibodies against neuronal surface antigens (i.e., LGI1, CASPR2 and VGKC-complex, NMDAR, γ-aminobutyric-acid receptor (GABABR), α-amino-3-hydroxy-5-methyl-4-isoxazolepropionic-acid receptor (AMPAR), and metabotropic-glutamate-receptor 5 (mGluR5) (Baumgartner et al. 2019; Dallmau and Graus 2023).

Genetic testing is indicated in juvenile stroke-associated aphasia for diagnosing rare conditions such as CADASIL (NOTCH3 mutations), Fabry's disease (deficiency of α-galactosidase), and other genetic causes of stroke (Dichgans et al. 2019) and the mitochondrial encephalopathies. The MELAS syndrome (mitochondrial myopathy, encephalopathy, lactic acidosis, and stroke-like episodes), generally due to maternally transmitted mitochondrial tRNA (Leu) A3243G mutations, is an infrequent cause of acquired aphasia in children. In the case of primary progressive aphasia, multiple mutations have been described, the most frequent of which involve progranulin (GRN) and C9ORF72 genes (Ramos et al. 2019).

Cerebrospinal fluid analysis is required on suspicion of inflammatory disease. In the case of primary progressive aphasia, a CSF study of the quantity of beta amyloid and Tau protein in CSF is helpful for the differential diagnosis between AD (low beta/high tau) and non-Alzheimer pathologies (Paraskevas et al. 2017). Plasma biomarker for Alzheimer disease are in the course of validation and will soon reach clinical availability (Hansson et al. 2023). The measurement of 14-3-3 protein is useful for the diagnosis of prion disease (Johnson et al. 2013).

## 23.7 CT/MRI of the Brain and Other Radiologic Imaging (See Section 23.11)

Gregor Kasprian, Antonio Schindler and Silvia Rosa

### 23.7.1 Introduction

The diagnostic work-up of patients with a neurological disease leading to dysarthria usually includes the application of brain imaging techniques, which generally provide sufficient contrast to differentiate normal brain anatomy from pathological changes. As normal radiography of the skull does not directly resolve details on the human brain, multiplanar cross-sectional imaging techniques are used to diagnose structural abnormalities of the human brain radiologically. These techniques nowadays comprise computed tomography (CT) and magnetic resonance imaging (MRI). Furthermore, they can be combined with nuclear medicine techniques such as positron emission tomography (PET) or single-photon emission tomography (SPECT) in the form of PET-CT or PET-MRI.

### 23.7.2 Computed Tomography of the Brain

The technique of computed tomography was introduced in the early 1970s and is nowadays the workhorse for rapid head imaging (Ambrose and Hounsfield 1973). CT scanning uses a series of

X-rays of the head taken from many different directions. Technically there are one (single source) or multiple (dual source) X-ray beam-emitting tubes rotating around the head of the patient. The X-rays or photons are detected originally by a single ring of electronic detectors. Increasing the number of detector rings for photon detection around the patient ("multi-detector row CT"—usually up to 64, but sometimes even 256 rows) has allowed an incredible increase in scanning speed, and generated submillimetre "image slices" of the human head and body. The most recent developments in CT technology use two rotating X-ray tubes (called "dual source" CT technology), which cover more imaged tissue within an even smaller amount of time. If the two tubes are operated at different voltages and the detectors can absorb different energy spectra, a more specific characterisation of the imaged tissue is possible (for further details see Kaza et al. 2012). For instance, this now allows the differentiation of extravascular iodine contrast agent and haemorrhage (which both appear "hyperdense" or bright on CT images—Fig. 23.1). These technical improvements have additionally provided better and more robust image quality with fewer movement artefacts than possible before. The typical effective radiation dose of a head CT nowadays lies in the range of 1.6 mSv, which approximately equals the amount received in 7 months of naturally occurring background radiation (Jaffe et al. 2010).

The combination of X-ray tubes and detectors alone does not automatically produce an image. CT scanning uses a computer programme that performs a numerical integral calculation on the measured X-ray series to estimate how much of the X-ray beam is absorbed in a small volume of the brain. Thereby digital data are produced and typically presented as grey-scale images of cross-sections of the head. The collected image is always in 3D and thus allows a reconstruction of the scanned object in three dimensions.

In approximation, the denser a material is, the brighter "whiter" a volume of it will appear on the scan, just as in the more familiar "flat" X-rays, where dense bone appears white. If an iodine-based contrast agent is administered intravenously, vessels can also be visualised non-invasively—an examination called "CT angiography" (Fig. 23.2). If CT angiography examinations are ordered, the side effects of iodine-based contrast agents need to be taken into account. The most feared adverse reaction is anaphylactic shock, nowadays occurring in

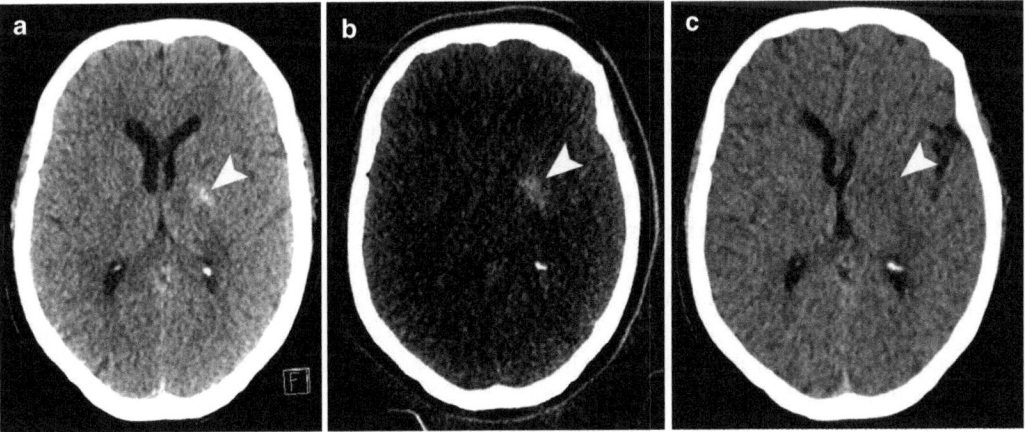

**Fig. 23.1** Dual Energy CT image of a patient who underwent thrombectomy after an ischaemic stroke of the left middle cerebral artery perforators. The arrowhead indicates a hyperdense lesion in the left basal ganglia (**a**), suggestive of haemorrhagic transformation of the ischaemic area. By using Dual Energy CT technology, the hyperdense change can be further differentiated with the iodine image (**b**) and the virtual non-contrast image (**c**). The brightness seen on the iodine image (**b**) indicates the presence of contrast agent in this area, which is not visible on the virtual non-contrast image (**c**). This helps the radiologist to differentiate between contrast agent leakage into ischaemia (as in this case) and haemorrhage. Kasprian © 2021

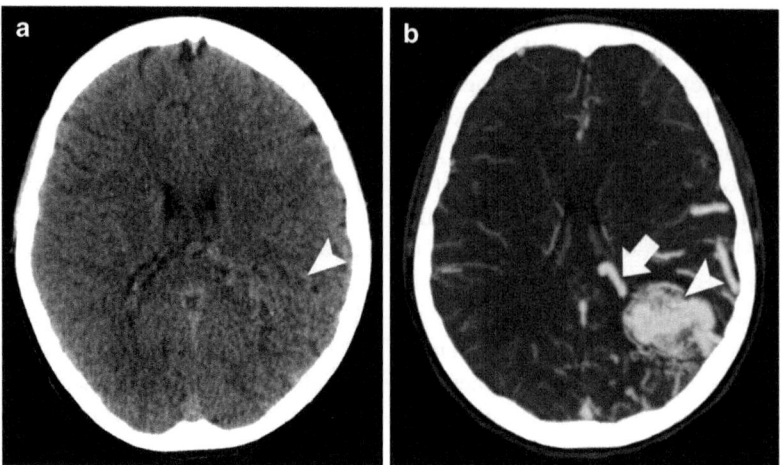

**Fig. 23.2** Non-contrast head CT (**a**) of a patient with recurrent therapy-resistant seizures (ictal aphasia) shows very subtle hyperdense structures in the left parietal lobe (arrowhead). CT Angiography with iodine-based intravenously administered contrast agent (**b**) allows the visuali- sation of the large arterio-venous malformation in the left parietal lobe. The arrow indicates a large draining vein. The arrowhead in (**b**) indicates the nidus of the vascular malformation. Kasprian © 2021

0.01–0.04% of i.v. iodinated contrast agent administrations with 1–3 deaths per 100,000–1,000,000 administrations (Kim et al. 2014; Wysowski and Nourjah 2006). The second-most common associated condition is contrast-induced nephropathy. In patients with pre-existing renal disease (multiple myeloma, renal transplant, nephrotic syndrome), intake of potentially nephrotoxic medication or application of other conditions with the potential to affect negatively renal function (diabetes mellitus, congestive heart failure, hypertonia, cirrhosis), iodinated contrast agent should be used with caution.

### 23.7.3 Strengths and Weaknesses of CT in the Diagnoses of Neurological Disease

The practical strengths of CT specifically lie in its rather wide availability and fast results. As the CT suite can be accessed without taking specific safety precautions, it grants fast patient logistics and a quick imaging procedure, mostly completed within 15 min. As a rule of thumb, CT is the imaging modality of choice in an acute setting. Patients with an acute onset of aphasia, are thus most likely to receive head CT imaging, as in most hospitals CT scanners are easily available

for acute patients, whereas the logistics of MR scanners are usually more difficult.

The most common indication for acute head CT imaging is the exclusion or diagnostic proof of an intracranial haemorrhage. This presents itself bright/"white" on a non-contrast head CT. Despite contrast agents not having been used, extravascular blood appears bright on non-contrast-enhanced CT, as blood contains haemoglobin-bound iron, which absorbs radiation. Owing to these characteristics, head CT is the "reference standard" for the detection of an acute intracranial haemorrhage (Wintermark et al. 2013).

A major benefit of CT is the indirect ability to quantify the "radiodensity"—corresponding to its attenuation coefficient—of local tissue, in "Hounsfield" units (HU). These are comparable in all CT scanners (which is substantially different from MRI quantifications, which are known to differ a lot between scanners). As a rule of thumb, certain tissue characteristics present with distinct changes on non-contrast head CT: "hypodense" (dark) regions indicate the presence of a local increase of water, commonly in the form of oedema. Distilled water shows a HU of 0 (in every CT scanner in the world). If a lesion contains primarily fat it appears very dark on CT and has negative radiodensity, from −120 to −90

HU. If a lesion contains clotted blood, it usually appears bright on CT with values around +50 to +75 HU. Tumours usually contain many proliferating cells, leading to a higher local cell density, resulting in an increase in brightness ("hyperdensity") on non-contrast head CT. Calcifications are strongly hyperdense with values over +300 HU and are frequently encountered in "physiological" locations, such as the pineal gland, but also commonly occur in cavernoma (small hyperdense lesions, mostly without surrounding oedema) or calcified brain tumours.

Compared with MRI, the most eminent weakness of head CT is its relative insensitivity to acute physiological tissue changes and reduced capacity to resolve tissue contrasts, which are not resolvable by photon attenuation alone (for instance, the difference between cortex and white matter of the brain, particularly in regions such as the brainstem). This weakness is particularly relevant if early changes during ischaemic stroke need to be detected. The early signs of cerebral ischaemia on head CT are loss of grey-white differentiation, sulcal effacement and a hyperdense clot in the proximal vessels—as seen in the patient presenting with acute aphasia in Fig. 23.3 (Wintermark et al. 2013). However, these signs are frequently invisible during the early acute stage of cerebral ischaemia (within the first 3 h, Fig. 23.3b). Moreover, their identification is highly dependent on the experience of the assessing radiologist. Furthermore, some brain regions, such as the brainstem, are generally poorly contrasted by CT. It is not uncommon that patients

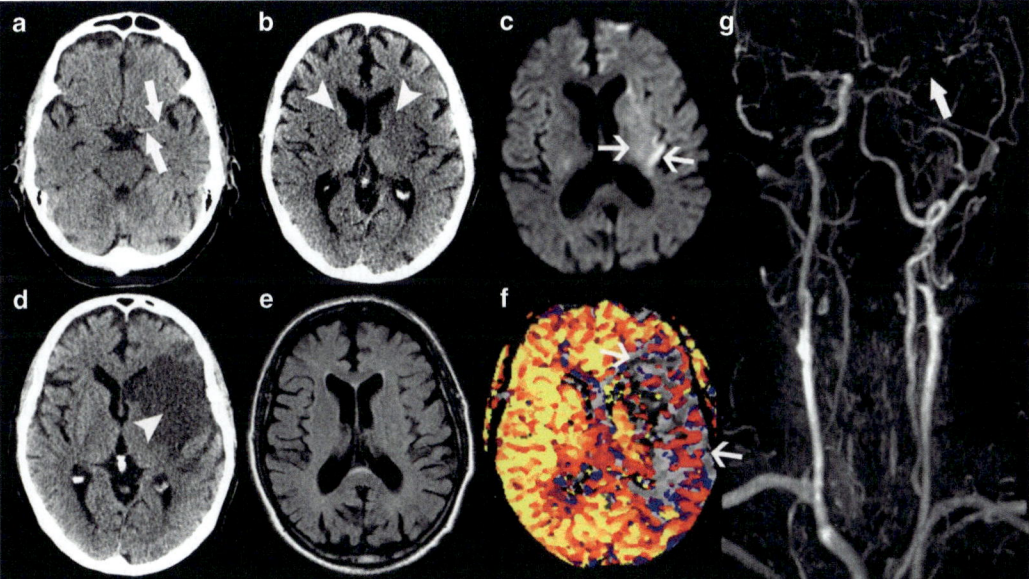

**Fig. 23.3** Evolution of an acute ischaemic stroke due to large vessel occlusion on non-contrast head CT (**a**, **b**, **d**) and MRI (**c**, **e**, **f**, **g**): 1 h after symptom onset (aphasia) an increased brightness of the left middle cerebral artery is noted on non-contrast CT (**a**, arrows)—the hyperdense media sign. At the same time point, extremely subtle CT findings are present in the middle cerebral artery territory, with a subtle loss of density in the region of the left caudate nucleus (left arrowhead compared with normal right arrowhead). About 1.5 h after the onset of symptoms contrast-enhanced MR angiography (**g**) depicts an occlusion of the left internal carotid artery and middle cerebral artery (arrow). Highly ischaemia-sensitive diffusion-weighted sequences (DWI) (**c**) shows diffusion restriction in the core area of the infarction (arrows, **c**), whereas no changes are seen in Fluid Attenuated Inversion Recovery Sequences (FLAIR) (**e**). Contrast-enhanced MR perfusion imaging allows the depiction of the tissue at risk (greyish colour code) in the middle cerebral artery territory (**f**, MR Perfusion tool; Dr. Christian Nasel, Univ. Clinics Tulln). Owing to contra-indications against thrombectomy, the ischaemia progressed and demarcated at late (12 h after clinical onset) non-contrast head CT (**d**). Note that the final extent of ischaemic tissue (**d**) corresponds to the amount of tissue at risk as predicted by MR perfusion (Fig. 23.3). Kasprian © 2021

with acute and severe neurological symptoms present with normal head CT findings for these reasons. Another weakness (which is also associated with MRI) is the occurrence of artefacts. Metals cause "streak" artefacts, which often interfere with the contrast of the surrounding tissue, leading to the inability to extract meaningful diagnostic information from the region surrounding the metal implant. In head CT, this is of particular relevance if patients with aneurysm clips or coils, or patients with dental implants, are imaged. Although to a lesser degree than MRI, CT is sensitive to patient motion, resulting in image series that do not cover the entire target regions and producing incorrect, negative results.

## 23.7.4 Magnetic Resonance Imaging (MRI) of the Brain

The technique of MRI evolved during the early 1980s and was soon established as a major diagnostic neuroimaging technology. In addition to providing structural images of the human brain, MRI nowadays also provides insights into human brain function.

The technique of magnetic resultant imaging is based on the magnetic properties of protons/water molecules. A strong static magnetic field ranging from originally 0.5 Tesla (T) to the nowadays clinically used 1.5 T and 3 T (to experimentally used 7 T to 11 T) is combined with an electromagnetic impulse. The resulting electromagnetic wave emitted back by the patient is measured by coils that are positioned close to the patient. As water comprises 70–90% of most tissues, the characterisation of the distinct electromagnetic properties of water enables the differentiation of certain tissue types owing to their water content and distribution. Tissues with low water content (such as bone), usually provide low MR signals, whereas water-rich structures—such as the human brain and especially the brain of a neonate—provide a large MR signal. Certain techniques even allow the visualisation of water motion within a tissue, providing impressive visualisation of the architecture of the human brain white matter.

Gradients are used to locate the MR signals coming from the imaged tissue. Gradients are slight spatial variations in the magnetic field strength across the patient. Coils are used to receive the signals coming from the patient. Most neuroradiological MR examinations use a head coil with a certain number of channels. To put it simply, the more channels are built into a coil, the more images per time period can be collected. For spine imaging, cervical, thoracic and lumbar coil arrays are used. In addition to aspects of field strength, the quality of gradients and coils is crucial for the technical capabilities of a MR scanner.

Nowadays, MRI of the brain is the most commonly performed MR technology examination. For characterising different tissue types, and elaborating the characteristics of brain pathology, different sequences are used. A sequence is a combination of high-frequency impulses and gradients, which are deployed in a predefined spatio-temporal pattern, resulting in a characteristic appearance of certain tissues. A variety of technical parameters of each sequence can be modified by the operator before examining a patient, leading to different possibilities and options to optimise the detection and characterisation of brain pathologies (for further details see McRobbie et al. 2006).

In the following section the more commonly used neuro-MR sequences and their resulting contrast of the human brain grey and white matter are described.

**T1-Weighted Sequences**

These images provide excellent contrast between fluid-rich tissues and fat-containing tissues. On T1-weighted images the anatomy of the adult human brain is visualised as depicted in an anatomy textbook: the grey matter of the human brain is dark, the white matter appears bright. All grey matter nuclei, as well as the basal ganglia, are thus visualised rather greyish/dark, and all white matter tracts and structures—such as the corpus callosum—appear bright/white. Fluids and water such as the cerebrospinal fluid (CSF) do not result in a strong MR signal on T1-weighted sequences, and appear very dark/black (Fig. 23.4).

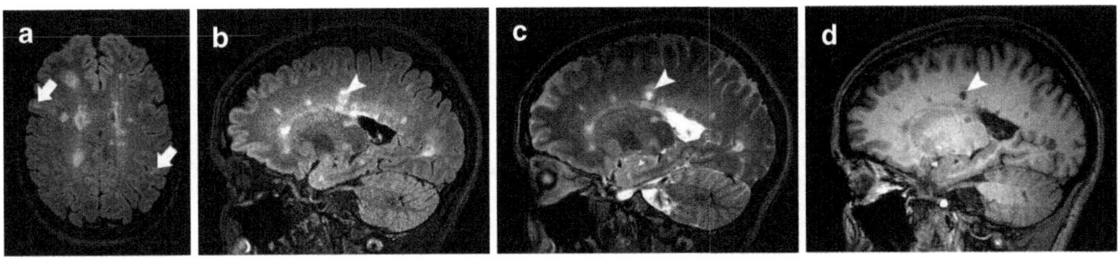

**Fig. 23.4** Patient suffering from relapsing-remitting Multiple Sclerosis (MS). FLAIR 3D sequence with axial (**a**) and sagittal (**b**) reconstructions. Sagittal T2-weighted 3D sequence (**c**) and T1-weighted sequence (**d**). The arrowhead marks a periventricular demyelinating lesion, which appears T2-weighted bright and T1-weighted hypointense (**d**). Marked T1 hypointensity indicates a long-standing lesion. The arrows (**a**) point to a juxtacortical MS lesion. Both demyelinating lesions are considered "characteristic" according to the MS diagnostic criteria (Filippi et al. 2016). Kasprian © 2021

**T2-Weighted Sequences**

These cause an inverted contrast compared with T1 (and thus are not brain "anatomy"-like). Thus T2-weighted sequences depict grey matter structures as rather bright, and white matter structures as rather dark. Fluids such as water or CSF appear very bright on T2-weighted sequences. Consequently, oedema or fluid collections will result in a hyper-intense or bright signal on T2-weighted sequences (Figs. 23.4 and 23.7).

**Fluid Attenuated Inversion Recovery Sequences**

FLAIR sequences are commonly used in head MRI and constitute the workhorse of most neuro-MR examinations. FLAIR uses the possibility of suppressing the signal of CSF combined with a T2-weighted sequence, resulting in a basic T2-weighted contrast, however, the CSF is visualised very dark (rather than on conventional T2-weighting, where CSF is typically bright). This property enhances the contrast between brain pathologies, which mostly appear hyperintense on T2 and FLAIR, and the surrounding brain tissue. As normal brain tissue is darker than brain lesions or pathologies (Figs. 23.4, 23.5, and 23.7), the conspicuousness of brain tissue abnormalities is elevated. This helps radiologists identify lesions and pathologies relatively easily.

**Diffusion-Weighted Sequences (DWI)**

DWI is a technique that is sensitive to water and proton motion. By using different radiofrequency impulses at different time points, DWI enables the measurement of protons within the visualised tissue in a certain time period. This is particularly practical in imaging acute ischaemic stroke, as early changes on a cellular level, leading to intracellular oedema and cell swelling, can be sensitively picked up by DWI (Figs. 23.3 and 23.5). If cells swell during the early stages of ischaemia owing to loss of osmotic regulation, DWI detects the local changes due to locally increasingly restricted proton motion. As of now, DWI is the most sensitive MRI imaging technique for visualising early ischaemia-related tissue damage (Figs. 23.3 and 23.5).

**Diffusion Tensor Imaging (DTI) and Tractography**

Since DWI assesses microstructural changes in the brain parenchyma, the technique allows the characterisation of the microstructure of the human brain. The DWI technique of DTI provides DWI data covering a variety of directions in space, allowing geometrical covering and description of three-dimensional structures such as fibre tracts (tractography). A variety of mathematical approaches can be used, when postprocessing raw DTI data (for technical details see Jones 2012), resulting in the in vivo reconstruction and dissection of the three-dimensional fibre architecture of the human brain (Catani et al. 2002). For assessing the aphasic patient, knowledge about the involvement of structural language networks can provide information about the extent and nature of an individual pathology (Fig. 23.7). According to the recently evolved

**Fig. 23.5** MRI of a patient with post-stroke apraxia of speech. The arrowhead on FLAIR (**a**, **c**) and T1-weighted (**d**) images indicates the large post-ischaemic left hemispheric area (in neuroradiology all axial images are assessed as if the physician were looking from below) involving the inferior frontal gyrus in combination with the precentral gyrus (motor) in its lateral aspect. The arrow indicates the more acute ischaemic area in the right precentral gyrus region. DWI (apparent diffusion coefficient image) shows cytotoxic oedema confirming that the ischaemia was a recent event (dark areas in **b**). Kasprian © 2021

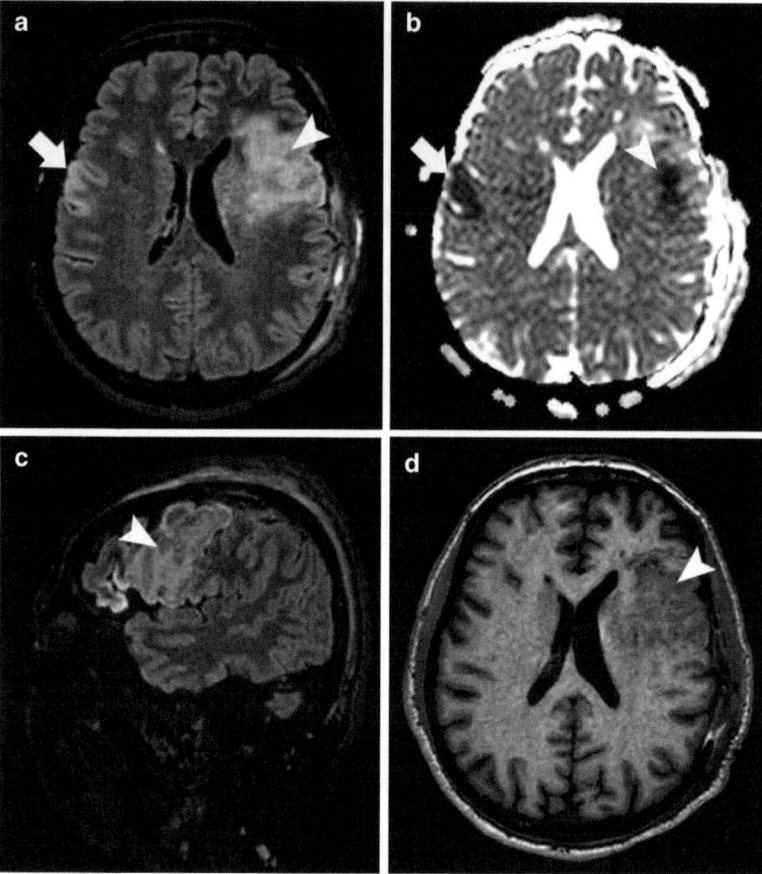

model of cortical language processing proposed by Hickok and Poeppel (2007), the neural architecture of phonemic processing is mainly related to two "streams" of neural activity. The ventral stream is represented by the inferior fronto-occipital and uncinate fascicles (Fig. 23.6), while the structural pathway of the dorsal stream is the arcuate and parts of the superior longitudinal fascicle (Fig. 23.6). With appropriate technical and neuroanatomical expertise, local deviations and alterations of language-related pathways (Fridriksson et al. 2018) can be depicted non-invasively. Intactness and microstructure of these pathways, moreover, correlate well with diverse aspects of language function (Catani et al. 2007).

## Functional MRI (fMRI)

A special mode of sequence acquisition—"echo planar imaging" or EPI—is particularly sensitive to the magnetic effects of iron. Thus this method is capable of non-invasively detecting the level of

oxygenation of blood haemoglobin. Owing to cerebral autoregulation of local brain blood supply, brain areas that are more active during certain functional processes tend to show an increase in blood supply and perfusion (neuronal activation and blood flow are "coupled"). The increase of oxygenated blood in a specific area of the human brain correlates with its local functional activity at the neuronal level and can be measured indirectly by MRI. This measurement is frequently corrupted by noise from various sources and hence statistical procedures are used to extract the underlying signal. The resulting brain activation can be presented graphically by colour-coding the strength of activation across the brain or the specific region studied (Kent 1998).

By using fMRI it is possible to visualise brain regions that are active during certain cognitive tasks. Thus the characteristic areas associated with language comprehension and production can be non-invasively identified (Fig. 23.8). By

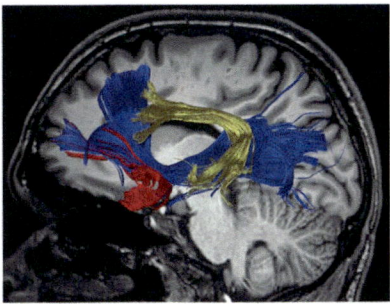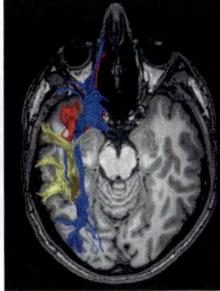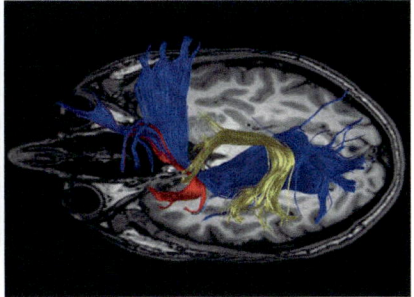

**Fig. 23.6** Diffusion tensor imaging (DTI)-based white matter pathway reconstructions of language-related pathways following the dual stream model of language processing: structural depiction of the ventral and dorsal stream in phonological processing. The ventral stream from the lateral and posterior temporal lobe follows the inferior fronto-occipital fascicle (blue) and the uncinate fascicle (red). The dorsal stream mainly follows the arcuate fascicle (yellow) connecting the inferior frontal gyrus to the supramarginal and superior and middle temporal gyri. Kasprian © 2021

using more advanced post-processing techniques on fMRI data, it is now possible to describe large parts of language-related brain activations as "language networks". These show lesion-specific alterations with different brain pathologies (tumours, malformations, epileptogenic lesions) leading to different patterns of language network changes (Foesleitner et al. 2020a). Network changes related to elective neurosurgical procedures can also be better understood by visualising the extensive alterations in these patients (Foesleitner et al. 2020b). This opens new ways of assessing clinically subtle aphasia and clinical understanding of the severity of language deficits at the individual level.

### 23.7.5 Structural Pathology of the Brain

Computed tomography (CT) and magnetic resonance imaging (MRI) allow assessment of the site and size of focal, multifocal and diffuse brain damage. Depending on the setting (acute or chronic) and patient presentation, both CT and MRI are instrumental examinations in the neurological diagnostic process. From a phoniatrician's point of view, CT and MRI bring two key pieces of information: the impaired domain of the speech motor system (cortico-bulbar system, extrapyramidal system, cerebellar system, brainstem) and the presence of damage in the non-motor system (diffuse cortical or subcortical damage, multifocal lesions, language areas lesions) (Figs. 23.4, 23.5, 23.6, 23.7, and 23.8). Knowledge of the domain of the motor system is necessary for the classification of dysarthria subtypes, as perceptual assessment alone might be misleading (Fig. 23.4). Information on the non-motor brain structures is equally important, as it allows the suspicion of potential impairment in linguistic or cognitive functions, both important in rehabilitation (Figs. 23.6 and 23.8). Communication approaches and augmentative alternative approaches (AAC) assume that verbal or cognitive skills for communication are preserved.

Overall, the neuroradiological assessment of potential brain abnormalities requires detailed knowledge about the underlying neuroanatomical functional architecture to be able to assess patients with dysarthria or aphasia appropriately.

## 23.8 Differential Diagnosis in Respect of Various Neurological Diseases and Subtypes of Language Disorder

Stefano Cappa

Differential diagnosis of the multiple diseases that can be associated with an acquired language disorder is based foremost, as in any other area of

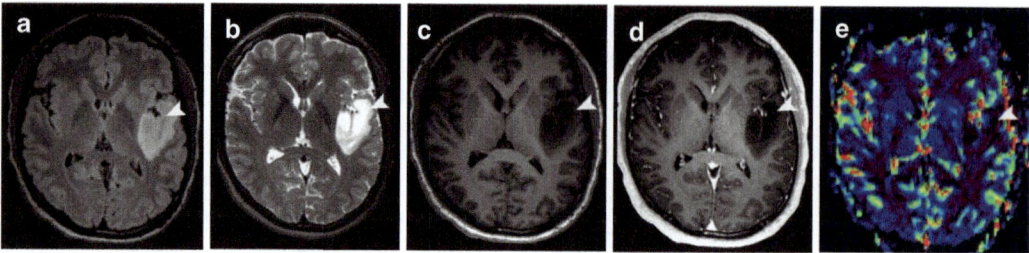

**Fig. 23.7** Axial series of FLAIR (**a**), T2-weighted (**b**), T1-weighted (**c**), T1-weighted with gadolinium-based contrast agent (**d**), perfusion-weighted/cerebral blood volume map (**e**) MRI in a patient with a low-grade glioma of the left superior temporal gyrus and insular region. The lesion (arrowhead) is FLAIR and T2-weighted hyperintense/bright and T1-weighted hypointense. As a rather characteristic of low-grade glioma, there is no clear contrast agent uptake (**d**). MR perfusion map indicates no significant hypervascularisation of the tumour also consistent with its low tumour grade. Kasprian © 2021

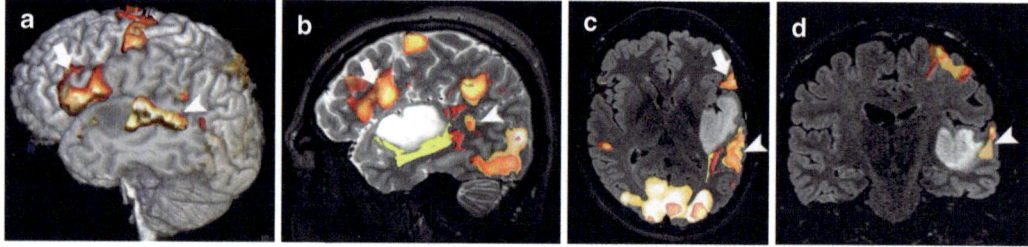

**Fig. 23.8** Functional language fMRI with a verb generation and a sentence completion task in the same patient as shown in Fig. 23.7. The orange and yellow areas mark those regions linked to increased blood flow due to neural activity. The Broca area in the left inferior frontal region (arrow) and the Wernicke regions in the left posterior temporal lobe (arrowhead) are significantly correlated with overt language comprehension and production tasks. The glioma shows a very close association with language activation and the language-associated pathways (inferior longitudinal fascicle in yellow and arcuate fascicle in red). Kasprian © 2021

clinical neurology, on an accurate clinical history, followed by the neurological examination and diagnostic tests. The aetiological diagnosis in neurology follows the topographical diagnosis, which, in the case of language disorders, is relatively straightforward, pointing to the language networks of the dominant hemisphere.

The modality of onset is a first, crucial clue for the differential diagnosis. Any acute focal lesion to the brain, involving the multiple cortical and subcortical regions associated with language processing (see Sect. 21.5) can result in language impairment. An acute onset in most cases is compatible with the diagnosis of stroke, the most common cause of acquired aphasia. The ischaemic or haemorrhagic nature of the lesion is evident on the CT scan or MRI investigation. Other frequent causes, prevalent in the younger

population, are the consequences of traumatic brain injury.

On the other hand, a progressive onset is compatible with a number of hypotheses, with tumours and neurodegenerative disorders ranking in the first place. Of course, the presence of other signs and symptoms, and the age of the patient, are other factors to be considered in the differential diagnosis. Not to be neglected, in particular in the elderly population, is the possibility of a chronic subdural haematoma, often unrelated to any known head injury, compressing the language areas of the left hemisphere. In this case, a CT or MRI scan is sufficient to diagnose the presence of a space-occupying lesion.

On the other hand, the structural imaging methods in general do not allow a definite diagnosis of the neurodegenerative condition that may be responsible for a primary progressive aphasia in individual subjects in the early stages. Functional imaging, in particular positron emission tomography (PET), allowing the assessment of local metabolism (Fluorodeoxyglucose-PET FDG-PET) or molecular pathology (amyloid and tau scans), is a powerful method for the diagnosis of neurodegeneration (Chandra et al. 2019). PET imaging is particularly useful in the diagnosis of primary progressive aphasia and its variants (Tee and Gorno-Tempini 2019). Aphasia can be observed as a rare presentation of Creutzfeldt-Jakob disease (Riancho et al. 2016).

A special case to be considered is transient aphasia, with sudden onset and complete recovery, usually within 24 h. The most frequent cause is a transient ischaemic attack, most often in the left internal carotid artery territory. It is always important to consider three "stroke mimics" that can be associated with sudden onset of aphasia, i.e., epilepsy, migraine and hypoglycaemia. A partial seizure, often from a left temporal lobe focus, can manifest as a transient language disorder (Trebuchon et al. 2018). The differential diagnosis is largely based on a careful clinical history and may not always be simple. Structural brain imaging is usually normal or shows unspecific features. The inter-ictal electro-encephalography (EEG), recorded when the patient is not having a clinical seizure, may also be uninformative. Prolonged EEG recording and video-EEG may unusually be required for the differential diagnosis. Aphasia can also be observed in the aura phase of a migraine attack, often following visual disturbances in the right visual hemi-field, reflecting spreading cortical depression (Mishra et al. 2009). The possibility of hypoglycaemia needs to be considered in any diabetic patient on insulin treatment.

Finally, mention should be made of language disorders in psychiatric conditions. Mutism is very seldom observed in aphasia, except in the first few hours after a major stroke. Persistent mutism usually points to a psychiatric disorder. On the other hand, fluent, meaningless production with defective comprehension, in many ways similar to severe Wernicke's aphasia with jargon, has been reported in schizophrenia (Little et al. 2019). Again, the diagnosis should not be difficult on purely clinical grounds, supplemented, if necessary, by brain imaging.

## 23.9 Clinical Neurophysiology

Stefano Cappa

While neurophysiological methods are applied extensively to language research, their clinical diagnostic role in the assessment of acquired language disorders in adults is currently limited. The presence of a focal or degenerative brain process can be routinely assessed by neuroimaging methods, including structural and functional brain imaging, limiting the diagnostic usefulness of clinical neurophysiology to a few specific clinical instances.

The role of electro-encephalography (EEG) remains crucial only for the assessment of paroxysmal language disorders. Aphasia during an epileptic seizure is not uncommon, but only rarely is it an isolated clinical manifestation. It has been reported with left temporal lobe foci. A rare condition is aphasic status epilepticus, a form of isolated status epilepticus (Trinka et al. 2015) that is characterised by the acute onset of aphasic symptoms, correlating with an EEG showing continuous left hemispheric epileptic activity. It can be due to a variety of conditions, including focal brain lesions (usually tumours) or systemic disorders, such as non-ketotic hyperglycaemia (Tsai et al. 2018). Speech and language disorders can also be observed in the context of the complex behavioural manifestations of a non-convulsive status epilepticus due to frontal seizures. An important condition in paediatric neurology in which EEG plays a central role is the Landau-Kleffner syndrome, characterised by aphasia and continuous spike-and-wave activity during sleep, which is now considered to be part of an epilepsy-aphasia spectrum (Tsai et al. 2013). The typical triphasic periodic complexes on EEG are diagnostic of the unusual presentation of Creutzfeldt-Jakob disease as a rapidly progressive aphasia (Mandell et al. 1989).

The recording of evoked responses in visual, auditory, and somatosensory modalities is part of the diagnostic evaluation of multiple-sclerosis patients, in which aphasia is a very rare clinical presentation (Lacour et al. 2004). Finally, EMG is used to assess the presence of lower motor neuron involvement in patients with Primary Progressive Aphasia (PPA) due to pathology belonging to the FTD-MND spectrum (Vinceti et al. 2019).

While the clinical applications of neurophysiology to language disorders are now limited, advanced neurophysiological techniques, including magneto-encephalography, are widely used as a research tool in the field of psycholinguistics and neuropsychology. Their main contribution is to provide a high temporal resolution counterpart to the structural and functional brain imaging techniques, allowing a precise temporal analysis of the brain mechanism involved in language processing, such as auditory comprehension (Friederici 2011) and reading (Salmelin 2010).

Invasive recording of brain activity during language tasks (electrocorticography) as well as intra-operative direct electrical stimulation of the language cortex are now extensively used in the evaluation of patients undergoing awake surgery for the treatment of brain tumours and malformations (Babajani-Feremi et al. 2016; Schuerman and Leonard 2023). Besides the obvious clinical importance, these tools are providing invaluable new information about the brain mechanism responsible for language processing (Martin et al. 2019).

Neuromodulation methods (transcranial magnetic and electrical stimulation) are the focus of intensive investigation as potential tools to improve language recovery in stroke aphasia and PPA. Several meta-analytic studies have reviewed the available evidence about effectiveness (Georgiou et al. 2019; Cotelli et al. 2020; Mimura et al. 2023).

## 23.10  Interpretation of Results of (Neuro-)Psychological Examinations

Stefano Zago and Edoardo Nicolò Aiello

Neuropsychological assessment has to be approached both qualitatively and quantitatively. Individuals' psychometric outcomes are indeed complemented with signs detected during both test execution (e.g., phonemic conduites d'approche during a confrontation naming task) and clinical interviews (e.g., uncriticised incorrect verb inflections), as well as with referred symptoms (e.g., tip-of-the-tongue phenomena in spontaneous speech) (Hannay and Lezak 2004). Qualitative clinical features also happen to be susceptible to a form of scoring (e.g., perseverance during a constructional-praxis task)—thus possibly becoming quantifiable (Somerville et al. 2000). However, although still inherently probabilistic, an accurate interpretation of potential qualitative markers of cognitive/behavioural dysfunctions is more dependent on practitioners' applied (e.g., clinical) background than it is on their methodological expertise (Monti et al. 2008; Kolakowsky-Hayner and Caplan 2011). By contrast, when it comes to drawing clinical judgements from test scores, care should be paid to the adopted statistical frameworks.

Practitioners have first to bear in mind fundamental psychometric properties that tests have to possess in order for them to be applicable—and thus test scores to be interpretable (Barr 2001). A test has to be valid—i.e., to measure what it is intended to (systematic error variability will be lower than the portion reflecting the target construct)—and reliable—i.e., to yield similar results on different administrations, other predictors remaining constant (random error variability will be lower than systematic components) (Willmes 2010). Epidemiological statistics have also to be addressed, such as sensitivity—i.e., the ability of a test to label a pathological performance as impaired—and specificity—i.e., labelling a normal performance as unimpaired (Rohling et al. 2017; Trevethan 2017). For instance, one would not uncritically regard a defective score on the Paced Auditory Serial Addition Test (PASAT) (Gronwall 1977) per se as supportive of a relevant attentive/executive deficit in an individual with suspected logopenic aphasia (Gorno-Tempini et al. 2011). Indeed, highly demanding and thus sensitive tests (e.g., the PASAT) may be inadequate as screeners or as the sole means through which a clinical inference is made (Brooks et al. 2011). Moreover, caution should be exerted when interpreting scores whose systematic error variability is possibly high—e.g., both linguistic (i.e., phonological) and extra-linguistic (e.g., short-term memory) components may underlie the performance on the PASAT (Strub and Gardner 1974).

Given that a test is psychometrically satisfactory, raw scores (RSs) yielded by its administration have to be quantitatively attributed a clinical, qualitative judgement (Willmes 2010). Performance levels are defined according to a comparison of RSs against point/interval norms—often by converting them into a common metric (Capitani 1997). When standardising RSs, one should pay attention to both the nature of the data and the adequacy of norm-inferring methods. Those requiring distributional assumptions (e.g., z-transformations, which assume that data converge to a normal distribution) should be cautiously adopted (Crawford 2003), as these criteria are often not met by neuropsychological data (e.g., normality and homogeneous variance violations owing to ceiling/floor effects and high inter-individual variability) (Malek-Ahmadi et al. 2017). Non-parametric approaches to RSs standardisation have therefore been traditionally preferred (e.g., Equivalent Scores, ESs) (Capitani and Laiacona 1997, 2017)—this being relevant for practitioners not falling into errors when interpreting results (e.g., underestimation of cognitive deficits severity) (Scherr et al. 2016). It has to be noted that not all standardisation procedures provide checks for inferential errors (Willmes 2010). For instance, the cut-off computed within the ESs method corresponds to the outer one-sided non-parametric lower tolerance limit, i.e., the highest observation in the "worst" 5% of a healthy sample that yields a $\geq 95\%$ probability that at most 5% of the population performs below it (Capitani and Laiacona 2017). This allows practitioners to keep the error risk at 5% when judging a performance as defective (ibidem): the same precaution, however, is not considered when adopting as cut-off, e.g., either a percentile or a z-score (Crawford 2003; Willmes 2010;

Capitani and Laiacona 2017). The representativeness of the normative sample from which norms are derived has also to be accounted when judging their quality (Willmes 2010).

Therefore, when it comes to fruition of both novel tests and updated norms—the latter being needed owing to socio-demographic changes (Siciliano et al. 2019), practitioners should always take into consideration methodological-statistical correctness of works (Bush 2010).

When interpreting RSs and standardising them, one should also bear in mind the statistical unit under investigation (Hambleton and Jones 1993). Although global test scores are often regarded as the only outcome (e.g., Classical Test Theory), single-item level approaches (e.g., Item Response Theory) are gaining ground (Martins et al. 2020). This last assertion happens to be true especially in the aphasiological field, where adaptive testing techniques happen to be intuitively applicable (e.g., a clinician administering only "difficult" items of a naming task to a patient clinically diagnosed with mild anomic aphasia after suffering a traumatic brain injury) (Edmonds and Donovan 2012).

A final remark has to be made on intervening constructs possibly bringing error variability into test scores—such as individual features (e.g., age, educational attainment, sex), psychological functioning (e.g., state of anxiety, personality traits) or environmental variables (e.g., background noises during the examination) (Kessels and Brands 2009). For example, regression-based norm-inferring methods (e.g., ESs) allow accounting for the influence of systematic variables such as age and education, by adjusting RSs via ad hoc equations—i.e., by computing Ass (adjusted scores) (Willmes 2010, Capitani and Laiacona 2017). Less trivial would be to control quantitatively for stochastic confounding factors (e.g., situational mood fluctuations)—which should nonetheless be qualitatively kept in mind by practitioners when interpreting results of neuropsychological examinations (Kessels and Brands 2009; Kolakowsky-Hayner and Caplan 2011).

## 23.11 Interpretation of Results of Speech-Language Examination

Lisa Gerhards, Jana Quinting and Kristina Jonas

### 23.11.1 Introduction

A comprehensive assessment (analogue or digital/remote) is the beginning of every speech and language therapy intervention. Before deciding how to interpret a particular test result of a person with aphasia (PwA), clinicians should take a step back and ask: what was the purpose of the diagnostics?

The aim of a well-founded diagnosis is not only to differentiate between pathological and non-pathological language use and to give a name to the identified (combination of) symptoms. It is much more about a meaningful description and identification of underlying performance deficits, as well as the identification of individual resources of the PwA. This enables the speech and language therapist in collaboration with the PwA to derive individual and meaningful goals for the subsequent planning of speech-language therapy (Elston et al. 2021; Hersh et al. 2012; Keil and Kaszniak 2002; Thiele 2013).

A comprehensive evaluation of diagnostic information should therefore consider the following factors:

- Case history
- Formal diagnostic information
- Informal diagnostic information

These factors do contribute individually to diagnosis and intervention planning, but can also influence each other constantly during the interpretation process (e.g., knowledge about pre-morbid performance influences the interpretation of formal test results). Moreover, they are essential for the interpretation of all diagnostic results against the background of the patient's individu-

ally perceived constraints and needs, in order to define relevant therapy goals (Brown et al., 2022; Elston et al., 2021; Hersh et al. 2012; National Institute for Health and Care Excellence 2013). See Fig. 23.9 for an overview of all components that are relevant during the interpretation process.

### 23.11.2 Information of Case History

Case history information as well as demographic data is of particular importance when interpreting diagnostic results. Information on the medical history of the PwA, such as that on aetiology, severity or post-onset time (acute, post-acute, chronic state) has a relevant impact on the interpretation of test results. For example, in acute aphasia fluctuating symptoms predominate, and therefore symptomatology can be strongly affected by general signs of illness or neuropsychological impairments (e.g., fatigue, reduced alertness), whereas in post-acute and chronic aphasia, typical combinations of symptoms (i.e., syndromes) are manifested; thus, core impairments can be reliably identified. Henceforth, the focus of diagnostics in acute aphasia lies in identifying the linguistic impairment (aphasia: yes or no), on differential diagnosis including the differentiation from concomitant symptoms, as well as on the general patient's ability to endure therapeutic sessions (Nobis-Bosch et al. 2013).

Moreover, the diagnostic results should be analysed against the background of concomitant impairments of vision, attention, executive functions or memory, as well as concurrent motor speech disorders such as dysarthria and apraxia of speech (ASHA 2020; Raymer and Gonzalez Rothi 2018). Demographic variables such as age, education, and pre-morbid performance level should also be taken into account. Not least, case history data (e.g., family environment, social network, professional requirements) can be used to identify possible support factors or barriers to speech-language rehabilitation, as well as parameters that influence vocational (and school) rehabilitation (Raymer and Gonzalez Rothi 2018).

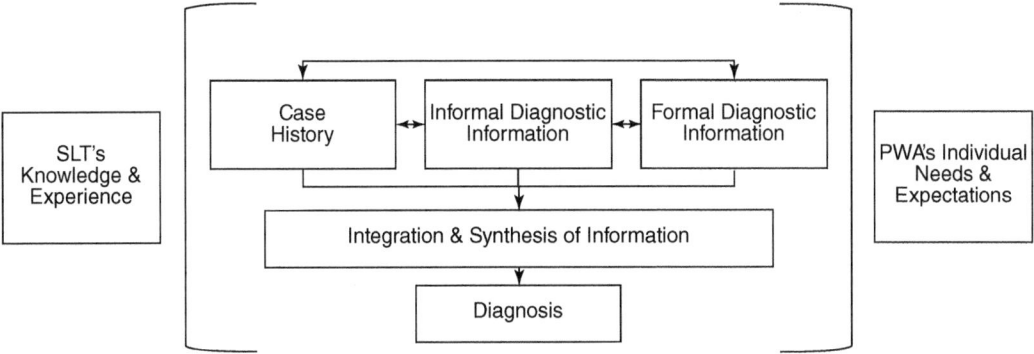

**Fig. 23.9** Components of the Interpretation Process. (Modified from Pindzola et al. 2015.) *SLT* Speech-Language Therapist, *PwA* Person with Aphasia

### 23.11.3 Interpretation of Formal Assessment Data

A comprehensive formal assessment includes standardised and psychometrically evaluated test procedures, and elicits language performance in a structured context (Murray and Coppens 2013). It thus enables a reliable measurement of language function in this particular setting in order to derive a diagnosis that permits a prediction of performance in real-life settings. The strong structuring of the test situation enables, for example, a comparison of the PwA's test performance over time, but carries the risk of misjudging communicative performance in everyday life. Generally, owing to their artificial and abstract nature, test scores need to be considered only as an approximation of real-life performance (Lezak et al. 2004).

#### 23.11.3.1 Interpretation of Test Scores

Different types of test score can be observed as outcomes for standardised and normed language assessments. The raw score reflects the obvious performance of the examinee (e.g., a PwA) and mostly derives from the total number of correct answers, for example: 23 out of 30 items could be named correctly during a picture naming test, resulting in a raw score of 23. However, this raw score is not informative per se, as it does not analyse the examinee's score compared with an age-, gender-, or education-matched reference group. Hence, in order to classify the raw score and get

an impression of its relative value, it must be converted into a norm-referenced test score (Dancey and Reidy 2020; Field 2018; Moosbrugger and Kelava 2020; Lezak et al. 2004). Therefore, standardised assessments always include information on normed data.

One possibility for comparing an individual's test scores to the norm are percentile ranks. A percentile rank indicates the percentage of the norm (i.e., test score outcomes of the norm group) that fall at or below the examinees performance level (raw score).

Example: A PwA achieves a percentile rank of 63 in the Scenario Test (Nobis-Bosch et al. 2020). This indicates that the PwA scores are as good as or better than 63% of the norm group.

A more precise possibility of comparing an individual test score to the norm is the conversion of the raw into a standard score from the assumption that the test results are normally distributed. This means that most of the people of a norm sample would achieve average test scores whereas only a few people would demonstrate extreme scores. For an illustration of a normal distribution see Fig. 23.10.

The peak of the curve illustrates the mean (score) (M) of the norm sample. The standard deviation (SD) indicates the amount of variability as the dispersion of test scores within the norm sample in relation to the mean. These, the mean and the standard deviation either side, include 68% of the norm group (1 SD comprises 34%). A test score that deviates two standard deviations from the mean is often determined as statistically significant and therefore indicates (if lower than two SD below the mean) a pathological performance (Dancey and Reidy 2020; Field 2018). There are different kinds of standard scores or scales that can be found in language and communication assessments. These differ in their respective mean score and the standard deviation (see Fig. 23.10 for an illustration of the z-score, t-score, stanine, and percentile ranks).

Example T-score: The mean of the t-score is 50 and the standard deviation is 10. Imagine that a PwA achieves a raw score of 46 on the auditory comprehension subtest of the Aachen Aphasia Test (Huber et al. 1983). According to the norm tables of the AAT, a raw score of 46 corresponds to a t-score of 55: this is to be interpreted as average performance.

Furthermore, to interpret formal diagnostic information of speech and language assessments the following methodological considerations must be taken into account.

**Quality of the Test Procedure**

The interpretation of the results always depends on the quality of the test used to examine language and communication skills. In this context, not (only) the classic psychometric criteria of objectivity, reliability, and validity, or the sensitivity or specificity of a test (Keil and Kaszniak 2002, Jonas and Jaecks 2021, Lezak et al. 2004, Moosbrugger and Kelava 2020, see Table 23.1 for definitions) are of particular importance, but rather the concept of ecological validity, which is relevant in order to be able to make a therapy-relevant prediction about everyday life performance of a PwA (Lezak et al. 2004).

**Interfering or Influencing Factors During Diagnostics**

In order to obtain an unbiased impression of the language and communication abilities of the PwA, test results should always be evaluated against the background of unsystematic error sources or possible interfering variables [(e.g., daily form, stress, fluctuations in attention and motivation during the assessment, performance inconsistency, pain, medication, fatigue, depression/frustration, (Moosbrugger and Kelava

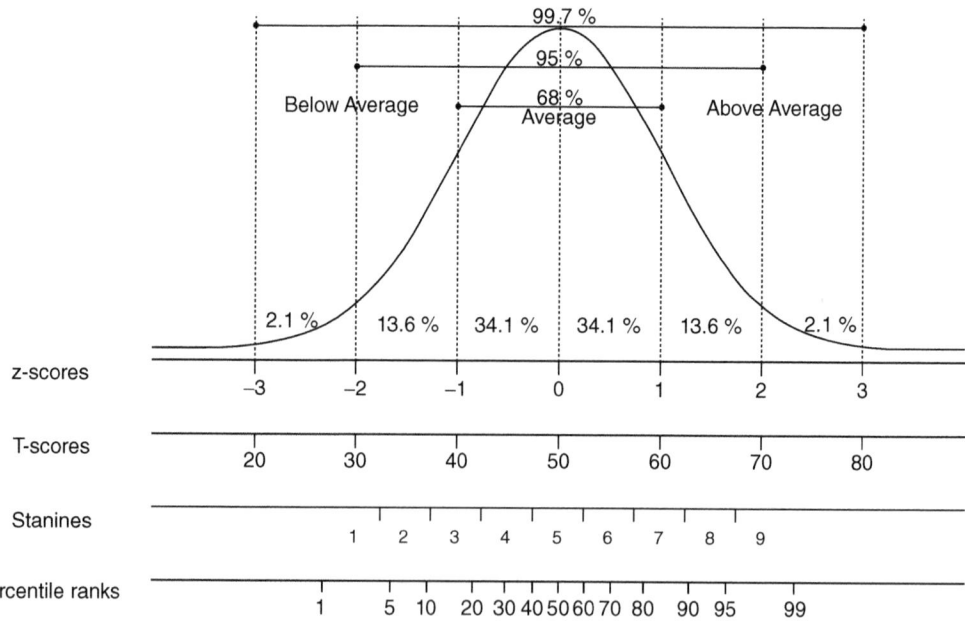

**Fig. 23.10** Normal curve and associated standard scores. (Modified from Moosbrugger and Kelava 2020)

**Table 23.1** Definitions: psychometric criteria and measures of classification accuracy

| | |
|---|---|
| Objectivity | The objectivity of a test is met when the analysis of performance is independent of test administrators or scorers |
| Reliability | The reliability of a test indicates the consistency with which a performance is recorded (with little measuring error) |
| Validity | The validity of a test is met when it measures the performance it is intended to measure and no other |
| Sensitivity | Sensitivity is a measure of the probability with which a test will identify an impairment when an impairment is actually present |
| Specificity | Specificity is a measure of the probability with which a test will not detect an impairment when there is no (or another) impairment |

Definitions based on Moosbrugger and Kelava (2020)

2020)]. In the particular context of remote diagnostics (e.g., telepractice), the impact of eHelpers (e.g., significant others) on the diagnostic outcome must be considered, as inappropriate support or feedback could be given during the testing process (Kester 2020).

**Common Interpretation Errors**

When interpreting test results, the examiners should constantly reflect on their hypotheses and expectations on the PwA's performance, to avoid unconscious interpretation errors. Common interpretation errors that tend to occur during the interpretation process (Lezak et al. 2004) are for example:

- Confirmatory Bias: exclusion of findings that contradict the suspected hypothesis or diagnosis.
- Over- or under-interpretation of results: e.g., an over-interpretation of a single prominent finding (e.g., low performance in one subscore) while performance in other subscores is within normal range.
- False negatives: the absence of low scores in a speech-language assessment does not necessarily mean the absence of a speech and language disorder. A test may not detect impaired performance even though it exists. For exam-

ple, subtle language deficits often cannot be reliably detected by standardised procedures, as symptoms tend to show up in challenging everyday situations. The examiner should always reflect on the assessment tool chosen and its ability to detect present difficulties.

**Evaluation Issues**

In general, the determination of standard scores is not acceptable if the norming sample does not adequately represent the PwA and his or her demographic profile (ASHA 2020). Given that most language tests do not provide separate norms adjusted for such demographic variables as age, sex, education, etc. (Rohde et al. 2018), the examiner should consider the existing norms cautiously. Therefore, test performance should always be reflected against the background of pre-morbid functioning (Lezak et al. 2004).

**ICF-Related Considerations**

From the interpretation of formal assessment data, linguistic and communicative performance (difficulties and resources) at the level of Body Structures and Functions (World Health Organization 2001) can be detected in expressive and receptive abilities in spoken and written language at all linguistic levels, e.g., phonology, morphology, semantics, syntax, and pragmatics (Rubi-Fessen 2017). From the diagnostic results, well-preserved functions as well as impairments can be identified. For example, if a PwA shows impaired understanding of dates (times), but performs well in sight-reading of words, the use of written words/times can be used as a resource in therapy. Intact or well-preserved linguistic abilities could then be used as resources in therapy for the learning of new skills and for establishing compensatory strategies (e.g., Augmentative and Alternative Communication) (cf. Rose et al. 2003, 2011). Finally, a comprehensive formal diagnosis should also address the effects of language impairment on activity, participation and quality of life (cf. Canadian Stroke Best Practice 2019; Worrall et al. 2011; ASHA 2020) and determine which functional impairments have the strongest impact.

### 23.11.4 Interpretation of Informal Diagnostic Information

Compared with formal methods, informal ones (e.g., observations during test sessions) help to include individual strategies or compensation mechanisms in the derivation of therapy goals (Thomson et al. 2018). In her process-orientated approach, Kaplan (1988) emphasises that for the assessment and characterisation of a performance deficit, not only the test result is of importance. The testing process as well as a compound diagnosis also involves the observation of behaviour during the performance of a specific task or in everyday communication (Lezak et al. 2004; Whitworth et al. 2013). This is especially important because the same test score can be obtained in different ways, meaning by qualitative different performances. Thus, the steps that led to the result or the behaviour during the test should also be taken into account when assessing performance (Kaplan 1988). The example of word fluency tasks (e.g., "Name as many animals as possible within one minute") illustrates this quite well. This type of task traditionally uses the number of correct responses as a performance measure (cf. Thiele 2013; Thiele et al. 2016). If, for example, the result is five correct answers, this number of answers can have been obtained in different ways: (i) the PwA named only five animals within 1 min, (ii) the PwA produced a total of 12 different words, but only five of these were animals.

### 23.11.5 Conclusion

The challenge for the speech-language therapist is to integrate and synthesise all the outlined information in order to derive a comprehensive diagnosis and thus be able to propose a therapeutic intervention to the PwA. Drawing a coherent picture of the language disorder with its impact on the individual's everyday life requires, ultimately, the speech-language therapist's knowledge and clinical experience (Pindzola et al. 2015, see Fig. 23.9). It is the therapist's responsibility to build up this experience and constantly re-evaluate his or her own behaviour in the interpretation process.

### 23.12 Occupational Therapist as a Team Member Supporting Adults with Acquired Language Disorders

Anne Escher and Sue Berger

### 23.12.1 Occupational Therapy for Adults with Acquired Language Disorders

Occupational therapists assist people to participate in meaningful everyday activities, referred to as occupations. Adults with acquired language disorders experience decreased participation in their life activities. Those with post-stroke aphasia often experience additional sequelae, for instance cognitive changes, hemiparesis, sensory loss or visual perceptual challenges. Communication impairment can have an impact on many areas of occupation, such as social participation, work or education. The addition of a physical, cognitive or perceptual limitation can exacerbate the impact on the client's participation in daily activities. For instance, someone who has experienced a left-sided stroke may experience right-sided motor weakness or paralysis along with aphasia, making daily activities such as cooking challenging. The International Classification of Function (ICF) provides a framework for organising and understanding a client's functional status. Occupational therapy outcomes focus on the areas of activity—"the execution of a task or action by an individual"—and participation—"involvement in a life situation" (World Health Organization 2002, p. 11). Within the Activities and Participation section of the ICF, communication, interpersonal interactions and relationships, and community, social and civic life directly relate to the desire of people with aphasia to participate more fully in valued life activities. Given that the scope of occupational therapy practice supports the use of occupation-based interventions to increase participation of individuals post-stroke (Wolf et al. 2015), occupational therapy is uniquely suited to assist clients with aphasia to re-engage in valued occupations affected by their communication and possible additional impairments. Through activity and task analysis, occupational therapists are able to assess the holistic impact of acquired language disorders on participation in daily activities.

The goals of occupational therapy intervention for adults with aphasia are focused on improving an individual's ability to perform daily activities that often require communication. Consider the example of cooking dinner. Even if cooking alone, one uses multiple language skills to complete this activity. Understanding a recipe, reading measurements and setting the oven temperature all require language abilities. Through activity analysis, occupational therapists identify the areas of challenge, and with adaptations and education help support re-engagement in this activity. Cooking dinner can also take on a social dimension for many people as well—cooking together may be common in some households. Supporting the person with aphasia to be able to participate in the cooking of a meal may also include education of communication partners. Cooking is just one of many daily tasks that involve communication. Occupational therapists play a key role in supporting participation in many daily occupations for adults with communication impairment.

### 23.12.2 Evaluation of Daily Activities Impacted by Aphasia

Occupational therapists use multiple types of assessment to evaluate the impact of impairments on daily life activities. When available, results from the speech and language pathologist's (SLP) evaluation guide the occupational therapist's approach to evaluation and intervention for clients with aphasia. Occupational therapy evaluations may be standardised or non-standardised. Non-standardised evaluation includes skilled observation and interviews. Occupational therapists are trained in skilled observation of clients performing daily activities, and these observations provide much information regarding how the client is functioning and their strengths and challenges.

Standardised outcome measures are based on the practitioner's observations, or client self-report. Patient-reported outcomes have become increasingly important in the health care environment (National Quality Forum 2021; National Quality Forum 2015). Although completing self-report standardised assessments may be challenging for people with communication impairments, there are ways to adapt administrative styles to make participation in self-report measures possible for this population. For instance, offering scaled levels of support with self-reported measures, such as repeating the question and the answer choices, simplifying the question, re-explaining the choice scale, and combining a yes/no question with the scale, have been found to be effective with clients with aphasia (Australian Aphasia Rehabilitation Pathway 2014; Hagelskjaer et al. 2019; Herbert et al. 2012; Tucker et al. 2012).

Goal-setting is done in collaboration with the client. Occupational therapy practitioners use adapted materials and strategies to ensure that the client understands the occupational therapist's role and that the client can be a part of the collaborative goal-setting process. These adapted strategies may include providing choice, using pictures, simplifying language and facilitating multimodal ways to communicate (Berger et al. 2017). The collaborative occupational therapy goals should focus on the client's ability to re-engage in valued daily activities.

### 23.12.3 Therapeutic Interventions

Occupational therapists use a variety of strategies to support individuals with acquired language disorders (Escher et al. 2022; Escher et al. 2020). Some examples of therapeutic interventions within the scope of occupational therapy practice are listed below.

#### 23.12.3.1 Augmentative and Alternative Communication

From multiple systematic reviews, there is strong evidence that augmentative and alternative communication (AAC) is effective in supporting communication in functional situations (Pedrozo Campos Antunes et al. 2018; Russo et al. 2017). Speech and language pathologists and occupational therapists recommend, and train individuals in, the use of AAC. The context, the individual's abilities and the therapeutic goals all influence which discipline might be most appropriate to support the use of AAC, and often professionals from both disciplines collaborate to determine the most effective strategy.

Occupational therapists can determine if the individual has enough fine motor coordination to use a hand or finger to operate technology or whether a joystick, eye gaze, optical pointers or visual scanning would be more appropriate. Occupational therapists collaborate with the client to determine the best positioning of the device to support proper body mechanics, along with figuring out how AAC fits into daily routines. For example, does the client wear clothing with pockets to carry a device, for them to be able to access it when needed, or is there proper lighting in the area where they use device?

High-tech options to support communication have increased significantly over the past 20 years with a wide variety of cell phones, tablets, and computers to choose from, all with accessibility features. Because options and technology often change, it may be necessary to refer to an assistive technology specialist, often an occupational therapist or speech and language pathologist, who specialises in this practice.

Stigma, inadequate training and lack of support from care partners are just a few of the reasons people abandon AAC (Chavers et al. 2021; Mindel 2020). Occupational therapists play an important role in supporting the continued use of AAC by assuring a good match of the device to the user's physical, cognitive, and communication abilities; providing adequate training for users, family, and caregivers; offering realistic expectations; and providing opportunities to practise use of the device in the natural environment (Moorcroft et al. 2019).

### 23.12.3.2 Social Participation as Intervention

Improving communication skills can lead to increased social participation, but just as importantly, participation in meaningful occupations

can improve communication (Escher et al. 2020). Daily activities, especially those performed with others, such as social, leisure, work, and volunteer activities provide those with communication impairment the opportunity and motivation to communicate. Occupational therapists can support individuals to resume activities that are important to them through adaptation of the environment or the task or both.

Participation in groups, including therapy groups, supports socialising for people with aphasia (Lanyon et al. 2018). While therapy groups often focus on improving specific skills, many individuals participate in therapy groups primarily to meet other people and develop friendships (Lanyon et al. 2018). Beyond participating in therapy groups, occupational therapists can support the participation of people with aphasia in social activities within their community. Engaging in topics that are relevant, motivating, and authentic can improve communication skills, self-confidence, and overall participation (Garrett and Lasker 2013).

### 23.12.3.3 Additional Compensatory and Adaptive Strategies

Many post-stroke clients have motoric, sensory or cognitive challenges that limit their ability to engage in their daily occupations. Aphasia is an additional challenge that can severely affect their ability to do the things they need or want to do. Some adaptive strategies that occupational therapists might employ to support participation at home and in the community for people with decreased communication include the following:

- Evaluating where individuals choose to socialise and collaborating on ways for them to continue to socialise effectively, such as dining with one friend versus a group of friends. Finding activities to do with others that don't involve extensive oral communication skills (e.g., playing checkers versus reading a book with grandchildren) may make engaging with others easier
- Observing clients cooking a meal. Do they struggle to follow a recipe or read the instructions on the back of a frozen food packet?

Occupational therapists can adapt recipes or directions to support comprehension by using plain language, an organised layout, and photos, as appropriate

- Assuring proper positioning of both the individual and equipment to support communication. Proper ergonomic set-up is important for everyone, but especially those who might be sitting for extended periods of time. Determining the need for tablet stands, a stylus and lighting is all within the scope of occupational therapy practice
- Discussing daily routines and providing strategies to support social participation. For example, socialising at times of day when one is least tired
- Determining strategies to support daily activities that facilitate communication. For example, practising and devising ways that clients can independently change batteries and insert hearing aids, despite hemiparesis
- Teaching one-handed typing skills for clients who use a tablet or computer to communicate/ type but have hemiparesis. Recommending and testing a variety of keyboards that can facilitate one-handed typing
- Exploring strategies to facilitate financial management. Brainstorming and testing a variety of options, such as using large-print cheques, setting up automatic bill paying, using an ATM machine, paying with virtual options such as Venmo or ApplePay, and using credit or debit cards

Most importantly, occupational therapists collaborate with speech and language pathologists to support clients' goals. Working together, occupational therapists learn which communication strategy might work best for each client. For example, for some, providing written material along with verbal communication might be most effective. For others, using short sentences and pauses are ideal. Occupational therapists need to learn the best strategy to communicate with their client to support the evaluation and goal-setting process and guide intervention. To meet the needs of clients with communication impairment and their care partners, occupational therapists should collaborate with SLP.

## 23.12.4 Conclusion

Ultimately, occupational therapists work with people with aphasia to ensure their ability to participate in the everyday life activities that are most important to them. Through interprofessional collaboration with SLP and the rest of the team involved in the client's care, occupational therapists evaluate performance, set collaborative goals, and provide interventions that take into account the client's full environmental context. Interventions may be adaptive or compensatory and often involve environmental adaptations and training with communication partners. Consider one example of a client who wants to take the bus. The SLP might work with the client on reading the timetable and developing scripts for greeting the bus driver. The occupational therapist might support the client in using money to buy a ticket and ensuring physical access to get on and off the bus. Occupational therapy brings a unique and important perspective to the care of adults with acquired language impairment—the "doing" of life activities.

## References

Allibrio G, Gori A, Signorini G et al (2009) Esame del linguaggio al letto del malato (Examination of speech at the bedside). Giornale di psicologia 3(1):7–21

Ambrose J, Hounsfield G (1973) Computerized transverse axial tomography. Br J Radiol 46(542):148–149

American Psychiatric Association (2013) Diagnostic and statistical manual of mental disorders, 5th edn. American Psychiatric Association, Washington

Andreetta S, Cantagallo A, Marini A (2012) Narrative discourse in anomicaphasia. Neuropsychologia 50(8):1787–1793

Andreetta S, Marini A, Menichelli A, Furlanis G, Vincis E, Caruso P, Naccarato M, Manganotti P (2024) Language assessment in persons with aphasia early after thrombolysis: the utility of multilevel procedures of discourse analysis. Aphasiology 1–32. https://doi.org/10.1080/02687038.2024.2340797

Angeleri R, Bara BG, Bosco FM et al (2019) ABaCo assessment battery for communication, II edn. Giunti Editore, Firenze

Arcara G, Bambini V (2016) Test for the Assessment of Pragmatic Abilities and Cognitive Substrates (APACS): normative data and psychometric properties. Front Psychol 7:70. https://doi.org/10.3389/fpsyg.2016.00070. Accessed 20 Aug 2021

Armstrong E (2000) Aphasic discourse analysis: the story so far. Aphasiology 14(9):875–892

Arnett PE (2013) Secondary influences on neuropsychological test performance. Oxford Academic Press, New York

ASHA (American Speech-Language-Hearing Association) (2020) Aphasia (practice portal). Available via www.asha.org/Practice-Portal/Clinical-Topics/Aphasia/. Accessed 1 Jan 2020

ASHA (American Speech-Language-Hearing Association) (2020) Assessment tools, techniques, and data sources. Available via https://www.asha.org/practice-portal/clinical-topics/late-language-emergence/assessment-tools-techniques-and-data-sources/. Accessed 1 Jan 2020

ASHA (American Speech-Language-Hearing Association) website (2020) Augmentative and alternative communication (AAC). Available via https://www.asha.org/public/speech/disorders/aac/. Accessed 2 Aug 2021

Australian Aphasia Rehabilitation Pathway (2014) Best practice for aphasia services across the continuum of care. Available at: http://www.aphasiapathway.com.au/

Babajani-Feremi A, Narayana S, Rezaie R et al (2016) Language mapping using high gamma electrocorticography, fMRI, and TMS versus electrocortical stimulation. Clin Neurophysiol 127(3):1822–1836

Bara BG (1999) Pragmatica cognitiva. Bollati Boringhieri, Torino

Barr WB (2001) Methodologic issues in neuropsychological testing. J Athl Train 36(3):297–302

Battista P, Miozzo A, Piccininni M et al (2017) Primary progressive aphasia: a review of neuropsychological tests for the assessment of speech and language disorders. Aphasiology 31(12):1359–1378

Baumgartner A, Rauer S, Hottenrott T et al (2019) Admission diagnoses of patients later diagnosed with autoimmune encephalitis. J Neurol 266(1):124–132

Baxter SEP, Evans PJS (2012) Barriers and facilitators to the use of high-technology augmentative and alternative communication devices: a systematic review and qualitative synthesis. Int J Lang Commun Disord 47(2):115–129

Bechara A, Damasio AR, Damasio H et al (1994) Insensitivity to future consequences following damage to human prefrontal cortex. Cognition 50(1-3):7–15

Berg EA (1948) A simple objective technique for measuring flexibility in thinking. J Gen Psychol 39(1):15–22

Berger S, Escher A, Hildebrand M et al (2017) Modifying outcome measures to support participation for people with aphasia. OT Pract 22(10):10–13

Biniek R, Huber W, Glindemann R et al (1992) The Aachen Aphasia Bedside Test-criteria for validity of psychologic tests. Nervenarzt 63(8):473–479

Brainin M, Heiss W-D (2019) Textbook of stroke medicine, 3rd edn. Cambridge University Press, Cambridge

Broca P (1861) Remarques sur le siège de la faculté du langage, suivie d'une observation d'aphémie (perte de la parole) (Remarks on the seat of the faculty of language, followed by an observation of aphemia (loss of speech)). Bulletins de la Sociètè anatomique 6:330–357

Brooks JBB, Giraud VO, Saleh YJ et al (2011) Paced auditory serial addition test (PASAT): a very difficult test even for individuals with high intellectual capability. Arq Neuropsiquiatr 69(3):482–484

Brown K, Worrall LE, Davidson B et al (2011) Living successfully with aphasia: a qualitative meta-analysis of the perspectives of individuals with aphasia, family members, and speech-language pathologists. Int J Speech Lang Pathol 14(20):141–155

Brown SE, Scobbie L, Worrall L et al (2022) Access G-AP: development of an accessible goal setting and action planning resource for stroke survivors with aphasia. Disability and Rehabilitation 45(13):2107–2117. https://doi.org/10.1080/09638288.2022.2085331

Bryant L, Ferguson A, Spencer E (2016) Linguistic analysis of discourse in aphasia: a review of the literature. Clin Linguist Phon 30(7):489–518

Burgess PW, Shallice T (1997) The Hayling and Brixton tests. Harcourt Assessment, London

Buschke H (1984) Cued recall in amnesia. J Clin Exp Neuropsychol 6(4):433–440

Bush SS (2010) Determining whether or when to adopt new versions of psychological and neuropsychological tests: ethical and professional considerations. Clin Neuropsychol 24(1):7–16

Bushnell CD, Johnston DB, Goldstein LB (2001) Retrospective assessment of initial stroke severity comparison of the NIH Stroke Scale and the Canadian Neurological Scale. Stroke 32(3):656–660

Canadian Stroke Best Practice (2019) Rehabilitation and recovery following stroke. Rehabilitation to improve language and communication. Available via https://www.strokebestpractices.ca/recommendations/stroke-rehabilitation/rehabilitation-to-improve-language-and-communication. Accessed 1 Jan 2020

Capasso R, Miceli G (2001) Esame Neuropsicologico per l'afasia (ENPA) (Neuropsychological examination for aphasia (ENPA)). Springer, Berlin/Heidelberg

Capitani E (1997) Normative data and neuropsychological assessment. Common problems in clinical practice and research. Neuropsychol Rehabil 7(4):295–310

Capitani E, Laiacona M (1997) Composite neuropsychological batteries and demographic correction: standardization based on equivalent scores, with a review of published data. J Clin Exp Neuropsychol 19(6):795–809

Capitani E, Laiacona M (2017) Outer and inner tolerance limits: their usefulness for the construction of norms and the standardization of neuropsychological tests. Clin Neuropsychol 31(6-7):1219–1230

Catani M, Howard RJ, Pajevic S et al (2002) Virtual in vivo interactive dissection of white matter fasciculi in the human brain. NeuroImage 17(1):77–94

Catani M, Allin MP, Husain M et al (2007) Symmetries in human brain language pathways correlate with verbal recall. Proc Natl Acad Sci USA 104(43):17163–17168

Catricalà E, Gobbi E, Battista P et al (2017) SAND: a screening for aphasia in neurodegeneration. Development and normative data. Neurol Sci 38(8):1469–1483

Catricalà E, Boschi V, Cuoco S et al (2019) The language profile of progressive supranuclear palsy. Cortex 115:294–308

Chandra A, Valkimadi PE, Pagano G et al (2019) Applications of amyloid, tau, and neuroinflammation PET imaging to Alzheimer's disease and mild cognitive impairment. Hum Brain Map 40(18):5424–5442

Chavers T, Cheng C, Koul R (2021) AAC interventions in persons with aphasia. In B.T. Ogletree (Ed.), Augmentative and alternative communication: Challenges and solutions (pp.141–168). PluralPublishing. https://web-p-ebscohost-com. ezproxy.bu.edu/bsi/ebookviewer/ebook/bmxlYmtfXzI 3MzA4MjNfX0FO0?sid=1706a383-8909-47f5-a83d-9dafe4b80f91@redis&vid=0&format=EB&rid=1

Cipolotti L, Warrington EK (1995) Neuropsychological assessment. J Neurol Neurosurg Psychiatry 58(6):655–664

Ciurli P, Marangolo P, Basso A (1996) In: Giunti OS (ed) Esame del Linguaggio II (Examination of language II), Firenze

Cotelli M, Manenti R, Ferrari C et al (2020) Effectiveness of language training and non-invasive brain stimulation on oral and written naming performance in Primary Progressive Aphasia: a meta-analysis and systematic review. Neurosci Biobehav Rev 108:498–525

Crary MA, Haak NJ, Malinsky AE (1989) Preliminary psychometric evaluation of an acute aphasia screening protocol. Aphasiology 3(7):631–618

Crawford JR (2003) Psychometric foundations of neuropsychological assessment. In: Goldstein LH, McNeil J (eds) Clinical neuropsychology: a practical guide to assessment and management for clinicians. Wiley, Chichester, pp 121–140

Dalmau J, Graus F (2023) Diagnostic criteria for autoimmune encephalitis: utility and pitfalls for antibody-negative disease. The Lancet Neurology 22(6):529–540.

Dancey C, Reidy J (2020) Statistics without maths for psychology. Pearson Education Limited, Harlow

De Renzi A, Vignolo LA (1962) Token test: a sensitive test to detect receptive disturbances in aphasics. Brain 85:665–678

Diamond A (2013) Executive functions. Ann Rev Psychol 64:135–168

Dichgans M, Pulit SL, Rosand J (2019) Stroke genetics: discovery, biology, and clinical applications. Lancet Neurol 18(6):587–599

Dodich A, Cerami C, Inguscio E et al (2019) The clinico-metabolic correlates of language impairment in corticobasal syndrome and progressive supranuclear palsy. Neuroimage Clin 24:102009. https://doi.org/10.1016/j.nicl.2019.102009

Doesborgh SJ, van de Sandt-Koenderman WM, Dippel DW et al (2003) Linguistic deficits in the acute phase of stroke. J Neurol 250:977–982

Edmonds LA, Donovan NJ (2012) Item-level psychometrics and predictors of performance for Spanish/English bilingual speakers on an object and action naming battery. J Speech Lang Hear Res 55(2):359–381

Ekman P, Friesen WV (1969) The repertoire of nonverbal behavior: categories, origins, usage, and coding. Semiotica 1:49–98

El Hachioui H, Visch-Brink EG, de Lau LM et al (2017) Screening tests for aphasia in patients with stroke: a systematic review. J Neurol 264(2):211–220

Elston A, Barnden R, Hersh D et al (2021) Developing person-centred goal setting resources with and for people with aphasia: a multi-phase qualitative study. Aphasiology 36(7):761–780. https://doi.org/10.1080/02687038.2021.1907294

Enderby P, Crow E (1996) Frenchay Aphasia Screening Test: validity and comparability. Disabil Rehabil 18(5):238–240

Escher A, Berger S, Carney A (2020) Communication assessment and intervention. In: Dirette DP, Gutman SA (eds) Occupational therapy for physical dysfunction, 8th edn. Wolters Kluwer, Philadelphia, pp 343–365

Escher A, McKinnon S, Berger S (2022) Effective interventions within the scope of occupational therapy practice to address participation for adults with aphasia: A systematic review. British Journal of Occupational Therapy 85(2):99–110.

Faiz A (2016) Lothian assessment for screening cognition in aphasia (LASCA): a new nonverbal assessment of cognition. Procedia Soc Behav Sci 217:1052–1062

Field A (2018) Discovering statistics using IBM SPSS statistics, 5th edn. SAGE, Los Angeles

Filippi M, Rocca MA, Ciccarelli O et al (2016) MRI criteria for the diagnosis of multiple sclerosis: MAGNIMS consensus guidelines. Lancet Neurol 15(3):292–303

Fitch-West J, Ross-Swain D, Sands ES (1998) Best-2: Bedside Evaluation Screening Test. Pro-Ed, Austin

Flamand-Roze C, Falissard B, Roze E et al (2011) Validation of a new language screening tool for patients with acute stroke: the Language Screening Test (LAST). Stroke 42(5):1224–1229

Foesleitner O, Nenning KH, Bartha-Doering L et al (2020a) Lesion-specific language network alterations in temporal lobe epilepsy. Am J Neuroradiol 41(1):147–154

Foesleitner O, Sigl B, Schmidbauer V et al (2020b) Language network reorganization before and after temporal lobe epilepsy surgery. J Neurosurg 134(6):1694–1170

Folstein MF, Folstein SE, McHugh PR (1975) "Mini-mental state": a practical method for grading the cognitive state of patients for the clinician. J Psychiatr Res 12(3):189–198

Folstein MF, Folstein SE, McHugh PR (2010) 5.2 Mini-mental state examination (MMSE). In: Manual of screeners for dementia. Springer, p 51

Frattali C, Thompson C, Holland A et al (eds) (2017) Functional assessment of communication skills for adults (ASHA FACS). American Speech-Language-Hearing Association, Rockville

Frattali CM, Thompson CM, Holland AL, et al (1995) The FACS of life ASHA facs--a functional outcome measure for adults. ASHA 37(4):40–6. PMID: 7733997.

Fridriksson J, den Ouden DB, Hillis AE et al (2018) Anatomy of aphasia revisited. Brain 141(3):848–862

Friederici AD (2011) The brain basis of language processing: from structure to function. Physiol Rev 91(4):1357–1392

Fujii D (2017) A mini-compendium of neuropsychological tests with cross-cultural validity. In: Fujii D (ed) Conducting a culturally informed neuropsychological evaluation. American Psychological Association, Washington, DC, pp 145–196

Gainotti G, Marra C, Villa G (2001) A double dissociation between accuracy and time of execution on attentional tasks in Alzheimer's disease and multi-infarct dementia. Brain 124(4):731–738

Galetto V, Andreetta S, Zettin M et al (2013) Patterns of impairment of narrative language in mild traumatic brain injury. J Neurolinguistics 26(6):649–661

Garrett KL, Lasker JP (2013) Adults with severe aphasia and apraxia of speech. In: Beukelman DR, Mirenda P (eds) Augmentative and alternative communication: supporting children and adults with complex communication needs, 4th edn. Brookes, Baltimore, pp 405–445

Georgiou AM, Lada E, Kambanaros M (2019) Evaluating the quality of conduct of systematic reviews on the application of transcranial magnetic stimulation (TMS) for aphasia rehabilitation post-stroke. Aphasiology 34(5):540–556

Glosser G, Deser T (1990) Patterns of discourse production among neurological patients with fluent language disorders. Brain Lang 40(1):67–88

Goodglass H, Kaplan E, Barresi B (2000) Boston Diagnostic Aphasia Evaluation (BDAE-3), 3rd edn. The Psychological Corporation, San Antonio

Gorno-Tempini ML, Hillis AE, Weintraub S et al (2011) Classification of primary progressive aphasia and its variants. Neurology 76(11):1006–1014

Gronwall DMA (1977) Paced auditory serial-addition task: a measure of recovery from concussion. Percept Mot Ski 44(2):367–373

Hagelskjaer V et al (2019) Canadian Occupational Performance Measure supported by Talking Mats: An evaluation of the clinical utility. Occupational Therapy International 28(1):1–13

Hambleton RK, Jones RW (1993) Comparison of classical test theory and item response theory and their applications to test development. Educ Meas Issues Pract 12(3):38–47

Hannay HJ, Lezak MD (2004) The neuropsychological examination: interpretation. In: Lezak MD et al (eds) Neuropsychological assessment, 4th edn. Oxford University Press, New York, pp 133–155

Hansson O et al (2023) Blood biomarkers for Alzheimer's disease in clinical practice and trials. Nature aging 3(5):506–519

Harvey PD (2012) Clinical applications of neuropsychological assessment. Dialogues Clin Neurosci 14(1):91–99

Herbert R et al (2012) Accessible information guidelines: Making information accessible for people with aphasia. Stroke Association. Available at: https://www. stroke.org.uk/sites/default/files/accessible_information_guidelines.pdf1_.pdf

Hersh D, Worrall L, Howe T et al (2012) SMARTER goal setting in aphasia rehabilitation. Aphasiology 26(2):220–233

Hickok G, Poeppel D (2007) The cortical organization of speech processing. Nat Rev Neurosci 8(5):393–402

Hilari K, Galante L, Huck A et al (2018) Cultural adaptation and psychometric testing of the Scenario Test UK for people with aphasia. Int J Lang Commun Disord 53(4):748–760

Hillis AE (2005) Stages and mechanisms of recovery from aphasia. Jap J Neuropsychol 21:35–43

Höglinger GU, Respondek G, Stamelou M et al (2017) Clinical diagnosis of progressive supranuclear palsy: the movement disorder society criteria. Move Disord 32(6):853–864

Holland A (1980) CADL Communicative Abilities of Daily Living. University Park Press, Baltimore

Hsieh S, Schubert S, Hoon C et al (2013) Validation of the Addenbrooke's Cognitive Examination III in frontotemporal dementia and Alzheimer's disease. Dement Geriatr Cogn Disord 36(3-4):242–250

Huber W, Poeck K, Weniger D et al (1983) Aachener Aphasie Test (AAT) (Aachen Aphasia Test (AAT)). Verlag für Psychologie Hogrefe, Göttingen, Zurich

Huber W, Poeck K, Willmes K (1984) The Aachen Aphasia Test. Adv Neurol 42:291–303

Indefrey P (2011) The spatial and temporal signatures of word production components: a critical update. Front Psychol 2:255. https://doi.org/10.3389/fpsyg.2011.00255

Jaffe TA, Hoang JK, Yoshizumi TT et al (2010) Radiation dose for routine clinical adult brain CT: variability on different scanners at one institution. Am J Roentgenol 195(2):433–438

Johnson DY, Dunkelberger DL, Henry M et al (2013) Sporadic Jakob-Creutzfeldt disease presenting as primary progressive aphasia. JAMA Neurol 70(2):254–257

Jonas K, Jaecks P (2021) Digitale Diagnostik: Innovative Wege für die Sprachtherapie (Digital diagnostics: innovative ways for speech and language therapy). In: Fritzsche T et al (eds) Klick für Klick. Schritte in der digitalen Sprachtherapie (Click by click. Steps in digital speech and language therapy). Spektrum Patholinguistik, Universitätsverlag Potsdam (in press)

Jones DK (2012) Diffusion MRI: theory, methods, and applications. Oxford University Press, Oxford

Jones RD, Benton AL (1995) Use of the multilingual aphasia examination in the detection of language disorders. J Int Neuropsychol Soc 1:364–364

Kagan A (1998) Supported conversation for adults with aphasia: methods and resources for training conversation partners. Aphasiology 12(9):816–830

Kagan A, Black ES, Felson Duchan JF et al (2001) Training volunteers as conversation partners using "Supported Conversation for Adults with Aphasia" (SCA): a controlled trial. J Speech Lang Hear Res 44:624–638

Kagan A, Winckel J, Black S et al (2004) A set of observational measures for rating support and participation in conversation. Top Stroke Rehabil 11(1):67–83

Kagan A (2011) A-FROM in action at the Aphasia Institute. Seminars in speech and language 32,03, pp. 216–228.

Kalbe E, Reinhold N, Brand M et al (2005) A new test battery to assess aphasic disturbances and associated cognitive dysfunctions—German normative data on the aphasia check list. J Clin Exp Neuropsychol 27(7):779–794

Kaplan E (1988) The process approach to neuropsychological assessment. Aphasiology 2(3-4):309–311

Kaplan E, Goodglass H, Weintraub S (1983) Boston Naming Test. Lea and Febiger, Philadelphia

Kay J, Lesser R, Coltheart M (1996) Psycholinguistic Assessments of Language Processing in Aphasia (PALPA): an introduction. Aphasiology 10(2):159–180

Kaza RK, Platt JF, Cohan RH et al (2012) Dual-energy CT with single- and dual-source scanners: current applications in evaluating the genitourinary tract. Radiographics 32(2):353–369

Keil K, Kaszniak AW (2002) Examining executive function in individuals with brain injury: a review. Aphasiology 16(3):305–335

Kent RD (1998) Neuroimaging studies of brain activation for language, with an emphasis on functional magnetic resonance imaging: a review. Folia Phoniatr Logop 50:291–304

Kertesz A (2006) Western Aphasia Battery-Revised (WAB-R). Pearson, New York

Kessels RP, Brands AM (2009) Neuropsychological assessment. In: Biessels G, Luchsinger J (eds) Diabetes and the brain. Contemporary diabetes. Humana Press, New York, pp 77–102

Kester E (2020) Conducting student speech-language evaluations via telepractice. The ASHA Leader Live. Available via https://leader.pubs.asha.org/do/10.1044/leader.SCM.25062020.36/full/?fbclid=IwAR1ZMYmK0mZIer9IP4GFpUieiADxUELMP7-Vmik0ytTHevZp50f_EWxOCYc. Accessed 11 Nov 2020

Kim M-H, Lee S-Y, Lee S-E et al (2014) Anaphylaxis to iodinated contrast media: clinical characteristics related with development of anaphylactic shock. PLoS One 9(6):e100154. https://doi.org/10.1371/journal.pone.0100154

Kiran S (2012) What is the nature of post-stroke language recovery and reorganization? IRSN Neurol 786872. https://doi.org/10.5402/2012/786872

Kolakowsky-Hayner SA, Caplan B (2011) Qualitative neuropsychological assessment. In: Kreutzer JS et al (eds) Encyclopedia of clinical neuropsychology. Springer, New York, pp 2098–2099

Lacour A, De Seze J, Revenco E et al (2004) Acute aphasia in multiple sclerosis a multicenter study of 22 patients. Neurology 62(6):974–977

Lanyon L, Worrall L, Rose M (2018) Combating social isolation for people with severe chronic aphasia through community aphasia groups: consumer views on getting it right and wrong. Aphasiology 32(5):493–517

Lapointe L, Stierwalt JAG (2018) Aphasia and related neurogenic language disorders, 5th edn. Thieme Medical Publisher, New York

Larfeuil C, Le Dorze G (1997) An analysis of the word-finding difficulties and of the content of the discourse of recent and chronic aphasic speakers. Aphasiology 11(8):783–811

Lezak MD, Howieson DB, Loring DW (2004) Neuropsychological assessment, 4th edn. Oxford University Press, Oxford

Lezak MD, Howieson DB, Bigler ED et al (2012) Neuropsychological assessment, 5th edn. Oxford University Press, New York

Linnik A, Bastiaanse R, Höhle B (2015) Discourse production in aphasia: a current review of theoretical and methodological challenges. Aphasiology 3(7):765–800

Little B, Gallagher P, Zimmerer V et al (2019) Language in schizophrenia and aphasia: the relationship with non-verbal cognition and thought disorder. Cogn Neuropsychiatry 24(6):389–405

Mahieux F, Michelet D, Manifacier MJ et al (1995) Mini-Mental Parkinson: first validation study of a new bedside test constructed for Parkinson's disease. Behav Neurol 8(1):15–22

Malek-Ahmadi M, Mufson EJ, Perez SE (2017) Statistical considerations for assessing cognition and neuropathology associations in preclinical Alzheimer's disease. Biostat Epidemiol 1(1):92–104

Mandell AM, Alexander MP, Carpenter S (1989) Creutzfeldt-Jakob disease presenting as isolated aphasia. Neurology 39(1):55–58

Marangolo P, Fiori V, Calpagnano MA et al (2013) tDCS over the left inferior frontal cortex improves speech production in aphasia. Front Hum Neurosci 7:539. https://doi.org/10.3389/fnhum.2013.00539

Marini A, Boewe A, Caltagirone C et al (2005) Age-related differences in the production of textual descriptions. J Psycholing Res 34(5):439–463

Marini A, Caltagirone C, Pasqualetti P et al (2007) Patterns of language improvement in adults with non-chronic non-fluent aphasia after specific therapies. Aphasiology 21(2):164–186

Marini A, Andreetta S, Del Tin S et al (2011) A multilevel approach to the analysis of narrative language in Aphasia. Aphasiology, Special Issue on Discourse in Aphasia 25(11):1372–1392

Marini A, Urgesi C, Fabbro F (2012) Clinical neurolinguistics of bilingualism. In: Faust M (ed) The handbook of the neuropsychology of language, vol 2. Blackwell Publishing Group, Chichester, pp 738–759

Martin S, Millán JDR, Knight RT et al (2019) The use of intracranial recordings to decode human language: challenges and opportunities. Brain Lang 193:73–83

Martins PS, Barbosa-Pereira D, Valgas-Costa M et al (2020) Item analysis of the Child Neuropsychological Assessment Test (TENI): classical test theory and item response theory. Appl Neuropsychol Child 1–11. https://doi.org/10.1080/21622965.2020.1846128

Mathew R, Bak TH, Hodges JR (2012) Diagnostic criteria for corticobasal syndrome: a comparative study. J Neurol Neurosurg Psychiatry 83(4):405–410

McRobbie DW, Moore EA, Graves MJ et al (2006) MRI from picture to proton, 2nd edn. Cambridge University Press, Cambridge

Miceli G, Laudanna A, Burani C et al (1994) Batteria per l'analisi dei deficit afasici (BADA) (Battery for the analysis of aphasic deficits (BADA)). CEPSAG Editore, Rome

Miller N, Willmes K, De Bleser R (2000) The psychometric properties of the English language version of the Aachen Aphasia Test (EAAT). Aphasiology 14(7):683–722

Mimura Y et al (2023) Transcranial magnetic stimulation neurophysiology in patients with non-Alzheimer's neurodegenerative diseases: a systematic review and meta-analysis. Neuroscience & Biobehavioral Reviews 105451

Mindel M (2020) Talk like me: Supporting students who are African American using augmentative and alternative communication. Perspectives of the ASHA Special Interest Groups 5(6):1586–1592. https://doi.org/10.1044/2020_PERSP-20-00041

Mioshi E, Dawson K, Mitchell J et al (2006) The Addenbrooke's Cognitive Examination Revised (ACE-R): a brief cognitive test battery for dementia screening. Int J Geriatr Psychiatry 21(11):1078–1085

Mishra NK, Rossetti AO, Ménétrey A et al (2009) Recurrent Wernicke's aphasia: migraine and not stroke! Headache 49(5):765–768

Miyake A, Friedman NP, Emerson MJ et al (2000) The unity and diversity of executive functions and their contributions to complex "frontal lobe" tasks: a latent variable analysis. Cogn Psychol 41(1):49–100

Monti A, Poletti B, Zago S (2008) 'Cogmarkers' for the diagnosis of dementia of Alzheimer's type. In: Galimberti D, Scarpani E (eds) Biomarkers for early diagnosis of Alzheimer's disease. Nova Science Publishers, New York, pp 11–28

Moorcroft A, Scarinci N, Meyer C (2019) Speech pathologist perspectives on the acceptance versus rejection or abandonment of AAC systems for children with complex communication needs. Augmentative and Alternative Communication 35(3):193–204. https://doi.org/10.1080/07434618.2019.1609577

Moosbrugger H, Kelava A (2020) Testtheorie und Fragebogenkonstruktion (Test theory and questionnaire construction). Springer, Heidelberg

Murray L, Coppens P (2013) Formal and informal assessment of aphasia. In: Papathanasiou I et al (eds) Aphasia and related neurogenic communication disorders. Jones and Bartlett Learning, Burlington, pp 67–91

Nakase-Thompson R, Manning E, Sherer M et al (2005) Brief assessment of severe language impairments: initial validation of the Mississippi aphasia screening test. Brain Inj 19(9):685–691

Nasreddine ZS, Phillips NA, Bédirian V et al (2005) The Montreal Cognitive Assessment, MoCA: a brief screening tool for mild cognitive impairment. J Am Geriatr Soc 53(4):695–699

National Institute for Health and Care Excellence (2013) Stroke rehabilitation in adults (NICE clinical guideline 162). Available via https://www.nice.org.uk/guidance/cg162/resources/stroke-rehabilitation-in-adults-pdf-35109688408261. Accessed 1 Dec 2020

National Quality Forum (2015) NQF-Endorsed measures for person- and family-centered care: phase I technical report. Available via https://www.qualityforum.org/projects/person_family_centered_care/. Accessed 15 Sept 2020

National Quality Forum (2021) Building a roadmap from patient-reported outcome measures to patient-reported outcome performance measures: Technical guidance – final draft. https://www.qualityforum.org/WorkArea/linkit.aspx?LinkIdentifier=id&ItemID=96460

Nicholas L, Brookshire R (1993) A system for quantifying the informativeness and efficiency of the connected speech of adults with aphasia. J Speech Hear Res 36(2):338–350

Niven E, Newton J, Foley J et al (2015) Validation of the Edinburgh Cognitive and Behavioural Amyotrophic Lateral Sclerosis Screen (ECAS): a cognitive tool for motor disorders. ALS-FTD 16(3–4):172–179

Nobis-Bosch R, Schrey-Dern D, Rubi-Fessen I et al (eds) (2013) Forum Logopädie. Diagnostik und Therapie der akuten Aphasie: 52 Tabellen (Assessment and therapy of acute aphasia: 52 tables). Thieme, Stuttgart

Nobis-Bosch R, Bruehl S, Krzok F et al (2020) Szenario-Test: Testung verbaler und nonverbaler Aspekte aphasischer Kommunikation (The Scenario Test: testing verbal and non-verbal aspects of aphasic communication). Pro Log, Cologne

Nykänen A, Nyrkkö H, Nykänen M et al (2013) Communication therapy for people with aphasia and their partners (APPUTE). Aphasiology 27:1159–1179

Paradis M, Libben G (1987) The assessment of bilingual aphasia. Erlbaum, Hillsdale

Paraskevas GP, Kasselimis D, Kourtidou E et al (2017) Cerebrospinal fluid biomarkers as a diagnostic tool of the underlying pathology of primary progressive aphasia. J Alzheimers Dis 55(4):1453–1461

Parsons TD, Duffield T (2019) National Institutes of Health initiatives for advancing scientific developments in clinical neuropsychology. Clin Neuropsychol 33(2):246–270

Patel N, Peterson KA, Ingram R et al (2020) The Mini Linguistic State Examination (MLSE): a brief but accurate assessment tool for classifying primary progressive aphasias. medRxiv. https://doi.org/10.1101/2020.06.02.20119974. Accessed 4 Aug 2021

Pedrozo Campos Antunes T, Bulle S, de Oliveira A, Hudec R et al (2018) Assistive technology for communication of older adults: a systematic review. Aging Ment Health 23(4):417–427

Pierce JE, O'Halloran R, Togher L et al (2019) What is meant by "multimodal therapy" for aphasia? Am J Speech Lang Pathol 28:706–716

Piervincenzi C, Petrilli A, Marini A et al (2016) Multimodal assessment of hemispheric lateralization for language and its relevance for behavior. NeuroImage 142:351–370

Pindzola RH, Plexico LW, Haynes WO (2015) Diagnosis and evaluation in speech pathology. Pearson, Boston

Prutting C, Kirchner D (1987) A clinical appraisal of the pragmatic aspects of language. J Speech Hear Disord 52:105–119

Ramos EM, Dokuru DR, Van Berlo V et al (2019) Genetic screen in a large series of patients with primary progressive aphasia. Alzheimers Dement 15(4):553–560

Randolph C, Tierney MC, Mohr E et al (1998) The Repeatable Battery for the Assessment of Neuropsychological Status (RBANS): preliminary clinical validity. J Clin Exp Neuropsychol 20(3):310–319

Rautakoski P (2011) Training total communication. Aphasiology 25(3):344–365

Raymer AM, Gonzalez Rothi LJ (eds) (2018) The Oxford handbook of aphasia and language disorders. Oxford University Press, Oxford

RCSLT (2005) Royal College of Speech and Language Therapists clinical guidelines. Routledge

Rey A (1941) L'examen psychologique dans les cas d'encephalopathie traumatique. Arch Psychol (Geneve) 28:286–340

Riancho J, Delgado-Alvarado M, Fernández-Torre JL et al (2016) Subacute progressive aphasia: a rare presentation of Creutzfeldt–Jakob disease. J Neurol 263(3):600–602

Rohde A, Worrall L, Godecke E et al (2018) Diagnosis of aphasia in stroke populations: a systematic review of language tests. PLoS One 13(3):e0194143. https://doi.org/10.1371/journal.pone.0194143. Accessed 20 Aug 2021

Rohling ML, Axelrod BN, Langhinrichsen-Rohling J (2017) Fundamental forensic statistics: statistics every forensic neuropsychologist must know. In: Bush SS et al (eds) APA handbook of forensic neuropsychology. American Psychiatric Association Publishing, Washington, pp 3–22

Rose T, Worrall L, McKenna K (2003) The effectiveness of aphasia-friendly principles for printed health education materials for people with aphasia following stroke. Aphasiology 17(10):947–963

Rose TA, Worrall LE, Hickson LM et al (2011) Aphasia-friendly written health information: content and design characteristics. Int J Speech Lang Pathol 13(4):335–347

Roth C (2011) American Speech-Language-Hearing Association functional assessment of communication skills for adults. In: Kreutzer JS et al (eds) Encyclopedia of clinical neuropsychology. Springer, New York

Rubi-Fessen I (2017) Aphasietherapie (Aphasia therapy). Neuroreha 2(9):49–82

Russo MJ, Prodan V, Meda NN et al (2017) High-technology augmentative communication for adults with post-stroke aphasia: a systematic review. Expert Rev Med Devices 14(5):355–370

Saffran EM, Berndt RS, Schwartz MF (1989) The quantitative analysis of agrammatic production: procedure and data. Brain Lang 37(3):440–479

Salmelin R (2010) MEG and reading: from perception to linguistic analysis. In: Hansen PC et al (eds) MEG: an introduction to methods. Oxford University Press, Oxford, pp 346–371

Salter K, Jutai J, Foley N et al (2006) Identification of aphasia post stroke: a review of screening assessment tools. Brain Inj 20(6):559–568

Scherr M, Kunz A, Doll A et al (2016) Ignoring floor and ceiling effects may underestimate the effect of carotid artery stenting on cognitive performance. J Neurointerv Surg 8(7):747–751

Schroeder RW, Martin PK, Walling A (2019) Neuropsychological evaluations in adults. Am Fam Physician 99(2):101–108

Schuerman WL, Leonard MK (2023) Human Intracranial Recordings for Language Research. In Language Electrified: Principles, Methods, and Future Perspectives of Investigation. Springer US, New York, NY pp. 285–309

Shallice T (1982) Specific impairments of planning. Philos Trans R Soc Lond Ser B Biol Sci 298(1089):199–209

Siciliano M, Chiorri C, Battini V et al (2019) Regression-based normative data and equivalent scores for Trail Making Test (TMT): an updated Italian normative study. Neurol Sci 40(3):469–477

Simmons-Mackie N, Raymer A, Cherney L (2016) Communication Partner Training in Aphasia: an updated systematic review. Arch Phys Med Rehabil 97:2202–2221

Somerville J, Tremont G, Stern RA (2000) The Boston Qualitative Scoring System as a measure of executive functioning in Rey–Osterrieth Complex Figure performance. J Clin Exp Neuropsychol 22(5):613–621

Spinnler H, Tognoni G (1987) Italian Group on the neuropsychological study of ageing: Italian standardization and classification of neuropsychological tests. Ital J Neurol Sci 6(Suppl 8):1–120

Streiner D, Norman R (2000) Health measurement scales: a practical guide to their development and use. Oxford University Press, Oxford

Stroop JR (1935) Studies of interference in serial verbal reactions. J Exp Psychol 18(6):643–662

Strub RL, Gardner H (1974) The repetition defect in conduction aphasia: mnestic or linguistic? Brain Lang 1(3):241–255

Swinburn K, Porter G, Howard D (2004) Comprehensive Aphasia Test (CAT). Psychology Press, New York

Tan RH, Guennewig B, Dobson-Stone C et al (2019) The underacknowledged PPA-ALS: a unique clinico-pathologic subtype with strong heritability. Neurology 92(12):e1354–e1366

Tee BL, Gorno-Tempini ML (2019) Primary progressive aphasia: a model for neurodegenerative disease. Curr Opin Neurol 32(2):255–265

Thiele K (2013) Evaluation von Wortgenerierungsleistungen zur Diagnose kommunikativ-kognitiver Defizit (Evaluation of word generation performances to diagnose communicative-cognitive deficits). Doctoral dissertation. Universität Bielefeld, Bielefeld

Thiele K, Quinting JM, Stenneken P (2016) New ways to analyze word generation performance in brain injury: a systematic review and meta-analysis of additional performance measures. J Clin Exp Neuropsychol 38(7):764–781

Thommessen B, Thoresen GE, Bautz-Holter E et al (1999) Screening by nurses for aphasia in stroke: the Ullevaal Aphasia Screening (UAS) Test. Disabil Rehabil 21(3):110–115

Thomson J, Gee M, Sage K et al (2018) What 'form' does informal assessment take? A scoping review of the informal assessment literature for aphasia. Int J Lang Commun Disord 53(4):659–674

Trebuchon A, Lambert I, Guisiano B et al (2018) The different patterns of seizure-induced aphasia in temporal lobe epilepsies. Epilepsy Behav 78:256–264

Trevethan R (2017) Sensitivity, specificity, and predictive values: foundations, pliabilities, and pitfalls in research and practice. Front Public Health 5:307. https://doi.org/10.3389/fpubh.2017.00307

Trinka E, Cock H, Hesdorffer D et al (2015) A definition and classification of status epilepticus–report of the ILAE Task Force on Classification of Status Epilepticus. Epilepsia 56(10):1515–1523

Tsai MH, Vears DF, Turner SJ et al (2013) Clinical genetic study of the epilepsy-aphasia spectrum. Epilepsia 54(2):280–287

Tsai JP, Sheu JJ, Hsieh KLC (2018) Unusual magnetic resonance imaging abnormality in nonketotic hyperglycemia-related epilepsiapartialis continua. Ann Indian Acad Neurol 21(3):225–227

Tucker FM, Edwards DF, Mathews LK et al (2012) Modifying health outcome measures for people with aphasia. Am J Occup Ther 66(1):42–50

Ulatowska HK, Freedman-Stern R, Doyel AW et al (1983) Production of narrative discourse in aphasia. Brain Lang 19(2):317–334

van der Meulen I, van de Sandt-Koenderman WME, Duivenvoorden HJ et al (2010) Measuring verbal and non-verbal communication in aphasia: reliability, validity, and sensitivity of the Scenario Test. Int J Lang Commun Disord 45(4):424–435

Vinceti G, Olney N, Mandelli ML et al (2019) Primary progressive aphasia and the FTD-MND spectrum disorders: clinical, pathological, and neuroimaging correlates. ALS-FTSD 20(3–4):146–158

Vogel A, Maruff P, Morgan A (2010) Evaluation of communication assessment practices during the acute stages post stroke. J Eval Clin Pract 16(6):1183–1188

Wechsler D (1939) The measurement of adult intelligence. Williams and Witkins, Baltimore

Wechsler D (2008) Wechsler adult intelligence scale (WAIS-IV), 4th edn. NCS Pearson, San Antonio

Wernicke C (1874) Der aphasische Symptomencomplex. Eine psychologische Studie auf anatomischer Basis (The aphasic symptom complex. A psychological study on an anatomical basis). Cohn und Weigert, Breslau

Whitworth A, Webster J, Howard D (2013) A cognitive neuropsychological approach to assessment and intervention in aphasia: a clinician's guide, 2nd edn. Psychology Press, Hove

Willmes K (2010) The methodological and statistical foundations of neuropsychological assessment. In: Gurd J, Kischka U, Marshall J (eds) The handbook of clinical neuropsychology, 2nd edn. Oxford University Press, New York, pp 28–49

Wintermark M, Sanelli PC, Albers GW et al (2013) Imaging recommendations for acute stroke and transient ischemic attack patients: joint statement by the American Society of Neuroradiology, the American College of Radiology, and the Society of NeuroInterventional Surgery. Am J Neuroradiol 34(11):E117–E127

Wolf TJ, Chuh A, Floyd T et al (2015) Effectiveness of occupation-based interventions to improve areas of occupation and social participation after stroke: an evidence-based review. Am J Occup Ther 69(1):6901180060. https://doi.org/10.5014/ajot.2015.012195. Accessed 20 Aug 2021

Woolley SC, York MK, Moore DH et al (2010) Detecting frontotemporal dysfunction in ALS: utility of the ALS Cognitive Behavioral Screen (ALS-CBS™). Amyotroph Lateral Scler 11(3):303–311

World Health Organization (1993) The ICD-10 classification of mental and behavioural disorders: diagnostic criteria for research. World Health Organization, Geneva

World Health Organization (2001) International classification of functioning, disability and health (ICF). World Health Organization, Geneva

World Health Organization (2002) Towards a common language for functioning, disability and health ICF. Available via https://www.who.int/classifications/icf/icfbeginnersguide.pdf. Accessed 14 Sept 2020

Worrall L, Sherratt S, Rogers P et al (2011) What people with aphasia want: their goals according to the ICF. Aphasiology 25(3):309–322

Wysowski DK, Nourjah P (2006) Deaths attributed to X-ray contrast media on U.S. death certificates. Am J Roentgenol 186(3):613–615

# Prevention of Acquired Language Disorders: Aphasia

# 24

Laura Perucca

## 24.1 Understanding the Importance of Early Diagnosis of Aphasia Due to Neurological Disorders

Laura Perucca

Animal and clinical research suggests that early, intensive and focused rehabilitation in aphasia has significant impact on long-term functional results (Krakauer et al. 2012). Early diagnosis ensures a focus on early rehabilitation, which should therefore be pursued. Early diagnosis is also critical for understanding the severity of the injury and monitoring recovery and changes in the patient's condition. Growing evidence shows the need for early rehabilitation in aphasia, even if the large majority of clinical trials that testify to the efficacy and validity of rehabilitation have been carried out on chronic patients.

It is possible to identify three phases after aphasia onset: acute, sub-acute and chronic. Language rehabilitation has different aims and tools for evaluating the cognitive deficits' evolution and identifying the most appropriate therapeutic interventions for each phase. The Italian guidelines on stroke management (SPREAD 2012; Plowman et al. 2012) define the acute phase of aphasia as a period (about 1 week after lesion onset) during which neurological deficits can worsen. In this regard, it is worth noting that questionnaires and tests of gross neurological impairment, such as the NIHSS score (National Institute of Health 2003), include items investigating the cognitive deficits after stroke. These tests should not be used to differentiate between the different types of aphasia or grade the aphasia according to its severity. These tests are rather sensitive tests for aphasia identification and can help the clinician to choose the most appropriate rehabilitation regimen. Unfortunately, in the acute phase, tests for aphasia evaluation are often administered by a clinician with no formal training, eventually leading to a large number of false-positive diagnoses (Thommessen et al. 1999; Lazar et al. 2008). However, aphasia over-diagnosis is tolerated so that no "real" aphasic patient is lost.

The critical point is the availability of diagnostic instruments, first to identify the presence of aphasia and then to evaluate its severity, given that the initial degree of aphasia is one of the determinants of the prognosis of the aphasic patient (Crosson et al. 2019; Flamand-Roze et al. 2011). For this reason, rehabilitation has to begin as soon as possible. It must be noted that aphasic patients will have a lengthy hospital stay and are most frequently discharged to a rehabilitation centre. It has been hypothesised that a time win-

L. Perucca (✉)
Department of Biomedical Sciences for Health, University of Milan, Milan, Italy
e-mail: laura.perucca@unimi.it

© The Author(s), under exclusive license to Springer Nature Switzerland AG 2025
A. am Zehnhoff-Dinnesen et al. (eds.), *Phoniatrics III*, European Manual of Medicine,
https://doi.org/10.1007/978-3-031-48091-1_9

dow of increased responsiveness to training exists, resulting from heightened cerebral plasticity, as demonstrated in animal models. To date, there is no clear evidence that this possibility also exists in humans (Doesborgh et al. 2003).

Aphasia screening tests must have appropriate characteristics. First, they need to be short (maximum 15 min) and simple, suitable to be administered at the bedside in early acute stages. Moreover, they must evaluate the principal aspects of aphasia (spontaneous speech, written and auditory comprehension, writing and reading), highlight the necessity of further analyses, and guide adequate aphasia rehabilitative treatment. In a recent systematic review, El Hachioui et al. (2017) identified available tests for differentiating between aphasic and non-aphasic patients and evaluated test accuracy, reliability, and feasibility. An electronic search was performed on the most widely used bibliographic databases of published literature, and experts in the field of aphasia research detected additional published studies. A total of 1021 papers were selected. After the first screening of all titles and abstracts, 956 articles were excluded. Among other things, reasons for the exclusion were duplicates, other topics, no report of an aphasia screening test, conference abstract only, one letter. Other 54 full-text articles were excluded after the second screening because they did not meet the criteria of eligibility. For example, no aphasia screening test evaluation was present, no differentiation between aphasics and non-aphasics was detected, differentiation was performed only between aphasics and healthy controls. Other reasons for exclusion were different or unspecified aetiology, sensitivity and specificity could not be estimated, a post hoc scoring system and not a screening test. Eventually, only 11 papers, including 1 review, were selected. They contained eight screening tests for aphasia.

Only validation studies performed on stroke patients with and without aphasia were included. Among the selected studies with an intermediate or low risk of bias, two tests resulted in having the best diagnostic properties: the language screening test (LAST) (Flamand-Roze et al. 2011) and the ScreeLing (Crary et al. 1989). The

first requires 2 min to be administered, while the second requires 15 min, but it gives more detailed information for language treatment. Other frequently used tests are the Aphasia Screening Protocol (Crary et al. 1989), the Aachen Aphasia Bedside Test (Biniek et al. 1992) and the Bedside Western Aphasia Battery (Kertesz 2006), but there are no studies in which these tests are examined in stroke patients with and without aphasia. The token test is also widely used in clinical practice, but it exists in different versions (De Renzi and Vignolo 1962).

Evidence exists that patients do not always improve in the early post-stroke period because the interaction between frequency and intensity of the rehabilitative treatment is complex (Zeiler et al. 2016; Bernhardt et al. 2016). A recent case series confirmed that recovery from aphasia might not progress linearly with the post-onset time, so rehabilitative treatment may not be limited to the immediate period after stroke (Moss and Nicholas 2006).

In the sub-acute phase, lasting from the second week until 2–6 months after brain damage, specific tests such as the AABT (Biniek et al. 1992) can be administered, even at the bedside. Although the sub-acute phase is characterised by large symptom variability and ongoing spontaneous recovery, it is possible to identify the main characteristic of the language disorder and eventually choose the best rehabilitative intervention.

During both the acute and sub-acute phases, aphasia and the other cognitive deficits come after the patient's medical condition is evident. Thus, the patient has already become an aphasic person, inserted in a few hours into a world where his or her role has drastically changed. Awareness of the dramatic changes caused by aphasia and the chronicity of this new condition develops slowly in both the patient and his or her family. For this reason, when aphasia is diagnosed, it is fundamental to look at the future of the aphasic patient. Clinicians should have different roles in aphasic patient management: diagnosis, severity evaluation, education of both patient and his or her family about aphasia, and provision of tools to ease communication. Early intervention could lead to "false-positive" aphasic patients since low vigilance, severe dysarthria, loss of vision, campimetric alterations and different cognitive impairments or apraxia can mimic aphasia. However, early rehabilitation could be beneficial for these deficits, too. Published trials support the idea that patients who have rehabilitation improve more than patients who have not. This improvement is reported in all three phases and is more pronounced in the acute phase (Robey 1998).

**Key recommendation** If your patient is alert, take a short language evaluation (about 15 min) 4 days after the stroke onset and consider your patient for language rehabilitation.

## References

Bernhardt J, Churilov L, Ellery F et al (2016) Prespecified dose-response analysis for A Very Early Rehabilitation Trial (AVERT). Neurology 86(23):2138–2145

Biniek R, Huber W, Glindemann R et al (1992) The Aachen Aphasia Bedside Test—criteria for validity of psychologic tests. Nervenarzt 63:473–479

Crary MA, Haak NJ, Malinsky AE (1989) Preliminary psychometric evaluation of an acute aphasia screening protocol. Aphasiology 3:611–618

Crosson B, Rodriguez AD, Copland D et al (2019) Neuroplasticity and aphasia treatments: new approach for old problem. J Neurol Neurosurg Psychiatry 90(10):1147–1155

De Renzi E, Vignolo LA (1962) The token test: a sensitive test to detect receptive disturbances in aphasics. Brain 85:665–678

Doesborgh SJ, van de Sandt-Koenderman WM, Dippel DW et al (2003) Linguistic deficits in the acute phase of stroke. J Neurol 250:977–982

El Hachioui H, Visch-Brink EG, de Lau LML et al (2017) Screening tests for aphasia inpatients with stroke: a systematic review. J Neurol 24:211–220

Flamand-Roze C, Falissard B, Roze E et al (2011) Validation of a new language screening tool for patients with acute stroke: the Language Screening Test (LAST). Stroke 42(5):1224–1229

Kertesz A (2006) Western Aphasia Battery Revised. Harcourt Assessment, San Antonio

Krakauer JW, Carmichale ST, Corbett D et al (2012) Getting neurorehabilitation right: what can be learned from animal models? Neurorehabil Neural Repair 26:923–931

Lazar RM, Speizer AE, Festa JR et al (2008) Variability in language recovery after first-time stroke. J Neurol Neurosurg Psychiatry 79:530–534

Moss A, Nicholas M (2006) Language rehabilitation in chronic aphasia and time postonset: a review of single-subject data. Stroke 37(12):3043–3051

National Institutes of Health (2003) National Institute of Neurological Disorders and Stroke: free version of the NIH Stroke Scale, 2003. www.ninds.nih.gov/doctors/NIH_Stroke_Scale.pdf. Accessed 11 Jun 2021

Plowman E, Hentz B, Ellis C (2012) Post-stroke aphasia prognosis: a review of patient-related and stroke-related factors. J Eval Clin Pract 18:689–694

Robey RR (1998) A meta-analysis of clinical outcome in the treatment of aphasia. J Speech Lang Hear Res 4:172–187

SPREAD - Stroke Prevention and Educational Awareness Diffusion (2012) Ictus cerebrale: Linee guida italiane. Pubblicazioni Pierrel Research Italy SpA, Milano

Thommessen B, Thoresen GA, Bautz-Holter E et al (1999) Screening by nurses for aphasia in stroke—the Ullevaal Aphasia Screening (UAS) test. Disabil Rehabil 21:110–115

Zeiler SR, Hubbard R, Gibson EM et al (2016) Paradoxical motor recovery from a first stroke after induction of a second stroke: reopening a postischemic sensitive period. Neurorehabil Neural Repair 30(8):794–800

# Rehabilitation Measures and Prognosis of Acquired Language Disorders: Aphasia

Katharina M. Albrecht, Elisabetta Banco,
Charles Ellis, Anne Hüsgen, Fatima Jebahi,
Matti Lehtihalmes, Francesco Mozzanica,
Rossella Muò, Karel Neubauer, Rebekka Niepelt,
Ilona C. Rubi-Fessen, Beatrice Travalca Cupillo,
and Rosemary Varley

Elisabetta Banco, Rossella Muò and Beatrice Travalca
Cupillo shared first authorship.

K. M. Albrecht (✉)
Special Education and Rehabilitation of Speech and
Language Disabilities, Faculty of Human Sciences,
University of Cologne, Cologne, Germany
e-mail: katharina.albrecht@uni-koeln.de

E. Banco
Unità Operativa di Riabilitazione Neuromotoria,
Istituto Auxologico Italiano, IRCCS, San Luca, Italy

C. Ellis
University of Florida, Department of Speech
Language and Hearing Sciences,
Gainesville, USA
e-mail: ellisch@phhp.ufl.edu

A. Hüsgen · I. C. Rubi-Fessen
Faculty of Human Sciences, Department of Education
and Therapy for Speech and Language Disorders,
University of Cologne, Cologne, Germany
e-mail: anne.huesgen@uni-koeln.de; Ilona.Rubi-
Fessen@uni-koeln.de

F. Jebahi
Department of Communication Sciences and
Disorders, East Carolina University, 3310AA Health
Sciences Building, Greenville, NC, USA
e-mail: fjebahi@arizona.edu

M. Lehtihalmes
Faculty of Humanities, Research Unit of Logopedics,
University of Oulu, Oulu, Finland
e-mail: matti.lehtihalmes@oulu.fi

F. Mozzanica
San Giuseppe Hospital, Milan, Italy
e-mail: francesco.mozzanica@unimi.it

R. Muò
Recupero e Rieducazione Funzionale, ASL Città di
Torino, Turin, Italy
e-mail: rossella.muo@unito.it

K. Neubauer
Clinic of Phoniatrics of University Hospital Prague,
Charles University Faculty of Medicine,
Prague 2, Czech Republic
e-mail: Karel.Neubauer@lf1.cuni.cz

R. Niepelt
Faculty of Health and Therapy, DIPLOMA
University of Applied Sciences,
Bad Sooden-Allendorf, Germany
e-mail: rebekka.niepelt@diploma.de

B. Travalca Cupillo
Unit of Phoniatrics, IRCCS Polyclinic Hospital San
Martino, Genoa, Italy

R. Varley
Language & Cognition, Psychology & Language
Sciences, University College London, London, UK
e-mail: rosemary.varley@ucl.ac.uk

## 25.1 Coordination of Rehabilitative Measures: Aphasia

Matti Lehtihalmes

### 25.1.1 Importance of Defining Aphasia

The classic, but still very commonly used, definitions of aphasia derived from the symptoms of patients with stroke (e.g., Kertesz 1985) or traumatic brain injury (Luria 1970). Clinically these are still the more common aetiologies of aphasia. According to classic definitions, aphasia refers to acquired disorders of language, with language being understood as a system consisting of phonology, morphology, syntax and semantics. Today, natural language refers to a system that also includes prosody, voice quality, speech pauses, gaze, gestures, body movements and the ability to use language appropriately in different situations, i.e., pragmatic skills (Vigliocco et al. 2014). It follows that in addition to classical cases with obvious aphasia, patients with, for example, right hemisphere damage (Ferré et al. 2011), dementia (Swan et al. 2018) or schizophrenia (Little et al. 2019) will have language-related cognitive communication disorders, and they should also be referred to a speech and language therapist for assessment and rehabilitation. In these disorders, the core problems of communication are in such cognitive skills as attention, memory, executive functions, organisation, reasoning and social cognition (MacDonald 2021).

Today, however, patients with these disorders are still rarely sent to the speech and language therapist. One reason for this might be that many professionals in neurological rehabilitation teams think of aphasia as a narrow, traditional issue as described at the beginning of this paragraph. Often the content of the term *cognitive communication disorders*, beyond the traditional definition of aphasia, is not clear for them either (Thompson et al. 2010). In addition, standardised tests for assessing cognitive communication disorders are usually available only in a few languages (Turkstra et al. 2005). However, the use of language-independent checklists (e.g., MacDonald 2021) gives speech and language therapists some information to help formulate the nature of the disorder and find specific methods of a more detailed assessment and appropriate forms of rehabilitation. Increased cooperation in the rehabilitation team should increase knowledge of the contribution and competence of the different professions working with patients who have various types of neurological disease and damage. Optimal neurological rehabilitation should be provided by a multidisciplinary team with a high nursing ratio and specialists in at least neurology, neuroradiology, neuropsychology, speech and language therapy, physiotherapy, occupational therapy and nutrition (Hurford et al. 2020).

Damage to the right hemisphere can cause problems in speech prosody, narrative discourse and conversational skills (Ferré et al. 2011; Lindell 2006). Prosody of speech covers pitch, stress and rhythm, which allows the expression of, e.g., emotions in conversation. Problems in narrative discourse may appear as less informative and more incoherent speech. Interpretation of humour and figurative language, such as sarcasm and metaphors, is often disordered, as patients tend to assume their literal interpretation. All these features of right hemispheric damage may cause mild to serious problems in everyday conversation. A speech and language therapist must also evaluate these problems when performing a comprehensive aphasia assessment and evaluation of functional communication beyond classical aphasia (MacDonald 2017).

Communication disorders associated with various forms of dementia have been the subject of increasing research in recent years. However, only a small proportion of patients in this group are referred to a speech and language therapist, and most of them suffer from problems in swallowing. The type of the disease in dementia patients has to be determined, and the speech and language therapist should make an assessment of communication skills and rehabilitation needs of patients and their family members (El-Wahsh et al. 2021; Swan et al. 2018). Cooperation of the speech and language therapist with a neurologist, geriatrician and neuropsychologist is suggested.

A large variation of language-related problems in abstract and figurative language, narrative and pragmatic skills, is also common in patients with psychiatric diseases, e.g., schizophrenia (Pawełczyk et al. 2018). Patients with schizophrenia may also have strokes. Therefore, differential diagnosis between stroke-induced aphasia and formal thought disorder-related language impairment in schizophrenia is required (Little et al. 2019). It has been suggested that a rehabilitation programme aimed at improving communication could significantly help to improve the cognitive problems of schizophrenic patients (Nakamura et al. 2020). Cooperation between a speech and language therapist, (neuro) psychiatrist and neuropsychologist will be of value when planning their rehabilitation programme.

## 25.1.2 Rehabilitation from the Acute Phase

Stroke is the leading cause of neurological disability, including aphasia. In the acute phase, intravenous thrombolysis is an effective treatment, but it needs to be performed within 4.5 h of the onset. Endovascular thrombectomy is an effective treatment as well, and it can be performed a few hours later. However, public knowledge of the red flag signs of possible stroke, and the immediate transfer to an acute stroke emergency unit, are crucial for a good outcome. It is important to have a team specialised in acute stroke treatment, including neurologists, speech and language therapists, physiotherapists, occupational therapists, as well as high quality nursing facilities, because patients need continuous monitoring during the first days after stroke (Hurford et al. 2020). In most centres a neurologist or a certified research nurse applies the National Institutes of Health Stroke Scale (NIHSS) as soon as the patient enters the emergency room. This scale can indicate patients with severe aphasia, but some patients may be misclassified as having dysarthria (Mitchell et al.

2020), and other patients with mild aphasias may be misclassified as not having aphasia (Grönberg et al. 2021). This may exclude patients with minor stroke, but with isolated aphasia, from effective acute stroke treatments (Khatri et al. 2010). Aphasia is a symptom predictive of poor recovery in minor stroke (isolated aphasia without hemiparesis), but these patients may benefit of recanalisation treatments (Denier et al. 2016; Nesi et al. 2014). The speech and language therapist should perform at least one screening test for aphasia and other neurogenic communication disorders, as well as for dysphagia. Stroke-related pneumonia occurs in up to 40% of patients with acute stroke, most often owing to aspiration (Zhu et al. 2020). It is crucial for the speech and language therapist to check the ability of acute stroke patients to swallow safely, before providing any oral intake to them.

## 25.1.3 Rehabilitation in the Subacute Phase of Stroke

When the acute phase has stabilised, patients have undergone basic assessments of functional capacity, and a preliminary rehabilitation plan has been designed for the subacute phase 2–11 weeks after the stroke, which is the period of major improvement. In the optimal situation, patients are referred to a neurological rehabilitation unit where, with the support of a multiprofessional team, they receive intensive rehabilitation supported by a neurologist, speech and language therapist, physiotherapist, occupational therapist, music therapist, neuropsychologist, social worker and nursing staff. A decisive issue in rehabilitation is the intensity of the treatment. Several studies have recently shown that during the subacute phase (Ali et al. 2021) intensive treatment, including a massed practice, will lead to good improvement in patients, even those with chronic aphasia (e.g., Breitenstein et al. 2017). However, it should be recognised that what is needed for good recovery is the intensity and extent of therapy, i.e., the number of treatment hours per week, for impairment-level improvement, and the total number of hours/sessions over the whole rehabilitation period, for long-lasting activity- and participation-level recovery (Doogan et al. 2018). However, there is currently insufficient evidence to determine how much treatment is optimal for specific targets of aphasia recovery (Godecke et al. 2020; Harvey et al. 2020).

Music therapy has a long history in aphasia rehabilitation. However, in recent years, the use of musical elements (listening, singing, playing, melodic intonation therapy) in the context of various rehabilitation methods, as in speech and language therapy, physiotherapy and occupational therapy, has increased significantly (Sihvonen et al. 2017; Zumbansen and Tremblay 2019). In its simplest form, listening to music for 1–2 h a day has been shown to enhance recovery of aphasia and cognition after stroke (Särkämö et al. 2008).

Computer-assisted methods have been a part of aphasia therapy for many decades. This is an area where speech and language therapists should cooperate with computer scientists and researchers in information technology. With these methods, it is possible to create personalised, self-managing and game-type programmes for aphasia therapy. In a recent systematic review, self-delivered exercises or practising with the help of family members were proven to be effective for aphasia therapy, and the daily number of therapeutic activities could be significantly higher than possible with face-to-face therapy with a speech and language therapist (Repetto et al. 2020). Virtual reality (VR) has been used with 2D screen technology more than 20 years in different fields of neurological rehabilitation (Grechuta et al. 2019). VR-based therapy programmes have also been used in teletherapy (Maresca et al. 2019)—a field growing fast, especially now during the COVID-19 pandemic. New technology with 3D head-mounted VR-devices makes exercises even more immersive. This technology can also be used when moving the goals of therapy from body functions towards the activity and participation levels of the International Classification of Functioning, Disability and Health (World Health Organization 2001). Jane Marshall and her group have designed the EVA-Park programme for aphasia therapy, where it is possible to participate in a discussion group in different VR-environments regardless of the location of the members (Carragher et al. 2021).

Combinations of conventional but intensive speech-language therapy and various methods of non-invasive brain stimulation have been the subject of a sharp increase in research in recent years (Bucur and Papagno 2019). Non-invasive brain stimulation alone seems not to be as effective as when combined with intensive speech and language therapy (Bai et al. 2021). Repetitive transcranial magnetic stimulation (rTMS) (Hartwigsen and Volz 2021; Yao et al. 2020) and transcranial direct current stimulation (tDCS) (Zheng et al. 2016) appear to increase interhemispheric connectivity between contralateral homologous regions; interactions between differentially specialised intra-hemispheric networks; and the importance of more general networks that are involved in the reorganisation of disordered specific functions. tDCS is a simpler and significantly cheaper stimulation method than rTMS, and it has also been shown to enhance recovery from aphasia (Elsner et al. 2020; Marangolo 2020). Targeting, designing and implementing the stimulation for best results need a multiprofessional team, comprising a speech and language therapist, neuropsychologist, neurologist and neurophysiologist.

Pharmacotherapy combined with conventional aphasia rehabilitation has been overshadowed in recent years, especially by brain stimulation therapies. Despite active research on pharmacotherapy in aphasia rehabilitation (more than 1000 studies in total and about 400 in the 2010s), no "aphasia pills" have been found. This is mainly because aphasia is a highly diverse disorder in its symptom profile, aetiology and pathophysiology. These are all factors that differ significantly pharmacologically (Llano and Small 2016). In his comprehensive review on pharmacotherapy research in rehabilitation of aphasic patients, Berthier (2021) suggests combining pharmacotherapy with speech and language therapy and non-invasive brain stimulation. In addition, he points out that in most studies the outcome measures have been restricted to improvement of naming, but of even more importance would be finding out the effect of pharmacotherapy on functional communication skills and quality of life.

## 25.1.4 Rehabilitation in the Chronic Phase of Stroke

Too often active therapy is discontinued when the patient has entered a chronic phase of the stroke. However, it is strongly suggested, from scientific evidence, for rehabilitation of stroke patients to continue during the chronic phase (Teasell et al. 2012). At this stage, as earlier, the multiprofessional treatment should be intensive, working the whole day, with 2 h of speech-language therapy per day (Stahl et al. 2018). It has been shown that intensive communication treatment can reduce depressive symptoms in patients with severe aphasia (Mohr et al. 2017). It is quite common that the speech functions of some patients with only fragmentary or short periods of proper treatment will deteriorate when the treatment has ended. This might be due to "learned non-use of speech" (Berthier and Pulvermüller 2011)—when speaking is felt too difficult, it is easier to avoid it. At some point, however, regular rehabilitation will have to be ended, but at this point, various patient- and volunteer-based organisations can play significant roles. They organise aphasia clubs with social and leisure activities and various rehabilitation courses. Aphasia is not just a patient's problem, it affects the whole community around him or her, and therefore the cooperation between the speech and language therapist and the patient's family at all phases of rehabilitation is necessary (Brown et al. 2011). Adaptive life-coaching, in the context of peer support activities together with the family members, prevents neuropsychiatric symptoms and improves the quality of life (Worrall et al. 2010). In this way, patients with aphasia can gradually move towards independent and successful living with aphasia.

## 25.1.5 Conclusion

Aphasia is no longer seen only as a disorder according to its classical definition. The understanding of language as a broad system of different elements of communication has brought to the concept of aphasia numerous "new" diseases, such as different forms of dementia, damage of the right brain hemisphere and some psychiatric disorders such as schizophrenia. These types of communication problem are called cognitive communication disorders. This means that speech-language therapists should also have a wide selection of specific methods for assessment and treatment of these problems (Doedens and Meteyard 2020). The current problem is that even the most used standardised tests are available in only a few languages. The knowledge among rehabilitation team professionals about the possibilities of speech and language therapists' use of language and communication treatments with these groups of patients should be increased.

Not so long ago it was very typical to offer one weekly therapy session to patients with aphasia. In some rehabilitation studies that examined the effect of a method or the intensity of rehabilitation, such a therapy is allowed for the control group "because therapy at this low frequency is unlikely to have a significant influence on the course of aphasia" (Goldenberg and Spatt 1994, pp. 685–686). Today, national and international guidelines recommend intensive and comprehensive models for aphasia therapy. There is still variation in the intensity of current rehabilitation methods and the use of technology in different countries. However, there is a clear trend towards scientifically based, intensive and technology-intensive therapies for patients with aphasia (Trebilcock et al. 2019).

Therapists working in aphasia rehabilitation teams need to be familiar with international guidelines for aphasia therapy, although only in a few countries are national guidelines for aphasia rehabilitation available. Nina Simmons-Mackie and a group of leading professionals in aphasia rehabilitation reviewed guidelines from different countries and summarised ten best practice recommendations for aphasia therapy (Simmons-Mackie et al. 2017). These can be used to harmonise clinical practice for aphasia around the world. In addition, as aphasia therapy involves human interactions, personality and professional skills play an important role in the effectiveness of rehabilitation. Linda Worrall (2019) presents in her review seven habits of highly successful aphasia therapists. She describes how patients with aphasia trust an expert therapist, but they value his or her behavioural skills the most. The ability to understand and create a functional relationship between a therapist and a patient should come first. Patients should be made to feel that they have participated in a goal-setting and planning of therapy. In addition, at the beginning of therapy, a therapist and a patient should have a clear vision of how to continue through the different stages of the therapy—and how to end it. All speech and language therapists and other professionals working in aphasia rehabilitation teams should be familiar with these excellent guidelines.

## 25.2 Planning and Monitoring of Speech and Language Therapy Executed by Logopaedists/Speech and Language Therapists

Rebekka Niepelt, Anne Hüsgen,
Katharina M. Albrecht and Ilona C. Rubi-Fessen
This section focuses on individual therapeutic intervention, namely, on the definition of therapeutic goals, the achievement and the examination of these goals in people with aphasia (PwA). The basic principles that will be introduced are those of evidence-based-practice, specific aspects of therapy structure, ideas for therapeutic settings and efficacy testing of the individual intervention.

### 25.2.1 Evidence-Based Practice

Evidence-based practice (EBP), derived from the idea of evidence-based medicine (EBM), is "the conscientious, explicit and judicious use of cur-

rent best evidence in making decisions about the care of individual patients" (Sackett 1997, p. 3). To fulfil that aim, the clinician's experience, the patient's personal beliefs and the best available scientific information have to be integrated to guide decisions about clinical management (Sackett 1997; Reynolds 2000; Beushausen 2016; Law and MacDermid 2024). Hence, therapeutic management involves the consideration of different scientific approaches, the evaluation of the research evidence and the selection of the most suitable approach before adopting the right therapeutic intervention. Consequently, through the EBM perspective three areas of EBP in speech and language therapy can be identified: the clinician, the patient and research evidence (Reynolds 2000; Beushausen and Walther 2010).

Therefore, within the process of clinical decision-making in the areas of diagnosis and therapy, speech and language therapists (SLT's) should consult and trust their individual evidence-based clinical expertise (Law and MacDermid 2008; Beushausen and Walther 2010; Haring and Siegmüller 2018; Greenwell and Walsh 2021). They should base their therapeutic management on their own research-informed and technical competence, as well as interpersonal abilities and the motivation of self-reflection; though, knowledge received through research evidence should be central to therapeutic practice (Schulte 2020). Henceforth, most current research outcomes, such as studies and articles, should be used in the process of decision-making, in accordance with the patient's expectations (Dollaghan 2007).

Furthermore, the patient-orientated transfer from diagnosis to treatment and daily life should be supported by clinical reasoning (CR), which underlies the clinical argumentation, conclusion and use of evidence from the SLT (Higgs et al. 2008; Beushausen and Walther 2010). CR is used to ensure the best possible outcome for the individual patient through therapeutic and diagnostic procedures. Thereby, it constitutes a strategy to make therapeutic action transparent and objective. Characteristics of CR are the constant description, questioning, reflecting and justifying of actions on different levels (Schell and Schell 2008). Additionally, incorporating CR into clinical practice can ensure successful aftercare and long-term rehabilitation of patients, by focusing and reflecting on their individual needs.

Besides these principles, therapy must be based on suitably chosen assessments. These provide information about linguistic and communicative skills of PwA (see Sect. 23.1) and can be classified within the framework of the *International Classification of Functioning, Disability and Health* (ICF) (WHO 2001). A combination of impairment-based and functional assessments guarantee a comprehensive picture of the patient's abilities at different linguistic levels, but also on individual participative functions. Impairment-based tools evaluate linguistic skills at the ICF level of body functions and structure, for example word retrieval in a naming task, whereas functional assessment tools measure communication at the level of activity and participation, such as word finding while making a telephone call. Furthermore, assessments are disease phase-specific and should be chosen accordingly.

Since acquired language and communication disorders such as aphasia result from brain damage from which recovery is greatest during the first 2–6 weeks after the incident, an early start of intervention during the acute phase is recommended to support spontaneous recovery (e.g., Godecke et al. 2014). Therapy during this phase aims to reactivate and stimulate the impaired brain areas that are only temporarily affected, and thereby supports spontaneous remission. In the chronic stage of aphasia, therapy focuses on relearning and compensating for the persistent loss of language knowledge and impaired associated activities (Allen et al. 2012). However, the exact starting time of an intervention is dependent on the patient's general condition, their individual attention abilities (Worrall et al. 2017), as well as service-related variables (e.g., Breitenstein et al. 2022).

To reach optimal intervention intensity, five dimensions reflecting quantitative and qualitative aspects of the patient's learning experiences must be considered, both within and across therapy units (Baker 2012); i.e., dose, dose form, dose frequency, total intervention duration and cumu-lative intervention intensity (Warren et al. 2007). The overall duration of an intervention, though, usually depends on external factors, for example, the conditions of inpatient and outpatient care. Recent studies have proven the efficacy of intensive therapy on communicative abilities regardless of the duration of aphasia (e.g., Breitenstein et al. 2017). Therefore, the phases of high-intensity intervention can generally be recommended with PwA, also in the chronic stage of aphasia.

## 25.2.2 Therapeutic Goals

The overarching aim of speech and language therapy is to improve language and communication abilities of a patient and to enable the person to participate in everyday life. Planning and structuring an evidence-based therapy requires the SLT to set up specific and individual goals in collaboration with the PwA (e.g., Worrall et al. 2017). These are necessary to plan the exact intervention gradually, including appropriate exercises and materials, and to evaluate the efficacy of the treatment (e.g., Breitenstein et al. 2022). Regarding the content of therapeutic goals, the ICF framework helps the therapist to take a holistic perspective on the communication problem by addressing the levels of participation, communicative activities and cognitive-linguistic functions (WHO 2001). Knowing the language and communication profile, as well as the expectations of the patient, the therapist further has to determine realistic points in time for achieving the different goals. This can be implemented by formulating short-, middle- and long-term goals (Worrall et al. 2017). The time frame for these depends on a variety of different factors, such as the given therapy setting with regard to the frequency and duration of the sessions, as well as personal and environmental factors including individual resources. Furthermore, other factors, for example, individual comorbidities, language profile, severity of the impairment and rehabilitation phase, influence the rehabilitation process (e.g., Raymer and Gonzalez Rothi 2017).

Establishing therapeutic goals is dependent on the stage of aphasia. Based on the underlying physiological processes (e.g., reduction of penumbra and diachisis) during the acute phase, the aim is primarily to reactivate temporarily affected language skills (Wittler 2009). Owing to the strong effect of spontaneous recovery, therapeutic goals have to be adjusted daily in a very flexible way and are therefore short-term goals. They can be located at the ICF level of body (psychological) functions, because the patient's limitations in everyday life are not yet reliably foreseeable.

If there are less-fluctuating symptoms and a decrease of spontaneous recovery in the post-acute phase, the intervention focus shifts to supporting the functional reorganisation by specifically training the impaired cognitive-linguistic functions during the chronic phase. Since there is no further spontaneous recovery to be expected in chronic aphasia, other communication-orientated intervention approaches might become relevant to optimise the use of the remaining verbal and non-verbal abilities, besides the continuing and intensive training of specific language functions. Compensatory strategies could also be relevant for the patient (e.g., Raymer and Gonzalez Rothi 2018; Aphasia United 2020); hence, middle- and long-term goals are defined. The individual perception of the language disorder, as well as the needs of the patient and his or her relatives, are of particular importance (e.g., Worrall et al. 2011).

To address the superordinate aim of participation, the therapist has to deduce communicative activities that underlie the target situation and that have to be improved. Furthermore, cognitive-linguistic functions underlying those communicative activities have to be considered (Worrall et al. 2017; Hanne and Stadie 2019).

Specific and measurable goals are inevitable regarding an evidence-based therapy (Brown et al. 2023). To formulate such goals, the SMART-rules (Bovend'Eerdt et al. 2009; Hersh et al. 2012) are helpful. Following these, therapeutic goals should always be **s**pecific, **m**easurable, **a**chievable, **r**elevant and **t**imed (Hersh et al.

2012). Furthermore, goal attainment scaling may help to define specific goals and evaluate the treatment outcome. After a predetermined time frame that was defined during goal formulation, the patient and therapist rate the therapy outcome on a five-step scale (Bovend'Eerdt et al. 2009; Wade 2009).

### 25.2.3 Structure and Content of Therapy Sessions

The session-specific goals include the methodological design of the session. In addition to an appropriate approach, (psycho-)linguistically controlled material, relevant for the everyday life of the PwA, has to be chosen (e.g., Stadie and Schröder 2009; Renvall et al. 2013a, b). The methodological design is based on several factors and principles. Approaches for acute aphasia, focusing on activation and stimulation, differ from function-specific and model-orientated methods in post-acute and chronic aphasia, and from the more communicative-pragmatic approaches that are especially relevant for the chronic rehabilitation phase (e.g., Worrall et al. 2017; Raymer and Gonzalez Rothi 2018; Monnelly et al. 2023). When selecting an appropriate approach, the therapist should always consider the existing evidence (e.g., Brady et al. 2016a).

Moreover, a hierarchy of relevant cues should be defined. Depending on the stage of aphasia, the methodological procedure and the hierarchy differ. In the acute phase, maximum support and decreasing cues are used, whereas the hierarchy (choice) of cues in the chronic phase is derived from the individual language profile of the PwA (Nobis-Bosch et al. 2013). Different types of cues can be used to elicit a certain utterance, for example, phonological, semantic, graphematic or gesticulative. In addition, the therapist has to plan different opportunities to increase the level of exercises. Such an increase may refer to the linguistic criteria of the material, the contextual complexity or the situational context (Hanne and Stadie 2019). Furthermore, criteria to interrupt the selected exercises have to be defined.

To plan a therapeutic session, its overall structure should also be taken into account. Dwight (2006) proposes a tripartite structure including the introduction, the body and the closing. Finally, counselling of the patient and his or her partners is an important element during all phases of aphasia. Whilst in the acute phase, basic information about the disease and simple communication strategies are conveyed; counselling in the chronic phase additionally serves to train and establish effective communication strategies, for example, between the PwA and the partner or in challenging daily life situations.

## 25.2.4 Efficacy Testing

Eventually, the careful planning and delivery of therapy should be followed by the testing of its efficacy (Haring and Siegmüller 2018; Volkmer et al., 2023). In this way, the process of monitoring speech and language therapy can be successfully achieved. The aim of efficacy testing is to study the therapeutic intervention in an individual patient and its effectiveness systematically (Stadie and Schröder 2009). For this the use of single-case study designs has become an important device within the evaluation of daily therapy. A single-case study requires the SLT to formulate hypotheses and expected outcomes before therapeutic intervention and to compare them with the actual outcomes (Field 2013). This method of analysis facilitates and ensures the adjustment of the previously planned therapeutic goals and of the therapy procedure as a whole. Different predicted effects should be investigated when evaluating intervention (ASHA 2004). These effects measure the success of therapy intervention on different levels. They are described as the training effect (*pre-* versus *post-therapy performance on trained items*), the generalisation effect (*pre-* versus *post-therapy performance on untrained items*), the therapeutic specific effect (*control tasks measuring unrelated skills before and after therapy*), the transfer effect (*pre- and post-therapy performance on comparable skills*) and the long-term effect (*post-therapy performance*

versus *performance after a therapy pause*) (Stadie and Schröder 2009). In order to measure the described therapy effects correctly, a number of different variables should be considered, such as linguistic and psycholinguistic features of the items used (e.g., syllable amount, word type, frequency and semantics) (Caravolas and Bruck 1993; Stokes and Surendran 2005; New et al. 2006). Practised and unpractised items, as well as items for the control task should always mirror the same characteristics, so as to provide valid results.

The last step of successful planning and monitoring of intervention is a statistical evaluation of its effectiveness/efficacy (Field 2013; Oleson et al. 2019). Whereas it is difficult to evaluate statistically the small amount of data a single-case study usually provides, it is suggested that descriptive statistics can help to identify specific outcomes. Furthermore, measured outcomes should be compared to expectations of the SLT.

## 25.2.5 Conclusion

This section has provided an overview of the elements that should be included in the strategic planning and monitoring of speech and language therapy executed by SLTs. It has especially highlighted the necessity for grounding therapeutic action on evidence-based theory, the individual needs of the patient and the professional knowledge of the therapist. Hereby, a transparent method is vital. Underpinning formulated therapeutic goals and documenting the patient's progress in a professional and objective manner allows the SLT to frame hypotheses about expectations and to evaluate these hypotheses after the completion of the treatment. Consequently, the individual steps presented above can make speech and language therapy more accessible and transparent; a practice that can be monitored from the very beginning to the very end (even at an aftercare/long-term rehabilitation stage), whilst always considering the personal and situational context of the patient and the logopaedist/SLT.

## 25.3 Principles of Aphasia Rehabilitation

Ilona C Rubi-Fessen

### 25.3.1 Introduction

Aphasia can affect and restrict enormously the social life of people with aphasia (PWA) and their relatives (Hilari et al. 2015). Thus, the ultimate goal of aphasia rehabilitation is to improve communicative skills in order to facilitate participation in everyday life. In recent years, the perspective on aphasia and its rehabilitation has been widened by new findings. In fact, imaging studies have shown that language processing is much more than the effective functioning of few specialised language centres, and modern approaches consider language processing in terms of distributed networks (e.g., Hartwigsen and Saur 2019). Secondly, behavioural treatment of aphasia has shifted from training with an exclusive impairment-based treatment of linguistic deficits to considering all aspects of the framework of the International Classification of Functioning, Disability and Health (ICF) (World Health Organization 2001)—that is, body functions, activities and participation, and environment. Finally, newly developed techniques of non-invasive brain stimulation (NIBS) have been used successfully to enhance neural plasticity (e.g., Breining and Sebastian 2020) and therefore increased rehabilitation outcomes after stroke.

Because other sections of this manual address various aspects of aphasia, the approaches and options for therapy and treatment, and the holistic view of the ICF in more detail, the present section provides an overview of overall principles underlying rehabilitation in aphasia. These principles relate primarily to the neurophysiological basis of language processing, as well as to the recovery from aphasia in different stages, in which modern imaging techniques provide new insights. Accordingly, this section will first summarise both long-established and new findings of the physiological and neural basis of aphasia and its recovery, followed by the "10

principles of aphasia rehabilitation" (Kleim and Jones 2008). The latter will be presented with reference to current therapy research. For more in-depth information, the reader is referred to the basic literature cited or to the excellent detailed book chapters by, for example, Raymer and Gonzalez Rothi (2018) and Papathanasiou et al. (2017).

Planning of rehabilitative care therapy requires the integration of knowledge about both the above-mentioned principles and adequate behavioural therapy approaches, accompanied by individual information about the stage and severity of aphasia, the cognitive resources, information about the person's participation in social life, and above all the specific needs and goals of each individual. Therefore, this section offers a foundation for the understanding of specific therapeutic approaches (see following sections) by highlighting the "10 principles" in the light of their implications and consequences for speech and language therapy (SLT).

### 25.3.2 Physiological Aspects of Aphasia

#### 25.3.2.1 Aphasia: A Network Disorder? Aphasia—A Network Disorder!

Recent imaging studies have shown that language processing is much more than the effective functioning of a few specialised language centres, such as Broca's area in the inferior frontal gyrus and Wernicke's area in the middle and superior temporal gyrus. Modern approaches assume language processing to be a collaboration of distributed networks. This connectionist concept, which was first formulated in a rudimentary form in the Wernicke-Lichtheim model in 1885 (Lichtheim 1885), has been systematically refined in recent years. In addition to language-specific components and their well-known connection, the arcuate fascicle, the language network has been extended by new pathways, for example, the ventral pathway (Poeppel 2014; Friederici and Gierhan 2013; Saur et al. 2008) and extended by domain-general networks that control, coordinate and integrate the individual processes of language processing (Hartwigsen and Volz 2021; Geranmayeh et al. 2014). Therefore, damage to different parts of these overlapping networks may cause aphasic symptoms (Saur et al. 2006; Geranmayeh et al. 2016; Turkeltaub et al. 2016; Hillis et al. 2002). Conversely, network plasticity and reorganisation allow the brain to compensate focal brain lesions after stroke dynamically, and may lead to different patterns of recovery, depending on factors such as the stage of aphasia and the location and size of the lesion (Hartwigsen and Volz 2021; Stockert et al. 2020).

**Implications for Speech and Language Therapy (SLT)** Therapists and physicians should be aware of communication disorders in lesions independent of the typical language regions. It should be clarified by differential diagnosis whether the observed symptoms result from a loss of language knowledge or represent the expression of a disruption of access to language knowledge due to disturbances of other components of the (language) network or their connections.

## 25.3.2.2 Modes of Recovery

Functional reorganisation of language involves both intra-hemispheric interactions between the damaged left hemisphere and peri-lesional sites, and inter-hemispheric interactions between the lesioned left hemispheric language areas. The functional contribution of left and right hemispheric areas to language recovery is not yet fully understood, but it seems certain that it changes over time (Stockert et al. 2016, 2020; Hartwigsen and Saur 2019; Hamilton et al. 2011; Saur et al. 2006). In the post-acute and chronic stages of aphasia, the reintegration of peri-lesional, undamaged areas in the language-dominant hemisphere leads to a most favourable outcome in recovery from aphasia (Crosson et al. 2019; Thiel and Zumbansen 2016; Torres et al. 2013; Hamilton et al. 2011; Heiss and Thiel 2006). However, during the acute stage of aphasia the transient activation of right hemispheric areas seems to support

normalisation of left hemispheric network activity (Stockert et al. 2020; Saur et al. 2006).

In an early longitudinal fMRI study with 14 patients with aphasia, Saur and collaborators (2006) investigated the temporal dynamics of language-related brain activation changes. They found that the reorganisation of network activity follows a specific pattern of language-related brain activation changes: in the acute phase (2–4 days after stroke), a complete breakdown of left-hemispheric language-related activation was observed, while in the subacute phase (about 2 weeks post onset) increased recruitment of homologous language areas in the right hemisphere was found. In the chronic stage of aphasia (more than 4 months after onset) participants showed normalisation of activation with a re-shift of activation to left-hemispheric language areas. Stockert et al. (2020) replicated and extended this study with the same design, but with a greater and more controlled sample, consisting of two subgroups of patients with circumscribed lesions of either the left frontal or temporo-parietal cortex. Results showed that involvement of the lesion-homologous cortex was only observed in the subgroup with left frontal lesions, whereas both groups showed increased activation of bilateral domain-general networks and the peri-lesional cortex in the subacute stage. Finally, irrespective of lesion location, language reorganisation during recovery predominantly occurred in pre-existing networks, which was similar to activation patterns of healthy controls. In summary, the study elaborated the phase-specific mechanisms and contribution to language recovery for different lesion locations. Stockert et al. (2020) emphasise that these time- and lesion-specific activation patterns also provide different options for therapeutic approaches and supportive therapies as non-invasive brain stimulation, which will be addressed later in this section.

Nevertheless, it is still an open question whether this early contra-lesional activation is associated with language-specific or domain-general processes such as attentional resources or executive capacities (Hartwigsen and Saur 2019; Geranmayeh et al. 2014). The contribution of persistent (over-)activation to recovery is discussed controversially (e.g., Szaflarski et al. 2013). In cases of extended lesions, a permanent right hemispheric activation might be beneficial to compensate for damaged left hemispheric language areas but will be associated with a limited recovery from aphasia. Otherwise, a persistent (over-)activation of right hemispheric areas is considered a disruptive factor that compromises the physiological function of the brain regions that are normally involved in performing a task. It is hypothesised that the stroke lesion may disrupt the interaction and balance of the hemispheres in the manner of an increased inhibitory impact from the right intact to the left lesioned hemisphere. Thus, this inhibition prevents favourable reorganisation of peri-lesional areas (Tscherpel and Grefkes 2020; Thiel and Zumbansen 2016).

**Implications for SLT**  A crucial point is to tailor the approach of behavioural therapy to the stage and severity of aphasia and the expected pattern of recovery—an aspect that will be considered several times in the following sections.

### 25.3.2.3  What Induces (Positive) Neuroplasticity?

**Behavioural Therapy**  Recent neuroimaging developments that allow measurement of structural and functional changes have demonstrated that behavioural aphasia therapy promotes neuroplastic changes and modulates the remaining language network in PWA. Depending on the therapeutic approach, neuroplasticity (coupled with linguistic and communicative improvement) can be achieved in different areas of the brain. In the majority of studies, enhancement of activation has been observed in the left hemisphere, such as in Fridriksson and colleagues' study (2012) in which subjects underwent intensive computer-assisted naming therapy. Marcotte et al. (2012) found a significant correlation between improved naming and activation in the left precentral gyrus after naming therapy intervention using the method "semantic feature analysis" (SFA). In contrast, after an intensive therapy phase with melodic intonation therapy (MIT),

Schlaug et al. (2009) observed a significant increase in the number of fibres and volume of the arcuate fasciculus in the right hemisphere.

Crosson et al. (2019) add non-language behaviour as a further neuroplasticity-inducing activity. They attribute behaviour that activates specific regions of the brain and thereby modulates neuroplasticity, such as executing specific hand movements, which are associated with better word finding (Altmann et al. 2014), or watching videos involving manipulation of objects, which improves naming performance in PWA (Chen et al. 2015), to the engagement of the mirror neuron system.

**Non-invasive Brain Stimulation**  To boost the recovery of language function and optimise rehabilitation outcome, techniques of non-invasive brain stimulation (NIBS) have been established and refined during recent years. Repetitive transcranial magnetic stimulation (rTMS) and transcranial direct current stimulation (tDCS) can modulate cortical excitability and neuroplasticity. When using rTMS, a coil is held over the scalp, delivering a changing magnetic field that induces electrical currents in focal regions of the brain. Therefore, depending on the frequency, duration and intensity of the stimulation, the excitability of the stimulated cortex is changed by depolarisation or hyperpolarisation of neurons (Nerantzini et al. 2020). During tDCS, a weak electrical current (1–2 mA) is administered through electrodes attached to the scalp. By means of a polarity-dependent change of the resting membrane potential of the nerve cells within the targeted brain region, tDCS can increase or decrease cortical excitability (Breining and Sebastian 2020; Stagg et al. 2018). One advantage of rTMS is that, owing to its high spatial accuracy, specific areas of the brain can be targeted precisely. However, to benefit from this spatial accuracy, expensive equipment, such as neuronavigation systems, are required. Depending on the size of the electrodes, tDCS stimulates larger areas of the brain than rTMS, but less precisely, but it can easily and inexpensively be integrated in everyday clinical practice.

The use of high-definition tDCS, which allows a more focused stimulation than traditional tDCS, has shown promising effects on verb naming in chronic aphasia (Fiori et al. 2019). However, a superiority of high-definition tDCS over traditional tDCS has not been demonstrated so far (Richardson et al. 2015). When administered according to the manufacturer's guidelines, both TMS and tDCS are largely free of undesirable side effects (Rossi et al. 2021).

Both tDCS and rTMS can be applied to excite or inhibit specific regions of the brain and can be delivered with or without behavioural therapy. When coupled with speech and language therapy (online or offline with tDCS, or directly after (r) TMS stimulation), synergies can be generated and the effectiveness of the behavioural therapy increased. While there are still inhomogeneous study results for rTMS and tDCS relating to the (sub)acute phase of aphasia (Rubi-Fessen et al. 2024; Stockbridge et al. 2023; Spielmann et al. 2018; Rubi-Fessen et al. 2015; Seniów et al. 2013), there is converging evidence that NIBS can induce or enhance neuroplastic changes and support functional reorganization in aphasia, especially when associated with speech therapy (Ding et al. 2022; Kielar et al. 2022; Nerantzini et al. 2020; Breining and Sebastian 2020; Elsner et al. 2019). Additionally, NIBS methods have shown that they can not only have a positive impact on linguistic functions, such as word retrieval (Chai et al. 2024; Elsner et al. 2020), but can also improve communicative skills (Stockbridge et al. 2023; Meinzer et al. 2016; Rubi-Fessen et al. 2015; Medina et al. 2012). Crosson et al. (2019) provide an excellent overview on the integration of behavioural aphasia therapy and NIBS-methods and outline a model of how individual imaging data could be used phase-specifically to identify and determine a personalised combination of NIBS and aphasia therapy approaches in the future. The fMRI-guided procedure to identity suitable stimulation sites was successfully applied by Stockbridge et al. (2023) or Fridriksson et al. (2018). A recent review by Sloane and Hamilton (2024) provides an excellent overview of the application of tDCS as an intervention for augmenting cognitive recovery (including aphasia) after stroke.

**Implications for SLT**  To build synergisms, it makes sense to coordinate the stimulation location and type with the therapy method; for example, excitatory left-hemispheric tDCS coupled with systematic naming therapy relying on left hemispheric structures (Meinzer et al. 2016). Right hemispheric tDCS has been coupled with melodic intonation therapy (MIT), which has been shown to engage right hemispheric structures (Vines et al. 2011).

### 25.3.3 Ten Principles of Aphasia Rehabilitation

Healthy and damaged brains continuously remodel their neuronal circuitry, which enables behavioural change (Grossman et al. 2002). Irrespective of the "hardware" (brain structures) used, there are established learning principles that govern the learning of healthy individuals and that can be (partially) transferred to relearning in aphasia.

On the basis of findings derived from studies on rodent models, Kleim and Jones (2008) presented ten basic principles (see also quotations below which are all from Kleim and Jones 2008), which (most likely) influence neuroplasticity in healthy and brain-damaged individuals and which are summarised in the following passage:

1. **"Use it or Lose it"** ("Failure to drive specific brain functions can lead to functional degradation") refers to the fact that neural circuits not actively engaged in task performance for an extended time begin to degrade and may lead to a further degradation or even loss of function (Robbins et al. 2007; Coslett and Saffran 1989). This principle applies equally to the (sub)acute and chronic phases of aphasia. During the acute stage of aphasia, therapy will focus on enhancing temporarily impaired language functions and reactivating dormant information stores by direct or indirect stimulation and de-blocking cues, as the therapeutic

overall goal is to stimulate the patient, by all available means, to communicate as appropriately as possible (Papathanasiou et al. 2017).

To overcome the so-called learned non-use (Taub 2000), especially in the chronic stage, among other approaches constraint-induced therapies for motor and language deficits (CIMT: constraint-induced motor therapy, and CILT: constraint-induced language therapy) were developed (Taub et al. 2003; Pulvermüller et al. 2001). These approaches force the individual to use the non-used limb or language function. For aphasia, this means pushing the patient to his or her linguistic and communicative limits in order to reactivate, and thus possibly strengthen, the language circuits that have survived a lesion. The positive effects of intensive specific training support the second principle.

2. **"Use it and improve it"** ("Training that drives a specific brain function can lead to an enhancement of that function.") is confirmed for both the chronic and acute phases of aphasia. It does not only count for the constraint-induced therapies (Pulvermüller et al. 2001; Woldag et al. 2017), but also for traditional (e.g. multi-, unimodal and model-oriented) therapy approaches (Rose et al 2022; Breitenstein et al. 2017).

**Implications for SLT** Although there is no clear evidence for a single therapy approach in the very early stage of aphasia, it is common best practice (Springer 2008; Papathanasiou et al. 2017) to administer multimodal stimulation to facilitate, for example, meaningful word retrieval and to avoid possible learned non-use. For the chronic stage of aphasia (see also 5 "Intensity Matters") there are many well-established and evidence-based therapy approaches (besides those of CILT) that directly address the disturbed language function such as verbal word retrieval (see Sects. 25.4 and 25.5).

3. **"Specificity"** ("The nature of the training experience dictates the nature of the plasticity") describes the third principle, which applies especially in the chronic stage of aphasia with a stable language profile. In fact,

it characterises therapy goals and contents during that stage, which are derived from phase-specific assessments (see for example Sect. 25.2). Accordingly, therapy methods are specifically adapted to the goals and the resources and deficits of each PWA.

**Implications for SLT** It is important to note that in aphasia therapy a "one-size-fits-all" approach is not applicable, as each person with aphasia shows an individual linguistic and pragmatic disorder profile with individual personal parameters, and furthermore each pursues personal goals (see, e.g., Sect. 25.2).

4. **"Repetition matters"** ("Induction of plasticity requires sufficient repetition") **and (5) "Intensity matters"** ("Induction of plasticity requires sufficient training intensity") are principles that have been proven for both successful motor learning and cognitive-linguistic improvements (Johnson 2017; Pulvermüller et al. 2001; Breitenstein et al. 2018). Successful (re)learning implies the implementation of neuroplasticity that is driven by changes in behavioural, sensory and cognitive experiences (Kleim and Jones 2008).

Repetition of relearned or newly learned behaviour is required to induce neuroplasticity and the lasting neural changes needed to obtain a level of improvement that is resistant to decay. Intensity within training sessions is a factor implemented in many therapy programmes (e.g., Melodic Intonation Therapy MIT) (Albert et al. 1973), Sound Production Treatment (SPT, Wambaugh and Nessler 2004), Lee Silverman Voice treatment (LSVT, Sapir et al. 2011)), and refers to the number of opportunities to produce a specific behaviour within a single therapy session. Breitenstein et al. (2018) compared the specificity of daily training of linguistic items versus non-trained control items during an intensive speech therapy period. The results revealed a clear benefit for items with daily training over control items presented at study assessments only.

The term intensity is also used to describe the number of therapy sessions within a defined period of time. Many meta-analyses have been conducted in an attempt to provide evidence for treatment intensity in aphasia rehabilitation (Boghal et al. 2003; Ali et al. 2021). There is growing evidence, especially in the chronic stage of aphasia, that high intensive therapy (a high total number of therapy sessions) leads to favourable therapy outcome and has the potential to achieve relevant clinical changes in linguistic and communicative abilities (Brady et al. 2016a). In a randomised controlled trial, Breitenstein et al. (2017) demonstrated the effectiveness and sustainability of intensive speech therapy (3 weeks $\geq$10 h per week). Significant improvements in functional communication were observed regardless of severity and duration of illness. Rose et al. (2022) investigated the effectiveness of two intensive therapy programmes (Constraint-Induced Aphasia Therapy (CIAT) and Multimodality Aphasia Therapy (M-MAT)). Both programmes showed equally to be effective for word retrieval, functional communication, and quality of life compared to "usual care" with a low therapy intensity.

For the acute stage, the results were less consistent (Husak et al. 2023), and the optimal time window for initiating intensive speech therapy after stroke has not been identified empirically. Although intensive therapy has been shown to be feasible and effective in early stage aphasia (Van Der Meulen et al. 2016; Martins et al. 2013), Godecke et al. (2020) and Nouwens et al. (2017) failed to demonstrate the superiority of intensive therapy over a less intensive treatment programme or the usual care for acute and subacute aphasia. However, the contribution of spontaneous recovery to the outcome of these studies in these early stages of aphasia remains elusive. Furthermore, high-intensity and high-dose interventions may not be acceptable to all PWA in the vulnerable early stage of aphasia.

**Implications for SLT** Intensive therapy approaches have proven to be highly effective, particularly in the chronic phase of aphasia. In the (sub)acute phase, the intensity should depend on the patient's resilience in avoiding symptoms of overload or overuse symptoms, such as perseverations and speech automatisms.

5. **"Time matters"** ("Different forms of plasticity occur at different times during training") A very recent individual participant data meta-analysis observed the greatest improvement for enrolment within 1 month after stroke across all language domains (Ali et al. 2021). Although behavioural therapy should support neural restructuring in any stage of aphasia, there might be time windows in which certain therapeutic approaches and forms of therapy can be particularly effective in enhancing neuronal plasticity. Summarising evidence from animal and human motor stroke recovery models, Krakauer et al. (2012) suggest that the first 90 days after stroke are the most favourable time window with the greatest potential to enhance spontaneous recovery. Furthermore, Stockert et al. (2020) showed that during this period different patterns of activity can be observed.

**Implications for SLT** Therapy should be initiated in the acute stage of aphasia. Nevertheless, the behavioural treatment approach and a potential additive method of NIBS have to take into account and complement the underlying physiological processes. This requires the use of both phase-specific and severity-specific behavioural methods.

6. **"Salience matters"** ("The training experience must be sufficiently salient to induce plasticity") describes another principle that influences the rehabilitation process importantly (Kleim and Jones 2008). As each individual has to weigh the importance of any given experience, the content of therapy has to be salient and worth being encoded and remembered. Therefore, saliency detection is considered a key attentional mechanism that facilitates learning. The salience network composed of the dorsal anterior cingulate cortex and bilateral insula (Ham et al. 2013) seems to be involved in detecting and filtering salient stimuli, as well as in recruiting relevant functional networks (Menon and Uddin 2010).

**Implications for SLT** To enable PWA to attend their possibly limited perceptual and cognitive resources to the most relevant set of the available sensory data, and to induce plasticity, therapy items should be useful, familiar and of high functional and personal relevance.

7. **"Age matters"** ("Training-induced plasticity occurs more readily in younger brains") Language abilities and cognitive functions deteriorate while neuroplastic responses in the aged brain alter, possibly related to decreased functional and structural connectivity within specialised brain networks (Antonenko et al. 2013; Nieto-Sampedro and Nieto-Diaz 2005; Park et al. 1996). Although normal ageing is associated with neuronal atrophy and reduced neuroplasticity (Salat 2011), the aged brain is capable of learning. Plasticity may occur more slowly and less effectively though than in younger brains (van Praag et al. 2005). Nonetheless, poorer performance found in studies conducted under laboratory conditions may not be manifested in difficulties in everyday life activities (Park 1999). It has been shown that measures of semantic memory (e.g., world knowledge) are spared or even increase with age (Nilsson 2003; Hopper and Holland 2005). In PWA, world knowledge may be intact, but impaired comprehension and retrieval processes can result in difficulty accessing this knowledge or sharing it (Hopper and Holland 2005). Despite single studies identifying age as a negative predictor of rehabilitation outcome in aphasia (e.g., Laska et al. 2001), recent meta-analyses have not revealed significant differences between therapy outcome of younger and older PWA (Ali et al. 2021; Watila and Balarabe 2015).

**Implications for SLT** Performance in tasks that require less effortful processing and those that depend on acquired world knowledge may be relatively preserved in older adults (Craik and Jennings 1992; Park 1999). Consequently, approaches to therapy with PWA should use the spared cognitive abilities as much as possible and include preserved conceptual and procedural knowledge about the world (Hopper and Holland 2005).

8. **"Transference"** ("Plasticity in response to one training experience can enhance the acquisition of similar behaviour") describes the ability of plasticity within one set of neural circuits to promote concurrent or subsequent plasticity (Kleim and Jones 2008). At the neuronal level, transference is regarded as an expansion of cortical representation and an improvement of the related function that can be induced by behavioural training or the techniques of non-invasive brain stimulation that influence and modulate cortical excitability. In linguistic terms "transfer" and "generalisation" are often used synonymously (Webster et al. 2015). Generalisation has been used to refer to cross-modality generalisation, e.g., from verbal production to reading (Madden et al. 2020) or generalisation from trained to untrained items. Additionally, the term "stimulus generalisation" refers to the "transfer of trained behaviours to stimulus conditions or situations that differ from those in which training takes place" (Thompson 1989, p. 196).

The largest empirical evidence may be found for within-level generalisation and extend to the improvement to untreated words or nouns. In treatments targeting strategic approaches, e.g., sublexical processes in writing or reading, generalisation to untreated items is expected, as the PWA acquires phoneme-to-grapheme or grapheme-to-phoneme correspondence rules, which can be applied to all regularly spelled words and non-words (Shea et al. 2020; Luzatti et al. 2000; Kendall et al. 1998). For other approaches, for instance, "script training," there is evidence for transfer that refers to establishing a limited, personally relevant, highly overlearned and automatised set of words or phrases in daily life conversation of PWA. The "mechanism" for transfer in the latter case is the attainment of item-based automaticity by practising in a holistic manner and a high-frequency recall of the learned phrases in various changing conversational demands (Youmans et al. 2011; Cherney et al. 2008).

**Implications for SLT** The expected transfer is largely dependent on the choice of the therapy method. It should be tailored to the resources and needs of the individual PWA. Whilst more mildly affected patients may benefit more from process-orientated approaches, more severely affected patients with extended lesions may achieve better participation through item-based strategies.

9. **"Interference"** ("Plasticity in response to one experience can interfere with the acquisition of other behaviour") is explained as "the ability of plasticity within a given neural circuitry to impede the induction of new, or expression of existing, plasticity within that same circuitry" (Kleim and Jones 2008, p. 233) and can also impede or inhibit learning. For example, the aforementioned "learned non-use" of the physiological behaviour and the extensive use of easy to perform compensatory strategies can lead to further degradation of function, and thereby hinder optimal rehabilitation, while neural circuits not actively engaged in task performance begin to degrade. This obviously does not mean that compensatory behaviour is always negative. In cases where the loss of brain tissue is so extensive that the physiological function can no longer be retrieved, the required function must either be taken over by other brain areas or replaced by another function.

**Implications for SLT** The selection of the appropriate therapeutic approach requires knowledge of the physiology of the process of recovery, and an understanding of the effects of different therapeutic approaches, and possibly supportive adjuvant procedures of NIBS.

The review of the ten principles has shown that rehabilitation in aphasia is guided by determined physiological processes, from which the derivation of suitable therapy methods results. However, these must take into account the individual needs and goals of people with aphasia. Altogether, this section has placed special emphasis on presenting the physiological basis of the rehabilitation process and creating a link to appropriate therapeutic approaches and therapeutic action. As future research will provide even more detailed insights, the principles will be further refined. At present, structural and functional imaging studies, as well as therapeutic research, focus on the identification of predictors for an optimal recovery from aphasia (Crosson et al. 2019; Ali et al. 2021). However, it is essential to implement the new findings into clinical therapeutic practice, as the goal of all basic research is to improve the quality of life and participation of people with aphasia.

## 25.4 Linguistic Approaches to Rehabilitation of Aphasia Patients

Elisabetta Banco and Rossella Muò

### 25.4.1 Introduction

Language rehabilitation for people with aphasia (PwA) has been either the unique or the core intervention for several decades. During those years, many rehabilitation approaches have been proposed to improve receptive and expressive language through the different rehabilitation phases (from the acute to the chronic) and within different rehabilitation settings (for example, individual or group therapy and, more recently, face-to-face or tele-rehabilitation therapy).

In PwA, four primary areas can be impaired: spoken language expression, spoken language comprehension, written expression and reading comprehension (ASHA 2021). The language impairment may involve the form of language (phonology, morphology, syntax), the content of language (semantics) or the function of language in communication (pragmatics) either in a selective way or in any combination of two or more areas and with different degrees of severity. The main aim of the assessment conducted by Speech-Language Therapists (SLTs) is to identify which functions are still spared and which ones the brain lesion has damaged, in order to set appropriate rehabilitation goals. It is a rehabilitation competence of SLTs to individualise the treatment plan, taking into account the severity of the disorder, the nature of the impairment, the phase of intervention and the preferences of PwA and their significant others. The rehabilitation based on the recovery of language impairment is particularly needed during the post-acute and the rehabilitation phases, as neuroplasticity has been showed to be particularly relevant in the immediate post-stroke months (Coleman et al. 2017). It is also particularly suggested for people with mild to moderate aphasia, as they generally have more chances of recovery, as well as for PwA treated with specific medical interventions such as thrombolysis during the immediate post-stroke hours (Menichelli et al. 2019). During the chronic phase or when language is severely impaired, other approaches such as communication partner training or compensatory approaches have been shown to be more relevant, although some studies suggest that language improvement is still possible during the chronic phase (Simmons-Mackie et al. 2016). In fact, it is a shared idea that the ultimate goal of aphasia treatment should be to help PwA improve their communicative ability and achieve the highest level of independent function for participation in daily living (Martin et al. 2008; ASHA 2021). This goal is often achieved with a combination of restorative and compensatory approaches through different rehabilitation phases. Simmons-Mackie et al. (2017) identified the top ten best practice recommendations for PwA. According to those recommendations, PwA need to be offered intensive and individualised aphasia therapy, designed to have a meaningful impact on communication and life (Recommendation Level from A to GPP, depending on approach, intensity, timing). Every intervention should be designed and delivered under the supervision of a qualified professional. Mentioned therapies include impairment-orientated therapy, compensatory training, conversation therapy, functional/participation orientated therapy, environmental intervention and training in communication support or augmentative and alternative communication (AAC). The rehabilitation of language lies, to some extent, within impairment-orientated therapy and conversation therapy. Modes of delivery might include individual therapy, group therapy, tele-rehabilitation and computer-assisted treatment, either in a selective way or in combination of two or more.

In this section the authors aim to provide an overview of the main linguistic approaches to rehabilitation of PwA.

## 25.4.2 Impairment-Orientated Therapy

Impairment-orientated therapies are based on a "restorative" approach that focuses on the recovery of impaired processes, rather than on the use of compensatory strategies (Cicerone et al. 2005, 2011). Traditionally, the rehabilitation of language was directed at either comprehension tasks (for example, comprehension of nouns and sentences) or production tasks (typically repetition, naming and picture description) on the basis of the categorisation of aphasia (for example, Broca's aphasia vs. Wernicke's aphasia). Nowadays, the introduction of recent cognitive neuropsychological models of language processing, based on the theory of a modular organisation of cognitive processes, have inspired more specific and individualised tasks for the rehabilitation of language in PwA. One of the better known and used models is the Lexical-Semantic model. According to this model (Fig. 25.1) each domain (semantic system, phonology, lexicon, sublexical processes and buffers) and each mode of input and output (written, object/picture, auditory) may be selectively impaired and need to be rehabilitated with specific tasks. As a consequence, rehabilitation approaches can be grouped, according to the specific language impairment targeted, into:

- Semantic rehabilitation.
- Input and output lexical rehabilitation.
- Phonological and articulatory rehabilitation.

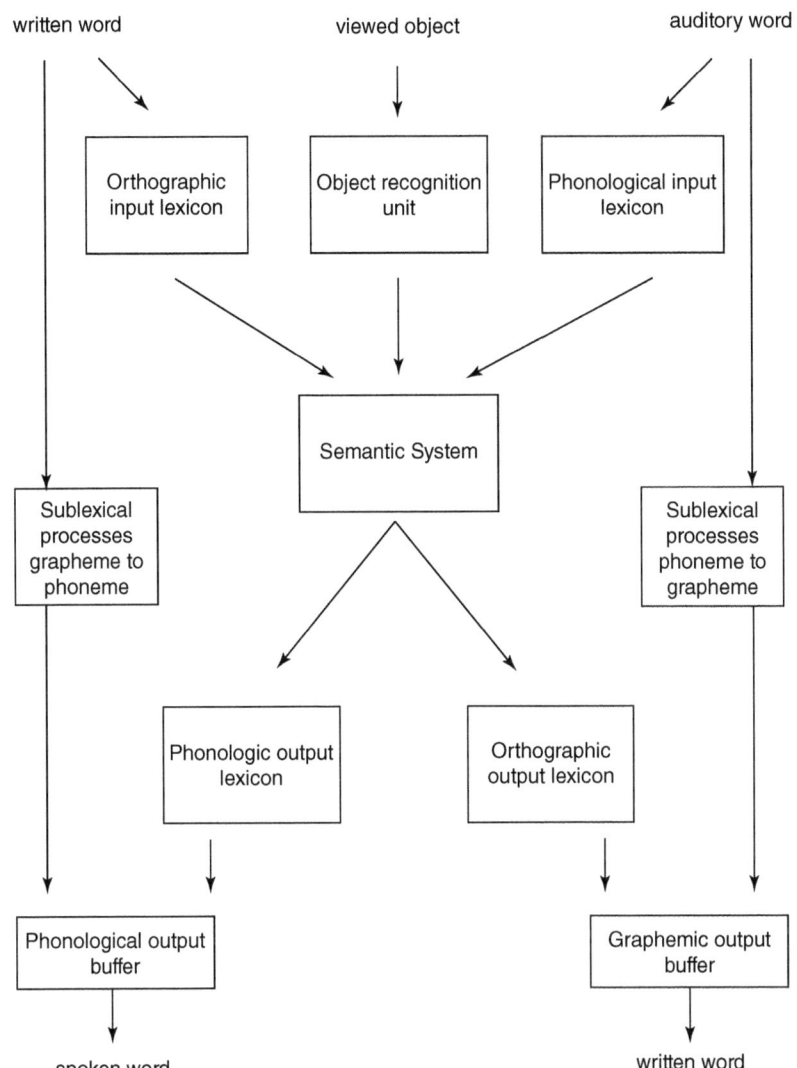

**Fig. 25.1** Lexical-semantic model. (Modified from Caramazza and Hillis 1990)

### 25.4.2.1 Semantic Rehabilitation

According to the Lexical-Semantic model, the Semantic System contains the word's meaning and its conceptual knowledge, and it is involved every time a task of word comprehension or word production is performed. A word's meaning can be thought of as a sum of several semantic traits that describe the object's perceptual characteristics (such as shape, colour, dimension, etc.) and functional characteristics (such as information on context and use). Words are also organised into complex networks of superordinate and subordinate semantic categories. The aim of the rehabili-

tation of the semantic system is to help PwA improve their organisation of semantic categories through associative, exclusion and sorting tasks, and stimulating mental representation of a single object through use, copying and recognition. The rehabilitation of the semantics system should be based on non-linguistic tasks, but few treatments exploit iconographic materials exclusively without requiring lexical processing (Basso 2003). As a consequence, non-linguistic tasks for the rehabilitation of the semantic system are generally preferred for people with severe impairment, while linguistic tasks are usually associated during the rehabilitation of people with mild to moderate impairment.

### 25.4.2.2 Lexical Rehabilitation

The Lexical-Semantic model distinguishes between input and output lexical components. The Lexicon is organised into grammatical classes and each class can be impaired to different degrees of severity (Luzzatti et al. 2006). It is therefore useful for patients to perform exercises that train all grammatical classes or, in the case of selective deficits, the most affected category. SLTs should manage the complexity of the exercises by changing factors such as the frequency of word use, the conceptual proximity and the number of stimuli and distractors used for each task.

Exercises that address specifically the lexical level include, for example, lexical decision tasks where PwA need to discriminate words from non-words. A progression of difficulty can start from illegal non-words (XCOVFGLE) to pseudo-words that differ only by one sound/letter from an existing word.

Other activities, such as word-to-picture matching or word/sentence comprehension tasks, involve both semantic and lexical levels, as well as other language levels (for example, visual and phonological input lexicons, and phonological and graphemic output lexicons). SLTs should carefully consider the language levels involved in any task they use during rehabilitation sessions, in order to calibrate the task difficulty according to the person's specific impairments. Although widely used, the extent to which lexical therapy has an impact on everyday communication remains unclear. At present, lexical comprehension exercises in a sentence context seem to be more advisable (Herbert et al. 2014).

Phonological output lexicon rehabilitation can be divided into two main approaches. The first one aims to recover vocabulary through repetition tasks and relearning of words. PwA are invited to identify words in a dictionary, read them and write them. Then they are asked to repeat daily the previously learned words, and progressively add two or three words every day, in order to increase their personal vocabulary. The advantage of this approach includes the possibility of working autonomously and performing many hours of rehabilitation without a therapist's constant presence.

The second approach focuses on facilitating the restoration of connections in the semantic-lexical network through exercises of lexical retrieval, based on phonological, semantic or grammatical criteria. For example, two quite recent therapeutic techniques include *Semantic Feature Analysis* (SFA) (Boyle and Coelho 1995) and *Phonological Components Analysis* (PCA) (Leonard et al. 2008).

SFA (Fig. 25.2) aims to facilitate word retrieval through semantic features of the concept. PwA are provided with a picture and are asked to name it. If they show naming difficulties, they are prompted to describe salient features, such as group, use, action, properties, location and associations. In case of failure, repetition is required.

Modelled on SFA, PCA treatment (Fig. 25.3) consists of showing a target picture in the centre of a chart and asking the participant to name it (Van Hees et al. 2013). Regardless the PwA's ability to name the picture, they are asked either to provide or choose, on the basis of their language skills, five phonological components related to the target: a word that rhymes with it, the first sound, another word starting with the same first sound, the last sound, and the number of syllables. Once this task is completed, the patient is asked to name the target again. The examiner then reviews all the phonological components and asks the patient to name the target a third time.

Another typical task to improve naming is the picture naming task, with semantic or phonological cueing or both. During this task the therapist provides aids in a progressively facilitating order to enable the PwA to name the picture. For example, in order to obtain the production of the word "train" the therapist would suggest semantic cues, such as "It's a vehicle", "It travels on rails", "You get it at the station" and finally "At the station you get the …". Similarly, the therapist may offer phonological cues, such as "It rhymes with rain", "It starts with the letter /t/" or

**Fig. 25.2** An example of the Semantic Features Analysis chart (SFA). (Modified from Snodgrass and Vanderwart 1980)

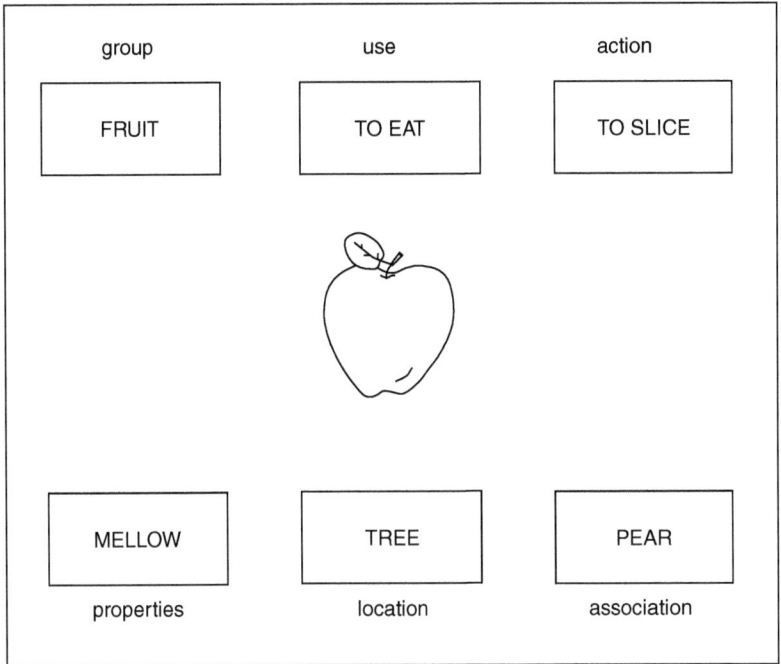

**Fig. 25.3** An example of the phonological components analysis chart (PCA). (Modified from Snodgrass and Vanderwart 1980)

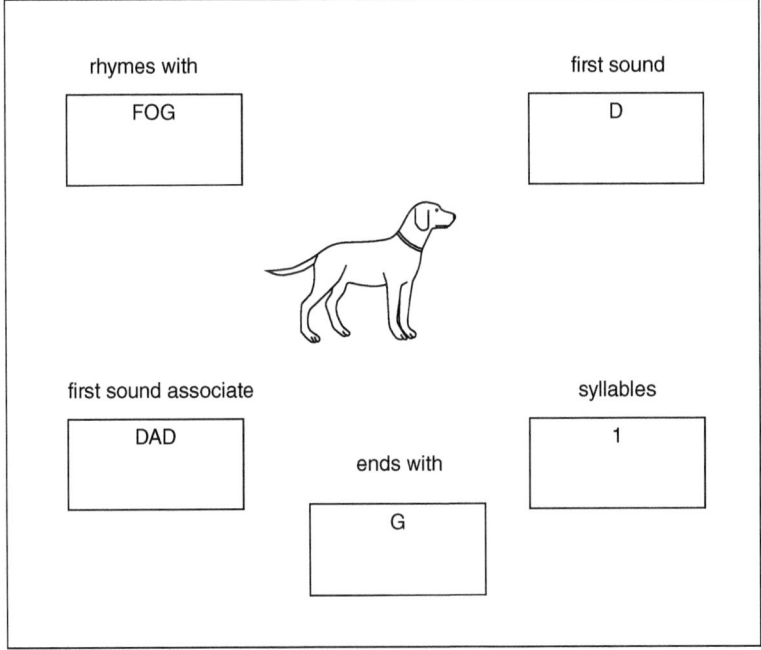

"The word rhymes with rain and it starts with a /t/…".

Both facilitation methods progressively lead to an automatic retrieval of the word. However, untreated items do not seem to improve signifi- cantly so the use of this method is not supported by current evidence (Efstratiadou et al. 2018).

Lastly, repetition is an exercise used in many rehabilitative contexts both for lexical retrieval and for deficits of phonological buffer output.

However, the international guidelines do not recommend the exclusive use of repetition as an effective treatment because there is little convincing evidence of generalisation to lexical retrieval (Vallar et al. 2012).

### 25.4.2.3 Phonological Rehabilitation

At the phonological level, both input and output phonology tasks can be proposed. Phonological rehabilitation is based on the principle of "minimal phonological pair" and on the enhancement of phonological awareness on both input and output sides. Tasks usually require the discrimination or the production of syllables in minimal pairs, presented in rapid succession (drills). The treatment plan proceeds according to the selectivity of the deficit, varying the distinctive features that differentiate trained phonemes (Table 25.1). These activities are usually proposed in cases of phonological deficits that arise at the level of the phonemic output buffer (conduction aphasia). The training material consists of written syllables and words: the ability to read is therefore a requirement for treatment.

Evidence indicates that task-specific semantic therapy and task-specific phonological therapy improve semantic and phonological language activities, respectively. A growing body of evidence (Vallar et al. 2012) indicates that intervention should include tasks that focus on lexical retrieval on the basis of different criteria (phonological, semantic or grammatical).

### 25.4.2.4 Articulatory Rehabilitation

Articulatory deficits are a main component of a specific communication disorder termed Apraxia of Speech (AoS) (Ballard et al. 2000; Basso et al. 2011; Wambaugh et al. 2013). For mildly apraxic patients, poor prosody may be the primary speech deficit and therefore therapeutic procedures designed to improve intonation and stress may be the most appropriate. There are at least two approaches to articulation therapy: one (Table 25.2) is aimed at the relearning of oral positions required to produce speech sounds, following a progression of complexity, as reported in Table 25.2. The other approach allows the patient access to a lexicon, stimulating an automatic retrieval of words. This approach is strictly related with AoS severity. For people with severe AoS the use of compensatory strategies (e.g., gesturing, writing, drawing) and alternative or augmentative communication devices is strongly suggested.

### 25.4.2.5 Syntactic and Morphological Rehabilitation

The Lexical-Semantic model offers a theoretical guide for the rehabilitation of language at the word level. Unfortunately, we still do not have a well recognised model as a basis for rehabilitation at the sentence level. The rehabilitation should include both comprehension and production tasks. Treatment of morphological and syntactic aspects of sentence production requires careful analysis of how, and in what ways, the sentence processing/production system has been affected by brain damage. The most commonly used methods are *Mapping Therapy* (MT) (Schwartz et al. 1994) and a treatment based on the analysis of the movement, using Wh-word questions (those requiring who, what, where, when, why and how) (Thompson et al. 1997).

**Table 25.1** Treatment plan for phonological rehabilitation (based on Luzzatti et al. 2015)

| Repetition, comprehension and reading (drill) |
| --- |
|   – Syllable |
|   – Two-syllable words |
|   – Consonant clusters |
|   – Polysyllabic words and non-words |
| Picture naming |
| Sentence repetition |
| Sentence reading |
| Scene description |
| Generalisation at spontaneous oral speech |

**Table 25.2** Steps of articulatory therapy (based on Basso et al. 2011)

| Practice exercises targeted at articulatory movement |
| --- |
| Voiceless, with/without visual feedback |
| Voiced articulatory treatment (vowels—syllable CV) |
| Two-syllable word treatment—repetition, reading and visual naming |
| Polysyllabic word treatment—repetition, reading and visual naming |
| Visual naming and sentence reading |
| Articulatory control in spontaneous oral speech |

In the MT paradigm, subjects perform comprehension exercises that require them to identify grammatical parts of a written sentence, such as subject and verb. The work is carried out in stages, on the basis of sentence complexity (active or passive sentences, for instance). Production activities involve an increasing level of task difficulty, from the SV (subject-verb) phrase to more complex structures, requiring an increasing coherence between the meanings of sentence constituents.

A second approach is based on Wh-questions, both in comprehension and production. The scientific literature reports positive results and generalisation to untreated sentences if similar in structure to the that of treated ones.

It is helpful to use a graphical representation of the sentence, making it more complex as the work progresses. Table 25.3 illustrates how a configuration can be used at an early stage (SV) up to a higher level.

During treatment, the therapist puts a verb—initially an intransitive one—in the V box; then the patient is required to name a subject or to choose one in case of anomia. The successive phase consists of the opposite task: the therapist puts a noun in the subject box, asking the patient to retrieve a verb. Only at the third step does the therapist require the patient to generate autonomously an SV phrase. The next steps involve the inclusion of a direct object and lastly the diversification between article and noun, with the aim of improving the generative awareness of the patient.

### 25.4.2.6 Acquired Dyslexia and Dysgraphia Rehabilitation

Several treatments are available in the literature to improve reading and writing deficits, especially for English, a language characterised by low transparency. Some treatments focus on the sublexical unit, with the aim of rebuilding the ability to convert graphemes into phonemes and vice versa, whereas other treatments focus on the word or sentence level. For the English language several approaches proposed for the treatment of the sublexical route show good generalisation in the lexical; the generalisation is even more evident in languages with high transparency (i.e., Italian, Spanish). A recent systematic review (Purdy et al. 2019) reported two principal reading comprehension treatments: the *Oral Reading for Language in Aphasia* (ORLA) and the *Modified Multiple Oral Re-reading* (MMOR). Both approaches involve the participant orally reading text-level material, either in unison with the clinician or independently. Moreover, other approaches have been described, such as the hierarchical treatment approach for reading, and specific strategies, such as moving a card to hide text above and below the target text, stopping at the end of each paragraph, and verbally summarising the main points, highlighting the main characters' names and key words, writing important plot developments in the margin of the book, creating "mind-maps" to track who, where and what happened in the text, and writing summaries at the end of each chapter.

The rehabilitation of writing deficits can be approached at both lexical and sublexical levels, often concurrently, with the aim of restoring the damaged pathways. It is useful to remember that the above-mentioned activities of lexical rehabilitation, such as writing and reading single words, can be regarded as a compensatory method for the acquired dyslexia and dysgraphia, orientated to an ecological use of treated materials without restorative intent or the possibility of generalisation.

### 25.4.3 Conversation Therapies

Conversation therapies for PwA include a great variety of several different approaches. A descriptive taxonomy has been provided by Simmons-Mackie et al. (2014). Reviewed therapies have been shown to differ for type of participants

Table 25.3 An exercise scheme for the rehabilitation of agrammatism (based on Rochon et al. 2005)

| THE CHILD | | RUNS | | |
|---|---|---|---|---|
| Subject | | Verb | | |

| THE | CHILD | READS | A | BOOK |
|---|---|---|---|---|
| Article | Subject | Verb | Article | Direct object |

(PwA only, communication partner only or dyads), type of service delivery (individual or group therapy), their principal roots (for example, Conversation Analysis, functional or behavioural, social model or relationship orientated therapies), the main focus of intervention, as well as training methods, activities proposed and outcomes. Among those different approaches that share the same aim of improving participants' conversational skills, some therapies may be more "language-orientated", as a consequence of the severity of participants' language impairment, the phase of the rehabilitation and the theoretical background of the therapist. Techniques such as modelling of strategies, natural reinforcement, scaffolding, subtle prompting and reinforcement of successful conversational behaviour are employed to improve conversation.

### 25.4.4 Other Approaches

#### 25.4.4.1 Melodic Intonation Therapy (MIT)

MIT (Zumbansen et al. 2014) is a therapeutic procedure that attempts to improve lexical retrieval through repetition with melodic facilitation. This method can be applied when there is a lack of repetition but at the same time the patient is able to pronounce some words correctly when he or she sings a familiar song. The method involves a series of exercises aimed at the repetition of high-frequency words in unison with the therapist through the use of the melody. The task can be made progressively more difficult by introducing latency between therapist production and patient repetition, until an autonomous production of the word is achieved, even in an ecological context. The programme is dedicated to patients with severe non-fluent aphasia and requires good collaboration and adequate attention functions.

#### 25.4.4.2 Constraint-Induced Therapy (CIT)

CIT (Meinzer et al. 2012; Pulvermüller et al. 2001) is orientated towards a linguistic approach that considers language as a whole, rather than intervening on specific deficits of language subsystems. Inspired by motor rehabilitation, CIT relies on the "learned non-use" phenomenon. Learned non-use is a phenomenon commonly associated with post-stroke cortical reorganisation. From a motor perspective, patients have been shown not to use their impaired arm, because of unsuccessful prior attempts, even when the progressive recovery of motor function would allow it. As a consequence of the decreased use during the cortical reorganisation process, the hand region of the motor cortex is invaded by areas representing more proximal arm control. Thus, a persistent cycle of decreased use leading to disadvantageous cortical reorganisation may be established (Field-Fote 2015). From a linguistic perspective, the same trend can be observed, with a difficulty in oral communication leading to a loss of language skills. By suppressing compensatory modalities, such as drawing and writing, CIT requests that a patient's communication modality be restricted to spoken language (constraint induction). Modifications to communication behaviour are introduced gradually (shaping) in a group therapy setting, when patients are required to exchange oral messages. During a session, the therapist may distribute different cards depicting objects. The task consists of communicating to another subject the content of the card or asking another participant for information about his or her own card. Through gradual shaping, the participants are encouraged to use the best language within their real skills. Therapy is carried out in a communicative setting that is similar to an ecological situation, in order to promote generalisation.

#### 25.4.4.3 Non-invasive Brain Stimulation (NIBS) Techniques

These techniques, such as transcranial magnetic stimulation (TMS) and transcranial direct current stimulation (tDCS), have been studied in the last decades and have been shown to improve language recovery for PwA due to stroke, facilitating neuroplastic changes (Norise and Hamilton 2017). Although NIBS techniques are used in research protocols but are not yet introduced as a regular clinical practice, experimental results seem promising and deserve attention in the following years.

### 25.4.5 Conclusion

Several approaches for the treatment of language impairment have been proposed and reviewed. Despite most of them showing improved language in PwA, their long-term effects, generalisation and impact on everyday communication and quality of life need to be further investigated. It is, however, the authors' opinion that those drawing up treatment plans for PwA should carefully consider how to integrate different approaches to help clients reach a successful life with aphasia.

## 25.5 Pragmatic Approaches to Rehabilitation of People with Aphasia

Rossella Muò and Beatrice Travalca Cupillo

### 25.5.1 Introduction

Under the umbrella term of "pragmatics" several aspects related to verbal and non-verbal communication have been considered and reported by researchers and clinicians from different areas (linguistics, psychology, sociology, etc.). Providing a complete definition of the term is difficult, and a shared definition wholly adequate on all occasions has not yet been reached (Cummings 2009).

Three different but related conceptual approaches to the study of pragmatics have been reported (Olness and Ulatowska 2017). The first one, a *component view* of pragmatics, emphasises the contribution of language skills to pragmatic abilities. It focuses mainly on studies exploring how language is used in pragmatic concepts such as deixis, implicature and presupposition. The second one, a *perspectivist view* of pragmatics, focuses on sociological, cultural and psychological perspectives on the natural variation and adaptation of language, as language activities operate pragmatically in context. It focuses mainly on studies exploring how language is used in specific contexts, such as maintaining code-switching abilities for bilingual speakers, engaging in an argumentative repartee, or testifying in legal proceedings. The last one, a *functional view* of pragmatics, considers how human expressions function as a means of social togetherness, rather than simply as a means of transmitting impersonal information. This approach has the fundamental potential to bring together both the component and the perspectivist views, as it includes the range of available linguistic techniques and describes those typically used within communicative contexts (which are described cognitively, socially and culturally) to the functional satisfaction of the interlocutors involved.

Recently the concept of *clinical pragmatics* has been introduced. This has been defined as

> the study of various ways in which an individual's use of language to achieve communication purposes can be disrupted… Developmental and acquired pragmatic disorders have diverse aetiologies and may be the consequences of, related to or perpetuated by a range of cognitive and linguistic factors. (Cummings 2009)

During recent decades the aphasia concept has been deeply transformed, moving from a closely linguistic point of view to a broader communicative one, and finally to a more extensive social and environmental framework. What has been called the "pragmatic revolution 1975–2000" (Duchan 2001) and the publication of the International Classification of Functioning, Disability and Health (ICF 2001) have both supported this development. Despite new frameworks, there is still no universal agreement upon a definition of aphasia in research and clinical practice, neither has a consensus on a new definition of aphasia been reached. The two issues that continue to prevent a consensus are the types of lesion (focal vs. diffuse) that cause aphasia, and whether the term aphasia should be defined as a communication disability or as a language impairment (Berg et al. 2020).

In this manuscript, a functional view within the context of clinical pragmatics will be considered and aphasia will be defined as a communication disability due to a focal lesion. As a consequence, the concepts of "pragmatic competence" and "communication competence" will be considered as overlapping.

Pragmatic approaches to rehabilitation of people with aphasia are based on the consideration that communication is more than language itself, that is, language use in different contexts (including conversations, discourses, social interactions and participation in language events) and also non-linguistic communication strategies have to be considered in the assessment and rehabilitation programmes of persons with aphasia (LaPointe 2003). Language plays a pivotal role in our understanding of the pragmatic abilities of people who have aphasia and we should include pragmatic assessment designs that include both linguistic and non-linguistic sources of pragmatic information when examining how speakers with aphasia may or may not be able to vary and adapt linguistic forms to align them pragmatically with specific contexts of communication (Olness and Ulatowska 2017). In contrast to other clinical conditions, where the linguistic function is mainly preserved while the pragmatic use of language is impaired (see, for example, traumatic brain injury, mild to moderate major neuro-cognitive disorder with the exclusion of early stage primary progressive aphasia or high-functioning autism spectrum disorders), for people with aphasia pragmatic disability can be considered as related to the language impairment (Cummings 2009). It is generally manifested in contexts where the linguistic demands are high and other contributing sources of pragmatic information, such as prosody, gesture-shared world knowledge and immediate textual and environmental context, are minimal or unavailable, as well as in highly demanding contexts where specific pragmatic and linguistic abilities are required, such as engaging in argumentative repartee or testifying in a legal proceedings (Olness and Ulatowska 2017). On the other hand, pragmatic competence plays a fundamental role in conveying messages through non-verbal means, allowing communication when the linguistic function is severely or completely impaired.

Aphasia is often a chronic condition, so that a complete language recovery is often impossible, and language impairment may range from very mild to very severe. Functional rehabilitation outcomes should consider achieving the highest possible communication competence (including preserved linguistic skills) in the patient's own environmental and daily living social context with his or her own significant communication partners. Linguistic and communicative difficulties can influence both the quality and quantity of daily conversations, resulting in changed relationships and reduced quality of life and psychological well-being (Brown et al. 2012), so that persons with aphasia are often excluded from full participation in communication and social interactions (Simmons-Mackie and Damico 2007).

Pragmatic approaches to aphasia rehabilitation have been introduced to help people with aphasia, and their significant others, improve language and communication skills, and to meet the goal of successful participation in daily life situations. Among these approaches, "Promoting Aphasics Communication Effectiveness" (PACE) is suggested for people with moderate to severe aphasia, while conversational approaches may be useful for the rehabilitation of people with mild to moderate aphasia. Life participation approaches to aphasia and social models will be briefly described, as they represent an indispensable knowledge to frame the aims of the pragmatic abilities rehabilitation. A functional communication concept, defined as "the ability to receive or to convey a message, regardless of the mode, to communicate effectively and independently in a given natural environment" (Frattali et al. 1995), should also be considered as it permeates all pragmatic approaches.

## 25.5.2 The Life Participation Approach to Aphasia and Social Models

Social models of aphasia have grown since the year 2000. In particular, in 2001, the American Speech-Language and Hearing Association (ASHA) promoted the "Life Participation Approach to Aphasia" (LPAA) workgroup. The

LPAA is a general philosophy and model of service delivery, a "consumer-driven service delivery approach that supports individuals with aphasia and others affected by it in achieving their immediate and longer term life goals". The person with aphasia is considered the centre of all decision-making and has to be given the opportunity to select and participate in the recovery process and to collaborate in the design of interventions that aim for a more rapid return to active life (Chapey et al. 2000). LPAA focuses on re-engagement in life, through real-life rehabilitation goals, beginning with initial assessment and intervention, and continuing after hospital discharge until the consumer no longer elects to have communication support.

Influenced by the ICF framework (ICF 2001), "Living Successfully with Aphasia", which is a full own-life participation scheme, is recognised as the main goal of the entire rehabilitation project. As a consequence, environmental and personal factors of persons with aphasia, caregivers and social partners have to be taken into account carefully and included in the rehabilitation programme. In particular, in the LPAA framework the assessment has to include determining the relevant life participation needs and discovering the range of competence of clients (without and with support), and treatment programmes should include any event for which aphasia is a barrier to life participation (even if the activity is not directly related to communication). From this framework, it follows that clinicians might train both the person with aphasia (enhancing their linguistic and non-linguistic communication abilities) and communication partners (to reduce barriers to making the environment more "aphasia-friendly"). In fact, a highly supportive environment can lessen the consequences of aphasia on one's life, whatever the language impairment, while a non-supportive environment can substantially increase the chance of aphasia affecting daily routines.

Following LPAA suggestions, Aura Kagan et al. elaborated the "Living with Aphasia: Framework for Outcome Measurement" (A-FROM). A-FROM is a broad, non-prescriptive conceptual approach to outcome measurement

that takes into account the impact of aphasia on life areas deemed important by people with aphasia and their families. The A-FROM model simplifies the ICF framework, narrowing the focus to elements of practical interest in aphasia. Four main domains are considered in A-FROM around the person who lives with aphasia: (1) aphasia severity, (2) participation in real-life situations, (3) communication and language environment, and (4) personal attitude and feelings; all these domains influence each other, resulting in a better or worse quality of life with aphasia, in terms of full engagement in life situations and social participation (Kagan et al. 2008).

Within this social model, the conversational partners of persons with aphasia play a role that is at least as important for communication as is the language disorder. Social approaches emphasise the need for multimodal communication (including pragmatic and non-linguistic abilities and augmentative and alternative communication); the need for communication partner training, for them to become an effective communication ramp for the person with aphasia; and the need for opportunities to promote social interaction, in order to increase social participation (Kagan et al. 2004). A growing amount of evidence supports the view that social models are effective in reaching a significant rehabilitation outcome.

### 25.5.3 Promoting Aphasics' Communication Effectiveness

"Promoting Aphasics Communication Effectiveness" (PACE) (Carlomagno 2002) is a rehabilitation treatment conceived by Davis and Wilcox (1981), specifically designed to improve pragmatic and conversational skills for people with moderate to severe aphasia. The main aim is to create a rehabilitation setting where the fundamental rules of a real conversation are maintained. As opposed to traditional treatment sessions, where the conversational partner can see the image that the person with aphasia has to name or describe, twin images (usually eight for each participant) are placed on a both sides of a lectern, so that both the conversational partner and the person with aphasia share the same content and context but are not able to see the partner's images directly. In turn, they are asked to choose an image and describe it, to allow their partner to determine which one has been chosen. All communication modalities and strategies are accepted in conveying the message. In this way, conversations take place in a real communicative situation, where both the person with aphasia and the conversational partner take turns as message sender and receiver, share the same context, are engaged in a real understanding task as they need to find out the correct image, and are stimulated to use all the communication strategies they are able to. At the end of each turn, both participants are asked to display the chosen image to verify that the message has been correctly sent and received, providing a real feedback about the conversation effectiveness.

PACE treatments promote active participation of people with aphasia and enhance pragmatic and conversational competence. The speech and language therapist may gradually increase or decrease the task difficulty through selection of images (for example, very similar images require better descriptive and comprehension abilities) and through a strategic selection of the characteristics of their messages (for example, using verbal/non-verbal messages, complete/partial sentences, positive/negative sentences, active/passive sentences, and so on).

## 25.5.4  Conversation Approaches

Conversation has been described as the heart of human communication (Simmons-Mackie et al. 2014) and as an important arena for the use of pragmatic language skills (Cummings 2009).

A recent qualitative review of conversation therapies for people with aphasia (Simmons-Mackie et al. 2014) identified several different approaches under the conversational label. Among the key elements identified as categorising relevant studies, the authors listed the following: participants (people with aphasia, communication partner, dyads), principal roots

(social models, conversation analysis, functional or behavioural treatment), service delivery (individual or group), focus of intervention (individualised, problem/solution orientated, compensatory), training methods, activities, outcomes and research design.

Among all the existing approaches, communication partner training and conversation analysis will be briefly described.

### 25.5.4.1  Communication Partner Training

As there is no communication without a conversational partner, the communication partner training approach is based on the idea that people with aphasia have an inherent competence, masked by their language impairment, which can be revealed through the skill of a conversation partner. A skilled conversational partner can provide conversational support to the person with aphasia (that is, to be an effective communication ramp), helping that person to overcome barriers to participation in conversation and reach a full life participation (Kagan et al. 2004). In order to train volunteers and partners, a new intervention called "Supported Conversation for Adults with Aphasia" (SCA) was developed in 2001 (Kagan et al. 2001) and now "Communication Partner Training" (CPT) methods are widespread (see Simmons-Mackie et al. 2016 for a review). Through CPT methods, conversational partners are encouraged to use their communication abilities, including verbal and non-verbal strategies, and resources such as pictographic booklets, to help the partner understand the message, to provide the partner a means to respond and to verify that they have understood correctly what the person with aphasia wanted to say. CPT is particularly useful for all people with communication disorders who know more than they can say, including people with severe aphasia.

An increasing amount of evidence supports the view that CPT is effective in reaching a significant rehabilitation outcome. In particular, CPT can enhance conversational skills and increase social participation for individuals with aphasia (Teasell et al. 2003) and can improve communication activities/participation for individuals with chronic aphasia, with improvements maintained over time (Simmons-Mackie et al. 2016). CPT should address environmental barriers of individuals with aphasia and promote access and inclusion through aphasia-friendly formats and other environmental adaptations (National Stroke Foundation 2010; Stroke Foundation of New Zealand and New Zealand Guidelines Group 2010).

Rehabilitation treatments are recommended for training the conversation partner in both verbal and non-verbal strategies to improve communication interactions and functional communication abilities of individuals with aphasia (Taylor-Goh 2005), and speech and language therapists are encouraged to consider "increasing the conversation partner's awareness of their own skills and the communication strengths and needs of the person with aphasia and training the conversation partner on verbal and non-verbal strategies to improve communication interactions and conversations" (Taylor-Goh 2005).

### 25.5.4.2  Conversation Analysis

Much literature has emerged that focuses on improving conversation in aphasia, guided by "Conversation Analysis" (CA). CA is a rigorous approach to analysing naturally occurring talk, with particular attention paid to the structural features and resources that people use to achieve conversational goals, such as collaboratively negotiating meaning, taking turns and repairing communicative breakdowns (Simmons-Mackie et al. 2014).

CA was developed in the 1960s, and is used in sociology, anthropology, linguistics, speech communication and psychology. The main principles of this method include the compilation of a natural database, without preconceived theoretical categories of analysis, through expanding its realm to face-to-face interactions, and including non-verbal communication, through the use of video recording. There are three central characteristics of CA: (1) all the data must be considered, including minimal utterance such as "uh", micro pauses, sound prolongations, coughs and laughter; (2) each utterance or non-verbal occur-

rence has a significance that is sequentially constructed by the conversational partner step by step and (3) the analyst interprets the exchange though the participants' own behaviour and not by pre-defined categories or an observer's judgement of success.

Unlike traditional functional approaches, CA applies structures drawn from data and uses the participants themselves as judges of success, rather than by using invented samples or focusing on patients' failures and successes. As a consequence, it draws implications from therapies that are inherently individualised to the particular dyad (Lesser 2003). Particular attention is given to the study of turn-taking, repair strategies and overlap management. Certainly the communication partners' role in facilitating communicative exchange cannot be neglected, as has been highlighted above, since the conversational partner of a person with aphasia usually carries the greater part of the conversational burden. Therapy usually includes regular communication partners such as family members, and may target the behaviour of either person in the conversational dyad. The emphasis is on creating conversational interactions that help participants achieve the goal of co-constructing meaning, and on managing their social relationship, but does not necessarily entail traditional linguistic or grammatical "accuracy" (Simmons-Mackie et al. 2014).

Although CA has considerable potential, its practical use remains difficult both for research purposes, given the problem of quantifying results, and for clinical purposes, given the laborious transcriptions needed.

### 25.5.4.3  Supporting Partners of People with Aphasia in Relationships and Conversation (SPPARC)

A growing amount of evidence highlights the importance of targeting aphasia therapy directly at the everyday conversations between people with aphasia and their significant partners (Simmons-Mackie et al. 2016). The SPPARC Conversation Training Programme was adapted from CA techniques for use in clinical setting.

It is designed to help clinicians implement conversation training and provides a framework for assessing and working directly on conversation.

The SPPARC Conversation Training Programme (Lock et al. 2001) is structured into six steps, which cover assessment and treatment: (1) preparation, as assessment and training are based on video-(or audio-)taped conversations between couples in their own homes, participants need to be prepared for taping; (2) recording the conversation, lasting at least 10 min; (3) preliminary viewing of the recording and transcription, to enable the clinician to become familiar with their conversation; (4) conversation assessment, focused on three main areas of conversation that are identified as the most pertinent to aphasia (repair and turns, topic and emotions); (5) moving from assessment to training, identifying the occurrences of the main conversational patterns of the couple and the areas that cause discomfort or stress; (6) conversation training, which is articulated into the following three stages: to enable the partner or couple to gain or develop their awareness of (a) the general area of conversation being focused on, (b) their own pattern of conversation, and (c) to enable participants to identify and use strategies for changing their everyday conversations.

### 25.5.5 Conclusion

In order to meet the rehabilitation outcome needs of a given person with aphasia, and to enhance language skills, communication abilities and social participation for them to reach a better quality of life, one or more rehabilitation approaches may be needed and can be integrated. Pragmatic approaches are shown to be really useful in all phases of recovery and rehabilitation, not only in the last phase, when no other linguistic changes can be expected. Therefore, their use is highly recommended, particularly for people with moderate to severe aphasia, where nonverbal abilities are a fundamental means of reaching communication goals and pragmatic approaches offer tools for their training.

## 25.6 Domain-General Mechanisms in Aphasia Rehabilitation

Rosemary Varley

### 25.6.1 Introduction

Aphasia rehabilitation does not, and should not, sit in isolation from other trends and influences in cognitive neuroscience. Through the 1970s to more recent times, the theory, evaluation and treatment of aphasia was influenced by approaches that emphasised the independence of language from other cognitive domains. For example, approaches such as generative grammar stressed the specialisation of the language faculty, reflected in ideas such as innate specification of language (Chomsky 1965). Similarly, Fodor's influential modular approach to the human mind, although allowing some interaction between language and other cognitive mechanisms, emphasised the autonomy of language in many important respects from other systems (Fodor 1983). The impact of these ideas can be found in aphasia interventions with the development of very specific therapies directed at "language-internal" processes. For example, in remediation of grammatical deficits Thompson and Shapiro (2005) designed an intervention—Treatment of Underlying Forms—that aimed to rebuild the syntactic operation movement, in order to support comprehension and production of non-canonical structures (i.e., sentences that do not conform to standard word order for a language). In lexical retrieval, interventions were devised to enhance representation and mapping between hierarchical modules within the word processing system, such as facilitating associations between semantic and phonological representations (e.g., Nickels et al. 2002).

These system-internal approaches led to significant advances in aphasia therapy; however, other cognitive capacities, and in particular domain-general mechanisms, were little addressed. Domain-general systems are multipurpose or generalist mechanisms and, unlike a modular approach to language, they are not specialised for processing a specific type of information. Capacities such as executive function, selective attention/inhibition and working memory are typically described under the heading of domain-general or multiple-demand systems (Shallice 1988; Duncan 2010). Increased interest in domain-general processes in aphasia rehabilitation is consistent with a change in neuroscience where narrowly modular approaches to language are no longer the dominant tradition. At a neurological level, there is widespread recognition that the biological underpinnings of language are not restricted to focal regions of cortex such as Broca's and Wernicke's areas, but rather there is massive interconnectivity and interaction between multiple neural sites (Hauk et al. 2004; Price 2010). Similarly, in the field of language development, many scientists now emphasise the interdependence of language learning with other cognitive mechanisms such as social cognition, selective attention, categorisation and memory (Tomasello 2005; Ibbotson 2020).

## 25.6.2 Domain-General Systems

One of the early systematic approaches to domain-general/executive function processes was developed by Shallice (1988) and labelled as the "Supervisory Attentional System" (SAS). Shallice proposed that these resources intervened in cognitive processing when domain-specific mechanisms, such as auditory comprehension or sentence production, were failing or operating under conditions of high challenge. For example, when attempting to decode an unknown foreign language, the entrained processing system that maps auditory phonological inputs to meaning will fail. In consequence, additional domain-general resources are required in order to interpret the speaker's communicative intentions. These might include increased attention to and maintenance of the novel string in working memory, social cognitive mechanisms to determine the speaker's likely purpose, and problem-solving resources to interpret the situation and decide an optimal course of behaviour when responding.

Given this focus on novelty and cognitive challenge, the links to aphasia therapy are clear: the person with aphasia faces the constant challenge of interpreting and signalling meaning and intentions with damaged language mechanisms.

A more recent approach to domain-general cognition, developed by Duncan (2010), describes the "multiple demand" system (MD) and elaborates its neural basis. The MD system represents a large-scale brain network involving regions of dorso-lateral prefrontal and parietal cortex. Importantly, the MD network is more bilaterally organised than language networks and, although parts of it are adjacent to language zones, the two systems appear to be independent both functionally and anatomically (Fedorenko et al. 2011; Fedorenko and Varley 2016). This offers the possibility that intact tissue within the MD network is available to support language processing following aphasic stroke. In a functional neuro-imaging study, Geranmayeh et al. (2017) revealed that activity within MD networks was one of the factors that predicted the degree of recovery from aphasia. They suggest that targeting these regions through neuro-stimulation techniques such as transcranial magnetic stimulation might assist recovery. Similar findings are reported in behavioural investigations: aphasic participants with the best response to interventions have more executive function capacity (Nicholas et al. 2005; Fillingham et al. 2006; Simic et al. 2019).

### 25.6.2.1 Domain-General Abilities in Aphasia

Typically, the performance of people with aphasia is lower on measures of domain-general abilities than those of non-brain injured (neurotypical) people. For example, Baldo et al. (2015) reported lowered scores for a group of aphasic participants on the Wisconsin Card Sort Test (Grant and Berg 1993), a standard measure of executive function. However, not all aphasic individuals are impaired in measures of domain-general capacities, and there are reports of dissociations between impaired language and residual non-linguistic cognition, particularly when tests are adapted to reduce language demands (Varley et al. 2001;

Keil and Kaszniak 2002; Purdy 2002; Fucetola et al. 2009). Furthermore, if scores of aphasic people are compared with those of other groups with atypical neuro-cognitive profiles, rather than with only healthy controls, then an uneven cognitive profile emerges in aphasia. For example, Little et al. (2019) compared performance of aphasic participants with people with schizophrenia on a range of cognitive and language tasks. Although the aphasic group had markedly lower scores than both neurotypical and schizophrenic participants on measures of lexical and syntactic ability, they were not as impaired as schizophrenic groups on tests of non-linguistic cognition such as matrix reasoning.

In the face of lowered performance in domain-general tests of cognition in many people with aphasia, one possibility is to target intervention at capacities such as working memory, attention or executive function. Improvement in these processes might substantially enhance therapy outcomes, particularly with regard to achieving behavioural gains that might generalise across communicative tasks (Fridriksson et al. 2006). For example, a therapy aimed at improving working memory might result in enhanced comprehension not only for sentences used in training, but across all communicative tasks and situations. Similarly, strategy use is seen as a component of executive function. A problem-solving strategy directed at resolving word-finding difficulty, such as encouraging circumlocution around an inaccessible target word, might assist communication across a range of contexts.

### 25.6.3 Cognitive Therapies for Aphasia

#### 25.6.3.1 Working Memory (WM)
WM is a cognitive workspace and short-term memory (STM) system in which information is maintained and manipulated (Baddeley 1990). All sensory modalities are supported by WM mechanisms, but auditory/phonological and visuo-spatial WM are particularly important in human cognition, with phonological WM (pWM) implicated in language learning (Gathercole and

Baddeley 1993). A standard pWM task is digit span, where a participant listens to, and then repeats, a string of numbers. Digit recall can be in a forward direction (i.e., in the same sequence in which the digits were heard) or backwards recall (i.e., recall in reverse sequence). Backwards recall requires more executive resource than reproducing the original sequence. The amount of information maintained in WM is limited, with typical span of seven items (Miller 1956), and WM capacity appears to be reduced with age (Park et al. 2002).

The role of WM in neurotypical language processing has been much debated (Just and Carpenter 1992; Caplan and Waters 1999; Caplan et al. 2013). Although pWM may be required for maintenance of syntactically complex and information-loaded sentences ("before putting the small blue circle to the right of the large green triangle, touch the blue square"), it appears to have a minimal role in the understanding of the types of sentences heard in everyday language. However, what may be true for neurotypical listeners/speakers may not hold for aphasic people—perhaps even everyday sentences are information-heavy for the aphasic listener. Most individuals with aphasia have reduced pWM span and a commonly encountered therapy for aphasia, particularly for auditory comprehension impairments, is training of word span. Salis et al. (2017) provides a valuable review of interventions directed at STM in aphasia and reports the results of a well-controlled intervention study. The therapy involved listening to words in lists, and judging if they were in the same serial order across two presentations. Despite relatively high-dose intervention (27–30 sessions), little change was observed in either an untrained digit span task or sentence comprehension. This is an important result and indicates that training in recall of unordered word lists may have little impact on everyday sentence comprehension.

#### 25.6.3.2 Attention/Inhibition
Capacities such as WM are closely related to attention. In order for information to be maintained in WM it has to remain at the centre of attention, and if attention shifts there is rapid

decay of that content. Attention is also a key element of the MD system: we live in complex sensory environments and the capacity to attend to the most salient signals and inhibit competing information that is not central to current goals, is critical for adaptive behaviour. Erickson et al. (1996) provided an influential demonstration of impaired auditory attention in aphasia. Participants with non-fluent, Broca's type aphasia displayed no difference from those in a neurotypical group in a non-linguistic auditory task that involved detecting an odd-ball sound in a string of pure tones. However, when the aphasic participants had to perform an additional non-linguistic sorting task (categorising cards by colours), auditory vigilance of the aphasic group was significantly lower than that of controls. These results fit well with the accounts of well-recovered aphasic people who report that, while their ability in quiet and controlled situations is adequate, their language performance deteriorates when in complex environments, such as listening and contributing to group interactions in noisy settings.

The results of Erickson et al. (1996) might suggest that attention training would be a valuable therapy for aphasia. However, there is need for caution. First, notice that the study involved attention to two non-linguistic tasks, and there is limited evidence that training attention with non-linguistic stimuli assists language processing (Murray et al. 2006). Second, not all of the aphasic participants displayed a decrement in auditory attention in the dual-task condition. Two of the ten participants showed only a small change, and thus demonstrated a dissociation between language and general attentional capacities. Although the remaining participants showed an association between impairments, this does not entail a causal relationship between impaired non-linguistic attention and aphasia. The association might arise from the anatomical proximity of the anterior and posterior components of the MD system and regions of cortex that are typically damaged in aphasia. Careful evaluation of causal mechanisms is especially important when designing therapy: if the relationship between capacities is not causal, treatment directed at, for example, non-linguistic auditory or visual attention may have minimal impact on language ability. The need for caution is confirmed by a single-case study reported by Murray et al. (2006). Despite extensive attention training in tasks involving auditory-linguistic stimuli, the participant showed limited transfer of behavioural gains to spoken language comprehension.

### 25.6.3.3 Executive Function

Capacities such as working memory and attention are inter-related with executive function (Keil and Kaszniak 2002; Kendrick et al. 2019). A standard clinical task for the evaluation of language-linked executive function is verbal fluency. In this lexical task, the participant is asked to recall as many members of a category (e.g., "Animals") as possible in a short time span. Individuals who achieve high scores maintain the overarching category label, engage in strategic recall of words from sub-categories of animals (e.g., found in a jungle/farm), discard a sub-category when retrieval slows and switch attention and recall to a new sub-category. Previously retrieved items and sub-categories have to be inhibited to avoid repetition. One possibility is that these same processes of selective attention, maintenance and inhibition are employed not only in these meta-linguistic tasks such as verbal fluency, but also in language-internal computations. For example, retrieval of lexical items to fit into a sentence frame might involve selective attention to the desired word, inhibition of semantically/phonologically similar forms, followed by rapid decay of the target item to avoid perseveration. However, the relationship between the executive processes involved in highly conscious cognition, such as those employed in a verbal fluency task, and the selection/inhibition dynamics intrinsic to language computations is unclear. The issue here is of the granularity of these mechanisms: is the language system so interconnected with domain-general resources that it employs macro-level processes to perform its computations, or are capacities such as selection and inhibition intrinsic to lexical and syntactic networks such that they operate in relative autonomy from domain-general processes? Recent evidence from functional neuro-imaging indicates a separation of these systems in neurotypical listeners. Diachek et al. (2020) report robust activation of left hemisphere language networks (i.e., cortex surrounding the perisylvian fissure) in passive listening to sentences, while MD network activation was not evident in passive listening but was present in meta-linguistic/conscious tasks. Furthermore, MD activation was observed in response to unconnected word lists rather than everyday sentences.

Despite the apparent separation of MD activation and language-internal computations in neurotypical people, there is considerable interest in developing interventions directed at executive function for people with aphasia. One possibility is that conscious, meta-linguistic strategies may support compensations, such as using alternative modalities to communicate when linguistic resources are impaired (Nicholas et al. 2005; Mayer et al. 2017). Spitzer et al. (2020) describe an innovative study that combined a lexical intervention with linguistic-executive training. The intervention targeted cognitive flexibility, for example, monitoring the interlocutor for communicative breakdown and solving difficulties through use of gesture, writing or drawing. Importantly, the training was within the language/communicative domain, as opposed to training executive skills in non-communicative contexts and with non-linguistic materials, in the hope that they might transfer to language. Across all the domain-general systems reviewed here—WM, attention and executive function—a similar pattern emerges, in which direct transfer from non-linguistic tasks to communicative function cannot be assumed, and interventions employing structured language content are more likely candidates for effective therapies.

### 25.6.4 Conclusions

This section summarises approaches to domain-general interventions in aphasia rehabilitation. As in many areas of neuro-rehabilitation, the evidence for effective intervention regimes is still fragmentary. Many investigations employ single-case study or case-series designs and, as a result, a robust evidence-base that allows generalisable conclusions regarding treatment effectiveness is not yet available. Key themes that emerge are that lowered performance in tests of domain-general capacities are common in aphasia, particularly if scores are compared with those of neurotypical controls. However, dissociations are also reported where aphasic individuals display marked impairment on language probes, but normal or near-normal performance in other cognitive domains, particularly where tests do not have complex instructions, language stimuli or require verbal responses. These dissociations suggest that there is no direct relationship between the processing of everyday language and domain-general cognition. Until clearer evidence of functional benefit in language processing, some caution is needed in using therapy approaches that train non-linguistic capacities with non-linguistic materials if the goal of the intervention is to improve everyday communicative ability.

## 25.7 Augmentative and Alternative Communication for People with Aphasia

Rossella Muò

### 25.7.1 Introduction

Augmentative and Alternative Communication (AAC) is an area of clinical practice that addresses the needs of individuals with significant and complex communication disorders characterised by impairments in speech-language production or comprehension or both, including spoken and written modes of communication. AAC is augmentative when used to supplement existing speech, and alternative when used in place of speech that is absent or not functional. AAC may be temporary, as when used by patients postoperatively in intensive care, or permanent, as when used by an individual who will require the use of some form of AAC throughout his or her lifetime (ASHA Practice Portal 2020). AAC involves a variety of techniques and tools to help the individual express thoughts, wants and needs, feelings and ideas. It is typically divided into two broad categories: unaided, when no external tools are required (for example, the use of gestures, manual signs, facial expressions, vocalisations; body language is included in this area), or aided, when some form of external support is required. External support can be either non-electronic or low-tech (such as the use of pictures, objects, photographs, writing, communication boards), or electronic or high-tech (such as speech-generating devices or AAC apps or software) (ASHA Practice Portal 2020). The design of an AAC system incorporates each individual's strengths and needs, so that people often use both aided and unaided AAC strategies, depending on the communication context of the situation (i.e., topic, listener, time of day) and disease progression or recovery (Dietz et al. 2020). A well-designed AAC system should be flexible and adaptable, to allow for changes in vocabulary and mode of access, as the individual's language and physical needs change over time. Romski and Sevcik (2005) identified six common myths about the use of AAC for children with communication difficulties. Some of them may also affect the use of AAC for adults, such as the statement that "AAC is a 'last resort' in speech-language intervention" or that "AAC hinders or stops further speech development". The authors reported that available research does not support these myths (Romski and Sevcik 2005). On the contrary, an AAC system is designed to maximise the individual's abilities to communicate effectively and efficiently across environments and with a variety of communication partners. The ultimate goal of AAC should not be to find a technological solution to communication problems, but to enable individuals efficiently and effectively to engage in a variety of interactions and participate in activities of their choice (Beukelman and Mirenda 2013, p. 8).

### 25.7.2 Augmentative and Alternative Communication and Aphasia

The use of AAC as compensation for expressive communication impairments in aphasiology has a long history, beginning in 1989 when Garrett documented how a low-tech AAC system could be implemented for People with Aphasia (PWA) (Dietz et al. 2020). Since then, both AAC implementation, as well as many common myths that can potentially affect an individual's or family member's willingness and motivation to use AAC, have increased. For example, a quite common misconception is that a person with aphasia should learn the sign language used by people with deafness in order to communicate, although brain lesions that cause aphasia compromise language competence and consequently also the possibility of learning a new language (even a sign language). AAC approaches for aphasia typically involve multimodal communication strategies. Communicators with aphasia are encouraged to use natural communication modalities, such as residual speech, gestures and writing, as well as externally represented messages, or AAC (Garrett and Lasker 2013). AAC can serve many functions for PWA, such as (1) enhancing the comprehension of individuals with auditory comprehension deficits; (2) providing a means of expressing preferences, needs or basic personal information; (3) serving as a word or phrase bank for more elaborate topics; (4) serving as a comprehensive communication tool to generate both spoken and written language and (5) offering a specific technique to enable some individuals to participate with more independence in an important life activity (Garrett and Lasker 2013).

### 25.7.3 Assessment Tools for Planning AAC Intervention

Determining which AAC strategies are the most useful for particular individuals with severe aphasia can be challenging. In order to plan an AAC intervention, Speech-Language Pathologists (SLPs) need a clear understanding of several types of competence possessed by the PWA and required by a specific AAC intervention to achieve optimal improvement in communication.

Body functions such as cognitive, linguistic, sensory and motor need to be included in the assessment, as should representational and communicative competence. Systematic methods for evaluating communication needs and participation contexts before selecting AAC interventions have also been underlined (Garrett and Lasker 2013). The assessment should also include a system to help SLPs differentiate between individuals who can communicate independently with AAC strategies, and those who function best when AAC is used in partner-supported contexts. Within these two groupings, the AAC intervention varies with the communicators' optimal participation levels, communication needs or specific cognitive-linguistic competence (Garrett and Lasker 2013). Garrett and Lasker (2005a) identified the following categories of communicators, which constitute an ascending hierarchy of cognitive and linguistic competence, independence and need:

1. Partner-dependent Communicators, divided into
   (a) Emerging communicators
   (b) Contextual choice communicators
   (c) Transitional communicators
2. Independent Communicators, divided into
   (a) Stored message communicators
   (b) Generative message communicators
   (c) Specific needs communicators

The AAC Aphasia Categories of Communicators Checklist (Garrett and Lasker 2005a) delineates the characteristics of each communicator category and sub-category, helping SLPs identify skills and challenges for each communicator type.

Another useful tool for assessing the PWA's communication abilities and for differentiating independent communicators from communicators who require partner support, is the Multimodal Communication Screening Task for Persons with Aphasia (MCST-A). The MCST-A (Garrett and Lasker 2005b) consists of eight tasks

aimed at revealing how a communicator answers situational questions by gesturing, spelling, pointing to locations on a map or locating pictorial symbols. The test is administered by presenting each page of the picture stimulus manually to the person with aphasia, and then asking them to communicate a specific message. It also provides information on the person's ability to categorise and to point referentially when telling a story. The MCST-A stimulus book contains several resources in order of increasing complexity, from concrete concepts represented with pictures, photos and words, through graphic symbols representing descriptors, to slightly more abstract concepts that can be combined with other items to represent complex meanings in sets of written words and phrases, to an alphabet board to communicate highly specific names by spelling or pointing to the first letter. The scoring form documents the accuracy of message transmission via use of the symbols in the stimulus book, as well as the types of cues that the clinician uses to help the communicator achieve communication success.

Among the assessment tools, the Scenario Test (van der Meulen et al. 2010, cultural adaptation for UK in Hilari et al. 2018) has been specifically designed to assess multimodal communication in an interactive setting, by examining the ability to convey a message, verbally or non-verbally or both, in daily life scenarios. The test comprises 18 items, representing daily life communicative situations, grouped into 6 scenarios (shopping, visiting the doctor, taxi, visiting a friend, domestic help, restaurant), each of them consisting of logical sequences of 3 communicative situations. The assessment scale reflects both the amount of information conveyed by the PWA and the amount of help needed from the communication partner. The quantitative overall score does not provide qualitative information on how a patient communicates the information; therefore, the Scenario Test also allows a qualitative analysis to include information about which communication mode a PWA uses predominantly, how effective these communication modes are, the PWA's flexibility in switching from one communication mode to another, the amount and type of help needed from the communication partner, and comprehension of the scenarios. These ratings provide a profile of communicative performance that can be used for planning treatment.

The Social Network (Blackstone and Hunt Berg 2012) is an assessment and intervention planning tool that helps SLPs determine appropriate communication strategies and technologies for PWA and their communication partners. It includes an inventory that presents the social network of the communicator by using a series of concentric circles to denote level of involvement (from life partners to unknown communication partners). For each level, communication tools and strategies as well as communication efficacy are explored.

Finally, the Aphasia Needs Assessment (Garrett and Beukelman 2006) assists clinicians to obtain information about the PWA's communication needs in a systematic manner. Included in the questionnaire are questions about how well the PWA is communicating, reading and writing; which situations are perceived as the most difficult; which topics are preferred for conversations, reading and writing; which strategies are perceived as the most useful to support conversations.

### 25.7.4 AAC Interventions for People with Aphasia

Recent developments highlight the need for AAC to be better integrated into the rehabilitation plans for PWA. Background frameworks that underline the importance of providing PWA with an alternative or augmentative way to communicate include, for example, the Communication Bill of Rights (Brady et al. 2016b) and the best Practice Recommendations for Aphasia (Simmons-Mackie et al. 2017, p. 139). These documents outline the right to maintain and develop relationships, which may be accomplished through AAC interventions that extend beyond the communication of basic needs, and the recommendation that no PWA should be discharged from services without some means of communicating needs and wishes (for example, by using AAC).

Although assistive, communication technology can change people's lives, AAC technology alone does not make one a competent, proficient communicator without appropriate support, instruction, practice and encouragement. Therefore, SLPs have to provide AAC options in a timely manner so that PWA can become competent and proficient with AAC strategies (Dietz et al. 2020).

In the early stages of recovery, SLPs should help PWA to re-establish meaningful communication as rapidly as possible. AAC strategies can be extremely beneficial during this period, particularly if natural speech is slow to emerge or comprehension is severely impaired. During rehabilitation, clinicians begin to determine whether individuals are likely to regain natural speech and functional comprehension. Restorative therapy approaches are often emphasised in this phase. However, as the individuals transition to home health, outpatient or long-term care phases of treatment, AAC strategies and interventions may merit increased attention if aphasia continues to restrict an individual's ability to participate in important life activities (Garrett and Lasker 2013).

Low-tech AAC strategies can assist partner-dependent emerging AAC communicators with aphasia both to comprehend and control their personal environment by making basic choices, symbolised with real objects, within the context of familiar routines (for example, dressing or eating). Treatment for the emerging AAC communicator focuses on developing basic communication skills, such as turn-taking, choice-making ability with tangible objects or photographs, referential skills, and clear signals for agreement and rejection. Contextual choice AAC communicators do not have the linguistic ability to initiate or add to a conversation on their own, but usually can spontaneously point to objects or recognise visual symbols such as photographs, labels, written names and signs. AAC interventions are typically embedded within conversations about familiar topics. The primary expressive language goals involve consistently teaching PWA to refer to (point to) what they are talking about, understand the meaningfulness of graphic symbols, make choices to answer conversational questions, and begin to ask questions by pointing or using exaggerated intonation. Written choice conversation strategies can be introduced to support conversation abilities.

Transitional AAC communicators demonstrate an ability to use external symbols and strategies for communicating, such as gestures, drawing or speaking to start an interaction with the communication partner. They may begin to search through their notebooks for written choices from prior conversations to find relevant information for the present discussion, so communication notebooks or speech-generating devices (SGDs) containing message sets for common situations can be introduced. However, they typically need cues from the partner to use an external strategy to supplement their spoken communication.

Independent AAC communicators can learn to support their abilities with augmented strategies to communicate effectively in multiple environments with a variety of partners. Strategies may include the use of stored-messages within low- or high-tech AAC systems, use of synthesised voice-output, pointing to elements of a picture to elaborate on a topic, spelling the first letter on an alphabet card (Garrett and Lasker 2013).

Typically, AAC treatment is multimodal, a combination of aided and unaided AAC components, and ideally should be implemented alongside traditional restorative interventions that serve to achieve the same life participation goals. This approach allows PWA to recover as much language as possible, reducing overall aphasia severity. However, AAC also provides a backup plan for PWA, to be used when the language impairment limits the interactions of the desired activity. In addition, AAC may be used to enhance natural language ability, as AAC treatment has the potential simultaneously to strengthen the communication and language environment and to reduce the pressure of relying solely on independent retrieval of the target concept (Dietz et al. 2020).

A comprehensive view of AAC for aphasia incorporates communication partners as key contributors. When PWA are dependent communicators, it is essential that clinicians actively work to adapt the environment and identify AAC facilitators who can be trained as communication partners (Garrett and Lasker 2013). On the other hand, even when the PWA is an independent communicator, the role of the communication partner has been shown to be crucial both to acknowledge and reveal the PWA's competence and to support and facilitate the use of available communication strategies (Kagan et al. 2004). A recent survey (Elman et al. 2016) revealed that only 50% of caregivers reported receiving education about AAC approaches from the speech-language pathologist during the first 3 months after a stroke.

Although current evidence does not identify a superior model of AAC intervention for improving functional communication skills, and evidence is still scant (Koul and Corwin 2011; Russo et al. 2017), some AAC intervention strategies have proved to be useful. The use of AAC strategies for individuals with communication disorders due to aphasia has been shown to improve quality and effectiveness of communication (Johnson et al. 2008). High-technology devices with AAC systems can be used as a compensatory strategy for enhancing communication and social participation in adults with chronic aphasia post-stroke (Russo et al. 2017).

### 25.7.4.1 Conclusions

Dietz et al. (2020) reported three common issues related to the implementation of AAC in PWA: (a) the use of strategies to support expression of basic needs, without regard for other purposes of communication; (b) the use of AAC only with people with the most severe aphasia and (c) prioritisation of traditional restorative treatment over compensatory/combined approaches. AAC strategies are recommended for people with complex communication needs, such as PWA. The implementation of AAC strategies provided early in rehabilitation alongside traditional therapy should help dispel the myth that AAC is used solely for people who will not recover speech ability and may result in increased acceptance of AAC and better long-term participation outcomes. Access to AAC strategies may empower PWA to participate actively in their health care decision-making, to experience increased participation in life events and to reclaim or discover new social roles.

## 25.8 Efficacy of Drug Treatment in Acquired Motor Speech and Language Disorders

Francesco Mozzanica

The generally poor prognosis of the severe forms of post-stroke aphasia (PSA) treated with language and communication therapies alone has stimulated the search for alternative treatments. It has been well demonstrated in a number of randomised controlled trials (RCTs) that aphasia can be treated both in the acute and chronic stages by using technological interventions, constraint-induced aphasia therapy (CIAT), brain stimulation techniques and pharmacological treatments. The rationale for pharmacological intervention is based on the notion that re-establishing the activity of specific neurotransmitters in dysfunctional, but not irretrievably damaged, brain regions may strengthen neural activity in networks mediating attention, word learning and memory (Berthier and Pulvermüller 2011).

During recent decades, several pharmacological treatments have been analysed: piracetam, bromocriptine, bifemelane, donepezil and memantine. Piracetam, a γ-aminobutyric acid derivative with effects on acetylcholine and glutamate action, is one of the more studied treatment options since it may improve cognitive function or act as neuroprotector owing to its metabolic activation (De Deyn et al. 1998). In addition, it increases cerebral blood flow, enhances oxygen extraction, restores membrane fluidity and modulates neurotransmission (Zhang et al. 2016). This nootropic drug has a positive effect on overall language measures and written language, and this effect emerges within a short period (Zhang et al. 2016). These improvements appear correlated with an increase in blood flow in the left peri-Sylvian cortex. However, except for the written language ability, piracetam seems to determine poor long-term benefits (Enderby et al. 1994; Greener et al. 2001; Liepert 2008; Tanaka et al. 1997). Positive effects have been demonstrated with bromocriptine, a dopaminergic agent, which appears useful in the treatment of transcortical motor aphasia and adynamic aphasia. However, variable outcomes in the treatment of Broca's aphasia, and a lack of positive effects in severe cases, have also been reported (De Deyn et al. 1998; Sabe et al. 1995; Berthier et al. 2006). Moreover, in a recent systematic review Zhang et al. (2018) concluded that bromocriptine showed no significant improvements in the treatment of aphasia after stroke. Positive effects on naming, comprehension and repetition, but not in fluency, have been reported with bifemelane, a cholinergic agent. In this case, the language improvements also appear related to an increase in blood flow in the left peri-Sylvian cortex (Berthier et al. 2009).

Interesting results have been reported with donepezil. This is a dose-dependent acetylcholinesterase inhibitor with a selective central action (mainly on post-synaptic pyramidal cell bodies of cortical layers) and a vascular action dilating cerebral parenchymal arterioles (De Deyn et al. 1998). Positive effects on aphasia severity and everyday functional communication, and significant benefits on spontaneous speech, comprehension and naming in chronic aphasia have been demonstrated (Berthier et al. 2011). Memantine, a glutamatergic activity modulator, is effective in the reduction of aphasia severity. Significant benefits on spontaneous speech, comprehension and naming have also been demonstrated, especially if used in combination with CIAT (Huber et al. 1997; Berthier et al. 2009).

These preliminary data suggest that combining neuroscience-based intensive aphasia techniques and drugs acting on cholinergic and glutamatergic neurotransmitter systems might engender better outcomes than other strategies. However, the literature supporting this claim is still limited and further studies are needed.

Nonetheless, the current state of the evidence suggests that drug therapy may play a key role in the treatment of PSA and other forms of acquired aphasia.

## 25.9 Group Therapy for People with Neurogenic Communication Disorders

Karel Neubauer

### 25.9.1 Introduction

The presence of serious persistent illness or the consequences of CNS trauma that cause persistent restrictions on communication, reactive mental health problems and social isolation, is the source of psychic traumatisation of such affected persons. Especially for adults and ageing persons with neurogenic communication disorders, it is desirable to include forms of psychotherapy in individual and group-supportive psychotherapeutic practices throughout the process of recovery and stimulating of communication skills. The aim of this text is to describe the forms of group therapy for people with neurogenic communication disorders that link speech therapy and psychotherapeutic group therapy programmes, with emphasis on the author's own clinical practice (Neubauer 2007, 2014, 2017, 2018).

Such a therapeutic attitude supports current approaches to effective therapeutic intervention for persons with neurogenic communication disorders, including those suffering from dysarthria, aphasia, manifestations of cognitive communication disorder after trauma or degenerative disease of the CNS. These are the efforts to understand the manifestations of communication disorder, to help friends, family and nursing professionals to achieve the maximum possible success in communication with a person with acquired neurogenic speech communication disorder and to induce a natural and friendly environment for interpersonal communication (Gravell 1988; Lubinski 1995; Nadeau et al. 2000; Thompson

2005; Neubauer 2016; Carozza 2016; Elman 2018).

Group therapy programmes using the concept of supportive psychotherapy and a cognitive-behavioural approach for the benefit of people with neurogenic speech communication disorders are based on group dynamics (Brookshire and McNeil 2015; Elman 2018). Prof. Stanislav Kratochví – the founder of Czech psychotherapeutic group psychotherapy – states in accordance with internationally recognized assumptions (Yalom and Leszcz 2008), that group therapy is a procedure that uses group dynamics for therapeutic goals, i.e., relationships and interactions between members and a therapist, and among members of the group (Kratochvíl 1978, 2005). Group dynamics is thus understood as the sum of group events and group interactions. It is created by interpersonal relationships and the interaction of the personalities of the group members with external forces from the social environment. This has its positive and complicating factors.

Effective factors of group psychotherapy include:

- Belonging to a group of people who have a similar problem (one does not feel excluded and lonely).
- The possibility of helping other people (one feels useful, it increases one's self-confidence).
- The possibility of reliving past experiences constructively.
- The possibility of learning new behaviour.
- An opportunity to create new hopes for the future.

Complications of group-therapeutic work can be:

- The formation of pairs or closed subgroups of participants who withhold secrets from the rest of the group.
- The presence of a member wishing to acquire a monopoly on speaking.
- The tendency of several members of a group to engage in highly intellectual or specialised

debates that are incomprehensible to or undermine other members of the group.

- Long-term silence of one or more group members.
- Absence of one or more members of the group at sessions (Kratochvíl 1978, 2005; Praško et al. 2019).

### 25.9.2 Group Therapy in Persons with Neurogenic Communication Disorders

Intensive individual speech therapy, which is applied in the early period of care for people with persistent motor speech, language (aphasia) or cognitive communication disorder, should be gradually supplemented with a group therapy programme. Recent developments in group activities for people with neurogenic communication disorders, in club programmes and in self-help groups for persons with aphasia demonstrate the usefulness and necessity of this form of therapeutic assistance, its importance, and the professional integrity of a number of clinical speech-language therapists (SLTs). An inspirational review of the group programmes presented is the publication *Group Treatment of Neurogenic Communication Disorders* (Elman 2006), which presents selected university and expert group programmes in the English-speaking parts of the world.

Neubauer (2007) applies the benefits of group therapy to the group of people with acquired neurogenic disorders and draws attention to the need to apply a psychotherapeutic approach based on the concept of supportive cover-up psychotherapy in group communication activities. For persons with severe neurogenic communication disorders the use of the concept of so-called communication groups is recommended, and for people with residual disorders, who need to work more to restore their self-confidence in communication situations, the so-called therapeutic relaxation and conversational groups are recommended. Engaging in group activities in the therapeutic process in clinical SLT pursues three dominant objectives:

- To create an interactive group environment for the use of induced communication strategies that have been mastered at some level in previous individual therapy and which a person with global aphasia, for example, will use within the group with the possible assistance of a therapist. A communication table with pictograms can be used during group activity.
- To initiate specific group stimulation activities, e.g., using an approach that stimulates the practical exchange of information between group members, in group speech and through language activating gaming activities, etc. More often, these procedures are first applied to group members already in previous individual therapy.
- To instruct the use and appropriate guidance of procedures for psychotherapeutic activity on group members, to stimulate positive development of group dynamics and its stability (Neubauer 2007, p. 158).

### 25.9.3 Supportive Cover-Up Psychotherapy and Group Therapy

When discussing psychotherapeutic activity in group-therapeutic activities, two points should be highlighted:

- Psychotherapy, especially targeted uncovering psychotherapy (revealing traumas or addiction sources), is not the dominant form of therapeutic approach for people with aphasia or other neurogenic communication disorders. (This form of therapy has a dominant position in psychogenic related disorders.) The psychological problems of these persons, if they did not suffer from psychogenic diseases before the development of a communication disorder, are reactive in nature and are a manifestation of coping with the difficult life situation. For these patients it is appropriate to focus on the psychotherapeutic approach and supportive cover-up psychotherapy.

- Psychotherapeutic influence is not a selective activity, one that can either be performed or avoided. Just as it is impossible not to communicate in human contact, so in the therapeutic process the mental state of others is always affected. In the therapeutic group created there are mutual interactions and group dynamics. The therapist may or may not register, understand or direct these relationships, but uses them to help group members (Neubauer 2007).

In facing the reality of a severe CNS disease or trauma, the accepted view is that a psychotherapeutic approach, with individual and group-supportive psychotherapy procedures, is needed in the entire process of restoring, stimulating and stabilising speech abilities in the treatment of aphasia (Neubauer 2007, 2017, 2018). This has the support of psychologists:

> The need to involve psychotherapeutic support and guidance is particularly evident in speech fluency disorders and aphasia. The psychotherapeutic guidance provided by the SLTs is therefore necessary not only for their own cooperation in the practice of correct speaking, but also to prevent neurotic personality development. (Vymětal 1989, p. 29)

The inspiration for supporting cover-up psychotherapy is primarily humanist-orientated psychotherapy—non-directive psychotherapy by either Rogers or Frankl logotherapy. Finding the meaning of life's situation now and in the future from experiencing the current situation are essential (Frankl 1984, 1995; Rogers 2007; Vymětal 1996, 2007; Graber 2004). Another coexisting source of inspiration in this area is the currently increasingly popular cognitive-behavioural therapeutic direction in psychotherapy (Beck and Beck 2011; Pešek et al. 2012) and the concept of short dynamic therapy (Levenson 2017; Burns 2010).

The differences in targeted uncovering psychotherapy and cover-up supportive psychotherapy, and the effective components of these approaches, are reported by Beran (1992) and Neubauer (2007), both of whom also articulate the broader goals of supportive cover-up psychotherapy as:

- Strengthening psychological defences (counteracting reactive depression, strengthening

active adaptation to a given state and performing therapeutic assignments, supporting the patient's own beliefs about their importance).
- Restoring previous mental balance (life activities, previous interests, encouraging the search for new leisure activities appropriate to the situation).
- Reducing anxiety and fear (to contribute therapeutically to stabilise the condition and alleviate the difficulties, to strengthen the sense of belonging to the environment, to provide continued support).
- Helping withstand difficult life situations better (to contribute to a sense of confidence that the patient can withstand future changes in situation on the basis of existing therapy results) (Beran 1992, 2002, 2010).

When seeking group therapeutic assistance for a wider group of people with neurogenic disorders, two types of group activity have proved successful in clinical SLT practice (Neubauer 2007):

- Communication group.
- Therapeutic relaxation and conversation group.

### 25.9.3.1 Communication Group

This is an open group for persons with severe speech communication disorders. Most often it includes persons with severe aphasia, dysarthria or cognitive communication disorders, from the beginning of intensive rehabilitation to the development of neurogenic disability and may also include persons with chronic persistent severe communication deficits. They are therefore persons with seriously impaired speech intelligibility, significantly reduced ability to express themselves in multiple words, and difficulties in communicating their feelings. It is preferable to form a group from those with similar types of communication disorder (e.g., people with severe motor aphasia), but this situation is rather rare in clinical practice; more often the groups are quite heterogeneous in terms of types of disorder, which makes it difficult but definitely does not impede their activity. The group usually has four to six members; a higher number blocks the effectiveness of group activities. In such a conceived group, there are always one or more persons who are in a stage that can be called that of initial restoration of social contact with the help of a therapist.

Thus the therapist must facilitate each person's communication efforts, by using, e.g., phonemic and rhythmic hints for the beginning of words, or completing the beginning of a message that this group member wants to communicate to others, helping him or her to use a communication table, etc. An experienced therapist can handle this demanding activity with two people who are seated in the group at their side, but according to our experience, this is the maximum load. The frequency of meetings is most often once to twice a week, depending on the nature of the therapy. The programme involves the use of techniques to strengthen the cohesiveness of group members, to reflect the current experience of neutral emotional content, PACE techniques (Promoting Aphasics' Communication Effectiveness: Shewan and Bandur 1991; Roth and Worthington 2019) and the use of storyline description, passive music therapy procedures and music-based imagination (Grocke and Wigram 2006).

### 25.9.3.2 Therapeutic Relaxation and Conversation Group

The inclusion of persons with mild speech deficits or residual difficulties in speech communication in a group programme of persons with severe communication deficits is not entirely optimal in terms of therapeutic assistance. Creating a group that is more psychotherapeutically and conversationally focused is a suitable form of group activity, especially for people with chronically persistent mild speech deficits or for people with good recovery from communication disorders and difficulties in adapting to a new life situation. These people often suffer from persistent low self-esteem of their communication and their ability to re-engage in social relationships. Some people experience a situation where, despite a good level of practical communication skills, the inner feeling of inadequacy and disability in verbal communication with the environment persists.

This perception seems to preserve the feelings experienced by the person in a period of loss or severe restriction of their own communication, and for those with a disposition to develop feelings of inferiority and disability causes the attitude to the surroundings to be fixed. This situation leads to the possibility of applying the full range of the above-mentioned psychotherapeutically effective components of the supporting cover-up psychotherapy, in particular abreaction and clarification. This increases the demand for psychotherapeutic action and the use of group interactions for appropriate therapeutic purposes.

The therapist's ability to lead members to mutual respect and self-reflection through a professional approach can play a key role in the success of the group. The frequency of meetings is most often once to twice a week, depending on the nature of the therapy. The programme involves the use of techniques to strengthen the mutual cohesion of group members, by reflection and reliving traumatic experiences from the past and present (Levenson 2017), passive music therapy procedures and imagination based on music and procedures of relaxation activities (Kast 1999, 2012).

### 25.9.4 Conclusion: Social and Psychological Dimensions of Neurogenic Communication Disorders

Organic lesions of the CNS are a frequent cause of chronic persistent deficits in interpersonal communication, in many cases at the level of loss of speech ability, severe verbal code misunderstanding, with limited compensation for these losses in partial or complete mobility and coordination deficits. The consequences of cerebral vascular diseases, brain tumours or degenerative diseases are also mostly sudden and maximum traumatic interventions in the lives of some adults and ageing people.

Comprehensive therapy of communication disorders by clinical SLTs necessarily includes, besides their own methods of speech and language therapy, some form of psychological approach and influence on cognitive, especially verbal, memory functions and attention. The term "psychological approach" means, in accordance with the concept of supportive psychotherapy in clinical practice (Beran 1992, 2002, 2010; Winston et al. 2012), the application of a psychologically beneficial effect from the behaviour of health professionals, manifested by the involvement of experiences of reciprocity, trust and hope. The psychological approach is an integral part of the therapeutic relationship, supporting the therapy process. Targeted development of the professional competence of clinical speech therapists in this field is highly desirable, e.g., in the form of self-experience psychotherapeutic training, to increase the ability of empathy, and to induce motivation and long-term therapeutic guidance. Comprehensive psychotherapeutic education is an essential factor for a therapist trying to involve group forms of therapy in helping people with neurogenic speech communication disorders. Its significance does not lie primarily in the adoption of some exclusive methodologies of psychotherapeutic activity.

> Having a long-term training and education program is, first and foremost, a fundamental experience for each person in knowing himself. As a member of a training group, he gradually learns about his/her own possibilities and limits, about getting to know himself/herself in stressful situations, gaining information about how others see him/her, how he/she perceives and evaluates his/her person and behaviour. To put it simply, if I know myself and my limits, I can better understand others and manage such demanding and responsible activities as group therapy of people with any disability. (Neubauer 2007, p. 158)

## 25.10 Post-stroke Aphasia Prognosis

Charles Ellis and Fatima Jebahi

### 25.10.1 Introduction to Post-stroke Aphasia Prognosis

Clinicians are frequently faced with considering a complex set of factors known to influence apha-sia recovery, and accordingly formulate a prediction about aphasia recovery. According to Cheng et al. (2020) prognostication about aphasia recovery is a critical aspect of patient-centred care, as clinicians are required to formulate and deliver information to Persons with Aphasia (PWA) and their families. Prognostication in general attempts to provide answers to a common question among PWA and their families: what is the likely aphasia outcome given their current status (Croft et al. 2015)? Prognostication is not an easy process and requires a prediction about the course of aphasia recovery based on experience, intuition and a wealth of evidence-based information related to the factors that influence aphasia outcomes (Brookshire and McNeil 2014). There is no clearly established and simple process to derive an aphasia prognosis, as ample information concerning patient-related variables (age, handedness, sex, educational attainment, socio-economic status, access to healthcare and beliefs and attitudes regarding health care) and clinical variables (initial aphasia severity, aphasia type, site of lesion, size of lesion and the presence of comorbid conditions) must be carefully considered to generate an accurate prognosis (Plowman et al. 2011). In this section we shall explore the patient-related and clinical variables believed most salient to aphasia recovery.

### 25.10.2 Patient-Related Predictors of Aphasia Recovery

Understanding aphasia recovery is a critical first step in knowing who should be treated and how to best personalise treatment programmes to achieve optimal outcomes (Doogan et al. 2018). One of the difficulties associated with aphasia prognostication is that language recovery is a non-linear process that is associated with the interplay of a range of variables all differing among individuals recovering from aphasia (Kiran and Thompson 2019). In this section, the patient-related factors believed to influence aphasia outcomes will be explored and their predictive value for aphasia prognosis will be discussed.

### 25.10.2.1 Age

A review of literature completed by Plowman et al. (2011) regarding the impact of age on aphasia outcomes, and including 40 studies and almost 15,000 participants, found that PWA after stroke are typically older than stroke survivors without aphasia. In addition, those PWA who exhibited non-fluent or Broca's type of aphasia were younger than those with other types of aphasia. However, studies that have investigated the role of age in aphasia recovery have yielded mixed results. Plowman et al. (2011) concluded that studies designed to examine the impact of age on aphasia recovery did not demonstrate a clear relationship between age and aphasia outcomes. A later review by Ellis and Urban (2016) found that stroke patients with aphasia were typically older than stroke with patients without aphasia and that age primarily influenced the likelihood of aphasia and aphasia type rather than recovery patterns. In contrast, Nakagawa et al. (2019) followed 121 patients with aphasia for at least 2 years after onset with cognitive-based linguistic treatment and found that younger age was correlated with better aphasia outcomes. However, other studies examining the impact of age on aphasia recovery have yielded the same inconclusive relationship (Watila and Balarabe 2015; Neves and Catrini 2017). In conclusion, the role of age in aphasia recovery is yet to be conclusively determined.

### 25.10.2.2 Handedness

Evidence suggests that left-handed and ambidextrous individuals may have a more bi-hemispheric representation for language, which offers a greater opportunity for aphasia recovery (Ferro et al. 1999). However, studies examining handedness and aphasia recovery have shown that language representation in left-handed and right-right handed PWA exhibits a large degree of overlap during lesion symptom mapping (Baldo and Dronkers 2014) and handedness has not been shown to predict aphasia recovery (Pickersgill and Lincoln 1983; Pedersen et al. 1995; Watila and Balarabe 2015).

### 25.10.2.3 Sex

A higher incidence of aphasia has been reported among women than men (female/male ratio of 1.1–1.14) (Engelter et al. 2006; Wallentin 2018). However, studies of sex differences in aphasia outcomes have been mixed. Early studies of sex differences found none (Lendrem and Lincoln 1985; Sarno et al. 1985; Neves and Catrini 2017). A more recent study including almost 300 PWA, utilising data from the AphasiaBank, found that men presented with more severe aphasia than women on the Western Aphasia Battery-Revised (WAB-R) and their lower scores were in the areas of information content, fluency, repetition, sentence completion, responsive speech and tests of comprehension (Sharma et al. 2019). Collectively, the evidence regarding sex and aphasia recovery is equivocal.

### 25.10.2.4 Educational Attainment

Education is a commonly collected variable that is associated with better health (Zajacova and Lawrence 2018). Education as an outcome variable can be confounded by literacy levels, general intelligence, coexistence of learning disability and other hard-to-measure variables such as cultural influence (Plowman et al. 2011). Despite these confounding issues, educational attainment and aphasia recovery have shown no clear association (Connor et al. 2001; Lazar et al. 2008; Watila and Balarabe 2015; Neves and Catrini 2017).

### 25.10.2.5 Other Variables Associated with General Stroke Recovery

A range of patient-related variables known to have an impact on general stroke recovery, such as socio-economic status, access to healthcare, and beliefs and attitudes regarding health care, have been hypothesised to affect aphasia recovery. Socio-economic status and its link to the presence or absence of health insurance, and subsequently access to rehabilitation care for aphasia, are regularly discussed in relationship to aphasia recovery. Although socio-economic status has been associated with initial aphasia severity (Connor et al. 2001) there is no clear evidence to show its relationship with aphasia recovery. Similarly, commonly collected variables such as access to healthcare, as measured by the presence of insurance or beliefs and attitudes about healthcare, have not been shown to be related to aphasia recovery (Plowman et al. 2011; Neves and Catrini 2017).

### 25.10.3 Clinical Predictors of Aphasia Recovery

Like patient-related predictors of aphasia recovery, the neuropathological aspects of the underlying condition causing aphasia (e.g., stroke), the significance of those conditions, as well as initial aphasia profiles, are believed to influence aphasia recovery. In this section the clinical factors believed to influence aphasia outcomes and their predictive value for aphasia prognosis will be explored.

#### 25.10.3.1 Initial Aphasia Severity

Studies of aphasia have consistently shown that initial aphasia severity is a strong predictor of aphasia recovery. Studies by Laska et al. (2001) and Pedersen et al. (2004) showed that aphasia outcomes can be predicted by initial aphasia severity as measured by standardised aphasia batteries. They further noted that PWA with milder aphasia symptomology have greater aphasia recovery. More recent studies have shown similar findings (Maas et al. 2012; Benghanem et al. 2019; Kim et al. 2019; Osa García et al. 2020). Kim et al. (2019) examined 235 individuals with stroke by using the Frenchay Aphasia Screening Test (K-Fast) and found that initial aphasia severity was a strong predictor of aphasia recovery. Likewise, Lahiri et al. (2020) concluded that initial aphasia severity was the strongest determining factor of aphasia recovery, among other patient-related and lesion-related factors. Osa García et al. (2020) utilised a composite score based on subscale measures from the Montreal-Toulouse aphasia battery (MT-86), the revised version of the Token Test, the semantic fluency task of the Protocole Montréal d'Évaluation de la Communication, a naming task; either the test

Dénomination Orale d'images (DO-80) for French speakers or the Boston Naming Test for English speakers, to measure aphasia outcomes, and also found that initial aphasia severity was the best predictor of aphasia recovery. Similarly, Maas et al. (2012) measured initial aphasia severity with the National Institutes of Health Stroke Scale (NIHSS) and also found that PWA with "mild" initial NIHSS scores (<5) were most likely to experience resolution of symptoms within 6 months. Likewise, Tábuas-Pereira et al. (2020) found that the NIHSS baseline score predicts well the Aphasia Handicap Score at 6 months. Both these findings align with reports in the general stroke literature indicating stroke survivors with higher NIHSS scores are at increased risk of poor stroke outcomes (Sablot et al. 2011; Saif and Fazal 2014; Jia et al. 2016). Finally, at least three comprehensive reviews of the literature by Berthier (2005), Watila and Balarabe (2015) and Neves and Catrini (2017) have all concluded that initial aphasia severity is a strong predictor of aphasia recovery.

#### 25.10.3.2 Aphasia Type

The literature regarding aphasia type and recovery patterns is quite mixed. Comprehensive reviews of aphasia recovery generally report that individuals with Broca's and conduction aphasia are more likely to experience better recovery than those with global and anomic aphasia (Watila and Balarabe 2015; Neves and Catrini 2017). However, studies of aphasia type are limited by the transitioning of aphasia type over time particularly with a final endpoint of anomic aphasia. Similarly, those with anomic aphasia frequently are limited by the ceiling effects of standardised tests. Nevertheless, Laska et al. (2001) found that individuals with fluent aphasia regained a higher level of recovery than those with non-fluent aphasia. Similarly, Jung et al. (2011) found that individuals with less-severe fluent aphasia improved to a greater degree than those with non-fluent aphasia. Examination of aphasia recovery by El Hachioui et al. (2013a) indicated that aphasia recovery is characterised by different recovery patterns that vary across different language domains (semantics, phonology and syntax).

Consequently, with such changes, aphasia types may not be a strong predictor of aphasia recovery.

### 25.10.3.3 Site of Lesion

Longstanding studies of aphasia have shown that there are specific brain locations that can result in substantial language impairment and poor recovery. An early study by Hojo et al. (1985) showed that lesions involving Broca's area and the lower part of the precentral gyrus, in combination with lesions in the opercular and insular regions, resulted in severe naming deficits. Knopman et al. (1983) found that persistent non-fluency was associated with large lesions located in the Rolandic cortical regions extending into underlying white matter. In contrast, lesions in the left superior temporal gyrus resulted in global aphasia and poor recovery patterns (Hanlon et al. 1999).

Significant advances in imaging techniques have offered greater precision regarding the importance of lesion location to aphasia recovery. For example, Benghanem et al. (2019) found that poor aphasia outcomes were commonly associated with lesions in the left temporoparietal junction. Sul et al. (2019) found that injuries to Broca's area, the inferior prefrontal gyrus and premotor cortex were associated with slower aphasia recovery. Nakagawa et al. (2019) found that lesions in the left superior temporal gyrus inclusive of Wernicke's area were associated with poor aphasia recovery. Benghanem et al. (2019) found that damage to the left temporo-parietal junction was associated with poor aphasia recovery. Additionally, Sul et al. (2019) identified more specific regions associated with poor aphasia recovery. Specifically, (a) poor fluency recovery was associated with lesions of the inferior triangularis and inferior operculum of the frontal cortex, supramarginal cortex and insula; (b) poor comprehension recovery was associated with lesions of the parietal cortex, angular cortex, temporal middle cortex, sagittal stratum and temporal superior cortex; (c) poor naming recovery was associated with lesions to the angular cortex, supramarginal cortex, posterior corona radiata, superior longitudinal fasciculus, internal capsule, temporal superior cortex and temporal middle cortex and (d) poor repetition recovery was associated with lesions to the superior temporal cortex, posterior corona radiata and superior longitudinal fasciculus. Finally, studies have shown that individuals who experience subcortical lesions have better outcomes than those with cortical lesions (Kang et al. 2010). Collectively, the current evidence indicates that lesions to certain area of the brain critical to language recovery can be predictors of aphasia recovery.

### 25.10.3.4 Size of Lesion and Brain Structural Disconnection

As with lesion location, the advances in imaging techniques have offered substantial insights into the role that lesion size has on aphasia recovery. It is notable that Maas et al. (2012) reported that better general stroke outcomes were associated with clinically and radiographically smaller strokes, as well as lower disability before the onset of stroke. Specific to aphasia, Benghanem et al. (2019), using magnetic resonance imaging (MRI), found that large lesion size (volume $\geq 50$ mL or intersection index $\geq 20\%$) predicted poor aphasia recovery. Similarly, Tábuas-Pereira et al. (2020) found that larger infarct volumes on a CT scan were associated with poorer aphasia recovery at 6 months as measured by the Aphasia Handicap Score. In contrast, Kim et al. (2019) found that individuals with larger lesions experienced greater language improvement. The authors concluded that larger lesion volume may be associated with global brain function, which ultimately results in greater initial aphasia severity yet greater room for improvement because of initially lower scores.

Continued advances in imaging have resulted in the hypothesis that aphasia recovery is tied to disruption of white matter pathways critical to language. Hope et al. (2018) examined this issue in 818 individuals with a history of stroke and found no evidence that connectivity disruption predicted aphasia outcomes. Moulton et al. (2019) argued that language recovery relies upon the preservation of white matter tracts in the brain. Consequently, an examination of post-stroke damage to these white matter fasciculi of the language network tracts may offer prediction information about aphasia recovery. They found that axial diffusivity of the arcuate fasciculus was also an independent predictor of aphasia outcome at 3 months after stroke onset. Marebwa et al. (2017) hypothesised that white matter loss and cortical disconnection may be an independent predictor of naming impairments and aphasia recovery. They found that greater left hemisphere network fragmentation and disintegration of peri-Sylvian networks were associated with more severe chronic aphasia. The collective evidence indicates size of lesion and structural disconnection of white matter networks are likely critical predictors of aphasia recovery. More importantly, predictions of aphasia recovery are enhanced by considering lesion location, lesion size and disruption of white matter tracts critical to language.

### 25.10.3.5 Presence of Comorbid Conditions

It is not uncommon for aphasia to coexist with other neurological or medical conditions. In fact, in their sample of almost 3000 acute stroke patients, Guyomard et al. (2009) reported that 28% of PWA had coexisting dysphagia. Similarly, Ali et al. (2015) reported that 29.6% of their 8904 patient sample had both dysphagia and aphasia. They also found that having both conditions was associated with worse prognosis, higher mortality and longer acute hospital stay (Guyomard et al. 2009). Furthermore, Trapl et al. (2004) documented that 10% of their sample of 91 patients with acute ischaemic strokes had both aphasia and dysarthria. Additionally, in Rogers et al. (2014)'s sample of 2154 patients with acquired speech or language disorders, 13% had both aphasia and apraxia of speech. The presence of disorders interfering with motor activities accompanying aphasia has been associated with poorer prognosis, impairing functional recovery (Mayo et al. 1991). Moreover, infection during hospitalisation was found to have a negative effect on aphasia recovery at 6 months, as measured by the Aphasia Handicap Score (Tábuas-Pereira et al. 2020). In summary, the coexistence of other neu-

rological and medical conditions is a negative predictor of aphasia recovery.

### 25.10.3.6 Predictors of Long-Term Aphasia Recovery

There was a long-standing belief that aphasia recovery ceases at 1 year after aphasia onset. However, more recent evidence suggests aphasia recovery can continue for many years after initial diagnosis, although at a much slower rate (Holland et al. 2017). A number of studies have identified predictors of aphasia recovery 1 year and beyond. Pedersen et al. (1995) measured aphasia recovery in 881 patients with acute stroke and found that initial aphasia severity was the primary predictor of recovery at 1 year. El Hachioui et al. (2013b) found that aphasia recovery at 1-year can be predicted by a measure of phonology derived from the ScreeLing, a screening test that includes measures of semantics (word meaning), phonology (word sound) and syntax (sentence structure). Finally, Nakagawa et al. (2019) reported that a combination of age of onset, lesion location, aphasia severity, phonological functions and semantic functions were significant predictors of aphasia recovery beyond 2 years. Although some studies have identified predictors of long-term aphasia recovery, additional study is needed to clarify which predictors are most informative.

### 25.10.4 Summary

A prognosis represents a clinician's "best guess" about recovery, based upon current available evidence integrated with the clinician's experience observing patient recovery patterns (Brookshire and McNeil 2014). A range of variables should be considered all together to reach an appropriate informed aphasia prognosis. However, according to the evidence, it seems that different variables contribute differently to aphasia recovery. The current available evidence suggests clinical variables that are primarily related to stroke or the neuropathological aspects of stroke (initial aphasia severity, site of lesion, size of lesion, degree of brain structural disconnection and the pres-

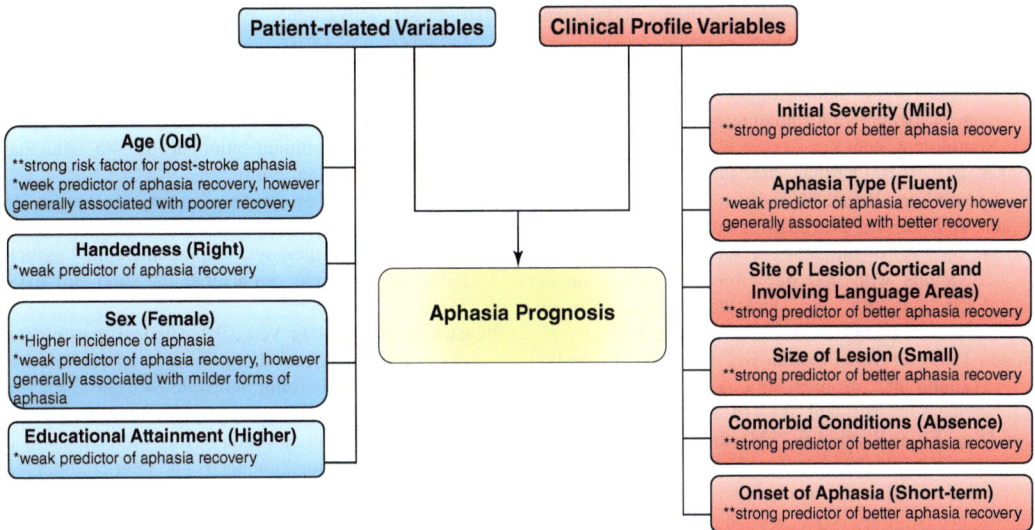

**Fig. 25.4** Patient-related and clinical profile variables with prognostic impact. (©Ellis and Jebahi 2020)

ence of comorbid conditions) are stronger than traditional patient-related variables (age, handedness, sex and educational attainment) (see Fig. 25.4).

Consequently, greater emphasis should be placed on the consequences of stroke that contribute to aphasia than on the sociodemographic characteristics of stroke survivors. We note that the variables included here are not the only hypothesised variables predictive of aphasia recovery. Other potential predictors include auditory processing, personality and attitudinal actors, social integration and social support (Tompkins et al. 1990; Watila and Balarabe 2015), emotional characteristics, mood disorders, premorbid intelligence, bilingualism, socioeconomic status, personal values, beliefs/attitudes about health, treatment quality/intensity (Neves and Catrini 2017). In summary, a wide range of behavioural variables, initial language performance variables and stroke-related clinical outcome variables are critical to generating an accurate aphasia prognosis (de Riesthal and Wertz 2004). Clinicians and researchers must also consider the potential inter-relationships between the wide range of variables known to influence aphasia outcomes when making prognoses as aphasia outcomes can differ significantly across PWA.

# References

Albert ML, Sparks RW, Helm NA (1973) Melodic intonation therapy for aphasia. Arch Neurol 29(2):130–131

Ali M, Lyden P, Brady M (2015) Aphasia and dysarthria in acute stroke: recovery and functional outcome. Int J Stroke 10(3):400–406

Ali M, Van den Berg K, Williams LJ et al (2021) Predictors of poststroke aphasia recovery: a systematic review-informed individual participant data meta-analysis. Stroke 52:1778–1787

Allen L, Mehta S, Andrew McClure J et al (2012) Therapeutic interventions for aphasia initiated more than six months post stroke: a review of the evidence. Top Stroke Rehabil 19(6):523–535

Altmann LJP, Hazamy AA, Carvajal PJ et al (2014) Delayed stimulus-specific improvements in discourse following anomia treatment using an intentional gesture. J Speech Lang Hear Res 57(2):439–454

Antonenko D, Brauer J, Meinzer M et al (2013) Functional and structural syntax networks in aging. NeuroImage 83:513–523

Aphasia United (2020) Aphasia united: best practice recommendations. http://www.aphasiaunited.org/best-practice-recommendations. Accessed 13 Dec 2020

ASHA (2021) Aphasia. https://www.asha.org/practice-portal/clinical-topics/aphasia/. Accessed 31 Aug 2021

ASHA (American Speech-Language-Hearing Association) (2004) Preferred practice patterns for the profession of speech-language pathology (preferred practice patterns). www.asha.org/policy. Accessed 26 Jan 2021

ASHA Practice Portal (2020) Augmentative and alternative communication. https://www.asha.org/practice-portal/professional-issues/augmentative-and-alternative-communication/. Accessed 16 Jun 2021

Baddeley A (1990) Human memory: theory and practice. Lawrence Erlbaum, London

Bai G, Jiang L, Ma W et al (2021) Effect of low-frequency rTMS and intensive speech therapy treatment on patients with nonfluent aphasia after stroke. Neurologist 26:6–9

Baker E (2012) Optimal intervention intensity. Int J Speech Lang Pathol 14(5):401–409

Baldo J, Dronkers N (2014) Does handedness affect the cerebral organization of speech and language in individuals with aphasia? Front Psychol. Frontiers Media SA, 5th edn. https://doi.org/10.3389/conf.fpsyg.2014.64.00073. Accessed 27 Aug 2021

Baldo JV, Paulraj SR, Curran BC et al (2015) Impaired reasoning and problem-solving in individuals with language impairment due to aphasia or language delay. Front Psychol 6:1523. https://doi.org/10.3389/fpsyg.2015.01523. Accessed 26 Aug 2021

Ballard KJ, Granier JP, Robin DA (2000) Understanding the nature of apraxia of speech: theory, analysis, and treatment. Aphasiology 10:969–995

Basso A (2003) Aphasia and its therapy. Oxford University Press, Oxford

Basso A, Cattaneo S, Girelli L et al (2011) Treatment efficacy of language and calculation disorders and speech apraxia: a review of the literature. Eur J Phys Rehabil Med 47:101–121

Beck J, Beck A (2011) Cognitive behavior therapy, 2nd edn: basics and beyond. The Guilford Press, New York

Benghanem S, Rosso C, Arbizu C et al (2019) Aphasia outcome: the interactions between initial severity, lesion size and location. J Neurol 266(6):1303–1309

Beran J (1992) Psychoterapeutický přístup v klinické praxi (Psychotherapeutic approach in clinical practice). H & H, Prague

Beran J (2002) Základy psychoterapie pro lékaře (Basics of psychotherapy for physicians). Grada, Prague

Beran J (2010) Lékařská psychologie v praxi (Medical psychology in practice). Grada, Prague

Berg K, Isaksen J, Wallace SJ et al (2020) Establishing consensus on a definition of aphasia: an e-Delphi study of international aphasia researchers. Aphasiology 36:385. https://doi.org/10.1080/02687038.2020.1852003. Accessed 26 Aug 2021

Berthier ML (2005) Poststroke aphasia: epidemiology, pathophysiology and treatment. Drugs Aging 22(2):163–182

Berthier ML (2021) The key reasons for continuing research on pharmacotherapy for post-stroke aphasia. Aphasiology 35:824–858

Berthier ML, Pulvermüller F (2011) Neuroscience insights improve neurorehabilitation of poststroke aphasia. Nat Rev Neurol 7:86–97

Berthier ML, Green C, Higueras C et al (2006) A randomized placebo controlled study of donepezil in post-stroke aphasia. Neurology 67:1687–1689

Berthier ML, Green C, Lara JP et al (2009) Memantine and constraint-induced aphasia therapy in chronic poststroke aphasia. Ann Neurol 65:577–585

Berthier ML, Pulvermüller F, Dávila G et al (2011) Drug therapy of post-stroke aphasia: a review of current evidence. Neuropsychol Rev 21(3):302–317

Beukelman DR, Mirenda P (2013) Augmentative & alternative communication. Supporting children & adults with complex communication needs, 4th edn. Paul Brookes Publishing, Baltimore

Beushausen U (2016) Evidenz-basiert arbeiten in der Sprachtherapie (Evidence-based working in speech an language therapy). Sprachtherapie aktuell: Schwerpunktthema: Sprachtherapie und Inklusion 3(1):1–9

Beushausen U, Walther W (2010) Clinical reasoning in der Logopädie (Clinical reasoning in speech and language therapy). Forum Logopädie 24(4):30–37

Blackstone S, Hunt Berg M (2012) Social networks: a communication inventory for individuals with complex communication needs and their communication partners. Attainment Company, Verona

Boghal SK, Teasell R, Speechley M (2003) Intensity of aphasia therapy, impact on recovery. Stroke 34:987–993

Bovend'Eerdt TJ, Botell RE, Wade DT (2009) Writing SMART rehabilitation goals and achieving goal attainment scaling: a practical guide. Clin Rehabil 23(4):352–361

Boyle M, Coelho CA (1995) Application of semantic feature analysis as a treatment for aphasic dysnomia. Am J Speech Lang Pathol 4:94–98

Brady MC, Kelly H, Godwin J et al (2016a) Speech and language therapy for aphasia following stroke. Cochrane Database Syst Rev 2016(6):CD000425. https://doi.org/10.1002/14651858.CD000425.pub4. Accessed 4 Sep 2021

Brady NC, Bruce S, Goldman A et al (2016b) Communication services and supports for individuals with severe disabilities: guidance for assessment and intervention. Am J Intellect Dev Disabil 121(2):121–138

Breining BL, Sebastian R (2020) Neuromodulation in post-stroke aphasia treatment. Curr Phys Med Rehabil Rep 8:44–56

Breitenstein C, Grewe T, Flöel A et al (2017) Intensive speech and language therapy in patients with chronic aphasia after stroke: a randomised, open-label, blinded-endpoint, controlled trial in a health-care setting. Lancet 389(10078):1528–1538

Breitenstein C, Abel S, Baumgaertner A et al (2018) Impact of daily item training on short- and long-term success of intensive cognitive-linguistic therapy in chronic aphasia. Aphasiology 32(Supp 1):26–29

Breitenstein C, Hilari K, Menahemi-Falkov M, L. Rose M, Wallace SJ, Brady MC. … Willmes K (2022) Operationalising treatment success in aphasia rehabilitation. Aphasiology, 37(11):1693–1732. https://doi.org/10.1080/02687038.2021.2016594

Brookshire RH, McNeil MR (2014) Introduction to neurogenic communication disorders, 8th edn. Mosby, St. Louis

Brookshire R, McNeil M (2015) Treatment of aphasia and related disorders. In: Brookshire R, McNeil M (eds) Introduction to neurogenic communication disorders, 8th edn. Elsevier Mosby Inc., St. Louis, pp 211–252

Brown K, Worrall L, Davidson B et al (2011) Living successfully with aphasia: family members share their views. Top Stroke Rehabil 18:536–548

Brown K, Worral LE, Davidson B et al (2012) Living successfully with aphasia: a qualitative meta-analysis of the perspectives of individuals with aphasia, family members, and speech-language pathologists. Int J Speech Lang Pathol 14:141–155

Brown SE, Scobbie L, Worrall L, Brady MC (2023) A multinational online survey of the goal setting practice of rehabilitation staff with stroke survivors with aphasia. Aphasiology, 37(3):479–503

Bucur M, Papagno C (2019) Are transcranial brain stimulation effects long-lasting in post-stroke aphasia? A comparative systematic review and meta-analysis on naming performance. Neurosci Biobehav Rev 102:264–289

Burns K (2010) Solution focused brief therapy for people with acquired communication impairments. In: Brumfitt S (ed) Psychological well being and acquired communication impairment. Wiley-Blackwell, Chichester, pp 204–215

Caplan D, Waters GS (1999) Verbal working memory and sentence comprehension. Behav Brain Sci 22(1):77–94

Caplan D, Michaud J, Hufford R (2013) Short-term memory, working memory, and syntactic comprehension in aphasia. Cogn Neuropsychol 30(2):77–109

Caramazza A, Hillis AE (1990) Where do semantic errors come from? Cortex 26(1):95–122

Caravolas M, Bruck M (1993) The effect of oral and written language input on children's phonological awareness: a cross-linguistic study. J Exp Child Psychol 55(1):1–30

Carlomagno S (2002) Approcci pragmatici alla terapia dell'afasia. Dai modelli empirici alla tecnica P.A.C.E. Springer-Verlag Italia, Milano

Carozza L (2016) Communication and aging. Plural Publishing Inc., San Diego

Carragher M, Steel G, Talbot R et al (2021) Adapting therapy for a new world: storytelling therapy in EVA Park. Aphasiology 35:704–729

Chai L, Huang Y, Guo X, Xiong A, Lin B, Huang J (2024) Does SLT combined with NIBS enhance naming recovery in post-stroke aphasia? A meta-analysis and systematic review. NeuroRehabilitation, 54(4):543–561. https://doi.org/10.3233/NRE-240065

Chapey R, Duchan JF, Elman RJ et al (2000) Life participation approach to aphasia Dai modelli empirici alla tecnica P.A.C.E—a statement of values for the future. The ASHA Leader. https://doi.org/10.1044/leader. FTR.05032000.4. Accessed 25 Aug 2021

Chen W, Ye Q, Ji X et al (2015) Mirror neuron system based therapy for aphasia rehabilitation. Front Psychol 6:1665. https://doi.org/10.3389/fpsyg.2015.01665. Accessed 24 Aug 2021

Cheng BBY, Worrall LE, Copland DA et al (2020) Prognostication in post-stroke aphasia: how do speech pathologists formulate and deliver information about recovery? Int J Lang Commun Disord 55:520. https://doi.org/10.1111/1460-6984.12534. Accessed 27 Aug 2021

Cherney R, Halper AS, Holland A et al (2008) Computerized script training for aphasia: preliminary results. Am J Speech Lang Pathol 17(1):19–34

Chomsky N (1965) Aspects of the theory of syntax. MIT Press, Cambridge

Cicerone KD, Dahlberg C, Malec JF et al (2005) Evidence-based cognitive rehabilitation: updated review of the literature from 1998 through 2002. Arch Phys Med Rehabil 86:1681–1692

Cicerone KD, Langenbahn DM, Braden C et al (2011) Evidence-based cognitive rehabilitation: updated review of the literature from 2003 through 2008. Arch Phys Med Rehabil 92:519–530

Coleman ER, Moudgal R, Lang K et al (2017) Early rehabilitation after stroke: a narrative review. Curr Atheroscler Rep 19(12):59. https://doi.org/10.1007/s11883-017-0686-6. Accessed 2 Sep 2021

Connor LT, Obler LK, Tocco M et al (2001) Effect of socioeconomic status on aphasia severity and recovery. Brain Lang 78(2):254–257

Coslett HB, Saffran EM (1989) Evidence for preserved reading in "pure alexia". Brain 112(2):327–359

Craik FIM, Jennings JM (1992) Human memory. In: Craik FIM, Salthouse TA (eds) The handbook of aging and cognition. Lawrence Erlbaum Associates, Inc., Hillsdale, pp 51–110

Croft P, Altman DG, Deeks JJ et al (2015) The science of clinical practice: disease diagnosis or patient prognosis? Evidence about "what is likely to happen" should shape clinical practice. BMC Med 13:20. https://doi.org/10.1186/s12916-014-0265-4. Accessed 27 Aug 2021

Crosson B, Rodriguez AD, Copland D et al (2019) Neuroplasticity and aphasia treatments: new approaches for an old problem. J Neurol Neurosurg Psychiatry 90(10):1147–1155

Cummings L (2009) Clinical pragmatics. Cambridge University Press, Cambridge

Davis GA, Wilcox MJ (1981) Incorporating parameters of natural conversation aphasia treatment. In: Chapey R (ed) Language intervention strategies in adult aphasia. Williams & Wilkins, Baltimore

De Deyn PP, Orgogozo JM, De Reuck J (1998) Acute treatment of stroke. PASS group. Piracetam acute stroke study. Lancet 352(9124):326. https://doi.org/10.1016/s0140-6736(05)60306-6. Accessed 4 Sep 2021

de Riesthal M, Wertz RT (2004) Prognosis for aphasia: relationship between selected biographical and behavioural variables and outcome and improvement. Aphasiology 18(10):899–915

Denier C, Chassin O, Vanderdries C et al (2016) Thrombolysis in stroke patients with isolated aphasia. Cerebrovasc Dis 41:163–169

Diachek E, Blank I, Siegelman M et al (2020) The domain-general multiple demand (MD) network does not support core aspects of language comprehension: a large-scale fMRI investigation. J Neurosci 40(23):4536–4550

Dietz A, Wallace SE, Weissling K (2020) Revisiting the role of augmentative and alternative communication in aphasia rehabilitation. Am J Speech Lang Pathol 29(2):909–913

Ding X, Zhang S, Huang W, Zhang S, Zhang L, Hu J, Li J, Ge Q, Wang Y, Ye X, Zhang J (2022) Comparative efficacy of non-invasive brain stimulation for post-stroke aphasia: a network meta-analysis and meta-regression of moderators. Neurosci Biobehav Rev 140:104804. https://doi.org/10.1016/j.neubiorev.2022.104804

Doedens WJ, Meteyard L (2020) Measures of functional, real-world communication for aphasia: a critical review. Aphasiology 34:492–514

Dollaghan CA (2007) The handbook for evidence-based practice in communication disorders. Paul H Brookes Publishing, Baltimore, MD

Doogan C, Dignam J, Copland D et al (2018) Aphasia recovery: when, how and who to treat? Curr Neurol Neurosci Rep 18(12):90. https://doi.org/10.1007/s11910-018-0891-x. Accessed 27 Aug 2021

Duchan J (2001) The pragmatic revolution 1975-2000. History of speech and language in America. http://www.acsu.buffalo.edu/~duchan/1975-2000.html. Accessed 25 Aug 2021

Duncan J (2010) The multiple-demand (MD) system of the primate brain: mental programs for intelligent behaviour. Trends Cogn Sci 14(4):172–179

Dwight DM (2006) Here's how to do therapy. Hands-on core skills in speech-language pathology. Plural Publishing, San Diego, CA

Efstratiadou EA, Papathanasiou I, Holland R et al (2018) A systematic review of semantic feature analysis therapy studies for aphasia. J Speech Lang Hear Res 61:1261–1278

El Hachioui H, Lingsma HF, Van De Sandt-Koenderman MWME et al (2013a) Long-term prognosis of aphasia after stroke. J Neurol Neurosurg Psychiatry 84(3):310–315

El Hachioui H, Lingsma HF, Van De Sandt-Koenderman ME et al (2013b) Recovery of aphasia after stroke: a 1-year follow-up study. J Neurol 260(1):166–171

Ellis C, Urban S (2016) Age and aphasia: a review of presence, type, recovery, and clinical outcomes. Top Stroke Rehabil 23(6):430–439

Elman R (ed) (2006) Group treatment of neurogenic communication disorders. Plural Publishing Inc., San Diego

Elman R (2018) Social and life participation approaches to aphasia intervention. In: LaPointe L (ed) Aphasia and related neurogenic language disorders, 5th edn. Thieme Medical Publishers Inc., New York

Elman RJ, Cohen A, Silverman A (2016) Perceptions of speech-language pathology services provided to persons with aphasia: a caregiver survey. Paper presented at the Clinical Aphasiology Conference, May 2016, Charlottesville, Virginia

Elsner B, Kugler J, Pohl M et al (2019) Transcranial direct current stimulation (tDCS) for improving aphasia in patients after stroke. Cochrane Database Syst Rev (5):CD009760. https://doi.org/10.1002/14651858.CD009760.pub4. Accessed 24 Aug 2021

Elsner B, Kugler J, Mehrholz J (2020) Transcranial direct current stimulation (tDCS) for improving aphasia after stroke: a systematic review with network meta-analysis of randomized controlled trials. J Neuroeng Rehabil 17(1):88. https://doi.org/10.1186/s12984-020-00708-z. Accessed 4 Sep 2021

El-Wahsh S, Monroe P, Kumfor F et al (2021) Communication interventions for people with dementia and their communication partners. In: Low LF, Laver K (eds) Dementia rehabilitation. Evidence-based interventions and clinical recommendations. Academic Press, London, pp 35–56

Enderby P, Broeckx J, Hospers W et al (1994) Effect of piracetam on recovery and rehabilitation after stroke: a double-blind, placebo-controlled study. Clin Neuropharmacol 17(4):320–331

Engelter ST, Gostynski M, Papa S et al (2006) Epidemiology of aphasia attributable to first ischemic stroke: incidence, severity, fluency, etiology, and thrombolysis. Stroke 37(6):1379–1384

Erickson RJ, Goldinger SD, LaPointe LL (1996) Auditory vigilance in aphasic individuals: detecting nonlinguistic stimuli with full or divided attention. Brain Cogn 30(2):244–253

Fedorenko E, Varley R (2016) Language and thought are not the same thing: evidence from neuroimaging and neurological patients. Ann NY Acad Sci 1369(1):132–153

Fedorenko E, Behr MK, Kanwisher N (2011) Functional specificity for high-level linguistic processing in the human brain. Proc Natl Acad Sci U S A 108(39):16428–16433

Ferré P, Ska B, Lajoie C et al (2011) Clinical focus on prosodic, discursive and pragmatic treatment for right hemisphere damaged adults: what's right? Rehabil Res Pract 2011:131280. https://doi.org/10.1155/2011/131820. Accessed 4 Sep 2021

Ferro JM, Mariano G, Madureira S (1999) Recovery from aphasia and neglect. Cerebrovasc Dis 9(Suppl 5):6–22

Field A (2013) Discovering statistics using IBM SPSS statistics. Sage, Thousand Oaks, CA

Field-Fote EC (2015) Exciting recovery: augmenting practice with stimulation to optimize outcomes after spinal cord injury. Progr Brain Res 128:103–126

Fillingham JK, Sage K, Lambon Ralph MA (2006) The treatment of anomia using errorless learning. Neuropsychol Rehabil 16(2):129–154

Fiori V, Nitsche MA, Cucuzza G et al (2019) High-definition transcranial direct current stimulation improves verb recovery in aphasic patients depending on current intensity. Neuroscience 406:159–166

Fodor J (1983) Modularity of mind. MIT Press, Cambridge

Frankl V (1984) Man's search for meaning: an introduction to logotherapy, 3rd edn. Touchstone, New York

Frankl V (1995) Lékařská péče o duši. Základy logoterapie a existenciální analýzy (Medical care for the soul. Basics of logotherapy and existential analysis). Cesta, Brno

Frattali CM, Thompson CM, Holland AL et al (1995) The FACS of life ASHA facs—a functional outcome measure for adults. ASHA 37(4):40–56

Fridriksson J, Nettles C, Davis M et al (2006) Functional communication and executive function in aphasia. Clin Linguist Phon 20(6):401–410

Fridriksson J, Richardson JD, Fillmore P et al (2012) Left hemisphere plasticity and aphasia recovery. NeuroImage 60(2):854–863

Fridriksson J, Elm J, Stark BC, Basilakos A, Rorden C, Sen S, George MS, Gottfried M, Bonilha L (2018) Bdnf genotype and tDCS interaction in aphasia treatment. Brain Stimul 11(6):1276–1281. https://doi.org/10.1016/j.brs.2018.08.009

Friederici AD, Gierhan SME (2013) The language network. Curr Opin Neurobiol 23(2):250–254

Fucetola R, Connor LT, Strube MJ et al (2009) Unravelling nonverbal cognitive performance in acquired aphasia. Aphasiology 23(12):1418–1426

Garrett KL, Beukelman DR (2006) Aphasia needs assessment. https://cehs.unl.edu/documents/secd/aac/assessment/aphasianeeds.pdf. Accessed 16 Jun 2021

Garrett KL, Lasker JP (2005a) AAC aphasia categories of communicators checklist. https://cehs.unl.edu/documents/secd/aac/assessment/aphasiachecklist.pdf. Accessed 16 Jun 2021

Garrett KL, Lasker JP (2005b) The multimodal communication screening task for persons with aphasia (MCST-A). https://cehs.unl.edu/documents/secd/aac/assessment/score.pdf. Accessed 16 Jun 2021

Garrett KL, Lasker JP (2013) Adults with severe aphasia and apraxia of speech. In: Beukelman DR, Mirenda P (eds) Augmentative and alternative communication: supporting children and adults with complex communication needs. Brookes Publishing, Baltimore, pp 405–445

Gathercole SE, Baddeley A (1993) Working memory and language. Lawrence Erlbaum, Hove

Geranmayeh F, Wise RJS, Mehta A et al (2014) Overlapping networks engaged during spoken language production and its cognitive control. J Neurosci 34(26):8728–8740

Geranmayeh F, Leech R, Wise RJS (2016) Network dysfunction predicts speech production after left hemisphere stroke. Neurology 86(14):1296–1305

Geranmayeh F, Chau TW, Wise RJS et al (2017) Domain-general subregions of the medial prefrontal cortex contribute to recovery of language after stroke. Brain 140(7):1947–1958

Godecke E, Ciccone NA, Granger AS et al (2014) A comparison of aphasia therapy outcomes before and after a very early rehabilitation programme following stroke. Int J Lang Commun Disord 49(2):149–161

Godecke E, Armstrong E, Rai T, et al on behalf of the VERSE Collaborative Group (2020) A randomized control trial of intensive aphasia therapy after acute stroke: the Very Early Rehabilitation for SpEech (VERSE) study. Int J Stroke 16(5):556–572

Goldenberg G, Spatt J (1994) Influence of size and site of cerebral lesions on spontaneous recovery of aphasia and on success of language therapy. Brain Lang 47:684–698

Graber AV (2004) Viktor Frankl's logotherapy: meaning-centered counseling. Wyndham Hall Press, Lima

Grant DA, Berg EA (1993) Wisconsin card sorting test. Psychological Assessment Resources, Tampa

Gravell R (1988) Communication problems in elderly people. Chapman and Hall, London

Grechuta K, Ballester BB, Munne RE et al (2019) Augmented dyadic therapy boosts recovery of language function in patients with nonfluent aphasia. A randomized study. Stroke 50:1270–1274

Greener J, Enderby P, Whurr R (2001) Pharmacological treatment for aphasia following stroke (Review). Cochrane Database Syst Rev 2001(4):CD000424

Greenwell T, Walsh B (2021) Evidence-based practice in speech-language pathology: where are we now? Am J Speech Lang Pathol. 30(1):186–198. https://doi.org/10.1044/2020_AJSLP-20-00194. Epub 2021 Jan 21. PMID: 33476190; PMCID: PMC8758319

Grocke D, Wigram T (2006) Receptive methods in music therapy. Jessica Kingsley Publishers, London

Grönberg A, Henriksson I, Lindgren A (2021) Accuracy of NIH Stroke Scale for diagnosing aphasia. Acta Neurol Scand 143:375–382

Grossman AW, Churchill JD, Bates KE et al (2002) A brain adaptation view of plasticity: is synaptic plasticity an overly limited concept? Prog Brain Res 138:91–108

Guyomard V, Fulcher RA, Redmayne O et al (2009) Effect of dysphasia and dysphagia on inpatient mortality and hospital length of stay: a database study. J Am Geriatr Soc 57(11):21011–22106

Ham T, Leff A, de Boissezon X et al (2013) Cognitive control and the salience network: an investigation of error processing and effective connectivity. J Neurosci 33(16):7091–7098

Hamilton RH, Chrysikou EG, Coslett B (2011) Mechanisms of aphasia recovery after stroke and the role of noninvasive brain stimulation. Brain Lang 118(1–2):40–50

Hanlon RE, Lux WE, Dromerick AW (1999) Global aphasia without hemiparesis: language profiles and lesion distribution. J Neurol Neurosurg Psychiatry 66(3):365–369

Hanne S, Stadie N (2019) Therapie lexikalischer und semantischer Störungen (Therapy of lexical and semantic dysfunctions). In: Stadie N et al (eds) Lexikalische und semantische Störungen bei Aphasie (Lexicon and semantic dysfunctions in aphasia). Georg Thieme Verlag, Stuttgart

Haring R, Siegmüller J (2018) Evidenzbasierte Praxis in den Gesundheitsberufen (Evidence-based practice in health professions). Springer, Berlin

Hartwigsen G, Saur D (2019) Neuroimaging of stroke recovery from aphasia—insights into plasticity of the human language network. NeuroImage 190:14–31

Hartwigsen G, Volz LJ (2021) Probing rapid network reorganization of motor and language functions via neuromodulation and neuroimaging. NeuroImage 224:117449. https://doi.org/10.1016/j.neuroimage.2020.117449. Accessed 24 Aug 2021

Harvey S, Carragher M, Dickey MW et al (2020) Dose effects in behavioural treatment of post-stroke aphasia: a systematic review and meta-analysis. Disabil Rehabil 44(12):2548–2559. https://doi.org/10.1080/09638288.2020.1843079. Accessed 4 Sep 2021

Hauk O, Johnsrude I, Pulvermüller F (2004) Somatotopic representation of action words in human motor and premotor cortex. Neuron 41(2):301–307

Heiss WD, Thiel A (2006) A proposed regional hierarchy in recovery of post-stroke aphasia. Brain Lang 98(1):118–123

Herbert R, Gregory E, Best W (2014) Syntactic versus lexical therapy for anomia in acquired aphasia: differential effects on narrative and conversation. Int J Lang Commun Disord 49:162–173

Hersh D, Worrall L, Howle T et al (2012) SMARTER goal setting in aphasia rehabilitation. Aphasiology 26(2):220–233

Higgs J, Jones MA, Loftus S et al (eds) (2008) Clinical reasoning in the health profession. Elsevier Health Sciences, Amsterdam

Hilari K, Cruice M, Sorin-Peters R et al (2015) Quality of life in aphasia: state of the art. Folia Phoniatr Logop 67(3):114–118

Hilari K, Galante L, Huck A et al (2018) Cultural adaptation and psychometric testing of the Scenario Test UK for people with aphasia. Int J Lang Commun Disord 53(4):748–760

Hillis AE, Wityk RJ, Barker PB et al (2002) Subcortical aphasia and neglect in acute stroke: the role of cortical hypoperfusion. Brain 125(5):1094–1104

Hojo K, Watanabe S, Tasakin H et al (1985) Localization of lesions in aphasia—clinical-CT scan correlations (Part III): paraphasia and meaningless speech (Article in Japanese). No to shinkei [Brain and nerve] 37(2):117–126

Holland A, Fromm D, Forbes M et al (2017) Long-term recovery in stroke accompanied by aphasia: a reconsideration. Aphasiology 32(2):152–165

Hope TMH, Leff AP, Price CJ (2018) Predicting language outcomes after stroke: is structural disconnection a useful predictor? Neuroimage Clin 19:22–29

Hopper T, Holland A (2005) Aphasia and learning in adults: key concepts and clinical considerations. Top Geriatr Rehabil 21(4):315–322

Huber W, Wilmes K, Poek K et al (1997) Piracetam as an adjuvant to language therapy for aphasia: a randomized double-blind placebo controlled pilot study. Arch Phys Med Rehabil 78(3):245–250

Hurford R, Sekhar A, Hughes TAT et al (2020) Diagnosis and management of acute ischemic stroke. Pract Neurol 20:306–318

Husak RS, Wallace SE, Marshall RC, Visch-Brink EG (2023) A systematic review of aphasia therapy provided in the early period of post-stroke recovery. Aphasiology, 37(1):143–176. https://doi.org/10.1080/02687038.2021.1987381

Ibbotson P (2020) What it takes to talk: exploring developmental cognitive linguistics. De Gruyter Mouton, Boston

ICF (2001) World Health Organization international classification of functioning, disability and health. WHO, Geneva

Jia XY, Huang M, Zou Y-F et al (2016) Predictors of poor outcomes in first-event ischemic stroke as assessed by magnetic resonance imaging. Clin Invest Med 39(3):E95–E104

Johnson RK (2017) Motor learning guided treatment for acquired apraxia of speech. Speech Lang Hear 21(4):202–212

Johnson RK, Hough MS, King KA et al (2008) Functional communication in individuals with chronic severe aphasia using augmentative communication. Augment Altern Commun 24(4):269–280

Jung IY, Lim JY, Kang EK et al (2011) The factors associated with good responses to speech therapy combined with transcranial direct current stimulation in post-stroke aphasic patients. Ann Rehabil Med 35(4):460–469

Just M, Carpenter P (1992) A capacity theory of comprehension: individual differences in working memory. Psychol Rev 99(1):122–149

Kagan A, Black SE, Duchan FJ et al (2001) Training volunteers as conversation partners using "Supported conversation for adults with aphasia" (SCA): a controlled trial. J Speech Lang Hear Res 44:624–638

Kagan A, Winckel J, Black S et al (2004) A set of observational measures for rating support and participation in conversation between adults with aphasia and their conversation partners. Top Stroke Rehabil 11(1):67–83

Kagan A, Simmons-Mackie N, Rowland A et al (2008) Counting what counts: a framework for capturing real-life outcomes of aphasia intervention. Aphasiology 22:258–280

Kang EK, Sohn HM, Han M-K et al (2010) Severity of post-stroke aphasia according to aphasia type and lesion location in Koreans. J Korean Med Sci 25(1):123–127

Kast V (1999) Imaginace jako prostor setkání s nevědomím (Imagination as a meeting place with the unconscious). Portál, Prague

Kast V (2012) Imagination: Zugänge zu inneren Ressourcen finden (Imagination: find access to internal resources). Patmos-Verlag, Einbeck

Keil K, Kaszniak AW (2002) Examining executive function in individuals with brain injury: a review. Aphasiology 16(3):305–335

Kendall DL, McNeill MR, Small SL (1998) Rule-based treatment for acquired phonological dyslexia. Aphasiology 12(7–8):587–600

Kendrick LT, Robson H, Meteyard L (2019) Executive control in frontal lesion aphasia: does verbal load matter? Neuropsychologia 133:107178. https://doi.org/10.1016/j.neuropsychologia.2019.107178. Accessed 26 Aug 2021

Kertesz A (1985) Aphasia. In: Fredriks JAM (ed) Handbook of clinical neurology, vol 45: clinical neuropsychology. Elsevier, Amsterdam, pp 298–331

Khatri P, Kleindorfer DO, Yeatts SD et al (2010) Strokes with minor symptoms. An exploratory analysis of the National Institute of Neurological Disorders and stroke recombinant tissue plasminogen activator trials. Stroke 41:2581–2586

Kielar A, Patterson D, Chou Y (2022) Efficacy of repetitive transcranial magnetic stimulation in treating stroke aphasia: systematic review and meta-analysis. Clin Neurophysiol 140:196–227. https://doi.org/10.1016/j.clinph.2022.04.017

Kim KA, Lee JS, Chang WH et al (2019) Changes in language function and recovery-related prognostic factors in first-ever left hemispheric ischemic stroke. Ann Rehabil Med 43(6):625–634

Kiran S, Thompson CK (2019) Neuroplasticity of language networks in aphasia: advances, updates, and future challenges. Front Neurol 10:295. https://doi.org/10.3389/fneur.2019.00295. Accessed 27 Aug 2021

Kleim JA, Jones TA (2008) Principles of experience-dependent neural plasticity: implications for rehabilitation after brain damage. J Speech Lang Hearing Res 51(1):225–239

Knopman DS, Selnes OA, Niccum N et al (1983) A longitudinal study of speech fluency in aphasia: CT correlates of recovery and persistent nonfluency. Neurology 33(9):1170–1178

Koul RK, Corwin M (2011) Augmentative and alternative communication intervention for persons with chronic severe aphasia: bringing research to practice. EBP Briefs 6(2):1–8

Krakauer JW, Carmichael ST, Corbett D et al (2012) Getting neurorehabilitation right: what can be learned from animal models? Neurorehabil Neural Repair 26(3):923–931

Kratochvíl S (1978) Skupinová psychoterapie neuros (Group psychotherapy). Avicenum, Prague

Kratochvíl S (2005) Skupinová psychoterapie v praxi (Group psychotherapy in practice). Galén, Prague

Lahiri D, Dubey S, Ardila A (2020) Determinants of aphasia recovery: exploratory decision tree analysis. Lang Cogn Neurosci 36(1):25–32. https://doi.org/10.1080/23273798.2020.1777314. Accessed 27 Aug 2020

LaPointe LL (2003) Functional and pragmatic directions in aphasia therapy. In: Papathanasiou I, De Bleser R (eds) The science of aphasia: from therapy to theory. Pergamon, Amsterdam, pp 163–172

Laska AC, Hellblom A, Murray V et al (2001) Aphasia in acute stroke and relation to outcome. J Intern Med 249(5):413–422

Law MC, MacDermid J (eds) (2008) Evidence-based rehabilitation: a guide to practice. Slack Incorporated, Thorofare

Law M, MacDermid, J (2024) Evidence-based rehabilitation: A guide to practice. Taylor & Francis, London, United Kingdom

Lazar RM, Speizer AE, Festa JR et al (2008) Variability in language recovery after first-time stroke. J Neurol Neurosurg Psychiatry 79(5):530–534

Lendrem W, Lincoln NB (1985) Spontaneous recovery of language in patients with aphasia between 4 and 34 weeks after stroke. J Neurol Neurosurg Psychiatry 48(8):743–748

Leonard C, Rochon E, Laird L (2008) Treating naming impairments in aphasia: findings from a phonological components analysis treatment. Aphasiology 22:923–947

Lesser R (2003) Conversation analysis and aphasia therapy. In: Papathanasiou I, De Bleser R (eds) The science of aphasia: from therapy to theory. Pergamon, Amsterdam, pp 173–185

Levenson H (2017) Brief dynamic therapy. American Psychological Association, Washington, DC

Lichtheim L (1885) On aphasia. Brain 7:433–484

Liepert J (2008) Pharmacotherapy in restorative neurology. Curr Opin Neurol 21(6):639–643

Lindell AK (2006) In your right mind: right hemisphere contributions to language processing and production. Neuropsychol Rev 16:131–148

Little B, Gallagher P, Zimmerer V et al (2019) Language in schizophrenia and aphasia: the relationship with non-verbal cognition and thought disorder. Cogn Neuropsychiatry 24(6):389–405

Llano DA, Small SL (2016) Pharmacotherapy for aphasia. In: Hickok G, Small SL (eds) Neurobiology of language. Academic Press/Elsevier, Amsterdam, pp 1067–1083

Lock S, Wilkinson R, Bryan K et al (2001) Supporting partners of people with aphasia in relationships and conversation (SPPARC). Int J Lang Commun Disord 36(Suppl):25–30

Lubinski R (1995) Dementia and communication. B. C. Decker, Philadelphia

Luria AR (1970) Traumatic aphasia. Mouton, Haag

Luzatti C, Colombo C, Frustaci M et al (2000) Rehabilitation of spelling along the sub-word level routine. Neuropsychol Rehabil 10(3):249–278

Luzzatti C, Aggujaro S, Crepaldi D (2006) Verb-noun dissociation in aphasia: theoretical and neuroanatomical foundations. Cortex 42:875–883

Luzzatti C, Molinari AL, Zanobio ME et al (2015) Phonological rehabilitation in acquired aphasia. Front Psychol. In: Conference abstract: academy of aphasia 53rd annual meeting. https://doi.org/10.3389/conf.fpsyg.2015.65.00036. Accessed 4 Sep 2021

Maas MB, Lev MH, Ay H et al (2012) The prognosis for aphasia in stroke. J Stroke Cerebrovasc Dis 21(5):350–357

MacDonald S (2017) Introducing the model of cognitive-communication competence: a model to guide evidence-based communication interventions after brain injury. Brain Inj 31:1760–1780

MacDonald S (2021) The cognitive-communication checklist for acquired brain injury: a means of identifying, recording, and tracking communication impairments. Am J Speech Lang Pathol 30:1074–1089

Madden EB, Torrence J, Kendall DL (2020) Cross-modal generalization of anomia treatment to reading in aphasia. Aphasiology 35:875. https://doi.org/10.1080/0268 7038.2020.1734529. Accessed 24 Aug 2021

Marangolo P (2020) The potential effects of transcranial direct current stimulation (tDCS) on language functioning: combining neuromodulation and behavioral intervention in aphasia. Neurosci Lett 719:133329. https://doi.org/10.1016/j.neulet.2017.12.057. Accessed 4 Sep 2021

Marcotte K, Adrover-Roig D, Damien B et al (2012) Therapy-induced neuroplasticity in chronic aphasia. Neuropsychologia 50(8):1776–1786

Marebwa BK, Fridricsson J, Yougovan G et al (2017) Chronic post-stroke aphasia severity is determined by fragmentation of residual white matter networks. Sci Rep 7(1):8188. https://doi.org/10.1038/s41598-017-07607-9. Accessed 27 Aug 2021

Maresca G, Maggio MG, Latella D et al (2019) Toward improving poststroke aphasia: a pilot study on the growing use of telerehabilitation for the continuity of care. J Stroke Cerebrovasc Dis 28(10):104303. https://doi.org/10.1016/j.strokecerebrovasculardis.2019.104303. Accessed 4 Sep 2021

Martin N, Thompson CK, Worrall L (2008) Aphasia rehabilitation. The impairment and its consequences. Plural Publishing, San Diego

Martins IP, Leal G, Fonseca I et al (2013) A randomized, rater-blinded, parallel trial of intensive speech therapy in sub-acute post-stroke aphasia: the SP-I-R-IT study. Int J Lang Commun Disord 48(4):421–431

Mayer JF, Mitchinson SI, Murray LL (2017) Addressing concomitant executive dysfunction and aphasia: previous approaches and the new brain budget protocol. Aphasiology 31(7):837–860

Mayo NE, Korner-Bitensky NA, Becker R (1991) Recovery time of independent function post-stroke. Am J Phys Med Rehabil 70(1):5–12

Medina J, Norise C, Faseyitan O et al (2012) Finding the right words: transcranial magnetic stimulation improves discourse productivity in non-fluent aphasia after stroke. Aphasiology 26(9):1153–1168

Meinzer M, Rodriguez AD, Rothi LJ (2012) First decade of research on constrained-induced treatment approaches for aphasia rehabilitation. Arch Phys Med Rehabil 93:35–45

Meinzer M, Darkow R, Lindenberg R et al (2016) Electrical stimulation of the motor cortex enhances treatment outcome in post-stroke aphasia. Brain 139(4):1152–1163

Menichelli A, Furlanis G, Sartori A et al (2019) Thrombolysis' benefits on early post-stroke language recovery in aphasia patients. J Clin Neurosci 70:92–95

Menon V, Uddin LQ (2010) Saliency, switching, attention and control: a network model of insula function. Brain Struct Funct 214(5–6):655–667

Miller G (1956) The magical number seven, plus or minus two: some limits on our capacity for processing information. Psychol Rev 63(2):81–97

Mitchell C, Gittins M, Tyson S et al (2020) Prevalence of aphasia and dysarthria among inpatient stroke survivors: describing the population, therapy provision and outcomes on discharge. Aphasiology 32(Suppl1):145–146

Mohr B, Stahl B, Berthier ML et al (2017) Intensive communicative therapy reduces symptoms of depression in chronic nonfluent aphasia. Neurorehabil Neural Repair 31:1053–1062

Monnelly K, Marshall J, Dipper L, Cruice M (2023) Intensive and comprehensive aphasia therapy—a survey of the definitions, practices and views of speech and language therapists in the United Kingdom. International Journal of Language & Communication Disorders, 58(6):2077–2102

Moulton E, Magno S, Valabregue R et al (2019) Acute diffusivity biomarkers for prediction of motor and language outcome in mild-to-severe stroke patients. Stroke 50(8):2050–2056

Murray LL, Keeton RJ, Karcher L (2006) Treating attention in mild aphasia: evaluation of attention process training-II. J Commun Disord 39(1):37–61

Nadeau S, Rothi L, Crosson B (eds) (2000) Aphasia and language. Theory and practice. The Guilford Press, New York

Nakagawa Y, Sano Y, Funayama M et al (2019) Prognostic factors for long-term improvement from stroke-related aphasia with adequate linguistic rehabilitation. Neurol Sci 40(10):2141–2146

Nakamura R, Asami T, Yoshimi A et al (2020) Illness management and recovery program induced neuroprotective effects on language network in schizophrenia. Schizophr Res 230:101–103

National Stroke Foundation (2010) Clinical guidelines for acute stroke management. National Stroke Foundation, Melbourne

Nerantzini M, Savoulidou D, Stavrakaki S et al (2020) Transcranial magnetic stimulation in aphasia rehabilitation. In: Argyropoulos G (ed) Translational neuroscience of speech and language disorders. Contemporary clinical neuroscience. Springer, Cham

Nesi M, Lucente G, Nencini P et al (2014) Aphasia predicts unfavorable outcome in mild ischemic stroke patients and prompts thrombolytic treatment. J Stroke Cerebrovasc Dis 23:204–208

Neubauer K (2007) Terapeutická pomoc osobám se ZNPŘK (Therapeutic assistance to persons with physical disabilities). In: Neubauer K et al (eds) Neurogenní poruchy komunikace u dospělých. (diagnostika a terapie) (Neurogenic communication disorders in adults (diagnostics and therapy)). Portál, Prague, pp 117–174

Neubauer K (2014) Získané neurogenní poruchy řečové komunikace (ZNPŘK) (Acquired neurogenic disorders of speech communication). In: Neubauer K, Dobias S (eds) Neurogenně podmíněné poruchy řečové komunikace a dysfagie (Neurogenic disorders of speech communication and dysphagia). Gaudeamus, Hradec Kralove, pp 9–205

Neubauer K (2016) Speech-language therapy and neurogenic disorders of communication. P. Mervart a PdF Univerzity of Hradec Králové, Červený Kostelec

Neubauer K (2017) Assessment and treatment of adult persons with acquired disorders of communication and neurogenic dysphagia. Internationale Stiftung Schulung, Kunst

Neubauer K (2018) Vývojové hledisko a psychoterapeutický přístup v klinické praxi. (Developmental point of view and psychotherapeutic approach in clinical practice). In: Neubauer K et al (eds) Kompendium klinické logopedie (Compendium of clinical speech therapy). Portál, Prague, pp 87–94

Neves C, Catrini M (2017) O olhar clínico sobre os fatores prognósticos das afasias (The clinical view on the prognostic factors of aphasia). Distúrbios da Comunicação 29(2):208–217

New B, Ferrand L, Pallier C et al (2006) Reexamining the word length effect in visual word recognition: new evidence from the English Lexicon Project. Psychon Bull Rev 13(1):45–52

Nicholas M, Sinotte M, Helm-Estabrooks N (2005) Using a computer to communicate: effect of executive function impairments in people with severe aphasia. Aphasiology 19(10–11):1052–1065

Nickels L, Best W, Biedermann R et al (2002) Therapy for naming disorders: revisiting, revising, and reviewing. Aphasiology 16(10–11):935–979

Nieto-Sampedro M, Nieto-Diaz M (2005) Neural plasticity: changes with age. J Neural Transm 112:3–27

Nilsson L-G (2003) Memory function in normal aging. Acta Neurol Scand 107(Suppl 179):7–13

Nobis-Bosch R, Rubi-Fessen I, Biniek R et al (2013) Diagnostik und Therapie der akuten Aphasie (Assessment and therapy of aphasia in the acute phase). Georg Thieme Verlag, Stuttgart

Norise C, Hamilton RH (2017) Non-invasive brain stimulation in the treatment of post-stroke and neurodegenerative aphasia: parallels, differences, and lessons learned. Front Hum Neurosci 10:675. https://doi.org/10.3389/fnhum.2016.00675. Accessed 31 Aug 2021

Nouwens F, de Lau LM, Visch-Brink EG et al (2017) Efficacy of early cognitive-linguistic treatment for aphasia due to stroke: a randomized controlled trial (Rotterdam Aphasia Therapy Study-3). Eur Stroke J 2:126–136

Oleson JJ, Brown GD, McCreery R (2019) The evolution of statistical methods in speech, language, and hearing sciences. J Speech Lang Hear Res 62(3):498–506

Olness GS, Ulatowska HK (2017) Aphasias. In: Cummings L (ed) Research in clinical pragmatics. Springer International Publishing, New York

Osa García A, Brambati SM, Brisebois A et al (2020) Predicting early post-stroke aphasia outcome from initial aphasia severity. Front Neurol 11:120. https://doi.org/10.3389/fneur.2020.00120. Accessed 27 Aug 2021

Papathanasiou I, Coppens P, Durand E et al (2017) Plasticity and recovery in aphasia. In: Papathanasiou I, Coppens P (eds) Aphasia and related neurogenic communication disorders. Jones & Bartlett Learning, Burlington, pp 109–127

Park DC (1999) The basic mechanisms accounting for age related decline in cognitive function. In: Park DC, Schwarz N (eds) Cognitive aging: a primer. Psychology Press, New York, pp 3–21

Park DC, Smith AD, Lautenschlager G et al (1996) Mediators of long-term memory performance across the age span. Psychol Aging 11(4):621–637

Park DC, Lautenschlager G, Hedden T et al (2002) Models of visuospatial and verbal memory across the adult life span. Psychol Aging 17(2):299–320

Pawełczyk A, Łojek E, Żurner N et al (2018) High-order language dysfunctions as a possible neurolinguistic endophenotype for schizophrenia: evidence from patients and their unaffected first degree relatives. Psychiatry Res 267:63–72

Pedersen PM, Jørgensen HS, Nakayama H et al (1995) Aphasia in acute stroke: incidence, determinants, and recovery. Ann Neurol 38(4):659–666

Pedersen PM, Vinter K, Olsen TS (2004) Aphasia after stroke: type, severity and prognosis: the Copenhagen aphasia study. Cerebrovasc Dis 17(1):35–43

Pešek R, Praško J, Štípek P (2012) Kognitivně behaviorální terapie v praxi (Cognitive behavioural therapy in practice). Portál, Prague

Pickersgill MJ, Lincoln NB (1983) Prognostic indicators and the pattern of recovery of communication in aphasic stroke patients. J Neurol Neurosurg 46(2):130–139

Plowman E, Hentz B, Ellis C (2011) Post-stroke aphasia prognosis: a review of patient-related and stroke-related factors. J Eval Clin Pract 18(3):689–694

Poeppel D (2014) The neuroanatomic and neurophysiological infrastructure for speech and language. Curr Opin Neurobiol 28:142–149

Praško J, Grambal A, Šlepecký M et al (2019) Skupinová kognitivně-behaviorální terapie (Group cognitive-behavioral therapy). Grada Publishing, Prague

Price CJ (2010) The anatomy of language: a review of 100 fMRI studies published in 2009. Ann N Y Acad Sci U S A 1191:62–88

Pulvermüller F, Neininger B, Elbert T et al (2001) Constraint-induced therapy of chronic aphasia after stroke. Stroke 32:1621–1626

Purdy M (2002) Executive function ability in persons with aphasia. Aphasiology 16(4–6):549–557

Purdy M, Coppens P, Brookshire Madden E et al (2019) Reading comprehension treatment in aphasia: a systematic review. Aphasiology 33:625–691

Raymer AM, Gonzalez Rothi LJ (2018) Principles of aphasia rehabilitation. In: Raymer AM, Gonzalez Rothi AJ (eds) The Oxford handbook of aphasia and language disorders. Oxford University Press, New York, pp 309–326

Renvall K, Nickels L, Davidson B (2013a) Functionally relevant items in the treatment of aphasia (part I): challenges for current practice. Aphasiology 27(6):636–650

Renvall K, Nickels L, Davidson B (2013b) Functionally relevant items in the treatment of aphasia (part II): further perspectives and specific tools. Aphasiology 27(6):651–677

Repetto C, Paolillo MP, Tuena C et al (2020) Innovative technology-based interventions in aphasia rehabilitation: a systematic review. Aphasiology 35:1623. https://doi.org/10.1080/02687038.2020.1819957. Accessed 4 Sep 2021

Reynolds S (2000) The anatomy of evidence-base practice: principles and methods. In: Trinder L, Reynolds S (eds) Evidence-based practice: a critical appraisal. Blackwell Science Ltd, Oxford

Richardson J, Datta A, Dmochowski J et al (2015) Feasibility of using high-definition transcranial direct current stimulation (HD-tDCS) to enhance treatment outcomes in persons with aphasia. NeuroRehabilitation 36(1):115–126

Robbins J, Butler SG, Daniels S et al (2007) Neural plasticity, swallowing and dysphagia rehabilitation: translating principles of neural plasticity into clinically oriented evidence. J Speech Lang Hear Res 50(1):276–300

Rochon E, Laird L, Bose A et al (2005) Mapping therapy for sentence production impairments in nonfluent aphasia. Neuropsychol Rehabil 15(1):1–36

Rogers C (2007) Counseling and psychotherapy. Rogers Press, Cambridge

Rogers MA, Roye F, Mullen R (2014) Measuring outcomes in aphasia and apraxia of speech in the context of a learning health care system. In: 44th clinical aphasiology conference, St. Simons Island, GA

Romski M, Sevcik RA (2005) Augmentative communication and early intervention. Myths and realities. Infants Young Child 18(3):174–185

Rose ML, Nickels L, Copland D et al (2022) Results of the COMPARE trial of Constraint-induced or Multimodality Aphasia Therapy compared with usual care in chronic post-stroke aphasia. Journal of Neurology, Neurosurgery & Psychiatry, 93(6):573–581. https://doi.org/10.1136/jnnp-2021-328422

Rossi S, Antal A, Bestmann S et al (2021) Safety and recommendations for TMS use in healthy subjects and patient populations, with updates on training, ethical and regulatory issues: expert guidelines. Clin Neurophysiol 132(1):269–306

Roth FP, Worthington CK (2019) Treatment resource manual for speech-language pathology. Plural Publishing Inc., New York

Rubi-Fessen I, Hartmann A, Huber W et al (2015) Add-on effects of repetitive transcranial magnetic stimulation on subacute aphasia therapy: enhanced improvement of functional communication and basic linguistic skills. A randomized controlled study. Arch Phys Med Rehabil 96(11):1935–1944

Rubi-Fessen I, Gerbershagen K, Stenneken P, Willmes K (2024) Early boost of linguistic skills? individualized non-invasive brain stimulation in early post-acute aphasia. Brain Sciences, 14(8):789. https://doi.org/10.3390/brainsci14080789

Russo MJ, Prodan V, Meda NN et al (2017) High-technology augmentative communication for adults with post-stroke aphasia: a systematic review. Expert Rev Med Devices 14(5):355–370

Sabe L, Salvarezza F, Cuerva G et al (1995) A randomized, double-blind, placebo-controlled study of bromocriptine in nonfluent aphasia. Neurology 45(12):2272–2274

Sablot D, Belahsen F, Vuiller F et al (2011) Predicting acute ischaemic stroke outcome using clinical and temporal thresholds. ISRN Neurol 2011:354642. https://doi.org/10.5402/2011/354642. Accessed 27 Aug 2021

Sackett DL (1997) Evidence-based medicine. Semin Perinatol 21(1):3–5

Saif S, Fazal N (2014) Association between NIH Stroke Scale score and functional outcome in acute ischemic stroke. Forces Med J 64(4):585–590

Salat DH (2011) The declining infrastructure of the aging brain. Brain Connect 1(4):279–293

Salis C, Hwang F, Howard D et al (2017) Short-term and working memory treatments for improving sentence comprehension in aphasia: a review and a replication study. Semin Speech Lang 38(1):29–39

Sapir S, Ramig LO, Fox CM (2011) Intensive voice treatment in Parkinson's disease: Lee Silverman Voice Treatment. Expert Rev Neurother 11(6):815–830

Särkämö T, Tervaniemi M, Laitinen S et al (2008) Music listening enhances cognitive recovery and mood after middle cerebral artery stroke. Brain 131:866–876

Sarno MT, Buonaguro A, Levita E (1985) Gender and recovery from aphasia after stroke. J Nerv Ment Dis 173(10):605–608

Saur D, Lange R, Baumgaertner A et al (2006) Dynamics of language reorganization after stroke. Brain 129(6):1371–1384

Saur D, Kreher BW, Schnell S et al (2008) Ventral and dorsal pathways for language. Proc Natl Acad Sci U S A 105(46):18035–18040

Schell BAB, Schell JW (eds) (2008) Clinical and professional reasoning in occupational therapy. Lippincott Williams & Wilkins, Philadelphia

Schlaug G, Marchina S, Norton A (2009) Evidence for plasticity in white matter tracts of chronic aphasic patients undergoing intense intonation-based speech therapy. Ann N Y Acad Sci 1169(1):385–394

Schulte MC (2020) Evidence-based medicine—a paradigm ready to be challenged? How scientific evidence shapes our understanding and use of medicine. Springer, Berlin

Schwartz MF, Saffran EM, Fink RB et al (1994) Mapping therapy: a treatment programme for agrammatism. Aphasiology 8:19–54

Seniów J, Waldowski K, Leśniak M et al (2013) Transcranial magnetic stimulation combined with speech and language training in early aphasia rehabilitation: a randomized double-blind controlled pilot study. Top Stroke Rehabil 20(3):250–261

Shallice T (1988) From neuropsychology to mental structure. Cambridge University Press, Cambridge

Sharma S, Briley PM, Wright HH et al (2019) Gender differences in aphasia outcomes: evidence from the AphasiaBank. Int J Lang Commun Disord 54(5):806–813

Shea J, Wiley R, Moss N et al (2020) Pseudoword spelling ability predicts response to word spelling treatment in acquired dysgraphia. Neuropsychol Rehabil 32:231. https://doi.org/10.1080/09602011.2020.1813596. Accessed 24 Aug 2021

Shewan C, Bandur D (1991) Treatment of aphasia: language-oriented approach. Pro Ed, Austin

Sihvonen AJ, Särkämö T, Leo V et al (2017) Music-based interventions in neurological rehabilitation. Lancet Neurol 16:648–660

Simic T, Rochon E, Greco E et al (2019) Baseline executive control ability and its relationship to language therapy improvements in post-stroke aphasia: a systematic review. Neuropsychol Rehabil 29(3):395–439

Simmons-Mackie N, Damico JS (2007) Access and social inclusion in aphasia: interactional principles and applications. Aphasiology 21:81–97

Simmons-Mackie N, Savage MC, Worrall L (2014) Conversation therapy for aphasia: a qualitative review of the literature. Int J Commun Disord 49:511–526

Simmons-Mackie N, Raymer A, Cherney LR (2016) Communication partner training in aphasia: a systematic review. Arch Phys Med Rehabil 97:2202–2221

Simmons-Mackie N, Worrall L, Murray LL et al (2017) The top ten: best practice recommendations for aphasia. Aphasiology 31(2):131–151

Sloane KL, Hamilton RH (2024) Transcranial direct current stimulation to ameliorate post-stroke cognitive impairment. Brain Sciences, 14(6). https://doi.org/10.3390/brainsci14060614

Snodgrass JG, Vanderwart M (1980) A standardized set of 260 pictures: norms for name agreement, image agreement, familiarity, and visual complexity. J Exp Psychol Hum Learn 6(2):174–215

Spielmann K, van de Sandt-Koenderman WME, Heijenbrok-Kal MH et al (2018) Transcranial direct current stimulation does not improve language outcome in subacute poststroke aphasia. Stroke 49(4):1018–1020

Spitzer L, Binkofski F, Willmes K et al (2020) The novel cognitive flexibility in aphasia therapy (CFAT): a combined treatment of aphasia and executive functions to improve communicative success. Int J Speech Lang Pathol 23(2):168–179

Springer L (2008) Therapeutic approaches in aphasia therapy. In: Stemmer B, Whitacker H (eds) Handbook of the neuroscience of language. Elsevier, London, pp 397–406

Stadie N, Schröder A (2009) Kognitivorientierte Sprachtherapie: Methoden, Material und Evaluation für Aphasie, Dyslexie und Dysgraphie (Cognitive-

orientated speech and language therapy: methods, materials and evaluation for aphasia, dyslexia and dysgraphy). Urban Fischer Verlag, München

Stagg CJ, Antal A, Nitsche MA (2018) Physiology of transcranial direct current stimulation. J ECT 34(3):144–152

Stahl B, Mohr B, Büscher V et al (2018) Efficacy of intensive aphasia therapy in patients with chronic stroke: a randomized controlled trial. J Neurol Neurosurg Psychiatry 89:586–592

Stockbridge MD, Elm J, Breining BL et al (2023) Transcranial direct-current stimulation in subacute aphasia: a randomized controlled trial. Stroke, 54(4):912–920. https://doi.org/10.1161/STROKEAHA.122.041557

Stockert A, Kümmerer D, Saur D (2016) Insights into early language recovery: from basic principles to practical applications. Aphasiology 30(5):517–541

Stockert A, Wawrzyniak M, Klingbeil J et al (2020) Dynamics of language reorganization after left-temporal and frontal stroke. Brain 143(3):844–861

Stokes SF, Surendran D (2005) Articulatory complexity, ambient frequency, and functional load as predictors of consonant development in children. J Speech Lang Hear Res 48(3):577–591

Stroke Foundation of New Zealand and New Zealand Guidelines Group (2010) New Zealand clinical guidelines for stroke management. Stroke Foundation of New Zealand. https://books.google.de/books?id=kDUS0AEACAAJ

Sul B, Lee KB, Hong BY et al (2019) Association of lesion location with long-term recovery in post-stroke aphasia and language deficits. Front Neurol 10:766. https://doi.org/10.3389/fneur.2019.00776. Accessed 27 Aug 2021

Swan K, Hopper M, Wenke R et al (2018) Speech-language pathologist interventions for communication in moderate-severe dementia: a systematic review. Am Speech Lang Pathol 27:836–852

Szaflarski JP, Allendorfer JB, Banks C et al (2013) Recovered vs not-recovered from poststroke aphasia: the contributions from the dominant and non-dominant hemispheres. Restor Neurol Neurosci 31(4):347–360

Tábuas-Pereira M, Beato-Coelho J, Ribeiro J et al (2020) Single word repetition predicts long-term outcome of aphasia caused by an ischemic stroke. J Stroke Cerebrovasc Dis 29(2):104566. https://doi.org/10.1016/j.jstrokecerebrovasdis.2019.104566. Accessed 27 Aug 2021

Tanaka Y, Miyazaki M, Albert ML (1997) Effects of increased cholinergic activity on naming in aphasia. Lancet 350(9071):116–117

Taub E (2000) Constraint-induced movement therapy and massed practice. Stroke 31(4):986–988

Taub E, Uswatte G, Morris DM (2003) Improved motor recovery after stroke and massive cortical reorganization following constraint-induced movement therapy. Phys Med Rehabil Clin N Am 14(Supp 1):S77–S91

Taylor-Goh S (ed) (2005) Royal College of Speech and Language Therapists Clinical Guidelines.

Routledge, London. ISBN 10: 0863885055 ISBN 13: 9780863885051

Teasell RW, Foley NC, Salter K et al (2003) An evidence-based review of stroke rehabilitation. Top Stroke Rehabil 10:29–58

Teasell R, Mehta S, Pereira S et al (2012) Time to rethink long-term rehabilitation management of stroke patients. Top Stroke Rehabil 19:457–462

Thiel A, Zumbansen A (2016) The pathophysiology of post-stroke aphasia: a network approach. Restor Neurol Neurosci 34(4):507–518

Thompson C (1989) Generalization research in aphasia. In: Prescott T (ed) Clinical aphasiology, vol 18. College Hill Press, Boston, pp 195–222

Thompson C (2005) Social and life participation approaches to aphasia intervention. In: LaPointe L (ed) Aphasia and related neurogenic language disorders. Thieme Medical Publishers Inc., New York

Thompson CK, Shapiro LP (2005) Treating agrammatic aphasia within a linguistic framework. Aphasiology 19(10–11):1021–1036

Thompson CK, Shapiro LP, Ballard KJ et al (1997) Training and generalized production of wh- and NP-movement structures in agrammatic aphasia. J Speech Lang Hear Res 40:228–244

Thompson I, Yastrubetskaya O, Lautenschlager N et al (2010) Assessing speech and communication impairments in cognitive disorders: an innovative development in a memory clinic. Int Psychogeriatr 22:341–345

Tomasello M (2005) Constructing a language: a usage-based theory of language acquisition. Harvard University Press, Cambridge

Tompkins CA, Jackson ST, Schulz R (1990) On prognostic research in adult neurologic disorders. J Speech Hear Res 33(2):398–401

Torres J, Drebing D, Hamilton R (2013) TMS and tDCS in post-stroke aphasia: integrating novel treatment approaches with mechanisms of plasticity. Restor Neurol Neurosci 31(4):501–515

Trapl M, Eckhard R, Bosak P et al (2004) Früherkennung von sprachlichen und sprachassoziierten Störungen nach akutem Schlaganfall (Early recognition of speech and speech-associated disorders after acute stroke). Wien Med Wochenschr 154(23–24):571–576

Trebilcock M, Worrall L, Ryan B et al (2019) Increasing the intensity and comprehensiveness of aphasia services: identification of key factors influencing implementation across six countries. Aphasiology 33:865–887

Tscherpel C, Grefkes C (2020) Funktionserholung nach Schlaganfall und die therapeutische Rolle der nicht-invasiven Hirnstimulation. Klinische Neurophysiologie 51(4):214–223

Turkeltaub PE, Swears MK, D'Mello AM et al (2016) Cerebellar tDCS as a novel treatment for aphasia? Evidence from behavioral and resting-state functional connectivity data in healthy adults. Restor Neurol Neurosci 34(4):491–505

Turkstra LS, Coelhom C, Ylvisaker M (2005) The use of standardized tests for individuals with cognitive-communication disorders. Semin Speech Lang 26:215–222

Vallar G, Cantagallo A, Cappa S et al (2012) La riabilitazione neuropsicologica. Un'analisi basata sul metodo evidence-based medicine. Springer-Verlag, Milan

van der Meulen I, van de Sandt-Koenderman WME, Duivenvoorden HJ et al (2010) Measuring verbal and non-verbal communication in aphasia: reliability, validity, and sensitivity of the Scenario Test. Int J Lang Commun Disord 45(4):424–435

Van Der Meulen I, Van de Sandt-Koenderman WME, Heijenbrok MH et al (2016) Melodic Intonation Therapy in chronic aphasia: evidence from a pilot randomized controlled trial. Front Hum Neurosci 10:533. https://doi.org/10.3389/fnhum.2016.00533. Accessed 24 Aug 2021

Van Hees S, Angwin A, McMahon K et al (2013) A comparison of semantic feature analysis and phonological components analysis for the treatment of naming impairments in aphasia. Neuropsychol Rehabil 23:102–132

van Praag H, Shubert T, Zhao C et al (2005) Exercise enhances learning and hippocampal neurogenesis in aged mice. J Neurosci 25(38):8680–8685

Varley R, Siegal M, Want S (2001) Severe impairment in grammar does not preclude theory of mind. Neurocase 7(6):489–493

Vigliocco G, Perniss P, Vinson D (2014) Language as a multimodal phenomenon: implications for language learning, processing and evolution. Philos Trans Roy Soc B Biol Sci 369(1651):20130292. https://doi.org/10.1098/rstb.2013.0292. Accessed 4 Sep 2021

Vines B, Norton A, Schlaug G (2011) Non-invasive brain stimulation enhances the effects of Melodic Intonation Therapy. Front Psychol 2:230. https://doi.org/10.3389/fpsyg.2011.00230. Accessed 24 Aug 2021

Volkmer A, Cartwright J, Ruggero L et al (2023) Principles and philosophies for speech and language therapists working with people with primary progressive aphasia: an international expert consensus. Disabil Rehabil. 45(6):1063–1078. https://doi.org/10.1080/09638288.2022.2051080. Epub 2022 Mar 30. PMID: 35352609

Vymětal J (1989) Psychoterapie. Pomoc psychologickými prostředky (Psychotherapy. Help by psychological means). Horizont, Prague

Vymětal J (1996) Rogerovská psychoterapie (Roger's psychotherapy). Český spisovatel, Prague

Vymětal J (2007) Speciální psychoterapie (Special psychotherapy). Grada, Prague

Wade DT (2009) Goal setting in rehabilitation: an overview of what, why and how. Clin Rehabil 23(4):291–295

Wallentin M (2018) Sex differences in post-stroke aphasia rates are caused by age. A meta-analysis and database query. PLoS One 13(12):e0209571. https://doi.org/10.1371/journal.pone.0209571. Accessed 27 Aug 2021

Wambaugh J, Nessler C (2004) Modification of sound production treatment for apraxia of speech: acquisition and generalisation effects. Aphasiology 18(5–7):407–427

Wambaugh JL, Nessler C, Rosalea C et al (2013) Treatment for acquired apraxia of speech: examination of treatment intensity and practice schedule. Am J Speech Lang Pathol 22:84–102

Warren SF, Fey ME, Yoder PJ (2007) Differential treatment intensity research: a missing link to creating optimality effective communication interventions. Ment Retard Dev Disabil Res Rev 13(1):70–77

Watila MM, Balarabe B (2015) Factors predicting post-stroke aphasia recovery. J Neurol Sci 352(1–2):12–18

Webster J, Whitworth A, Morris J (2015) Is it time to stop "fishing"? A review of generalisation following aphasia intervention. Aphasiology 29(11):1240–1264

Winston A, Rosenthal E, Pinsker H (2012) Learning supportive psychotherapy: an illustrated guide (core competencies in psychotherapy). American Psychiatric Publishing, New York

Wittler M (2009) Rückbildungsprozesse in der Akut- und Postakutphase von Aphasien (Remissonprocesses in the acute and post-acute phase of aphasia). Evidenzen aus der neurologischen Forschung 6(23):12–18

Woldag MD, Voigt N, Bley M et al (2017) Constraint-induced aphasia therapy in the acute stage: what is the key factor for efficacy? A randomized controlled study. Neurorehabil Neural Repair 31(1):72–80

World Health Organization (WHO) (2001) International classification of functioning, disability and health: ICF. WHO, Geneva. https://www.who.int/standards/classifications/international-classification-of--functioning-disability-and-health. Accessed 17 Aug 2021

Worrall L (2019) The seven habits of highly effective aphasia therapists: the perspective of people living with aphasia. Int J Speech Lang Pathol 21:438–447

Worrall L, Brown K, Cruice M et al (2010) The evidence for a life-coaching approach to aphasia. Aphasiology 24:497–514

Worrall L, Sherratt S, Rogers P et al (2011) What people with aphasia want: their goals according to the ICF. Aphasiology 25(3):309–322

Worrall L, Sherratt S, Papathanasiou I (2017) Therapy approaches to aphasia. In: Papathanasiou I, Coppens P (eds) Aphasia and related neurogenic communication disorders. Jones & Bartlett Learning, Burlington, pp 109–127

Yalom I, Leszcz M (2008) The theory and practice of group psychotherapy. Basic Books, New York

Yao L, Zhao H, Shen C et al (2020) Low-frequency repetitive transcranial magnetic stimulation in patients with poststroke aphasia: systematic review and meta-analysis of its effect upon communication. J Speech Lang Hear Res 63:3801–3815

Youmans G, Youmans SR, Hancock AB (2011) Script training treatment for adults with apraxia of speech. Am J Speech Lang Pathol 20(1):23–37

Zajacova A, Lawrence EM (2018) The relationship between education and health: reducing disparities through a contextual approach. Annu Rev Public Health 39:273–289

Zhang J, Wei R, Chen Z et al (2016) Piracetam for aphasia in post-stroke patients: a systematic review and meta-analysis of randomized controlled trials. NS Drugs 30(7):575–587

Zhang X, Shu S, Zhang D et al (2018) The efficacy and safety of pharmacological treatments for post-stroke aphasia. CNS Neurol Disord Drug Targets 17(7):509–521

Zheng X, Dai W, Alsop DC et al (2016) Modulating transcallosal and intra-hemispheric brain connectivity with tDCS: implications for interventions in aphasia. Restor Neurol Neurosci 34:519–530

Zhu Y, Gao J, Lv Q et al (2020) Risk factors and outcomes of stroke-associated pneumonia in patients with stroke and acute large artery occlusion treated with endovascular thrombectomy. J Stroke Cerebrovasc Dis 29:11. https://doi.org/10.1016/j.jstrokecerebrovasdis.2020.105223. Accessed 4 Sep 2021

Zumbansen A, Tremblay P (2019) Music-based interventions for aphasia could act through a motor-speech mechanism: a systematic review and case-control analysis of published individual participant data. Aphasiology 33:466–497

Zumbansen A, Peretz I, Hébert S (2014) Melodic intonation therapy: back to basics for future research. Front Neurol 5:7. https://doi.org/10.3389/fneur.2014.00007. Accessed 31 Aug 2021

Editors: Patrick Zorowka, Antoinette am Zehnhoff-Dinnesen

Lectors: Jörg Bohlender, Irena Hočevar Boltežar, Sabine Crestani, Daniele Farneti, Pascale Fichaux-Bourin, Simone Graf, Michael Jungheim, Mari Markkanen-Leppänen, Tadeus Nawka, Christina Pflug, John Rubin, Carola Schön, Heidrun Schröter-Morasch, André Smout, Peter Sporns, Miro Tedla, Darija Vranisek, Virginie Woisard

# Basics of Dysphagia

**26**

Wolfgang Bigenzahn
and Doris-Maria Denk-Linnert

## 26.1 Definitions of Swallowing Disorders

Doris-Maria Denk-Linnert and
Wolfgang Bigenzahn

*Dysphagia* is defined as a disturbance of the oral intake or transport of food, liquids or saliva from the oral cavity to the stomach. From the differential diagnostic point of view dysphagia has to be distinguished from other swallowing difficulties, such as *odynophagia* or *globus sensation*. *Odynophagia* describes the painful swallowing that occurs in inflammatory diseases (e.g., acute tonsillitis, epiglottitis, etc.) or tumours of the upper aerodigestive tract. *Globus sensation (globus pharyngis)* is a feeling of a lump or foreign body in the throat and discomfort when swallowing saliva

**Supplementary Information** The online version contains supplementary material available at https://doi.org/10.1007/978-3-031-48091-1_11.

W. Bigenzahn (✉)
Formerly Division of Phoniatrics and Speech Language Therapy, Department of Otorhinolaryngology, now in Private Praxis, Vienna, Austria
e-mail: wolfgang.bigenzahn@chello.at

D.-M. Denk-Linnert
Division of Phoniatrics and Speech Language Therapy, Department of Otorhinolaryngology, Medical University of Vienna, Vienna, Austria
e-mail: doris-maria.denklinnert@meduniwien.ac.at

(see Sect. 27.4). In contrast to dysphagia, swallowing of food is not disturbed. The symptom mainly occurs during swallowing of saliva and decreases or vanishes while swallowing food.

A precondition for understanding the complexity of dysphagia is knowledge of anatomy and physiology of the upper aerodigestive tract, and swallowing physiology in particular. Swallowing belongs to the most frequent activities in the human body (between 580 and 2000 times a day: Garliner 1974; Logemann 1983). However, swallowing is not only a vital primary function to ensure adequate nutrition and hydration, but also contributes to quality of life and social integration.

Before swallowing begins, the food is looked at, smelled and put into the mouth (preoral anticipatory phase of the swallow: Leopold and Kagel 1997). The *normal swallowing process* consists of four phases:

- Oral preparatory (or chewing) phase
  The food is formed (sucking, chewing) into the so-called bolus, ready to be swallowed
- Oral (transit) phase
  By anterior-to-posterior propulsion the tongue moves the bolus into the pharynx. When sensory receptors, mainly at the base of the anterior faucial pillars, are stimulated, the swallowing reflex is triggered. From this point onwards, the swallow proceeds involuntarily as reflexive chain of events
- Pharyngeal phase

After the swallowing reflex has been elicited, a number of physiological activities occur nearly simultaneously in a very short time (duration about 1 s):

- Complete velopharyngeal closure
- Elevation and anterior movement of the hyoid and larynx
- Laryngeal closure (at three levels)
- Contraction of the pharyngeal wall
- Closure of the larynx
- Epiglottal tilting
- Contact of the tongue base with the posterior pharyngeal wall
- Complex opening of the upper oesophageal sphincter (UES)
- Oesophageal phase

The primary (induced by the swallow reflex) and secondary (induced by oesophageal distention) peristaltic contraction waves move the bolus into the stomach. When the lower oesophageal sphincter relaxes, the bolus can enter the stomach. The oesophageal transit takes approximately 4–20 s

The *central control of swallowing* is located in the supratentorial and infratentorial (brainstem) regions; in the latter the central "pattern generators" are located. From the anatomical point of view *oropharyngeal dysphagia* (disturbance of oropharyngeal swallowing) can be differentiated from *oesophageal dysphagia*. Both types of dysphagia may influence each other or can occur simultaneously.

*Dysphagia* is a syndrome, not a diagnosis itself, and can be present with or without aspiration. *Aspiration* means the entry of saliva, food *(anterograde aspiration)* or gastric secretion *(retrograde aspiration)* into the airway below the level of the vocal folds. It may be accompanied by coughing or appear without it (so-called *silent aspiration*) and is regarded a major risk factor for the development of a potentially life-threatening aspiration pneumonia.

The possible sequelae of dysphagia are malnutrition, dehydration, and life-threating aspiration pneumonia. Moreover, dysphagic patients may suffer from impaired quality of life and social isolation (Chen et al. 2001; Ekberg et al.

2002; Silbergleit et al. 2012; Speyer et al. 2014; Woisard and Sordes 2014).

Further components of impaired swallowing are as follows (Denk-Linnert 2012; Arens et al. 2015; Prosiegel and Weber 2018) (see also Sect. 26.3):

- Drooling: describes oral spills, i.e., the falling of food, liquid or saliva from the oral cavity
- Leaking (or spillage): defined as premature loss of the bolus over the tongue base into the pharynx before the swallowing reflex is triggered
- A delayed triggering is delayed pharyngeal swallowing after the bolus has entered the pharynx. It occurs in neurological diseases and when the anterior faucial pillars are damaged
- Retention (residue) of saliva or food may be localised in the oral cavity, valleculae, hypopharynx or larynx
- Nasal penetration defines the entry of food or secretions into the nasopharynx/nose
- Laryngeal penetration: food or saliva reaches the endolarynx as far as the glottis
- Pharyngeal regurgitation is described by parts of the already swallowed bolus flowing back in the pharynx
- Multiple swallows are present when the patient completes the swallowing of a small/medium bolus in more than two acts (piecemeal deglutition); for a bolus larger than 20 ml multiple swallows are not pathological (oral fragmentation)

Patients with dysphagia often cross speciality lines. To meet their diagnostic and therapeutic requirements a multidisciplinary and multiprofessional team approach is indispensable for evaluation of the aerodigestive tract and swallowing function from the oral cavity to the stomach (Farneti and Consolmagno 2007). Many patients often present with "swallowing difficulties" first to an otorhinolaryngologist/phoniatrician, who has to begin with the diagnostic work up and refer the patient—if necessary—for further diagnostics to reveal the underlying pathophysiology and aetiology, and to enable the appropriate treatment. Therefore, the ENT specialist/phoniatrician plays a key role in the multidisciplinary swallowing team, especially in case of oropharyngeal dysphagia.

## 26.2 Epidemiology of Dysphagia

Doris-Maria Denk-Linnert and
Wolfgang Bigenzahn

The prevalence of dysphagia is on the rise and varies widely. It depends on the underlying aetiology, age, environment of the patient, and the type of recording (subjective report, screening or instrumental diagnostics (Rommel and Hamdy 2016). In a large population-based survey, one of six adults reported experiencing the symptoms of dysphagia (Adkins et al. 2020). Dysphagia may occur at any age, but its prevalence is higher among elderly people (Lindgren and Jazon 1991; Baijens et al. 2016). This is because age-related changes in swallow anatomy and physiology reduce the functional reserve of the swallow, i.e., that the ability to compensate diminishes with increasing age (primary dysphagia, mainly due to sarcopenia). Furthermore, neurological diseases and dementia occur more frequently in older people (secondary dysphagia). Dementia is often associated with malnutrition and dysphagia. The prevalence data of dementia, which are expected to double within the next 30 years, highlight the need for adequate dysphagia management. For life expectancy, the nutritional status, independent oral feeding, and the prevention of aspiration-related pulmonary complications are of utmost prognostic relevance. Geriatric dysphagia is regarded as a syndrome owing to its multiple aetiological factors and association with comorbidities and poor prognosis. It needs a multidimensional approach, but sometimes it is still underdiagnosed or untreated (Baijens et al. 2016).

Epidemiological data are scarce. The overall dysphagia prevalence is from 6% to 50% (Roden and Altmann 2013). Oropharyngeal dysphagia affects between 27% and 91% of people 70 years of age or older (Ortega et al. 2017). About 16% of people from 70 to 80 years who live independently report dysphagia, 33% in the group aged 80 years or more. This percentage reaches up to 47% in frail elderly hospitalised patients and 50% in older nursing home residents (Clavé and Shaker 2015).

In acute care hospitals, 13–14% of patients are estimated to suffer from dysphagia, whereas in nursing homes/palliative care settings the percentage of dysphagic patients is much higher (up to 50%; Logemann 1995; Robbins et al. 2001). Aspiration pneumonia is the fourth most frequent cause of death among Japanese, of which 92% occurs in patients aged more than 65 years (Sasaki 1991). Rehabilitative measurements for aspiration pneumonia, especially in older patients, are indispensable (Momosaki 2017). After all, the management of the dysphagic patient has become of great clinical importance and a focus of scientific interest, especially with regard to the demographic changes.

As a consequence of medical progress, especially in intensive care medicine, neonatology and paediatrics, a greater number of patients surviving severe diseases suffer from swallowing impairment, which has become a great challenge for therapy and rehabilitation. Intensive Care Unit patients often suffer from dysphagia related to long-term intubation, critical illness neuropathy or to the underlying disease itself (Zuercher et al. 2019). The prevalence rate differs (86% aspiration, Partik et al. 2000; prevalence of dysphagia 35.9%, risk of aspiration 24.9%, Oliveira et al. 2018).

Owing to more surviving premature infants, some even born from the 23rd gestation week onwards, feeding and swallowing problems have to be managed. Often neurocognitive deficits and syndromes result in feeding and swallowing problems, aspiration or dyspnoea (Arvedson and Brodsky 2001; Dodrill 2014). Furthermore, organ-preserving concepts in head and neck cancer treatment contribute to the increased need for functional dysphagia therapy.

## 26.3 Symptomatic Profile of Dysphagia

Doris-Maria Denk-Linnert

### 26.3.1 Symptomatic Components of Dysphagia

The most important and dangerous dysphagia-related symptom is *aspiration*, which is defined as the entry of saliva, food or gastric secretion into the airway below the level of the vocal folds. In case of a lacking cough reflex, a silent aspiration is present.

Other components of dysphagia are *drooling, leaking, nasal penetration, laryngeal penetration, retention or pharyngeal regurgitation* (Denk-Linnert 2019; Arens et al. 2015; Prosiegel and Weber 2018).

**Drooling** describes complaints of oral spill, i.e., the falling of food, liquid or saliva from the mouth anteriorly when lip closure is incomplete. Sometimes saliva and secretions drool posteriorly (posterior drooling), possibly resulting in pre-swallow pooling.

**Leaking** is defined as premature loss of the bolus over the tongue base into the pharynx before the swallowing reflex is triggered. Consequently, the risk of aspiration occurs.

**Delayed Triggering of the Swallowing Reflex** occurs in neurological diseases (e.g., stroke) or after extensive surgical resection of the trigger points for the pharyngeal swallow, thus causing the risk of aspiration before the swallow.

**Retention** (residue) of saliva or food may be localised in the oral cavity, valleculae or hypopharynx (Fig. 26.1a, b, c). Retention in the anterior or lateral sulcus are due to reduced muscle tone in the labial or buccal musculature. Disturbed lingual function may result in retention on the floor of the mouth and in the valleculae. Weakness, paresis or scarring of pharyngeal muscles bring about pharyngeal retention, which bring about the risk of post-deglutitive aspiration. Scaling the extent of saliva retention helps classify the severity of saliva retention

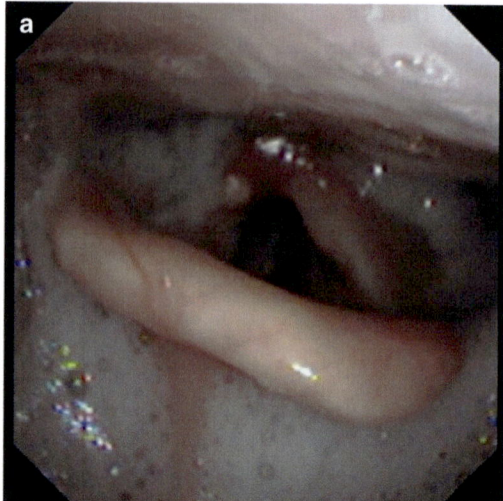
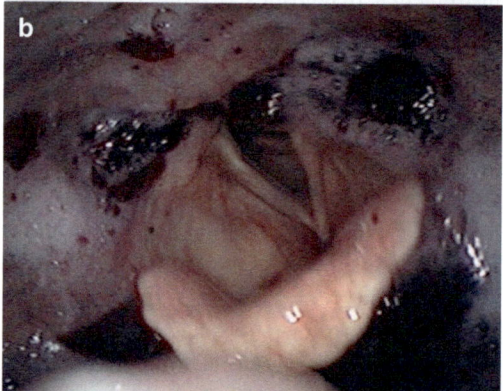
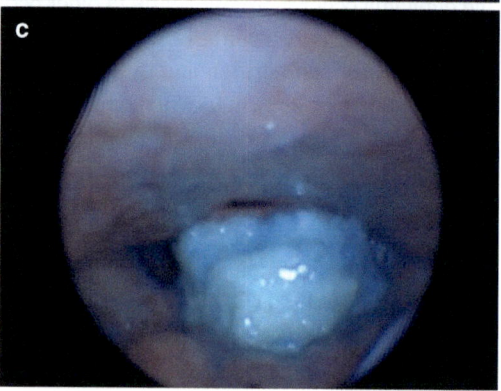

**Fig. 26.1** (from top to bottom) Retention of (**a**) saliva in the valleculae and piriform sinuses, (**b**) saliva and jelly in the valleculae, hypopharynx/piriform sinuses, (**c**) biscuit in the valleculae © Denk-Linnert 2019

(Murray et al. 1996; Hey et al. 2015; Farneti 2008).

**Nasal Penetration (Regurgitation)** describes the entry of food into the nose and may be caused by incomplete velopharyngeal closure or pharyn-

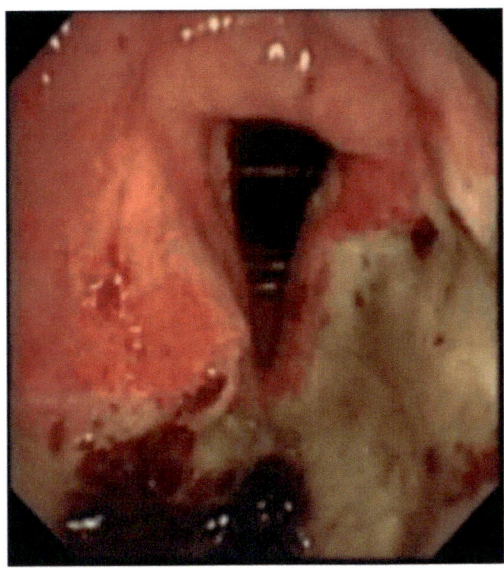

**Fig. 26.2** Laryngeal Penetration (videoendoscopic view) after transoral laser resection of a supraglottal tumour. Jelly has penetrated into the supraglottis © Denk-Linnert 2019

geal/oesophageal stopping of the bolus passage with subsequent overflow into the nasal cavity.

**Laryngeal Penetration** is characterised by food or saliva reaching the larynx to the level of the vocal folds (Fig. 26.2).

**Pharyngeal Regurgitation** is characterised by the (partial) flowing of the already swallowed bolus back into the pharynx. This may be, e.g., due to a Zenker's diverticulum or disturbed oesophageal bolus transport.

### 26.3.2 Aspiration and Scaling of Its Severity

The *main goal* of the diagnostic workup of dysphagic patients is to reveal or exclude aspiration and the risk of aspiration, which determines further patient management. In the case of absent or reduced cough reflex, aspiration does not induce coughing, but remains "silent" (*silent aspiration*) and is not immediately noticed. About 40% of aspirating patients are the so-called silent aspirators. Therefore, aspiration can only be proven or excluded by the dynamic instrumental methods of videoendoscopic swallowing study FEES(ST)— flexible (originally: fibreoptic)

evaluation of swallowing (with sensory testing); Langmore et al. 1988; Bastian 1991; Aviv et al. 1998, Denk-Linnert et al. 2023, Pizzorni et al. 2024) or videofluoroscopic swallowing studies (Logemann 1983, 1993, 1998; Ekberg 1992, 2012; Pokieser and Scharitzer 2019). Both dynamic instrumental GOLD standard- methods are complementary and may be used simultaneously, mainly for scientific purposes (Scharitzer et al. 2019).

*Aspiration* can be classified in relation to the triggering of the swallowing reflex. It may occur before (pre-deglutitive), during (intra-deglutitive), after (post-deglutitive) swallowing or in combined forms (Logemann 1983). *Aspiration before swallowing* may be present when the triggering of the swallowing reflex is absent or disturbed, e.g., after stroke. Incomplete laryngeal closure or reduced laryngeal elevation may give rise to *aspiration during the swallow*, as is the case, for example, in vocal fold paralysis or in laryngeal defects after partial laryngectomy. Reduced pharyngeal peristalsis, reduced laryngeal elevation and disturbed opening of the pharyngo-oesophageal sphincter possibly result in *aspiration after the swallow* (Fig. 26.3a, b), e.g., in fibrosis with "frozen" (immobile) larynx after radiation therapy or cricopharyngeal achalasia (i.e., disturbance of the opening of the upper oesophageal sphincter).

The severity of aspiration is not only influenced by the amount and type of the aspirated material, but also by the presence of cough reflex and the possibility of voluntary coughing and throat clearing. A deep aspiration of material into the distal airways is more dangerous than aspiration into the subglottis or upper portion of the trachea. Moreover, the physical properties of the aspirate are of great influence (acidic material and material including infectious organisms increase the risk of developing aspiration pneumonia).

Several severity scales are used for the grading of aspiration (Table 26.1). The clinical aspiration scale (Miller and Eliachar 1994) considers possible pulmonary consequences. In the videoendoscopic aspiration scale (Schröter-Morasch 1996) attention is paid to the cough reflex and voluntary coughing. The videofluoroscopic aspi-

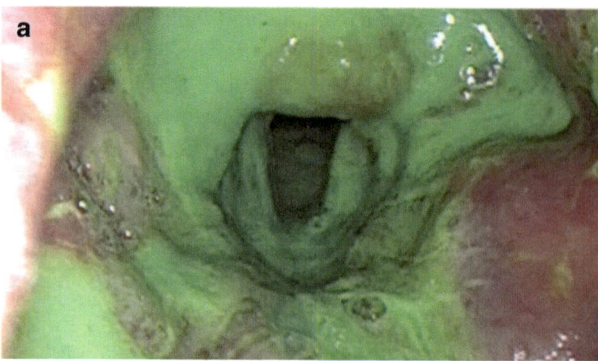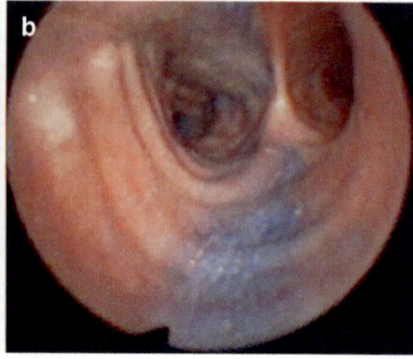

**Fig. 26.3** (from left to right) Aspiration (videoendoscopic view); (**a**) coloured yoghurt is passing below the level of the vocal folds; (**b**) blue aspirated liquid in the trachea above the bifurcation © Denk-Linnert 2019

**Table 26.1** Aspiration scales

| Clinical Scale (Miller and Eliachar 1994) |
| --- |
| I   Incidental aspiration without complications |
| II   Intermittent aspiration of liquids; saliva and solid boluses can be swallowed |
| III   No oral feeding possible, intermittent pneumonia |
| IV   Life-threatening aspiration; chronic pneumonia/ hypoxia |
| Videoendoscopic Scale (Schröter-Morasch 1996) |
| I   Incidental aspiration, intact cough reflex |
| II   Incidental aspiration, no cough reflex, voluntary coughing possible or Permanent aspiration, intact cough reflex |
| III   Permanent aspiration, no cough reflex, voluntary coughing possible |
| IV   Permanent aspiration, no cough reflex, no voluntary coughing |
| Videofluoroscopic Scale (Hannig et al. 1995) |
| I   Aspiration of material that has penetrated into the laryngeal vestibule or ventricle, intact cough reflex |
| II   Constant aspiration of less than 10% of the bolus, intact cough reflex |
| III   Constant aspiration of less than 10% of the bolus, reduced cough reflex or Constant aspiration of more than 10% of the bolus, intact cough reflex |
| IV   Constant aspiration of more than 10% of the bolus, reduced cough reflex |

Reprinted by permission from Springer Nature: from Denk-Linnert (2019) Evaluation of symptoms. In: Ekberg O (ed) Dysphagia. Diagnosis and Treatment. Springer, Berlin, Heidelberg, pp. 83–93

**Table 26.2** Penetration—Aspiration Scale

| Grade | |
| --- | --- |
| 1 | Material does not enter the airway |
| 2 | Material enters the airway, remains above the vocal folds and is ejected from the airway |
| 3 | Material enters the airway, remains above the vocal folds and is not ejected from the airway |
| 4 | Material enters the airway, contacts the vocal folds and is ejected from the airway |
| 5 | Material enters the airway, contacts the vocal folds and is not ejected from the airway |
| 6 | Material enters the airway, passes below the vocal folds and is ejected into the larynx or out of the airway |
| 7 | Material enters the airway, passes below the vocal folds and is not ejected from the trachea despite effort |
| 8 | Material enters the airway, passes below the vocal folds and no effort is made to eject |

Reprinted by permission from **Springer Nature Customer Service Centre GmbH from** Rosenbek et al. (1996) A penetration-aspiration scale. Dysphagia 11(2): 93–98

(Validation of German version, Hey et al. 2014) describes an 8-point scale. The severity of aspiration is determined by the level in the airway of the entered material and whether this material can be expelled (Table 26.2). This scale is recognised and used worldwide.

The individual tolerance of aspiration varies widely. Some patients tolerate aspiration of more than 10% of the bolus, whereas other patients develop aspiration pneumonia even after aspiration of their saliva. Therefore, not only aspira-

ration scale (Hannig et al. 1995) is based on the amount of aspirated material and the presence or absence of the cough reflex. The penetration-aspiration scale by Rosenbek et al. (1996)

tion, but additional risk factors play an important role. Langmore et al. (1998) found the following predictors for the development of aspiration pneumonia: dependent on feeding, dependent on oral care, number of decayed teeth, tube feeding, more than one medical diagnosis, number of medications and smoking.

### 26.3.3 Indirect and Direct Symptoms of Dysphagia/Aspiration

Dysphagic patients may present with *indirect and direct symptoms of dysphagia/aspiration* (Table 26.3), which are possible hints for suspecting dysphagia and aspiration. A major diagnostic problem is silent aspiration. The fact that the dysphagic patient does not cough/choke while eating cannot be regarded as a reliable symptom "clue" to exclude aspiration. *Direct symptoms* occur during swallowing of food and liquids, whereas *indirect symptoms* are not directly associated with the swallow as such but are due to dysphagia/aspiration.

**Table 26.3** Symptoms of dysphagia/aspiration

| |
|---|
| *Indirect symptoms* |
|   Weight loss |
|   Frequent occurrence of fever |
|   Coughing |
|   Bronchitis/pneumonia |
|   Changes of voice, articulation/speech or language |
|   Globus sensation |
|   Heartburn |
|   Non-cardiac chest pain |
| *Direct symptoms* |
|   Prolonged duration of swallowing |
|   Pain |
|   Fear of swallowing |
|   Changes of posture |
|   Avoidance of particular food consistencies |
|   Drooling |
|   Obstruction, stuck food |
|   Choking, coughing |
|   Spitting of food |
|   Regurgitation |

Adapted by permission from Springer Nature: from Denk-Linnert (2019) Evaluation of symptoms. In: Ekberg O (ed) Dysphagia. Diagnosis and Treatment. Springer, Berlin, Heidelberg, pp. 83–93 and after Schröter-Morasch (1993, 1996)

Among the *indirect symptoms*, weight loss is regarded as a reliable hint for judging the effects of swallowing impairment, because weight is usually directly related to the nutritional state. Frequent occurrence of fever, coughing, bronchitis or pneumonia may be clinical consequences of aspiration. Changes of voice (dysphonia), speech (dysarthria), and language (aphasia) should not be neglected, as they may be related to neurological diseases. Moreover, anatomical and functional deficits in the upper aerodigestive tract possibly also lead to dysphonia, altered resonance [e.g., hyper-rhinophonia (too much nasal resonance)] or impaired articulation [e.g., dysglossia (disturbed articulation due to changes in the peripheral organs of speech)]. Globus sensation, heartburn or non-cardiac chest pain often are present in gastro-oesophageal reflux disease or oesophageal motility disorders. Alterations of taste or mucosal dryness impair swallowing function and the pleasure from oral intake.

*Direct symptoms of dysphagia and aspiration* include choking or coughing during or immediately after the swallow owing to aspiration, prolonged duration of swallowing, pain (odynophagia) or fear of swallowing. Furthermore, changes in posture during oral food intake and changes in eating habits (e.g., avoidance of some food consistency) deserve clinical awareness. Other direct symptoms the patient may report are drooling, nasal regurgitation, spitting of food or regurgitation. The feeling of obstruction may occur not only in patients with tumours, strictures, Zenker's diverticulum, webs or cervical osteophytes (DISH, diffuse idiopathic skeletal hyperostosis), but also in neurological diseases because of pharyngeal muscle weakness, lack of coordination of the swallow or oesophageal motility disorder.

### 26.4 Aetiology/Pathogenesis of Dysphagia

Doris-Maria Denk-Linnert and Wolfgang Bigenzahn

## 26.4.1 Aetiology of Dysphagia

Dysphagia is a symptom of an underlying structural or neuromotor disorder or may be a side effect of treatment (e.g., ENT, skull base, thoracic, cardiac surgery, radio−/chemotherapy) or medication (e.g., central nervous system depressants/neuroleptics, antipsychotic medications, neuromuscular blocking agents, dopamine antagonists, anticholinergic medications, narcotics, xerostomia-causing drugs). It has to be distinguished from odynophagia, which is defined as painful swallowing. The aetiologies are diverse

(Palmer et al. 2000). With regard to the afflicted phases, one differentiates oropharyngeal from oesophageal dysphagia.

Dysphagia frequently occurs in elderly people and has been recognised as geriatric syndrome (Jungheim et al. 2014; Baijens et al. 2016; Ortega et al. 2017). Owing to its multiform aetiology and tendency to increased age-dependence and mortality, it is classified as a "geriatric giant" (Smithard 2016) (see Sect. 27.6). At the other end of the age spectrum, right after birth, the management of paediatric dysphagia and aspiration increasingly develop to be

**Table 26.4** Examples of dysphagia aetiology

| (a) Oropharyngeal Dysphagia | |
|---|---|
| Type of dysphagia | Aetiology |
| Mechanical dysphagia | |
| | Tooth loss |
| | Cleft lip palate |
| | Inflammatory diseases |
| | Malignant tumours in the upper aerodigestive tract |
| | Sequelae after tumour therapy (surgery, radiation, chemotherapy) |
| | Diseases/surgery of the cervical spine |
| | Long-term-intubation |
| | Tracheostomy |
| | Tracheo-oesophageal fistula |
| | Diverticula (Zenker's diverticulum) |
| | Disorders of the upper oesophageal sphincter |
| | Goitre |
| | Systemic diseases (scleroderma, amyloidosis) |
| | Graft-versus-host-disease |
| Neurogenic dysphagia | |
| Central nervous system | Stroke |
| | Amyotrophic lateral sclerosis |
| | Parkinson disease |
| | Multiple sclerosis |
| | Cerebral palsy |
| | Dementia, Alzheimer disease |
| | Post-polio syndrome |
| | Encephalitis |
| | AIDS |
| | Posterior fossa tumours |
| | Head trauma, cervical spine cord injury |
| | Intoxication |
| | Drug effects (sedatives, neuroleptics) |
| | Arnold Chiari malformation |
| Peripheral nervous system | Skull base tumours (chordoma, meningioma) |
| | Meningitis |
| | Guillain-Barré syndrome |
| | Neuropathy (alcoholic, diabetic) |

(continued)

**Table 26.4** (continued)

| | |
|---|---|
| Neuromuscular junction | Myasthenia gravis |
| | Botulism |
| | Lambert-Eaton syndrome |
| Muscles | Dermatomyositis, polymyositis |
| | Myopathy (endocrine/metabolic) |
| | Myotonia, muscular dystrophy |
| Psychogenic dysphagia | |
| | Phagophobia |

**(b) Oesophageal Dysphagia**
Tracheo-oesophageal fistula
Oesophageal atresia
Foreign body
Oesophageal perforation
Inflammation (e.g., eosinophilic oesophagitis)
Intrinsic obstructive oesophageal diseases (peptic, tumorous, stenosis)
Extrinsic obstructive oesophageal diseases (compression by mediastinal mass, vascular compression, cervical spine osteophytes)
Motility disorders (gastro-oesophageal reflux disease (GERD), non-propulsive contractions, achalasia,…)

Modified from Denk-Linnert (2019) and Denk and Bigenzahn (1999, 2005)

a multi-professional challenge. As a consequence of medical progress in neonatology and paediatrics, more very preterm infants und neonates suffering from syndromes survive, necessitating dysphagia management (Arvedson and Lefton-Greif. 2017; Horton et al. 2018) (see Sect. 27.1). Examples of dysphagia aetiology are displayed in Table 26.4.

### 26.4.1.1 Oropharyngeal Dysphagia
The aetiology of oropharyngeal dysphagia may be divided into the following three groups:

1. Diseases of the upper aerodigestive tract (peripheral "mechanical" dysphagia)
2. Neurological diseases (neurogenic dysphagia)
3. Psychogenic dysphagia

After exclusion of a peripheral or neurogenic dysphagia aetiology, psychogenic factors (e.g., phagophobia) have to be considered (see Sect. 27.4). In some cases, the distinction from eating disorders may be difficult.

**Mechanical Dysphagia**
Diseases of the upper swallowing and respiratory tract or surrounding structures may give rise to dysphagia and aspiration. In the oral phases,

tooth loss and mastication disorders may impair swallowing (Nozomi et al. 2012).

In any case, the symptom of dysphagia makes the exclusion of a malignant tumour necessary (see Sect. 27.5). Moreover, not only a tumorous disease of the oral cavity, pharynx or larynx itself, but also the sequelae of tumour therapy—surgical resection, radiation, chemotherapy—can impair bolus preparation or transfer, or airway protection, with consequent dysphagia and aspiration. The different tumour resections in the head and neck are known to create patterns of swallowing disorders, but the same resections need not necessarily result in the same form and degree of dysphagia and aspiration. The extent and localisation of the resections carried out are regarded as determining factors for the severity of dysphagia. Besides these local factors, general factors, e.g., the patient's general condition and individual capability of compensation, and postoperative therapy onset, also influence the outcome of swallowing rehabilitation (Denk and Kaider 1997).

Thyroid gland disease (e.g., goitre) or cervical osteophyte compression due to diffuse idiopathic skeletal hyperostosis (DISH) (Marks et al. 1998) may be responsible for obstructive dysphagic symptoms, which are typically worse for a solid than liquid bolus. Patients suffering from DISH mostly become symptomatic when an additional disease afflicting swallowing function diminishes the patient's functional compensatory capability.

**Neurogenic Dysphagia**

Nearly all neurological diseases potentially disturb the four levels of sensomotoric control of the swallow (central, peripheral nervous system, neuromuscular junction, muscles) and may cause dysphagia and aspiration or residue (see Sect. 27.3). For patient management it is important to distinguish between neurological lesions with recovery potential (e.g., stroke, head trauma, cervical spine cord injury, etc.) and progressive diseases.

For clinical aspects it has to be pointed out that laryngo-pharyngeal and oesophageal muscles are represented asymmetrically between the two cortical hemispheres, mostly in the dominant swallowing hemisphere (Hamdy et al. 1996). Therefore, oropharyngeal dysphagia may result from a unilateral cortical stroke (Hamdy et al. 1997). The medullary regions controlling swallowing are represented on both sides of the brainstem and are interconnected. Thus, a unilateral medullary lesion may cause a bilateral pharyngeal motor and sensory dysfunction (Aviv et al. 1997).

The most frequent cause of dysphagia is stroke (25%, Groher and Bukatman 1986 Smithard et al. 1997; Smithard 2002; Martino et al. 2005). The percentage of dysphagic stroke patients differs with the time from the onset of stroke (41% in the first 2 weeks after stroke, 16% in the chronic phase, Kuhlemeier 1994). Pneumonia incidence and mortality rate are higher in dysphagic stroke patients, underlining the need for appropriate dysphagia screening, diagnostics and management (Suntrup-Krueger et al. 2018, Labeit et al. 2024).

Besides the swallowing disturbance, neurological patients possibly show additional symptoms that have to be considered. Disturbances in the motor system bring about impaired posture and head control, and cognitive deficits lead to a lack of awareness of disease. Severely impaired speech and language (e.g., dysarthria, aphasia) impair communication with the patient.

### 26.4.1.2 Oesophageal Dysphagia

This is mainly caused by (Malagelada et al. 2007; Clavé and Shaker 2015):

- Mucosal (intrinsic) diseases (lumen narrowing/obstruction due to inflammation, fibrosis or neoplasia)
- Mediastinal (extrinsic) diseases (oesophageal obstruction due to direct invasion or lymph-node enlargement)
- Neuromuscular diseases (affecting the oesophageal muscle and its innervation, disturbed peristalsis or lower oesophageal sphincter disorder)

## 26.4.2 Pathogenesis of Dysphagia

After thorough diagnostics the aetiology and pathophysiology of dysphagia/aspiration should be overt. Possible impairments of swallowing function may be due to a disturbed bolus passage (caused by e.g. mechanical obstruction or muscular weakness), disturbed airway protection or disturbed breathing/swallowing coordination. For evaluation of the pathophysiological factors responsible, a meticulous analysis of the swallowing phases is necessary.

- If the visual presentation, smell, taste, and cognition (e.g., in dementia) are disturbed, the anticipatory phase is negatively influenced
- In the oral preparatory and oral phase, impairments of biting, mastication, lip closure, bolus formation and transport, tone of the cheek muscles, velar function, delay of the swallowing reflex or oral sensibility may lead to drooling, oral retention, leaking or aspiration before swallowing
- In the pharyngeal phase an impairment of velopharyngeal or laryngeal closure, laryngeal sensation, laryngeal elevation, delayed or insufficient opening of the upper oesophageal sphincter or pharyngeal weakness possibly result in nasal penetration, laryngeal penetration, aspiration during or after swallowing and pharyngeal residue
- Disturbed oesophageal bolus transport may give rise to pharyngeal regurgitation. Therefore, the oesophageal phase should also be given attention in oropharyngeal dysphagia

# References

Adkins C, Takakura W, Spiegel BMR et al (2020) Prevalence and characteristics of dysphagia based on a population-based survey. Clin Gastroenterol Hepatol 18(9):1970–1979

Arens C, Herrmann IF, Rohrbach S et al (2015) Positionspapier der DGHNO und der DGPP–Stand der klinischen und endoskopischen Diagnostik, Evaluation und Therapie von Schluckstörungen bei Kindern und Erwachsenen (Position paper of the German Society of Oto-Rhino-Laryngology, Head and Neck Surgery and the German Society of Phoniatrics and Pediatric Audiology–current state of clinical and endoscopic diagnostics, evaluation and therapy of swallowing disorders in children and adults). Laryngorhinootologie 94(Suppl 1):S306–S354

Arvedson JC, Brodsky L (2001) Pediatric swallowing and feeding: assessment and management. Early childhood intervention series, 2nd edn. Delmar Publishers, New York

Arvedson JC, Lefton-Greif MA (2017) Instrumental assessment of pediatric dysphagia. Semin Speech Lang 38(2):135–146

Aviv JE, Mohr JP, Blitzer A et al (1997) Restoration of laryngopharyngeal sensation by neural anastomosis. Arch Otolaryngol Head Neck Surg 123(2):154–160

Aviv JE, Kim T, Sacco RL et al (1998) FEESST: a new bedside endoscopic test of the motor and sensory components of swallowing. Ann Otol Rhinol Laryngol 107(5–1):378–387

Baijens LW, Clavé P, Cras P et al (2016) European Society for Swallowing Disorders–European Union Geriatric Medicine Society white paper: oropharyngeal dysphagia as a geriatric syndrome. Clin Interv Aging 11:1403–1428

Bastian RW (1991) Videoendoscopic evaluation of patients with dysphagia: an adjunct to the modified barium swallow. Otolaryngol Head Neck Surg 104(3):339–350

Chen AY, Frankowski R, Bishop-Leone J et al (2001) The development and validation of a dysphagia-specific quality-of-life questionnaire for patients with head and neck cancer: the MD Anderson Dysphagia Inventory. Arch Otolaryngol Head Neck Surg 127(7):870–876

Clavé P, Shaker R (2015) Dysphagia: current reality and scope of the problem. Nat Rev Gastroenterol Hepatol 12(5):259–270

Denk D-M, Bigenzahn W (1999) Oropharyngeale Dysphagien: Definitonen, Ursachen und Pathophysiologie (Oropharyngeal dysphagia: definitions, causes, and pathophysiology). In: Bigenzahn W, Denk D-M (eds) Oropharyngeale Dysphagien (Oropharyngeal dysphagia). Ätiologie, Klinik, Diagnostik und Therapie von Schluckstörungen (Aetiology, clinic, diagnosis and therapy of swallowing disorders). Thieme, Stuttgart

Denk D-M, Bigenzahn W (2005) Management oropharyngealer Dysphagien. Eine Standortbestimmmung (Management of oropharyngeal dysphagia. Current status.). HNO 53(7):661–672

Denk D-M, Kaider A (1997) Videoendoscopic biofeedback: a simple method to improve the efficacy of swallowing rehabilitation of patients after head and neck surgery. ORL J Otorhinolaryngol Relat Spec 59(2):100–105

Denk-Linnert DM (2012) Evaluation of symptoms. In: Ekberg O (ed) Dysphagia: diagnosis and treatment. Springer, Berlin/Heidelberg, pp 71–81

Denk-Linnert DM (2019) Evaluation of symptoms. In: Ekberg O (ed) Dysphagia: diagnosis and treatment. Springer, Berlin/Heidelberg, pp 83–94

Denk-Linnert DM, Farneti D, Nawka T et al. (2023) Position Statement of the Union of European Phoniatricians (UEP): Fees and Phoniatricians' Role in Multidisciplinary and Multiprofessional Dysphagia Management Team. Dysphagia 38(2):711-718

Dodrill P (2014) Feeding problems and oropharyngeal dysphagia in children. J Gastroenterol Hepatol Res 3(5):1055–1060

Ekberg O (1992) Radiologic evaluation of swallowing. In: Groher ME (ed) Dysphagia: diagnosis and management. Butterworth-Heinemann, Stoneham, pp 163–195

Ekberg O (2012) Imaging techniques and some principles of interpretation (including radiation physics). In: Ekberg O (ed) Dysphagia: diagnosis and treatment. Springer, Berlin/Heidelberg, pp 237–252

Ekberg O, Hamdy S, Woisard V et al (2002) Social and psychological burden of dysphagia: its impact on diagnosis and treatment. Dysphagia 17(2):139–146

Farneti D (2008) Pooling score: an endoscopic model for evaluating severity of dysphagia. Acta Otorhinolaryngol Ital 28(3):135–140

Farneti D, Consolmagno P (2007) The swallowing centre: rationale for a multidisciplinary management. Acta Otorhinolaryngol Ital 27(4):200–207

Garliner D (1974) Myofunctional therapy in dental practice. Bartel, New York

Groher ME, Bukatman R (1986) The prevalence of swallowing disorders in two teaching hospitals. Dysphagia 1(1):1–3

Hamdy S, Aziz Q, Rothwell JC et al (1996) The cortical topography of human swallowing musculature in health and disease. Nature Med 2(11):1217–1224

Hamdy S, Aziz Q, Rothwell JC et al (1997) Explaining oropharyngeal dysphagia after unilateral hemispheric stroke. Lancet 350(9079):686–692

Hannig C, Wuttge-Hannig A, Hess U (1995) Analyse und radiologisches Staging des Typs und Schweregrades einer Aspiration (Analysis and radiological staging of type and grade of aspiration). Radiologe 358:741–746

Hey C, Pluschinski P, Zaretsky Y et al (2014) Penetrations-Aspirations-Skala nach Rosenbek. Validierung der deutschen Version für die endoskopische Dysphagiediagnostik (Penetration-aspiration scale according to Rosenbek. Validation of the German version for endoscopic dysphagia diagnostics). HNO 62(4):276–281

Hey C, Pluschinski P, Stöver T et al (2015) Validierung der deutschen Kurzversion der Sekretbeurteilungsskala nach Murray (Validation of the German short version of the Murray Secretion Rating Scale). Laryngorhinootologie 94(3):169–172

Horton J, Atwood C, Gnagi S et al (2018) Temporal trends of pediatric dysphagia in hospitalized patients. Dysphagia 33(5):655–661

Jungheim M, Schwemmle C, Miller S et al (2014) Swallowing and dysphagia in the elderly. HNO 62(9):644–651

Kuhlemeier KV (1994) Epidemiology and dysphagia. Dysphagia 9(4):209–217

Labeit B, Michou E, Trapl-Grundschober M, Suntrup-Krueger S, Muhle P, Bath PM, Dziewas R. Dysphagia after stroke: research advances in treatment interventions. Lancet Neurol. 2024;23(4):418-428.

Langmore S, Schatz K, Olsen N (1988) Fiberoptic examination of swallowing safety: a new procedure. Dysphagia 2(4):216–219

Langmore SE, Terpenning MS, Schork A et al (1998) Predictors of aspiration pneumonia: how important is dysphagia? Dysphagia 13(2):69–81

Leopold NA, Kagel MC (1997) Dysphagia—ingestion or deglutition? A proposed paradigm. Dysphagia 12(4):202–206

Lindgren S, Jazon L (1991) Prevalence of swallowing complaints and clinical findings among 50–70 year old men and women in an urban population. Dysphagia 6(4):187–192

Logemann JA (1983) Evaluation and treatment of swallowing disorders. Pro-ed, Austin

Logemann JA (1993) Manual for the videofluorographic study of swallowing, 2nd edn. Pro-ed, Austin

Logemann JA (1995) Dysphagia: evaluation and treatment. Folia Phoniatr Logop 47(3):140–164

Logemann JA (1998) Evaluation and treatment of swallowing disorders, vol 6. Pro-ed, Austin, p 395

Malagelada JR, Bazzoli F, Elewaut A et al (2007) Dysphagia; World Gastroenterology Organisation practice guidelines. Available http://www.worldgastroenterology.org/UserFiles/file/guidelines/dysphagia-english-2014.pdf. Accessed 6 Feb 2022

Marks B, Schober E, Swoboda H (1998) Diffuse idiopathic skeletal hyperostosis causing obstructive laryngeal edema. Eur Arch Otolaryngol 255(5):256–258

Martino R, Foley N, Bhogal S et al (2005) Dysphagia after stroke: incidence, diagnosis, and pulmonary complications. Stroke 36(12):2756–2763

Miller FR, Eliachar J (1994) Managing the aspirating patient. Am J Otolaryngol 15(1):1–17

Momosaki R (2017) Rehabilitative management for aspiration pneumonia in elderly patients. J Gen Fam Med 18(1):12–15

Murray J, Langmore SE, Ginsberg S et al (1996) The significance of accumulated oropharyngeal secretions and swallowing frequency in predicting aspiration. Dysphagia 11(2):99–103

Nozomi Okamoto N, Kimiko Tomioka K, Keigo Saeki K et al (2012) Relationship between swallowing problems and tooth loss in community-dwelling independent elderly adults: the Fujiwara-kyo Study. J Am Geriatr Soc 60(5):849–853

Oliveira ACM, Friche AAL, Salomão MS et al (2018) Predictive factors for oropharyngeal dysphagia after prolonged orotracheal intubation. Braz J Otorhinolaryngol 84(6):722–728

Ortega O, Martín A, Clavé P (2017) Diagnosis and management of oropharyngeal dysphagia among older persons, state of the art. J Am Med Dir Assoc 18(7):576–582

Palmer JB, Drennan JC, Baba M (2000) Evaluation and treatment of swallowing impairments. Am Fam Physician 61(8):2453–2462

Partik B, Pokieser P, Schima W et al (2000) Videofluoroscopy of swallowing in symptomatic patients who have undergone long-term intubation. Am J Roentgenol 174(5):1409–1412

Pizzorni N, Rocca S, Eplite A et al. (2024) Fiberoptic endoscopic evaluation of swallowing (FEES) in pediatrics: A systematic review. Int J Pediatr Otorhinolaryngol 181:111983. Epub

Pokieser P, Scharitzer M (2019) The clinical and radiological approach to dysphagia. In: Ekberg O (ed) Dysphagia: diagnosis and treatment. Springer, Berlin/Heidelberg, pp 285–316

Prosiegel M, Weber S (2018) Dysphagie. Diagnostik und Therapie. Ein Wegweiser für kompetentes Handeln (Dysphagia. Diagnostics and therapy. A guide for competent action), 3rd edn. Springer, Berlin/Heidelberg

Robbins J, Langmore S, Hind JA et al (2002) Dysphagia research in the 21st century and beyond: proceedings from Dysphagia Experts Meeting, August 21, 2001. J Rehabil Res Dev 39(4):543–548

Roden DF, Altman KW (2013) Causes of dysphagia among different age groups: a systematic review of the literature. Otolaryngol Clin N Am 46(6):965–987

Rommel N, Hamdy S (2016) Oropharyngeal dysphagia: manifestations and diagnosis. Nat Rev Gastroenterol Hepatol 13(1):49–59

Rosenbek JC, Robbins JA, Roecker EB et al (1996) A penetration-aspiration scale. Dysphagia 11(2):93–98

Sasaki H (1991) Management of respiratory diseases in the elderly. Nippon-Kyobu-Shikkan-Gakkai-Zasshi 29:1227–1233

Scharitzer M, Roesner I, Pokieser P et al. (2019) Simultaneous Radiological and Fiberendoscopic Evaluation of Swallowing ("SIRFES") in Patients After Surgery of Oropharyngeal/Laryngeal Cancer and Postoperative Dysphagia. Dysphagia 34(6):852-861

Schröter-Morasch H (1993) Klinische Untersuchung der am Schluckvorgang beteiligten Organe (Clinical examination). In: Bartolome G et al (eds) Diagnostik und Therapie neurologisch bedingter Schluckstörungen. Gustav Fischer, Stuttgart, pp 73–108

Schröter-Morasch H (1996) Schweregradeinteilung der Aspiration bei Patienten mit Schluckstörung (Severity of aspiration in dysphagic patients). In: Gross VM (ed) Aktuelle phoniatrisch-pädaudiologische Aspekte

(Current phoniatric-paediatric audiological aspects). R. Gross Verlag, Berlin, pp 145–146

Silbergleit AK, Schultz L, Jacobson BH et al (2012) The Dysphagia Handicap Index: development and validation. Dysphagia 27(1):46–52

Smithard DG (2002) Swallowing and stroke. Neuro effects recovery. Cerebrovasc Dis 14(1):1–8

Smithard D (2016) Dysphagia: a geriatric giant? Med Clin Rev 2(1):5. https://doi.org/10.21767/2471-299X.1000014

Smithard DG, O'Neill PA, Park C et al (1997) Complications and outcome after acute stroke. Does dysphagia matter? Stroke 27(7):1200–1204

Speyer R, Cordier R, Kertscher B et al (2014) Psychometric properties of questionnaires on functional health status in oropharyngeal dysphagia: a systematic literature review. Biomed Res Int 2014:458678. https://doi.org/10.1155/2014/458678

Suntrup-Krueger S, Minnerup J, Muhle P et al (2018) The effect of improved dysphagia care on outcome in patients with acute stroke: trends from 8-year data of a large stroke register. Cerebrovasc Dis 45(3–4):101–108

Woisard V, Sordes F (2014) Health related quality of life and oropharyngeal dysphagia. J Gastroenterol Hepatol Res 3(10):1292–1300

Zuercher P, Moret CS, Dziewas R, Schefold JC. Dysphagia in the intensive care unit: epidemiology, mechanisms, and clinical management. Crit Care. 2019;28;23(1):103.

# Special Kinds of Dysphagia

27

Antoinette am Zehnhoff-Dinnesen,
Carl-Albert Bader, Liesbeth ten Cate,
Daniele Farneti, Pascale Fichaux-Bourin,
Gerrit J. M. Hemmink, Irena Hočevar Boltežar,
Mieke Moerman, Heidrun Schröter-Morasch,
Miroslav Tedla, Dirk Vanneste,
Melanie-Jasmin Vauth-Weidig, Virginie Woisard,
and Patrick G. Zorowka

The original version of the chapter has been revised. A correction to this chapter can be found at https://doi.org/10.1007/978-3-031-48091-1_18

A. am Zehnhoff-Dinnesen (✉)
Department of Phoniatrics and Pedaudiology,
University Hospital Münster,
Münster, Germany
e-mail: am.zehnhoff@uni-muenster.de

C.-A. Bader
Department of Otorhinolaryngology, University
Hospital Saarland Homburg, Homburg/Saar,
Germany
e-mail: c-a.bader@web.de

L. ten Cate
Stem en Spraak, Logopedie aan de Amstel,
Amsterdam, Netherlands
e-mail: ltencate@xs4all.nl

D. Farneti
Audiology Phoniatric Service, ENT Department,
"Infermi" Hospital Rimini, Rimini, Italy
e-mail: Italydaniele.farneti@auslromagna.it

P. Fichaux-Bourin
Centre de référence du syndrome de Prader-Willi,
Hôpital des Enfants, Toulouse, France
e-mail: fichaux-bourin.p@chu-toulouse.fr

G. J. M. Hemmink
Department of Gastroenterology, Isala, Zwolle,
The Netherlands
e-mail: g.j.m.hemmink@isala.nl

I. Hočevar Boltežar
Department of Otorhinolaryngology and
Cervicofacial Surgery, Faculty of Medicine, Ljubljana
University Medical Centre, Ljubljana, Slovenia
e-mail: irena.hocevar-boltezar@mf.uni-lj.si

M. Moerman
Petegem a/d Leie_Deinze, Belgium

H. Schröter-Morasch
Klinik für, nicht fuer Frührehabilitation und
Physikalische Medizin, München Klinik
Bogenhausen, Munich, Germany
e-mail: HSM@extern.LRZ-muenchen.de

M. Tedla
Faculty of Medicine, Department of ENT
and HNS, Comenius University,
University Hospital Bratislava,
Bratislava, Slovakia
e-mail: miroslav.tedla@unb.sk

D. Vanneste
Privatpraxis for Speech and Voice Therapy,
Kooigem (Kortrijk), Belgium

M.-J. Vauth-Weidig
Clinic of Phoniatrics and Pedaudiology,
University Hospital Muenster,
Muenster, Germany
e-mail: Melanie-Jasmin.Vauth-Weidig@ukmuenster.de

V. Woisard
Voice and Deglutition Unit in Larrey Hospital and
Onco-Rehabilitation Unit in Oncopole Hospital,
Larrey Hospital and Oncopole Hospital,
Toulouse, France
e-mail: woisard.virginie@iuct-incopole.fr

P. G. Zorowka
Department for Hearing, Voice and Speech Disorders,
Medical University Innsbruck, Innsbruck, Austria
e-mail: patrick.zorowka@i-med.ac.at

## 27.1 Paediatric Dysphagia

Pascale Fichaux-Bourin and Carl-Albert Bader

### 27.1.1 Introduction

Much attention has been paid to dysphagia of paediatric patients since the 1990s. This is reflected in an increasing number of publications on the subject, as well as in the establishment of special facilities for the diagnosis and treatment of dysphagia in children.

The special status of dysphagia in children is based on the fact that, in contrast to adult patients, it occurs in a person who is still growing and maturing (Dodrill and Gosa 2015). This developmental process is very fast during the perinatal time and reaches a plateau at 10 years of age. Throughout adulthood, the development remains stable until it degrades gradually during senescence. It is necessary to consider the fast transformation in infants because abnormal development will have a harmful effect on swallowing in adulthood, and also on other functions such as phonation and breathing. In addition to consequences seen in adult patients, such as malnutrition and respiratory distress, they can have serious consequences for the motor, intellectual, mental and social development of the child. In particular, owing to dysphagia, a disturbed psychosocial interaction between child and caregiver can be expected (Craig 2013), as well as effects on the quality of life of the caregivers (Lefton-Greif et al. 2015).

The phoniatrician has to diagnose the cause, the severity and the level of risk of the disorders. They will also have to ensure a coordinating role in management of the interdisciplinary team, including at least a speech therapist and dietician. But first of all let us reconsider the distinction between feeding and swallowing disorders.

### 27.1.2 Definition and Differentiation

The term *dysphagia in children* is used very broadly and is almost universally used for aetiologically very different disorders of nutritional intake in childhood. In particular, there is a lack or vague separation between feeding disorders (ICD F98.2) and dysphagia in children (see also the comments in Frey 2011a) even though both disorders in some cases may occur simultaneously. Another distinction needs to be made from myofunctional disorders in the orofacial area (ICD F82.2) (International Statistical Classification XE "Classification" of Diseases and Related Health Problems 2015).

> "Swallowing begins at the lips and ends in the stomach" (Arvedson and Brodsky 2002)

This statement marks on the one hand the anatomical sections in which dysphagia in children is manifested, and on the other also makes clear that the term *dysphagia in children* combines two disorder complexes, which should be differentiated, not only for systematic reasons but also with regard to diagnostic and therapeutic measures.

*Oesophageal* dysphagia falls within the field of the paediatrician specialized in gastroenterology, while *oropharyngeal* dysphagia, in addition to the neuro-paediatric field, is primarily the topic of phoniatrics, ENT and paediatric pulmonology. This article refers only to oropharyngeal dysphagia.

### 27.1.3 Some Recall of the Child's Development

Suckling begins rather early in embryonic life appearing as comparatively simple tongue movements starting from the 15th week of gestational age (WGA) (Sonies et al. 1981). Pharyngeal swallowing is noticed in ultrasonic studies as of the 12th WGA. Suckling and swallowing gradually join to become functional between the 34th and 37th WGA (Miller et al. 2003) taking part in the neural network activation of the central suckling pattern generation (Barlow and Estep 2006). Suckling and swallowing also play a role in the growth of the upper aerodigestive tracts, both from the mouth to the stomach and from the trachea to the alveoli. Amniotic fluid passes as much through the digestive as it does through the respiratory tract. The mother's womb is the place of the first sensory experiences for the baby about to be born. Olfactory and gustatory particles are transferred to the placenta. At birth the new-born must adapt quickly to extra-uterine life meaning that suckling and swallowing must already be coordinated and synchronised with breathing (Lau et al. 2003). During the first month, this activity is purely reflexive (Qureshi et al. 2002) depending on the brainstem and neuro-endocrine control for installing the primary learning rhythms and the wake-sleep and hunger-satiety cycles. All the motility of the baby is controlled by the brainstem. Gradually, the immature cortex will grow rich by various neuronal circuits linked to the first sensorimotor experiences. This encephalisation, or corticospinal takeover, is preceded by the apoptotic death of the unused neurons and refinement of the synaptic connections (Lagercrantz and Ringstedt 2001). It is thus easy to understand why this perinatal period is paramount in the infant's cerebral construction. While unused premotor patterns disappear those used evolve from gross to fine motility.

Similar maturation processes occur in the digestive maturation of oesophageal peristalsis (Staiano et al. 2008; Gupta et al. 2009) and gastric emptying which evolves with the rhythmicity of meals and the gradually increasing volumes of milk.

During this diversification the infant passes gradually from liquid to semi-solid food, suckling evolving to sucking then to chewing around 10–12 months of age. Concerning orofacial motility, the tongue becomes independent of the mandible, thus supporting the change in alimentary tract content texture from lumpy to soft pieces. A similar change is seen for the management of liquids from the feeding-bottle to the cup, with mouthful aspiration by a dissociated movement of the lips and the tongue. These various stages follow those of psychomotor development, with a stable head posture at 4 months, and sitting at 6 months when coordination and balance control begin. The baby at this stage picks up objects, turns the wrist to observe it, and attempts to pass it from one hand to the other side via the mouth. Eye-hand and hand-mouth control becomes increasingly refined. From the 8th to 9th month, the infant starts to want to eat by himself (Arvedson and Lefton-Greif 1996).

## 27.1.4 Aetiology of Paediatric Swallowing Disorders

Major diagnostic categories associated with swallowing disorders are defined as neurological, anatomical and structural, genetic, secondary to systemic illness, psychosocial and behavioural or secondary to a resolved medical condition (Arvedson and Brodsky 2002).

### 27.1.4.1 Non-developmental Central Neurological Causes

- They can be acquired and will have different consequences according to the location:

  - Encephalopathies (e.g., cerebral palsy or perinatal asphyxia): swallowing problems will depend on the severity of the cerebral lesions. They are mild in diplegia or hemiplegia; usually limited to a slight lack of bolus formation. In quadriplegia, the severity of the disorder is determined by the spasticity, the level of dependence and the associated disability. In most cases, only the oral phase is deficient, which explains the lack of diagnosis during the infant's first months of life. The pharyngeal phase is rarely deficient but if pharyngeal transport is affected swallowing disorders will be more severe (Rogers et al. 1994). Dysphagia is expected in 25–30% of di-or hemi-paresis patients, and 60% to over 90% of patients with tetra-paresis and in extra pyramidal movement disorders (Arvedson and Brodsky 2002; Calis et al. 2008).
  - Brainstem injury: this may occur secondary to anoxia by prolonged/obstructed labour causing severe swallowing disorders from birth onwards. Brainstem tumours associated with cranial nerve palsy also may cause swallowing disorders. Neonatal dysfunction of the brainstem has, e.g., been described by Abadie et al. (1996) in form of abnormal lingual posture, abnormal maxillofacial growth, disorders of pharyngo-laryngeal tone and motility, and

also upper digestive disorders such as gastro-oesophageal reflux (Abadie et al. 1999, 2002). The most outstanding example is the Pierre Robin sequence (Abadie and Couly 2013; Thouvenin et al. 2013).

- They can be structural brain abnormalities such as gyration anomalies. Often, they are associated with a microcephalus and intellectual disabilities but can also arise from agenesis of the corpus callosum or atrophy of the cerebellar vermis. These disorders depend on the extent of the lesions and are associated with lack of bolus propulsion and synchronisation. Sometimes cranio-cervical junction anomalies can cause swallowing disorders. In this case they can be congenital, such as the Chiari malformation with variable degrees of brainstem herniation or elongation, and of vermian herniation. They can be acquired such as traumatic cervical spine injury during dystocic delivery.

### 27.1.4.2 Developmental Central Neurological Causes

Because swallowing disorders will develop in the course of the underlying pathology it is necessary to instigate at least an annual functional follow-up according to the severity of the encephalopathy. Most cases are associated with a drug-resistant epilepsy or with encephalopathies (Fig. 27.1) caused by lysosomal storage disorders, such as Niemann-Pick disease, Gaucher's disease or Mucopolysaccharidosis.

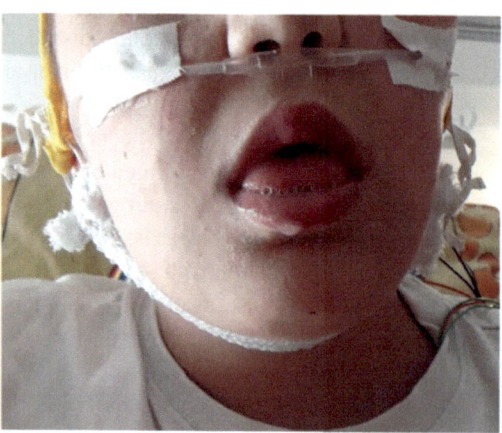

**Fig. 27.1** Encephalopathy and drooling

### 27.1.4.3 Peripheral Neurological Causes

- Cranial nerve injury: vagal nerve injury can be secondary to cardiac surgery, furthermore nervi IX, X, and XII can be injured by cervical tumour surgery.
- Neuromuscular disease:
  - Metabolic myopathies, lysosomal dysfunction of glycogenesis or lipogenesis, thyroid hormone deficiency or mitochondrial myopathies due to dysfunction of the respiratory chain.
  - Genetic myopathies such as the myotonic dystrophy of Duchesne, initially characterized by impaired oral control followed by a motility reduction progressing from oral to pharyngeal. By contrast, in the myotonic dystrophy of Steinert swallowing disorders are prominent and occur in the pharyngeal phase from the beginning of the disease.
  - Spinal Muscular Atrophy (SMA) with its three forms; the vital prognosis of the first two types is decided before the age of 2 years. For Type II SMA the first signs appear after 6 months, for Type III SMA after 18 months. They are associated with paralysis leading to lack of propulsion, velopharyngeal insufficiency and respiratory disorders.
  - Myasthenia gravis in infants: this can be a neonatal myasthenia gravis, by mothers who have myasthenia; if treated promptly, infants generally recover within 2 months after birth. On the other hand, it can be a rare hereditary form of myasthenia, called congenital myasthenic syndrome. The diagnosis is made by the association of progressive muscular weakness with fasting tiredness and partial or total recovery at rest.

### 27.1.4.4 Genetic Causes

Many genetic syndromes are associated with swallowing and feeding disorders. The first diagnosis to consider is the Prader-Willi syndrome, when newborn present severe hypotonia and poor sucking (Diène et al. 2007; Fichaux-Bourin et al.

2009; Tauber et al. 2017). Major axial hypotonia is associated with an oropharyngeal hypotonia causing nasopharyngeal reflux and pharyngeal residues. These fragile babies face an important risk of aspiration.

The other genetic causes can be classified in three groups:

- Those that present with hypotonia and intellectual disability such as Trisomy 21 or Trisomy 18, Fragile X syndrome or monosomy 5p, also known as "Cri du Chat syndrome". Here, swallowing disorders are the consequence of a delayed acquisition of the oral phase and lack of oral transport.
- Those that involve hypothalamic-pituitary axis dysregulation with loss of appetite control and other dysfunctions of the endocrine system. These growth disorders can occur before and after birth, such as in Russel-Silver syndrome. Mutations in the *HRAS* gene cause Noonan syndrome, Costello syndrome, and cardiofaciocutaneous syndrome (Lorenz et al. 2013). This gene codes for H-RAS, which is part of a pathway that helps to control cell growth, division and differentiation. Because of the abnormal H-RAS protein, many of the symptoms probably result from cell overgrowth and abnormal cell division responsible for both leukaemia and solid tumours, which can be associated with moderate to severe feeding disorders, dysmorphic facial and cutaneous signs, angiogenesis disorders, and heart disease.
- Those that associate with craniofacial abnormalities and cranial nerve impairment due to defects of the first, second and third branchial arches, such as Franceschetti syndrome and Goldenhar syndrome for the first branchial arch, Moebius syndrome for the second, and Pierre Robin sequence (Fig. 27.2) or 22q11 deletion for the third (Johnson et al. 2011a, b; Abadie and Couly 2013).

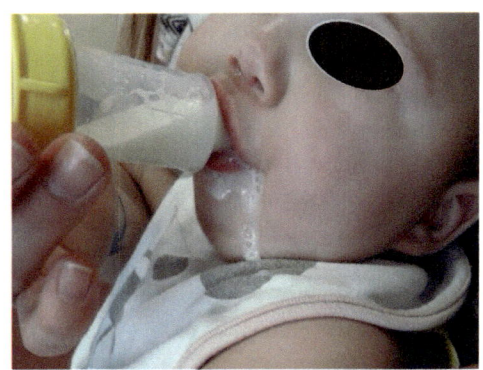

**Fig. 27.2** Pierre Robin sequence and drooling

### 27.1.4.5 Anatomical and Structural Causes

These can be congenital or acquired. Any anomaly of the aerodigestive tracts of the mouth to the duodenum can be the cause of swallowing disorders. The pathological mechanisms then will depend on the importance and the location of the anomaly.

- In the case of craniofacial anomalies, the most severe ones are the midface hypoplasia such as the craniosynostoses of Crouzon or Apert, due to premature closure of the cranial sutures. The phenotypic presentation is highly variable and comprises cranial synostosis, midface hypoplasia, ocular ptosis or cleft palate. Consequences manifest both in airway obstruction and oral feeding ability. In the case of facial clefts, the failure of facial fusion can affect the lip, philtrum, alveolus, hard and soft palate. In cleft lip/alveolus, lack of lip closure leads to failure to thrive. Usually, the primary cheiloplasty will resolve the difficulties in the first weeks of life. On the other hand, for clefts involving the hard and soft palate, feeding difficulties are due to failure in setting up a negative intra-oral pressure and in protecting the nasopharynx during sucking and swallowing. Palate orthosis and adapted feeding bottles can support feeding and swallowing skills during the first months before the secondary maxillofacial surgery of palatoplasty.

- Congenital tumours of the neck, oral cavity and tongue (lymphangiomas, teratomas, congenital cysts, etc.) are an obstacle to sucking, swallowing and breathing. Early management often requires a tracheotomy and feeding tube until surgical treatment is performed as soon as possible (Gupta et al. 2007). Macroglossia may also interfere with breathing, swallowing and speaking, e.g., in the case of a Beckwith-Wiedemann syndrome or a Down syndrome.
- Laryngeal anomalies can be morphological, dynamic or can reflect a tonus defect. They may present with stridor and feeding problems. Flexible nasopharyngoscopy with or without rigid direct laryngoscopy provides different sets of information for the diagnosis of laryngeal cleft, chronic reflux laryngitis, supraglottal cyst, vocal fold paralysis or paradoxical vocal fold motion and laryngomalacia.
- Tracheo-oesophageal fistulae need to be systematically looked for in a baby presenting with the triad of coughing, choking and cyanosis without a particular pathological context. In case of oesophageal atresia or diaphragmatic hernia, reduced oesophageal motility and gastro-oesophageal reflux (GER) persist even after specific surgery. They have a negative impact on eating and feeding skills, increasing the risk of eating and feeding disorders owing to early oral deprivation. Other upper digestive tract anomalies can comprise achalasia of the oesophagus (Pyun et al. 2015), microgastria (Giurgea et al. 2000) and pyloric stenosis. Their symptoms may vary from gagging to vomiting, associated with limited appetite and food refusal, driven by the lack of digestive clearance and the GER.
- Inflammatory or infectious causes (stomatitis, strep throat and epiglottitis) and anatomical injury by caustic ingestion.

### 27.1.4.6 Systemic Consequences of Pathologies

Infants are not able to maintain good homeostasis or an efficient synchronisation of sucking-swallowing with a respiratory illness (chronic lung disease, bronchopulmonary dysplasia, deficiency of surfactant protein) or congenital cardiac anomalies, which explains their frequent failure to thrive. Moreover, they are at high risk of aspiration because of the limited duration of apnoea.

Gastrointestinal (GI) illness, such as GI dysmotility constipation, can be a source of pain and may cause sudden anorexia in a child without a particular pathology. On the other hand, congenital or acquired short bowel syndrome, food allergies, gluten sensitivity or celiac disease, may all cause nutritional disorders more than swallowing or feeding disorders.

Nephrological pathologies involving a major lack of craving require enteral feeding support, although the child has no dysphagia.

Finally, the side effects of chemotherapy and radiotherapy for cancer in infants and children may have an impact on swallowing and feeding skills because of fatigue, pain, mucositis, nausea and vomiting.

### 27.1.4.7 Causes Secondary to Resolved Medical Condition

Prematurity by birth or weight is the leading cause (Sharma et al. 2016; Adams-Chapman et al. 2013). In addition, there are prolonged feeding difficulties, impaired maturation, and negative sensory stimulation in neonates by intubation, probes and tube feeding.

Hospitalisation as well as the consequences of prolonged parenteral or enteral feeding in turn may lead to an impaired acquisition of swallowing and feeding skills. Oral deprivation exacerbates these disorders.

### 27.1.4.8 Behavioural and Psychological Pathologies

Both can appear as side effect of a maternal psychopathology or a bonding or attachment disorder. They can also result from a child's psychopathology, such as infantile anorexia, food phobias or autism. They will be described in detail in a following chapter about feeding disorders.

## 27.1.5 Diagnostics

The diagnosis of oropharyngeal dysphagia in children ideally results from an interdisciplinary approach involving medical and non-medical professionals (Arvedson 2008).

### 27.1.5.1 Procedures

The procedures usually rely on:

- Medical history (anamnesis)
- Clinical examination
- Instrument-based diagnostics

Major topics of the *anamnesis* are general diseases of the child and pre-existing, potentially dysphagia-triggering conditions. In addition, key data of the overall development of the child need to be assessed as well as its family relationships. Further, information about the special food history is required such as the development of swallowing competence, the type of nutrition (oral, tube feeding), preferred food consistencies, the food and drink items consumed, and the position taken during eating and drinking.

Arvedson (2013) formulated four important aspects of the feeding history that should be clarified, such as:

- Feeding time
- Burden on parents and children through food intake
- Weight gain of the child
- Indications of respiratory problems

The author mentions as warning signs of relevant dysphagia a feeding time exceeding 30 minutes, stress in the child or the parents while eating, a lack of weight gain by the child over 2–3 months or even a loss of weight (especially within the first 2 years of life) as well as frequent (deep) respiratory infections, and a gurgling voice. The presence of these warning signals should be a reason for further clarification.

For the *clinical examination* of swallowing, no clear recommendations can yet be formulated with regard to a standardised procedure

(Heckathorn et al. 2016). This also applies to screening methods. Therefore, an approach based on individual ideas, intuition and experience will be used. Above all, the documentation of the following aspects can be regarded as relevant:

- General and nutritional status
- Torso and head posture
- Examination of oral motor skills (depending on the ability of the child to cooperate)
- Observation of spontaneous swallowing (and in particular of the spontaneous swallowing drive)

*Clinical examination*
- Observing the intake of food of different consistencies, including detecting auditory abnormal phenomena (such as a "wet voice", conspicuous swallowing sounds, stridor, coughing, clearing throat, etc.), as well as behavioural problems (such as refusing to eat) and observing the interaction between caregiver and child.

*Instrumental diagnostics* have significant importance in identifying the pathophysiological mechanisms that underly dysphagia in order to develop a suitable therapy. Following Schröter-Morasch (2005), there are three main aspects of impaired swallowing:

- Incomplete transport with oral or pharyngeal residues after swallowing
- Execution of a via falsa with the consequence of penetration or aspiration
- Retrograde transport with drooling, reflux or regurgitation phenomena

Basically, the same instrumented-based procedures as those used in adults are available in paediatric swallowing diagnostics. However, each of these procedures is typically limited in the child. In addition, age and developmental characteristics of the child's swallowing should be taken into account for the interpretation of all findings. Depending on the equipment and the individual experience of the examiner, the following procedures can be used in the diagnosis of oropharyngeal dysphagia:

- Flexible-endoscopic evaluation of swallowing (FEES), possibly also with sensory testing (FEESST)
- Videofluoroscopic swallow study (VFSS) or comparable radiological procedures
- Ultrasonographic examination
- Manometry
- Surface electromyographie (sEMG)

The *flexible-endoscopic evaluation* of the swallowing act uses the technique of transnasal endoscopy with a flexible light guide. Today, the findings are usually documented by computers. The method was first described by Langmore et al. (1988) as 'fiberoptic evaluation of swallowing' for use in adult patients, and subsequently considered suitable for the paediatric dysphagia patient (Willging 1995).Given a sufficient experience of the examiner and her/his compliance with safety measures, FEES can be considered as a safe and low-complication procedure when used in children (Bader and Niemann 2007). The food tests are performed after ensuring that the child is in a stable cardio-respiratory state and ready to be nourished. However, limitations of feasibility and accessibility must be expected, owing to a limited ability to cooperate, to anatomical and structural conditions and limited visibility (especially in the subglottal area) (Bader and Niemann 2010; Böckler 2015), see Fig. 27.3.

Digital video recording allows storage and retrieval of images from evaluations performed at different times.

The typical endoscopic examination procedure can be subdivided into different parts. After assessment of the anatomical structures, and functional testing without food, swallowing of food is tested with offering age-appropriate consistencies. Bolus volumes, timing and other characteristics are varied by the examiner. Depending on the individual situation and the state of therapy, therapeutic measures can also be tested endoscopically for their efficacy (Arens et al. 2015).

The *videofluoroscopic swallow study (VFSS)*, for which several synonyms are used, combines a dynamic radiological examination technique with video documentation. It was developed by

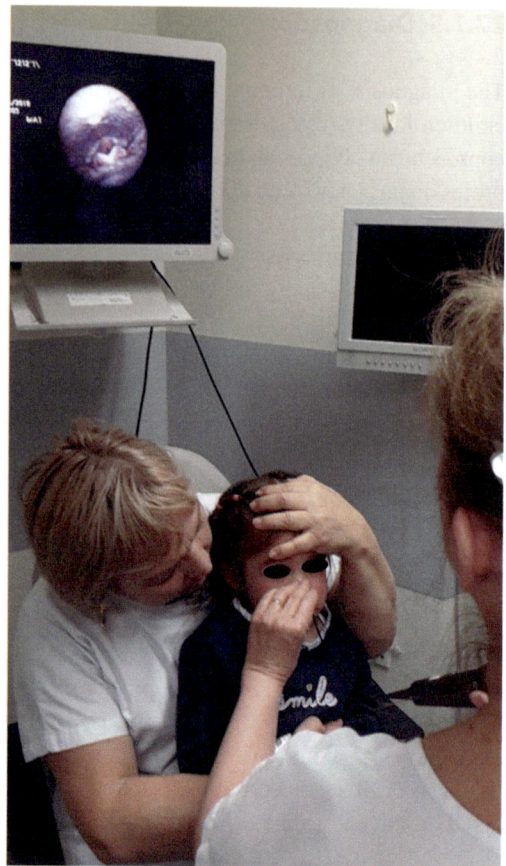

**Fig. 27.3** Child undergoing flexible laryngoscopy to assess swallowing

Logemann (1993) and has been used in the paediatric field for many years. The technique focuses on bone abnormalities (vertebrae, maxillary, and mandibular), on the oesophageal-gastric junction and the dynamics and synchronisation at various times of swallowing (Arvedson 2008). Videofluoroscopy comprises food-free swallowing tests and swallowing tests with food by using X-rays, whereby the food of interest must generate sufficient contrast. The use of videofluoroscopy is limited due to the exposure of the child to ionising radiation, especially if organs such as the thyroid gland and the bulbi are in the field of exposure. Hersh et al. (2016) calculated exposure doses for paediatric videofluoroscopy that were ten times higher compared with chest radiographs, but only 1/10 of the computed tomography exposure of the skull.

To obtain radiographic images of sufficient quality, the patient needs to be positioned accurately and has to stay stably within the beam path. The child's positioning is determined by his developmental age and his motor skills, sitting or lying down on a moulded-foam cushion for

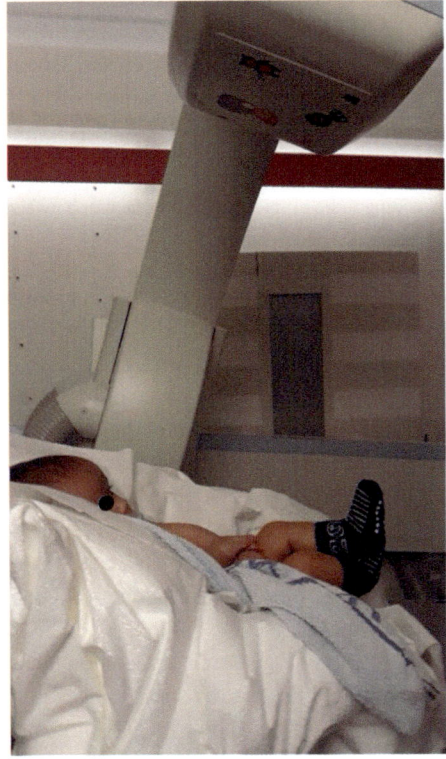

**Fig. 27.4** Example of an infant's positioning during videofluorosocopy of swallowing

babies or special seats for older children. Optionally, the contrast solution (Barium sulfate or iohexol) can be mixed with fruit juice or thickened water. Tests can also include a piece of cake for assessing the quality of oral preparation and of oral continence during chewing. For babies, the contrast solution is mixed with mineral water in the same proportions and is administered with a feeding bottle. See Figs. 27.4 and 27.5.

Despite their limitations, flexible endoscopic swallowing diagnostics and videofluoroscopy are established standard procedures, which in adult patients are considered to be complementary, rather than competing (Langmore 2003). For their application in children there are only few data available so far. To verify aspiration events, however, both methods seem to be equally suited in children (da Silva et al. 2010).

*Ultrasonography* has been used primarily to visualize the structures of the floor of the mouth and tongue, including the hyoid bone, and to depict oral movements. It is also able to reveal selected aspects of the pharyngeal phase (Barberena et al. 2014). However, owing to methodological limitations, it is not suitable for detecting aspiration.

The use of *manometric methods* was initially described in the paediatric patient only for use in oesophageal dysphagia. In the meantime, the method has also been succesfully used for the evaluation of the pharyngo-oesophageal transition in children (Ferris et al. 2016) and especially as high-resolution manometry (Rommel et al.

**Fig. 27.5** Example of an older child's positioning during videofluorosocopy of swallowing

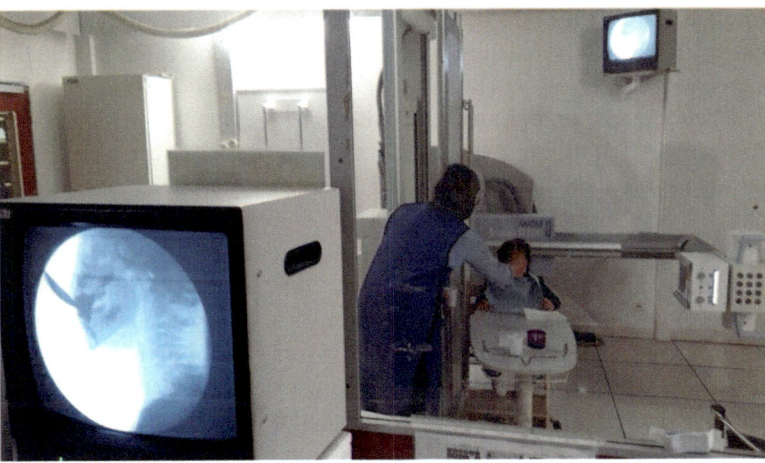

2011; Knigge et al. 2014). A final assessment of manometric methods is currently not possible.

*Electromyography* (EMG)- generally done as surface EMG (sEMG) - can be performed, e.g., in the event of ineffective suction alternatively to ultrasonography to visualize the oral phase and to determine the temporal synchronisation between oral movements and pharyngeal propulsion.

### 27.1.5.2 Interdisciplinary Evaluation

The converging views of the different actors enable the interdisciplinary team to better characterise the needs of the child with a swallowing disorder and of his parents.

**The Nurse's Assessment** The nurse collects the anthropometric data (height, weight, cranial circumference, etc.). She or he outlines the parents' tolerance, exhaustion and their desire for change. It is the first step in the educational diagnosis.

**Medical Evaluation** The clinical examination of the child will primarily search for signs suggesting the cause of the disorder, and will assess their consequences. Further, imaging assessment helps to verify the diagnosis and to define the therapeutic management as well as the follow-up regime. The therapeutic concept is mainly implemented by speech therapists and dieticians. Both, the rehabilitation and adaptation programmes are not conceived without the active participation of the parents and the care givers.

It is thus necessary to specify the handicap felt by the entourage to feed the child, the meal's duration, the signs raised by the parents testifying to the child's difficulties, but also to their own stress felt in front of possible aspiration, vomiting or ceaseless crying and tears.

**The Speech and Language Therapist's Assessment** The therapist evaluates the communication skills and the sensorimotor and training abilities of the child. In the paediatric dysphagia field there is a need for a validated non-instrumental evaluation of swallowing and feeding function. As recalled by Heckathorn, there is a high variability among the many assessments available to the clinicians in this field, and mostly those have not been evaluated for validity or reliability (Heckathorn et al. 2016). Some

standardised scales are available such as NOMAS (Neonatal Oral Motor Assessment Scale) for infants of less than six months (Palmer et al. 1993; da Costa and van der Schans 2008; da Costa et al. 2016) and SOMA (Schedule of Oral Motor Assessment) for children (Reilly and Skuse 1999). The difficulty lies in the accuracy of the clinical evaluation in detecting penetration or aspiration (DeMatteo et al. 2005).

In the feeding context, however, assessment of behaviour, environment and qualities of interactions between the child and his parents is required. As recalled by Chatoor:

"Feeding to be efficient needs interaction between giving-receiving" Chatoor et al. (1998a)

Regarding the importance of the interactional aspect, it is necessary to consider the three stages of feeding development: homeostasis until two months, when food intake is a reflex and the infant in total dependence; attachment until six months, when the child initiates the exchange and the meal becomes a social event; finally separation and individualisation, when the child can refuse food and wants to eat by himself.

**The Dietetic Assessment** It contains a quantitative and qualitative evaluation. The dietician appreciates the energy demand recommended for the age of the child and the specific needs of the associated pathology. She or he gets information about the weaning and diversification history of the child from his parents and asks for the context of the meals, the description of the child's appetite, his likes and dislikes. The discussion with the parents also outlines the parental concepts concerning food in general and of their child in particular; do they have strong concerns about diet?

The dietetic diagnosis thus determines the nutritional composition and will ensure that nutritional balance and daily recommended contributions are respected (protein, fatty acids, vitamins, minerals, not too many sweet products or polyunsaturated fats).

**Further Assessments** These include dental examination, tests by psychologists, paediatricians, neurologists, gastroenterologists, geneticists, etc.

**Synthesis of this Multidisciplinary Evaluation** The conclusions of the different assessments are presented and discussed with the family in order to define and explain with them the treatment planned.

At the end of this multidisciplinary evaluation, the following questions will have been answered:

- Is there a swallowing disorder? What is its nature? If a genetic disorder, neurological impairment, gastrointestinal dysfunction or psychopathology are suspected, it is necessary to ask other specialists for complementary opinions.
- Is oral feeding possible?
  - If so, we need to focus on what quantity, what frequency during the day, what enrichment is required.
  - Oral sensory approaches to feeding: adaptation to the sensory environment, physical handling techniques, modified textures of food and drinks, specific feeding utensils are usually needed.
  - Position and posture management to avoid aspiration or to enhance oral propulsion.
  - Direct oral sensorimotor treatment to help the child in the oral preparatory phase of swallowing which is focused on jaws, lips, tongue and cheeks. However, careful analysis of the child's responses is necessary to avoid adverse or stressful reactions.
  - If not, how to avoid negative impact on feeding and swallowing skills in case of an exclusive enteral feeding? Here, controlled oral feeding tests or simple gustatory and scent stimulations are important to maintain at least the ability to swallow saliva and secretions.
- What are the consequences? They can be infectious, requiring specific treatments; nutritional, requiring a food enrichment and sometimes enteral feeding support; or psychological, requiring specific management.
- Are specific programmes prescribed to enhance swallowing and feeding? Is a programme of rehabilitation indicated, involving parental accompaniment or weekly rehabilitation with a speech therapist? Is an occupational therapist needed for the child's positioning (adaptive seating, head support system, etc.) and the environmental adaptation? Should a psychiatric therapy be considered?
- Which functional follow-up is necessary? This will obviously depend on associated pathologies and the kind of disorders present. The interval can vary from 3 to12 months, according to the child's development. It should be carried out sooner in the case of exclusive tube feeding, in order to follow the development of the disorder and to change as soon as possible to oral feeding.

## 27.1.6 Therapy and Progress

Ensuring adequate nutrition with the best possible respiratory protection is a particularly important therapeutic goal in children with a swallowing disorder. Other aspects, such as the child's quality of life, the prognosis of his underlying disease and the individual parent–child relationship have to be considered as well.

From the *medical side*, both surgical and non-surgical procedures can be used (see overview in Tutor and Gosa 2012). Especially pharmacotherapy plays a role in reducing the production of saliva by administration of cholinergic drugs. The injection of botulinum toxin into the salivary glands is also possible.

Among the surgical options, tracheotomy or tracheostomy can be carried out under stringent indication, e.g., in cases of persistent saliva aspiration. It should be reserved for the experienced surgeon. In combination with a suitable cannula, it contributes to the protection of the respiratory tract if this cannot be achieved by other means.

In children, a tracheostoma is considered to be a more risky situation than in adults (Kremer et al. 2012). Therefore, both the tracheostoma and the trachea need regular and careful endoscopic checks. Especially in paediatric patients who have been tracheostomised over an extended period, the anterior wall of the trachea should be monitored thoroughly as lesions in this region — if they remain undetected— can lead to a lethal trachea-arterial fistula (Schaefer and Irwin 1995). However, this complication will be extremely rare if the tracheostomy tubes are adapted in their diameter, length, and material to the child's conditions.

A non-oral diet belongs to the field of medical intervention, if no safe and sufficient nutrition is possible per os. Alternative ways of fluid and caloric intake can be ensured by:

• Insertion of a nasogastric (possibly also an orogastric) tube
• Application of a gastrostomy [usually in the sense of a percutaneous endoscopic gastrostomy/PEG or jejunostomy/PEJ].
• Parenteral nutrition through an appropriate intravenous access.

For medium and long term periods, the PEG/PEJ plan is the most important, with typical complications to be considered (Baker et al. 2015).

Of great importance in the treatment of childhood dysphagia is the treatment provided by *non-medical therapist*s. Different professional groups (e.g., academic and non-academic speech therapists, occupational therapists, physiotherapists, and others) may be involved and a variety of therapeutic approaches may be used.

From a systematic view, the common treatment concepts can be divided into:

• Procedures that follow a specific "school" (such as Vojta Therapy, Bobath Neurodevelopmental Therapy, Kay Coombes Facial Oral Tract Therapy [FOTT®], Proprioceptive Neuromuscular Facilitation [PNF] by Kabat, Orofacial Regulation Therapy by Castillo-Morales etc.)
• Symptom-orientated procedures that combine, modify and reinterpret meaningful therapeutic approaches from different schools and, of course, contribute their own approaches (e.g., Frey 2011b; Bartolome and Schröter-Morasch 2014).

For children with cerebral palsy and oropharyngeal swallowing disorders the following therapeutic goals are particularly important :

• Improving the posture and positioning of the patient
• Reducing pathological motor activities in the orofacial area and the (re)establishment of physiological motor actions
• Reducing oral hypersensitivity
• Stimulating the frequency of spontaneous swallowing
• Instigating measures to improve mouth closure
• Adjusting the diet
• Using suitable drinking, eating and feeding aids
• Providing parental advice and support
• Informing those involved about any emergency measures to be taken

Although there are many positive evaluations for several treatment approaches, it has to be emphasised that until now there is no evidence-based proof for the efficacy of a specific therapy. Multicentre studies with large patient groups are urgently needed to obtain a valid comparison of the efficacy of different therapeutic procedures. These studies, of course, have to adhere to strict ethical criteria.

Prognostic information regarding the course of dysphagia in children is very difficult, especially since the number of affected children is low and the causes are inhomogeneous (Gisel 2008). Endoscopic findings alone can hardly be used to derive a reliable prognosis (Sitton et al. 2011). For tetra-paretic children with severe neurogenic dysphagia in particular, the prognosis is impossible to derive.

### 27.1.7 Management of Swallowing Disorders: Some Examples

The management will depend on the nature of the disorder, its severity, and its negative impact as well as associated pathology.

### 27.1.7.1 Feeding Developmental Delays

This occurs in cases of developmental retardation, brainstem immaturity or oral food deprivation. Speech and language intervention is prescribed to enhance oral sensorimotor functions in feeding as well as in speech. Nutritional support is rarely indicated, except in case of a Pierre Robin sequence. The functional follow-up is adapted then to the child's development, considering the underlying medical status, family dynamics, social environment and oral motor skills. It can span from 3 to 6 months until 2 years.

In young children, it is generally caused by a delay of sensory and oral motor development. The oral preparatory phase of swallowing is deficient without any bolus formation or chewing, and usually the child refuses to eat lumpy or hard solid food. Speech therapy is prescribed and the functional follow-up can be proposed in intervals from 8 to 12 months.

### 27.1.7.2 Deficiency by Neurological Impairment

A multidisciplinary team, comprising a physiotherapist, occupational therapist, and speech therapist is essential. The treatment is based on inhibition of pathological sensorimotor patterns and prevention of postural anomalies and spasticity-induced orthopaedic deformations, e.g., in cases of cerebral palsy. Interventions are combined or modified by the constraints induced by movement therapies intended to guide the development of the gross motor and oral motor functions. The child's developmental age should always be kept in mind, and adaptive equipment and interventions should be adaequately used to help the child achieve his milestones. The functional follow-up will make it possible to check the improved capabilities of handling different food consistencies and the absence of nutritional consequences. In the case of a fixed pathology, timing of functional follow-up varies according to the age of the child; from every 6 months until 2 years, then annually thereafter. It can be planned at shorter intervals in case of a progressive disease, that bears the risk of an accelerated sensorimotor skill degradation with consequences on swallowing and upper airway protection.

### 27.1.7.3 Incapacity by Structural Anomalies

The goal is to avoid the negative effects of oral deprivation. Rehabilitation must be coordinated with surgical planning, proposing sensorimotor stimulations to involve sucking-swallowing patterns followed by the establishment of chewing patterns, even if the oral feeding has not yet been authorised. After surgical procedures, the programme of rehabilitation will aim for avoiding penetration, aspiration and expulsion mechanisms such as nausea or vomiting, accompanied by gradual changes of food in its consistency, texture, volume, and quantity.

### 27.1.8 Summary

- Swallowing disorders in infants and children have multi-axial diagnoses and variable consequences.
- The special status of oropharyngeal dysphagia in children is mainly due to its negative effect on the development of the child and on the interaction between child and caregiver.
- The diagnosis of paediatric dysphagia may be based on established imaging techniques known from adult dysphagia diagnostics. However, they are subject to certain limitations in the application to children and require special knowledge and experience.
- Diagnostics need to be performed as soon as possible to avoid malnutrition and the negative impact on swallowing and feeding skills. It should be repeated to adapt intervention and rehabilitation programme to the child's development.
- Diagnostics and therapy are ideally based on an interdisciplinary approach and a close cooperation between medical and non-medical specialist groups. The parents are protagonists of this management and participate in the different decisions to be made.

## 27.2   Feeding Disorders

Melanie-Jasmin Vauth-Weidig

### 27.2.1 Definition of Feeding Disorders

Infants and children with feeding disorders fail to grow adequately, or lose weight, as a result of not being able to take in, or not having received, adequate nutrients to support growth. They may be irritable or apathetic. Feeding disorders can have medical causes such as cardiac, neurological and gastro-oesophageal diseases, metabolic disorders and anatomical abnormalities. Not only associated with medical disturbances, they can also have a remarkable behaviour- and emotional-social component, including lack of nutrition, failure to read the child's hunger and satiety cues accurately, poverty, or mental or psychiatric parental illness (Chatoor 2002). Feeding disturbances affect early infant development and are associated with cognitive developmental disorders, anxiety or eating disorders, and behavioural problems in childhood, adolescence and early adulthood (Chatoor 2002).

### 27.2.2 Aetiology of Feeding Disorders

Multifactorial physiological, environmental, behavioural and psychological factors interact and may include temperamental and regulatory characteristics of child and caregiver (caregiver–infant relationship), traumatic experiences of both infant and caregiver, health problems, sensory-perceptual problems and mealtime behaviour.

### 27.2.3 Epidemiology of Feeding Disorders

Twenty-five percentage to forty-five percentage of all healthily developing infants and about 80% of infants with developmental disorders are reported to have feeding problems such as colic, slow feeding, vomiting or refusal to eat (Chatoor 2002; Linscheid et al. 2003). Severe clinical feeding disorders are experienced by 3–10% of all infants (Kerwin 1999; Jenkins et al. 1984). These children fail to grow adequately or lose weight. Severe feeding disturbances tend to persist and worsen over time. They are more prevalent in children with physical disabilities (26–90%), mental retardation (23–43%), illness or low birthweight (10–49%) (Kerwin 1999; Sharp et al. 2010; Kroll 2011).

### 27.2.4 Clinical Symptoms of Feeding Disorders

Feeding disorders show a great variability of characteristics and have to be defined multi-dimensionally. It is necessary to classify clinical symptoms as feeding disturbances, differentiating feeding disorders from less severe subclinical feeding problems, including both currently uninterpretable phenomenology and useful diagnostic characteristics.

In cases of cardiac problems, oesophageal diseases, metabolic disorders, structural abnormalities of the nasopharynx, oropharynx, larynx and oesophagus, or neurodevelopmental disabilities, the infant may show distress over the course of feeding. Owing to drowsiness or strong agitation, the child may have difficulties in reaching, obtaining or maintaining a calm state of alertness during feeding. The difficulties occur during the newborn period and last for at least 2 weeks.

After exposure to a major adverse event, such as suctioning, intubation or tube feeding, and for children with medical problems or premature infants, food or feeding sessions may be reminders of the traumatic event that caused distress and are manifested by anticipatory distress causing food refusal.

In cases of specific nutritional deficiencies or hypersensitivity, and difficulties in or a delay of oral-motor-development, the child consistently refuses to eat food with specific tastes, textures or smells; it may show picky, choosy or selective eating and low variability in food intake. These distinctive features may occur during the introduction of a novel type of food (e.g., the child may drink one type of milk, but refuse another). Children who are affected by maternal deprivation, lack of nurturing and social reciprocity do not display developmentally appropriate signs of social reciprocity (e.g., visual engagement, smiling or babbling) with the caregiver during feeding.

The onset of complete food refusal or refusal to eat adequate amounts of food occurs before the child is 3 years old and lasts at least 1 month, when one or more of the following symptoms in the child may occur (Chatoor et al. 1997; Chatoor 2002):

- Feeding is only possible with pressure or distraction.
- Poor sucking.
- Breastfeeding is only possible if the child dozes.
- Daily vomiting and regurgitation.
- Problems with chewing and swallowing.
- Less appetite, less nutrition intake over more than 1 month.
- Refusal of food.
- Crying and symptoms of distress while feeding.

In 2008, Bryant-Waught and Piepenstock listed the common disturbances in feeding/eating seen in a clinical setting as follows:

- Delay or absence of development or lack of feeding/eating skills.
- Difficulty in managing or tolerating fluids or foodstuff.
- Reluctance or refusal to eat, on the basis of taste, texture and other sensory factors.
- Lack of interest/appetite.
- Use of feeding for self-soothing, self-stimulation or comfort.

## 27.2.5 History of Terminology of Feeding/Eating Disorders

For many years, there has been no consensus on terminology of feeding disorders. Eating disorders in infancy and early childhood were dichot-omised as "Organic Failure to thrive" or "Non-Organic Failure to Thrive" (Keren 2016). In 2002, Irene Chatoor-Koch developed a classification system including six subtypes of feeding disorder. Her pioneering work (Chatoor 2002; Chatoor and Egan 1983) demonstrated that the early dichotomous classification was misleading. In cooperation with the American Academy of Child and Adolescent Psychiatry and the American Psychiatric Association the six characteristics have been advanced and taken under the title "Feeding Behaviour Disorders" in the Diagnostic Classification of Mental Health and Developmental Disorders in Infancy and Early Childhood (DC:0-3R; Zero To Three 2005).

Describing four subtypes of behavioural feeding disorder (1–4) occurring during infant development, Chatoor (2002) also underlined two types caused by medical disturbances (5–6):

1. Feeding disorder of State Regulation (Feeding disorder of Homeostasis)
2. Feeding disorder of Caregiver-Infant Reciprocity.
3. Infantile Anorexia.
4. Sensory Food Aversion.
5. Feeding disorder associated with insults to the gastrointestinal tract / Post-traumatic Feeding. Disorder of Infancy.
6. Feeding disorder with a concurrent medical condition.

In 2015, Kerzner et al. proposed a practical approach to identifying, classifying and managing feeding difficulties in infants. Their concept can be represented by a pyramid (Fig. 27.6). Kerzner et al. (2015) classify children on the basis of the parents' expressed concerns about their feeding behaviour, which fall into three categories: those not eating enough (limited appetite), those eating an inadequate variety or an inadequate amount of food (selective intake) and those afraid to eat (fear of feeding). Each category has subcategories, which indicate that such concerns may be a misperception on the part of the parents, or primarily behavioural or organic, each with a spectrum ranging from mild to severe. Because feeding is a transaction influenced by both the child's behaviour and the parents' feeding technique, the categories also include the four fundamental feeding styles that have the potential

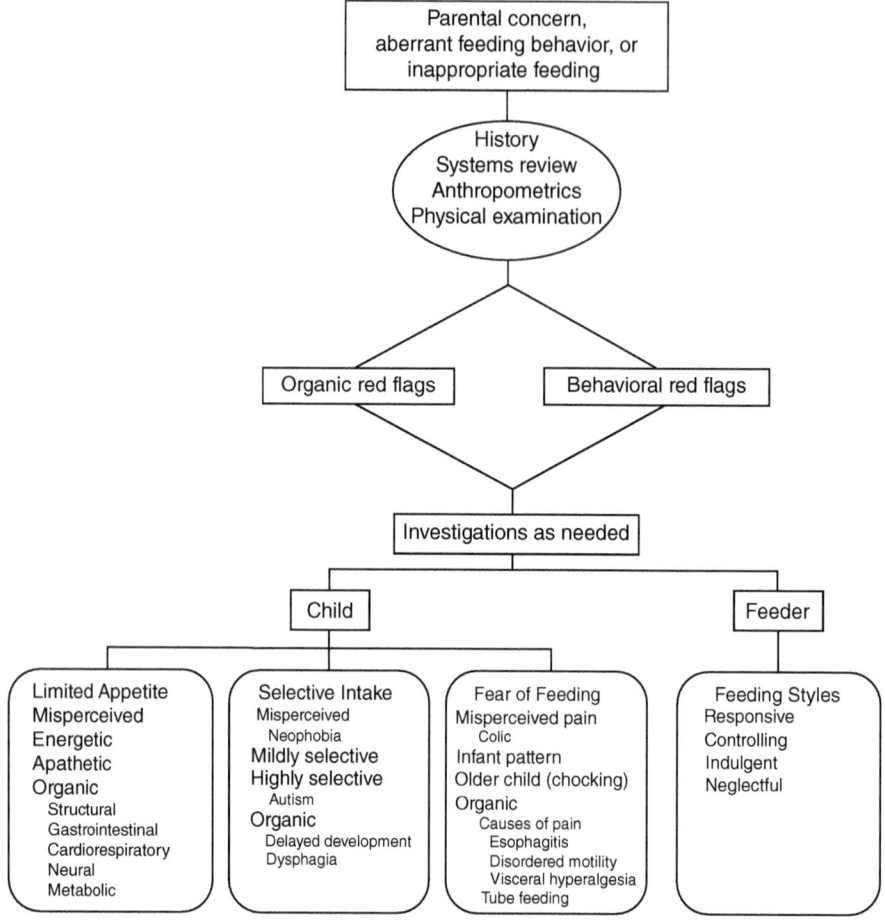

**Fig. 27.6** An approach to identifying and managing feeding difficulties. (Republished with permission of American Academy of Pediatrics from Kerzner et al. (2015), permission conveyed through Copyright Clearance Center, Inc. chocking should be choking)

to affect every feeding problem positively or negatively.

Since 2013 the DC:0–3 has been updated and revised (APA 2013). This ended in the publication of DC:0–5 (2016): Diagnostic Classification of Mental Health and Developmental Disorders of Infancy and Early Childhood: Zero to Five in 2016, specifically dealing with eating disorders in the first 5 years of life. The main changes include changes in terminology, such as "Eating Disorders" instead of "Feeding Behaviour Disorders", focusing on the child's observed eating problems that are observed beyond any specific caregiver–child relationship context and those that are associated with one specific rela-

tionship. DC:0–5 (2016) describes the following categories.

### 27.2.5.1 Overeating Disorder

Overeating disorder in the young child is manifested by a pattern of seeking food between mealtimes or scheduled feedings, persistently asking for excessive amounts of food during meals, taking food from others or foraging from garbage bins. The child becomes distressed if prevented from engaging in this behaviour and it may show non-specific symptoms of anxiety, irritability or anger. Overeating is rarely seen in children under the age of two, because some degree of autonomy is required. Overfeeding, in contrast, occurs during the first year of life. Diagnostic procedures have to rule out food unavailability and hunger, medical conditions (e.g., Prader-Willi syndrome or hypothyroidism, etc.) and medication side effects. If overeating is a manifestation of an early parent–infant relational disorder, an Axis I diagnosis *Relationship Specific Disorder* is warranted (Keren 2016).

### 27.2.5.2 Under-Eating Disorder

It is reported that 25–40% of infants and toddlers have under-eating problems in the early years. They mainly show colic, vomiting, slow feeding, selective eating and refusal to eat (McDermott et al. 2008). Under-eating disorder is diagnosed whenever the child consistently eats less than expected for his or her age, exhibits a maladaptive eating behaviour, such as a fearful avoidance of eating, shows a difficult regulation state during feeding, eats only when specific conditions imposed by him or her are fulfilled by the caregiver (e.g., in front of television, with toys and stories) or is an extremely picky-eater (e.g., in case of hypersensitivity or a delay in oral-motor-skills). In complex cases in which there is an underlying medical diagnosis, one has to make sure that the under-eating pattern is not fully explained by it or from a medication side effect. It is necessary to differentiate between feeding (interaction with caregiver and caregiver's behaviour) and eating (child's own behaviour with food) components of the problem. Physical morbidity and decreased exploratory behaviour are often observed among infants with persistent under-eating behaviour.

### 27.2.5.3 Atypical Eating Disorders

Publications on atypical eating behaviour are rare and additional research is needed. They include pica, rumination disorder, hoarding and pouching. Their respective prevalence is unclear. Both pica and rumination disorder may be seen in association with mental retardation and autism spectrum disorder (Bryant-Waught and Piepenstock 2008) (see Table 27.1).

**Pica** This describes persistent eating of non-food substances such as paper, soap, paint, earth, hair, ice, metal or plastic objects. Pica is not associated with general aversion of food and neither is it accompanied by weight or growth deficits.

**Rumination** This describes the repeated regurgitation of food that follows feeding or eating. A minimum duration of 3 months and an onset at 3–12 months of age, a lack of distress in the infant together with poor interaction with others and its absence during sleep are reported (Rasquin et al. 2006). Common medical conditions in infancy need to be ruled out before the diagnosis of regurgitation is made.

**Hoarding** This describes the child's storing of food in unusual places (under the pillow, in clothes, in a desk, etc.). Depending on what they do with the hidden food, some of the children are overweight, others are underweight. It has not been described in children under the age of 2 years. It is necessary to rule out hunger, maltreatment, neglect, etc.

**Table 27.1** Eating Disorders of Infancy/Early Childhood: an overview of diagnostic manuals (from Crosswalk from DC:0–5™ to DSM-5 and ICD-10 (www.zerotothree.org)) Zero to Three (2005) with kind permission from Zero to Three

| DC:0–5™ | DSM-5 | ICD-10 | ICD-10 Code |
|---|---|---|---|
| Overeating Disorder | Unspecified feeding Or eating disorder | Overeating associated with other Psychological disturbances | F50.4 |
| Under-eating disorder | Unspecified feeding Or eating disorder | Other eating disorders | F50.8 |
| Pica | Pica | Pica of infancy and childhood | F98.3 |
| Rumination | Rumination disorder | Feeding Disorders of infancy and early Childhood/rumination disorder of infancy | F98.21 |
| Hoarding | Other specified Feeding and Eating disorder | Feeding Disorders of infancy And early childhood | F98.2 |

**Pouching** Here the child holds food in his or her mouth for a long time without swallowing. It happens daily for several hours; dental caries is an often associated sign (Bhargav et al. 2014). From clinical experience, pouching may develop in the process of tube weaning in infants who have received a nasogastric (NG) tube or percutaneous endoscopic gastrostomy (PEG). Traumatic events that involve painful medical conditions may also play a role as risk factors. Any medical conditions that prevent the child from swallowing should be sought before diagnosis of pouching is manifested.

### 27.2.6 Diagnostic Procedures for Feeding Disorders

These include:

**Medical history**: this should include pre-, peri-, and post-natal history, family history of feeding problems, underlying illnesses and (traumatic) manipulation around the oropharynx, such as tube feeding, suctioning or intubation. The chronology of feeding disturbances, introduction of solids, absence of oral exploration, food aversions, quantities eaten and length of meals should be enquired into.

**Psychosocial history**: feeding disorders have multi-factorial causes and mostly a substantial behavioural component so that children's and parents' behaviour around mealtimes, emotional climate during the meals and great stress factors in the family need to be documented. If possible, parent–child interactions during mealtimes should be video-recorded for analysis. Parent-child-interaction also has to be recorded and documented if parents are suffering from any mental or psychiatric illness, such as depressive disorders or schizophrenia.

**Physical examination**: this should seek physical and craniofacial abnormalities and signs of systematic disease. A neurological status is mandatory, as is an evaluation of orofacial status and psychomotor development. A growth and weight curve should have been documented since birth.

Regardless of the types and causes of eating disorders, Birch and Davison (2001) suggest five key elements that should be considered in diagnostic procedures:

- How does the problem manifest itself?
- Is the child suffering from any medical disease?
- Have the child's weight, nutritional status and development been affected?
- What is the atmosphere during meals?
- Is the family under stress?

### 27.2.7 Therapy of Feeding Disorders

Successful interventions should be conducted at various levels and in various settings (hospital admissions together with parents; outpatient clinics; at home). Treatment involves dietary, behavioural, social and psychological intervention by a multidisciplinary team of health professionals such as paediatricians, psychologists, pedagogues, logopedists and dieticians (Steinberg 2007). Infants suffering from any physical disease, unable to take in food because of a concurrent medical problem (mostly orofacial or gastro-oesophageal abnormalities), should be supported by any tube feeding system to ensure adequate nutrition intake. Treatment always has to be discussed interdisciplinarily. Studies show that multidisciplinary treatment holds benefits for children with severe feeding difficulties (Sharp et al. 2017).

In cases of avoidance or refusal to eat caused by an underlying behavioural component, the aim is to activate the inner regulation of hunger and satiety cues. Psychological intervention is based on the *model of transaction of infantile anorexia* (Chatoor et al. 1997). Infants with low food intake or food refusal trigger their parent's anxiety. As a result, parents show inadequate behaviour such as feeding while playing or urging the child to eat by opening its mouth forcibly, in attempts to compensate for bad nutrition intake. Both parents and children are irritated, unable to build a supporting relationship which is necessary for any parental–infant interaction.

Parental–infant interaction can be additionally affected by general family conflicts, and conflicts around food (Davies et al. 2006). Studies show a link between maternal anxiety, distress or depression and non-responsive feeding styles (Stein et al. 2001). Benoit has reported that maternal depression and anxiety have been consistently associated with child feeding difficulties (Benoit 2002; Blissett et al. 2007; Chatoor et al. 1998b).

Intervention provides parental psychological treatment and infant–parental interaction analysis as well as therapeutically accompanied feeding sessions in a calm, warm atmosphere in which behavioural changes of the caregivers can be experienced.

In Bernard-Bonnin 2006, Bernard-Bonnin proposed food rules applicable to children beyond infancy, including
how parents should behave:

- Mealtime is not playing time.
- Mealtimes should not last longer than 30 min.
- Place a spoon or food into your child's mouth, not only before the child accepts food intake.
- Prepare child-friendly food appropriate to its age.
- Look for a daily routine with regular meals; nothing should be offered between meals.
- Make compromises in terms of the child's favourite food and remain consistent in offering healthy food.
- Don't let nutritional information on packages confuse you; children need different amounts of nutrition.
- Wait until your child turns its head to the spoon and stop feeding if the child turns aside, closing its mouth.
- Don't let your child walk around permanently with a baby bottle, even small amounts of sweet tea or juice could decrease your child's appetite.
- Only offer small portions of food and don't let your child drink right before a meal.
- Avoid any emotional pressure; no forcing of food.
- Spend mealtimes sitting together in a neutral and friendly atmosphere, avoid verbal disputes and controversy in front your child.
- Never give food as a reward or present.
- Offer solids first, fluids last.

## 27.2.8 Case Study

P., 1 year, 2 months of age and only child of a young couple, was born prematurely and was diagnosed at birth with a diaphragmatic hernia that necessitated immediate surgery. He stayed in hospital because of persistent respiratory problems and was discharged with diagnoses of left hemiplegia due to cerebral palsy, bronchopulmonary dysplasia and poor eating. Being at home after discharge was extremely stressful for the parents.

The mother herself was diagnosed with a mixed anorexia and bulimia eating disorder. Her eating disorder started shortly after her father died in an accident when she was 14 years old. Because of body changes, pregnancy had been difficult for her.

Observation of the mother-child interaction revealed a highly ambivalent relationship, with child breath-holding spells especially frequent at mealtimes. At a day-care centre, P. ate well and his breath-holding spells were limited to situations of frustration. They disappeared within a short time after the teacher learned to ignore them.

In DC:0–5, there is no diagnosis of eating disorder, but a mother–child relationship specific disorder of early childhood with symptoms of eating and breath-holding spells of the child, because the eating symptoms were observed only in the context of the mother-child interaction.

## 27.2.9 Conclusion

Feeding disorders have multi-factorial causes, including physiological and environmental factors and mostly a substantial behaviour component. They show a great variability of characteristics and have to be defined multidimensionally. Medical and family history, underlying illnesses and the chronology of feeding disturbances should be carefully reported. Successful interventions should be conducted at various levels and in various settings by a multidisciplinary team of health professionals.

## 27.3 Neurogenic Dysphagia

Heidrun Schröter-Morasch and
Irena Hočevar Boltežar

### 27.3.1 Introduction

Disturbances of the swallowing function as a result of neurogenic diseases are called "Neurogenic Dysphagia (ND)". Swallowing function in patients with ND may be impaired by an alteration in muscular tone, range and regularity of movements, and their initiation and coordination, as well of disturbances of sensibility and reflex activity.

Neurogenic swallowing deficits are not normally isolated symptoms but are seen together with general motor disorders such as disturbances of posture and movement, cognitive impairments and behavioural alterations, as well as speech and language disorders. In some cases, however, they might be the main symptoms (e.g., after small brainstem lesions or after posterior fossa tumour surgery) or the first sign of a neuro-myogenic disease (e.g., polymyositis). Swallowing disorders are a major determinant of the degree of severity of a neurogenic disease and the outcome of rehabilitation, as they can lead to serious morbidity, in particular malnutrition and dehydration, as

well as aspiration with resulting pulmonary complications, mainly aspiration pneumonia (Murray et al. 2014; Bray et al. 2017). Moreover, they result in a considerable reduction in the quality of life and high costs for the healthcare system. Since the symptoms of dysphagia may be subtle (above all aspiration without a cough reflex, the "silent aspiration") and some patients are not aware of their restrictions in swallowing, they are often overlooked.

### 27.3.2 Overview of Functional Neuroanatomy Related to Swallowing

In order to understand the different symptoms of patients with ND and the underlying pathophysiology, and to develop a functionally based therapy, a basic knowledge of the neuroanatomy of the swallowing system is required. Figure 27.7 shows a top–down approach to the nervous system in which sensory and motor components are described at each level.

Peripheral sensations (feeling of touch, smelling, tasting, usually attributed to positive feelings, "joy of eating") are transmitted as stimuli through afferent peripheral nerves to the brain stem and are processed in the nucleus tractus solitarii (NTS). Through conduction and activation of the so-called swallowing centres (two cell

**Fig. 27.7** Levels of the nervous system. (Reprinted from Nishino (2013) The swallowing reflex and its significance as an airway defensive reflex. Front Physiol 07 January 2013. © 2013 Nishino)

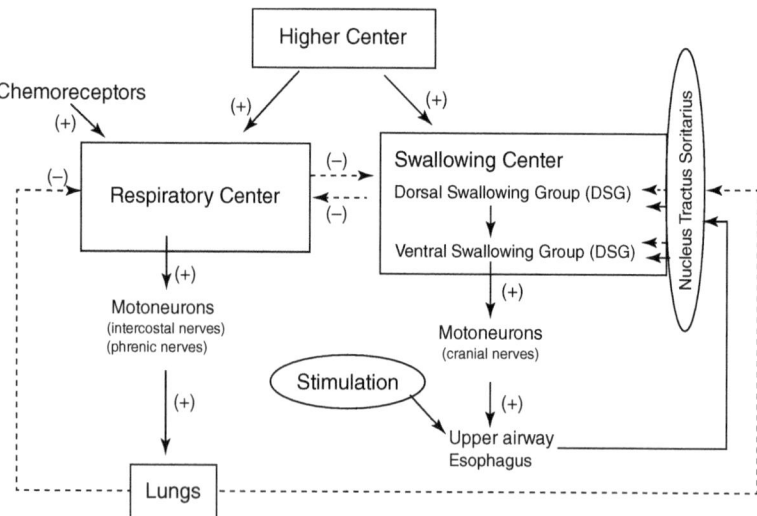

groups in the medulla, located dorsomedially and ventrolaterally) the switch to the cranial nerve motor nuclei takes place. These nuclei activate the swallowing muscles through the efferent cranial nerves. Thus, the act of swallowing is possible at the brainstem level. However, cortical and subcortical factors modulate the activation and the process of swallowing.

Swallowing disorders resulting from damage to the sensorimotor system may vary in response depending on the location of the lesion, extent of the lesion and whether the neurological damage is unilateral or bilateral. Lesions in the region of the upper motor neuron result in central or pseudobulbar symptoms, lesions of the lower motor neuron result in peripheral or bulbar symptoms (Table 27.2).

A thorough evaluation of these specific signs in the oropharyngeal and laryngeal region can frequently contribute to the diagnosis of the underlying neurological disease.

### 27.3.2.1 Cortical and Subcortical Structures Involved in Swallowing

Voluntary and automatic swallowing is represented within distributed networks of functionally distinct cortical areas that participate

**Table 27.2** Symptoms of central and peripheral paresis Reprinted from: Schröter-Morasch et al. (2018) Klinische und video-pharyngo-laryngoskopische Untersuchung der Schluckfunktion (Clinical and video-pharyngo-laryngoscopic evaluation of swallowing). In: Bartolome G, Schröter-Morasch H (eds) Schluckstörungen—Interdisziplinäre Diagnostik und Rehabilitation (Swallowing disorders—interdisciplinary diagnostics and rehabilitation). sixth edition. Elsevier, Urban & Fischer, Munich, with permission from Elsevier

| Central Paresis | Peripheral Paresis |
| --- | --- |
| Disturbed voluntary control of movements | Disturbed voluntary and reflexive movements |
| Increased muscle tone (hypertonus) | Decreased muscle tone (hypotonus) |
| No atrophy of the muscles | Muscle atrophy, sometimes lateral sulcus of the tongue |
| Dysdiadochokinesia | Fasciculations possible |
| Hyperkinesias (tremor, myoclonus) possible | |
| Impaired coordination | |

differentially in the control of swallowing (Martin et al. 2001). Cortical areas involved in motor control of swallowing are the lateral frontal cortex, the inferior frontal lobule and the insula (Fig. 27.8). Studies have indicated that swallowing has a bilateral but asymmetrical interhemispheric representation. Damage to the hemisphere that has the greater swallowing output appears to predispose the individual to swallowing problems (Li et al. 2009; Hamdy et al. 1998a). If the dominant swallowing cortical area is impaired, the contralateral area may be available to facilitate recovery ("cortical plasticity" Barritt and Smithard 2009), which can be supported by use of stimulation techniques (Bath et al. 2016; Suntrup-Krueger et al. 2018). From cortical areas, the corticonuclear pathways project ipsilaterally and contralaterally via the internal capsule to the nuclei of the cranial nerves in the brainstem (Fig. 27.8). Cortical areas for recognition and interpretation of sensory stimuli are located in the parietal lobe regions. Subcortical structures, the basal ganglia, the limbic-hypothalamic system and the cerebellum are also involved in the swallowing control mechanism (Zald and Pardo 1999; Michou and Hamdy 2009; Reed et al. 2019).

### 27.3.2.2 Brainstem Structures Involved in Swallowing and Peripheral Nerves

The more important structures for swallowing are located within the brainstem: the so-called "central pattern generators" (CPG), with a dorsomedial swallowing group (dmCPGs) and a ventrolateral swallowing group (vlCPGs). They receive sensory input by way of CN V, IX and X (see Table 27.3). They are responsible for initiation, coordination and integration of the complex swallowing act and activation of the motor nuclei of CN V, VII, IX, X and XII, also located in the brainstem, and the nuclei of the cervical nerves I–III in the spinal cord. The motor nuclei and the peripheral motor nerves (see Table 27.4) represent the lower motor neuron. It is important to stress a particular condition of the sensorimotor control of the swallowing system (as well as the system for respiration, voice and speech func-

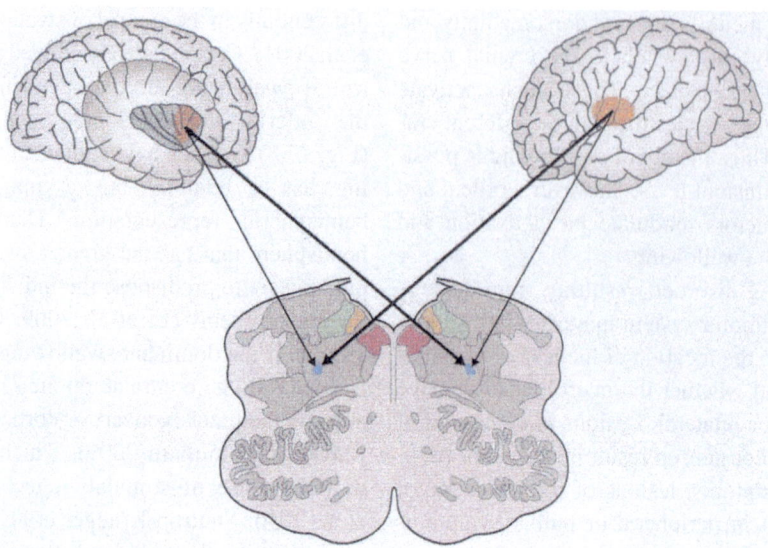

**Fig. 27.8** Swallowing cortex, corticobulbar fibres, brainstem. Top right: the fronto-parietal operculum (orange) of the left cerebral hemisphere Top left: right cerebral hemisphere, after removal of the operculum the insula can be seen, both cortical structures with corticobulbar fibres projecting in this example to the ipsilateral and contralateral nucleus ambiguous (the nucleus of CN X, vagus nerve) within the lower brainstem, the medulla. Reprinted from Prosiegel (2018a) Neuroanatomie des Schluckens (Neuroanatomy of swallowing). In: Bartolome G, Schröter-Morasch H (eds) Schluckstörungen—Diagnostik und Rehabilitation (Swallowing disorders—diagnostics and rehabilitation). (sixth edn) Elsevier, Urban & Fischer, Munich, with permission from Elsevier

**Table 27.3** Peripheral sensory input, afferent controls of swallowing. Modified from: Groher ME and Crary MA (2016) Dysphagia. Clinical management in adults and children. Elsevier, St. Louis, Missouri, with permission from Elsevier

| Region of Sensory Function | Innervation (Cranial Nerves) | |
|---|---|---|
| General sensation, anterior two-thirds of the tongue | Trigeminal N. (V) | |
| Taste, anterior two-thirds of the tongue | Chorda tympani, facial N. (VII) | |
| | Taste and general sensation, posterior third of the tongue | Glossopharyngeal N. (IX) |
| | Valleculae | Internal branch of superior laryngeal nerve vagus N. (X) |
| | Tonsils, soft palate | Glossopharyngeal N. (IX), trigeminal N. (V), |
| | Pharynx, larynx | Glossopharyngeal N. (IX), trigeminal N. (V), laryngeal branches of vagal N. (X) |

**Table 27.4** Peripheral efferent (motor) controls of swallowing. Modified from: Groher ME and Crary MA (2016) Dysphagia. Clinical management in adults and children. Elsevier, St. Louis, Missouri, with permission from Elsevier

| Structure | Innervation (Cranial Nerves) |
|---|---|
| *Oral structures* | |
| Muscles of mastication, buccinators, floor of the mouth | 3.2.3. Trigeminal N. (V); facial N. (VII) |
| Lip muscles | Facial N. (VII) |
| Tongue | Hypoglossal N. (XII) |
| *Pharyngeal and laryngeal structures* | |
| Pharyngeal constrictor muscles, m. Stylopharyngeus | Vagus N. (X), glossopharyngeal N. (IX) |
| Palatal muscles, laryngeal muscles | Vagus N. (X) |
| *Oesophageal structures* | |
| Oesophageal muscles | Vagus N. (X) |

tion), in contrast to the sensorimotor control of the limbs. For example, the roots of the cranial nerves, the cranial nerve nuclei, are comparable to the anterior horn cells in the spinal cord. Therefore, they are part of the lower motor neuron, although they are located in the brain within the skull.

The sensorimotor brainstem control system is governed by influences of the cortical as well as subcortical structures such as the basal ganglia, cerebellum and the limbic-hypothalamic system (Daniels and Huckabee 2014; Michou and Hamdy 2009; Martin et al. 2001). Therefore, the brainstem is much like a "junction box" (Groher and Crary 2016) (Figs. 27.7, 27.8) between the:

- Peripheral sensory input.
- Elicitation and coordination of swallowing activity (pattern generators).
- Central motor activation from the cortex, subcortical structures, cerebellum.
- Peripheral innervation, beginning in the cranial nerve nuclei.

### 27.3.3 Neurogenic Dysphagia Characteristics Seen in Diseases Affecting Various Levels of the Nervous System

According to the site of the lesion, diseases can be divided into four groups:

- Diseases of the central nervous system (e.g., stroke, inflammatory and degenerative diseases, tumours, traumatic brain injury TBI).
- Diseases of the peripheral nerves (cranial nerves, CI-III) (e.g., polyradiculitis, Guillan-Barré-syndrome, tumours, injury after surgery).
- Diseases of the neuromuscular junction (myasthenia gravis).
- Muscular diseases (inflammatory: polymyositis, dermatomyositis, inclusion body myositis, sarcoidosis; non-inflammatory: muscular dystrophies).

The prevalence of dysphagia in different types of neurogenic disease is listed in Table 27.5.

**Table 27.5** Prevalence of dysphagia in neurogenic diseases as percentages. Reprinted from Prosiegel (2018b) Mit Schluckstörungen assoziierte neurologische Erkrankungen (Neurological disorders associated with dysphagia). In: Bartolome G, Schröter-Morasch H (eds) Schluckstörungen—Diagnostik und Rehabilitation (Swallowing disorders—diagnostics and rehabilitation). (sixth edn) Elsevier, Urban & Fischer, Munich, with permission from Elsevier

| Disease | Frequency |
|---|---|
| Stroke | The most frequent cause of dysphagia in general! Early stage: > 50% Chronic stage: Ca. 30% |
| Parkinson's disease | > 50% |
| Progressive Supranuclear palsy (PSP) | Ca. 80% |
| Traumatic brain injury (TBI) | 30–70% |
| Multiple sclerosis (MS) | Ca. 30–40% |
| Amyotrophic lateral sclerosis (ALS) Motor neuron disease (MND) | Bulbar onset with dysarthria and dysphagia 25%, Later disease stages 100% |
| Spinobulbar muscular atrophy (SBMA) type Kennedy | In the process of disease 100% |
| Guillain-Barré syndrome (GBS) | Up to 60% (Mengi et al. 2017) |
| Critical-illness-Polyneuromyopathy (CIPNM), After long-term intubation | Up to 80% (Ponfick et al. 2015) |
| Myasthenia gravis | As a first symptom ca. 20%, during progress >50% |
| Lambert-Eaton syndrome (LES) | Ca. 30% |
| Dystrophia myotonica Curschmann-Steinert-batten | Ca. 70% |
| Oculopharyngeal muscular dystrophy (OPMD) | 100% |
| Polymyositis (PM), dermatomyositis (DM), Inclusion body myositis (IBM) | > 50%; frequent first symptom in IBM |
| Dementia | During the disease progress: 84–93% (Affoo et al. 2013) |

#### 27.3.3.1 Dysphagia in Diseases of the Central Nervous System

*Dysphagia after Stroke (Cerebral Vascular Accident CVA)* Stroke is the most frequent cause of dysphagia (incidence 250/100,000; prevalence 1200/100,000 (Prosiegel 2018b). In the acute stage, nearly 55% of patients exhibit symptoms of dysphagia, even more than 80% in cases of involvement of the brainstem (Martino et al. 2005; Nakao et al. 2019). These patients have a higher probability and incidence of pneumonia than non-dysphagic patients after stroke (18.8% versus 6.5%), as well as a higher mortality rate (10.5% versus 4.8%) 1 year after stroke (Ho et al. 2018), demonstrating the potential danger to these patients (Doggett et al. 2002). In nearly 25% of the patients, dysphagia persists in the chronic stage with abnormal oral intake of food and risk of aspiration.

*Swallowing Deficits in Hemispheric Stroke Syndromes* In recent years, extensive research has attempted to correlate the location of brain damage with the specific symptoms of dysphagia and to predict acute or protracted dysphagia (Suntrup et al. 2012; Wan et al. 2016; Seo et al. 2017).

Swallowing deficits in patients following hemispheric stroke include:

- Reduced ability to initiate volitional swallowing (frequently followed by drooling of saliva and liquids/food).
- Reduced oral transport and pharyngeal constriction owing to lesions of the upper motor neuron characterised by spastic weakness and associated movement impairments (central paresis) with resulting oral and pharyngeal residues.
- Delayed triggering of the swallowing reflex owing to reduced sensitivity.
- Incoordination of oral movements and pharyngeal swallowing (Prosiegel 2018b; Groher and Crary 2016; Oommen et al. 2011; Power et al. 2007).
- Decreasing of velocity variables (Wan et al. 2016).
- Reduced laryngeal closure (Power et al. 2007).

In cases of bilateral lesions of the cortex or the corticonuclear pathways "pseudobulbar palsy" results. After bilateral lesions of the frontoparietal operculum (bilateral anterior operculum syndrome, Foix-Chavany-Marie syndrome) patients are not able to speak, chew or swallow, owing to complete paresis of the oral and pharyngeal musculature.

After lesions of the cerebellum, the pons and the olivo-ponto-cerebellar pathway's involuntary rhythmic movements in the pharynx and larynx may occur ("symptomatic palatal tremor" Deuschl et al. 1990; Riva et al. 2024) and reduce velo-pharyngeal closure and pharyngeal contraction and impair an appropriate laryngeal closure during phonation as well as during swallowing (Schröter-Morasch and Hoole 1998; Barkmeier-Kraemer and Clark 2017; van de Loo et al. 2010).

*Swallowing Deficits after Brainstem Stroke* Since the swallowing structures in the brainstem are located very close together, even small unilateral lesions may result in severe disturbances of swallowing ("incomplete swallow", Groher and Crary 2016). The reasons for severe dysphagia after brainstem lesions are:

- Involvement of the swallowing centres, resulting in disturbances of the reflexive parts of swallowing (the pharyngeal phase and partly the oesophageal phase) with absent or delayed elicitation of the swallowing reflex as well as generalised disturbed coordination of swallowing stages and coordination of swallowing and respiration.
- Involvement of the corticobulbar pathways and cranial nerve nuclei may lead to combined central and peripheral neurological symptoms (combined lesions of the upper and lower motor neuron).
- Disturbance of the upper oesophageal sphincter (UES) opening (Wan et al. 2016).

These typical symptoms are frequently seen after the obliteration by a thrombus or embolus of the posterior inferior cerebellar artery (PICA), the "Wallenberg syndrome" after infarction of the dorsolateral medulla with the resulting damage of both central pattern generators, as well as of cranial nerve nuclei (Fig. 27.9). Predominant symptoms are peripheral paresis of cranial nerves, reduced or absent elicitation of the swallowing reflex, and frequently a long-lasting disturbance of the upper oesophageal sphincter opening.

Dysphagia after bilateral brainstem lesions exhibits the most severe symptoms with a poor prognosis and outcome ("bulbar paralysis").

*Dysphagia and Dementia* Dementia is another form of cortical impairment that can impair swal-

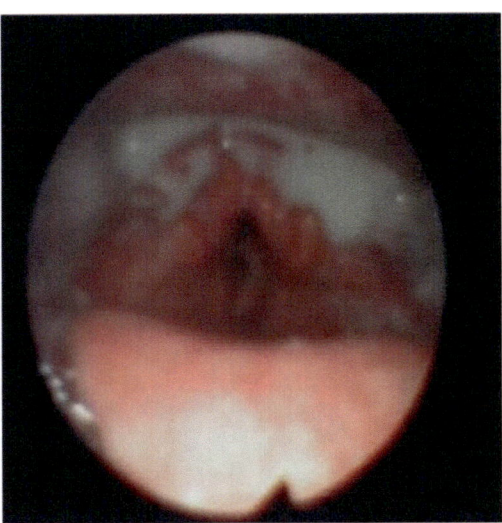

**Fig. 27.9** Male, age 66, 3 weeks after PICA infarction, peripheral paresis of CN IX, X on the left side, residues in the valleculae and piriform sinus with penetration and (silent) aspiration (bolus is seen in the subglottis)

**Table 27.6** Nutritional problems arising in different disease stages Reprinted from Volkert D, Chourdakis M, Faxen-Irving G et al. (2015) ESPEN guidelines on nutrition in dementia. Clin Nutr 34(6):1052–1073, with permission from Elsevier

| Nutritional Problems | Stage of Dementia |
| --- | --- |
| Olfactory and taste dysfunction | Preclinical and early stages |
| Attention deficit | Mild to moderate |
| Executive functions deficit (shopping, preparing food) | Mild to moderate |
| Impaired decision-making ability (slowdown in food Choice, reduced intake) | Mild to moderate |
| Dyspraxia (coordination disorder, loss of eating skills) | Moderate to severe |
| Agnosia[a] | Moderate to severe |
| Behavioural problems (wandering, agitating, disturbed Eating behaviour) | Moderate to severe |
| Oropharyngeal dysphagia | Moderate to severe |
| Refusal to eat | Severe |

[a]Loss of ability to recognise objects or comprehend the meaning of objects, which means that food may not be distinguished from non-food and eating utensils are not recognised as what they are

lowing ability and is on the rise worldwide in ageing societies (Alagiakrishnan et al. 2013; Affoo et al. 2013; Volkert et al. 2015). This progressive disease caused by neurodegenerative processes in specific brain regions leads to gradual deterioration of cognitive abilities including memory, orientation, judgement and problem-solving, as well as personality changes. Other cortical disturbances such as apraxia and aphasia may also occur. There are different causes of dementia syndromes: Alzheimer's disease (50–70%) and cerebrovascular diseases (15–20%) are the more common. In Parkinson's disease, Pick's syndrome, Huntington's disease or Lewy-body syndrome dementia also frequently occurs, especially in later stages (Warnecke and Dziewas 2018). Nutritional problems, arising in different disease stages, are listed in Table 27.6 (Volkert et al. 2015).

The prevalence of swallowing difficulties in patients with dementia ranges from 13% to 57% (Alagiakrishnan et al. 2013). The oropharyngeal motor and sensory functions are mostly affected with lack of swallowing initiation, uncoordinated oral control of food and liquid, disturbed mastication, as well as reduced swallowing reflex elicitation and reduced bolus clearing from the pharynx with retentions and possibly penetration and aspiration. Therefore, owing to cognitive, behavioural and swallowing restrictions, patients with dementia are at high risk of malnutrition, which may trigger a vicious circle for patients with dementia: malnutrition and weight loss are associated with sarcopenia and frailty, as well as with disease progression and cognitive decline. Therefore, early and appropriate interventions are required: routine screening for malnutrition, clinical and if possible instrumental assessment of dysphagia, periodic weight control, attractive, high-quality food according to individual needs, adequate nursing or caregiver support, functional treatment and oral nutritional supplements (Bartolome 2018). In patients with advanced dementia artificial nutrition is not recommended (Volkert et al. 2015).

*Dysphagia in Traumatic Brain Injury (TBI)*
The prevalence of dysphagia in acute or subacute TBI ranges from 60% to more than 90% with a high risk for aspiration pneumonia (30% in the acute stage, 12% during rehabilitation) (Takizawa et al. 2016).

The lesions observed after TBI are multifactorial:

- Primary lesions: local haemorrhage, contusions, lacerations and "diffuse axonal injury" with diffuse white matter lesions.
- Secondary lesions: infarctions and brainstem lesions caused by an increased intracranial pressure.

As a result, the symptoms of dysphagia are even more complex than in patients after stroke, frequently associated with widespread comorbidities: severe dysarthrophonias; disturbances of posture and gait; cognitive impairments, such as reduction of attention and memory; and psychogenic disorder, such as lack of drive or depression. These comorbidities must be taken into account in management and therapeutic procedures.

The severity of the initial injury and its necessary treatment (including time of ventilation, need for tracheostomy and feeding tubes) emerges as a strong predictor of both the presence of dysphagia and time to recovery of swallowing ability (Groher and Crary 2016).

The most frequent symptoms after traumatic brain injury are described as follows (Logeman 2021; Logemann 1998):

- Pathological oral reflex activity.
- Hypertonus of oral muscles, reduced opening or closure of the mouth, drooling of saliva.
- Reduced tongue movements.
- Delayed and reduced triggering of the swallowing reflex.
- Reduced velopharyngeal closure.
- Reduced laryngeal elevation.
- Reduced sensitivity of the larynx causing no elicitation of a cough reflex in the case of penetration / aspiration (Fig. 27.10).

The symptoms change with the course of time. Pathological reflexes can regress. The spasticity of the oral, and frequently of the neck, muscles with over-flexion of the head can increase. This can further impair the oral intake.

### 27.3.3.2 Dysphagia in Inflammatory Neurological Diseases

These have various origins and result in encephalitis and meningitis. The most severe symptoms are seen after the involvement of the brainstem (e.g.,

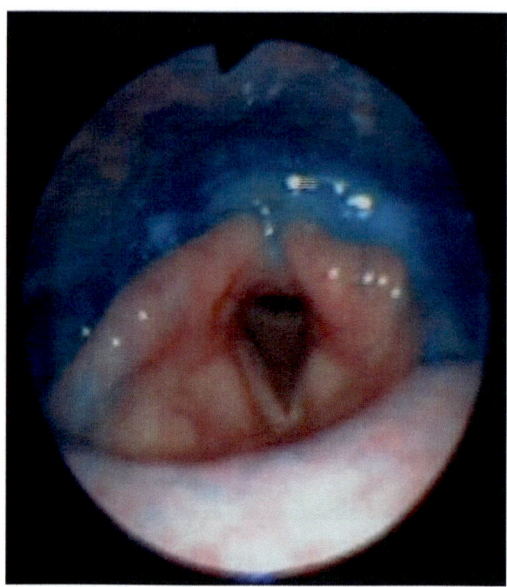

**Fig. 27.10** Male, age 28, 3 months after TBI. Accumulation of saliva in the entire hypopharynx with overflow into the laryngeal vestibule and the glottis without elicitation of a cough reflex (silent aspiration) or an attempt to clear the hypopharynx

in patients with Borrelia infection). Following a tetanus infection, swallowing disorders may be the initial symptoms or develop during the course of the disease. The cranial nerves may also be involved, e.g., in herpes virus infections.

*Polioencephalomyelitis* is a virus infection, mainly of the cranial nerve nuclei and the anterior horn cells of the spinal cord, resulting in peripheral paresis with corresponding swallowing disorders in nearly 30% of cases. However, even 20–40 years later, muscle weakness and atrophy may occur and cause or worsen dysphagic symptoms (post-polio-syndrome) (Soderholm et al. 2010).

*Multiple Sclerosis* is an autoimmune, inflammatory neurological disease affecting all parts of the central nervous system (incidence 6/100,000; prevalence 100/100,000). Dysphagia is seen in 30–65% of the patients, corresponding to the degree of severity of the disease and the involvement of the brainstem (Restivo et al. 2006). Depending on the location and the extent of lesions within the brain and spinal cord, sensory and motor disturbances appear, as well as vegetative and cognitive impairments.

*Severe Acute Respiratory Syndrome Coronavirus 2 (SARS-CoV-2)* Since December 2019 an infection with the new coronavirus has led to a previously unknown clinical picture, which is known as COVID-19 (COrona VIrus Disease 2019) (Berlit et al. 2020). Although the respiratory system complications have been the most frequent and life-threatening, the involvement of the central and peripheral nervous system may also lead to severe neurological manifestations with dysphagia: encephalopathy, meningo-encephalitis, ischaemic stroke, acute necrotising encephalopathy and Guillan–Barré Syndrome (Paterson et al. 2020), frequently with the need for intensive care unit admission, intubation or tracheostomy or both, as well as prolonged mechanical ventilation owing to acute respiratory distress syndrome and vasopressor treatment for septic shock. These measurements are key risk factors for the development of the critical illnesses polyneuropathy and myopathy, again, with the risk of severe swallowing disorders. Therefore "a careful assessment of safety and efficacy of swallowing including management of pharyngeal secretions seems of utmost importance in COVID survivors" (Dziewas et al. 2020).

Owing to the presence of the virus in the nasal cavity and the pharynx of infected individuals and possible aerosol generation, healthcare providers, above all ENT surgeons and phoniatricians, are at high risk of contracting the SARS-CoV-2 virus during the examination and treatment of the nose, throat, larynx and trachea. The Union of the European Phoniatricians therefore developed a series of recommendations to offer clinicians precepts on safe clinical practice in different settings (Geneid et al. 2020).

### 27.3.3.3 Dysphagia in Degenerative Neurological Diseases of the CNS

*Parkinson's Disease* (PD) is one of the more common neurological disorders worldwide. The prevalence increases with age from about 40/100,000 in 40–49-year-old subjects to nearly 1900/100,000 in over 80-year-old subjects! (Suttrup and Warnecke 2016). PD is a degenerative slowly progressive disease of the basal ganglia with the classic features of resting tremor, bradykinesia and rigidity of the musculature, accompanied by changes in body posture and gait, dysarthria and micrographia, as well as vegetative and cognitive impairments, psychogenic disorders and dementia. Dysphagia may be the first symptom of the disease or occur during the course of the disease. In later disease stages, 90–100% of the patients suffer from considerable swallowing problems, including silent aspiration. Therefore, aspiration pneumonia is the most frequent cause of death in PD patients (Rodrigues et al. 2011). Pflug et al. (2018) demonstrate in their study of 119 patients (1) a high prevalence of dysphagia, (2) a discrepancy between objective FEES-based results and self-reported swallowing problems, and (3) the presence of dysphagia already in early stages of the disease. Commonly observed characteristics during the oral and pharyngeal phase, caused by sensory and motor deficits are:

- Difficulty in retaining food in the mouth until masticated.
- Repetitive tongue pumping.
- Buccal retention.
- Delayed triggering of the swallowing reflex.
- Reduced pharyngeal peristalsis and laryngeal elevation.
- Hypopharyngeal retention, laryngeal penetration, (silent) aspiration.
- Pharyngo-oesophageal segment dysfunction.
- Drooling of saliva, or sialorrhoea, which may be related to the presence and severity of dysphagia, a reduced swallowing frequency and a higher risk of respiratory infections (Groher and Crary 2016).

Swallowing deficits in PD may extend to the oesophageal phase (oesophageal spasticity). Moreover, gastrointestinal motility can also be affected and result in gastroparesis or defaecation dysfunctions. PD-related dysphagia is associated with malnutrition, dehydration and loss of quality of life. Moreover, medicine administration and swallowing safety are particularly critical for patients with Parkinson's disease, where there is a dependence on timely and accurate medicine use. Healthcare professionals, patients and their family members must therefore work together to avoid medicine administration-related errors (Suttrup and Warnecke 2016; Oad et al. 2019).

*Amyotrophic Lateral Sclerosis (ALS)* is a progressive degenerative motor neuron disease (prevalence of about 7/100,000) of unknown cause with a life expectancy of three to 5 years. It is characterised by progressive degeneration of upper and lower motor neurons in the motor cortex, brainstem and spinal cord (Kühnlein et al. 2008). The neurological deficits result from involvement of the upper motor neuron with spastic weakness (pseudobulbar symptoms) as well as the lower motor neuron with flaccid weakness, atrophy and fasciculations (bulbar or spinal symptoms). Clinical signs are progressive limb weakness, respiratory insufficiency, spasticity, hyper-reflexia and bulbar symptoms such as dysarthria and dysphagia. Bulbar onset with dysarthria and dysphagia can be observed in up to 30% of patients, with fasciculations of the tongue or the lateral pharyngeal wall as an early symptom. In later disease stages, up to 100% of patients with predominantly corticospinal involvement demonstrate bulbar involvement with dysphagia as well (Warnecke et al. 2021; Buchholz 1997). Swallowing deficits in ALS are progressive and widespread and reflect the weakness of the oropharyngeal muscles involved in preparation and transportation of the bolus, leading to drooling of saliva, leakage of fluids and food, retention in the mouth and oropharynx, nasopharyngeal regurgitation, hypopharyngeal residues and airway spillage, as well as ineffective airway clearance with increasing risk for aspiration pneumonia. The use of botulinum toxin injections in the major salivary glands may be helpful in reducing the distressing symptom of drooling (Squires et al. 2014). In the final stage a tracheostomy with insertion of a cuffed tube is frequently needed to prevent aspiration, to allow suctioning of aspirated material and artificial ventilation because of respiratory muscle insufficiency.

Additionally, less frequent neurodegenerative diseases such as progressive supranuclear palsy (Warnecke et al. 2008), Chorea Huntington (Heemskerk and Roos 2011; Brotherton et al. 2012) and some types of dystonia may also cause severe swallowing disorders (Rosenbek and Jones 2009).

### 27.3.3.4 Dysphagia in Patients with Brain Tumours

Dysphagic symptoms in patients with tumours of the CNS may arise as a primary effect of local mass changes that damage brain tissue by compressing and displacing it because of increased intracranial pressure. Furthermore, dysphagic symptoms can occur as a secondary effect of tumour therapy by surgery (removal of tissue, lesions of cranial nerves and vessels) or the effects of radiation therapy and chemotherapy with subsequent sensory and motor functions loss (Newton et al. 1994; Thakkar et al. 2020; Wesling et al. 2003).

Again, the most severe impairments of swallowing are seen in tumours of the brainstem region, e.g., in patients with neurinoma of the cranial nerves VIII, IX or X (Best et al. 2018).

### 27.3.3.5 Dysphagia in Peripheral Nerve Diseases

The tumours mentioned above may also affect peripheral cranial nerves with resulting paresis, sensory loss and lack of reflex activity. The clinical and endoscopic findings may be similar to brainstem lesions with damage to the cranial nerve nuclei (see Fig. 27.9).

*Dysphagia in Guillain-Barré Syndrome* This is an immune-mediated demyelination of peripheral and cranial nerves with a distal-to-proximal pattern of ascending flaccid paresis, which may also affect swallowing and respiratory muscles, as well as the limbs (incidence 1.5/100,000). In more than 70% of the cases it occurs with a latency of about 10 or more days after respiratory or gastrointestinal infection (most commonly *Campylobacter jejuni*). Spontaneous recovery is possible; however, because of severe impairments of respiration and swallowing, mechanical ventilation and even tracheostomy may be necessary (Ogna et al. 2017).

*Dysphagia and Critical Illness Polyneuropathy/Myopathy* This is a common neurological complication of critical illness (Doherty and Steen 2010). After several weeks of treatment in the intensive care unit (ICU) with long-term ventilation owing to multiple organ dysfunction syndrome or systemic inflammatory response syndrome, 70–80% of patients with different underlying diseases develop flaccid paresis including muscle weakness and atrophy of the swallowing system with the high risk of aspiration (Leder et al. 1998; Brodsky et al. 2019; Skoretz et al. 2014; Ponfick et al. 2015). Perren et al. (2019) describe post-extubation dysphagia as the result of the "combination of oropharyngeal trauma, neuromuscular ICU acquired weakness, reduced sensation/sensorium, dyssynchronous breathing and gastrointestinal reflux".

While Ponfick et al. (2015) assume a good prognosis with regression of the symptoms within 4 weeks, other authors describe the disease as probably responsible for a worse outcome of long-term ventilated patients. Early after extubation a flexible-endoscopic evaluation of swallowing (FEES) should be performed in order to detect a possible aspiration (Brodsky et al. 2019; Leder et al. 1998).

### 27.3.3.6 Dysphagia in Neuromuscular Junction Disease

*Myasthenia Gravis* is an autoimmune disease process caused by auto-antibodies against the postsynaptic membrane at the neuromuscular junction, mostly against acetylcholine receptors (Meriggioli and Sanders 2009). Thereby fewer receptors are available on the muscle part of the neuromuscular junction leading to a more gradual neurotransmitter occupation with muscle use, leading to fatigue of muscular activity (Logemann 2021; Logemann 1998). At the beginning of a meal, chewing and swallowing muscle activity seems to be normal; however, after repeated movements muscle fatigue and reduced function result in oral and pharyngeal deficits including signs of aspiration. In addition, the oesophageal transit is often compromised. As reported by some authors and observed by FEES, injection of Tensilon (edrophonium chloride) may reduce the symptoms within a short time (Warnecke et al. 2008).

### 27.3.3.7 Dysphagia in Muscle Disease

*Polymyositis/Dermatomyositis/Inclusion Body Myositis (IBM)* These are inflammatory muscle diseases of the immune system. In 20–70% of the cases dysphagia may be the first sign of the disease with particular impairment of swallowing solid food substances, sticking of food in the throat, coughing during swallowing, owing to a general weakness of the oropharyngeal muscles, and a reduced opening of the upper oesophageal sphincter (Oh et al. 2007; Mulcahy et al. 2012; Olthoff et al. 2016). In some cases, swallowing of saliva and secretions may also be impaired (Schröter-Morasch et al. 2018) (Fig. 27.11a, b).

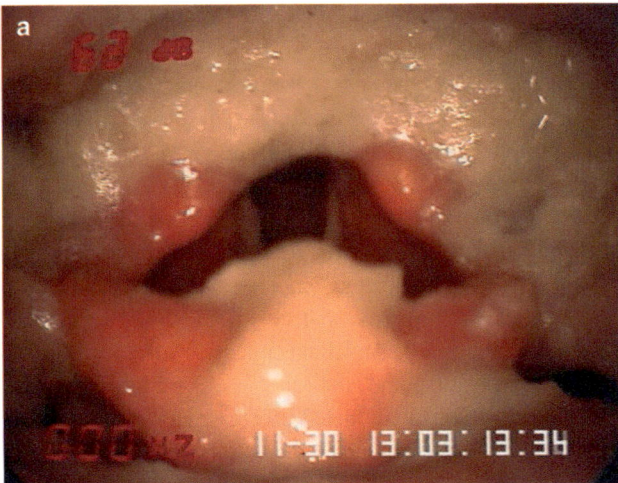
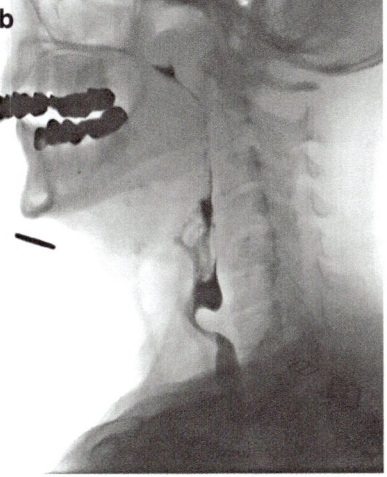

**Fig. 27.11** Female, age 72, presenting with polymyositis. (**a**) Left side: Videoendoscopy: massive hypopharyngeal retentions of food with penetration. (**b**) Right side Videofluoroscopy: disturbed opening of the upper oesophageal sphincter

Later in the disease process, no oral intake of food may be possible, and tube feeding may be required. After failure of medical and functional therapy, the opening of the UES can be improved by Botox injection, dilatation or myotomy (Kocdor et al. 2015b).

Inflammatory myopathy is an especially important consideration in cases of undiagnosed neurogenic dysphagia because immunosuppressant treatment with corticosteroids, intravenous immunoglobulin and other agents can be highly effective (Warnecke et al. 2021; Buchholz 1997).

*Myotonic Dystrophy* is characterised by prolonged contraction and difficulty in relaxation of involved muscles (muscles of mastication, the cricopharyngeal sphincter), resulting in disturbances of the oral phase, upper and anterior laryngeal movement and opening of the UES (Logemann 2021; Logemann 1998).

*Oculopharyngeal Dystrophy* is a muscular dystrophy affecting the ocular and pharyngeal muscles, characterised by dysphagia and ptosis. Owing to reduced strength of pharyngeal constrictors and reduced relaxation of the UES, the patients cannot propel material through the pharynx into the oesophagus and are at high risk of aspiration (Logemann 2021; Logemann 1998).

Case Study: A female patient, 38 years, prolonged mealtime and sticking of the bolus in the pharynx in the last 6 months, frequent ineffective cough during meals, weak and breathy voice, vocal fatigue, pneumonia in the last month, weight loss of 5 kg in the last 2 months. Flexible nasolaryngoscopy: practically immobile vocal folds with a 3-mm gap between them, accumulation of saliva in both valleculas, both pyriform sinuses and above the upper oesophageal sphincter, aspiration (spillage) over the posterior commissure when swallowing a bolus of 2 mL (Fig. 27.12).

Generally, compensatory strategies are best for management of these kinds of swallowing disorder. In case of failure of conservative therapy, dilation or myotomy of the UES can also be successful (Coiffier et al. 2006; Nagano et al. 2009; Manjaly et al. 2012).

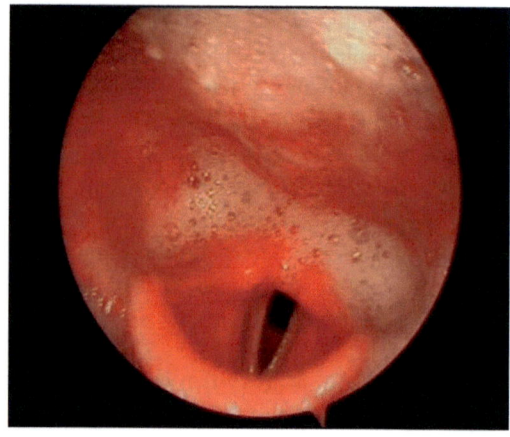

**Fig. 27.12** Female, 38 years, with oculopharyngeal dystrophy. Immobile both vocal folds, accumulation of saliva in both pyriform sinuses and above the upper oesophageal sphincter

### 27.3.3.8 Iatrogenic Oral/Pharyngeal Dysphagia

Treatment-related, or iatrogenic, dysphagia can arise from different mechanisms: medication related, (Buchholz 1997; Warnecke et al. 2021; Schwemmle et al. 2015; Prosiegel 2017), post-surgical or after radiochemotherapy (Kotz et al. 2004; Nguyen et al. 2006; Hutcheson et al. 2012). Many active agents can have an adverse effect on swallowing. Therefore, when dysphagia appears to result from neurological dysfunction in the absence of overt neurological disease, medication-induced dysphagia should be considered, especially in patients with poly-medication in older age. Sedative medications that decrease the level of arousal or directly suppress brain stem functions can cause or exacerbate dysphagia. Dopamine antagonists, including neuroleptics, can cause extrapyramidal reactions (involuntary movement disorders), as well as tardive dyskinesia and lingual or laryngeal dystonia. After medication of corticosteroids, myopathic symptoms of the swallowing musculature may reduce swallowing safety and efficiency. Anticholinergic side effects of antidepressants and antihistamines, as well as other medications, may include decreased salivation and dry mouth with impaired bolus preparation and propulsion (Schwemmle et al. 2015).

As a side effect, after injection of botulinum toxin for torticollis or other focal dystonias affecting the neck, or for treatment of disturbed UES opening, an inadvertent pharyngeal weakness and laryngeal dysfunction may occur and even cause aspiration (Bledsoe and Comella 2016).

A variety of forms of surgery of the neck can be associated with neurogenic dysphagia (Groher and Crary 2016). Most importantly anterior cervical fusion and resection of cervical osteophytes, possibly because of oesophageal retraction, prominence of the cervical plate and prevertebral swelling, but also due to disconnection of the plexus pharyngeal nerve fibres from the pharyngeal constrictor muscles as well as intra-operative traction and manipulation of all nerves involved in swallowing, can cause neurogenic dysphagia (Cho et al. 2013; Rosenthal et al. 2007; Warnecke et al. 2021; Buchholz 1997).

Surgery of the posterior fossa (Prosiegel et al. 2005; Wadhwa et al. 2014; Schröter-Morasch et al. 1995) or base of the skull may result in damage to cranial nerves and brainstem structures owing to intra-operative contusion or ischaemia. In addition, cardiac and thoracic surgery may cause dysphagia following lesions of nerves involved in swallowing, frequently misdiagnosed or related to endotracheal intubation (Skoretz et al. 2014).

After head and neck tumour treatment with radiochemotherapy, neurogenic dysphagia may occur as a result of brainstem structures or peripheral nerve involvement, sometimes seen years or even decades after the end of therapy (Crawley and Sulica 2015).

## 27.3.4 Associated Symptoms (Comorbidities)

In addition to the effects of neurogenic disease on the swallowing mechanism, patients may exhibit a number of comorbidities, which must be considered in rehabilitation strategies:

- Movement disorders of the limbs, including apraxia with disturbances in preparation and intake of food.
- Decreased level of consciousness in the acute stage; later on, changes in mental status with

deficits in memory, concentration, attention, perception, alertness, reasoning and judgement, behaviour and personality.

- Communication disorders such as aphasia and dysarthria with an inability to describe swallowing complaints and restrictions.
- Structural damage after intubation, as well as tracheostomies and nasogastric tube feeding, may cause oedema, inflammation, granuloma, ulcers and scar tissue and therefore additionally influence or restrict speech and swallowing functions.

## 27.3.5 Summary

Neurogenic dysphagia is a major symptom in more than 50% of neurological diseases, above all in stroke, dementia and Parkinson's disease with a high prevalence in older age (Wirth et al. 2016a, b). Its incidence is expected to increase further by demographic development. The results of dysphagia—malnutrition and dehydration on the one hand, and aspiration with risk of aspiration pneumonia on the other—may be life-threatening, and frequently responsible for the course of the underlying disease, the duration of being treated in hospital and the rehabilitation outcome, therefore also for increasing costs of healthcare (Burgos et al. 2018; Wirth et al. 2016a, b; Murray et al. 2014). During recent years considerable efforts have been made to establish appropriate diagnostic and therapeutic tools for improving the diagnosis and management of dysphagia, not only in hospitals (stroke units, IUC, rehabilitation settings) and in nursing homes, but also for outpatient settings and healthcare establishments. Among patho-physiologically orientated diagnostic procedures, the endoscopic examination of swallowing has emerged within the past 20 years as an indispensable standard examination with high sensitivity and specificity in neurogenic dysphagia (Langmore et al. 1991; Dziewas et al. 2013, 2017; Warnecke and Dziewas 2018). Symptoms of neurogenic dysphagia that can be directly observed reflect the underlying sensorimotor characteristics of the neurological deficit, which may change over time, showing recovery (normally after TBI) or deterioration of function in degenerative diseases such as PD or ALS. Symptoms in neurogenic dysphagia are characterised by disturbances in muscular activity, sensitivity and reflex activity, resulting in a reduction of swallowing efficiency and safety. A thorough evaluation of the specific deficits in the oropharyngeal and laryngeal region frequently allows a diagnosis of the underlying neurological disease. At the same time, associated comorbidities and structural damage must not be overlooked. These complex patterns of disturbance need to be identified as early as possible by a thorough phoniatric examination and close cooperation with neurologists and speech therapists, as well as radiologists, gastroenterologists and other healthcare specialists to develop individually tailored therapies.

## 27.4    Psychogenic Dysphagia

Daniele Farneti

This section was written in memory of Docent Dirk Deuster, an honourable colleague and highly esteemed physician, who wanted to contribute to it, but passed away at a young age after a severe illness.

### 27.4.1 Introduction

The brain is involved in organic pathologies by compromising, in unpredictable and variously combined ways, not only its main motor and sensory functions, but also cognition and behaviour. It is also possible that frankly psychiatric pathologies, foreseen by the DSM-V (2013), are associated with neurological symptoms or with pharmacological therapeutic associations (Cicala et al. 2019).

### 27.4.2 Neurological Disorders

Multiple neurological pathologies involve motor and sensory functions, and the cognitive and behavioural domains. Physical and psycho-

pathological symptoms of illness can variously be combined: (1) physical symptoms come to light through complex psychological processes; (2) the psychological disorder itself is manifested by physical symptoms; (3) organic diseases cause a secondary psychological reaction; (4) a category of organic diseases that affect the brain, can give rise, more or less directly, to psychological manifestations (Butler and Zeman 2005).

The association between cognitive, psychological and behavioural sequelae in organic CNS pathology underlies several factors:

- **Time of onset:** acute pathologies (trauma, metabolic disorders, drugs, infections, for example) are particularly associated with "delirium" or confusional states; slowly progressive diseases are more often responsible for "chronic brain syndromes", such as dementia.
- **Site of lesion:** ischaemic lesions of the right hemisphere are associated with mania while those on the left (especially frontal) with disinhibition. Cortical and subcortical cognitive deficits are differentiated by the different expression of praxic, executive and communicative-linguistic systems.
- **Neurotransmitters:** acetylcholine deficiency characterises the initial stages of Alzheimer's disease; impaired serotonin, noradrenergic and dopaminergic transmission characterise depression in Parkinson's disease.
- **Individual differences:** age, sex, educational level and history of psychiatric pathologies can influence the likelihood of brain pathology giving rise to psychopathological symptoms.
- **Inheritance:** hereditary factors are often associated with neuropsychiatric as well as neurological manifestations. Examples are Huntington's disease, which associates depression, apathy, aggression up to psychosis; Wilson's disease, manifesting mainly as neuropsychiatric symptoms; acute intermittent porphyria which can give rise to acute psychosis, often associated with abdominal pain.

- **Acquired pathologies:** potentially all the main acquired pathologies of the CNS can be associated with psychiatric or neuropsychological alterations. An examination of them would lead away from the objective of this section.

## 27.4.3 Psychiatric Disorders

Mental health refers to a state of social, physical and mental well-being, which can be affected by biological, individual and social influences and perspectives. Mental illness, comprising a wide range of conditions with different symptoms, is usually characterised by a combination of abnormal thoughts, emotions, behaviour and relationships with others (WHO 2021). These include schizophrenia, depression, mental retardation and drug-abuse disorders. Among the more common major psychopathologies, apart from schizophrenias and bipolar syndromes, can be noted anxiety and depression.

Anxiety is a psychic state of an individual, predominantly conscious, characterised by a feeling of intense concern or fear, related to a specific environmental stimulus, associated with a failure of the organism to adapt in a given situation, leading to stress for the individuals themselves (DMS-V 2013).

Anxiety disorders include:

- **Generalised anxiety disorder:** worry about many events and routine life circumstances (e.g., health, finances, children or other family members, job responsibilities, appointments).
- **Specific phobias:** fear a specific situation or object and desire to avoid it.
- **Panic disorder:** recurrent panic attacks, which are characterised by intense anxiety or discomfort of sudden onset and brief duration.
- **Anxiety disorder due to another medical condition:** a disorder that can be best explained as a physiological effect of that condition.

Depression can be defined as a psychiatric pathology or mood disorder described by depressed mood episodes accompanied mainly by low self-esteem and loss of interest or pleasure in normally pleasant activities (anhedonia).

Depression disorders include:

- **Major depression:** melancholic mood and loss of interest in activities once enjoyed, weight loss and decreased appetite, sleeping problems, loss of energy, problems with concentration, and possible suicidal thoughts.
- **Persistent depressive disorder (dysthymia):** sustained depressed mood over a two-year period or more. Symptoms of dysthymia are less intense than those of major depressive disorders but still affect daily life.
- **Depressive disorder due to another medical condition:** comparable to those of anxiety disorders due to other medical conditions.
- **Somatic symptom disorder:** physical symptoms that cannot be explained by a somatic medical condition and are not attributable to another psychiatric condition.

A swallowing disorder is often reported in adult patients with mental illness, with a higher incidence than in the general population, in which dysphagia is estimated to be around 6% (Aldridge and Taylor 2012). Table 27.7 summarises the main swallowing disorders reported by patients with mental illness.

Possible causes of dysphagia in the mentally ill adult population include effects related to the use of antipsychotic drugs, including neurolep-

**Table 27.7** Main Swallowing Disorders Reported by Patients with Mental Illness (based on Aldridge and Taylor 2012 and Cicala et al. 2019)

| |
| --- |
| Fear of swallowing |
| Globus |
| General difficulty in swallowing |
| Breathing problems |
| Fear of choking |
| Weight loss |
| Avoidance of eating |
| Malnutrition |
| Presentation of small boluses |
| Multiple tongue movements |
| Complex oral motion: Rocking, swirling, bunching, pumping |
| Pharyngeal swallow delay without bolus propulsion |

tics, behavioural changes associated with the psychiatric disorder itself, concomitant and institutionalisation-related neurological disorders (Bazemore et al. 1991). An important contribution to this topic came from Cicala et al. (2019), who specifically considered the development of pneumonia and choking in association with these drugs. They reported: (1) a limited literature with only 45 case reports of antipsychotic (AP)-induced dysphagia with pharmacological mechanisms, (2) a systematic review of APs as a risk factor for dysphagia, (3) reviews suggesting adult patients with intellectual disability and dementia are prone to dysphagia (APs are a risk factor among multiple others), (4) studies of the increased risk of choking in patients with mental illness (APs are a contributing factor), (5) naturalistic pneumonia studies suggesting that pneumonia may contribute to AP-increased death in dementia, and (6) naturalistic studies suggesting that pneumonia may be a major cause of morbidity and mortality in clozapine patients.

The action of these drugs on swallowing can be summarised according to the following schemes:

- **Antidepressant side effects** (monoamine oxidase inhibitors (MAOIs), tricyclic, tetracyclic, serotonin reuptake inhibitors).
  - Sedation: mental or physical abilities, loss of appetite and attention to eating, drowsiness (first 2 weeks).
  - Anticholinergic: xerostomia, difficulty initiating swallowing, abnormal peristalsis of smooth visceral muscle; deglutitive inhibition on the oesophageal striated or smooth muscle.
  - Gastrointestinal: loss of appetite and attention to eating, nausea, vomiting, diarrhoea, impaired gastrointestinal motility and constipation.
- **Anti-anxiety side effects** (sedatives, hypnotics, benzodiazepines).
  - Sedation, coordination disorders, decreased concentration (inattention to meals, difficulty in eating), heartburn, nausea, vomiting, diarrhoea, constipation, gastrointestinal pain, anorexia, taste alterations, dry mouth,

cricopharyngeal incoordination, hypopharyngeal incoordination, aspiration.
- **Anti-psychotic side effects** (anticholinergic).
  - Sedation: loss of appetite and attention to eating, drowsiness (first two weeks).
  - Extra-pyramidal: rigidity, tremor, masked facies, dysarthria, akathisia, restless, dystonia in term of "Acute extra-pyramidal syndrome" or "Tardive dyskinesia".
  - Neuroleptic-associated choking: risk of asphyxiation in psychiatric hospital is 100 times that in the normal population.

As regards this last condition, Nagamine (2011) reported a history of aspiration in which pneumonia did not predict choking. Dysphagia induced by antipsychotics has been reported to increase the risk of both aspiration pneumonia and choking. Aspiration pneumonia arises from micro-aspiration causing the entry of small amounts of food and oral indigenous microbial flora into the trachea. It is often attributable to silent aspiration, and a major mechanism for its onset is reduction in pharyngeal reflex mediated by antipsychotic-induced decrease of Substance P. It is not always accompanied by extra-pyramidal symptoms. Respiratory arrest in cases of choking is not, however, caused by entry of food into the trachea but by obstruction of the pharynx with food mass.

Another recent review, by Fonta and Salsench (2017), reported after exclusion of clinical cases 18 clinical studies of dysphagia related to antipsychotics: 12 were related both to typical and atypical antipsychotics, four to atypical antipsychotics and two to typical antipsychotics. According to the clinical studies included, the prevalence of patients with swallowing problems taking antipsychotics ranges from 21.9 to 69.5% whereas that of patients without swallowing problems taking antipsychotics ranges from 5 to 30.5%. The available evidence suggests considering an aetiology of dysphagia in patients with swallowing problems who are taking antipsychotics, even if no other symptoms are present. Although few general conclusions can be drawn from current evidence, both typical and atypical antipsychotics can be associated with oropharyngeal dysphagia.

Data from older case histories are available in the literature. Barofsky and Fontaine (1998) reported only 3% of patients complaining of swallowing disorders in a large sample with normal results of a videofluoroscopic swallowing study (VFSS). Ekberg et al. 2002 (10) studying 1110 patients in a VFSS during 2002–2006 found 12 cases of psychogenic dysphagia (0.01%). The historical case report of the Johns Hopkins Swallowing Center reported 13% of globus hystericus (see below) in 1989 (Ravich et al. 1989). In the Rimini Swallowing Center (Farneti and Consolmagno 2007) during 2018, 27 of 1092 patients evaluated (3.7%) had no instrumental signs of dysphagia and 34.5% of these had a bolus complaint. During 2019, 41 of 1157 patients evaluated (3.5%) had no instrumental signs of dysphagia and the 32.8% had a bolus complaint.

These latest data are of interest, since increasing numbers of patients with indistinct or non-specific symptoms, or without anatomical or pathophysiological correlates of dysphagia, are making use of our services. In the past, these cases of dysphagia were variously labelled as globus, functional dysphagia, swallowing phobia, psychogenic dysphagia or phagophobia. These terms are listed in the DSM-V (specific phobia) and defined as abnormal sensations during swallowing, sometimes accompanied by behavioural abnormalities during swallowing examination. Phagophobia in also used to define functional somatic disorders, often a comorbidity of anxiety and depression or other clinical features that have to be distinguished from globus hystericus, choking phobia, a sudden inability to swallow solid foods (Jain 2016).

It should also be remembered and specified that reflux symptoms occur more frequently in patients with a diagnosed psychiatric disorder than those without. The reflux symptoms may not necessarily be associated with any specific type of medication (apart from antidepressants) and may reflect a generally reduced threshold or a distorted perception of symptoms. There have also been a few reports that dysphagia/oesophageal motility disorders are likely to be "inherent" in psychiatric disorders, more so in schizophrenia (Baheshree and Jonas 2012; Regan et al. 2006).

A more recent terminology and approach comes from Verdonschot et al. (2019), who introduced the term Medically Unexplained Oropharyngeal Dysphagia (MUNOD) to indicate those symptomatological and clinical conditions that are not clear or not clearly definable according to the usual diagnostic deglutological schemes. The study included 14 patients with dysphagic complaints who had no detectible structural or physiological abnormalities upon swallowing examination. All patients underwent a standardised examination protocol, with examination by fibre-optic endoscopic evaluation of swallowing (FEES), the Hospital Anxiety and Depression Scale (HADS) and the Dysphagia Severity Scale (DSS). The authors found that six patients (42.8%) had clinically relevant symptoms of anxiety or depression. The DSS scores did not differ significantly between patients with or without affective symptoms. None of the 14 patients showed any structural or physiological abnormalities during FEES examination, apart from abnormal piecemeal deglutition. Affective symptoms are common in patients with MUNOD, and their psychiatric conditions could be related to their swallowing problems. The authors concluded that a consultation with a psychiatrist for patients with MUNOD be recommended as part of a pathway towards multidisciplinary integrated care. They also recommended the screening of patients for anxiety and depression.

The correlation of anxiety and depression with dysphagia has been evaluated in operated head-and-neck cancer patients by Nguyen et al. (2005). They retrospectively evaluated 73 of 104 patients who complained of dysphagia after primary radiotherapy (RT), chemoradiotherapy or postoperative RT for head-and-neck malignancies. All patients underwent a modified barium swallowing examination to assess the severity of dysphagia, graded on a scale of 1–7. Quality of Life (QOL) was evaluated by the University of Washington (UW) and Hospital Anxiety and Depression questionnaires. The UW and HAD scores were reduced and elevated, respectively, in the dysphagia group compared with the no dysphagia group ($p = 0.0005$). They concluded that dysphagia is a significant morbidity of head-and-neck cancer treatment, and that the severity of dysphagia was correlated with a compromised QOL, anxiety and depression. Patients with moderate to severe dysphagia require a team approach involving nutritional support, physical therapy, speech rehabilitation, pain management and psychological counselling.

The association between subjective and objective symptoms requires careful evaluation by the clinician. Whatever the perspective from which this association is considered, there must always be a correlation between signs and symptoms: if this is not so, particular attention must be paid to the study of the patient before defining a swallowing disorder as functional and consulting a specialist before defining it as pertaining to psychiatry.

A possible evaluation protocol, in case of patients with these characteristics, can be summarised as follows in Table 27.8.

The dilemma between functional and organic origins of dysphagia still remains. The Johns Hopkins Swallowing Center reported 13% of globus hystericus in 1989, and in the same year Ravich et al. stated that two-thirds of this group was later found to have an organic aetiology for dysphagia (Ravich et al. 1989). Thus particular attention has to be given to patients with blurred or indistinct symptoms of dysphagia, mainly to patients with severe subjective symptoms but with no or modest objective instrumental findings. Worthy of attention, from the opposite point

**Table 27.8** Clinical Approach to Patients with Possible Psychologist./.Psychiatrist Substratum

| |
|---|
| Clinical evaluation: ENT, Phoniatrician |
| Instrumental evaluation: Fibre-optic endoscopic evaluation of swallowing (FEES), videofluoroscopic swallowing study (VFSS) |
| Functional scales: penetration/aspiration scale (PAS: Rosenbek et al. 1996), Pooling score (p-score: Farneti et al. 2014), functional oral intake scale (FOIS: Crary et al. 2005), Dysphagia Outcome and Severity Scale (DOSS: O'Neil et al. 1999) |
| Hospital Anxiety and Depression Scale (HADS scale: Zigmond and Snaith 1983) |
| QOL questionnaires (dysphagia severity scale, DSS) |
| Body mass index (BMI; http//www.calculator.net/bmi-calculator.html) |
| Mini Mental State Exam (MMSE: Folstein et al. 1975) |
| Low dysphagia (submit to gastroenterologist specialist) |

of view, are psychiatric patients with multi-drug therapies, who complain less of dysphagia symptoms and for whom the risks of pulmonary complications or choking are elevated.

## 27.5 Dysphagia After Head and Neck Tumour Treatment

Virginie Woisard,Antoinette am Zehnhoff-Dinnesen and Miroslav Tedla

### 27.5.1 Introduction

Head and neck cancer (HNC) is the sixth-most common cancer worldwide, accounting for 7% of all malignancies (GLOBOCAN 2012). The main treatment modalities are surgery and (chemo-) radiotherapy. The choice of modality is dependent on patient variables, primary site, clinical stage and resectability of the tumour. Patients presenting with early stage disease can be managed by single modality- curative surgery or radiotherapy. Patients presenting with loco-regionally advanced disease may be treated with surgical resection followed by postoperative (chemo) radiotherapy or with concomitant chemoradiotherapy. Neoadjuvant chemotherapy may also be used.

Head and neck cancer has an enormous impact on the quality of life (QoL) of patients. The most important physical symptoms are voice and speech problems, changed appearance, trismus, dry mouth and swallowing problems (De Boer et al. 1999). Distress is often present in spouses and patients (Verdonck-de Leeuw et al. 2007).

An altered swallow function can be secondary to the mechanical effects of a tumour, invading the normal anatomy needed for deglutition, or as a direct sequela of cancer treatment. At the time of diagnosis, almost 50% of HNC patients present with dysphagia. Severe dysphagia is a strongest independent predictor of survival (Shune et al. 2012). Pre-treatment swallowing problems also constitute a factor negatively influencing radiation-induced acute and late dysphagia (Dirix et al. 2009; Brown et al. 2013; Mortensen et al. 2013).

Key factors to consider regarding influence of the treatment on swallowing outcomes include site and extent of resection, neck dissection, laterality of radiotherapy fields, target volumes, radiotherapy technique, radiotherapy dose and concurrent chemotherapy (Hutcheson et al. 2019).

After treatment, swallowing disorders are frequent; the percentage depends on the tumour site. Nguyen et al. (2009) found swallowing disorders in 5%, 29%, 33% and 52% of oral cavity, laryngeal, oropharyngeal and hypopharyngeal tumours, respectively. During follow-up, in some of these patients (33%) dysphagia severity increased and only 3% patients achieved normalisation of swallowing. Campbell et al. (2004) found that almost half of long-term non-laryngectomy head and neck cancer survivors (>5 years) presented at least some degree of aspiration. Swallowing problems should be considered when determining appropriate cancer-directed treatment and post-treatment care. Approximately one third of dysphagic patients develop aspiration pneumonia requiring treatment, with mortality rates ranging between 20% and 65% (Pikus et al. 2003). Of the patients who aspirated, 55% had no protective cough reflex (silent aspiration) (Garon et al. 2009). Despite these data, the tolerance of aspirations may be surprisingly good (Simonelli et al. 2010) and some complications do not occur until after 5 years (Payakachat et al. 2013).

The management of swallowing disorders is driven by the associated life-threatening situation. For this reason, the benefit–risk balance concerning swallowing disorders and other sequelae, is in favour of benefit compared with the major risk of death without treatment.

Because of dysphagia's high incidence rate and association with survival, a swallowing specialist should be involved to ensure routine diagnostic and therapeutic swallowing interventions. Patients with moderate-to-severe dysphagia require a team approach involving nutritional support, physical therapy, speech rehabilitation, pain management and psychological counselling.

## 27.5.2 Dysphagia After Head and Neck Tumour Surgery

Surgical interventions on HNC might cause specific damage conditioning site-specific patterns of dysphagia; anatomical changes, scarring, sensoric and motor damage. In general oral transit time can be prolonged, manipulation with bolus in the pharynx is negatively affected as well as the strength and range of motion of the tongue. Constriction of the pharyngeal sphincter might be not effective, the hyolaryngeal movement might be reduced and laryngeal sphincter incompetent.

In spite of surgery being rarely performed alone, it can provoke a swallowing "shock", followed by a recovery phase. The risk of aspiration during the postoperative period is of particular concern. Knowledge of swallowing dysfunction mechanisms is a basic requirement for understanding the risk of complications during the treatment, providing the best recovery and reducing the swallowing disorders long-term after the end of the treatment (Woisard and Puech 2010). The consequences for swallowing will be described for the different types of surgery and the importance of some anatomical structures will be identified.

### 27.5.2.1 Oral and Oropharyngeal Surgery

**Lip Resection**, depending on the site and extent of the resection, can negatively affect labial closure and can present with sensor and motor deficit. The consequence can be drooling and poor bolus control.

Whenever possible full thickness skin flaps (skin, muscle and mucosa) should be used. The repair should provide sufficient mucosa contiguous to the commissure to avoid contracture (Kerawala et al. 2016).

**Floor of Mouth (FOM) Resection** Anterior FOM resection patients have problems with preparation for the swallow and oral transit (Logemann and Bytell 1979). The severity of swallowing dysfunction depends on the geniohyoid or mylohyoid muscle resection. The role of these muscles in the elevation and antero-propulsion of the larynx determines the risk of aspiration. The swallowing deficits can also vary according to the type of reconstruction. Direct closure shows better functional outcome than loco-regional and free flaps when it is possible (Hirano et al. 1992). Larger mass of the flap for the reconstruction of oral and oropharyngeal defects appears to improve swallowing outcomes (Kao et al. 2016).

**Oral Tongue Resection** Swallowing problems depend of the resected volume of the tongue. Oral tongue resection slows oral transit, reduces the capacity to control the bolus inside the oral cavity during chewing and oral phase, provoking retention of bolus and risk of aspiration (Logemann and Bytell 1979).

The long-term follow-up of patients after the surgical treatment of tongue carcinomas shows an acceptable QoL in partial resection, despite poor swallowing efficiency assessed by videofluoroscopy (Tei et al. 2012). Hirano et al. (1992) described the type of food and the degree of aspiration after total and partial glossectomy. Patients with tongue cancer who had hemiglossectomy without reconstruction could eat normal food without aspiration within a week after operation. Patients who had undergone a half to three-quarter glossectomy for tongue cancer could eat gruel with no or occasional liquid aspiration. Of patients who had near-total or total glossectomy for tongue cancer, three quarters could eat thin gruel or liquid with occasional aspiration, one quarter could not eat orally because of consistent severe aspiration. The probability of aspiration increases as the percentage of resected tongue increases (Russi et al. 2012), introducing the necessity to use a flap reconstruction. Larger mass of the flap for the reconstruction of oral and oropharyngeal defects appears to improve swallowing outcomes (Kao et al. 2016).

Only in small resections of the oral tongue (<30%) does primary defect closure give equal or better functional results than flap reconstruction (Zuydam et al. 2005).

**Oropharyngectomy** Tonsil/base of tongue resection patients have a slowing in the preparation for the swallow and in the oral and pharyngeal stages (Logemann and Bytell 1979). For tonsil resection, the severity of dysphagia is related to the extent of the resection affecting other anatomical structures. Isolated tonsillectomy is usually followed by complete and fast recovery. This is the same for the limited resection of the base of the tongue when less than 15% is resected. Extensive removal of the tongue base, extension to the pharyngeal wall, to the soft palate, to the floor of the mouth, and removal of a part of the mandibula are worsening factors, leading to the risk of not recovering oral feeding.

**Palate Resection** Surgical resection of the hard palate and maxillary sinus leads to surgical defects in with a large oronasal and oromaxillary communication. Tongue movements are not able to drive the bolus gathered on the dorsal surface of the tongue because of a deficient hard palate, thus material enters the nose through the oronasal fistula during swallowing. Prosthetic implants or free flap reconstruction allow a return to a normal diet with good swallowing QoL. In contrast, soft palate tumour resection might result in incomplete closure of the nasopharynx with nasal regurgitation at the end of the oral phase. The soft palate is very adaptive to structural changes with sufficient recovery time and intensive speech therapy, but dysphagia strongly depends on the degree of tissue loss. Defects involving the lateral aspect of the soft palate are more likely to result in persistent dysphagia as they are much more difficult to fill in than midline defects (Russi et al. 2012).

Some tumours of the oral cavity and approaches to access oropharyngeal tumours have impact on the mandible. The alveolar ridge can be infiltrated, requiring resection. Mandibular fracture and unilateral luxation may be performed to access the tumour. Simple transection with osteosynthesis, rim or marginal resection of the mandible will not disrupt the continuity of the mandibular arch and has little impact on swallowing function, but it limits the extent of mouth opening and presents a risk of trismus. Moreover, mandibulotomy can cause damage to the genioglossus muscles, the inferior alveolar nerve and to occlusion. The loss of occlusion causes dysphagia because of loss of stability during deglutition and loss of correct larynx elevator muscle action. Thus, in the case of mandibulectomy the reconstruction of the mandible at the time of initial surgical resection is recommended (Kronenberger and Meyers 1994).

Teeth and dentures are important for chewing and for jaw stabilisation by occlusion of the posterior teeth or dentures (Kronenberger and Meyers 1994). Suprahyoid musculatures pivoting on the immobilised mandible can pull the larynx forwards and permit the tongue base to cover it. Thus, the occurrence of laryngeal penetration might be nearly three times more likely for older patients swallowing without dentures (Yoshikawa et al. 2006).

The swallowing deficits can also vary according to the type of reconstruction. The degree of impairment in these patients is related to the volume of the resection leading to the indication of a flap for the reconstruction, the volume and the adynamic character of the flap itself. The volume of the flap affects the outcome differently according to the anatomical site (thin for FOM, thicker for the tongue). Sensory return in reinnervated free grafts might improve functional outcome in intraoral reconstruction (Mah et al. 1996).

### 27.5.2.2 Laryngeal Surgery

The knowledge of laryngeal closure levels is vital for understanding laryngeal compensation abilities. The larynx closes sequentially from the bottom upwards. It includes four levels and behaves like a cardboard box with side shutters (vocal folds and false vocal folds), a posterior shutter (arytenoids) and an anterior shutter (epiglottis). To each level a function can be assigned: voice production, coughing, forceful glottal closure, swallowing (Fig. 27.13) (Woisard and Puech 2010).

After partial laryngeal resection inadequate laryngeal closure can lead to aspiration. The compensation depends on the efficient action of the structures in the remaining levels.

**Open Surgery** The following surgical procedures belong to the open surgery:

### Total Laryngectomy

After total laryngectomy, the loss of the closure function is irrelevant to the swallowing process, as the airway is separated from the digestive tract. The confidence to eat in public and normality of diet in the long-term decreases in 50% of patients after total laryngectomy (Chone et al. 2011).

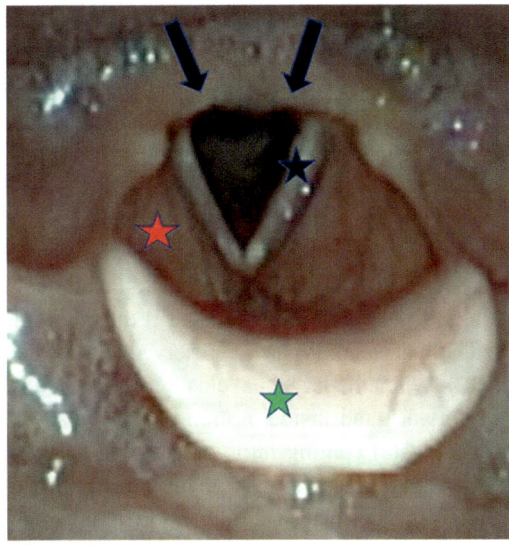

**Fig. 27.13** The levels of laryngeal closure: green asterisk, epiglottis; red asterisk, vestibular folds, black asterisk, glottis, arrows: arytenoids

Dysphagia may be a result of impaired pharyngeal propulsive contractile forces and increased resistance to bolus flow across the pharyngo-oesophageal segment or a benign stricture (Manikantan et al. 2009). Voice prostheses inserted after total laryngectomy can lead to aspiration/aspiration pneumonia or aspiration of the prosthesis itself (Tong et al. 2020).

### Vertical Partial Laryngeal Resection

This includes resection of the vocal cord, up to the anterior commissure, is resected with underlying cartilage extending posteriorly to include part of the arytenoid if necessary. Asymmetric elevation of the hyolaryngeal complex and compromised laryngeal closure increases risk of aspiration. Dysphagia is more prevalent in the early postoperative period. Early intervention can assist in the management of secretions and allows safe regain of the oral feeding (Messing et al. 2019).

### Supracricoid Partial Laryngectomy

This includes the removal of bilateral true and false folds, the paraglottal space, the thyroid cartilage and occasionally the epiglottis. The hyoid bone and both or at least one correctly functioning cricoid–arytenoid units need to be preserved in order to create a neoglottis, which retains the closure function. Early modified barium swallow assessment shows that all patients aspirated initially and had impaired base of tongue and laryngeal movements. Postoperative re-education is crucial in many cases, but patients with functional deglutition may present a well-tolerated degree of chronic silent aspiration and do not have to limit their oral intake of food (Simonelli et al. 2010). Outcomes are better if the epiglottis and both arytenoids can be preserved (Russi et al. 2012). When the laryngeal closure is achieved by the forward and inside motion of the remaining arytenoids(s) coming into contact with the base of the epiglottis, this movement corresponds to the closure performed during effortful swallowing with closed glottis. When the epiglottis is resected, the arytenoids can contact the base of the tongue. This has three consequences: (1) there is only one level of neoglottal closure, (2) the neoglottal closure depends on extra-laryngeal structures and (3) the mobilisation of the base of the tongue in the laryngeal closure decreases its role in the transport of the bolus. For deglutition the stepwise sequence of the different neuromuscular events needs a complete reorganisation. In the case that this reorganisation fails, aspiration and penetration might represent serious sequelae (Woisard et al. 1996).

### Supraglottal Partial Laryngeal Resection

This involves the removal of the epiglottis, ary-epiglottic folds, ventricular folds and one or both superior laryngeal nerves. These anatomical modifications lead to a supraglottic area bounded ventrally by the base of the tongue, at the bottom by the glottal plane and dorsally by the arytenoids. This is called the "glosso-laryngeal recess". Aspiration can occur because of incomplete airway closure, secondary to pharyngeal residues spilling into the airway, inadequate laryngeal elevation or weak propulsive forces (Logemann et al. 1994). In order to avoid any laryngeal penetration, the supraglottal closure should be compensated for by the complete closure of the glosso-laryngeal recess. This is achieved by an increasing forward motion of the arytenoids and an increasing backward movement of the base of the tongue. This may explain why patients have a slight slowing of the oral and pharyngeal transit. When the supraglottal laryngectomy involves the tongue base or arytenoids, aspiration is more likely. The functional outcomes can be bad. Suarez et al. (1996) reported that total laryngectomy for aspiration was required in 9.8% and in 21.4% of patients with supraglottal and base-of-tongue carcinomas, respectively.

**Endoscopic Surgery** Trans-oral laser surgery (TOLS) with the use of $CO_2$ laser has been introduced into clinical practice for decades. Monopolar microelectrodes or other types of lasers can be used instead of $CO_2$ laser. In recent years, the robotic systems are used to control endoscopic instruments during surgical procedures, this approach can be used also for some type of laryngeal resections. These approaches allow the transformation of open surgical management to trans-oral minimally invasive surgery, limiting functional damage and has an advantage for saving the swallowing process (Manakantan et al. 2009).

Endoscopic laser surgery for small glottal tumours usually causes glottal impairment, quickly compensated for by the upper levels of closure. Aspirations are rare and disappear quickly with re-education within a few days after the procedure.

TOLS for advanced glottal or supraglottal carcinoma of the larynx is an option in selected cases. In a study by Hinni et al. (2007), out of the 68 patients with T2-T4 glottal or supraglottal carcinoma resected with TOLS, on the latest follow-up, 44% had a normal function with episodic or daily symptoms of dysphagia, 49% had compensated abnormal function manifested by significant dietary modifications or prolonged mealtimes (without weight loss or aspiration) and 7% were feeding tube-dependent.

### 27.5.2.3 Neck Dissection and Skull Base Surgery

Neck dissection and the skull base surgery can jeopardise several structures important for deglutition. Cranial nerves as vagal, hypoglossal, glossopharyngeal, facial nerves are at risk. Cervical structures such as sternocleidomastoid muscle, other muscles, nerves or vessels may be damaged or sacrificed. Multiple damage of the cranial nerves can lead to severe aspiration with the need for non-oral feeding (Woisard and Puech 2010; Manakantan et al. 2009). Deglutition can be further affected in patient after chemoraciotherapy (Hutcheson et al. 2016).

### 27.5.2.4 Tracheostomy

Tracheostomy may be used as a short- or long-term solution when the tumour occludes the airway, for postoperative oedema or where the airway has to be secured during chemoradiation. A study performed by Leder et al. (2005) found that occlusion status of the tracheotomy tube did not influence the prevalence of aspiration in the immediate postoperative period. Moreover, neither the presence of a tracheotomy tube nor decannulation affected aspiration status in early post-surgical head and neck cancer patients. The impact of cuff-inflated cannula on swallowing is dramatically different. Ding and Logemann (2005) demonstrated that the frequencies of reduced laryngeal elevation and silent aspiration were significantly higher in the cuff-inflated condition than in the cuff-deflated.

The causes of aspiration with tracheostomy present can be divided into mechanical and neurophysiological (Nash 1988). One of the mechanical factors is decreased laryngeal elevation that reduces airway protection and cricopharyngeal opening. Other mechanical factors are local compression forces exerted by the inflated cuff, which lead to the retention of secretions in the upper airway and the cervical oesophagus. The neurophysiological factors are desensitisation of the protective cough reflex and a loss of coordination of laryngeal closure. An inflated cuff is not protective against aspiration in tracheostomised patients. In conclusion, it is not necessary to keep the tracheotomy tube in the postoperative period for swallowing rehabilitation. Keeping an open cannula with inflated cuff limits the recovery of the swallowing function.

### 27.5.2.5 The Anatomical Structures to Be Spared

Surgical experience has determined some limits to the procedures, compatible with sufficient functional outcomes, particularly for avoiding aspirations.

Tongue base resection is the main factor stressed in the literature. Patients with resection of more than a quarter (Zuydam et al. 2005) to half (Smith et al. 2008) of the tongue base are at high risk of having early postoperative aspiration. The conservation of lingual innervation is an important prognostic factor.

In the case of partial laryngectomies, chronic aspirations are correlated to the loss of more than two levels of laryngeal closure (Woisard and Puech 2010; Halczy-Kowalik et al. 2012). In the case of total laryngectomy, pharyngeal mucosal preservation is a keypoint of the procedure. Residual mucosa of pharyngeal tissue of more than 1.5 cm (relaxed) and 2.5 cm (stretched) are correlated with no dysphagia complaints (Hui et al. 1996).

Aspects of reconstructive surgery in head and neck are presented in Hanasono et al. (2016).

## 27.5.3 Dysphagia After Head and Neck Tumour Radiotherapy

Head and neck cancers can be treated with radiation therapy alone, by surgery or with chemotherapy or targeted therapies.

For many years, the standard approach in the majority of HNC patients involved opposed lateral fields encompassing the primary tumour sites and regional lymph nodes. The conventional radiotherapy dosage for cure in HNC is usually daily fractions of 1.8–2.0 Gray (Gy), up to total doses of 66–70 Gy over 6–7 weeks. Alterations in the fractionation schedule, as well as concomitant chemotherapy, significantly improve tumour responses. However, this aggressive treatment regimen has lead to significant sequelae including dysphagia (Manakantan et al. 2009).

New radiotherapy techniques available for HNC allow delivery of a curative dose to the tumour volume while sparing healthy tissues, thereby decreasing radiation-induced sequelae. Unlike conventional approaches, intensity-modulated radiation therapy (IMRT) restricts the radiation dose to the shape of the target tissues in three dimensions, reducing the dose delivered to the nearby normal tissues. IMRT has been shown to be associated with excellent outcomes with less damage to the salivary glands. Efforts have been made to identify dosimetric parameters important for dysphagia and hence the possibility of dose reduction or structure avoidance. Predictive models for swallowing dysfunction have been developed with the potential of improved intensity-modulated radiotherapy to reduce the risk of swallowing dysfunction.

Nevertheless, many dysphagic patients treated with conventional techniques suffer from long-term dry mouth (xerostomia), and there is poor knowledge of the incidence of long-term side effects with the new techniques. For Mortensen et al. (2013) QoL data showed a lower degree of dysphagia than objective measures. The most frequent swallowing dysfunction is retention; penetration and aspiration are less common.

### 27.5.3.1 Swallowing Consequences of (Chemo-)Radiotherapy

Definitive chemoradiotherapy is now a widely accepted treatment option for patients with HNC and it has become difficult to isolate the consequences of radiotherapy alone, especially when the publications deal with late effects.

**Pathophyiology** Radiation-induced dysphagia has a complex aetiopathogenesis (King et al. 2016). Lesions can be schematically classified into two main pathophysiological processes affecting all tissues: inflammation (and the resulting oedema) and fibrosis. Microvascular changes, atrophy of muscle fibres and vessels, and collagen deposits are also observed, with consequent neurological or muscular injury (Russi et al. 2012; Manakantan et al. 2009; Servagi-Vernat et al. 2014).

In early radio-induced dysphagia, oedema causes the obliteration of vallecula and piriform sinus for the bolus to flow down. Thus, the bolus can be directed into the airway instead of beyond it. In late dysphagia, fibrosis prevails over oedema and fibrotic tissue accumulates diffusely. Considering radiation-induced fibrosis, the normal wound healing process is deregulated. This issue is noteworthy for peri-mucosal structures

since fibrosis secondary to acute intense mucositis might spread to the underlying pharyngeal constrictor muscles (PCM), laryngeal muscles and para-pharyngeal and paraglottal spaces (Eisbruch et al. 2004).

The variability of the timing and intensity of radiation-induced swallowing defects depends on the intensity of acute reactions, as well as intrinsic radiation-sensitivity to fibrosis based on genetics and comorbidities (Rødningen et al. 2008). Certain patients can experience a progressive onset of fibrosis soon after radiation therapy, others a delayed onset, yet others need to undergo a further event (trauma-surgery, addition of comorbidity, exhaustion of compensatory mechanisms with age) to experience fibrosis. Thus, radio-induced fibrosis may cause atrophic changes in the tongue with or without fasciculation, vocal fold palsy, velopharyngeal incompetence with premature leakage, and poor pharyngeal constriction. These events may cause swallowing disorders, but there are no clear boundaries between what is considered a "normal" sequela and what is a complication of radiotherapy. The insidious aspect of this advancing process leads to the appearance of severe complications many years after the end of the treatment, sometimes up to 10 years.

**Swallowing Impact of Radiotherapy** Assessments of the swallowing process after radio-therapy reveal (Lazarus et al. 1996)

- Decreased pharyngeal peristalsis and poor synchronisation between pharyngeal contractions, opening of the upper oesophageal sphincter and closure of the larynx.
- Decreased or defective backward motion of the base of the tongue towards the posterior pharyngeal wall.
- Incomplete or delayed closure of the larynx with decreased laryngeal adduction during swallowing.
- Decreased elevation of the hyoid bone and larynx and decreased inversion of the epiglottis.
- Delayed opening of the upper oesophageal sphincter. Lack of coordination during the swallow and decreased oropharyngeal swallow efficiency.

All of these abnormalities are responsible for a risk of aspiration or persistence of residues of the bolus in the oropharynx, valleculae and hypopharynx at the end of the swallowing phase, which may then subsequently be inhaled. The cough reflex is also often deficient or even absent after radiotherapy.

The estimated frequency of aspiration after chemoradiotherapy is from 40 to 80% in recent studies evaluating swallowing disorders by videoendoscopy (Eisbruch et al. 2002; Nguyen et al. 2006; Schwartz et al. 2010). In a study (Nguyen et al. 2006) on 22 patients evaluated by videofluoroscopy before, at the end of, and 6–12 months after radiation, aspirations were reported by 14% of patients before, 62% at the end, and 65% from 6 to 12 months after radiotherapy. Six patients (28%) developed aspiration pneumonia during follow-up, which was the cause of death in two patients (10%). Xu et al. (2015) found that nearly 25% of elderly patients will suffer from aspiration pneumonia within 5 years after receiving chemoradiotherapy for head and neck cancer.

Patients complain of different problems according to the site of the tumour, but the main problems reported are xerostomia and dysphagia (60%) and speech or voice disorders (80%). Patients with oral cancer report problems with opening the mouth (73%) (Weber et al. 2010). Although the main complaints of the patient are often about the change in saliva, Logemann et al. (2003) and Lango et al. (2009) demonstrated that reduced salivary weight is not correlated with slowed or inefficient swallowing. Xerostomia affects the sensory process and comfort of eating more than bolus transport. It may hide severe dysphagia.

**Evolution in Time** In clinical practice, we are faced with two periods after the radiation time: the period where the patient may recover from the early side effects, and the period where the late effects may occur with possible complications.

There are few longitudinal follow-up studies providing knowledge of the temporal link between the degree of early effects and complications related to late effects. Early effects are usually described when they appear during the treatment time. A long-term effect is one when dysphagia persists after 1 year. Late side effects are those that take months or even years to develop. But it is difficult without objective assessment to distinguish between a worsening long-term effect and a late effect, because of psychological adjustment (Cartmill et al. 2012) and deterioration in sensitivity (Nguyen et al. 2007).

Mortensen et al. (2013) observed a prevalence of acute dysphagia of up to 80% in patients receiving conventional therapy. Early effects on swallowing explored by videofluoroscopic study (VFS) were significantly worse 3 months post-treatment but improved by 6 months post-treatment. After chemoradiation, there was an improvement from 3 to 12 months (Frowen et al. 2010). The prevalence of chronic dysphagia at 1, 2, 3, 4 and 5 years was, respectively, 46%, 32%, 29%, 24% and 23%. From this information we have chosen a cut-off of 1 year for describing the data in the literature.

### Early Effects

Acute side-effects of radiotherapy are mucositis, dysphagia, hoarseness, erythema and desquamation of the skin. The prevalence of severe acute dysphagia is about 40% of patients receiving conventional radiotherapy (Mortensen et al. 2013). Sensation of the epiglottis and arytenoid deteriorates significantly one and three months after radiotherapy and recovers in most cases within one year after radiotherapy (Ozawa et al. 2010). Maruo et al. (2014) also observed significantly reduced laryngeal sensation one month after (chemo-)radiotherapy, which by trend returned after one year with maintained swallowing reflex and function.

### Late Sequelae and Complications

The potential late sequelae of high radiation doses include dysarthria/dysphonia, cranial neuropathy, osteonecrosis, dental decay, trismus, hypogeusia, subcutaneous fibrosis, thyroid dysfunction, oesophageal stenosis, hoarseness and damage to the middle or inner ear (Manikantan et al. 2009; Hutcheson et al. 2012). Late sequelae can cause impairment of different structures involved in the swallowing process. Late radiation-induced mucositis comprises loss of colour, thinning and rigidity of the mucosa, induration of the subcutaneous tissues, and can be complicated by ulceration and necrosis. These disorders are due to ischaemia secondary to fibrosis and occlusion of small vessels. These effects are progressive and irreversible and may be observed between six months and five years after radiotherapy (Hutcheson et al. 2012).

– Pharyngo-oesophageal stricture after radiotherapy including IMRT and chemotherapy treatment, is not uncommon (odds ratio: 3.3) (Wang et al. 2012). Radiotherapy induces loss of mobility. About half of the patients who undergo primary treatment for oral and oropharyngeal cancer develop a limitation of mouth opening similar to that in a trismus (Weber et al. 2010). Neuropathy with such a severe complication as paralysis of the cranial nerves are described after radiation treatment for nasopharyngeal carcinoma but also pharyngeal and lingual tumours. The paralysis might begin more than 5 years after radiation treatment.
– Rarely delayed progressive cervicobulbar neuronopathy with myokymia (involuntary, spontaneous, localised quivering of a few muscles or bundles within a muscle) is observed as an uncommon complication of radiotherapy for nasopharyngeal carcinoma (Rison and Beydoun 2011).
– Radiotherapy deteriorates sensation. Patients tested before and 1 year after treatment for intraoral sensation, shape recognition and hole size identification show diminished intraoral sensation and shape recognition (Jäghagen et al. 2008). The cough reflex in patients who aspirated following radiation for head and neck cancer is altered in 50% of patients (Nguyen et al. 2007).
– No paper is able to give the frequency of long-term late swallowing complications in head and neck cancer survivors (McDowell et al. 2018), but it seems that this frequency is about

5% for oropharyngeal cancer to 15% for nasopharyngeal cancer.

### 27.5.3.2 Predictive Factors of Radiotherapy-Induced Dysphagia

The development of multi-leaf collimators has allowed the replacement of lead shields for conformation of static X-ray beams. The possibility of modulating the dose in the same field has stimulated a whole field of research focused on the anatomical structures to spare and the doses to protect the functioning in the irradiated field and the quality of life of the patient. Prescription by beam optimisation is determined from calculation algorithms in which the volumes of interest (tumour target volumes and organs at risk), dose constraints and priorities for each volume are entered. The treatment planning system then optimises the intensity profile of each beam to comply with these parameters (Servagi-Vernat et al. 2014).Dysphagia-/Aspiration-related Structures The anatomical structures of the upper aerodigestive tract defined as dysphagia/aspiration-related structures, or those that correlate with pharyngo-oesophageal stricture or with weight of loss related to dysphagia are: the pharyngeal constrictor muscles, 'supraglottis' glottis (Dirix et al. 2009; Eisbruch et al. 2002; Caudell et al. 2010). Correlation between the dose delivered to the anterior oral cavity, oral mucosa, oesophageal inlet muscle, soft palate masseter and pterygoid muscles, and the reduction of swallowing function after radiotherapy, are described in few papers (Lazarus et al. 1996; Schwartz et al. 2010; Caudell et al. 2010; Sanguineti et al. 2011; Christianen et al. 2012; van der Molen et al. 2013). Of the three pharyngeal constrictors the superior muscle seems to be more determinant but this might be due to the presence of more nasopharyngeal tumours in these studies.

**Doses for Reducing Late Radiotherapy-induced Dysphagia** Regarding the radiation doses, Duprez et al. (2013) and Servagi-Vernat et al. (2014) analysed published dose-volume data of the structures related to late radiotherapy-induced swallowing disturbances in HNC. The mean dose and the volume receiving a dose of 65 Gy to the pharyngeal constrictor muscles appeared to be the most important dosimetric predictors of late swallowing disturbances (Eisbruch et al. 2004; McDowell et al. 2018). The most predictive dosimetric indices for the larynx are the mean dose (Dirix et al. 2009; Eisbruch et al. 2004; McDowell et al. 2018; Sanguineti et al. 2011) and the volume receiving a dose of 50 Gy (Zuydam et al. 2005; Manikantan et al. 2009). Oesophageal dose constraints have been described by many authors as a major risk factor for swallowing disorders, but these studies did not define the oesophageal volume in the same way (Zuydam et al. 2005; Mah et al. 1996; Manikantan et al. 2009). For the oral cavity and masseter and pterygoid muscles, there are not enough data. Before the appearance of intensity-modulated radiation therapy (IMRT), predictive factors of dysphagia were techniques (Dirix et al. 2009; Frowen et al. 2010; Lazarus et al. 1996) and mainly accelerated radiotherapy (Mortensen et al. 2013; Lango et al. 2009), total dose >50-Gy, extension of treatment volume, interfraction interval and fraction size. More recently, the functional units of muscles involved in hyolaryngeal elevation, tongue base retraction and tongue motion have been defined, useful for a greater understanding of dysphagia mechanisms: floor of mouth, thyrohyoid muscles, posterior digastric/stylohyoid muscles complex, longitudinal pharyngeal muscles, hyoglossus/styloglossus muscles complex, genioglossus muscles and intrinsic tongue muscles (Gawryszuk et al. 2018).

**Factors Predictive of Radiotherapy-induced Dysphagia** The appearance of severe side effects is not only related to the radiotherapy itself. Knowledge of all the prognostic factors will help to determine the exposed population, e.g. candidates for prophylactic measures against swallowing dysfunction. The variables negatively influencing radiation-induced acute and late dysphagia are summarised in Table 27.9.

**Table 27.9** Variables negatively influencing radiation-induced acute and late dysphagia

| Factors | Acute effects | Late effects |
|---|---|---|
| Age | Age = > 62 years (Mortensen et al. 2013) | >65 years (Christianen et al. 2012) |
| Smoking status | During and after RT (Frowen et al. 2010) | During and after RT (Frowen et al. 2010), correlated with stricture (Caglar et al. 2008) |
| Alcohol status | Ex-heavy alcohol consumption (Frowen et al. 2010) | Alcohol abuse (Gawryszuk et al. 2018) |
| Concomitant chemoradiation | Yes (Lango et al. 2009) | Yes (Van der Molen et al. 2013) |
| Weight loss at baseline | Yes (Lango et al. 2009) | No data |
| Dysphagia at baseline | Yes (Dirix et al. 2009; Frowen et al. 2010; Mortensen et al. 2013) | Yes (Mortensen et al. 2013) |
| Site of the primary tumour | Tumour localisation (Dirix et al. 2009), Non-glottal cancer (Mortensen et al. 2013), 5.3.3. Naso–/ oro-pharynx (Lango et al. 2009) | Non-glottal cancer (Mortensen et al. 2013), Naso–/ oro-pharynx versus other sites (Christianen et al. 2012) |
| Size of the primary tumour | T-classification (Dirix et al. 2009), T3-T4 tumours (Frowen et al. 2010; Mortensen et al. 2013; Lango et al. 2009) | T3-T4 (Mortensen et al. 2013) |
| Node status | N-positive disease (Mortensen et al. 2013), Bilateral neck irradiation (Lango et al. 2009) | N-positive disease (Mortensen et al. 2013) |

### 27.5.4 Combination of Head and Neck Tumour Therapies

**Chemotherapy** Chemotherapy (CT) worsens swallowing difficulties in the acute phase and is associated with more severe swallowing sequalae. The anti-metabolites methotrexate and 5-fluorouracil are the drugs most associated with the oral, pharyngeal and oesophageal symptoms of dysphagia, even though combined modality treatment significantly increases late toxicity (Gawryszuk et al. 2018). In the acute phase, CT causes mucositis more often resulting in swallowing difficulty (Manikantan et al. 2009).

The causes of long-term dysphagia could be the enhancement of radiation-induced fibrosis of the musculature or toxic effects on the neuromuscular junctions (Russi et al. 2012). The prevalence of aspiration is about 60%. They are often silent and the main cause of delayed pneumonia (Eisbruch et al. 2002; Nguyen et al. 2006; Aguilar-Ponce et al. 2003).

**Surgery** HNC patients, treated with postoperative RT, experience both postsurgical and radiation- induced swallowing dysfunction. The cumulative effect of both therapies worsens the incoordination of swallowing and may cause severe dysphagia and aspiration. These dysfunctions are probably due to xerostomia and radiation-induced fibrosis of the oropharyngeal musculature. Fibrosis of the pharyngeal musculature after completion of radiotherapy may have a negative impact on pharyngeal clearance. The preservation of the tongue base in the swallowing mechanism is very important for pharyngeal clearance by contact of the tongue base with the posterior pharyngeal wall (Nguyen et al. 2009; Russi et al. 2012; Lazarus et al. 1996). In clinical practice, the impact of radiation after surgery depends on the type of surgery. For example, in oropharyngeal cancer, multivariate analyses showed the following correlations between treatment modalities and swallowing function: percentage of tongue base resected and extent of closure type for liquids; percentage of tongue base resected and unreconstructed mandible for swallowing pastes; total volume resected, percentage of lateral floor of mouth resected, and postoperative radiotherapy dose for masticated boluses (Pauloski et al. 2004).

When surgery occurs after a first treatment with radiotherapy, the therapy is a risk factor predicting early postoperative aspiration. Moreover, neck dissection may contribute to chronic oropharyngeal dysphagia in patients treated with primary radiation or chemoradiation (Smith et al. 2008; Topaloglu et al. 2012). Finally, patients who receive radiotherapy after supracricoid laryngectomy with cricohyoidopexy have significantly increased retention and aspiration.

### 27.5.5 Special Aspects in Diagnostics and Therapy of Head and Neck Tumour Patients with Swallowing Disorders

The objective of the assessment may be different, depending on the foreseen treatment. If the protocol includes (chemo-)radiotherapy alone or for the first time, the main objective of the assessment may be (1) to screen the population at risk of acute and late dysphagia at the beginning of the treatment, (2) to screen the population at risk of long-term sequelae during the follow-up, (3) to assess the patient identified by the screening test or because of complaints or complications. If the protocol includes surgery, the risk of dysphagia is expected. The aim of assessment is (1) to lead the recovery process after the surgery, (2) to follow the patient with sequalae who did not recover a safety swallow. The total dysphagia risk score (TDRS) (Lango et al. 2009) is a method for predicting acute swallowing dysfunction in patients with head and neck cancers undergoing definitive chemoradiotherapy. Factors of the TDRS are: T-classification, neck irradiation, weight loss, primary tumour site and treatment modality. Mortensen et al. (2012) established a multivariate prognostic model for acute and late dysphagia after RT, on the basis of information from a prospective trial. Factors added to those of the TDRS are: N-positive disease, age > median, baseline dysphagia >1 and accelerated radiotherapy for severe acute dysphagia; and only N-positive disease and baseline dysphagia >1 for late dysphagia. These prognostic models may be useful in identifying patients at risk of dysphagia, for example candidates for prophylactic measures against swallowing dysfunction, such as preventive swallowing exercises during treatment or emerging IMRT techniques aiming at sparing anatomical structures that are involved in swallowing.

### 27.5.5.1 Questionnaires, Screening Tools, Test Procedures

Questionnaires for swallowing disorders, especially swallowing related quality of life (QoL) questionnaires are presented in detail in Sect. 28.8. QoL concepts and instruments in HNC patients were reviewed by Vartanian et al. (2017). Screening tools are described in Sect. 28.1. In this section the following two tests are amplified considering their relevance for HNC patients:

A *water screening test* using increasing volumes (Hey et al. 2013) and the 100 mL water swallow test (WST) (Patterson et al. 2011) have been evaluated post-surgically for patients with HNC and patients referred for (chemo-)radiotherapy, respectively. The results are concordant with the limits usually observed with this kind of test. Post-surgically, it is an accurate tool for the early identification of OD in general, with a sensitivity of 96.2% and a positive likelihood ratio of 5.4. Sensitivity of the WST for predicting aspiration is >67%, specificity >46%. These tests are a useful adjunct to a clinical examination, helping to highlight patients who require an instrumental assessment such as videofluoroscopy of swallowing (VFS).

The *Mann Assessment of Swallowing Ability for Cancer (MASA-C)* is a clinical swallowing assessment (Carnaby and Crary 2014)). It was first designed for and validated on stroke populations. Subsequently, this tool was modified for validation in HNC patients by comparison with VFS. It includes a quantifiable measure for each item of the scale, reflecting the severity of impairment of that item. The items are: neck palpation, oral mucous membrane, saliva, taste, smell, weight loss, current diet, chest status, bolus clearance, oral transit, cough voluntary, voice, pharyngeal phase, pharyngeal response, dysarthria, tongue movement, tongue strength, tongue coordination, oral preparation, auditory comprehen-

sion, palate, lip seal, mouth opening. The MASA-C reveals strong sensitivity and specificity (Se 83%, Sp 96%) and likelihood ratios (21.6). The development and refinement of this swallowing assessment tool for use in multidisciplinary HNC teams would facilitate earlier identification of patients with swallowing difficulties.

### 27.5.5.2 Clinical and Instrumental Assessment

*Four clinical parameters* are correlated significantly with aspiration and limitation of oral intake: dysglossia, wet voice, tongue motility and tongue strength. But the predictability of clinical parameters for aspiration and limitation of oral intake is limited by low positive likelihood ratios (Hey et al. 2013). *Capture of oral tongue pressure* is a non-invasive method that allows repeated measures for the follow-up. But the reliability and stability of oro-lingual swallowing pressures captured from HNC patients compared with healthy subjects are of lower reliability in HNC patients (White et al. 2009).

The most common procedures to evaluate swallowing safety and efficiency in HNC patients quantitatively and qualitatively are *FEES and VFS* (see Sects. 28.2–28.5). Both seem to be equivalent in predicting pneumonia outcome (Speyer et al. 2009). Specifically developed for head and neck cancer the new dynamic imaging grade of swallowing toxicity (DIGEST) tool offers five-point ordinal summary grade of pharyngeal swallowing as determined through results of a modified barium swallow (MBS) study (Deutschmann et al. 2013). However, psychometric properties of VFS (stability, test-retest reliability, construct and concurrent validity) vary as a function of bolus consistency and may not be adequate for clinical and research environments (Frowen et al. 2008).

*Cine-MRI* is a safe, non-invasive technique for the evaluation of dry (saliva) swallowing in all patients. Its results have been compared to those of FEES and appears as complementary to clinical evaluation of swallowing in patients with an abnormal pharyngeal phase of swallowing resulting from treatment of cancer (Hartl et al. 2010).

*Pharyngeal manometry* (see Sect. 28.6) complements videofluoroscopy (VFS) in diagnosing pressure-related causes of dysphagia. Increases in pressure wave amplitude are significantly correlated with increased duration of tongue base-to-pharyngeal wall contact, reduced bolus transit times and oropharyngeal residue. Pharyngeal residue is the most important VFS variable in reflecting pharyngeal pressure measurements (Pauloski et al. 2009).

*Radionuclide scintigraphy* is a technique that quantifies bolus flow (transit time) and the degree of aspiration. Several cases demonstrate the advantages of the method and its usefulness in evaluating pulmonary risk of aspiration (Muz et al. 1994).

### 27.5.5.3 Therapeutic Tools, Prevention and Follow-Up

**Conservative Measures** Details of conservative therapy measures are explained in Sects. 30.1–30.7. Here only additional information is amplified.

There is no standardised dysphagia therapy for head and neck cancer patients and scant evidence to support any particular protocol more than another. That is why there is only anecdotal evidence of efficacy. For example, Crary et al. (2012) showed that swallowing performances improve significantly and are maintained at the three-month follow-up after 3 weeks of an *intensive, exercise-based dysphagia therapy* (Sects. 30.1–30.3) conducted daily for 1 h per day, with additional activities completed by subjects each night between therapy sessions.

The efficacy of *prophylactic swallowing exercises* on swallowing function (see Sects. 29.1 and 30.1) is better validated for preventing dysphagia after chemoradiotherapy. Randomised clinical trials have given outcomes on early swallowing disorders. After treatment, the rehabilitation groups displayed a significant improvement in swallowing function. The functional swallowing, mouth opening, chemosensory acuity and salivation rate deteriorated less in the active swallowing exercise group (Crary et al. 2012). These results were confirmed by a meta-analysis performed by Greco et al. (2018) independently of the technique, as the Swallowing intervention Package (SiP). The interest of swallowing therapy before and after surgery in patients undergoing subtotal laryngectomy has also been reported (Cavalot et al. 2009).

*Botulinum toxin injection* (Sect. 30.5) may be an alternative to surgical or radiological dilation, or to surgical myotomy. Marchese-Ragona et al. (2003) performed percutaneous injection of botulinum toxin under electromyographic control in five supracricoid laryngectomees with swallowing disorders unresolved by speech therapy. A single session of botulinum toxin type A treatment resolved the dysphagia in all cases.

*Neuromuscular electrical stimulation (NMES)* has recently been found to improve swallowing function in patients with dysphagia following stroke. Several authors have reported an improvement in swallowing function and xerostomia in HNC patients (Pattani et al. 2010). There is no consensus about the electrode position, the kind of current, the session organisation or the association with traditional swallowing training. There is no physiological explanation about the mechanism of the improvement, but initiation of NMES in this challenging population may be feasible from an oncological standpoint (Linkov et al. 2012).

Different kinds of *prosthesis* are possible (see Sects. 5.8, 5.9, 20.11) With the absence of lower anterior dentition, support of the lower lip is lost and traction from surgical closure can cause the lower lip to collapse into the oral cavity. For improving oral anterior contention and chewing, prosthetic treatment is helpful (Pigno and Funk 2003). A palatal augmentation prosthesis can be used in postoperative patients with oral cancer as an intra-oral appliance to compensate for postoperative loss. The aim is to reduce the free space between the roof and floor of the oral cavity to permit stronger lingual propulsion during oral deglutition and better linguopalatal contact during articulation (Okayama et al. 2008). Maxillary prostheses are used if velopharyngeal competence reconstruction is not possible. Hypopharyngeal tubes are used to prevent hypopharyngeal stenosis following transoral laser micro-resection in hypopharyngeal carcinomas or after total laryngectomy.

In a randomised trial Teguh et al. (2013) compared the effect of *early hyperbaric oxygen therapy after radiotherapy* on QoL and side effects. Patients randomised for receiving hyperbaric oxygen after the RT had better QoL scores for swallowing, sticky saliva, xerostomia and pain in the mouth.

**Surgical Interventions** Details of surgical procedures are presented in Sect. 30.8. Some additional observations are presented here:stricture remodelling by *stents* has been proposed versus multiple dilations usually required. Although technically feasible, placement is associated with a high risk of complications. This procedure is not recommended (Silva et al. 2012).

*Injections in the base of the tongue* show an improvement in swallowing disorders and QoL of selected patients after partial laryngectomy or of patients treated with radiation therapy for nasopharyngeal carcinoma (NPC) (Navach et al. 2011).

The therapeutic effect of *combination therapy of neuromuscular electrical stimulation (NMES) and balloon dilation* in the treatment of radiation-induced dysphagia in NPC patients has shown higher improvement in swallowing function in the treatment group in comparison with the control group (Long and Wu 2013).

**Nutritional Management and Percutaneous Gastrostomy** These topics are covered in Sects. 30.6, 30.7, 30.9.

**Preventive Measures** Prophylactic therapeutical considerations are discussed in Sect. 29.1. McCaul (2012) presented a plan for oral care considering the balance between the risk of osteonecrosis of mandibula and the importance of dentures for swallowing. Pre-treatment depression may serve as a marker for patients with increased risk of swallowing impairment and reduced QoL. Early intervention is important for the patient, their family and for the caregiver (Chan et al. 2011).

**Telepractice and Follow-Up** The usefulness of telepractice options is commented in Sect. 31.1.

Follow-up is a key point in HNC patients regarding the high percentage of second tumour development localisation. How to associate the oncological follow-up requires a search-efficient system. The Patient Concerns Inventory is a holistic, self-reported screening tool for detecting unmet needs in head and neck cancer patients. Its use enables all patients with swallowing or speech problems to discuss these concerns in the clinic and to access appropriate multidisciplinary intervention (Ghazali et al. 2012). Computerised monitoring of speech and swallowing outcomes (Cnossen et al. 2012) and real-time internet-based protocols for remote telefluoroscopic evaluation of oropharyngeal swallowing (Malandraki et al. 2011) open the field of a telemedicine system for evaluating oropharyngeal swallowing. Finally, the development of predictive risk models can be used by clinicians to assess patient risks when deciding on follow-up strategies to prevent or reduce severe late side effects (Teguh et al. 2013). During follow-up, the possibilities of intercurrent factors—whether in relation to the oncological disease or not—requires some attention. Hypothyroidism and hypoparathyroidism are common postoperative complications of patients who have undergone a total laryngectomy or neck radiation. Moreover, dysphagia must be integrated in a holistic approach for screening or managing all the sequelae.

Dysphagia is found to be predictive of disease recurrence and disease-related deaths, adjusting for T and N classifications, Eastern Cooperative Oncology Group (ECOG) performance status (Oken et al. 1982), smoking status and weight loss, and accounting for competing risks of death. A dysphagia measure captures the effort of maintaining nutrition and identifies patients predisposed to disease recurrence and disease-related death (Lango et al. 2014), as in HNC patients a high mortality rate for aspiration pneumonia during and after the treatment may be caused (Russi et al. 2012). Dysphagia at baseline is a predictive factor of late dysphagia after (chemo-)radiotherapy (Lango et al. 2009; Van der Molen et al. 2013). A not well documented route of metastasis was described in two case reports of patients with upper aerodigestive tract squamous cell carcinomas who developed lung metastases due to aspiration (Vaideeswar and Ghodke 2012).

### 27.5.6 Conclusion

Swallowing disorder management at any time during the HNC patient's journey is a real challenge having an impact on survival rate and quality of life. Nurses may have an important part in the multidisciplinary team using swallow screening tools. The high percentage of silent aspiration, slow loss of weight and slow pulmonary deterioration after end of therapy require a systematic follow-up protocol to prevent late effects. Monitoring is essential (Patterson 2019). Ongoing assessment provides predictive models determining the degree of risk for the patient.

## 27.6 Dysphagia in the Elderly

Patrick G. Zorowka

### 27.6.1 Introduction

Eating and drinking are not only basic biological requirements for maintaining health and bodily functions; they are also major sources of subjective pleasure and enjoyment. In addition, they are social events: by eating and drinking in company, we experience social integration, togetherness and entertainment.

In elderly people, where bodily functions decrease and social integration loosens, an impairment of the swallowing capacity can have devastating consequences on their health, well-being and social life. In not a few cases it may even become a life-threatening condition. For these reasons, dysphagia in the elderly is an issue of high clinical significance.

### 27.6.2 Prevalence

The exact prevalence of dysphagia in aged people is not known. Indeed, it is difficult to determine, as it depends on definitions of "dysphagia" on the one hand, and on age categories on the other as the prevalence of dysphagia advances with increasing age (Madhavan et al. 2016). In addition, different types of patient (independently living, hospitalised, multimorbid, etc.) may exhibit different prevalence rates (Baijens et al. 2016). However, there is no doubt that swallowing problems are very common in elderly people. In the general population, about one third of seniors is assumed to experience problems with swallowing, at least sometimes (Lindgren and Janzon 1991; Roy et al. 2007). In a survey of primary care patients, 22.6% of them reported dysphagia occurring several times per month or more frequently (Wilkins et al. 2007). An even higher percentage (32%) of persons with severe swallowing dysfunction was found in a population of long-term care units (Siebens et al. 1986). Another study, which included patients over 65 years old who complained of dysphagia, found that 80% of them needed some type of treatment for their swallowing problems (Kocdor et al. 2015a). As the prevalence increases with increasing age (Madhavan et al. 2016), dysphagia may affect from one third to one half of the people aged above 80 years. Severe degrees of swallowing dysfunction are a major reason for loss of independence and the need for care.

Absolute numbers of elderly patients with dysphagia are expected to rise significantly in the future because of population ageing, a trend that has been continuing for several decades in large parts of the West and is assumed to continue for some more decades. While in 2018 101 million EU citizens were aged 65 years or older, this number is expected to rise to 149 million by 2050 (Eurostat 2019). If the prognosis is right, then from the 2030s onwards more than one quarter of the European population will be aged 65 years or older.

The fact that dysphagia is much more prevalent in old people than in young has two causes. The first is *presbyphagia*, i.e., age-related changes in the swallowing physiology that make old people more vulnerable to disturbances of the swallowing process. The second is the high prevalence of age-related disorders associated with dysphagia. These two points will be dealt with in detail below.

## 27.6.3 Presbyphagia

The term *"presbyphagia"* indicates alterations of the swallowing system that occur because of age-related changes in the anatomical and physiological properties of the body organs. Presbyphagia is not a disease, but a normal age-related phenomenon (sometimes termed "senescent swallowing"). It develops slowly and can be compensated for by an adjusted strategy of eating and drinking. If compensation is adequate and successful, presbyphagia remains without notable impact on the subject's swallowing capacity. It nevertheless makes old people more vulnerable to dysphagia; in the case that additional conditions occur that impinge on swallowing, old people will much more easily experience dysphagia.

Physiological alterations contributing to presbyphagia are raised thresholds of reflexes, prolonged reaction times, restricted muscle motility, decreased sphincter tonus, loss of sensory sensitivity, reduced saliva production, decreased tissue elasticity and a subtle slowing of all processes, including swallowing. In addition, loss of teeth or poor dental function can affect the efficacy of chewing.

In sum, these alterations make the swallowing process more vulnerable to "errors" that occur. For instance, the tongue loses its strength to push the bolus forcefully so that it quickly and completely slips into the oropharynx. Consequently, parts of the bolus may remain in the oral cavity or may even penetrate the airways. In addition, the lips do not any more close so tightly as to withstand high pressure in the oral cavity, leading to anterior leakage. Increased thresholds of the tactile and taste senses retard the timely motor response when food, liquid or saliva is pooling in the pharynx, increasing the risk of aspiration.

Presbyphagia is definitely a risk factor for dysphagia. Developing slowly but steadily, it leads to an increase in swallowing problems in old people. While these problems may be mild in many cases, the boundary between severe presbyphagia and dysphagia is thus fluent. For this reason, it has been proposed to view dysphagia in the elderly as a *geriatric syndrome* (Baijens et al. 2016). This syndrome is a

**Table 27.10** Clinical conditions frequently associated with dysphagia. Based on Prasse and Kikano (2004), Ney et al. (2009) and Sura et al. (2012)

| | |
|---|---|
| Neurological | Stroke |
| | Parkinson and other dyskinesias |
| | Amyotrophic lateral sclerosis |
| | Brain tumours and brain injuries |
| | Huntington, Wilson disease |
| | Myasthenia gravis |
| | Multiple sclerosis |
| | Torticollis |
| | Dementia |
| Head and neck | Zenker's diverticulum |
| | Struma |
| | Pharyngitis, esophagitis |
| | Mucosal lesions |
| | Intubation |
| | Head-neck-cancer |
| | Tissue scarring from radiation therapy |
| Medications | Anticholinergics |
| | Antipsychotics |
| Others | Diabetes |
| | Thyroid disorders |
| | Gastro-oesophageal reflux disease (GERD) |
| | Scleroderma |
| | Sjögren disease |

clinical condition in which symptoms develop when the accumulated effect of several impairments in multiple domains compromise compensatory ability and reserve and the final outcome is a single phenomenology (Baijens et al. 2016)

## 27.6.4 Risk Factors for Dysphagia in Aged Persons

The second reason that dysphagia is frequent in elderly people is the high prevalence of age-related diseases that are associated with dysphagia. Some of the most frequent are given in Table 27.10. Neurological and neuromuscular disorders are among the principal risks for dysphagia; followed by diseases affecting the head-neck region. In addition, impaired cognitive functions, including low alertness and mental orientation, as typical of Alzheimer's disease and other forms of dementia, must be recognised as major risk factors for dysphagia.

Apart from age-related diseases, a number of drugs are known for side effects interacting with swallowing. Presenting with presbyphagia, elderly people are especially vulnerable to *drug-induced* dysphagia. Drug-induced swallowing problems are mediated, e.g., by xerostomia (dry mouth), reduced muscle tonus or muscle motility, or reduced alertness (drowsiness). Among the drugs that are frequently prescribed to old people and which are known for their potential of causing swallowing problems are ACE-Inhibitors, SSRIs, diuretics, tricyclic antidepressants, antihistamines, anti-arrythmics, benzodiazepines, antipsychotics and others.

### 27.6.5 Symptoms and Sequelae of Dysphagia

The symptoms of dysphagia in the elderly are similar to those in young patients. At an early stage, they include frequent throat clearing, drooling and choking or coughing while eating. The patient may have sensations that the food is sticking in the throat, and that he or she is unable to swallow it. Later, he or she may experience pain when swallowing (odynophagia) or complain about retrosternal pressure or burning after eating. Affections of the voice, e.g., a weak or hoarse voice, are frequent. As dysphagia progresses, the patient may lose the pleasure of eating and even experience anxiety or panic during mealtimes. This will frequently result in reduced food and liquid intake, and in social withdrawal, i.e., the patient avoids eating in company not to embarrass others by his or her swallowing difficulties.

Dysphagia has a variety of clinical sequelae. In not a few cases these may be indicative of a swallowing problem of the patient, before the swallowing problem itself is detected. This applies especially to an unexplained weight loss, unclear fever or recurrent airway infections. Other typical consequences of dysphagia are dehydration, malnutrition, sarcopenia and fatigue. In very old people, an overall decline in health may be observed, leading to increased dependence and the need for long-term hospitalisation. Rapid weight loss (>5 kg in 1 year) and a very low body mass index (<20 kg/m²) are found to be relevant risk factors for the 6-month mortality of nursing home residents aged 65 years or above (Wirth et al. 2016a, b; Muhle et al. 2015)

(Fig. 27.14a,b,c). These symptoms should hence be given special attention.

Another important complication of dysphagia is aspiration pneumonia, which, especially in old people, is associated with a significantly increased mortality (Eisenstadt 2010). In case of hospitalisation, dysphagia has a significant impact on the length of hospital stay and is a bad prognostic indicator (Altman et al. 2014).

### 27.6.6 Diagnostic Management

The diagnostic evaluation of dysphagia is a complex task and requires a multidisciplinary approach. It includes (a) the confirmation of a swallowing dysfunction, (b) the identification of its anatomical level (oropharyngeal or oesophageal), (c) the recognition of the disturbed mechanisms, (d) the detection of the causes of the swallowing dysfunction, and (e) the appraisal of its degree of severity. Additionally, the patient's general health status, his or her alertness and mental orientation, other impairments, and his or her ability to cooperate must be determined. All of this information is needed to implement an effective therapeutic or rehabilitative strategy.

Diagnostic evaluation will always start with a thorough anamnesis, followed by a physical examination. The latter will focus on the examination of the oral cavity, pharynx and larynx, including assessment of the organs' sensitivity and motility, i.e., motility of the tongue, the velum and the lips, the larynx and the epiglottis. In addition, inspection of the mucosa, assessment of saliva production and of the teeth must follow. Examination of the head and neck as well as testing of the function of cranial nerves V, IIV, IX, X and XII is mandatory. The patient's nutritional and hydration status, cognitive status and additional clinical conditions such as tremor, cloni, pareses, etc. must also be registered. During anamnesis and clinical examination, the patient is being monitored for signs of dysphagia such as dysphonia, dysarthria, coughing or repeated throat clearing.

To assess swallowing function roughly, bedside swallowing tests can be carried out, which are mostly performed by specially trained nurses

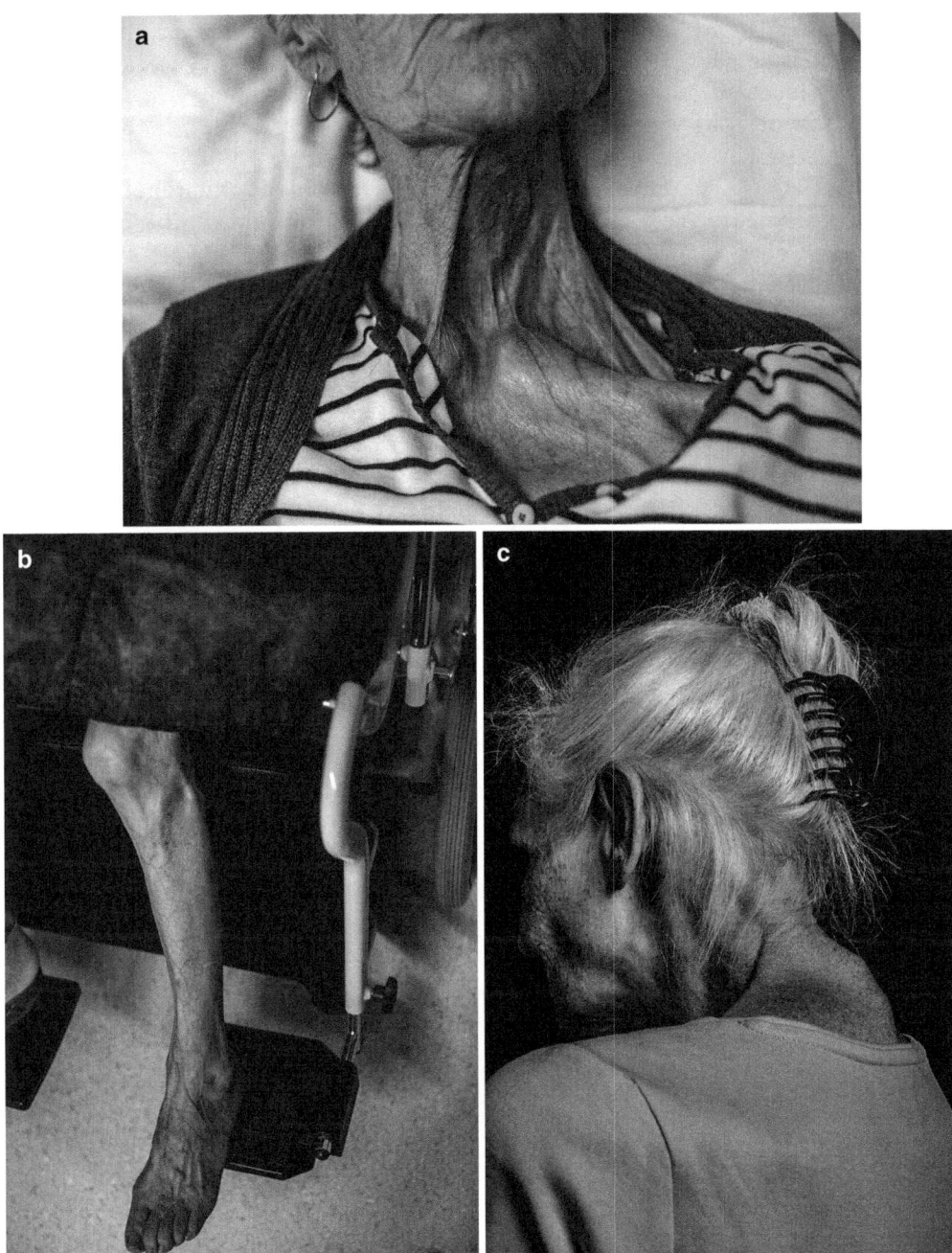

**Fig. 27.14**  (a–c) Examples of rapid weight loss as sequela of dysphagia

or logopaedists. Through these tests, swallowing problems can be identified and quantified to a certain degree. The degree of severity of swallowing problems is usually determined by clinical observation and by different scales and questionnaires, such as the Sydney Swallow Questionnaire (SSQ) (Wallace et al. 2000). For further details see Sects. 28.1, 28.4, 28.8.

For a more detailed and objective evaluation of dysphagia, specific diagnostic methods must be applied. Currently, there are several methods in use for determining and quantifying swallowing dysfunction: flexible optic endoscopic evaluation of swallowing (FEES); videofluoroscopic swallowing study (VFSS), upper endoscopy, barium radiography and oesophageal manometry. These methods supplement the clinical assessment and enable the clinician to evaluate further the function of the oral, pharyngeal, laryngeal and upper oesophageal swallowing physiology, as well as to estimate the benefit of compensatory and treatment strategies.

Whenever there is suspicion of oropharyngeal dysphagia, a flexible optic endoscopic evaluation of swallowing (FEES) should be performed. The FEES provides detailed information about the anatomy and physiology of the pharynx and larynx and allows for the assessment of the pharyngeal phase of swallowing. The FEES bears the advantage that it can be administered at the bedside, which may be required in hospitalised patients.

Apart from the FEES, the videofluoroscopic swallowing study (VFSS), also termed "modified barium swallow", is the most commonly used evaluation method, also in elderly people. VFSS allows inspection of the anatomical structures and the swallowing physiology of the oral cavity, pharynx, larynx and upper oesophagus during deglutition. It identifies the dysfunctional movement patterns of these tracts that cause ineffective deglutition. In addition, treatment strategies including different head positioning and swallow manoeuvres can be tested during the VFSS to determine whether swallowing efficiency can be increased or aspiration risk can be eliminated by them.

The other methods—barium radiography, upper endoscopy and oesophageal manometry—are preferably used in the evaluation of oesophageal dysphagia.

Considering that dysphagia is associated with several symptoms of a mainly subjective nature (e.g., pain, fear, aversion), patient-reported outcome measures (PROMs) may help evaluate the impact of a swallowing problem on the patient's everyday life. Several instruments have been developed for this purpose (Timmerman et al. 2014). Though all of them suffer from limitations, they can nevertheless be helpful tools in the assessment of dysphagia (Dorsey et al. 2021).

### 27.6.7 Treatment and Rehabilitation of Dysphagia in the Elderly

Treatment and rehabilitation of dysphagia in the elderly require the coordinated expertise of a number of health-care professionals, including phoniatricians, neurologists, general practitioners, logopaedists and nurses. The primary goal of the treatment—the restitution of the efficacy and safety of the oropharyngeal swallow—frequently cannot be achieved in old people. Hence, a variety of rehabilitative and compensatory measures may become necessary to achieve at least the secondary goal: to improve the swallowing function so far as to warrant oral nutrition, to minimise risk of aspiration, to prevent dehydration and malnutrition, and to enhance the quality of life by taking away anxiety or fear from eating and drinking.

Most elderly patients with dysphagia require swallowing therapy. The goal of swallowing therapy is to improve the swallowing function by enhancing the function of its subsystems. This goal is pursued by performing exercises that aim at strengthening the muscles involved in swallowing, at enhancing the control over them, and at improving their coordination. The exercises are intended to result in an increased strength of tongue and lips, in a more effective larynx elevation and airway protection, in the creation of a higher swallow pressure and, by this, in the reduction of leakage and penetration. Evidence shows that some of these exercises are very effective (Speyer et al. 2022).

Swallowing therapy requires the cooperation of the patient, which—in elderly or multimorbid persons—may be limited. As an alternative (or supplement) to swallowing therapy, compensatory strategies may be used that are less demanding on the patient. These strategies include inter-alia, postural manoeuvres, slowing the rate of eating, limiting bolus size and food modification.

Postural manoeuvres are simple techniques that improve the efficacy and safety of the swallow by biomechanical adjustment of the patient's position. Most important among them is the rule to eat in an upright position to facilitate the bolus flow by capitalising on gravitational forces. Other manoeuvres (like "chin up" or "chin down") aim at correctly directing the bolus flow, diminishing the probability of nasal regurgitation, or protecting the airways by better larynx elevation.

Additional important compensatory strategies include food modification, i.e., modifying the consistency of foods and liquids. Thickening of liquids has become a routine measure for preventing aspiration of fluids. In some patients, dysphagia may be caused by structural impairments that can be managed surgically. Patients with oesophageal strictures, a cricopharyngeal prominence or a Zenker diverticulum may immediately resume normal swallowing once the structure is repaired.

In cases where sufficient food intake by oral nutrition cannot be maintained, tube feeding must be taken in consideration. In patients with a short-term need for tube feeding (<4 weeks), nasogastric or naso-enteric feeding is the method of choice. In patients who require long-term tube feeding (>4 weeks), percutaneous endoscopic gastrostomy (PEG) can be considered. However, indications for PEG are not fully clear, as on the one hand its beneficial effect has not been demonstrated, while on the other, both complication rate and mortality after PEG are high (Mitchell and Tetroe 2000; Wirth 2018). In patients with severe dementia and malnutrition, PEG is not recommended; in all other patients an individual decision, based on clinical expertise, must be made (Wirth 2018).

Efficacy of a swallow rehabilitation programme in the elderly depends on many factors. It requires expertise of the professionals involved (who are many), cooperation of the patient and proper care. As of today, there is no standard approach for managing elderly patients with dysphagia. While there exist clear goals, the way to achieve them needs to be individualised and adjusted to the personal, social and environmental setting of the patient. Yet it is clear that management of dysphagia in elderly persons is not just treatment of a symptom: it is management of a condition that is ultimately destroying the patient's quality of life, ruining his or her health and threatening his or her life.

## 27.7 Supragastric Belching: Characteristics and Distinctive Features

Liesbeth ten Cate, Dirk Vanneste,
Gerrit J. M. Hemmink and Mieke Moerman

### 27.7.1 Definition of Gastric and Supragastric Belching

It is known that two patterns of belching mechanisms exist: gastric belching and supragastric belching.

The first, *gastric belching*, is a physiological phenomenon in which air escapes from the stomach by a physiological reflex, often shortly after swallowing food or carbonised drinks. Accumulation of swallowed air or gas causes distension of the proximal stomach which incites a transient lower oesophageal sphincter relaxation (TLESR). Subsequently, the air escapes into the oesophagus. Next, the distension of the oesophageal wall causes a relaxation of the upper oesophageal sphincter (UES) and the air flows into the pharynx towards the mouth. Accordingly to aerodynamic laws, a flow through a narrowing elicits a vibration. In this case vibration occurs at the UES level, resulting in a typical audible sound, the so-called belch. Frequently swallowing large quantities of air can result in aerophagia. Symptoms are bloating, (frequent) belching, flatulence, abdominal distension, constipation and abdominal pain (Bredenoord 2013).

The second, *supragastric belching* (SGB), has been studied during the last 20 years and differs from gastric belching as the air does not enter the stomach. The patient unconsciously and repeatedly forces air into the oesophagus by inducing a negative oesophageal pressure (air-inhalation) or by increasing pharyngeal pressure (air-injection). Immediately afterwards, within a second, air is expelled (Bredenoord et al. 2004). In patients with excessive belching as primary and predominant symptom, supragastric belches occur in impressive amounts. Excessive SGB is considered to be a behavioural disorder or a learned behaviour over which control is lost (Bredenoord 2013) and not a reflex mechanism. Lang et al. (2017) argue that human SGB is a learned voluntarily initiated reflex response. The exact reason some persons develop this behaviour is still uncertain, but some authors suggest that seeking relief of an unpleasant feeling, such as throat pressure, globus, heartburn, epigastric discomfort or bloating plays a major role (Bredenoord 2013; Hemmink et al. 2009). Bredenoord et al. (2006) reported that distracting the patient decreases the frequency of supragastric belches, stress being regarded as a precipitating factor. (Excessive) SGB can occur in isolation, but also in coexistence with other oesophageal conditions such as regurgitation, rumination, globus sensation and reflux symptoms (Hemmink et al. 2009; Koukias et al. 2015). Supragastric belches are also found in healthy volunteers. Koukias et al. (2015) defined the upper limit of "normal" SGB at 13 belches during 24 h, on the basis of observations in a control group. They reported a prevalence of excessive SGB in 3.4% of patients investigated for upper gastrointestinal complaints at their upper gastrointestinal physiology unit.

## 27.7.2 Diagnosis of Supragastric Belching

### 27.7.2.1 Clinical Observations

As belching is also a physiological phenomenon, it is important to distinguish normal belching patterns from pathological belching patterns, and to differentiate (frequent) gastric belching from (excessive) supragastric belching.

**History Taking** Excessive SGB is characterised by the occurrence of large numbers of belches during the day (hundreds is not an exception), independently of eating and drinking. Often, multiple episodes of continuous belching

(sometimes up to 20 times per minute) happen. Patients are often convinced that belching causes relief (ten Cate et al. 2018). Some patients report that belching remains absent during daily activities (working, talking), but that it starts when they are alone, feeling free to belch. In severe cases the patient cannot control the belching at all. This leads to avoiding social contact and activities with potential serious social impairment as a consequence (Bredenoord and Smout 2010).

Belching does not occur during sleep. Patients do not report weight loss, dysphagia or malnutrition. Mainly the belching itself and its social impact are the primary motives for seeking help.

**Clinical Examination** In case belching is the predominant symptom and undoubtedly excessive, the mechanism is mostly supragastric (Bredenoord 2013), involving air-inhalation or air-injection.

Clinical features of air-inhalation SGB are a sudden "high-thoracic" inspiration, often followed by a sudden breath stop by laryngeal (glottal) closure, tensioning of the muscles of the neck and a forward movement of the head. The air-injection mechanism is characterised by a tight mouth and laryngeal (glottal) closure and a simultaneous vertical laryngeal movement. The tongue and pharyngeal muscles contract, creating high pharyngeal pressure and injecting the air downwards through the UES (ten Cate et al. 2018; Kessing et al. 2014).

In both mechanisms there is a forced UES opening, permitting air influx into the oesophagus directly followed by an air expulsion (belch) because of the gastric and oesophageal pressure increase (Kessing et al. 2012a).

### 27.7.2.2 Technical Investigations
**Impedance Measurement and Manometry** Oesophageal impedance (electrical resistance) monitoring is the technical investigation of choice. A catheter with several electrodes is placed via the nose in the oesophagus and enables visualising the air passage through the oesophagus. The lowest electrode is situated at the level of the lower oesophageal sphincter (Fig. 27.15).

Air and liquid have different impedance characteristics. Air increases the impedance level

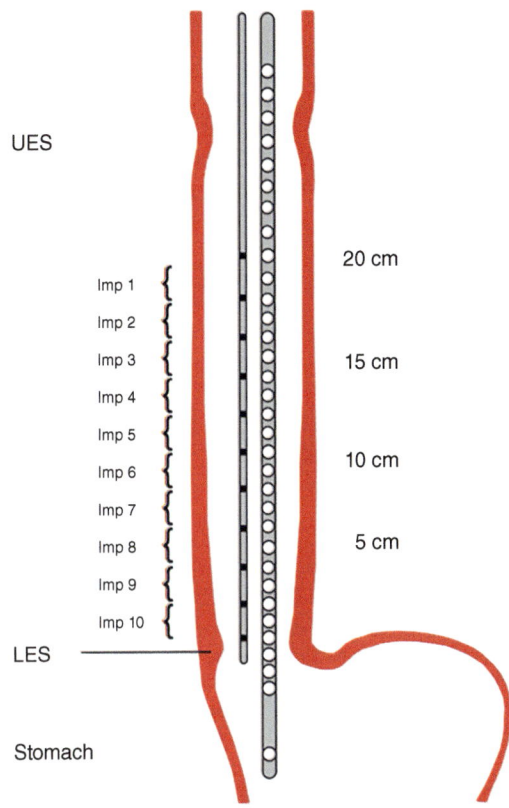

UES

Imp 1
Imp 2
Imp 3
Imp 4
Imp 5
Imp 6
Imp 7
Imp 8
Imp 9
Imp 10

20 cm

15 cm

10 cm

5 cm

LES

Stomach

**Fig. 27.15** Schematic example of localisation of an impedance catheter (left) and a manometry catheter (right) in the oesophagus. *LES* lower oesophageal sphincter, *UES* upper oesophageal sphincter. Hemmink©2019

whilst liquid decreases it. Furthermore, since the catheter is equipped with an array of electrodes, the direction in which the bolus (air or liquid) proceeds is monitored on the graph. In this way a differential diagnosis can be made between gastric belching and SGB.

Ambulatory 24-h pH-impedance measurements are regularly taken to evaluate belching symptoms, and can identify the frequency of supragastric belches, gastric belches (Fig. 27.16) and air swallows.

The two SGB mechanisms can be distinguished by combining impedance measurement with high-resolution manometry (HRM) (Kessing et al. 2012a) (Fig. 27.17). HRM provides a topographic mapping of the space-time patterns of hypopharyngeal and oesophageal pressures, represented by a coloured contour plot, and is highly

accurate for diagnosing oesophageal motility disorders (Dhawan et al. 2018). Similar to graphics used in meteorology, HRM colour plots represent pressure levels. Three-dimensional data are displayed on a two-dimensional planar surface: the pressure levels as colours (mm Hg) and the sensor position (cm) on the y-axis, the time (sec) on the x-axis.

During inhalation SGB, contracting the diaphragm creates a negative intra-thoracic pressure and hence a negative intra-oesophageal pressure. The opening of the UES permits air influx (Fig. 27.17).

Injection SGB, on the contrary, is characterised by a pharyngeal pressure rise due to a pumping action of the tongue against the pharynx (Fig. 27.18). This latter belching mechanism seems to be less common.

**Video-laryngoscopy** By examining a patient with an ENT specialist and a speech language pathologist (SLP) team, Ellegård and Nilsén (2016) showed that video-laryngoscopy can be supportive in diagnosing SGB - provided that the patient is performing this behaviour during the clinical assessment. During SGB the frequent opening of the oesophagus is visible. Moreover, the videorecording can be useful in explaining what is happening during belching. This feedback can be the first step in the treatment.

### 27.7.2.3 Differential Diagnosis
As stated above, if belching happens excessively and predominantly, the most likely diagnosis is SGB; especially when the patient suffers from severe social impairment and bothersome belching (pressure) in the throat, chest, or epigastric pain. Supragastric belches are associated with more severe belching complaints than gastric belches (Kessing et al. 2012b). Aerophagia is characterised by a bloated feeling and frequent belching, but not as excessive as in SGB (Bredenoord 2013) (Table 27.11). Moreover, in aerophagia the belching mainly occurs in relation to drinking or eating. The occurrence of both disorders together (SGB and aerophagia) complicates the differential diagnosis.

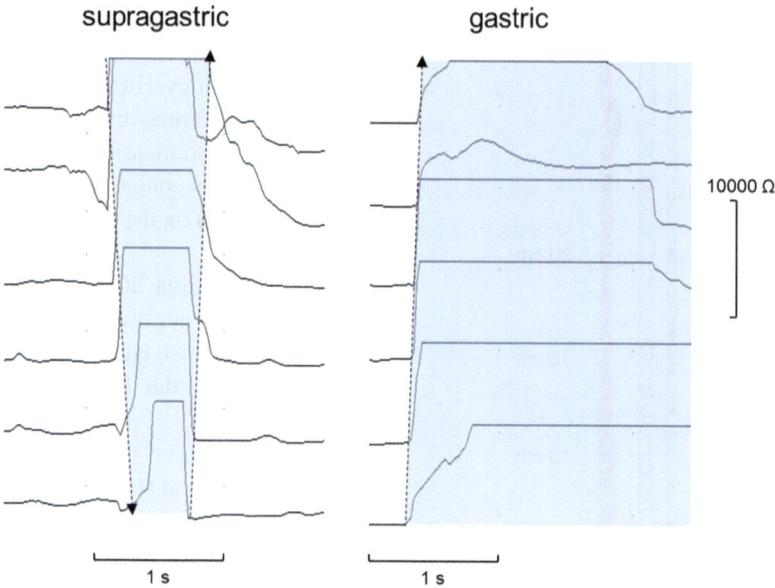

**Fig. 27.16** Example of a supragastric belch (left) and a gastric belch (right). A supragastric belch is characterised by rapid influx of air into the oesophagus from above causing an impedance increase moving proximally- to distally-located impedance segments. Within a second, the air is expelled in the opposite direction, causing a decrease of the impedance levels to baseline from distally upwards. A gastric belch, on the contrary, is defined as a rapid impedance rise from distally to proximally. Smout©2019

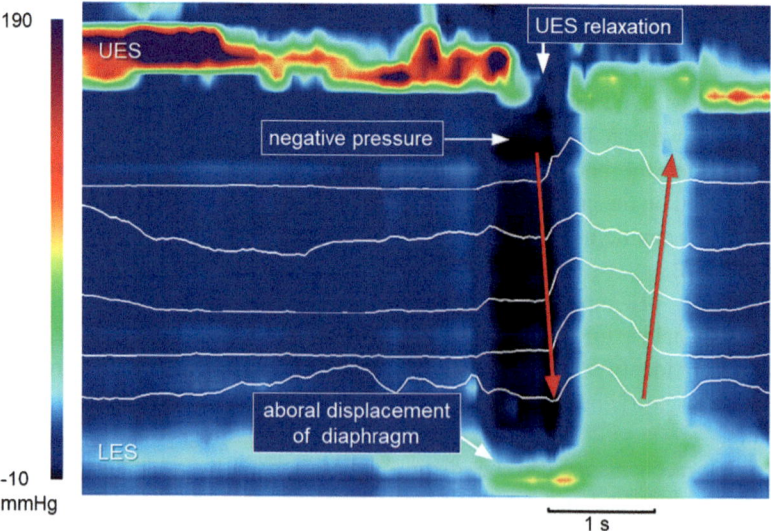

**Fig. 27.17** An example of a supragastric belch induced by negative pressure preceding the oesophageal airflow as revealed by high-resolution manometry. Clearly visible is the aboral movement of the diaphragm at the start of the pressure decrease and a subsequent relaxation (opening) of the upper oesophageal sphincter (UES). White lines are impedance signals. The V-shaped pattern (red arrows) indicates supragastric air movement (belch). *LES* lower oesophageal sphincter. Smout©2019

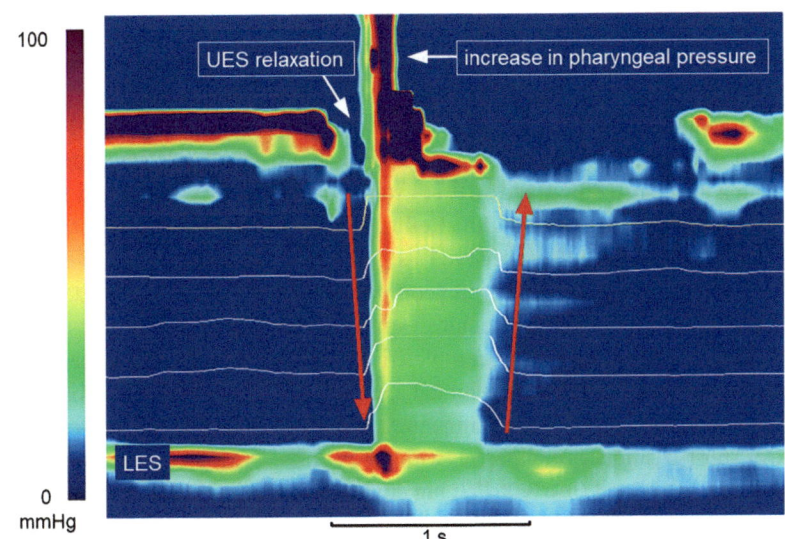

**Fig. 27.18** An example of a supragastric belch induced by pressure increase in the pharynx made by pumping movement of the tongue base against the pharynx, which serves as the driving force behind the air influx (high-resolution manometry). White lines are impedance signals. The V-shaped pattern (red arrows) indicates supragastric air movement (belch). *LES* lower oesophageal sphincter. Smout©2019

**Table 27.11** Distinctive features of supragastric belching and aerophagia. Based on Kessing et al. (2012b), Bredenoord (2013), Ten Cate et al. (2018), Sawada et al. (2020)

| Supragastric Belching | Gastric Belching caused by frequent or excessive air swallowing (Aerophagia) |
|---|---|
| *In history* | |
| Excessive belching, high numbers. Occurrence of repetitive, continuous belching episodes | Frequent belching, but not repetitive, continuous belching |
| Independent of food intake | Symptoms related to food intake, belching during or after meals or both |
| Supragastric belches are bothersome | Gastric belches are not bothersome |
| Unpleasant feeling (pressure) of chest, throat, stomach | Bloated feeling |
| Strongly convinced that air must be expelled, followed by relief | |
| No symptoms during sleeping | |
| *Clinical signs* | |
| Sudden breath stops by glottal closure, straining neck musculature *or* tight mouth and glottal closure, vertical laryngeal movement | Multiple swallows, suboptimal swallowing in the oropharyngeal transport phase |

### 27.7.3 Therapy of Supragastric Belching

Several studies have demonstrated that speech therapy helps to reduce excessive SGB (ten Cate et al. 2018; ten Cate 2022; Ellegård and Nilsén 2016; Ong et al. 2018; Hemmink et al. 2010). Ellegård and Nilsén (2016) described the success of speech therapy in a case study. Their therapy strategy consisted of explaining the features on video-laryngoscopy, creating awareness of the belching mechanism, and contrasting glottal closure and opening in relation to breathing exercises. In a waiting-list-controlled cohort study Ong et al. (2018) investigated the effectiveness of diaphragmatic breathing (DB) therapy on belching and gastro-oesophageal reflux symptoms. Fifteen patients were assigned to a treatment group and 21 patients to a waiting-list group (controls). The waiting-list group did not receive any form of therapy during 4 weeks. Belching severity and related aspects on belching was evaluated through self-assessment scales, namely a 100 mm visual analogue scale (VAS) and a non-validated short questionnaire. The latter contained questions regarding belching frequency and management. The authors reported a significant reduction of the mean ($\pm$ SD) belching severity VAS of $7.1 \pm 1.5$ to $3.5 \pm 2.0$ in the treatment group compared with the waiting-list group of 7.6 ± 1.1 to 7.4 ± 1.3 ($p < 0.001$). More than 50% of belching severity reduction was found in 60% of the patients receiving the DB treatment compared with 0% in the control group ($p < 0.001$), and the occurrence of belching diminished in 80% and 19%, respectively ($p = 0.001$). Moreover, the Reflux Disease Questionnaire results improved significantly ($p = 0.04$) in the treatment group compared with those of the waiting-list control group. The waiting-list controls finally completed their DB treatment as well, and demonstrated a significant reduction of belching VAS, frequency and control post-treatment compared with the post-waiting-list period ($p < 0.001$) (Ong et al. 2018).

Ten Cate et al. (2018) designed a specific therapy programme, based on an initial pilot study by Hemmink et al. in 2010. In the first stage the therapist explains the SGB mechanism and interviews the patients on their own ideas about the belching and its supposed cause. In the second stage the patient is taught to recognise the breath stops (laryngeal/glottal closure) preceding his or her specific SGB mechanism (air-inhalation or air-injection). Patients are encouraged to pay attention to the specific sensations predicting these acts. Then, the patient learns to interrupt and prevent the belching mechanisms through diaphragmatic breathing exercises. Extensive attention is given to management in daily life. The effectiveness of this therapy programme was evaluated in a retrospective study by comparing pre- and post-treatment VAS scores on six items, including social and physical aspects of belching. The scores of 48 patients were used for the outcome analysis. Of them, 30 had been diagnosed by impedance measurement and 18 by clinical assessment by a speech language pathologist without objective confirmation. The authors demonstrated a significant reduction in supragastric belching and its related symptoms (median total VAS score of 406 (291–463) pre-treatment and a median total VAS score of 125 (17–197) post-treatment ($p < 0.001$). Furthermore, significant improvements of all items separately were found. Forty patients (83%) had a sufficient or major improvement (total VAS score change), with a median therapy duration of 3 months and ten sessions. No significant difference

was found concerning the patient characteristics and therapy results between the impedance-confirmed and the clinically assessed SGB patients (ten Cate et al. 2018). Ten Cate (2022) performed a similar study in an enlarged group of patients ($N = 73$), treated from 2007 to 2021. The results showed a reduction of symptoms in the total median VAS scores of 395 (296–461) to 101 (30–195) ($p < 0.001$). In 84% of the patients the therapy had a positive effect. Interestingly, a significant difference ($p = 0.033$) in patient characteristics was found between the symptom duration of the impedance-confirmed group of patients (Mdn = 36 months) and the symptom duration of the clinically assessed patients (Mdn = 18 months), may be due to a longer period of medical investigations in the former group before the diagnosis SGB was made.

Glasinovic et al. (2018) investigated the results of cognitive behavioural therapy in a series of 39 patients, by using 24-h pH-impedance measurements and VAS scores. The therapy consisted of psycho-education, awareness training, identification of a 'warning signal' preceding SGB, and breathing exercises. Objectively, with pH-impedance, they found an SGB decrease of more than 50% in 16 of 31 patients. They calculated a mean of 116 supragastric belches (47–323) pre-treatment and 45 supragastric belches (22–139) post-treatment ($p = 0.0003$). Subjectively, from the VAS scores, the authors reported a significant reduction ($p < 0.0001$) in four items (from 260 (210–320) pre- to 140 (80–210) post-treatment), and an improvement in quality of life. The authors also reported a significant reduction of reflux episodes ($p = 0.0055$) (Glasinovic et al. 2018).

### 27.7.4 Conclusion

Excessive SGB is a disorder of behavioural origin that can be differentiated from frequent gastric belching caused by frequent air swallowing and aerophagia by its clinical presentation. For an objective assessment, impedance measurement is recommended. By adding HRM to impedance monitoring, the SBG mechanism (air-inhalation or air-injection) can be investigated in detail. Patients can successfully be treated by specialised speech language pathologists and specialised behavioural therapists/psychologists with attention to the cognitive and physical parts of the disorder. When excessive SGB coexists with frequent air swallowing or aerophagia, the experience of speech language pathologists specialised in treating swallowing disorders is preferable.

## 27.8 Post-Intubation Dysphagia

Miroslav Tedla and Žofia Korim

### 27.8.1 Introduction

Mechanical ventilation is the most used life support technique and is applied for a diverse spectrum of indications, from scheduled surgical procedures to organ failure. Endotracheal intubation with an orotracheal tube is usually applied during mechanical ventilation. Post-intubation dysphagia in critically ill patients is related to the duration of mechanical ventilation (De Vita and Spierer-Rundback 1990; de Larminat et al. 1995; Ajemian et al. 2001; Macht et al. 2011), negatively affects the return to oral intake, and is associated with prolonged hospitalisation (Barker et al. 2009). In patients requiring endotracheal intubation, the occurrence of dysphagia is due to multifactorial changes (Ajemian et al. 2001; Smithard 2013), mainly mechanical and cognitive (Kwok et al. 2013). The orotracheal tube passes through the oral cavity, oropharynx, larynx and trachea. Risks of laryngeal and tracheal injury, post-intubation voice disorder and dysphagia are present (Brodsky et al. 2020). The presence of dysphagia increases the risk of aspiration pneumonia.

However, dysphagia is not the only predictor of aspiration pneumonia in patients after extubation. The laryngeal sphincter is a key protective mechanism of the lower respiratory tract (Goldsmith 2000). The oral flora of intubated patients contains pathogenic bacteria (Macht et al. 2014). Shifting oral secretions through the larynx into the lower respiratory tract can cause infections and inflammatory pulmonary complications (Fernández-Carmona et al. 2012). Aspiration may lead to acute desaturation, pneumonia or pneumonitis, and the need for reintubation, which increases the length of stay in the hospital (Macht et al. 2013). Aspiration pneumonia is one of the 10 more common rehospitalisation diagnoses after severe sepsis (Prescott et al. 2015). The duration of endotracheal intubation is independently associated with aspiration, and the duration of intubation is positively correlated with the degree of dysphagia, which may help in identifying patients requiring examination of swallowing (Kim et al. 2015).

Predictive factors increasing the risk of dysphagia and aspiration after extubation include age, changes in voice quality and the degree of voice disorder (de Oliveira et al. 2018). Another factor that affects the incidence of dysphagia in critically ill patients is whether the patient has already had dysphagia before the intubation or developed it as a result of the current disease (Macht et al. 2013).

### 27.8.2 Incidence

Globally, 13–20 million patients are admitted to intensive care units (ICUs) each year (Adhikari et al. 2010). In the United States alone, there are five million ICU admissions yearly, with one million resulting in tracheal intubation. Information on the incidence of dysphagia in extubated patients varies. This is mainly due to methodological discrepancies, different methods of diagnosis and inconsistent evaluation intervals after extubation. In patients intubated for more than 48 h, the prevalence of dysphagia increases by 56%, of which 25% patients aspirate silently (Ajemian et al. 2001). Another study concludes that dysphagia is associated with intubation lasting more than 4 days (Leder et al. 2019). According to other studies, dysphagia occurs in 3–62% of patients recovering after critical illness (Macht et al. 2013). The possible mechanisms of dysphagia in extubated patients are described in more detail below.

### 27.8.3 Mechanisms of Development of Post-Intubation Dysphagia

Dysphagia developed as a consequence of intensive care and orotracheal intubation has six potential mechanisms of development:

- Oral, pharyngeal and laryngeal trauma.
- Neuromuscular weakness.
- Decreased laryngeal sensitivity.
- Altered sensorium.
- Gastro-oesophageal reflux.
- Impaired synchronisation of breathing and swallowing (Macht et al. 2013).

#### 27.8.3.1 Oropharyngeal and Laryngeal Trauma

The mechanical causes of post-intubation dysphagia are related to intubation itself, duration of intubation and endotracheal tube characteristics (Ajemian et al. 2001). Oropharyngeal trauma is associated with the oral and pharyngeal phase of swallowing. Injury to the lips may result in drooling of saliva and bolus (Komasawa et al. 2017). Dental damage occurs mainly in patients with known dental diseases, such as dental caries and periodontitis (Vogel et al. 2009).

Immediately after extubation, the oral cavity is frequently dry, with dried secretions around the lips, tongue and hard palate. In elderly patients, chewing may be impaired owing to the lack of dentition and possible cognitive deficits (Garcia and Chambers 2010). In the pharyngeal phase of swallowing, the impaired elevation of the hyolaryngeal complex and the laryngeal sphincter may increase the risk of aspiration (Goldsmith 2000). Impairment can be caused by oedema of oropharyngeal and laryngeal structures (Murry and Carrau 2006). Laryngeal oedema is one of the more frequent and serious complications of tracheal intubation (François et al. 2007). Endotracheal intubation may cause mucosal abrasion (Macht et al. 2012), inflammations, haematomas and ulcerations in the area of vocal folds, arytenoids, epiglottis and the base of tongue (Macht et al. 2013). Intubation may also result in dislocation (Kim et al. 2015) and sub-luxation of the arytenoid cartilage, which compromises the closure of the laryngeal vestibule (Lombardi and Arthur 2020). A specific situation is the injury of the recurrent laryngeal nerve; the endotracheal tube cuff can compress the branch of the recurrent laryngeal nerve (Macht et al. 2013). Vocal cord paresis may occur, depending on the type of tube (Tanaka et al. 2003), cuff size (Arts et al. 2013), pressure (Combes et al. 2001) and quality, and the duration of intubation (Matta et al. 2017). Laryngeal trauma raises the risk of insufficient laryngeal sphincter closing during swallowing, which leads to the likelihood of aspiration. Any type of laryngeal injury can be a risk factor for dysphagia (Brodsky et al. 2014). In an extubated patient, oropharyngeal and laryngeal trauma contribute to the development of respiratory distress, voice disorders and swallowing disorders (Matta et al. 2017).

#### 27.8.3.2 Neuromuscular Weakness

The swallowing act requires the involvement of more than 30 muscles and six cranial nerves. Intubation may cause atrophy of the structures involved in the swallowing act (Rassameehiran et al. 2015). The orotracheal intubation tube keeps the glottis open for extended periods of time, inhibiting the natural movement of the laryngeal and pharyngeal muscles. Movements of the intrinsic muscles of the larynx, which are necessary, e.g., in reflexive vocal fold closure, are also negatively affected by the presence of the orotracheal intubation tube (Fernández-Carmona et al. 2012).

Neuromuscular weakness may be a consequence of:

- Prolonged non-use of structures during long-term intubation (Rassameehiran et al. 2015).
- Prolonged analgosedation.
- Long-term use of neuromuscular blocking agents (Zuercher et al. 2019).

Neuromuscular weakness during the swallowing act leads to dyscoordination of muscles and nerves (Brodsky et al. 2018), is associated with the incidence of dysphagia and an increased risk of aspiration (Mirzakhani et al. 2013). In association with oropharyngeal or laryngeal trauma, it may cause a decrease in local sensitivity, leading to swallowing dysfunction. This was proved by the study of Brodsky et al. (2018), who identified significant changes in the pharyngeal phase of swallowing, specifically slowing of the muscles involved in swallowing, indicating neuromuscular weakness in Acute Respiratory Distress Syndrome (ARDS) patients.

### 27.8.3.3 Reduced Sensitivity

Reduced sensitivity of the upper respiratory tract is another potential factor of developing dysphagia in patients after extubation (Macht et al. 2013). Clinically, this is manifested when the bolus passes from the oral to the pharyngeal phase (Bradley 2000). Limited sensitivity to the bolus and secretions in the hypopharynx interferes with the protective reflexes of swallowing (Linden and Siebens 1983). Sensory deprivation causes rapid changes in chemoreceptors and mechanoreceptors of the upper respiratory tract and may last about 7 days after extubation (de Oliveira et al. 2018). If afferent input is impaired, aboral movement of the bolus through the reflection zone triggering swallowing will delay swallowing (Zuercher et al. 2019), resulting in pre-deglutive aspiration (Aviv 2000).

### 27.8.3.4 Altered Sensorium

The fourth mechanism of swallowing impairment is altered sensorium, related to the development of delirium (Macht et al. 2013). Qualitative or quantitative disorders of consciousness increase the risk of aspiration and may delay therapy for dysphagia (Zuercher et al. 2019). Sensory changes can also be attributed to the residual effect of narcotic and anxiolytic medication (Rassameehiran et al. 2015). The ability to answer orientation questions and follow simple verbal instructions provides information on the likelihood of liquid aspiration and the overall diet of the patient. Patients with impaired ability to answer questions and follow simple instructions are 31% more likely to aspirate liquids than patients who could answer questions and respond to instructions (Leder et al. 2009).

### 27.8.3.5 Gastro-Oesophageal Reflux (GERD)

Gastro-oesophageal reflux is the fifth possibility for the development of dysphagia in critically ill patients. The risk of developing GERD is increased by the presence of a nasogastric tube, the lying position, high doses of sedation, and the use of paralytic agents in therapy (Macht et al. 2013). GERD adversely affects laryngeal sphincter function, increasing the risk of aspiration (Mendell and Logemann 2002). Chronic GERD may contribute to the development of post-intubation dysphagia. The nasogastric tube often remains in place after extubation to supply a non-oral form of nutrition and hydration of the patient. Since an inserted nasogastric tube means a constant opening of the upper and lower oesophageal sphincter, there is a risk of aspiration of gastric content (Noordally et al. 2011).

### 27.8.3.6 Impaired Respiratory-Swallowing Coordination

The sixth mechanism of post-intubation dysphagia is associated with impairment of synchronisation between respiration and swallowing (Dziewas and Warnecke 2019). Swallowing and respiration are highly coordinated actions (Gross et al. 2009). During swallowing, breathing is briefly interrupted not only because of the laryngeal closure and elevation of the soft palate and epiglottal inversion; respiration is also suppressed at the brainstem level (Ertekin 2011). When drinking liquid, swallowing begins during exhalation. The respiratory pause lasts 0.5–1.5 s during swallowing; respiration usually starts during exhalation (Martin-Harris et al. 2005). This restoration is considered to be one of the mechanisms preventing the aspiration of bolus after swallowing (Goldsmith 2000). Eating solid food also changes the respiratory rhythm. The rhythm is impaired at the start of chewing. The duration of the respiratory cycle during chewing is reduced. The "exhale-swallow-exhale" relationship persists during eating. However, respiratory pauses are longer, usually starting before swallowing (Matsuo and Palmer 2008). Dysphagia may be related to tachypnoea. Prevention of aspiration depends on the accuracy of coordination of laryngeal closure, apnoea pauses and opening of the upper oesophageal sphincter.

The underlying patho-mechanism of post-intubation dysphagia is thought to determine its duration. Usually, oropharyngeal and laryngeal traumas normalise within a few days. However, neuromuscular weakness with muscle atrophy may persist over the long term and requires further intervention (Goldsmith 2000). Elderly patients may have more comorbidities and neuromuscular weakness owing to the ageing process. Therefore, they recover longer from post-intubation dysphagia (Tsai et al. 2016).

### 27.8.4 Evaluation of Swallowing in Patients after Orotracheal Intubation Tube Removal

Screening of swallowing is a quick way to identify the likelihood of dysphagia, the need for further swallowing examination, the safety of oral food intake, and the need for an alternative form of nourishment. The aim of the screening test is to identify as many patients at risk of dysphagia as possible before the clinical manifestation of dysphagia symptoms (Streiner 2003) and to minimise the risk of aspiration (de Oliveira et al. 2018). The screening of dysphagia involves testing of various consistencies of diet and fluid.

Early detection of post-intubation dysphagia is needed to reduce the incidence of complications (Rassameehiran et al. 2015). Systematic screening is crucial in identifying and monitoring patients at risk (Perren et al. 2019). In extubated patients, it is recommended that rapid, sensitive screening be carried out by a trained nurse in the ward. If the patient has a known history of neurological disease, head and neck surgery or prolonged mechanical ventilation, screening may be avoided and a detailed examination of swallowing by the speech and language therapist should be considered.

The timing of the swallowing assessment after patient extubation varies in studies and there is no consensus on screening. Screening takes place 1–5 days after extubation (Skoretz et al. 2010). Other studies suggest that swallowing assessment need not be delayed (Scheel et al. 2016;

Leder et al. 2019), with more than 82% of patients completing swallowing screening in the first hour after extubation (Leder et al. 2019). When screening 24 h after extubation, penetration and aspiration were significantly reduced, and respiratory protection was improved in 79% of patients compared with screening immediately after extubation. This suggests that swallowing function significantly improves during the first day after extubation. According to this study, patients may start with an oral intake of a consistency that is safe to swallow, but delayed screening (24 h after extubation) allows a faster return to a less restricted diet (Marvin et al. 2019).

Several screening tools have been developed for different groups of patients with neurological, structural and inflammatory disease (Schepp et al. 2012; Etges et al. 2014; Taveira et al. 2018). Some screenings have also been used in patients after extubation, but without demonstrating the sensitivity and specificity in this group of patients (Schefold et al. 2017). Swallowing screening has been developed for patients intubated for more than 48 h (Johnson et al. 2018). It contains specific items related to possible mechanisms of dysphagia after prolonged intubation. In the screening of swallowing after extubation, the risk of dysphagia is mainly associated with drooling, multiple swallowing, coughing and voice change during swallowing (de Medeiros et al. 2014). Screening should indicate the need for further clinical or instrumental examination of swallowing. If a speech therapist is available, a clinical swallowing examination may be performed.

The primary objective of a clinical swallowing examination is to determine the patient's ability to swallow, rather than the inability (Carnaby Mann 2012). Owing to the complexity of this method, the investigator can formulate a patient management plan, measure progress and guide the form and type of any other intervention options. In an extubated patient, the examination includes evaluation of saliva stasis, a cough during swallowing, the gag reflex and tongue movements. The presence of a cough after swallowing liquid or thickened liquid is the most reliable clinical sign of dysphagia (Noordally et al. 2011; de Medeiros et al. 2014). Coughing after swallowing liquid and thickened liquid is a contra-indication to oral intake. If the cough is only after a swallowing liquid, it is possible to modify the consistencies of the diet (Noordally et al. 2011). However, bedside examination may be partially unspecific in extubated patients, as patients recovering from a critical illness may have a cough and gargling voice for reasons other than the aspiration (Macht et al. 2014). In patients with other comorbidities, a history of neurological diseases, in geriatric patients and patients with known dysphagia, other mechanisms of swallowing impairment are also possible. Patients with prolonged intubation should have their swallowing assessed before the first oral intake. Understanding the pathophysiology of post-intubation dysphagia is crucial in choosing the appropriate procedure for further patient management.

## 27.8.5 Management of Post-Intubation Dysphagia

The body of evidence for the treatment of oropharyngeal dysphagia in dysphagia-positive ICU patients is limited. It is mainly focused on maintaining nutritional status, hydration and reducing morbidity from potential pulmonary consequences. From most studies, there are three major therapeutic options—dietary/texture modifications, postural changes/compensatory manoeuvres and interventions to improve swallowing function (therapeutic exercises, neuromuscular stimulation) (Rassameehiran et al. 2015; Zuercher et al. 2019). The patients receive treatment on the basis of the level of severity and the pattern of dysphagia after swallowing function assessment. Intervention usually consists of guidance, therapeutic techniques, airway protection and manoeuvres, orofacial myofunctional and vocal exercises and diet introduction. Double-blind Randomised Controlled Trials (RCT's) on extubated ICU patients with post-orotracheal intubation dysphagia identified an improvement of oropharyngeal dysphagia, with an early and safe return of oral intake. The intervention received was of 30-minute duration once a day for 10 days. The intervention methods were adjusted to each patient's needs and comprised the following strategies: individual therapeutic

planning; compensatory strategies (postural changes; diet modification; alternative texture/temperature/flavour of meals; thickening liquids); adjustment of environmental factors to improve deglutition/feeding abilities. Therapeutic strategies were also indicated, such as starting the swallowing response and the diet by mouth, strategies for airway protection and glottal cleaning manoeuvres, motoric and coordination exercises to improve the range of motion of the lips, tongue, jaw and improving vocal fold adduction, laryngeal elevation or tongue base retraction (three series of ten repetitions) (Turra et al. 2021).

Surface EMG of muscles involved in swallowing can assist in the assessment of the therapeutic progress (El Gharib et al. 2019). An intensive therapy approach with five training sessions a week seems to be more effective in the acute stage of swallowing dysfunction (Carnaby et al. 2006).

Surgically, upper oesophageal sphincter myotomy is an irreversible option in patients with a functional obstruction of the upper oesophageal sphincter, when done to facilitate pharyngo-oesophageal bolus propulsion (Shama et al. 2008; Kos et al. 2010). Medialisation thyroplasty can be applied to improve cough and throat clearance in patients with unilateral vocal fold paresis and suffering from aspiration (Flint et al. 1997). A laryngectomy poses a last resort for patients with persisting aspiration and suffering from repeated severe consequences. In doing this, breathing and alimentary pathways become completely separated.

Recently, pharyngeal electrical stimulation (PES) has been proposed as a novel treatment; a modality involving a nasogastric tube-like stimulation catheter to enhance neuromuscular pharyngeal stimulation, targeted to the individual patient. Stimulation levels are personalised at the start of the treatment to ensure that optimal levels of stimulation are delivered. PES is considered to target the afferent sensory feedback within the swallowing area that seems crucial for swallowing safety and efficacy of motor execution (Teismann et al. 2007). PES may involve two key modes of action: 1. Facilitation of corticobulbar pathways (Hamdy et al. 1998b) and 2. Increase of swallowing processing efficiency in the respective central nervous system areas (Suntrup et al. 2015), e.g., the right primary and secondary sensorimotor cortex and the right supplementary motor area. Data also demonstrate an increase of pharyngeal cortical representation and motor excitability for more than half an hour after 10 min of PES treatment. A dose-response study showed optimal cost-effectiveness when applying a PES protocol with one cycle of 10-min stimulation per day for a total of three consecutive days (Jayasekeran et al. 2010).

# References

Abadie V, Couly G (2013) Congenital feeding and swallowing disorders. Handb Clin Neurol 113:1539–1549

Abadie V, Chéron G, Lyonett S et al (1996) Isolated neonatal dysfunction of brainstem. Arch Pediatr 3(2):130–136

Abadie V, Champagnat J, Fortin G et al (1999) Sucking-deglutition-respiration and brain stem development genes. Arch Pediatr 6(10):1043–1047

Abadie V, Morisseau-Durand MP, Beyler C et al (2002) Brainstem dysfunction: a possible neuroembryological pathogenesis of isolated Pierre Robin sequence. Eur J Pediatr 161(5):275–280

Adams-Chapman I, Bann CM, Vaucher YE et al (2013) Association between feeding difficulties and language delay in preterm infants using Bayley scales of infant development. (3rd edn). J Pediatr 163(3):680–685

Adhikari NKJ, Fowler RA, Bhagwanjee S et al (2010) Critical care and the global burden of critical illness in adults. Lancet 376:1339–1346

Affoo RH, Foley N, Rosenbek J et al (2013) Swallowing dysfunction and autonomic nervous system dysfunction in Alzheimer's disease: a scoping review of the evidence. J Am Geriatr Soc 61(12):2203–2213

Aguilar-Ponce JL, Granados-García M, Cruz López JC et al (2003) Alternating chemotherapy: gemcitabine and cisplatin with concurrent radiotherapy for treatment of advanced head and neck cancer. Oral Oncol 49:249–254

Ajemian MS, Nirmul GB, Anderson MT et al (2001) Routine fiberoptic endoscopic evaluation of swallowing following prolonged intubation: implications for management. Arch Surg 136:434–437

Alagiakrishnan K, Bhanji RA, Kurian M (2013) Evaluation and management of oropharyngeal dysphagia in different types of dementia: a systematic review. Arch Gerontol Geriatr 56(1):1–9

Aldridge KJ, Taylor NF (2012) Dysphagia is a common and serious problem for adults with mental illness: a systematic review. Dysphagia 27:124–137

Altman KW, Yu GP, Schaefer SD (2014) Consequence of dysphagia in the hospitalized patient. Dysphagia 29:183–198. https://doi.org/10.1007/s00455-013-9511-8

APA (American Psychiatric Association) (2013) Diagnostic and statistical manual of mental disorders, 5th edn. APA, Washington, DC

Arens C, Herrmann IF, Rohrbach S et al (2015) Position paper of the German Society of Oto-Rhino-Laryngology, head and neck surgery and the German Society of Phoniatrics and Pediatric Audiology—current state of clinical and endoscopic diagnostics, evaluation, and therapy of swallowing disorders in children. GMS Curr Top Otorhinolaryngol Head Neck Surg 14:1–61

Arts MP, Rettig TCD, de Vries J et al (2013) Maintaining endotracheal tube cuff pressure at 20 mm hg to prevent dysphagia after anterior cervical spine surgery; protocol of a double-blind randomised controlled trial. BMC Musculoskelet Disord 14:280. https://doi.org/10.1186/1471-2474-14-280

Arvedson JC (2008) Assessment of pediatric dysphagia and feeding disorders: clinical and instrumental approaches. Dev Disabil Res Rev 14(2):118–127

Arvedson JC (2013) Feeding children with cerebral palsy and swallowing difficulties. Eur J Clin Nutr 67(Suppl 2):S9–S12

Arvedson JC, Brodsky L (2002) Pediatric swallowing und feeding. Assessment and management, 2nd edn. Singular Publishing Group, New York, NY

Arvedson JC, Lefton-Greif MA (1996) Anatomy, physiology, and development of feeding. Semin Speech Lang 17(4):261–268

Aviv JE (2000) Clinical assessment of pharyngolaryngeal sensitivity. Am J Med 108(Suppl 4a):68S–72S

Bader CA, Niemann G (2007) Dysphagien im Kindes—und Jugendlichenalter. Zum Stellenwert der fiberoptisch-endoskopischen Schluckdiagnostik (dysphagia in childhood and adolescence. On the importance of fibre-optic endoscopic swallowing diagnostics). HNO 56(4):397–401

Bader CA, Niemann G (2010) Dysphagie bei Kindern mit Infantiler Zerebralparese—Fiberoptisch-endoskopische Befunde (dysphagia in children with infantile cerebral palsy–fibre-optic endoscopic findings). Laryngol Rhino Otol 89(2):90–94

Baheshree RD, Jonas SS (2012) Dysphagia in a psychotic patient: diagnostic challenges and a systematic management approach. Indian J Psychiatry 54(3):280–282

Baijens LW, Clavé P, Cras P et al (2016) European Society for Swallowing Disorders—European Union geriatric medicine society white paper: oropharyngeal dysphagia as a geriatric syndrome. Clin Interv Aging 11:1403–1428

Baker L, Beres AL, Baird R (2015) A systematic review and meta-analysis of gastrostomy insertion techniques in children. J Pediatr Surg 50(5):718–725

Barberena LS, Brasil BC, Melo RM et al (2014) Ultrasound applicability in speech language pathology and audiology. Codas 26(6):520–530

Barker J, Martino R, Reichardt B et al (2009) Incidence and impact of dysphagia in patients receiving prolonged endotracheal intubation after cardiac surgery. Can J Surg 52:119–124

Barlow SM, Estep M (2006) Central pattern generation and the motor infrastructure for suck, respiration, and speech. J Commun Disord 39(5):366–380

Barofsky I, Fontaine KR (1998) Do psychogenic dysphagia patients have an eating disorder? Dysphagia 13:24–27

Barritt AW, Smithard DG (2009) Role of cerebral cortex plasticity in the recovery of swallowing function following dysphagic stroke. Dysphagia 24(1):83–90

Bartolome G (2018) Management von Schluckstörungen der Nahrungsaufnahme bei Demenz (Management of dysphagia of food intake in dementia). In: Bartolome G, Schröter-Morasch H (eds) Schluckstörungen—Diagnostik und rehabilitation (swallowing disorders—diagnostics and rehabilitation), 6th edn. Elsevier, Urban & Fischer, Munich

Bartolome G, Schröter-Morasch H (eds) (2014) Schluckstörungen. Diagnostik und rehabilitation (swallowing disorders. Diagnostics and rehabilitation), 5th edn. Elsevier Urban & Fischer, Munich

Bath PM, Scutt P, Love J et al (2016) Swallowing treatment using pharyngeal electrical stimulation (STEPS) trial investigators. Pharyngeal electrical stimulation for treatment of dysphagia in subacute stroke: a randomized controlled trial. Stroke 47(6):1562–1570

Barkmeier-Kraemer JM, Clark HM (2017) Speech-Language Pathology Evaluation and Management of Hyperkinetic Disorders Affecting Speech and Swallowing Function. Tremor Other Hyperkinet Mov (N Y) 7:489

Bazemore PH, Tonkonogy J, Ananth R (1991) Dysphagia in psychiatric patients: clinical and videofluoroscopic study. Dysphagia 6(1):2–5

Benoit D (2002) Feeding disorders, failure to thrive and obesity. In: Zeanah CH (ed) Handbook of infant mental health. Guilford Press, New York, NY, pp 339–352

Berlit P, Bösel J, Gahn G et al (2020) Neurological manifestations of COVID-19—guideline of the German Society of Neurology. Neurol Res Pract 2:51. https://doi.org/10.1186/s42466-020-00097-7

Bernard-Bonnin AC (2006) Feeding problems of infants and toddlers. Can Fam Physician 52(10):1247–1251

Best SR, Ahn J, Langmead S et al (2018) Voice and swallowing dysfunction in neurofibromatosis 2. Otolaryngol Head Neck Surg 158(3):505–510

Bhargav N, Hedge A, Chandra P et al (2014) Problematic eating and its association with early childhood caries among 46-71-month-old children using Children's eating behaviour questionnaire (CEBQ): a cross sectional study. Ind J Dent Res 25(5):602–606

Birch LL, Davison KK (2001) Family environmental factors influencing the developing behavioural controls of food intake and childhood overweight. Pediatr Clin N Am 48(4):893–907

Bledsoe IO, Comella CL (2016) Botulinum toxin treatment of cervical dystonia. Semin Neurol 36(1):47–53

Blissett J, Meyer C, Haycraft E (2007) Maternal mental health and child feeding problems on a non-clinical group. Eat Behav 8(3):311–318

Böckler R (2015) Dysphagie bei Säuglingen und Kleinkindern (Dysphagia in infants and toddlers). Logos 23(3):176–187

Bradley RM (2000) Sensory receptors of the larynx. Am J Med 108(Suppl 4a):47S–50S

Bray BD, Smith CJ, Cloud GC et al (2017) The association between delays in screening for and assessing dysphagia after acute stroke, and the risk of stroke-associated pneumonia. J Neurol Neurosurg Psychiatry 88(1):25–30

Bredenoord AJ (2013) Management of belching, hiccups, and aerophagia. Clin Gastroenterol Hepatol 11(1):6–12

Bredenoord AJ, Smout AJ (2010) Impaired health-related quality of life in patients with excessive supragastric belching. Eur J Gastroenterol Hepatol 22(12):1420–1423

Bredenoord AJ, Weusten BLAM, Sifrim D et al (2004) Aerophagia, gastric, and supragastric belching: a study using intraluminal electrical impedance monitoring. Gut 53(11):1561–1565

Bredenoord AJ, Weusten BLAM, Timmer R et al (2006) Psychological factors affect the frequency of belching in patients with aerophagia. Am J Gastroenterol 101(12):2777–2781

Brodsky MB, Gellar JE, Dinglas VD et al (2014) Duration of oral endotracheal intubation is associated with dysphagia symptoms in acute lung injury patients. J Crit Care 29:574–579

Brodsky MB, De I, Chilukuri K et al (2018) Coordination of pharyngeal and laryngeal swallowing events during single liquid swallows after oral endotracheal intubation for patients with acute respiratory distress syndrome. Dysphagia 33:768–777

Brodsky MB, Mayfield EB, Gross RD (2019) Clinical decision making in the ICU: dysphagia screening, assessment, and treatment. Semin Speech Lang 40(3):170–187

Brodsky MB, Pandian V, Needham DM (2020) Post-extubation dysphagia: a problem needing multidisciplinary efforts. Intensive Care Med 46:93–96

Brotherton A, Campos E, Rowell A et al (2012) Nutritional management of individuals with Huntington's disease: nutritional guidelines. Neurodegen Dis Manage 2(1):33–43

Brown TE, Spurgin AL, Ross L et al (2013) Validated swallowing and nutrition guidelines for patients with head and neck cancer: identification of high-risk patients for proactive gastrostomy. Head Neck 35:1385–1391

Bryant-Waught RJ, Piepenstock EHC (2008) Childhood disorders: feeding and related disorders of infancy and early childhood. In: Tasman AJ (ed) Psychiatry, 3rd edn. John Wiley & Sons Ltd, New York, NY, pp 830–846

Buchholz D (1997) Neurologic disorders of swallowing. In: Groher ME (ed) Dysphagia, diagnosis and management, 3rd edn. Butterworth-Heinemann, Boston, MA

Burgos R, Breton I, Cereda E et al (2018) ESPEN guideline clinical nutrition in neurology. Clin Nutr 37(1):354–396

Butler C, Zeman AZJ (2005) Neurological syndromes which can be mistaken for psychiatric conditions. J Neurol Neurosurg Psychiatry 76(Suppl I):i31–i38

Caglar HB, Tishler RB, Othus M et al (2008) Dose to larynx predicts for swallowing complications after intensity-modulated radiotherapy. Int J Radiat Oncol Biol Phys 72:1110–1118

Calis EA, Veugelers R, Sheppard JJ et al (2008) Dysphagia in children with severe generalized cerebral palsy and intellectual disability. Dev Med Child Neurol 50(8):625–630

Campbell BH, Spinelli K, Marbella AM et al (2004) Arch Otolaryngol Head Neck Surg 130:1100–1103

Carnaby GD, Crary MA (2014) Development and validation of a cancer-specific swallowing assessment tool: MASA-C. Support Care Cancer 22:595–602

Carnaby Mann GD (2012) Food for thought. Perspectives on swallowing and swallowing disorders. Dysphagia 21:143–149

Carnaby G, Hankey GJ, Pizzi J (2006) Behavioural intervention for dysphagia in acute stroke: a randomised controlled trial. Lancet Neurol 5:31–37

Cartmill B, Cornwell P, Ward E et al (2012) Long-term functional outcomes and patient perspective following altered fractionation radiotherapy with concomitant boost for oropharyngeal cancer. Dysphagia 27:481–490

Caudell JJ, Schaner PE, Desmond RA et al (2010) Dosimetric factors associated with long-term dysphagia after definitive radiotherapy for squamous cell carcinoma of the head and neck. Int J Radiat Oncol Biol Phys 76:403–409

Cavalot AL, Ricci E, Schindler A et al (2009) The importance of preoperative swallowing therapy in subtotal laryngectomies. Otolaryngol Head Neck Surg 140:822–825

Chan JY, Lua LL, Starmer HH et al (2011) The relationship between depressive symptoms and initial quality of life and function in head and neck cancer. Laryngoscope 121:1212–1218

Chatoor I (2002) Feeding disorders in infants and toddlers: diagnosis and treatment. Child Adoles Psychiatr Clin N Am 11(2):163–183

Chatoor I, Egan J (1983) Nonorganic failure to thrive and dwarfism due to food refusal: a separation disorder. J Am Acad Child Psychiatr 22(3):294–301

Chatoor I, Hirsch R, Persinger M (1997) Facilitating internal regulation of eating: a treatment model for infantile anorexia. Inf Young Child 9(4):12–22

Chatoor I, Ganiban J, Colin V et al (1998a) Attachment and feeding problems: a reexamination of nonorganic failure to thrive and attachment insecurity. J Am Acad Child Adolesc Psychiatry 37(11):1217–1224

Chatoor I, Hirsch R, Ganiban J et al (1998b) Diagnosing infantile anorexia: the observation of mother-infant interactions. Child Adolesc Psychiatr 37(9):959–967

Cho SK, Lu Y, Lee DH (2013) Dysphagia following anterior cervical spinal surgery. Bone Joint J 95B(7):868–873

Chone CT, Spina AL, Barcellos IH et al (2011) A prospective study of long-term dysphagia following total laryngectomy. B-ENT 7:103–109

Christianen ME, Schilstra C, Beetz I et al (2012) Predictive modelling for swallowing dysfunction after primary (chemo)radiation: results of a prospective observational study. Radiother Oncol 105(1):107–114

Cicala G, Barbieri MA, Spina E et al (2019) A comprehensive review of swallowing difficulties and dysphagia-associated with antipsychotics in adults. Expert Rev Clin Pharmacol 12(3):219–234

Cnossen IC, de Bree R, Rinkel RN et al (2012) Computerized monitoring of patient-reported speech and swallowing problems in head and neck cancer patients in clinical practice. Support Care Cancer 20:2925–2931

Coiffier L, Périé S, Laforêt P et al (2006) Long-term results of cricopharyngeal myotomy in oculopharyngeal muscular dystrophy. Otolaryngol Head Neck Surg 135(2):218–222

Combes X, Schauvliege F, Peyrouset O et al (2001) Intracuff pressure and tracheal morbidity: influence of filling with saline during nitrous oxide anesthesia. Anesthesiology 95:1120–1124

Craig GM (2013) Psychosocial aspects of feeding children with neurodisability. Eur J Clin Nutr 67(Suppl 2):S17–S20

Crary MA, Carnaby-Mann GD, Groher ME (2005) Initial psychometric assessment of a functional oral intake scale for dysphagia in stroke patients. Arch Phys Med Rehabil 86:1516–1520

Crary MA, Carnaby GD, LaGorio LA et al (2012) Functional and physiological outcomes from an exercise-based dysphagia therapy: a pilot investigation of the McNeill dysphagia therapy program. Arch Phys Med Rehabil 93:1173–1178

Crawley BK, Sulica L (2015) Vocal fold paralysis as a delayed consequence of neck and chest radiotherapy. Otolaryngol Head Neck Surg 153(2):239–243

da Costa SP, van der Schans CP (2008) The reliability of the neonatal Oral-motor assessment scale. Acta Paediatr 97(1):21–26

da Costa SP, Hübl N, Kaufman N et al (2016) New scoring system improves inter-rater reliability of the neonatal Oral-motor assessment scale. Acta Paediatr 105(8):e339–e344. https://doi.org/10.1111/apa.13461

da Silva AP, Lubianca Neto JF, Santoro PP et al (2010) Comparison between videofluoroscopy and endoscopic evaluation of swallowing for the diagnosis of dysphagia in children. Otolaryngol Head Neck Surg 143(2):204–209

Daniels SK, Huckabee ML (2014) Dysphagia following stroke, 2nd edn. Plural, San Diego, CA

Davies WH, Satter E, Berlin KS et al (2006) Reconceptualizing feeding and feeding disorders in interpersonal context: role of the family environment. Br J Psychiatry 184:210–215

DC:0-5™ (2016) Diagnostic classification of mental health and developmental disorders of infancy and early childhood-zero to five. DC:0-5™, Washington, DC

De Boer MF, McCormick LK, Pruyn JF et al (1999) Physical and psychosocial correlates of head and neck cancer: a review of the literature. Otolaryngol Head Neck Surg 120:427–436

de Larminat V, Montravers P, Dureuil B et al (1995) Alteration in swallowing reflex after extubation in intensive care unit patients. Crit Care Med 23:486–490

de Medeiros GC, Sassi FC, Mangilli LD et al (2014) Clinical dysphagia risk predictors after prolonged orotracheal intubation. Clinics (São Paulo) 69:8–14

de Oliveira ACM, de Lima Friche AA, Salomão MS et al (2018) Predictive factors for oropharyngeal dysphagia after prolonged orotracheal intubation. Braz J Otorhinolaryngol 84:722–728

De Vita MA, Spierer-Rundback L (1990) Swallowing disorders in patients with prolonged orotracheal intubation or tracheostomy tubes. Crit Care Med 18:1328–1330

DeMatteo C, Matovich D, Hjartarson S (2005) Comparison of clinical and videofluoroscopic evaluation of children with feeding and swallowing difficulties. Dev Med Child Neurol 47(3):149–157

Deuschl G, Mischke G, Schenck E et al (1990) Symptomatic and essential rhythmic palatal myoclonus. Brain 113(6):1645–1672

Deutschmann MW, McDonough A, Dort JC et al (2013) Fiber-optic endoscopic evaluation of swallowing (FEES): predictor of swallowing-related complications in the head and neck cancer population. Head Neck 35:974–979

Dhawan I, O'Connell B, Patel A et al (2018) Utility of esophageal high-resolution manometry in clinical practice: first, do HRM. Dig Dis Sci 63(12):3178–3186

Diène G, Postel-Vinay A, Pinto G et al (2007) The Prader-Willi syndrome. Ann Endocrinol (Paris) 68(2–3):129–137

Ding R, Logemann JA (2005) Swallow physiology in patients with trach cuff inflated or deflated: a retrospective study. Head Neck 27:809–813

Dirix P, Abbeel S, Vanstraelen B et al (2009) Dysphagia after chemoradiotherapy for head-and-neck squamous cell carcinoma: dose-effect relationships for the swallowing structures. Int J Radiat Oncol Biol Phys 75:385–392

Dodrill P, Gosa MM (2015) Pediatric dysphagia: physiology, assessment, and management. Ann Nutr Metab 66(Suppl 5):24–31

Doggett DL, Turkelson CM, Coates V (2002) Recent developments in diagnosis and intervention for aspiration and dysphagia in stroke and other neuromuscular disorders. Curr Atheroscler Rep 4(4):311–331

Doherty N, Steen CD (2010) Critical illness polyneuromyopathy (CIPNM); rehabilitation during critical illness. Therapeutic options in nursing to promote recovery: a review of the literature. Intensive Crit Care Nur 26(6):353–362

Dorsey YC, Song EJ, Leiman DA (2021) Beyond the Eckardt score: patient-reported outcomes measures in esophageal disorders. Curr Gastroenterol Rep 23(12):29. https://doi.org/10.1007/s11894-021-00831-4

DSM-V (2013) American Psychiatric Association: diagnostic and statistical manual of mental disorders, 5th edn. American Psychiatric Association, Arlington, VA

Duprez F, Madani I, De Potter B et al (2013) Systematic review of dose-volume correlates for structures related to late swallowing disturbances after radiotherapy for head and neck cancer. Dysphagia 28:337–349

Dziewas R, Warnecke T (2019) ICU-related dysphagia. In: Ekberg O (ed) Dysphagia: diagnosis and treatment. Springer, Cham, pp 157–164

Dziewas R, Busse O, Glahn J et al (2013) FEES auf der Stroke-Unit (FEES on stroke unit). Nervenarzt 84:705–708

Dziewas R, Beck AM, Clave P et al (2017) Recognizing the importance of dysphagia: stumbling blocks and stepping stones in the twenty-first century. Dysphagia 32(1):78–82

Dziewas R, Warnecke T, Zurcher P et al (2020) Dysphagia in COVID-19—multilevel damage to the swallowing network? Eur J Neurol 27(9):e46–e47. https://doi.org/10.1111/ene.14367

Eisbruch A, Lyden T, Bradford CR et al (2002) Objective assessment of swallowing dysfunction and aspiration after radiation concurrent with chemotherapy for head-and-neck cancer. Int J Radiat Oncol Biol Phys 53:23–28

Eisbruch A, Schwartz M, Rasch C et al (2004) Dysphagia and aspiration after chemoradiotherapy for head-and-neck cancer: which anatomic structures are affected and can they be spared by IMRT? Int J Radiat Oncol Biol Phys 60:1425–1439

Eisenstadt SE (2010) Dysphagia and aspiration pneumonia in older adults. J Am Acad Nurse Pract 22(1):17–22

Ekberg O, Hamdy S, Woisard V et al (2002) Social and psychological burden of dysphagia: its impact on diagnosis and treatment. Dysphagia 17(2):139–146

El Gharib AZG, Berretin-Felix G, Rossoni DF et al (2019) Effectiveness of therapy on post-extubation dysphagia: clinical and electromyographic findings. Clin Med Insights Ear Nose Throat 12:117955061987336. https://doi.org/10.1177/1179550619873364

Ellegård E, Nilsén CH (2016) Supragastric belching—case report of a severe handicap. Acta Oto-Laryngol Case Rep 1(1):1–3

Ertekin C (2011) Voluntary versus spontaneous swallowing in man. Dysphagia 26:183–192

Etges CL, Scheeren B, Gomes E et al (2014) Screening tools for dysphagia: a systematic review. Codas 26:343–349

Eurostat (2019) Ageing Europe. Looking at the lives of older people in the EU. Publications Office of the European Union, Luxembourg, pp 14–15

Farneti D, Consolmagno P (2007) The swallowing Centre: rationale for a multidisciplinary management. Acta Otorhinolaryngol Ital 27:200–207

Farneti D, Fattori B, Nacci A et al (2014) The pooling-score (P-score): inter—and intra-rater reliability in endoscopic assessment of the severity of dysphagia. Acta Otorhinolaryngol Ital 34:105–110

Fernández-Carmona A, Peñas-Maldonado L, Yuste-Osorio E et al (2012) Exploration and approach to artificial airway dysphagia. Med Intensiva 36:423–433

Ferris L, Rommel N, Doeltgen S et al (2016) Pressure-flow analysis for the assessment of pediatric oropharyngeal dysphagia. J Pediatr 177:279–285

Fichaux-Bourin P, Diène G, Glattard M et al (2009) Early education for children with Prader-Willi syndrome. Rev Laryngol Otol Rhinol (Bord) 130(1):35–40

Flint PW, Purcell LL, Cummings CW (1997) Pathophysiology and indications for medialization thyroplasty in patients with dysphagia and aspiration. Otolaryngol Head Neck Surg 116:349–354

Folstein MF, Folstein SE, McHugh PR (1975) "Mini-mental state". A practical method for grading the cognitive state of patients for the clinician. J Psychiatr Res 12(3):189–198

Fonta MM, Salsench LR (2017) Antipsychotic medication and oropharyngeal dysphagia: systematic review. Eur J Gastroenterol Hepatol 29(12):1332–1339

François B, Bellissant E, Gissot V et al (2007) 12-h pretreatment with methylprednisolone versus placebo for prevention of postextubation laryngeal oedema: a randomised double-blind trial. Lancet 369:1083–1089

Frey S (2011a) Oropharyngeale Dysphagien (oropharyngeal dysphagia). In: Frey S (ed) Pädiatrisches Dysphagiemanagement (pediatric dysphagia management). Urban & Fischer, München, pp 106–122

Frey S (2011b) PÄDY Pädiatrisches Dysphagiemanagement–therapeutische Maßnahmen (Paediatric dysphagia management–therapeutic measures). In: Frey S (ed) Pädiatrisches Dysphagiemanagement (pediatric dysphagia management). Urban & Fischer, München, pp 259–301

Frowen JJ, Cotton SM, Perry AR (2008) The stability, reliability, and validity of videofluoroscopy measures for patients with head and neck cancer. Dysphagia 23:348–363

Frowen J, Cotton S, Corry J et al (2010) Impact of demographics, tumor characteristics, and treatment factors on swallowing after (chemo)radiotherapy for head and neck cancer. Head Neck 32:513–528

Garcia JM, Chambers EI (2010) Managing dysphagia through diet modifications. Am J Nurs 110:26–33

Garon BR, Sierzant T, Ormiston C (2009) Silent aspiration: results of 2,000 video fluoroscopic evaluations. J Neurosci Nurs 41:178–185

Gawryszuk A, Bijl HP, Holwerda M et al (2018) Functional swallowing units (FSUs) as organs-at-risk for radiotherapy. PART 1: physiology and anatomy. Radiother Oncol S0167-8140(18):33552–33557

Geneid A, Nawka T, Schindler A et al (2020) Union of the European Phoniatricians' position statement on the exit strategy of phoniatric and laryngological services: staying safe and getting back to normal after the peak of coronavirus disease 2019. Laryngol Otol 134(8):661–664

Ghazali N, Kanatas A, Scott B et al (2012) Use of the patient concerns inventory to identify speech and swallowing concerns following treatment for oral and oropharyngeal cancer. J Laryngol Otol 126:800–808

Gisel E (2008) Interventions and outcomes for children with dysphagia. Dev Disabil Res Rev 14(2):165–173

Giurgea I, Raqbi F, Nihoul-Fékété G et al (2000) Congenital microgastria with Pierre Robin sequence and partial trismus. Clin Dysmorphol 9(4):307–308

Glasinovic E, Wynter E, Arguero J et al (2018) Treatment of supragastric belching with cognitive behavioral therapy improves quality of life and reduces acid gastroesophageal reflux. Am J Gastroenterol 113(4):539–547

GLOBOCAN (2012) Estimated cancer incidence and mortality worldwide in 2012: IARC Cancer Base [web site]. International Agency for Research on Cancer, Lyon. http://globocan.iarc.fr. Accessed 11 Aug 2014

Goldsmith T (2000) Evaluation and treatment of swallowing disorders following endotracheal intubation and tracheostomy. Int Anesthesiol Clin 38:219–242

Greco E, Simic T, Ringash J et al (2018) Dysphagia treatment for patients with head and neck cancer undergoing radiation therapy: a meta-analysis review. Int J Radiat Oncol Biol Phys 101:421–444

Groher ME, Crary MA (2016) Dysphagia. Clinical management in adults and children, Elsevier, St. Louis, MO

Gross RD, Atwood CW, Ross SB et al (2009) The coordination of breathing and swallowing in chronic obstructive pulmonary disease. Am J Respir Crit Care Med 179:559–565

Gupta SP, Shivaji PR, Goyal M et al (2007) Congenital tumor of tongue. Indian J Surg 69(6):266–267

Gupta A, Gulati P, Kim W et al (2009) Effect of postnatal maturation on the mechanisms of esophageal propulsion in preterm human neonates: primary and secondary peristalsis. Am J Gastroenterol 104(2):411–419

Halczy-Kowalik L, Sulikowski M, Wysocki R et al (2012) The role of the epiglottis in the swallow process after a partial or total glossectomy due to a neoplasm. Dysphagia 27:20–31

Hamdy S, Aziz Q, Rothwell JC et al (1998a) Recovery of swallowing after dysphagic stroke relates to functional reorganization in the intact motor cortex. Gastroenterology 115(5):1104–1112

Hamdy S, Rothwell JC, Aziz Q et al (1998b) Long-term reorganization of human motor cortex driven by short-term sensory stimulation. Nat Neurosci 1:64–68

Hanasono MM, Robb GL, Skoracki RJ et al (2016) Reconstructive plastic surgery of the head and neck: current techniques and flap atlas. Thieme, Stuttgart

Hartl DM, Kolb F, Bretagne E et al (2010) Cine-MRI swallowing evaluation after tongue reconstruction. Eur J Radiol 73:108–113

Heckathorn DE, Speyer R, Taylor J et al (2016) Systematic review: non-instrumental swallowing and feeding assessments in pediatrics. Dysphagia 31(1):1–23

Heemskerk AW, Roos RAC (2011) Dysphagia in Huntington's disease: a review. Dysphagia 26(1):62–66

Hemmink GJM, Bredenoord AJ, Weusten BLAM et al (2009) Supragastric belching in patients with reflux symptoms. Am J Gastroenterol 104(8):1992–1997

Hemmink GJM, Ten Cate L, Bredenoord AJ et al (2010) Speech therapy in patients with excessive supragastric belching—a pilot study. Neurogastroenterol Motil 22(1):24–28

Hersh C, Wentland C, Sally S et al (2016) Radiation exposure from videofluoroscopic swallow studies in children with a type 1 laryngeal cleft and pharyngeal dysphagia: a retrospective review. Int J Pediatr Otorhinolaryngol 89:92–96

Hey C, Lange BP, Eberle S et al (2013) Water swallow screening test for patients after surgery for head and neck cancer: early identification of dysphagia, aspiration and limitations of oral intake. Anticancer Res 33:4017–4021

Hinni ML, Salassa JR, Grant DG et al (2007) Transoral laser microsurgery for advanced laryngeal cancer. Arch Otolaryngol Head Neck Surg 133:1198–1204

Hirano M, Kuroiwa Y, Tanaka S et al (1992) Dysphagia following various degrees of surgical resection for oral cancer. Ann Otol Rhinol Laryngol 101:138–141

Ho CH, Lin WC, Hsu YF et al (2018) One-year risk of pneumonia and mortality in patients with poststroke dysphagia: a nationwide population-based study. J Stroke Cerebrovasc Dis 27(5):1311–1317

Hui Y, Wei WI, Yuen PW et al (1996) Primary closure of pharyngeal remnant after total laryngectomy and partial pharyngectomy: how much residual mucosa is sufficient? Laryngoscope 106:490–494

Hutcheson KA, Lewin JS, Barringer DA et al (2012) Late dysphagia after radiotherapy-based treatment of head and neck cancer. Cancer 118(23):5793–5799

Hutcheson KA, Abualsamh AR, Sosa A et al (2016) Impact of selective neck dissection on chronic dysphagia after chemo-intensity-modulated radiotherapy for oropharyngeal carcinoma. Head Neck 38(6):886–893

Hutcheson KA, Warneke CL, Yao C et al (2019) Dysphagia after primary transoral robotic surgery with neck dissection vs nonsurgical therapy in patients with low- to intermediate-risk oropharyngeal cancer. JAMA Otolaryngol Head Neck Surg 145(11):1053–1063

ICD-10-GM (2015) International Statistical Classification of Diseases and Related Health Problems. Deutsches Institut für Medizinische Dokumentation und Information, Köln. German Institute for Medical Documentation and Information, Cologne

Jäghagen EL, Bodin I, Isberg A (2008) Pharyngeal swallowing dysfunction following treatment for oral and pharyngeal cancer—association with diminished intraoral sensation and discrimination ability. Head Neck 30:1344–13451

Jain S (2016) When the diagnosis is hard to swallow, take these management steps. Curr Psychiatr 15(8):67–68

Jayasekeran V, Singh S, Tyrrell P et al (2010) Adjunctive functional pharyngeal electrical stimulation reverses swallowing disability after brain lesions. Gastroenterology 138:1737–1746

Jenkins S, Owen C, Bax M et al (1984) Continuities of common behaviour problems in preschool children. J Child Psychol Psychiatr 25(819):75–89

Johnson JM, Moonis G, Green GE et al (2011a) Syndromes of the first and second branchial arches, part 1: embryology and characteristic defects. Am J Neuroradiol 32(1):14–19

Johnson JM, Moonis G, Green GE et al (2011b) Syndromes of the first and second branchial arches, part 2: syndromes. Am J Neuroradiol 32(2):230–237

Johnson KL, Speirs L, Mitchell A et al (2018) Validation of a postextubation dysphagia screening tool for patients after prolonged endotracheal intubation. Am J Crit Care 27:89–96

Kao SS, Peters MD, Krishnan SG et al (2016) Swallowing outcomes following primary surgical resection and primary free flap reconstruction for oral and oropharyngeal squamous cell carcinomas: a systematic review. Laryngoscope 126(7):1572–15780

Kerawala C, Roques T, Jeannon JP et al (2016) Oral cavity and lip cancer: United Kingdom National Multidisciplinary Guidelines. J Laryngol Otol 130(S2):S83–S89

Keren M (2016) Eating and feeding disorders in the first five years of life: revising the DC:0-3R diagnostic classification of mental health and developmental disorders of infancy and early childhood and rationale for the new DC:0-5 proposed criteria. Infant Ment Health 37(5):498–508

Kerwin R (1999) Empirically supported treatments in pediatric psychology: severe feeding problems. J Pediatr Psychol 24(3):193–214

Kerzner B, Milano K, Macleran WC et al (2015) A practical approach to classifying and managing feeding difficulties. Pediatrics 135(2):344–353

Kessing BF, Bredenoord AJ, Smout AJPM (2012a) Mechanisms of gastric and supragastric belching: a study using concurrent high-resolution manometry and impedance monitoring: gastric belching and supragastric belching. Neurogastroenterol Motil 24(12):e573–e579. https://doi.org/10.1111/nmo.12024

Kessing BF, Bredenoord AJ, Velosa M et al (2012b) Supragastric belches are the main determinants of troublesome belching symptoms in patients with gastro-oesophageal reflux disease. Aliment Pharmacol Ther 35(9):1073–1079

Kessing BF, Bredenoord AJ, Smout AJ (2014) The pathophysiology, diagnosis and treatment of excessive belching symptoms. Am J Gastroenterol 109(8):1196–1203

Kim MJ, Park YH, Park YS et al (2015) Associations between prolonged intubation and developing postextubation dysphagia and aspiration pneumonia in non-neurologic critically ill patients. Ann Rehabil Med 39:763–771

King SN, Dunlap NE, Tennant PA et al (2016) Pathophysiology of radiation-induced dysphagia in head and neck cancer. Dysphagia 31(3):339–351

Knigge MA, Thibeault S, McCulloch TM (2014) Implementation of high-resolution manometry in the clinical practice of speech language pathology. Dysphagia 29(1):2–16

Kocdor P, Siegel ER, Giese R et al (2015a) Characteristics of dysphagia in older patients evaluated at a tertiary center. Laryngoscope 125(2):400–405

Kocdor P, Siegel ER, Tulunay-Ugur OE (2015b) Cricopharyngeal dysfunction: a systematic review comparing outcomes of dilatation, botulinum toxin injection, and myotomy. Laryngoscope 126(1):135–141

Komasawa N, Komatsu M, Yamasaki H et al (2017) Lip, tooth, and pharyngeal injuries during tracheal intubation at a teaching hospital. Br J Anaesth 119:171–171

Kos MP, David EF, Klinkenberg-Knol EC et al (2010) Long-term results of external upper esophageal sphincter myotomy for oropharyngeal. Dysphagia 25:169–176

Kotz T, Costello R, Li Y et al (2004) Swallowing dysfunction after chemoradiation for advanced squamous cell carcinoma of the head and neck. Head Neck 26(4):365–372

Koukias N, Woodland P, Yazaki E et al (2015) Supragastric belching: prevalence and association with gastroesophageal reflux disease and esophageal Hypomotility. J Neurogastroenterol Motil 21(3):398–403

Kremer B, Botos-Kremer AI, Eckel HE et al (2012) Indications, complications, and surgical techniques for pediatric tracheostomies—an update. J Pediatr Surgery 37(11):1556–1562

Kroll M (2011) Interdisziplinäre Eltern-Kind Behandlung von schweren komplexen Fütterstörungen (interdisciplinary parent-child treatment of severe complex feeding disorders). Prax Kinderpsychologie/Kinderpsychiatry 60(6):452–465

Kronenberger MB, Meyers AD (1994) Dysphagia following head and neck cancer surgery. Dysphagia 9:236–244

Kühnlein P, Gdynia HJ, Sperfeld AD et al (2008) Diagnosis and treatment of bulbar symptoms in amyotrophic lateral sclerosis. Nat Clin Pract Neurol 4(7):366–374

Kwok AM, Davis JW, Cagle KM et al (2013) Post-extubation dysphagia in trauma patients: it's hard to swallow. Am J Surg 206:924–928

Lagercrantz H, Ringstedt T (2001) Organization of the neuronal circuits in the central nervous system during development. Acta Paediatr 90(7):707–715

Lang IM, Medda BK, Shaker R (2017) Characterization and mechanisms of the supragastric belch in the cat. Am J Physiol Gastrointest Liver Physiol 313(3):G220–G229

Langmore SE (2003) Evaluation of oropharyngeal dysphagia: which diagnostic tool is superior? Curr Opin Otolaryngol Head Neck Surg 11(6):485–489

Langmore SE, Schatz K, Olsen N (1988) Fiberoptic endoscopic examination of swallowing safety: a new procedure. Dysphagia 2(4):216–219

Langmore SE, Schatz K, Olsen N (1991) Endoscopic and videofluoroscopic evaluations of swallowing and aspiration. Ann Otol Rhinol Laryngol 100(8):678–681

Lango MN, Langendijk JA, Doornaert P et al (2009) A predictive model for swallowing dysfunction after curative radiotherapy in head and neck cancer. Radiother Oncol 90:189–195

Lango MN, Egleston B, Fang C et al (2014) Baseline health perceptions, dysphagia, and survival in patients with head and neck cancer. Cancer 120:840–847

Lau C, Smith EO, Schanler RJ (2003) Coordination of suck-swallow and swallow respiration in preterm infants. Acta Paediatr 92(6):721–727

Lazarus CL, Logemann JA, Pauloski BR et al (1996) Swallowing disorders in head and neck cancer patients treated with radiotherapy and adjuvant chemotherapy. Laryngoscope 106:1157–1166

Leder SB, Cohn SM, Moller BA (1998) Fiberoptic endoscopic documentation of the high incidence of aspiration following extubation in critically ill trauma patients. Dysphagia 13(4):208–212

Leder SB, Joe JK, Ross DA et al (2005) Presence of a tracheotomy tube and aspiration status in early, postsurgical head and neck cancer patients. Head Neck 27:757–761

Leder SB, Suiter DM, Lisitano Warner H (2009) Answering orientation questions and following single-step verbal commands: effect on aspiration status. Dysphagia 24:290–295

Leder SB, Lisitano Warner H, Suiter DM et al (2019) Evaluation of swallow function post-extubation: is it necessary to wait 24 hours? Ann Otol Rhinol Laryngol 128:619–624

Lefton-Greif MA, Okelo SO, Wright JM et al (2015) Impact of children's feeding/swallowing problems: validation of a new caregiver instrument. Dysphagia 29(6):671–677

Li S, Luo C, Yu B, Yan B, Gong Q, He C, He L, Huang X, Yao D, Lui S, Tang H, Chen Q, Zeng Y, Zhou D (2009) Functional magnetic resonance imaging study on dysphagia after unilateral hemispheric stroke: a preliminary study. J Neurol Neurosurg Psychiatry 80(12):1320–9

Linden P, Siebens AA (1983) Dysphagia: predicting laryngeal penetration. Arch Phys Med Rehabil 64:281–284

Lindgren S, Janzon L (1991) Prevalence of swallowing complaints and clinical findings among 50–79-year-old men and women in an urban population. Dysphagia 6(4):187–192

Linkov G, Branski RC, Amin M et al (2012) Murine model of neuromuscular electrical stimulation on squamous cell carcinoma:potential implications for dysphagia therapy. Head Neck 34:1428–1433

Linscheid TR, Budd KS, Rasnake LK (2003) Pediatric feeding disorders. In: Roberts MC (ed) Handbook of pediatric psychology. The Guilford Press, New York, NY, pp 481–498

Logemann JA (1993) Manual for videofluorographic study of swallowing, 2nd edn. Pro-Ed, Austin, TX

Logemann JA (1998) Evaluation and treatment of swallowing disorders, vol 6, 2nd edn. Pro-ed, Austin, TX, p 395

Logemann JA, Bytell DE (1979) Swallowing disorders in three types of head and neck surgical patients. Cancer 44:1095–1105

Logemann JA, Gibbons PJ, Rademaker AW et al (1994) Mechanisms of recovery of swallow after supraglottic laryngectomy. J Speech Hear Res 37:965–974

Logemann JA, Pauloski BR, Rademaker AW et al (2003) Xerostomia: 12-month changes in saliva production and its relationship to perception and performance of swallow function, oral intake, and diet after chemoradiation. Head Neck 25:432–437

Lombardi RA, Arthur ME (2020) Arytenoid subluxation. In: StatPearls. StatPearls Publishing, Treasure Island, FL

Logemann JA (2021) Logemann's Evaluation and Treatment of Swallowing Disorders. Pro-ed, Austin TX

Long YB, Wu XP (2013) A randomized controlled trail of combination therapy of neuromuscular electrical stimulation and balloon dilatation in the treatment of radiation-induced dysphagia in nasopharyngeal carcinoma patients. Disabil Rehabil 35:450–454

Lorenz S, Lissewski C, Simsek-Kiper PO et al (2013) Functional analysis of a duplication (p.E63_D69dup) in the switch II region of HRAS: new aspects of the molecular pathogenesis underlying Costello syndrome. Hum Mol Genet 22(8):1643–1653

Macht M, Wimbish T, Clark BJ et al (2011) Postextubation dysphagia is persistent and associated with poor outcomes in survivors of critical illness. Crit Care 15(5):R231. https://doi.org/10.1186/cc10472

Macht M, Wimbish T, Clark BJ et al (2012) Diagnosis and treatment of post-extubation dysphagia: results from a national survey. J Crit Care 27:578–586

Macht M, Wimbish T, Bodine C et al (2013) ICU-acquired swallowing disorders. Crit Care Med 41(10):2396–2405

Macht M, White SD, Moss M (2014) Swallowing dysfunction after critical illness. Chest 146(6):1681–1689

Madhavan A, LaGorio LA, Crary MA et al (2016) Prevalence of and risk factors for dysphagia in the community dwelling elderly: a systematic review. J Nutr Health Aging 20(8):806–815

Mah SM, Durham JS, Anderson DW et al (1996) Functional results in oral cavity reconstruction using reinnervated versus nonreinnervated free fasciocutaneous grafts. J Otolaryngol 25:75–81

Malandraki GA, McCullough G, He X et al (2011) Teledynamic evaluation of oropharyngeal swallowing. J Speech Lang Hear Res 54:1497–1505

Manikantan K, Khode S, Sayed SI et al (2009) Dysphagia in head and neck cancer. Cancer Treat Rev 35(8):724–732

Manjaly JG, Vaughan-Shaw PG, Dale OT et al (2012) Cricopharyngeal dilatation for the long-term treatment of dysphagia in oculopharyngeal muscular dystrophy. Dysphagia 27(2):216–220

Marchese-Ragona R, De Grandis D, Restivo DA et al (2003) Recovery of swallowing disorders in patients undergoing supracricoid laryngectomy with botulinum toxin therapy. Ann Otol Rhinol Laryngol 112:258–263

Martin RE, Goodyear BG, Gati JS et al (2001) Cerebral cortical representation of automatic and volitional swallowing in humans. J Neurophysiol 85(2):938–950

Martin-Harris B, Brodsky MB, Michel Y et al (2005) Breathing and swallowing dynamics across the adult lifespan. Arch Otolaryngol Head Neck Surg 131:762–770

Martino R, Foley N, Bhogal S et al (2005) Dysphagia after stroke: incidence, diagnosis and pulmonary complications. Stroke 36(12):2756–2763

Maruo T, Fujimoto Y, Ozawa K et al (2014) Laryngeal sensation and pharyngeal delay time after (chemo)radiotherapy. Eur Arch Otorrinolaringol 271:2299–2304

Marvin S, Thibeault S, Ehlenbach WJ (2019) Post-extubation dysphagia: does timing of evaluation matter? Dysphagia 34:210–219

Matsuo K, Palmer JB (2008) Anatomy and physiology of feeding and swallowing: normal and abnormal. Phys Med Rehabil Clin N Am 19:691–707

Matta RI, Halan BK, Sandhu K (2017) Postintubation recurrent laryngeal nerve palsy: a review. J Laryngol Voice 7(2):25–28

McCaul LK (2012) Oral and dental management for head and neck cancer patients treated by chemotherapy and radiotherapy. Dent Update 39(135–138):140

McDermott BM, Mamun AA, Najman JM et al (2008) Preschool children perceived by mothers as irregular eaters: physical and psychosocial predictors from a birth cohort study. J Dev Behav Pediatr 29(3):197–205

McDowell LJ, Rock K, Xu W et al (2018) Long-term late toxicity, quality of life, and emotional distress in patients with nasopharyngeal carcinoma treated with intensity modulated radiation therapy. Int J Radiat Oncol Biol Phys 102(2):340–352

Mendell DA, Logemann JA (2002) A retrospective analysis of the pharyngeal swallow in patients with a clinical diagnosis of GERD compared with normal controls: a pilot study. Dysphagia 17:220–226

Mengi T, Seçil Y, Incesu TK et al (2017) Guillain-Barré syndrome and swallowing dysfunction. J Clin Neurophysiol 34(5):393–399

Meriggioli MN, Sanders DB (2009) Autoimmune myasthenia gravis: emerging clinical and biological heterogeneity. Lancet Neurol 8(5):475–490

Messing BP, Ward EC, Lazarus C et al (2019) Establishing a multidisciplinary head and neck clinical pathway: an implementation evaluation and audit of dysphagia-related services and outcomes. Dysphagia 34(1):89–104

Michou E, Hamdy S (2009) Cortical input in control of swallowing. Curr Opin Otolaryngol Head Neck Surg. 7(3):166–71.

Miller JL, Sonies BC, Macedonia C (2003) Emergence of oropharyngeal, laryngeal and swallowing activity in the developing fetal upper aerodigestive tract: an ultrasound evaluation. Early Hum Dev 71(1):61–87

Mirzakhani H, Williams J-N, Mello J et al (2013) Muscle weakness predicts pharyngeal dysfunction and symptomatic aspiration in long-term ventilated patients. Anesthesiology 119:389–397

Mitchell SL, Tetroe JM (2000) Survival after percutaneous endoscopic gastrostomy placement in older persons. J Gerontol A Biol Sci Med Sci 55:M735–M739

Mortensen HR, Overgaard J, Jensen K et al (2012) Factors associated with acute and late dysphagia in the DAHANCA 6 & 7 randomized trial with accelerated radiotherapy for head and neck cancer. Acta Oncol 52:1535–1542

Mortensen HR, Jensen K, Aksglæde K et al (2013) Late dysphagia after IMRT for head and neck cancer and correlation with dose-volume parameters. Radiother Oncol 107:288–294

Muhle P, Wirth R, Glahn J et al (2015) Schluckstörungen im Alter. Physiologie und Pathophysiologie (swallowing disorders in old age. Physiology and pathophysiology). Nervenarzt 86(4):440–451

Mulcahy KP, Langdon PC, Mastaglia F (2012) Dysphagia in inflammatory myopathy: self-report, incidence, and prevalence. Dysphagia 27(1):64–69

Murray J, Miller M, Doeltgen S et al (2014) Intake of thickened liquids by hospitalized adults with dysphagia after stroke. Int J Speech Lang Pathol 16(5):486–494

Murry T, Carrau R (2006) The abnormal swallow: conditions and diseases. In: Clinical Management of Swallowing Disorders, 2nd edn. Plural Publishing, San Diego, CA, pp 17–32

Muz J, Hamlet S, Mathog R et al (1994) Scintigraphic assessment of aspiration in head and neck cancer patients with tracheostomy. Head Neck 16:17–20

Nagamine T (2011) Choking risk among psychiatric inpatients. Neuropsychiatr Dis Treat 7:381–382

Nagano H, Yoshifuko K, Kurono Y (2009) Polymyositis with dysphagia treated with endoscopic balloon dilatation. Auris Nasus Larynx 36(6):705–708

Nakao M, Oshima F, Maeno Y et al (2019) Disruption of the obligatory swallowing sequence in patients with Wallenberg syndrome. Dysphagia 34(5):673–680

Nash M (1988) Swallowing problems in the tracheotomized patient. Otolaryngol Clin N Am 21:701–709

Navach V, Calabrese LS, Zurlo V et al (2011) Functional base of tongue fat injection in a patient with severe postradiation dysphagia. Dysphagia 26:196–199

Newton HB, Newton C, Pearl D et al (1994) Swallowing assessment in primary brain tumor patients with dysphagia. Neurology 44(10):1927–1932

Ney DM, Weiss JM, Kind AJ et al (2009) Senescent swallowing: impact, strategies, and interventions. Nutr Clin Pract 24(3):395–413

Nguyen NP, Frank C, Moltz CC et al (2005) Impact of dysphagia on quality of life after treatment of head-and-neck cancer. Int J Radiat Oncol Biol Phys 61(3):772–778

Nguyen NP, Moltz CC, Frank C et al (2006) Evolution of chronic dysphagia following treatment for head and neck cancer. Oral Oncol 42(4):374–380

Nguyen NP, Moltz CC, Frank C et al (2007) Effectiveness of the cough reflex in patients with aspiration following radiation for head and neck cancer. Lung 185:243–248

Nguyen NP, Frank C, Moltz CC et al (2009) Analysis of factors influencing dysphagia severity following treatment of head and neck cancer. Anticancer Res 29:3299–3304

Nishino T (2013) The swallowing reflex and its significance as an airway defensive reflex. Front Physiol 3:489. https://doi.org/10.3389/fphys.2012.00489

Noordally SO, Sohawon S, De Gieter M et al (2011) A study to determine the correlation between clinical, fiber-optic endoscopic evaluation of swallowing and videofluoroscopic evaluations of swallowing after prolonged intubation. Nutr Clin Pract 26:457–462

Oad MA, Miles A, Lee A et al (2019) Medicine administration in people with Parkinson's disease in New Zealand: an interprofessional, stakeholder-driven online survey. Dysphagia 34(1):119–128

Ogna A, Prigent H, Lejaille M et al (2017) Swallowing and swallowing-breathing interaction as predictors of intubation in Guillain-Barré syndrome. Brain Behav 7(2):e00611. https://doi.org/10.1002/brb3.611

Oh TH, Brumfield KA, Hoskin TL et al (2007) Dysphagia in inflammatory myopathy: clinical characteristics, treatment strategies, and outcome in 62 patients. Mayo Clin Proc 82(4):441–447

Okayama H, Tamura F, Kikutani T et al (2008) Effects of a palatal augmentation prosthesis on lingual function in postoperative patients with oral cancer: coronal section analysis by ultrasonography. Odontology 96:26–31

Oken MM, Creech RH, Tormey DC et al (1982) Toxicity and response criteria of the eastern cooperative oncology group. Am J Clin Oncol 5:649–655

Olthoff A, Carstens PE, Zhang S et al (2016) Evaluation of dysphagia by novel real-time MRI. Neurology 87(20):2132–2138

O'Neil KH, Purdy M, Falk J et al (1999) The dysphagia outcome and severity scale. Dysphagia 14(3):139–145

Ong AM-L, Chua LT-T, Khor CJ-L et al (2018) Diaphragmatic breathing reduces belching and proton pump inhibitor refractory gastroesophageal reflux symptoms. Clin Gastroenterol Hepatol 16(3):407–416

Oommen ER, Kim Y, McCullough G (2011) Stage transition and laryngeal closure in poststroke patients with dysphagia. Dysphagia 26(3):318–323

Ozawa K, Fujimoto Y, Nakashima T (2010) Changes in laryngeal sensation evaluated with a new method before and after radiotherapy. Eur Arch Otorrinolaringol 267:811–816

Palmer MM, Crawley K, Blanc IA (1993) Neonatal Oral-motor assessment scale: a reliability study. J Perinatol 13(1):28–35

Paterson RW, Brown RL, Benjamin L et al (2020) The emerging spectrum of COVID-19 neurology: clinical, radiological and laboratory findings. Brain 143(10):3104–3120

Pattani KM, McDuffie CM, Morgan M et al (2010) Electrical stimulation of post-irradiated head and neck squamous cell carcinoma to improve xerostomia. J La State Med Soc 162:21–25

Patterson JM (2019) Late effects of organ preservation treatment on swallowing and voice; presentation, assessment, and screening. Front Oncol 9:401. https://doi.org/10.3389/fonc.2019.00401

Patterson JM, Hildreth A, McColl E et al (2011) The clinical application of the 100mL water swallow test in head and neck cancer. Oral Oncol 47:180–184

Pauloski BR, Rademaker AW, Logemann JA et al (2004) Surgical variables affecting swallowing in patients treated for oral/oropharyngeal cancer. Head Neck 26:625–636

Pauloski BR, Rademaker AW, Lazarus C et al (2009) Relationship between manometric and videofluoroscopic measures of swallow function in healthy adults and patients treated for head and neck cancer with various modalities. Dysphagia 24:196–203

Payakachat N, Ounpraseuth S, Suen JY (2013) Late complications and long-term quality of life for survivors (>5 years) with history of head and neck cancer. Head Neck 35:819–825

Perren A, Zürcher P, Schefold JC (2019) Clinical approaches to assess post extubation dysphagia (PED) in the critically ill. Dysphagia 34(4):475–486

Pflug C, Bihler M, Emich K et al (2018) Critical dysphagia is common in Parkinson disease and occurs even in early stages: a prospective cohort study. Dysphagia 33(1):41–50

Pigno MA, Funk JJ (2003) Prosthetic management of a total glossectomy defect after free flap reconstruction in an edentulous patient: a clinical report. J Prosthet Dent 89:119–122

Pikus L, Levine MS, Yang Y-X et al (2003) Videofluoroscopic studies of swallowing dysfunction and the relative risk of pneumonia. Am J Roentgenol 180:1613–1616

Ponfick M, Linden R, Nowak DA (2015) Dysphagia—a common, transient symptom in critical illness polyneuropathy: a fiberoptic endoscopic evaluation of swallowing study. Crit Care Med 43(2):365–372

Power ML, Hamdy S, Singh S et al (2007) Deglutitive laryngeal closure in stroke patients. J Neurol Neurosurg Psychiatry 78(2):141–146

Prasse JE, Kikano GE (2004) An overview of dysphagia in the elderly. Adv Stud Med 4:527–533

Prescott HC, Langa KM, Iwashyna TJ (2015) Readmission diagnoses after severe sepsis and other acute medical conditions. JAMA 313:1055–1057

Prosiegel M (2017) Neurology of swallowing and dysphagia. In: Ekberg O (ed) Dysphagia, diagnosis and treatment, 2nd edn. Springer, Cham, pp 95–121

Prosiegel M (2018a) Neuroanatomie des Schluckens (neuroanatomy of swallowing). In: Bartolome G, Schröter-Morasch H (eds) Schluckstörungen—Diagnostik und Rehabilitation (Swallowing disorders—diagnostics and rehabilitation), 6th edn. Elsevier, Urban & Fischer, Munich

Prosiegel M (2018b) Mit Schluckstörungen assoziierte neurologische Erkrankungen (Neurological disorders associated with dysphagia). In: Bartolome G, Schröter-Morasch H (eds) Schluckstörungen—Diagnostik und rehabilitation (swallowing disorders—diagnostics and rehabilitation), 6th edn. Elsevier, Urban & Fischer, Munich

Prosiegel M, Holing R, Heintze M et al (2005) Swallowing therapy—a prospective study on patients with neurogenic dysphagia due to unilateral paresis of the vagal nerve, Avellis' syndrome, Wallenberg's syndrome, posterior fossa tumours and cerebellar hemorrhage. Acta Neurochir Suppl 93:35–37

Pyun JE, Choi DM, Lee JH et al (2015) Achalasia previously diagnosed as gastroesophageal reflux disease by relying on esophageal impedance-pH monitoring: use of high-resolution esophageal manometry in children. Pediatr Gastroenterol Hepatol Nutr 18(1):55–59

Qureshi MA, Vice FL, Taciak VL et al (2002) Changes in rhythmic suckle feeding patterns in term infants in the first month of life. Dev Med Child Neurol 44(1):34–39

Rasquin A, Di Lorenzo C, Forbes D et al (2006) Childhood functional gastrointestinal disorders. Gastroenterology 130(5):1527–1537

Rassameehiran S, Klomjit S, Mankongpaisarnrung C et al (2015) Postextubation dysphagia. Proc (Bayl Univ Med Cent) 28(1):18–20

Ravich WJ, Wilson RS, Jones B et al (1989) Psychogenic dysphagia and globus: reevaluation of 23 patients. Dysphagia 4(1):35–38

Reed MD, English M, English C et al (2019) The role of the cerebellum in control of swallow: evidence of inspiratory activity during swallow. Lung 197(2):235–240

Regan J, Sowman R, Walsh I (2006) Prevalence of dysphagia in acute and community mental health settings. Dysphagia 21(2):95–101

Reilly S, Skuse D (1999) Schedule for Oral motor assessment (SOMA). Wiley, Hoboken, NJ

Restivo DA, Marchese-Ragona R, Patti F (2006) Management of swallowing disorders in multiple sclerosis. Neurol Sci 4(Suppl 4):338–340

Rison RA, Beydoun SR (2011) Delayed cervicobulbar neuronopathy and myokymia after head and neck radiotherapy for nasopharyngeal carcinoma: a case report. J Clin Neuromuscul Dis 12:147–152

Riva A, D'Onofrio G, Ferlazzo E, Pascarella A, Pasini E, Franceschetti S, Panzica F, Canafoglia L, Vignoli A, Coppola A, Badioni V, Beccaria F, Labate A, Gambardella A, Romeo A, Capovilla G, Michelucci R, Striano P, Belcastro V (2024) Myoclonus: Differential diagnosis and current management. Epilepsia Open 9(2):486–500

Rødningen OK, Børresen-Dale A-L, Alsner J et al (2008) Radiation-induced gene expression in human subcutaneous fibroblasts is predictive of radiation-induced fibrosis. Radiother Oncol 86:314–320

Rodrigues B, Nobrega AC, Sampaio M et al (2011) Silent saliva aspiration in Parkinsons disease. Mov Disord 26(1):138–141

Rogers B, Arvedson J, Bukc G et al (1994) Characteristics of dysphagia in children with cerebral palsy. Dysphagia 9(1):69–73

Rommel N, van Wijk M, Boets B et al (2011) Development of pharyngo-esophageal physiology during swallowing in the preterm infant. Neurogastroenterol Motil 23(10):e401–e408

Rosenbek JC, Jones HN (2009) Dysphagia in movement disorders. Plural Publishing, San Diego, CA

Rosenbek JC, Robbins JA, Roecker EB et al (1996) A penetration-aspiration scale. Dysphagia 11:93–98

Rosenthal LH, Benninger MS, Deep RH (2007) Vocal fold immobility: a longitudinal analysis of etiology over 20 years. Laryngoscope 117(10):1864–1870

Roy N, Stemple J, Merrill RM et al (2007) Dysphagia in the elderly: preliminary evidence of prevalence, risk factors, and socioemotional effects. Ann Otol Rhinol Laryngol 116(11):858–865

Russi EG, Corvò R, Merlotti A et al (2012) Swallowing dysfunction in head and neck cancer patients treated by radiotherapy: review and recommendations of the supportive task group of the Italian Association of Radiation Oncology. Cancer Treat Rev 38:1033–1049

Sanguineti G, Gunn GB, Parker BC et al (2011) Weekly dose-volume parameters of mucosa and constrictor muscles predict the use of percutaneous endoscopic gastrostomy during exclusive intensity-modulated radiotherapy for oropharyngeal cancer. Int J Radiat Oncol Biol Phys 79:52–59

Sawada A, Fujiwara Y, Sifrim D (2020) Belching in gastroesophageal reflux disease: literature review. J Clin Med 9(10):3360. https://doi.org/10.3390/jcm9103360

Schaefer OP, Irwin RS (1995) Tracheoarterial fistula: an unusual complication of tracheostomy. J Intensive Care Med 10(2):64–75

Scheel R, Pisegna JM, McNally E et al (2016) Endoscopic assessment of swallowing after prolonged intubation in the ICU setting. Ann Otol Rhinol Laryngol 125:43–52

Schefold JC, Berger D, Zürcher P et al (2017) Dysphagia in mechanically ventilated ICU patients (DYnAMICS): a prospective observational trial. Crit Care Med 45:2061–2069

Schepp SK, Tirschwell DL, Miller RM et al (2012) Swallowing screens after acute stroke. Stroke 43:869–871

Schröter-Morasch H (2005) Schluckstörungen (Swallowing disorders). In: Wendler J, Seidner W et al (eds) Lehrbuch der Phoniatrie und Pädaudiologie (textbook of Phoniatrics and pediatric audiology), 4th edn. Thieme, Stuttgart

Schröter-Morasch H, Hoole P (1998) Differenzialdiagnose hyperkinetischer Bewegungsstörungen des Kehlkopfs (differential diagnosis of hyperkinetic movement disorders of the larynx). In: Gross M (ed) Aktuelle phoniatrisch-pädaudiologische Aspekte 1997/1998 (current phoniatric-paediatric aspects 1997/1998). Median, Heidelberg

Schröter-Morasch H, Winkler R, Lumenta R (1995) Dysphagia after posterior fossa tumor surgery. Abstracts of scientific papers presented at the third annual dysphagia research society meeting McLean, Virginia, October 14–16, 1994. Dysphagia 10:135–141

Schröter-Morasch H, Liebmann E, Feussner H (2018) Klinische und pathophysiologische Aspekte der Dysphagie bei Myositis und ihre therapeutische Relevanz. 4. Dreiländertagung D-A-CH, 35. Wissenschaftliche Jahrestagung der DGPP (Clinical and pathophysiological aspects of dysphagia in myositis and their therapeutic relevance. 4th Three-Country Meeting D-A-CH, 35th Annual Scientific Meeting of the DGPP). Innsbruck, Austria, 20.-23.09.2018. German Medical Science GMS Publishing House, Duesseldorf, DocV20

Schwartz DL, Hutcheson K, Barringer D et al (2010) Candidate dosimetric predictors of long-term swallowing dysfunction after oropharyngeal intensity-modulated radiotherapy. Int J Radiat Oncol Biol Phys 78:1356–1365

Schwemmle C, Jungheim M, Miller S et al (2015) Medikamenteninduzierte Dysphagien—ein Überblick (Drug-induced dysphagia—an overview). HNO 63(7):504–510

Seo HG, Kim JG, Nam HS et al (2017) Swallowing function and kinematics in stroke patients with tracheostomies. Dysphagia 32(3):393–400

Servagi-Vernat S, Ali D, Roubieu C et al (2014) Dysphagia after radiotherapy: state of the art and prevention. Eur Ann Otorhinolaryngol Head Neck Dis S1879-7296(14):00070–00072

Shama L, Connor NP, Ciucci MR et al (2008) Surgical treatment of dysphagia. Phys Med Rehabil Clin N Am 19:817–835

Sharma D, Shastri S, Sharma P (2016) Intrauterine growth restriction: antenatal and postnatal aspects. Clin Med Insights Pediatr 10:67–83

Sharp WG, Jaques DL, Morton JF et al (2010) Pediatric feeding disorders: a quantitative synthesis of treatment outcomes. Clin Child Fam Psychol 13(4):348–365

Sharp WG, Volkert V, Scahill L et al (2017) A systematic review and meta-analysis of intensive multidisciplinary intervention for pediatric feeding disorders: how standard is the standard of care? J Pediatr 181:116–124

Shune SE, Karnell LH, Karnell MP et al (2012) Association between severity of dysphagia and survival in patients with head and neck cancer. Head Neck 34:776–784

Siebens H, Trupe E, Siebens A et al (1986) Correlates and consequences of eating dependency in institutionalized elderly. J Am Geriatr Soc 34(3):192–198

Silva RA, Mesquita N, Nunes PP et al (2012) Tracheobronchial Polyflex stents for the management of benign refractory hypopharyngeal strictures. World J Gastroenterol 18:551–556

Simonelli M, Ruoppolo G, de Vincentiis M et al (2010) Swallowing ability and chronic aspiration after supracricoid partial laryngectomy. Otolaryngol Head Neck Surg 142:873–878

Sitton M, Arvedson J, Visotcky A et al (2011) Fiberoptic endoscopic evaluation of swallowing in children: feeding outcomes related to diagnostic groups and endoscopic findings. Int J Pediatr Otorhinolaryngol 75(8):1024–1031

Skoretz SA, Flowers HL, Martino R (2010) The incidence of dysphagia following endotracheal intubation: a systematic review. Chest 137:665–673

Skoretz SA, Yau TM, Ivanov J et al (2014) Dysphagia and associated risk factors following extubation in cardiovascular surgical patients. Dysphagia 29(6):647–654

Smith JE, Suh JD, Erman A et al (2008) Risk factors predicting aspiration after free flap reconstruction of oral cavity and oropharyngeal defects. Arch Otolaryngol Head Neck Surg 134:1205–1208

Smithard DG (2013) Neuromuscular disease and extubation dysphagia. Crit Care 17(5):194. https://doi.org/10.1186/cc12762

Soderholm S, Lehtinen A, Valtonen K et al (2010) Dysphagia and dysphonia among persons with postpolio syndrome—a challenge in neurorehabilitation. Acta Neurol Scand 122(5):343–349

Sonies BC, Shawker TH, Hall TE et al (1981) Ultrasonic visualization of tongue motion during speech. J Acoust Soc Am 70(3):683–686

Speyer R, Baijens L, Heijnen M et al (2009) Effects of therapy in oropharyngeal dysphagia by speech and language therapists: a systematic review. Ysphagia 25:40–65

Speyer R, Cordier R, Sutt AL et al (2022) Behavioural interventions in people with oropharyngeal dysphagia: a systematic review and meta-analysis of randomised clinical trials. J Clin Med 11(3):685. https://doi.org/10.3390/jcm11030685

Squires N, Humberstone M, Wills A et al (2014) The use of botulinum toxin injections to manage drooling in amyotrophic lateral sclerosis/motor neurone disease: a systematic review. Dysphagia 29(4):500–508

Staiano A, Boccia G, Miele E et al (2008) Segmental characteristics of oesophageal peristalsis in paediatric patients. Neurogastroenterol Motil 20(1):19–26

Stein A, Woolley H, Murray L et al (2001) Influence of psychiatric disorder on the controlling behavior of mothers with 1-year-old infants. A study of women with maternal eating disorder, postnatal depression and a healthy comparison group. Br J Psychiatry 179(2):157–162

Steinberg C (2007) Feeding disorders of infants, toddlers, and preschoolers. BCMJ 49(4):129–136

Streiner DL (2003) Diagnosing tests: using and misusing diagnostic and screening tests. J Pers Assess 81:209–219

Suarez C, Rodrigo JP, Herranz J et al (1996) Complications of supraglottic laryngectomy for carcinomas of the supraglottis and the base of the tongue. Clin Otolaryngol Allied Sci 21:87–90

Suntrup S, Warnecke T, Kemmling A et al (2012) Dysphagia in patients with acute striatocapsular hemorrhage. J Neurol 259(1):93–99

Suntrup S, Marian T, Schröder JB et al (2015) Electrical pharyngeal stimulation for dysphagia treatment in tracheotomized stroke patients: a randomized controlled trial. Intensive Care Med 41:1629–1637

Suntrup-Krueger S, Ringmaier C, Muhle P et al (2018) Randomized trial of transcranial direct current stimulation for poststroke dysphagia. Ann Neurol 83(2):328–340

Sura L, Madhavan A, Carnaby G et al (2012) Dysphagia in the elderly: management and nutritional considerations. Clin Interv Aging 7:287–298

Suttrup I, Warnecke T (2016) Dysphagia in Parkinson's disease. Dysphagia 31(1):24–32

Takizawa C, Gemmell E, Kenworthy J et al (2016) A systematic review of the prevalence of oropharyngeal dysphagia in stroke, Parkinson's disease, Alzheimer's disease, head injury, and pneumonia. Dysphagia 31(3):434–441

Tanaka A, Isono S, Ishikawa T et al (2003) Laryngeal resistance before and after minor surgery: endotracheal tube versus laryngeal mask airway. Anesthesiology 99:252–258

Tauber M, Boulanouar K, Diène G et al (2017) The use of oxytocin to improve feeding and social skills in infants with Prader-Willi syndrome. Pediatrics 139(2):e20162976. https://doi.org/10.1542/peds.2016-2976

Taveira KVM, Santos RS, de la Leão BLC et al (2018) Diagnostic validity of methods for assessment of swallowing sounds: a systematic review. Braz J Otorhinolaryngol 84:638–652

Teguh DN, Levendag PC, Ghidey W et al (2013) Risk model and nomogram for dysphagia and xerostomia prediction in head and neck cancer patients treated by radiotherapy and/or chemotherapy. Dysphagia 8:388–394

Tei K, Sakakibara N, Yamazaki Y et al (2012) Does swallowing function recover in the long term in patients with surgically treated tongue carcinomas? J Oral Maxillofac Surg 70:2680–2686

Teismann IK, Steinstraeter O, Stoeckigt K et al (2007) Functional oropharyngeal sensory disruption interferes with the cortical control of swallowing. BMC Neurosci 8:62. https://doi.org/10.1186/1471-2202-8-62

ten Cate L (2022) Supragastric belching: speech therapy intervention reduces excessive belching symptoms. In: Manfredi C (ed) Proceedings e-report of the 12th international workshop models and analysis of vocal emissions for biomedical applications. Firenze University Press, Florence. https://doi.org/10.36253/978-88-5518-449-6

ten Cate L, Herregods TVK, Dejonckere PH et al (2018) Speech therapy as treatment for supragastric belching. Dysphagia 33(5):707–715

Thakkar P, Greenwald BD, Patel P (2020) Rehabilitation of adult patients with primary brain tumors: a narrative review. Brain Sci 29;10(8):492

Thouvenin B, Djadi-Prat J, Chalouhi C et al (2013) Developmental outcome in Pierre Robin sequence: a longitudinal and prospective study of a consecutive series of severe phenotypes. Am J Med Genet A 161A(2):312–319

Timmerman AA, Speyer R, Heijnen BJ et al (2014) Psychometric characteristics of health-related quality-of-life questionnaires in oropharyngeal dysphagia. Dysphagia 29(2):183–198

Tong JY, Pasick LJ, Benito DA et al (2020) Complications associated with tracheoesophageal voice prostheses from 2010 to 2020: a MAUDE study. Am J Otolaryngol 41(6):102652. https://doi.org/10.1016/j.amjoto.2020.102652

Topaloglu I, Köprücü G, Bal M (2012) Analysis of swallowing function after supracricoid laryngectom with cricohyoidopexy. Otolaryngol Head Neck Surg 146:412–418

Tsai MH, Ku SC, Wang TG et al (2016) Swallowing dysfunction following endotracheal intubation: age matters. Medicine (Baltimore) 95:e3871. https://doi.org/10.1097/MD.0000000000003871

Turra GS, Schwartz IVD, de Almeida ST et al (2021) Efficacy of speech therapy in post-intubation patients with oropharyngeal dysphagia: a randomized controlled trial. Codas 33:e20190246. https://doi.org/10.1590/2317-1782/20202019246

Tutor D, Gosa MM (2012) Dysphagia and aspiration in children. Pediatr Pulmonol 47(4):321–337

Vaideeswar P, Ghodke R (2012) Upper aerodigestive tract cancer and the lung: a tale of two aspirations. J Postgrad Med 58:290–293

van de Loo S, Somasundaram S, Wagner M et al (2010) Dysphagia in symptomatic palatal tremor. Mov Disord 25(9):1304–1305

van der Molen L, Heemsbergen WD, de Jong R et al (2013) Dysphagia and trismus after concomitant chemo-intensity-modulated radiation therapy (chemo-IMRT) in advanced head and neck cancer; dose-effect relationships for swallowing and mastication structures. Radiother Oncol 106:364–369

Vartanian JG, Rogers S, Kowalski LP (2017) How to evaluate and assess quality of life issues in head and neck cancer patients. Curr Opin Oncol 29:159–165

Verdonck-de Leeuw IM, Eerenstein SE, Van der Linden MH et al (2007) Distress in spouses and patients after treatment for head and neck cancer. Laryngoscope 117:238–241

Verdonschot RJCG, Baijens LWJ, Vanbelle S et al (2019) Medically unexplained oropharyngeal dysphagia at the university hospital ENT outpatient clinic for dysphagia: a cross-sectional cohort study. Dysphagia 34(1):43–51

Vogel J, Stübinger S, Kaufmann M et al (2009) Dental injuries resulting from tracheal intubation—a retrospective study. Dent Traumatol 25:73–77

Volkert D, Chourdakis M, Faxen-Irving G et al (2015) ESPEN guidelines on nutrition in dementia. Clin Nutr 34(6):1052–1073

Wadhwa R, Toms J, Chittiboina P, Tawfik T, Glenn C, Caldito G, Guthikonda B, Nanda A (2014) Dysphagia following posterior fossa surgery in adults. World Neurosurg 82(5):822–7

Wallace KL, Middleton S, Cook IJ (2000) Development and validation of a self-report symptom inventory to assess the severity of oral-pharyngeal dysphagia. Gastroenterology 118(4):678–687

Wan P, Chen X, Zhu L et al (2016) Dysphagia post subcortical and supratentorial stroke. J Stroke Cerebrovasc Dis 25(1):74–82

Wang JJ, Goldsmith TA, Holman AS et al (2012) Pharyngoesophageal stricture after treatment for head and neck cancer. Head Neck 34:967–973

Warnecke T, Dziewas R (2018) Neurogene Dysphagien, Diagnostik und Therapie (neurogenic dysphagia, diagnosis and therapy), 2nd edn. Kohlhammer, Stuttgart

Warnecke T, Teismann I, Zimmermann J et al (2008) Fiberoptic endoscopic evaluation of swallowing with simultaneous Tensilon application in diagnosis and therapy of myasthenia gravis. J Neurol 255(2):224–230

Warnecke Tobias, Rainer Dziewas, Susan Langmore (2021) Neurogenic Dysphagia. Springer International Publishing, New York NYC

Weber C, Dommerich S, Pau HW et al (2010) Limited mouth opening after primary therapy of head and neck cancer. Oral Maxillofac Surg 14:169–173

Wesling M, Brady S, Jensen M et al (2003) Dysphagia outcomes in patients with brain tumors undergoing inpatient rehabilitation. Dysphagia 18(3):203–210

White R, Cotton SM, Hind J et al (2009) A comparison of the reliability and stability of oro-lingual swallowing pressures in patients with head and neck cancer and healthy adults. Dysphagia 24:137–144

WHO (2021) Mental health. World Health Organization, Geneva. http://www.who.int/mental_health/en/. Accessed 5 July 2021

Wilkins T, Gillies RA, Thomas AM et al (2007) The prevalence of dysphagia in primary care patients: a HamesNet research network study. J Am Board Fam Med 20(2):144–150

Willging JP (1995) Endoscopic evaluation of swallowing in children. Int J Pediatr Otorhinolaryngol 32(Suppl):S107–S108

Wirth R (2018) Percutaneous endoscopic gastrostomy in geriatrics. Indications, technique and complications. Z Gerontol Geriat 51:237–245

Wirth R, Streicher M, Smoliner C et al (2016a) The impact of weight loss and low BMI on mortality of nursing home residents—results from the nutrition day in nursing homes. Clin Nutr 35(4):900–906

Wirth R, Dziewas R, Beck AM et al (2016b) Oropharyngeal dysphagia in older persons—from pathophysiology to adequate intervention: a review and summary of an international expert meeting. Clin Interv Aging 11:189–208

Woisard V, Puech M (2010) La rehabilitation de la deglutition chez l'adulte. Le point sur prise en charge fonctionnelle (Rehabilitation of swallowing in adults. Update on functional support), 2nd edn. Solal, Marseille, p 411

Woisard V, Puech M, Yardeni E et al (1996) Deglutition after supracricoid laryngectomy: compensatory mechanisms and sequelae. Dysphagia 11:265–269

Xu B, Boero IJ, Hwang L et al (2015) Aspiration pneumonia after concurrent Chemoradiotherapy for head and neck cancer. Cancer 121:1303–1311

Yoshikawa M, Yoshida M, Nagasaki T et al (2006) Influence of aging and denture use on liquid swallowing in healthy dentulous and edentulous older people. J Am Geriatr Soc 54:444–449

Zald DH, Pardo JV (1999) The functional neuroanatomy of voluntary swallowing. Ann Neurol 46(3):281–286

Zero to Three (2005) Diagnostic classification of mental health and developmental disorders of infancy and early childhood. Revised Edition. Zero to Three Press, Washington, DC

Zigmond AS, Snaith RP (1983) The hospital anxiety and depression scale. Acta Psychiatr Scand 67(6):361–370

Zuercher P, Moret CS, Dziewas R et al (2019) Dysphagia in the intensive care unit: epidemiology, mechanisms, and clinical management. Crit Care 23(1):103. https://doi.org/10.1186/s13054-019-2400-2

Zuydam AC, Lowe D, Brown JS et al (2005) Predictors of speech and swallowing function following primary surgery for oral and oropharyngeal cancer. Clin Otolaryngol 30:428–437

# Diagnosis and Differential Diagnosis of Dysphagia

# 28

Wolfgang Angerstein, Mohamed Farahat,
Daniele Farneti, Simone Graf, Michael Jungheim,
Devora E. Kiagiadaki, Khalid H. Malki,
Mieke Moerman, Frank Müller, Julie C. Nienstedt,
Christina Pflug, Martina Scharitzer,
and Antonio Schindler

Daniele Farneti and Michael Jungheim shared first authorship.

**Supplementary Information** The online version contains supplementary material available at https://doi.org/10.1007/978-3-031-48091-1_13.

W. Angerstein (✉)
Phoniatrie und Päedaudiologie, Universitätsklinikum Düsseldorf, Düsseldorf, Germany
e-mail: wolfgang.angerstein@uni-duesseldorf.de

M. Farahat
Department of Otolaryngology, Communication and Swallowing Disorders Unit, ENT Department, College of Medicine, King Saud University, Riyadh, Saudi Arabia
e-mail: mfarahat@ksu.edu.sa

D. Farneti
Audiology Phoniatric Service, ENT Department, "Infermi" Hospital Rimini, Rimini, Italy
e-mail: daniele.farneti@auslromagna.it

S. Graf
Clinic for Hearing, Speech and Voice Disorders, Innsbruck Medical University, Innsbruck, Austria
e-mail: simone.graf@i-med.ac.at

M. Jungheim
HNO Phoniatrie Bremen, Bremen, Germany
e-mail: info@hno-phoniatrie-bremen.de

D. E. Kiagiadaki
ENT Department, Chania General Hospital, Heraklion-Crete, Greece
e-mail: info@dkiagiadaki.gr

K. H. Malki
Communication and Swallowing Disorders Unit, ENT Department, King Saud University, Riyadh, Saudi Arabia
e-mail: kalmalki@ksu.edu.sa

M. Moerman
Petegem a/d Leie_Deinze, Belgium

F. Müller · J. C. Nienstedt · C. Pflug
Department of Voice, Speech and Hearing Disorders, University Medical Center Hamburg-Eppendorf, Hamburg, Germany
e-mail: f.mueller@uke.de; ju.nienstedt@uke.de; c.pflug@uke.de

M. Scharitzer
Department of Biomedical Imaging and Image-Guided Therapy, Medical University of Vienna, Vienna, Austria
e-mail: martina.scharitzer@meduniwien.ac.at

A. Schindler
Luigi Sacco Hospital, Department of Biomedical and Clinical Sciences "L. Sacco", Phoniatrics, University of Milan, Milan, Italy
e-mail: antonio.schindler@unimi.it

## 28.1 Dysphagia Screening and Clinical Swallowing Evaluation

Simone Graf

### 28.1.1 Introduction

Early identification and detection of dysphagia reduce not only morbidity but also the length of hospitalisation and thus health costs, owing to prompt intervention (Daniels et al. 2012). For example, within 3 days of stroke, 42–67% of patients present symptoms of dysphagia. Fifty percent of these patients aspirate and 33% of those develop an aspiration pneumonia (Perry 2001a, b).

The diagnosis of dysphagia is stepwise. First, dysphagia screening; second, clinical swallowing evaluation (CSE); third, visual dysphagia evaluation, such as videofluoroscopy (videofluoroscopic swallowing study, VFSS) and the Flexible Endoscopic Evaluation of Swallowing (FEES), are performed. Through VFSS and FEES, one is able to determine the specific swallowing impairment and therapeutic achievements of compensation mechanisms (Audag et al. 2019).

### 28.1.2 Dysphagia Screening

> Swallowing screening is a pass/fail procedure to identify individuals who require a comprehensive assessment of swallowing function or a referral for other professional and/or medical services (Donovan et al. 2013).

This screening is the first step in identifying the risk of dysphagia, aspiration and those patients who do not need a formal evaluation and who can safely take food and medications by mouth (Schepp et al. 2012). The advantages of the dysphagia screening for aspiration are that it is quick, cheap, minimally invasive and can be performed by educated personnel, not exclusively speech and language pathologists. It supports the decision-making of taking immediate measures such as diet, additional diagnostics and

therapy. The disadvantage is the lack of information concerning the cause of malfunction (Logemann et al. 1999; Audag et al. 2019).

What do we require from a good screening tool? We need a profound certainty of administration and interpretation of findings with good inter-rater and intra-rater reliability. Feasibility, standardisation, and validity of the screening test have to be guaranteed. Most studies use water, which makes the test easy to administer and to compare. A high test sensitivity is needed to provide definitely proof of aspiration in patients with possible swallowing impairment. A high specificity guarantees the exclusion of swallowing impairment if the screening test is negative.

To be a valid and reliable diagnostic tool, a sensitivity of >80–90% and a specificity of at least >50% are required (Bours et al. 2009; Doggett et al. 2002). Owing to the high percentage of silent aspiration (without coughing), estimated at 50% in dysphagia, the conceptual design of a valid clinical test is especially challenging (Garon et al. 2009). Because of the increased morbidity and mortality associated with definite aspiration, many swallowing screenings focus on a high test sensitivity (Odderson et al. 1995; Hinchey et al. 2005; Lakshminarayan et al. 2010).

A low specificity, giving false positive results, may lead to uncalled prolonged hospital stays, unnecessary withholding of oral feeding, or even the positioning of feeding tubes (Donovan et al. 2013). Furthermore, nasogastric feeding tubes are associated with an increase in medical complications in patients with acute stroke—stressing the need for viable tests (Nascimento et al. 2018).

This matter has been reviewed systematically (Bours et al. 2009; Daniels et al. 2012; O'Horo et al. 2015; Brodsky et al. 2016). Currently, no single screening test has proved superior to others and achieved consensus as a standard screening tool (Daniels et al. 2012). The absence of a broad agreement on the best screening instrument, however, does not mean that a clinical screening should not be performed, since the alternative of an instrumental swallowing diagnostic test is not available everywhere and at short notice (Donovan et al. 2013).

Broadly one differentiates between swallowing tests with water, with different food consistencies and tests for cannulated patients. Contraindications for dysphagia screening include severe impairment of consciousness and obvious signs of aspiration or pulmonary impairment.

### 28.1.3 Frequently Used Tests

In the following passage, frequently used clinical tests with relatively high test sensitivity and specificity are exemplarily described:

#### 28.1.3.1 Three-Ounce Water-Swallow Test

De Pippo et al. published the following screening test in 1992. In this protocol, patients suspected of aspiration are asked to drink 3 oz (90 cc) of water in one draw without interruption. The inability to complete that task without coughing and choking or a wet hoarse vocal quality—either during or within 1 min of the test—are the clinical criteria for referral to further assessments (DePippo et al. 1992). In 2008, Suiter and Leder validated this score by FEES in a large and heterogeneous population of 3000 patients (Suiter and Leder 2008). Leder et al. showed in 2011 that 58% of patients aspirating small bolus volumes silently coughed and choked with bigger boluses of 90 cc. Thus, it can be reasoned that patients showing no symptoms during and after the 3-oz Water-Swallowing Test will most probably not have an aspiration (Leder et al. 2011). Chen et al. (2016) also came to the same conclusion. In a systematic review, they compared different water tests with volumes of 3–90 mL. The 90 mL water 3-oz water-swallow test achieved the best sensitivity of 97%, but a low specificity of 49%, leading to false positive results causing the problems as described above.

#### 28.1.3.2 Gugging Swallowing Screen (GUSS)

Acute stroke patients are known to show a higher impairment of swallowing liquids than semisolid textures. Thus, the GUSS is a stepwise approach to minimise the risk of aspiration during the test and allowing a graded rating with distinct evalu-

ation of fluid and non-fluid food, starting with non-fluid textures. This test was validated by therapists and nursing staff on 50 stroke patients. A sensitivity of 100% and specificity of 50% were achieved (Trapl et al. 2007). A re-examination of 100 acute stroke patients showed similar results (Warnecke et al. 2017). The problem of the test is the high rate of false positive results. This means that almost all patients with aspiration risk are detected, but not all detected patients really have a swallowing disorder.

As for all other screening tests, this one is performed in an upright sitting position. The GUSS is divided in two parts. Part 1 is a preliminary assessment with an indirect swallowing test: successful saliva swallowing is observed and is the precondition for the second part of the test. In the first part, vigilance, voluntary cough, and throat clearing are also assessed. Part 2 is the direct swallowing test, consisting of three sequentially performed subtests with material of different consistencies. This sequence is started with semi-solids, then liquids, and finally solids. An advantage of the GUSS is the possibility of grading the findings with a scale of 20 reachable points, classifying 4 severity codes (Trapl et al. 2007).

#### 28.1.3.3 Modified Evans Blue Dye Test (MEBDT)

This test is a dysphagia screening test for patients with tracheotomy cannula (Brady et al. 1999). Food and fluid swallow probes are tainted with blue dye or the saliva is coloured. After distinct time intervals (5, 10, 20, 30 min), secretion is aspirated through the tracheotomy cannula. If the secretion is blue, it can be taken as a sign of aspiration.

A review article by Béchet et al. in (2016) showed that sensitivity estimates varied widely across the studies (38–95%), indicating that the MEBDT is unreliable in detecting oropharyngeal aspiration, but the studies emerge with overall high specificity values, ranging from 79% to 100%.

#### 28.1.3.4 Tests for Patients with Head and Neck Cancer

Aspiration tests for dysphagia in patients with head and neck cancers can be scored with the Frankfurt Dysphagia Screening Score (FraDySc) (Hey et al.

2013), the 3-oz water-swallow test (DePippo et al. 1992) or the Mann Assessment of Swallowing Ability-Cancer (MASA-C) (Carnaby and Crary 2014). Details are described in Sect. 27.5.

## 28.2 Functional Swallowing Examination with Flexible Endoscopes

Antonio Schindler, Julie C. Nienstedt, and Christina Pflug

### 28.2.1 Introduction

The endoscopic examination of the upper air digestive tract has a long history. Fibre-optic laryngoscopy was introduced in 1963 (Sawashima and Hirose 1963) and extended the laryngological diagnostics sustainably. It became commercially available in 1973 (Davies 1973) and now is used in everyday clinical practice to assess anatomical structures (Schindler et al. 2005). The spread of endoscopy to the upper aerodigestive tract during swallowing occurred later. In 1988, Susan E. Langmore established the fiber-optic endoscopic evaluation of swallowing (FEES), setting a milestone in dysphagia diagnostics (Langmore et al. 1988). Various acronyms currently exist, but it is most commonly referred to as FEES (flexible- or, according to original fiberoptics, fiberoptic-endoscopic evaluation of swallowing) (Pisegna and Murray 2018). The diagnosis of dysphagia up to this time was reserved for radiological techniques, especially videofluoroscopy, which is widely used in the USA. Studies have shown that the sensitivity of FEES is at least as sensitive as videofluoroscopy, or even superior to it (Colodny 2002). Today, the radiological swallowing diagnosis is therefore useful for individual questions (diverticula, cervical spine diseases, quantification of the aspirate) (Langmore 2003).

Flexible endoscopy of the upper aerodigestive tract has a key role in dysphagia diagnostics and is under constant evolution (Langmore 2017). Since the clinical picture of dysphagia may be multidimensional, the endoscopy requires differential diagnostic considerations by the examiner. A differentiated knowledge of the anatomical structures and their physiological function is a prerequisite, and thus the endoscopy of swallowing is the speciality of phoniatricians and otorhinolaryngologists. Complications—such as epistaxis (0.3–1.2%), syncope (0–0.03%), laryngospasm (0–0.03%), allergic reactions to anaesthetics (0.02%)—are rare, but the examiner should be able to manage them (Nacci et al. 2022; Langmore 2017).

### 28.2.2 FEES Protocol

FEES is not a screening exam merely to identify aspiration. The objective of FEES is to examine swallowing thoroughly to determine if there is a disorder, and the FEES report should clearly describe anatomical or physiological impairment of the pharynx and larynx (Langmore 2000). It has not undergone validity testing, so it remains a guideline. The FEES protocol includes three parts to the exam:

- Part 1: Assessment of anatomy, secretion management, physiology and movement, sensitivity of swallowing structures.
- Part 2: Direct evaluation of swallowing different bolus volumes and consistencies.
- Part 3: Interventional part—trial of postural, dietary, and behavioural changes as problems occur.

### 28.2.3 Innovations and Technical Advances

Numerous modifications have been described since the first publication of the FEES protocol. While some examinations need to be done completely and in a consistent order, this is not always necessary. Other publications have described different FEES protocols and scoring systems for particular patient populations (Warnecke et al. 2009a, 2010, 2014; Baijens et al. 2014).

Several new methods and technical advances have improved the diagnostic validity of endoscopy and swallowing evaluation (Rosen et al. 2009). To enhance the visibility of the test bolus, staining with food dye has become established. Some video-rhinolaryngoscopes have an integrated narrow band imaging (NBI) filter that can be switched on at the push of a button. NBI is an innovative endoscopic procedure that has been used for the detection of mucosal lesions and carcinomas in the head and neck since 2004 (Muto et al. 2004; Arens et al. 2016; Piazza et al. 2008). In FEES, NBI causes a green test bolus to stand out more strongly from the surrounding mucosa (Nienstedt et al. 2017; Niessen et al. 2023). This greatly improves the contrast and the detection of laryngeal penetration and aspiration (Fig. 28.1).

Modern "chip-on-the-tip" endoscopes in high-definition (HD) quality have replaced conventional fibre endoscopes in the ENT area. Therefore, it is contemporary to use the term "flexible endoscopy" instead of "fibre-optic", which is how it will be used here. The technical advances increase the image quality and facilitate the visualisation of laryngeal anatomy and swallowing (Rosen et al. 2009). In addition, small LED lightsources improve the illumination of the laryngopharynx. Even very thin rhinolaryngoscopes today have an excellent image quality, which allows transnasal endoscopy of infants or transnasal oesophagoscopy. Video documentation has increased the reliability of FEES by retrospective viewing in slow motion or "frame-by-frame" (Hey et al. 2015). All these improvements have made FEES the gold standard for dysphagia diagnostics in most European countries (Langmore 2017; Colodny 2002; Deutschmann et al. 2013).

### 28.2.4 Procedure for FEES

Before starting FEES, patients should be informed about the meaning and structure of the examination and properly positioned. First, the oral cavity, soft palate, and pharyngeal wall should be examined and assessed for structure, function, sensitivity, and reflexes. Oropharyngeal pathologies may not only have a direct impact on oral preparation and transport but may also indicate a deeper, pharyngeal disorder. Before transnasal endoscopy, nasal decongestants and local anaesthesia of the nasal mucosa should be administered. This increases the tolerance of the patient and promotes the examination situation without affecting the swallow at an economical dosage of the anaesthetic (0.2–0.5 mL 4% lidocaine) (Fife et al. 2015; O'Dea et al. 2015).

#### 28.2.4.1 Assessment of Anatomy, Secretion Management, Physiology and Movement, and Sensitivity

All swallowing structures, including the nasopharynx, oropharynx with velum, tongue base and valleculae, hypopharynx with pyriform sinuses and postcricoid region, larynx and upper part of the trachea should be fully observed at rest

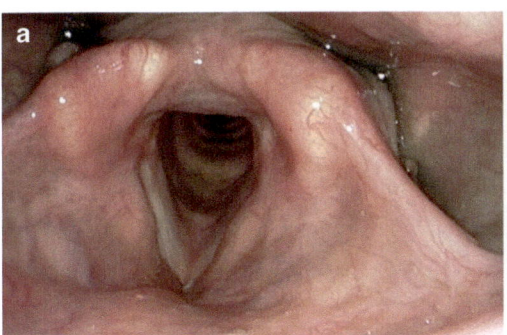 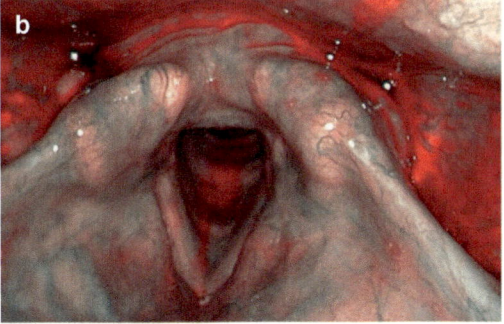

**Fig. 28.1** Examples for the enhanced visibility of aspiration of green water using NBI: (**a**) white light; (**b**) NBI-filter. (©C. Pflug 2022)

and in motion for pathologies of anatomy and physiology. The presence of secretions, their characteristics (serous, mucus), localisation (oro-/hypopharynx, larynx), and spontaneous or induced management are also of importance. Increased accumulations of saliva (salivary retention) may already indicate inadequate swallowing or laryngeal sensory disturbances. The assessment of the movement of the swallowing structures provides information about the neuro-motor functionality of the system. It includes specific manoeuvres that are rated by asking the patient to perform non-swallowing, breath-holding, and speaking tasks. After passing the nasal vestibule with the endoscope, velopharyn-geal closure can be inspected during an empty swallow or plosive phonation [kukuk].

Weakness of the soft palate occurs, for example, in cleft palate, tumours, and after operations, but also in many neurological diseases and paralyses. Diagnostically indicative for this is a tissue deficit or nasal penetration of saliva or food.

A view of the larynx at the empty swallow gives an impression of epiglottal retroflexion and laryngeal elevation, which is important for the opening of the upper oesophageal sphincter. The "pharyngeal squeeze manoeuvre", in which the patient has to phonate a high, strained [iii:], tests the pharyngeal constriction (Rodriguez et al. 2007) (Fig. 28.2).

Sufficient larynx closure is essential for aspiration protection by sealing the glottis and a strong cough for sufficient laryngeal clearing. The "Hi-Sniff manoeuvre"—a rapid change of [hi] and nasal inspiration—is suitable for assessing the mobility, the tone, and the closure of the vocal folds. Another method to check glottal occlusion is a slight breath-hold. The supraglottal closure can be tested by pressing.

Another important part of the endoscopic evaluation of swallowing is sensitivity testing of the laryngopharynx. This can be done with a light touch or tap of the laryngo-pharyngeal tissue with the tip of the endoscope, which normally causes the laryngeal adductor reflex. If available, sensory testing can also be performed with an air-puff generator, known as FEES with sensory testing (FEESST) (Aviv et al. 1998).

### 28.2.4.2 Direct Evaluation of Swallowing; Different Bolus Volumes and Consistencies

For the assessment of bolus transit, the endoscope may be positioned just below the velum (high position) for a general view of the pharynx and larynx or close to the laryngeal vestibule (low position) to detect laryngeal penetration or aspiration. If possible, different bolus consistencies with increasing volumes (liquids, puree, solid) and pills should be used. Depending on the question arising from the anamnesis and previous endoscopic findings, it is advisable to tailor the examination procedure and the selection of test consistencies individually to the patient without

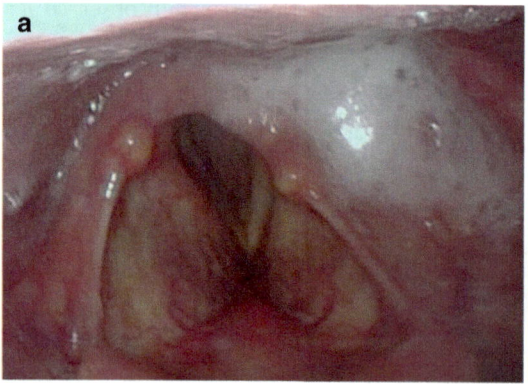
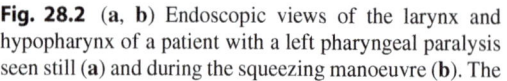
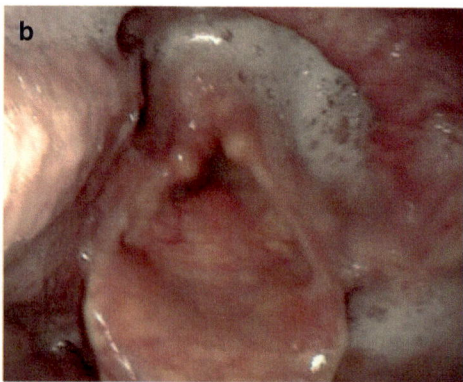

**Fig. 28.2** (**a**, **b**) Endoscopic views of the larynx and hypopharynx of a patient with a left pharyngeal paralysis seen still (**a**) and during the squeezing manoeuvre (**b**). The absence of left pharyngeal wall contraction is clearly visible. (©C. Pflug 2022)

following strict procedures. The patient can bring his own food of various consistencies (carrot juice, vegetable puree [lower in acid than fruit puree], biscuits, etc.). Alternatively, dyed water can be easily and quickly adjusted to the desired consistency by using commercially available thickening agents (e.g. Thick & Easy™—modified corn starch (E1442) + maltodextrin). A standardized terminology for describing food textures and liquid thicknesses is provided by the IDDSI framework, which consists of 8 levels (0–7; beverages: 0–4, food: 3–7) (Cichero et al. 2017).

It is advisable to start with the easiest to swallow consistency—generally puree—and gradually increase the level of difficulty, or to stop the examination if aspiration is severe. However, in patients with structural-motor deficits, such as head and neck cancer or mucositis and xerostomia after radiotherapy, pharyngeal transport of puree is usually more difficult than that of water. Since aspiration risk is underestimated in a limited number (three or four) of swallowing trials (Baijens et al. 2014), multiple trials should be made to obtain a realistic impression of the patient's actual swallowing function (e.g. "stress swallow" of 100 mL).

**Normal and Abnormal Findings**  Physiologically, no bolus should be visible during (intra-deglutitive), before (pre-deglutitive), or after swallowing (post-deglutitive) in the FEES.

**Pre-deglutitive Phase**  Before triggering the reflex pharyngeal phase, the following typical pathologies often can be diagnosed:

- Leakage (Spillage): The premature passage of the bolus from the oral cavity to the oro- and hypopharynx. Leakage indicates a poor oral control with insufficient linguo-velar sealing (of neurogenic or structural in origin) or a delayed reflex trigger.
- Pooling: The accumulation of bolus material in the oral cavity, valleculae, or hypopharynx. Pooling in general might be due to reduced strength of the muscles responsible for bolus propulsion (motor dysphagia, e.g. tongue base weakness, inadequate relaxation of the upper

oesophageal sphincter, reduced laryngeal elevation), to the presence of an obstruction (mechanical dysphagia, e.g. large osteophytes, oesophageal carcinoma) or to a delayed swallowing reflex (usually localised at the base of the tongue and anterior faucial pillar).

- Nasal Regurgitation: The bolus enters from the oropharynx into the nasopharynx. Nasal regurgitation may be due to a defect in the velopharyngeal valve (structural or neurogenic) or an inadequate timing of biomechanical events during the pharyngeal phase.
- Pre-deglutitive Laryngeal Penetration or Aspiration: The bolus enters the larynx or the trachea. Pre-swallowing penetration/aspiration is usually due to leakage or pooling.

**Intra-deglutitive Phase**  The endoscopic inspection of the glottis directly during swallowing is not possible. With the onset of the swallowing reflex and the beginning of the pharyngeal phase of swallowing, the pharynx changes its configuration from that of breathing to that of swallowing. The tongue base retracts and the pharyngeal wall is squeezed, resulting in a mucosal contact of the endoscope tip and hence loss of visibility (the so-called white-out phase).

Previous penetration or aspiration can easily be detected indirectly after swallowing by positioning the tip of the endoscope very near to the vocal folds or even in the upper trachea during long transnasal inspiration (dipping manoeuvre) (Rosen et al. 2009). For direct visualisation of the pharyngeal phase, videofluoroscopy is the superior method of examination. Intra-swallowing penetration/aspiration is usually due to insufficient laryngeal occlusion.

**Post-deglutitive Phase**  After swallowing, the following pathologies are of relevance:

- Residues with localisation in the valleculae, piriform sinuses, the postcricoid space or in the lateral pharyngeal walls are possibly caused by muscular weakness, reduced retraction of the tongue base, restricted laryngeal elevation or impaired opening of the upper oesophageal sphincter (Fig. 28.3).

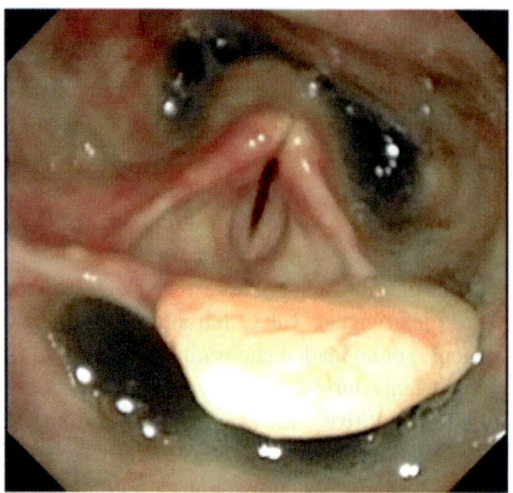

**Fig. 28.3** Endoscopic view of residues in the piriform sinus and valleculae after swallowing water. (©C. Pflug 2022)

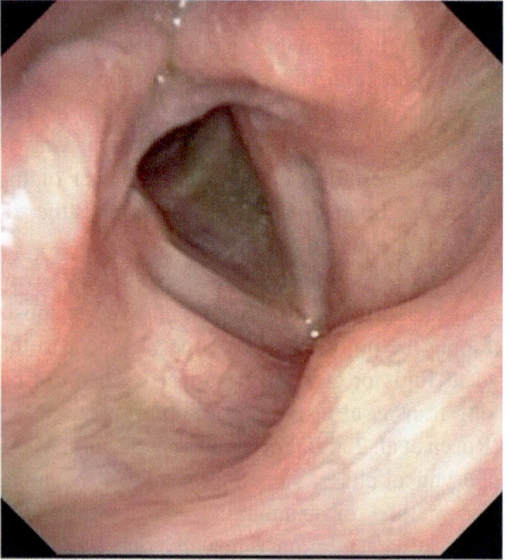

**Fig. 28.4** Aspiration of thickened water. The bolus is clearly visible in the subglottic area after the swallow (post-deglutitive). (©C. Pflug 2022)

• Post-Deglutitive Laryngeal Penetration/ Aspiration: It occurs frequently in sensory disorders from residues (Fig. 28.4). Even a regurgitation from the oesophagus into the pharynx due to a reflux disease, an expanding lesion in the oesophagus, inadequate relaxation of the upper oesophageal sphincter, or

Zenker's diverticulum can cause laryngeal penetration and aspiration.

**Observe Clearing** After swallowing, the patient's spontaneous clearing mechanisms, which provide evidence of sensitivity and muscle strength, should be observed. If no spontaneous clearing attempt is made, it is advisable to see whether it is possible after patient being asked.

### 28.2.4.3 Interventional Part: Trial of Postural, Dietary, and Behavioural Changes as Problems Occur

If dysphagia is present, the effects of modified food consistency, postural changes, and swallowing manoeuvres that permit safer or easier swallowing should be assessed (Table 28.1).

Therefore, FEES should be performed in tandem, i.e. by a physician together with a speech therapist. In selected cases, FEES can also be used for rehabilitation as a bio-feedback system (Logeman 1997).

**FEES Report** At the end of FEES, the findings must be documented and scored with special consideration of aspiration and bolus clearance or residue. The evaluation is facilitated by a video analysis and frame-by-frame mode. The different scoring systems are explained in Sect. 28.4. The FEES report should also include appropriate recommendations on nutrition (full oral, modified oral, non-oral) and rehabilitation (postural changes or modifications to the way the patient eats, or compensatory strategies, manoeuvre or strengthening exercises) or further examinations, such as videofluoroscopic swallowing examination, pharyngeal high-resolution manometry, or oesophago-gastroduodenoscopy.

For some patients, safe swallowing of pills is the biggest challenge. These often benefit from swallowing their oral medication with puree or special swallow gels (such as Gloup®, Rushwood B.V., Ottergeerde 30, 4941 VM Raamsdonksveer, Netherlands) that facilitate transport or protect against aspiration. This also has to be integrated into the recommendations.

**Table 28.1** Exemplary postural changes and swallowing manoeuvres as part of the FEES. Based on Logemann (2006), Schindler et al. (2021)

| Swallowing impairment | Posture/manoeuvre | Rationale |
|---|---|---|
| Insufficient oral transit | Head back | Use gravity to clear oral cavity |
| Delay in triggering the pharyngeal swallow | Chin down | Widens valleculae to prevent bolus entering airway; narrow airway entrance, reducing risk of aspiration |
| Reduced posterior motion of tongue base | Chin down | Pushes tongue base backwards towards pharyngeal wall |
| Unilateral vocal fold paralysis or surgical removal | Head rotated to damaged side | Places extrinsic pressure on thyroid cartilage, improving vocal fold approximation, and direct bolus down stronger side |
| Reduced pharyngeal contraction | Lying down on one side | Eliminates gravitation effect on pharyngeal residue |
| Unilateral oral and pharyngeal weakness on the same side | Head tilt to stronger side | Directs bolus down stronger side by gravity |
| Cricopharyngeal dysfunction | Head rotated | Pulls cricoid cartilage away from posterior pharyngeal wall, reducing resting pressure in cricopharyngeal sphincter |
| Unilateral pharyngeal paresis | Head rotated to the damaged side | Eliminates damaged side of pharynx from bolus path |
| Reduced or late vocal fold closure Delayed pharyngeal swallow | Supraglottal swallow | Voluntary breath-holding usually closes vocal folds before and during swallow |
| Reduced closure of the airway entrance | Super-supraglottal swallow | Effortful breath-holding tilts arytenoid forwards, closing airway entrance before and during swallow |
| Reduced posterior movement of the tongue base | Effortful swallow | Effort increases posterior tongue base movement |
| Reduced laryngeal elevation | Mendelsohn manoeuvre | Laryngeal movements open the UES; prolonging laryngeal elevation prolongs upper oesophageal sphincter opening |
| Uncoordinated swallow | Mendelsohn manoeuvre | Normalises timing of pharyngeal swallow events |

*UES* upper oesophageal sphincter

**Exact Description of the Deficits** An existing dysphagia can and should be treated. This prevents complications such as malnutrition and aspiration pneumonia and improves the patient's quality of life. In most cases, logopaedic dysphagia therapy can achieve significant results and protect patients against aspiration pneumonia, malnutrition, exsiccosis and cachexia, or avert invasive interventions such as PEG. In addition to the above, adaptation and compensatory strategies are of particular importance. Thus, even severe dysphagia with laryngeal penetration and aspiration can be effectively treated by special manoeuvres such as supraglottal swallowing. Important for the therapist is an accurate description of the deficits, for example: "Dysphagia with disturbed pharyngeal phase and residues in the right piriform sinus".

**Special Conditions** Many patient populations can benefit from FEES. The examination is usually possible in patients with physical limitations or suboptimal compliance, such as infants and babies, patients with dementia or bedridden conditions. If necessary, the procedure must be adapted accordingly. Even brief endoscopic views of the larynx can provide valuable information on anatomy, secretion management, and possibly bolus transport. Especially for very young children and babies, FEES has the advantages that they are not exposed to radiation and receive their usual food and liquids in their preferred position even while breastfeeding (Miller and Willging 2020; Miller et al. 2020).

In tracheostomy patients, assessment of bolus transit and the effects of swallowing manoeuvres can additionally be performed retrogradely, with the endoscope inserted through the tracheostomy. The retrograde vision is particularly useful to detect intra-deglutitive aspiration, which cannot be visualised directly through the transnasal access owing to the white-out phase (Ricci Maccarini et al. 2007).

### 28.2.5 Summary

Endoscopic swallowing diagnostics has a prominent position in dysphagia diagnostics and should always include expert endoscopy of the upper aerodigestive tract. As a classic domain of the ENT and phoniatrics speciality, it should be an integral part of specialist training (Graf et al. 2019). Continuous optimisation of methodology and technical progress improves the diagnostic validity of endoscopy and swallowing assessment. As a result, FEES is now considered the gold standard for swallowing evaluation in most European countries. It is advisable to proceed in accordance with the standard FEES protocol by S. Langmore described above. However, the examination procedure and the selection of the food or fluid consistencies to be tested should be individually tailored to the patient. The accurate detection and description of the deficits enable a targeted logopaedic swallowing therapy and thus prevent complications and improve the patients' quality of life.

## 28.3 Technical Background of Flexible Endoscopic Evaluation of Swallowing (FEES) and Digital Workstation Recording

Daniele Farneti and Christina Pflug

### 28.3.1 Introduction

Technology can help in evaluation of swallowing and some technological items are required for the standardised FEES described by Langmore

(2017): FEES is the first protocol, not yet validated, to evaluate swallowing endoscopically (see Sects. 28.2 and 28.4). Depending on the situation and location (e.g. bedside or in an outpatient setting) a video recording can be useful for a closer look after the examination and is an integral part of the FEES procedure according to Langmore; further analysis may include determination of inter-rater reliability, archiving, comparison with earlier examinations or frame-by-frame evaluation. Furthermore, valuable information can be drawn from still images (Farneti and Favero 2010; Schindler et al. 2009; Farneti 2014; Pluschinski et al. 2015).

### 28.3.2 The Technology of Endoscopic Evaluation of Swallowing

The following items are part of the technology in the field of endoscopic evaluation of swallowing

(a) Endoscopes
(b) Light sources
(c) Video equipment
  - Cameras
  - Video Recorders
  - Video Databases
  - Monitors

#### 28.3.2.1 Endoscopes

FEES requires flexible rhinolaryngoscopes that are inserted transnasally. Classical fiberoptic as well as modern chip-on-the-tip videoscopes are currently on the market for routine use (Eller et al. 2008). Fiberoptic endoscopes are limited in their spatial resolution (limited number of fibers in the package), whereas modern chip-on-the-tip endoscopes have the resolution of state-of-the-art camera chips, most of them high-definition (HD, $1929 \times 1080$ pixels) and in future 4K which is 4 times the resolution of HD ($3840 \times 2160$ pixels) (Woo 2016).

While fiberoptic endoscopes allow cost-effective area-wide use, distal chip endoscopes are superior in image quality and increase interrater-reliability (Plaat et al. 2014). HD quality portable videoendoscopy systems with an integrated LED light source are currently available. These are connected to a portable monitor or to a notebook via a USB. This enables mobile use with good quality. The HD endoscopes enable very good quality videos even with a small endoscope diameter. With these very thin endoscopes, even narrow anatomical structures (nose or airways) or infants can be examined very carefully. The resulting better compliance improves the examination. Thin, longer endoscopes of >60 cm can also be used transnasally for oesophagoscopy, bronchoscopy or panendoscopy.

### 28.3.2.2 Light Sources

Today LEDs are replacing classical halogen lights, that generate much heat, and xenon flash lights, that are noisy and limited in life-time. LEDs have a high efficiency, long life-time and include strobe flash (Steiger et al. 2009; Moreno and Sun 2008). Chip-in-scope and LED-in-scope technology, together with full HD image sensors, offer new possibilities in the endoscopic field.

Another innovation is the application of Narrow Band Imaging (NBI) to the deglutition field. NBI is widely used in gastrointestinal, laryngeal, and urological endoscopy. Its original purpose was to visualise blood vessels and epithelial irregularities. It has been observed and documented that the addition of the NBI to the common white light (WL) improves the contrast of the bolus test during FEES, increasing the detection of penetration and aspiration episodes in subjects with swallowing disorders, as well as the reliability of FEES (Nienstedt et al. 2017).

### 28.3.2.3 Video Equipment

The video images are normally displayed via video processor in real time on a monitor and stored in digital form. From the database the videos can be seen remotely, for discussion of a case with colleagues or collaborators, for facilitating video demonstrations for teaching and for feedback in a rehabilitation setting. Some workstations offer the possibility of implementing documentation systems, conceived to reduce editing time of reports and increase their completeness (Hey et al. 2011). Their usefulness on large samples has yet to be documented.

**Cameras** Classical fiberoptic endoscopes requires a separate video camera, which is mounted on the eyepiece of the endoscope.

After traditional video standard consumer TV technology, came an improvement in image quality with the introduction of high definition TV (HDTV), obtained by increasing the number of vertical lines of the image. This technology offers higher resolution and quality videos than standard definition (Tsunoda et al. 2008). Images with HD resolution can be projected onto large screens, providing excellent clarity and visibility for examiners.

A future option in endoscopic dysphagia diagnostics could be the three-dimensional technology (3D) (Bohr et al. 2016). This reproduces the principle of stereopsis, according to which each eye perceives the image of the object with a slightly different orientation: this allows the visual cortex to generate the third dimensional depth. According to this principle, the 3D system acquires images with a stereo-endoscope that receives the image of the right and left eye separately. These are instruments that require a dedicated and expensive technology; they were at first used for surgical purposes (robotic da Vinci Technology or the portable Aesculap Einstein Vision system), but more recently workstations applying this option are on the market: the third dimension is realised by wearing special glasses when viewing the monitor in the post-processing of images recorded by two cameras.

**Video Databases** Video databases allow the clinician to save videos, sounds and still images in a structured way together with patient information, and in a central patient database. The recorded material is easy to access and comparisons with a previous patient state can be made.

Many companies currently produce or distribute computerised workstations at affordable prices for endoscopic evaluation of swallowing. The video is digitised on the host computer, so that the physiological signals are presented synchronously with video images. A complete swallowing report with frames from the examination is easily generated and printed.

Special workstations offer optional tools. For example, video-synchronised movement sensors are able to identify pharyngeal swallowing events for measuring pharyngeal transit time. Special channels of analogue input can receive auxiliary signals such as surface EMG, tongue pressure transducers, solid-state pharyngeal/UES manometry, cervical auscultation, respiratory phases and speech. Finally, some workstations can also be implemented with programs used to record fluoroscopic studies analysers.

**Monitors** Medical monitors differ from usual ones by the possibility of colour calibration. Correct colour reproduction is important for a valid clinical evaluation. Medical monitors have features superior to those of consumer models. Colour calibration provides a colour impression close to that of the naked eye, which is essential in diagnostics. Brightness and colour saturation are less dependent on viewing angle, allowing experts to discuss cases in front of the screen. The devices are robust to daily cleaning procedures.

## 28.4 Rating of Flexible Endoscopic Evaluation of Swallowing (FEES)

Mohamed Farahat, Christina Pflug, Julie C. Nienstedt and Khalid H. Malki

### 28.4.1 Introduction

As described in Sect. 28.2, the FEES findings must be documented and evaluated at the end of the examination.

It is important to differentiate which bolus textures or consistencies (liquid, purée-like, solid), bolus volumes, and methods of delivery are safer to swallow than others (e.g. spoon, straw or cup, self-presented, or fed by someone else) (Logemann et al. 1995). It is also important to report whether the patient can sense penetration, aspiration, or residues, and whether he spontaneously initiates a throat-clearing manoeuvre.

Each rating sheet should include a detailed list of the normal and possible abnormal findings of all three parts of FEES. However, it is not assumed that every item will be scored for every examination. Some observations are critical, but others may be needed only for examinations that require detailed analysis of that aspect. The following section will guide the reader to a possible protocol that was adopted by Langmore (2001).

### 28.4.2 Assessment Protocol

#### 28.4.2.1 Anatomical-Physiological Assessment

The anatomical-physiological assessment includes the examination of anatomy, physiology and movement, secretion management, and sensitivity of swallowing structures, which are listed in Table 28.2.

#### 28.4.2.2 Direct Examination of Swallowing

The second part of FEES includes the rating of swallowing of different bolus volumes and consistencies as listed in Table 28.3.

The rating of the third part of FEES, intervention, involves the testing of postural, dietary, and behavioural changes when problems occur. The rating is done in analogy to the schemes mentioned above.

### 28.4.3 FEES Scoring Systems

In order to make the different FEES findings comparable, standardised scoring systems should be used. These should express the findings in statistically easy-to-evaluate numerical values. In particular, the parameters aspiration, bolus clearance and residues—and thus their scoring—have been the focus of dysphagia research in recent years. But there is so far no gold standard for a universal rating scale, since all previously published rating scales have their weaknesses (Nienstedt et al. 2018a; Langmore 2017). In addition, each swallow examination must be individually tailored to the patient, which compli-

**Table 28.2** Anatomical-physiological assessment

| | |
|---|---|
| A. Inspection of nasopharynx, oropharynx, hypopharynx, and larynx in resting position | • Abnormal anatomy/pathology<br>• Unusual features/normal variant<br>• Asymmetry<br>• Involuntary movement at rest<br>• Mucosal abnormalities: oedema, erythema, etc.<br>• Foreign body (feeding tube) impeding movement |
| B. Velopharyngeal closure (CN X and XI) | • Mobility<br>– Phonation<br>– Dry swallows<br>• Velar movement<br>– Completeness<br>– Exhaustibility<br>• Lateral wall movement<br>– Symmetry |
| C. Base of tongue (CN XII) function | • Movement<br>– Symmetry<br>– Range/amplitude<br>• Manoeuvre:<br>– Repeated "earl"<br>– Breathed (German) /h/<br>– "Hawking" sound<br>– Tongue pulling/pushing against resistance |
| D. Pharyngeal function, pharyngeal constrictor, and cricopharyngeal muscle (CN IX, X) | • Movement<br>– Symmetry<br>– Range/amplitude<br>• Manoeuvre:<br>– Strained loud high /ee/ (Bastian 1991)<br>– Pulling back/pressing the tongue against resistance |
| E. Laryngeal function (CN X) | • Respiration, phonation<br>– Normal finding<br>– Incompleteness<br>– Glottal gap<br>– Asymmetry<br>– Delayed onset<br>– Effort<br>– Hyperadduction<br>– Irregularity<br>• Airway protection<br>– Supraglottal and vocal fold closure<br>• Airway clearance<br>– Coughing via reflex or on request<br>– Cough strength |
| F. Secretions and their management | • Retained secretions<br>– Quantity<br>– Quality<br>– Localisation<br>• Sensitivity to retained secretions<br>– Spontaneous swallowing<br>– Coughing<br>– Clearing throat<br>• Clearing efficiency<br>• Frequency of spontaneous swallows |
| G. Sensitivity | • Reaction to presence of endoscope<br>• Reaction to light touch of tongue base (CN XII)/pharyngeal walls (CN IX and X)<br>• Reaction to light touch of epiglottis (CN IX, and X)<br>• Sensory threshold: response to direct air pulse on aryepiglottal rim (CN X) (Aviv et al. 1996)<br>• Reaction to secretions |

**Table 28.3** Rating of swallowing of different bolus volumes and consistencies

| A. Oral preparatory phase | • Inadequate mastication<br>– Unchewed bolus visible<br>– Anterior leakage (loss of bolus portions during chewing)<br>– Insufficient lingual/velar closure<br>• Phase duration<br>– Liquids (normal range, 0.5–2 s)<br>– Food (normal range, 4–14 s) (Palmer et al. 1992) |
|---|---|
| B. Oral transit | • Lingual propulsion of the bolus<br>• Asymmetry of tongue<br>– Bolus transport unilateral<br>• Repeated tongue pumping pre-swallow<br>• Bolus movement delayed<br>• Oral residue after swallow |
| C. Timing of swallow initiation | • Delay<br>• Pre-deglutitive leakage |
| D. Structural movements during swallow | • Clearing forces and laryngeal elevation base of tongue reverse movement<br>– Pharyngeal longitudinal movement<br>– Hyolaryngeal elevation<br>• Laryngeal closure<br>– Approach and forward tilt of the arytenoid cartilages<br>– Descent of the epiglottis<br>– Closure of the vocal folds with apnoea |
| E. Penetration or aspiration (Figs. 28.5, 28.6, and 28.7) | • Pre-/intra-/post-deglutitive (Rosenbek et al. 1996) |
| F. Residue (Figs. 28.8, 28.9, and 28.10) | • Amount<br>– None/small/medium/large<br>• Location<br>– Valleculae/pyriform sinus/larynx/subglottic space<br>• Clearing efficiency |
| G. Sensitivity | • Reaction to laryngeal penetration (CN X-SLN)<br>• Reaction to aspiration (CN X-RLN)<br>• Reaction to pharyngeal residue (CN IX and X) |

*CN* cranial nerve, *SLN* superior laryngeal nerve, *RLN* recurrent laryngeal nerve

**Table 28.4** Short version of the "secretion severity rating scale" (based on Murray et al. 1996, validated by Pluschinski et al. 2016)

| Rating | Description |
|---|---|
| 0 | Normal (moist) |
| 1 | Pooling in valleculae/piriform sinuses |
| 2 | Pooling in laryngeal vestibule transiently |
| 3 | Pooling in laryngeal vestibule consistently |

cates the standardisation of the examination process and rating of the findings. In the following, therefore, only the most common rating scales will be presented, without implying that they are officially guideline-compliant.

For the rating of retained pharyngeal secretions, the Murray score has prevailed (Murray et al. 1996; Pluschinski et al. 2016) (see Table 28.4). There is no validated method for the evaluation of material that passes beyond the base of the tongue into the deeper pharynx before swallowing, known as "leakage". The authors recommend the use of the "scale for bolus location" ranging from 0 to 4 (Langmore et al. 2007).

The most established rating scale for penetration and aspiration is the "penetration/aspiration scale" (PAS) (Rosenbek et al. 1996) (see Table 26.2). First described in the year 1996 by Rosenbek for VFSS, this rating scale has been proved to be reliable and valid for FEES scoring in different languages (Butler et al. 2015; Hey et al. 2014; Colodny 2002). ▶ It is important to mention that the PAS score alone is insufficient to describe dysphagia adequately. Other aspects, such as time of aspiration event (pre-/intra-/post-deglutitive) and bolus clearance, need to be described in detail.

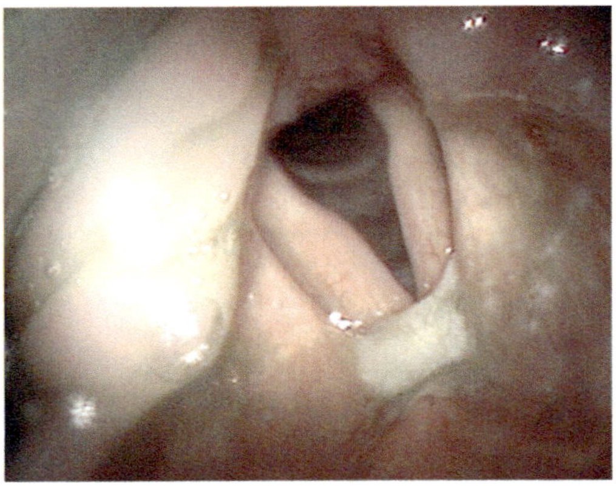

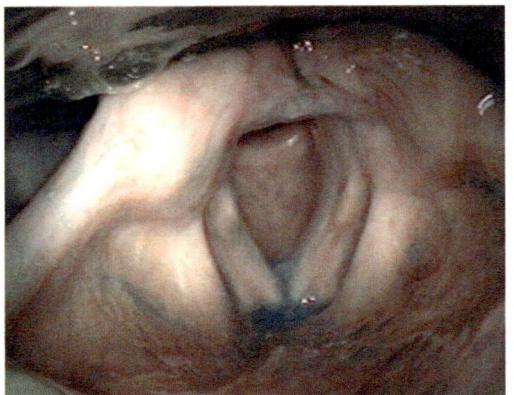

**Fig. 28.5** Penetration of purée consistency in the aditus laryngis 2019©Farahat

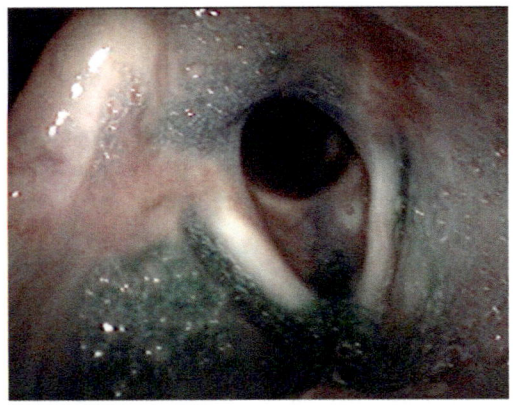

**Fig. 28.6** Penetration of thin liquids into the airways with contact to the vocal folds in the anterior commissure. 2019©Farahat

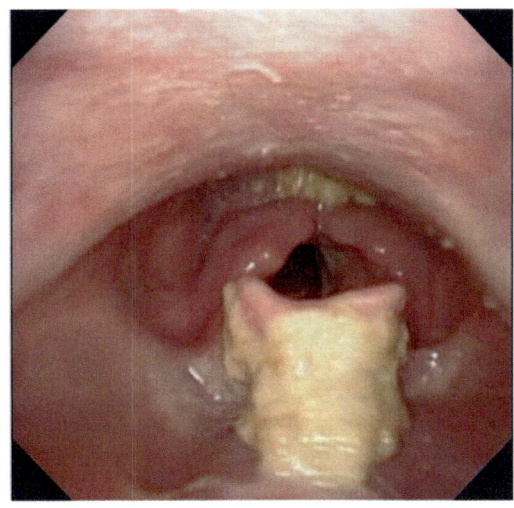

**Fig. 28.8** Post-swallow residue. Bread in the valleculae 2022©C. Pflug

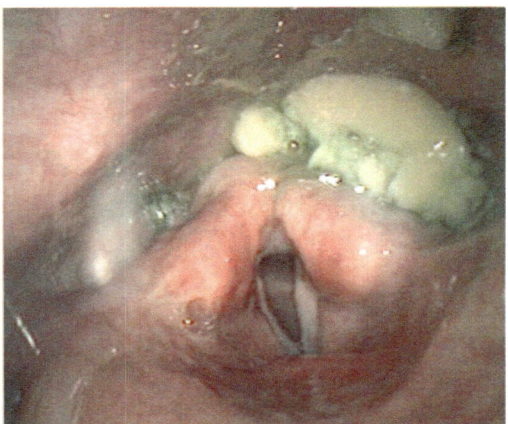

**Fig. 28.9** Residues of purée in the left piriform sinus 2019©Farahat

However, the use of a scale for the classification of residues is much more inhomogeneous. Numerous scales for residue severity have been published, including some for FEES exams such as the "Pooling Score" (Farneti 2008; Farneti et al. 2014), the "Boston Residue and Clearance Scale" (Kaneoka et al. 2013), and the "Yale Pharyngeal Residue Severity Rating Scale" (Neubauer et al. 2015; Gerschke et al. 2019). However, none of these has demonstrated excellent clinical validity or wide generalisability. Some scales also rate the location or the clearance of the residues or define the time of the eval-

**Fig. 28.7** Aspiration of thin and thick liquids 2019©Farahat

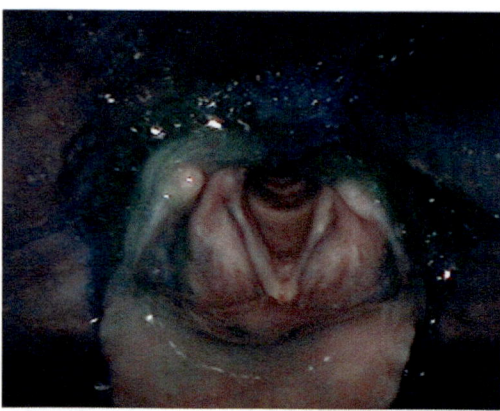

**Fig. 28.10** Residues of thin and thick liquids in both piriform sinus and lateral pharyngeal walls with penetration 2019©Farahat

**Table 28.5** Pill swallowing four-point scale FEES-based rating of ability to swallow pills (Buhmann et al. 2019). With permission from Elsevier

| Level | Difficulty in swallowing pills | Description |
|---|---|---|
| 0 | No | No problems swallowing oral medication |
| 1 | Mild | Oral medication remains initially in the oral cavity or pharynx but is felt by the patient and cleared spontaneously or by swallowing water |
| 2 | Moderate | Oral medication remains in the oral cavity or pharynx and is either not recognised or airway clearing is ineffective |
| 3 | Severe | Direct or indirect (coughing during or after swallowing) signs of aspiration. Oral medication can only be administered with purée or has to be crushed |

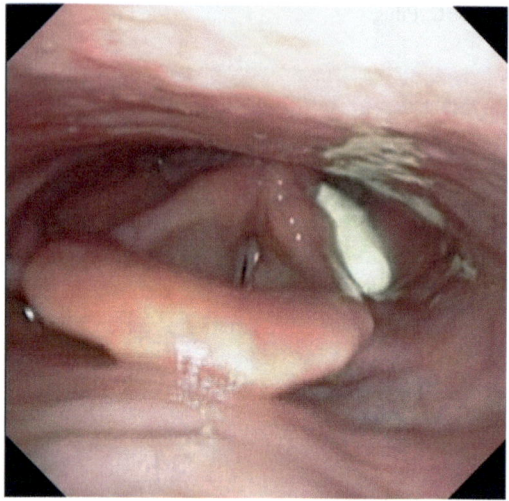

**Fig. 28.11** Capsule stuck in the right sinus piriform 2022©C. Pflug

**Table 28.6** Functional oral intake scale (FOIS) (Crary et al. 2005). With permission from Elsevier

| Level | Description |
|---|---|
| 1 | Nothing by mouth (NPO) |
| 2 | Tube-dependent with minimal attempts of food or liquid |
| 3 | Tube-dependent with consistent intake of liquid or food |
| 4 | Total oral diet of a single consistency |
| 5 | Total oral diet with multiple consistencies but requiring special preparation or compensation |
| 6 | Total oral diet with multiple consistencies without special preparation, but with specific food limitations |
| 7 | Total oral diet with no restriction |

uation (Kaneoka et al. 2013; Farneti 2008). Most of them are categorical scales, but differ in their classification levels (mild, moderate, severe, etc.). In a recent study, the benefits of an evaluation of residues by using a visual analogue scale (VAS), the "visual analogue residue scale" could be demonstrated (Pisegna et al. 2018).

Many patients have major problems with swallowing their pills safely (Fig. 28.11) (Buhmann et al. 2019; Nienstedt et al. 2018b). Therefore, it is recommended to check the ability to swallow pills of different formulations. In line with recent studies, the "pill swallowing four-point scale" ranges from 0 to 3: no, mild, moderate. And severe difficulties (Buhmann et al. 2019). Values ≥2 are to be considered pathological (Table 28.5).

In the end, the FEES report should also include appropriate therapeutic recommendations, particularly with regard to the nutrition (full oral, modified oral, non-oral).

The "functional oral intake scale" (FOIS) is an ordinal scale that reflects the functional oral intake of patients with dysphagia (Table 28.6) (Battel et al. 2018; Crary et al. 2005; Zhou et al. 2017). It is validated and widely applied in dysphagia research and clinical practice in English-speaking countries and recently was validated in Italian and Chinese (Battel et al. 2018; Zhou et al. 2017).

**Table 28.7** Fiberoptic endoscopic dysphagia severity scale (FEDSS) (Dziewas et al. 2008) (© Warnecke et al. 2009b; licensee BioMed Central Ltd.)

| | Main findings | Score | Possible clinical implications |
|---|---|---|---|
| Handling of secretions | Pooling with penetration/aspiration<br><br>No ↓     Yes | *6* | No oral food<br>Consider feeding via NGT<br>Watch out for respiratory distress |
| Purée consistency | Penetration/aspiration without or insufficient protective reflex<br>No ↓     Yes | *5* | No oral food<br>Consider feeding via NGT |
| | Penetration with sufficient protective reflex<br><br>No ↓     Yes | *4* | Consider feeding via NGT<br>Small amounts of purée during swallowing therapy |
| Liquids | Penetration without or insufficient protective reflex<br><br>No ↓     Yes | | |
| | Penetration with sufficient protective reflex<br><br>No ↓     Yes | *3* | Consider oral feeding with puréed food<br>Parenteral application of fluids |
| Soft solid consistency | Any penetration/aspiration massive residues in the valleculae or piriform sinus<br><br>No ↓     Yes | *2* | Consider oral feeding with puréed food and liquids |
| | No penetration/aspiration and no massive residues in the valleculae or piriform sinus | *1* | Consider oral feeding with soft solid food and liquids |

For patients with acute stroke the "Fiberoptic endoscopic dysphagia severity scale" (FEDSS), which classifies dysphagia into increasing severity levels 1–6, shown in Table 28.7, has been validated (Dziewas et al. 2008).

In addition, there are other nutrition outcome scales that are so far only available in one language, such as the "Bogenhausener Dysphagia-Score (BODS)" (Bartolome and Schröter-Morasch 2018; Prosiegel and Weber 2010).

## 28.4.4  Conclusion

Swallowing is a complex mechanism. Evaluating dysphagia by FEES is a comprehensive, diagnostic, and therapeutically valuable procedure. It provides visualisation of anatomical and temporal relationships within the pharyngeal mechanism relative to the bolus (Langmore et al. 1991; Rosenbek et al. 1996; O'Dea et al. 2015). The detailed presentation of the findings and classification of dysphagia is a substantial part of FEES (Hey et al. 2011; Arens et al. 2015). FEES implies much more than just detecting aspiration. Therefore, the FEES report should also clearly describe anatomical or physiological impairments of the pharynx and larynx (Langmore 2000).

The rating sheet should therefore include all three parts of FEES: (1) assessment of anatomy, physiology, and movement, secretion management, and sensitivity of swallowing structures, (2) direct assessment of swallowing of different bolus volumes and consistencies, (3) intervention part—testing of postural, dietary, and behavioural changes when problems occur.

The above procedure has not been subjected to validity testing and is just intended to serve as a suggestion until there are definitions for universally applicable rating sheets in corresponding guidelines. In the future, this will require broadly based validation studies and further interdisciplinary networking.

## 28.5  Radiological Examination

Martina Scharitzer

### 28.5.1  Introduction

A videofluoroscopic swallowing study (VFSS) is a dynamic radiological examination of the swallowing tract that also enables the analysis of functional and morphological abnormalities.

Fluoroscopy has been used since the early 1900s for the assessment of bones and soft tissues. It became a routinely used investigation tool in the 1980s, promoted by the group of Martin W. Donner and Bronwyn Jones (Jones and Donner 1989). The methods have been modified over the subsequent decades owing to the significant technological developments and increasing knowledge of swallowing physiology.

After administration of liquids and solids of varying consistencies, swallowing studies are recorded by using fluoroscopy in video or digitised format, enabling a detailed assessment of individual swallowing function by the use of slow motion and frame-by-frame analysis. Videofluoroscopy can be performed in children, as well as in adults of any age. Depending on individual clinical symptoms, a tailored examination that includes therapeutic swallowing manoeuvres, or the use of a tablet test, can be performed. Videofluoroscopy may serve as the initial basic evaluation of swallowing disorders, as well as a complementary method to other existing diagnostic tests for a comprehensive understanding of underlying symptoms. It can help to guide therapeutic recommendations for bolus modification, including specific volumes, textures, and consistencies, and the use of therapeutic rehabilitation strategies, such as postural manoeuvres. Disadvantages include the need for radiation exposure, problems with positioning the patient, and examination of unstable patients or patients who are unable to swallow.

## 28.5.2 Indications

Videofluoroscopy is a widely established assessment tool with which to determine the nature and extent of swallowing disorders, including difficulty in drinking and eating, the suspicion of aspiration, and globus sensation. It is indicated to observe the oral, pharyngeal, and oesophageal phase of swallowing in suspected morphological or functional abnormalities along the upper swallowing tract. The most common reason for referral for a videofluoroscopic swallowing study is the evaluation of the integrity of airway protection before, during, and after the swallow, and for concerns regarding the efficiency of swallowing function. In patients with a respiratory disorder, or a persistent nutrition or feeding problem, VFSS shows the characteristics of disturbed bolus movement. Patients with not only dysphagia, but also globus sensation, can be investigated by videofluoroscopy, which will show structural pathologies or functional disorders, such as signs of gastro-oesophageal reflux, abnormal upper oesophageal sphincter function, or oesophageal motor disorders. In particular, the timepoint of the occurrence of symptoms during the videofluoroscopic study in relation to bolus flow is helpful for a correct diagnosis. The presence of a medical condition or an underlying disease, with an associated high risk of swallowing disorders, is another indication for a VFSS. In addition, the effectiveness of therapeutic manoeuvres, bolus modifications, postures, or sensory enhancements to improve swallowing efficacy and safety can be tested.

Contraindications include unstable, uncooperative, or lethargic patients. If patients cannot be adequately positioned for imaging, the investigation cannot be performed. Limitations do exist owing to the use of radiation exposure, and thus there is the need for a time-restricted examination, as well as a limited ability to evaluate a possible fatigue effect on swallowing function, differences in viscosity and food composition between contrast material and natural foods, and the evaluation of single swallows as opposed to mealtime function.

## 28.5.3 Technical Considerations

The VFSS examination is performed with a fluoroscopy unit. Digital fluoroscopy offers higher spatial resolution in combination with lower radiation exposure than can be achieved by conventional fluoroscopy. Acquisition rates of 25–30 images per second are mandatory for a videofluoroscopic investigation. Studies have shown that higher image resolution results in fewer missed aspiration events, fewer swallows and therefore an overall shorter procedure length required for accurate decision-making, a better assessment of onset of aspiration in relation to initiation of swallowing, and a higher inter-rater agreement (Bonilha et al. 2024).

## 28.5.4 Radiation Dose

The radiation dosage amount should be "As Low as Reasonably Achievable (ALARA)", while ensuring that the accuracy of the swallowing study is not compromised. Radiation safety is important for all involved in the fluoroscopy suite room during the investigation. Minimising exposure time is fundamental in reducing the patient's dose by carefully planning the procedure and understanding the exact requirements and the clinical questions before beginning the VFSS. In addition, optimal collimation of the X-ray beam, avoidance of magnification modes, and the wearing of protective equipment, such as lead aprons, gloves, and thyroid collars by investigators, are important factors. Few studies have been published about the radiation dose to patients and physicians during a VFSS, but some have reported effective doses ranging from 0.2 to 1 mSv for patients—mainly depending on screening time—and a physician dose equivalent of 2.3 mSv/year (Morishima et al. 2016).

## 28.5.5 Examination Technique

The examination begins with a detailed exploration of each patient with regard to the nature and duration of symptoms and their relationship to the ingestion of food and liquids. Skilled history-taking is mandatory for tailoring the individual videofluoroscopic procedure and to include clinical information with radiological findings. Although most questionnaires cover the oral and pharyngeal symptoms of swallowing, all subtypes of dysphagia, and questions relating to problems attributable to oesophageal dysphagia (e.g. globus sensation, non-cardiac chest pain), should also be briefly covered prior to the examination to enable a full understanding of the patients' problems (Scharitzer et al. 2017a).

Optimally, a radiologist and a speech language pathologist should work together. In general, there are two different approaches (Ekberg and Pokieser 1997): one approach is to look for the correct diagnosis by searching for the worst swallow. This examination may include large bolus volumes or consistencies (solid food test) for decompensation of a compensated swallow. In contrast, in another approach for patients with known swallowing disorders, the VFSS may include testing of the effectiveness of manoeuvres, bolus modifications, and altering the patient's position to improve swallowing safety and to search for the best swallow.

Removing nasogastric tubes is not considered necessary for most patients. Although the duration of oropharyngeal swallowing, such as pharyngeal response, pharyngeal transit, or opening of the pharyngo-oesophageal segment may be prolonged, swallowing functions, such as bolus transit and clearance, are not altered by tubes (Huggins et al. 1999).

**Positioning** Patients are investigated in a standing position or seated in an upright position in a video-imaging chair, beginning with a lateral view to prevent superposition of the oesophagus and trachea. In some medical conditions, patients may also be positioned on their side or in the individual patient's representative eating position. Images should be centred at the relevant areas with proper collimation to reduce radiation exposure. Several swallows with boluses of different volumes and consistencies may be videorecorded, with a focus on the oropharyngeal region. Frontal views are necessary to assess swallow symmetry, to discriminate unilateral pharyngeal weakness or paresis, and to assess unilateral morphological pathologies. The evaluation of oesophageal function often needs to be performed with the patient in a recumbent position to eliminate bolus transport by gravity. Double-contrast images of the oesophagus can be performed to show subtle morphological pathologies.

**Contrast Media** Although several protocols tend to follow a uniform procedure, the strength of the modality is the possibility of a tailor-made approach, using foods similar to those the patient usually eats. This is especially important for VFSS of paediatric patients, when we start with the safest food being presented first and high-risk consistencies being presented afterwards. When there is a high clinical suspicion of severe aspiration, we prefer water-soluble, low-osmolar, non-ionic iodine contrast medium. A typical protocol includes thin liquid, thick liquid (nectar-like), puree and solids (a cracker coated with puree) as a standard, depending on individual circumstances or questions in the referral. In patients without severe aspiration, barium contrast medium should be used for better mucosal coating. Patients with a history of obstruction should be examined by a standardised solid-bolus test. A 13–14 mm tablet is helpful for demonstrating oesophageal strictures and estimating oesophageal residual lumen diameter (Scharitzer et al. 2017b). The tablet is also helpful when evaluation of the distal oesophagus is inadequate, or when over-distention may prevent the detection of symptomatic lower oesophageal rings or overlap of the distal oesophagus and an adjacent hiatal hernia. Provocation of clinical symptoms during tablet passage should be correlated with delayed tablet transport or impaction of the tablet.

**Therapeutic Manoeuvres** Visual examination of the effectiveness of therapeutic strategies in patients with dysphagia is another advantage of videofluoroscopy. These strategies may include postural changes for redirection of bolus flow, modification of bolus consistencies to improve clearance through the hypopharynx and oesophagus, techniques for sensory enhancement and swallowing manoeuvres to eliminate aspiration or reduce oral or pharyngeal residues, or alternating methods of the presentation of the bolus (such as spoons, modified cups, straws). The accurate realisation of rehabilitation strategies may be tested and imaging results can be shown to the patient.

### 28.5.6 Interpretation

Swallowing dysfunction may present as an impairment of any of the physiological components of swallowing, from the oral cavity to the oesophago-gastric junction. The most frequent findings include pharyngeal bolus retentions, laryngeal penetration or aspiration, and dysfunction of the pharyngo-oesophageal segment. In addition to functional disorders, videofluoroscopy has proven

to be an excellent method for the detection of structural abnormalities, which can be found in a large proportion of symptomatic patients (Scharitzer et al. 2002). When interpreting a VFSS, a visuo-perceptual evaluation, including temporal, spatial, and patient response factors, as well as quantitative measurements, can be used (Swan et al. 2019). Assessing each functional unit of swallowing allows a structured approach and improves the quality of radiological reporting (Fig. 28.12). Often several disorders of one functional unit in a patient can be found, as well as various combinations of findings in more than one functional unit, showing typical "patterns of findings" attributable to specific clinical symptoms. The radiological report should include a description of these videofluoroscopic findings with their

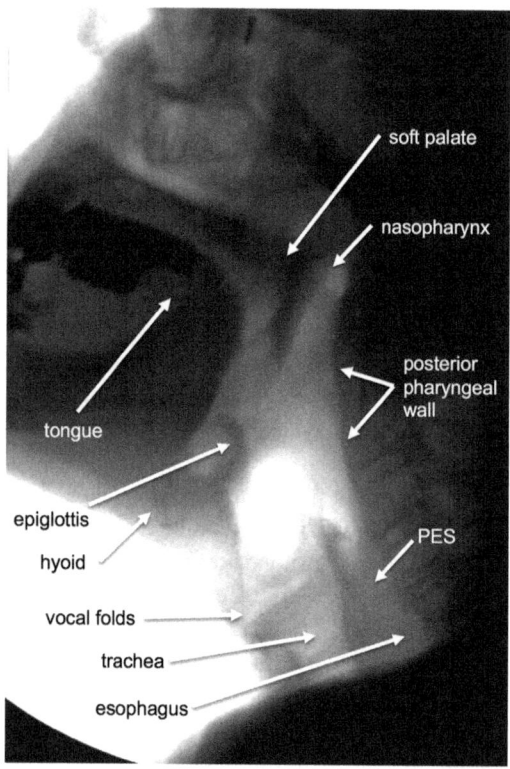

**Fig. 28.12** Normal anatomy of the swallowing tract. Lateral videofluoroscopic view of a young child showing the main anatomical landmarks that can be identified by VFSS. Within less than 1 s, six of the units complete the pharyngeal phase of swallowing. A complete barium swallow of 15 mL should reach the stomach within 10 s. *PES* pharyngoesophageal segment. (©Scharitzer2019)

effect on bolus transport, a comparison with the patient's symptoms, the final diagnosis, and further recommendations or comments. These include recommendations regarding oral versus non-oral intake, diet type, additional investigations or referrals to other specialists, and suggestions for treatment strategies. A simplified but accurate report is mandatory for effective communication with referring physicians and the patient. Since the VFSS may reveal several abnormalities along the swallowing tract that are not relevant for the individual clinical situation, the examiner needs considerable experience in dysphagia evaluation to put findings into an accurate clinical context.

**Oral Cavity** Normally, the bolus should rest on the dorsum of the tongue, controlled anteriorly by the lip seal and laterally and posteriorly by tongue-to-palatal contact. Insufficient lip closure is called "drooling". Bolus formation includes tongue movement in an efficient way without oral post-deglutitive retention. Impaired bolus formation with an inability to hold the bolus on the tongue surface, fragmentation of the bolus, and uncoordinated movements of the tongue can be observed. Inefficiencies, such as muscle weakness or a sensory loss, can be observed by contrast material that remains in the oral or pharyngeal cavity with the subsequent risk of inadequate nutrition or airway compromise. When initiating the swallow, the tongue base moves backward to come into contact with the pharynx and squeeze the bolus. Weakness of the tongue should be evaluated with thicker consistencies and is often combined with weakness of the pharyngeal muscles. An incompetent seal of the tongue and the palate leads to a leakage of the bolus into the oropharynx (Fig. 28.13).

**Soft Palate** In healthy people, the soft palate elevates to seal the nasopharynx, observable by videofluoroscopy. Incomplete elevation of the soft palate and lack of velopharyngeal closure, with reduced contraction of the upper pharyngeal sphincter muscles, is one of the more common findings and leads to "nasal regurgitation" (Fig. 28.14). This is especially evident in patients with Parkinson's disease, where there are pathologies of the oral phase of

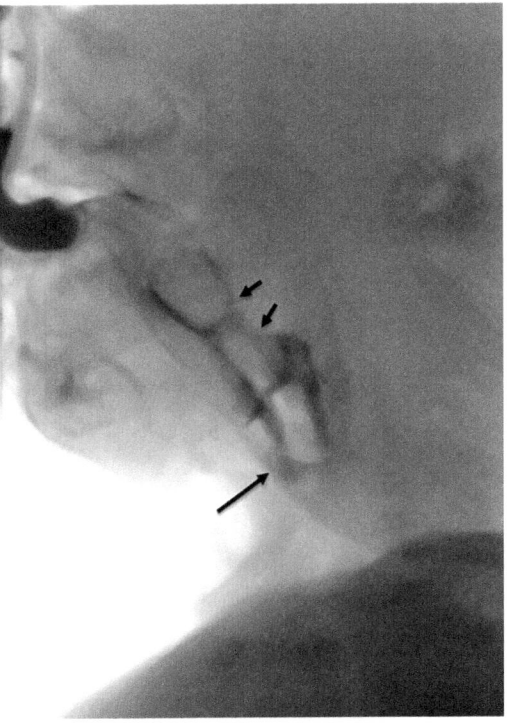

**Fig. 28.13** Posterior leaking. Videofluoroscopy of a child with cerebral palsy shows weakness of the tongue, insufficient dorsal closure of the oral cavity (short arrows), and contrast medium passing prematurely into the piriform sinus (arrow). (©Scharitzer2019)

swallowing and significantly delayed velopharyngeal junction closure, compared with healthy controls (Baijens et al. 2011). Initiation of an involuntary pharyngeal swallow reflex is often associated with elevation and retraction of the soft palate, but has been shown to be variable in time relative to the position of the bolus. Although the majority of patients show an onset of pharyngeal swallow initiation after the bolus head passes the posterior angle of the mandible, a trend towards later onset can be observed in older patients (Martin-Harris et al. 2007).

**Epiglottis** Epiglottal inversion is an important component of airway protection during swallowing. VFSS shows a horizontal position of the epiglottis first, followed by full epiglottal inversion. As shown by videofluoroscopy, impaired epiglottal tilting (Fig. 28.15) may be attributable to reduced tongue base retraction and laryngeal elevation (Pearson et al. 2016), with a

**Fig. 28.14** Nasal regurgitation. Young girl with congenital neurological disease and clinical suspicion of aspiration. Owing to insufficient closure between the elevating soft palate and the contraction of the upper pharyngeal sphincter, contrast material is seen in the nasopharynx (arrow). Additionally, penetration during deglutition can be observed (short arrow). (©Scharitzer2019)

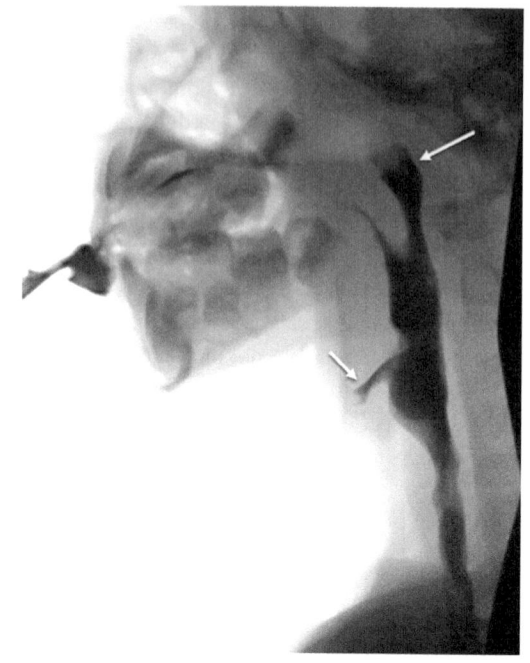

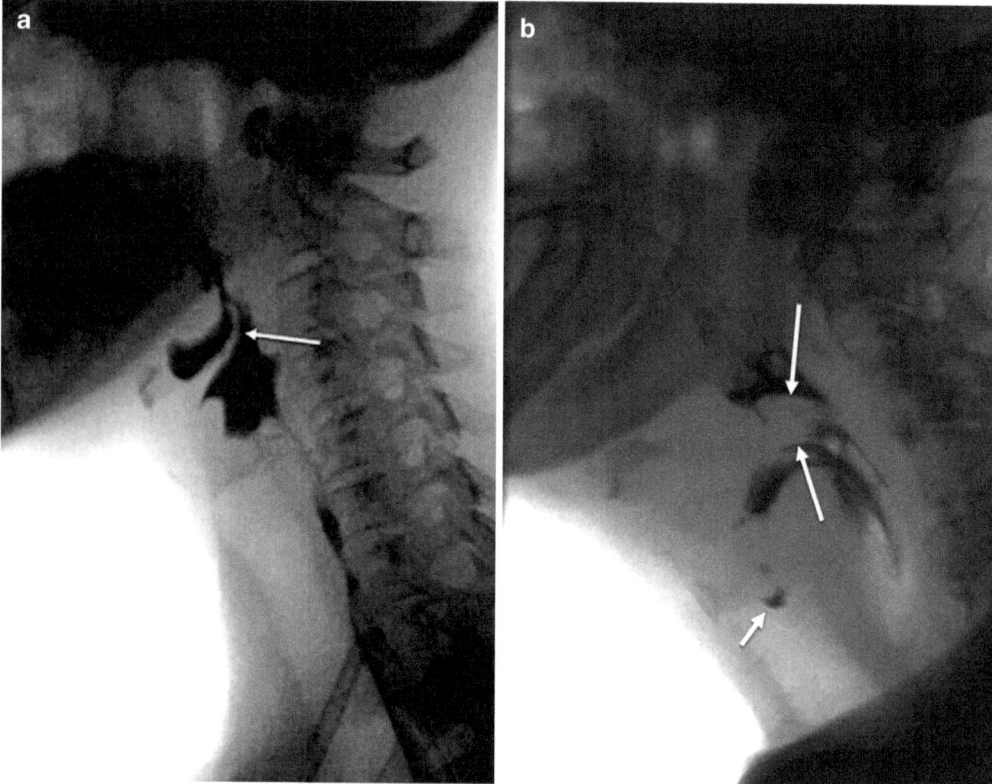

**Fig. 28.15** Epiglottis. **Left image** (**a**) The epiglottis is surrounded by contrast medium without showing an epiglottal tilt with the epiglottal tip still directing upwards (arrow). **Right image** (**b**) Patient with oropharyngeal can- cer and radiotherapy: the epiglottis is markedly swollen with diminished inversion (arrows), leading to contrast material entering the laryngeal vestibule below the vocal cords (short arrow). (©Scharitzer2019)

possible impact on therapeutic swallowing exercises. Important clues to the presence of incomplete tilting are retentions within the valleculae. Epiglottal swelling after radiation and inflammatory or tumorous pathologies could also be observed.

**Hyoid and Larynx**  The hyoid and larynx move superiorly and anteriorly, with laryngeal closure occurring from bottom to top. Incomplete laryngeal closure during bolus passage may lead to the bolus entering the laryngeal vestibule above the vocal cords (penetration, Fig. 28.16), or entering the airway below the vocal folds (aspiration). Transient or high penetration has been described in healthy people (Allen et al. 2010) and is followed by spontaneous clearance from the laryngeal vestibule. Penetration is usually a result of a discrepancy between bolus arrival at the entrance to the airway and closure of the laryngeal vestibule and may be caused by poor oral bolus control or a delayed initiation of the pharyngeal swallow.

Several factors are associated with an increased risk of aspiration, including respiratory factors, such as abnormalities in respiratory rates and oxygen saturation, reduced tongue pressure, reduced hyoid and laryngeal movement, and impaired laryngeal sensation. Aspiration can occur before the initiation of swallowing (pre-deglutitive), during pharyngeal bolus passage (intra-deglutitive) and after the involuntary act of swallowing (post-deglutitive) (Fig. 28.17). Causes and therapy of pre-, intra-, and post-deglutitive aspiration vary significantly, emphasising the need for an accurate assessment of aspiration in relation to the initiation of swallowing. A widely used grading system for the assessment of penetration and aspiration is the penetration-aspiration scale (PAS), which describes VFSS findings on an eight-point ordinal rating scale (Rosenbek et al. 1996). In addition to the identification of misdirected swallowing, it is important to note whether the patient coughs or observes any experience of a misdirected swallow, since silent aspiration is

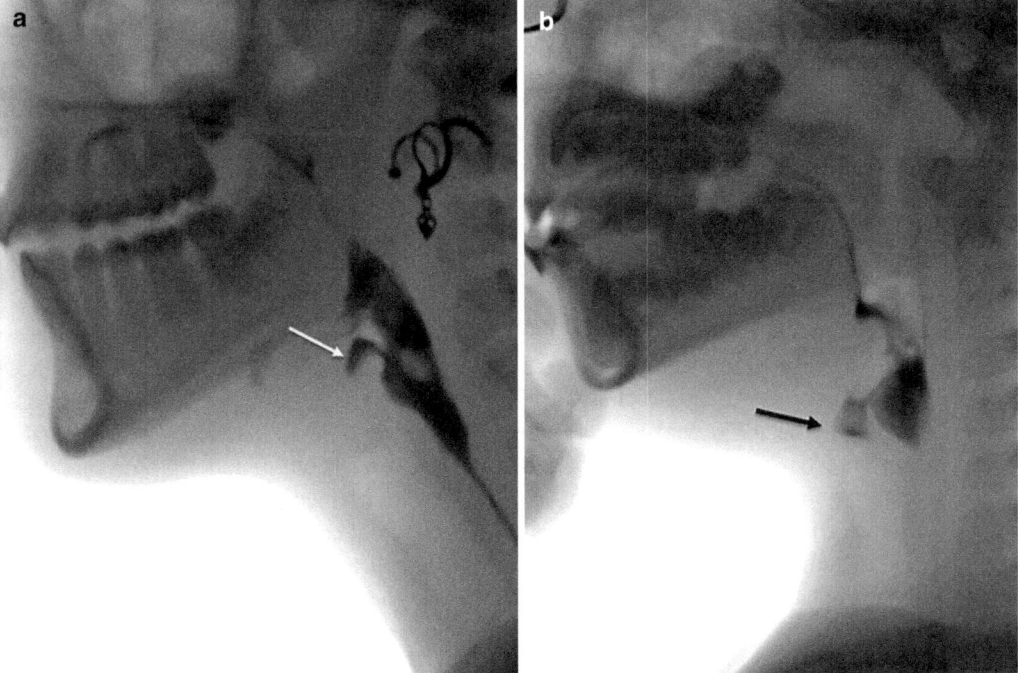

**Fig. 28.16**  Penetration. **Left image** (**a**) During swallowing, insufficient laryngeal closure leads to transient contrast medium entering the laryngeal vestibule (arrow). **Right image** (**b**) Deep penetration is characterised by contrast medium within the laryngeal vestibule reaching the upper vocal cords (arrow), indicative of a penetration-aspiration score of 4 or 5. (©Scharitzer2019)

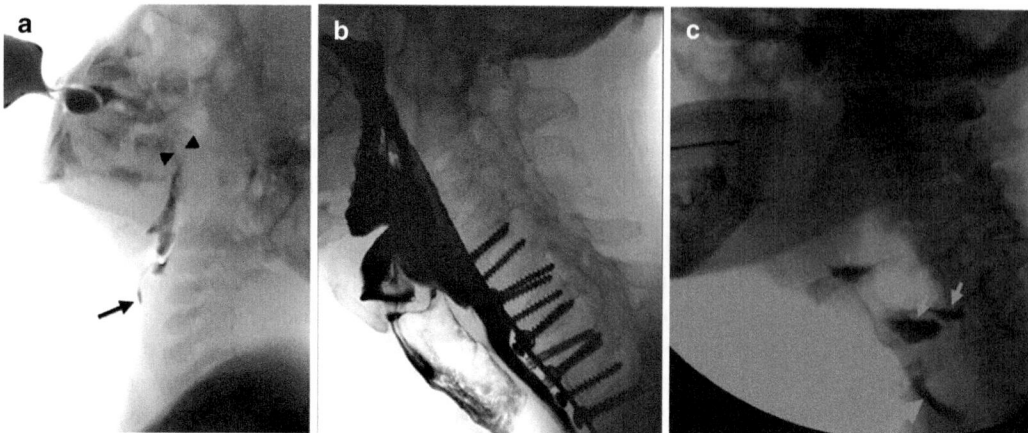

**Fig. 28.17** Three types of aspiration: **Left image** (**a**) before initiation of swallow, contrast medium enters the hypopharynx and runs into the trachea (pre-deglutitive, arrow). **Middle image** (**b**) In this patient after surgery of the vertebral spine, during bolus swallow incomplete laryngeal closure leads to aspiration during pharyngeal bolus passage (intra-deglutitive, arrow). **Right image** (**c**) Patient with pharyngeal paresis after stroke: after swallowing, severe retention within the valleculae and piriform sinus (short arrows) leads to overflow aspiration into the trachea (post-deglutitive, arrow). (©Scharitzer2019)

associated with an increased risk of airway disease. Silent aspiration can be easily detected by VFSS, especially in children with neurologically based dysphagia. Objective measurements, such as anatomically normalised hyoid movement, have shown a close relationship with the risk of penetration or aspiration (Steele and Cichero 2014). Although decreased fluoroscopic pulse rates reduce the radiation dose, aspiration events may occur for only parts of a second, as shown by Mercado-Deane, and therefore could be missed with pulse rates of 10/s (Mercado-Deane et al. 2001).

**Pharynx** The pharyngeal muscles should constrict and move anteriorly and medially, as seen in an approximation of both lateral pharyngeal walls to the middle on the frontal view. In the lateral view, contraction of the posterior pharyngeal wall from the top, moving downwards, can be observed. Objective measurements of pharyngeal function, including the pharyngeal constriction ratio and total pharyngeal transit time, can be related to airway closure duration and maximum and duration of pharyngeal opening. In addition to the safety of the pharyngeal phase of swallowing, which has been discussed in the previous paragraph, the efficacy of pharyngeal swallowing

is essential. Residues within the valleculae or the piriform sinus (Fig. 28.18) can be a sign of pharyngeal weakness or paresis and imply an increased risk of post-deglutitive aspiration with more severe pharyngeal residues (Eisenhuber et al. 2002). An estimation of the extent of retention within the valleculae and piriform sinus is helpful and various quantitative (Pearson et al. 2013; Dyer et al. 2008) and quantifiable (Rommel et al. 2015) scales have been published.

Additional structural defects that impair swallowing function should be excluded (Fig. 28.19).

**Pharyngo-oesophageal Segment** Incomplete or delayed opening at the pharyngo-oesophageal segment, a 2–5 cm-long region of elevated pressure between the pharynx and oesophagus, appears as a smooth posterior protrusion into the oesophageal lumen, leading to an indentation of the column of contrast material. By swallowing a 20 mL bolus, VFSS may discriminate between non-obstructive (Fig. 28.20a) and obstructive cricopharyngeal bars, by the use of a threshold of 6 mm (Leonard et al. 2004). Prolonged dysfunction of the cricopharyngeus muscle may lead to progressive dilation and weakness of pharyngeal constriction (Belafsky et al. 2010) (Fig. 28.20b).

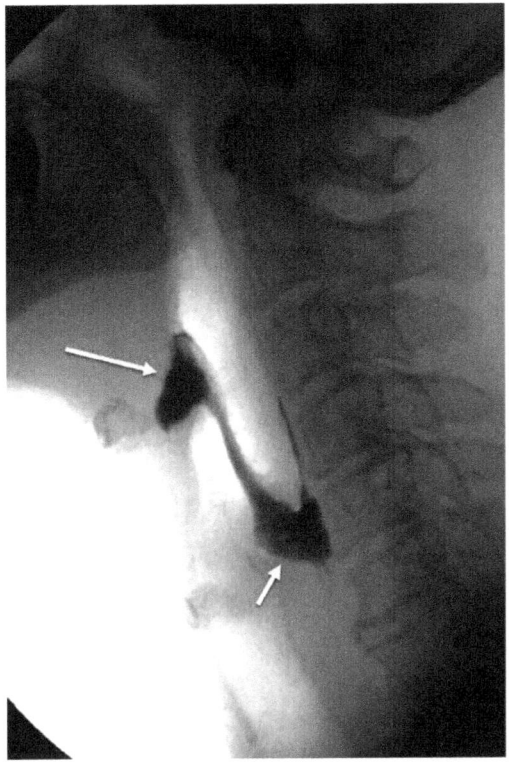

**Fig. 28.18** Pharyngeal retention. VFSS in this patient after brain stem infarct shows severe pharyngeal retention after swallowing of moderately thickened contrast material within the valleculae (arrow) and the piriform sinus (short arrow). (©Scharitzer2019)

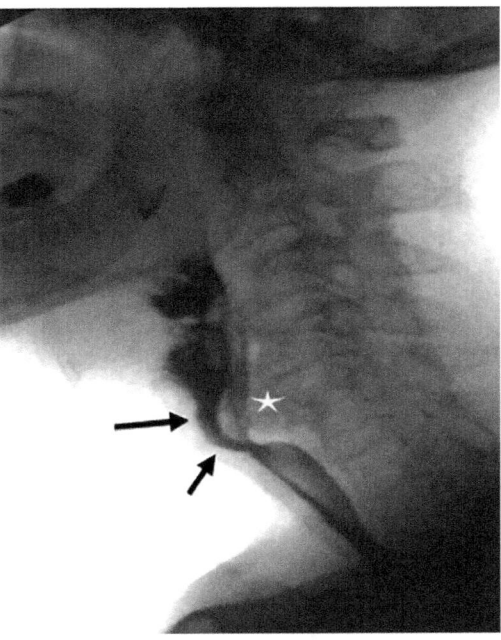

**Fig. 28.19** Cervical osteophytes. In this patient with severe solid food dysphagia, videofluoroscopy reveals a significant stenosis of bolus flow (arrows) owing to extensive ossification of the anterior longitudinal ligament of the cervical spine (asterisk). After surgical removal of osteophytic formations, dysphagia resolved. (©Scharitzer2019)

Additional findings can include a Zenker diverticulum, as well as a Killian–Jamieson diverticulum, and cervical oesophageal webs, which can be seen as thin, 2–3 mm membranes along the anterior wall of the lower hypopharynx and proximal cervical oesophagus, which may obstruct the lumen (Fig. 28.21).

**Oesophagus** During the overall investigation of swallowing, not only oropharyngeal but also oesophageal findings can be detected. This is very important, since the patient-perceived level of dysphagia is not reliable for the determination of the level of the underlying pathology and should not be used to tailor investigations (Ashraf et al. 2017). Mechanisms of oesophageal body motility and the oesophago-gastric junction are easy to study owing to the slow speed in relation to the oropharyngeal phase of swallowing. The bolus passes the oesophageal body via primary

and secondary oesophageal peristaltic contractions. Non-propulsive contractions (formerly called "tertiary") result in segmental oesophageal contractions that increase with age. The primary peristaltic contraction wave occludes the oesophageal lumen and leads to a "V"-shape of the proximal end of the bolus. The presence of a fluid level ("support level") indicates an altered motor function or a stenosis (Scharitzer et al. 2024). Videofluoroscopy is a good initial diagnostic test for the detection of achalasia, diffuse oesophageal spasm, nutcracker oesophagus, and other primary and secondary motility disorders. VFSS is also helpful in the detection of morphological findings, such as subtle rings or stenosis (especially when using a solid-bolus test), which can be missed by the passing endoscope (Scharitzer et al. 2017b) (Fig. 28.22). Extrinsic causes such as an enlarged thyroid gland, postoperative causes of dysphagia after surgery of the neck or thorax, and post-radiation strictures should be assessed. The lower spatial resolution of video recording than conventional radiographs should

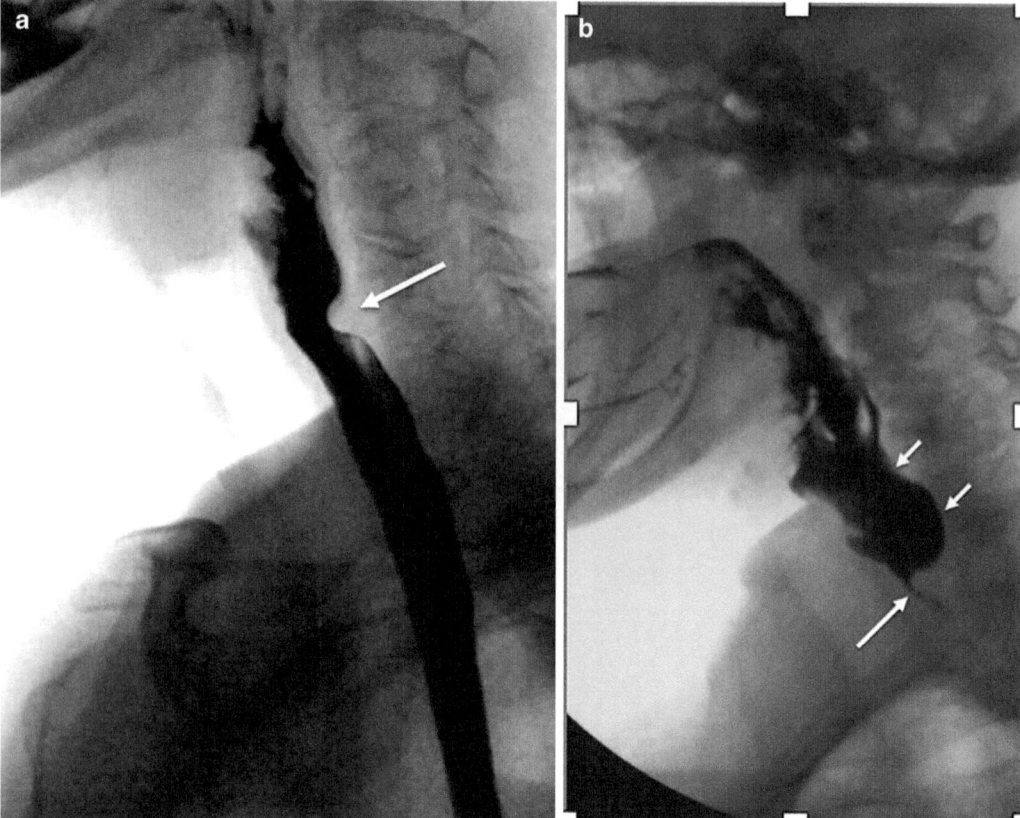

**Fig. 28.20** Dyskinesia of the pharyngoesophageal segment. **Left panel** (**a**) Small cricopharyngeal bar in this patient with suspicion of aspiration. This smooth, posterior bar-like protrusion into the lumen (arrow) can be seen in the lateral view at the junction of the hypopharynx and the cervical oesophagus and is found in 5–10% of asymptomatic patients. **Right panel** (**b**) In this patient with regurgitation and dysphagia, incomplete opening of the pharyngo-oesophageal segment (arrow) is seen with severely impaired bolus passage into the oesophagus and consecutive pharyngeal dilation and retention (short arrows). (©Scharitzer2019)

be considered when detecting subtle mucosal lesions. In these cases, an additional double-contrast examination should be included.

**Oesophago-gastric Junction** In a significant number of patients, symptoms referred proximally to the thoracic inlet or the throat can be attributed to gastro-oesophageal reflux disease. Including the oesophago-gastric junction in the swallowing study may reveal an abnormally configurated cardia, a hiatal hernia, spontaneous gastro-oesophageal reflux or associated oesophageal motility disorders (Levine et al. 2016). In addition, extra-oesophageal manifestations of gastro-oesophageal reflux disease, including impaired epiglottal tilting, pharyngeal paresis, or laryngeal penetration/aspiration, can be detected radiologically (Rubesin and Levine 2018). In a larger group of patients with hiatal hernia and videofluoroscopic signs of gastro-oesophageal reflux disease, dysfunction of the pharyngo-oesophageal segment can be found, which was reported by Nativ-Zeltzer et al. (2018) (Fig. 28.23).

## 28.5.7 Combined Investigations

Simultaneous videofluoroscopic and manometric investigations (video-manometry or manofluorography) provide an assessment of pressure topography and time-matched videofluoroscopic

**Fig. 28.21** Patient presenting with dysphagia and regurgitation of food after meals. Videofluoroscopy shows a large pouch developing from the posterior part of the hypopharynx, a Zenker's diverticulum (arrow) dislocating the cervical oesophagus anteriorly with obstruction for bolus passage (short arrows). (©Scharitzer2019)

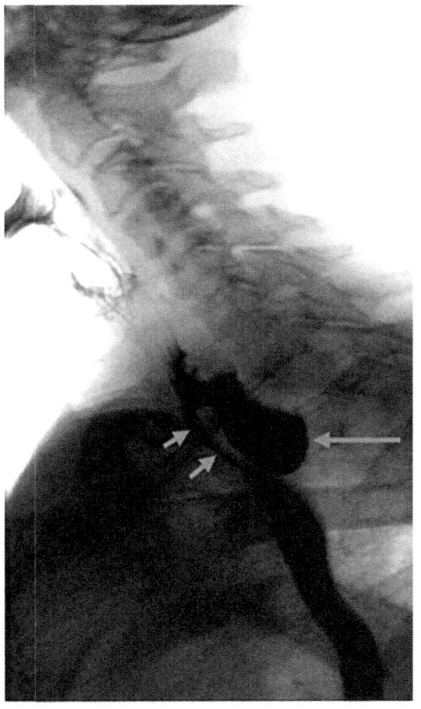

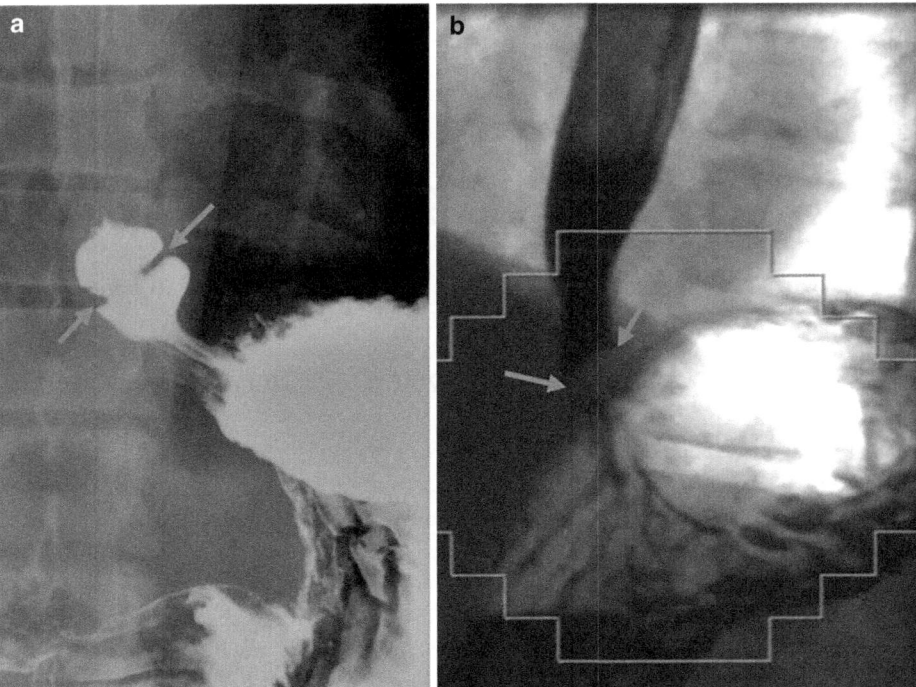

**Fig. 28.22 Left image (a)** Patient presenting with solid food dysphagia: videofluoroscopy reveals a thin circular ring-like stenosis in the distal oesophagus (arrows), a typical finding of a mucosal (or symptomatic Schatzki's ring).

**Right image (b)** A standardised 14 mm tablet was impacted (arrows), proving a significant stenosis of <14 mm. (©Scharitzer2019)

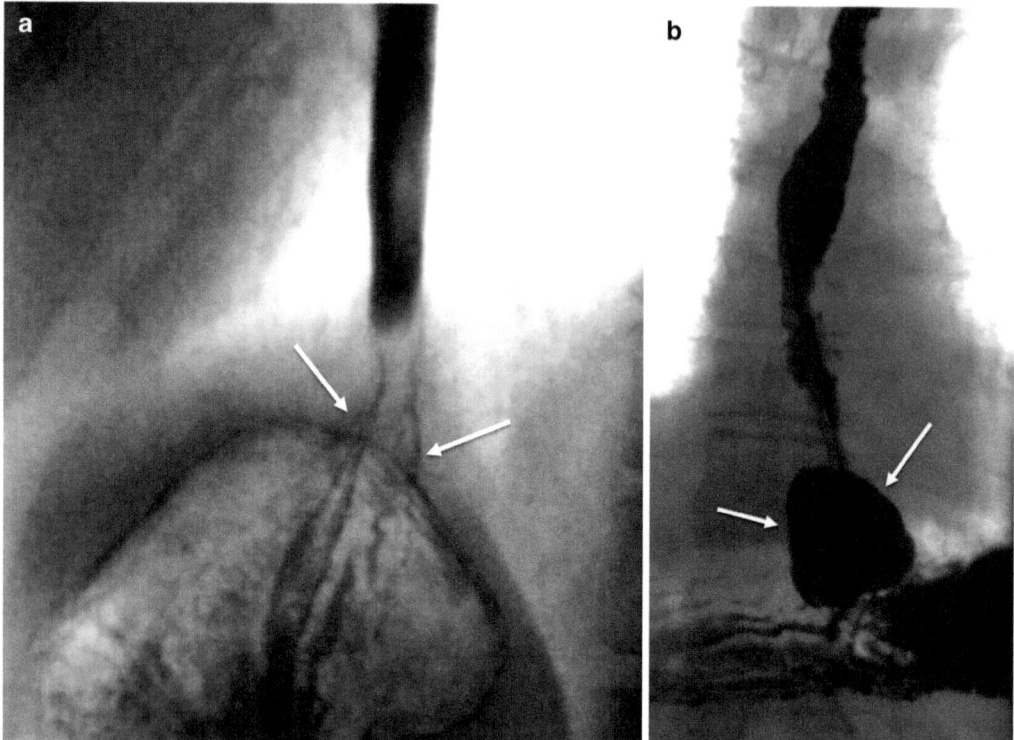

**Fig. 28.23** GERD **Left image** (**a**) In this patient with sensation of a lump in the throat, weakening of the ligaments around the cardia causes a funnel-shaped cardia (arrows) instead of the regular appearance with stellate folds radiating centrally ("cardiac rosette").

**Right image** (**b**) Additionally, a hiatal hernia (arrows) can be seen with non-propulsive oesophageal contractions. Oropharyngeal bolus passage was normal. (©Scharitzer2019)

imaging. Specifically designed computer software enables simultaneous recording of manometry and VFSS, with a clinical impact on the investigation of UES constriction (e.g. treatment outcomes after cricopharyngeal myotomy), surgery for anterior cervical osteophytes, identification of pharyngeal pressure elements or propulsion forces, or the characterisation of globus pharyngeus (Nativ-Zeltzer et al. 2012). The simultaneous assessment of FEES and VFSS enables an optimised investigation of oropharyngeal dysphagia by using the advantages and compensating disadvantages of both methods. Direct comparison in postoperative patients has shown significant differences when assessing the penetration-aspiration scale, with a tendency of higher scores from VFSS and the residue severity scores, with larger residues scores from FEES (Scharitzer et al. 2017b).

## 28.6 pH-Metry and Manometry

Daniele Farneti and Michael Jungheim

### 28.6.1 Introduction

Swallowing is a highly coordinated neuromuscular process involving both voluntary motor skills and reflexive muscular activities. These depend on sensory input and cortical and subcortical real-time modulations. The swallowing process involves the entire digestive tract from the oral cavity to the stomach. During clinical swallowing diagnostics, all of these components need to be assessed in order to determine any swallowing disorders. The swallowing process is divided into an oral, pharyngeal, and oesophageal phase. According to this classification, pathologies can be assigned precisely and adequate therapeutic measures initiated.

In addition to the swallowing process, the upper aerodigestive tract also fulfils further functions, e.g. breathing, phonation, and articulation. If pathologies occur, all functions can be affected and the clinical manifestations may be diverse. Consequently, a large number of symptoms and discomforts may result, which often cannot be accurately attributed to their origin (Farneti 2012). An important example is the laryngopharyngeal reflux (LPR) (Koufman et al. 2002) in delimitation to the cervical manifestation of the gastro-oesophageal reflux disease (GERD) (Kahrilas et al. 2008; Jungheim and Ptok 2011). Patients with reflux disease do not only complain of classic heartburn but also of other symptoms such as a globe sensation, dyscrinia, compulsory clearing of the throat or speech, and articulation disorders. In order to make an accurate diagnosis, a detailed medical history is crucial to observe all the subtle symptoms that patients often do not mention.

In addition to the history and radiological and endoscopic imaging procedures of the swallowing process (see Sects. 28.2 and 28.5), further instrumental techniques have been developed in recent decades to enable the functional evaluation of swallowing. Among the most relevant techniques are oesophageal and pharyngeal reflux monitoring (prolonged telemetry capsule pH monitoring and 24-h impedance pH-testing) and manometry studies (Kumar and Katz 2013).

## 28.6.2 Pharyngeal and Esophageal pH-Metry

Gastro-oesophageal reflux and laryngopharyngeal reflux are two disease entities that need to be differentiated. A GERD is present when gastral contents are regurgitated into the oesophagus. If passage through the upper oesophageal sphincter into the pharynx occurs, it is called an LPR. Different measuring techniques are used for diagnostics.

Oesophageal pH monitoring provides direct measurement of acidity in the oesophagus. This procedure has been considered the gold stan-dard for diagnosis of gastro-oesophageal reflux disease (GERD), in order to document reflux disease, to assess the severity, and to monitor the response to medical or surgical treatment. The first monitoring systems used catheters with single (distal) or dual (proximal and distal) pH sensors (Johnson and Demeester 1974). Newer systems use a capsule-based wireless technology, e.g. Bravo™ or OMOM™ pH monitoring systems (Pandolfino and Kwiatek 2008). In addition, methods for pharyngeal pH measurement were developed to assess extra-oesophageal reflux (Jungheim and Ptok 2011; Ayazi et al. 2009).

### 28.6.2.1 Catheter-Based Technology

In catheter-based oesophageal pH-metry, a flexible probe is inserted transnasally, passed through the pharynx, swallowed into the oesophagus, and fixed to the nose. If the probe has one measuring point, it is placed above the lower oesophageal sphincter. If there are two measurement points, the measurement is made in the distal and proximal oesophagus (Jungheim and Ptok 2011; Stein and Wehrmann 2006).

For pharyngeal pH measurement, the measuring probe is also inserted transnasally but is only advanced into the oropharynx. The correct position of the probe can be checked visually through the oral cavity. Patients usually become accustomed to the probe within an hour and the examination is often perceived as more pleasant, since no placement into the oesophagus is necessary (Jungheim and Ptok 2011; Ayazi et al. 2009).

In both systems, an external device records the measured values at intervals of 0.5–5 s (Fig. 28.24). With pharyngeal pH-metry, the transmission is wireless. The measurement can be performed for 24 or 48 h. These examinations are typically carried out as an outpatient examination in order to be able to take into account the individual circumstances of the patient.

### 28.6.2.2 Capsule-Based pH-Metry

Oesophageal pH measurement can also be performed without a catheter by using pH-metry capsules. These capsules (Fig. 28.25) are inserted into the oesophagus through an insertion catheter and attached to the mucosa by vacuum. The mea-

**Fig. 28.24** Example of catheter-based pH-metry: Dx-System (Restech) with kind permission from Restech Reflux Solutions, Houston TX, © 2021 Restech, Inc.

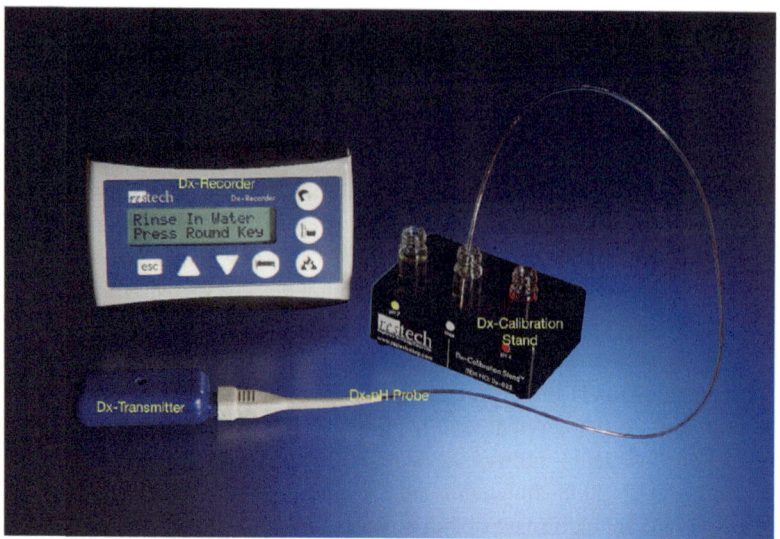

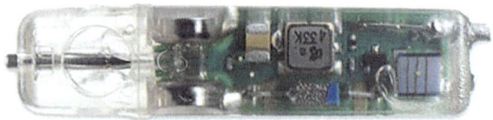

**Fig. 28.25** Example of capsule-based pH-metry: Bravo™ Reflux Capsule with kind permission from Medtronic France, Paris

sured data is transmitted wirelessly to a device that is worn on the belt. The measurement can also be performed over 24 or 48 h. After about 5 days, the capsule dissolves by itself and is excreted. The use of this measuring system avoids irritation by a catheter and allows the patient to have a normal diet and maintain regular activities (Pandolfino and Kwiatek 2008; Stein and Wehrmann 2006).

### 28.6.2.3 Evaluation of pH-Measurements

During the measurement procedure, the patient keeps a log of food intake and of reflux events, e.g. heartburn or coughing, which can be compared to the data collected. In oesophageal pH-metry, pH-values below 4 are considered pathological. After completion of the measurement, further parameters can be evaluated to estimate the extent of the reflux disease. The following parameters are evaluated regularly: total time pH < 4, upright time pH < 4, and supine time pH < 4 (in percentages, respectively), the number of reflux episodes, number of reflux episodes ≥5 min, longest reflux episode (in minutes) (Ward et al. 2004; Pandolfino et al. 2003; Streets et al. 2001). These parameters are also used to calculate the DeMeester-Score, which is used to quantify reflux disease (Jamieson et al. 1992).

In pharyngeal pH measurement, a pH value of 5.5 in the upright position and a pH value of 5 in the lying position are already considered pathological. Analogous to DeMeester-Score, the Ryan-Score can contribute to the quantification of reflux disease (Ayazi et al. 2009).

### 28.6.3 Manometry

#### 28.6.3.1 Multichannel Intraluminal Impedance Devices

Classical pH-metry provides good results in patients with acid reflux but is not sufficient in patients with neutral or basic reflux. This can occur, for example, when patients are on medication to reduce gastric acid, e.g. proton pump inhibitors (PPI). If reflux still occurs in these patients, symptoms such as coughing, heartburn, regurgitation, and chest pain may persist, although endoscopic findings may be unremarkable. To examine these patients, combined probe systems for simultaneous pH and impedance measurement are increasingly used. In fact, up to 35% of patients with non-acid reflux are missed when acidic reflux only is measured. The sensitivity of simple pH monitoring is below 71% and increases to 90% if impedance testing is performed additionally (Sifrim et al. 2004).

Multichannel intraluminal impedance (MII) was first introduced in 1991 (Silny 1991) and combined with pH monitoring (Tutuian et al. 2001). It is based on the measurement of changes in resistance to alternating electrical current (i.e. impedance) by a pair of metallic rings mounted on a catheter when a bolus passes. In the oesophagus, the electric current between the two rings has normally only a low conductivity, resulting in a high resistance. Liquid-containing boluses increase the conductivity when entering the impedance-measuring segment and reduce the impedance to a nadir value. The impedance stays low as long as the bolus is present, returning to baseline once the bolus is cleared by a contraction. Gas passing transiently by the impedance-measuring segments will produce a rapid and high (usually >3000 Ω) rise in the impedance since it offers poor electrical conductance (Boland et al. 2016).

#### 28.6.3.2 High-Resolution Manometry and Impedance

During the swallowing process, in addition to the spatial and temporal coordination of the muscles involved, a proper intraluminal pressure build-up ensures the physiological bolus propulsion. The intraluminal pressure can only be detected reliably by pharyngeal and oesophageal manometry. Manometry was initially used as a complementary diagnostic method in addition to endoscopy and radiological procedures but is now increasingly being used as a primary examination method.

In the beginning, perfusion manometry was used, in which capillaries of a polyvinyl-catheter are continuously perfused with water, so that conclusions can be made about the ambient pressures in the area of the capillary openings (Jungheim et al. 2013; Meyer et al. 2012; Fox and Bredenoord 2008). These systems have the disadvantage that they have to be laboriously calibrated, have a low measuring frequency, and often only a low resolution. Additionally, the permanent water perfusion may cause irritation, e.g. in the larynx. For these reasons, high-resolution manometry (HRM) is now widely used, which allows a high temporal and spatial resolution, owing to the use of electronic pressure transducers on the HRM catheter (Fox and Bredenoord 2008; Massey 2013). In addition, an impedance measurement can be integrated into the HRM probes in order to obtain information about the position of the bolus.

HRM is aimed at examining the structural integrity, the peristaltic function, and the bolus transport in order to detect pathologies in the swallowing process. For accurate diagnosis, the HRM study is evaluated together with the symptoms of the patient (Massey 2013).

In order to carry out the measurement, the HRM probe (Fig. 28.26) is introduced transna-

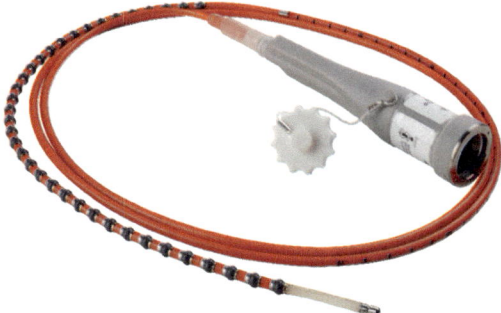

**Fig. 28.26** High-Resolution Manometry Probe Catheter Oe-S-36KI with kind permission by Standard Instruments GmbH, Karlsruhe, Germany

sally and, depending on the length of the probe, positioned so that the measurement area covers the oesophagus first. In a second measurement phase, the probe is pulled back to cover the pharyngeal structures.

Isolated measurements of the oesophagus or pharynx are also possible. The upper and lower oesophageal sphincter can be directly identified owing to their permanent resting pressure; the other structures can only be visualised during swallowing activity (Fox and Bredenoord 2008; Massey 2013). The sphincters can be used to

determine the optimal position of the probe. The acquired data can be displayed in a continuous graph for each pressure sensor or as a spatiotemporal-pressure plot (Fig. 28.27) (Clouse and Staiano 1993).

With the HRM data, the motor function of the involved muscles can be examined precisely. Pathologies, such as motility disorders, hyper- or hypo-contractility, and interruptions in the peristaltic wave can be detected on the spatiotemporal-pressure plot (e.g. see Figs. 28.28, 28.29, and 28.30). A large number

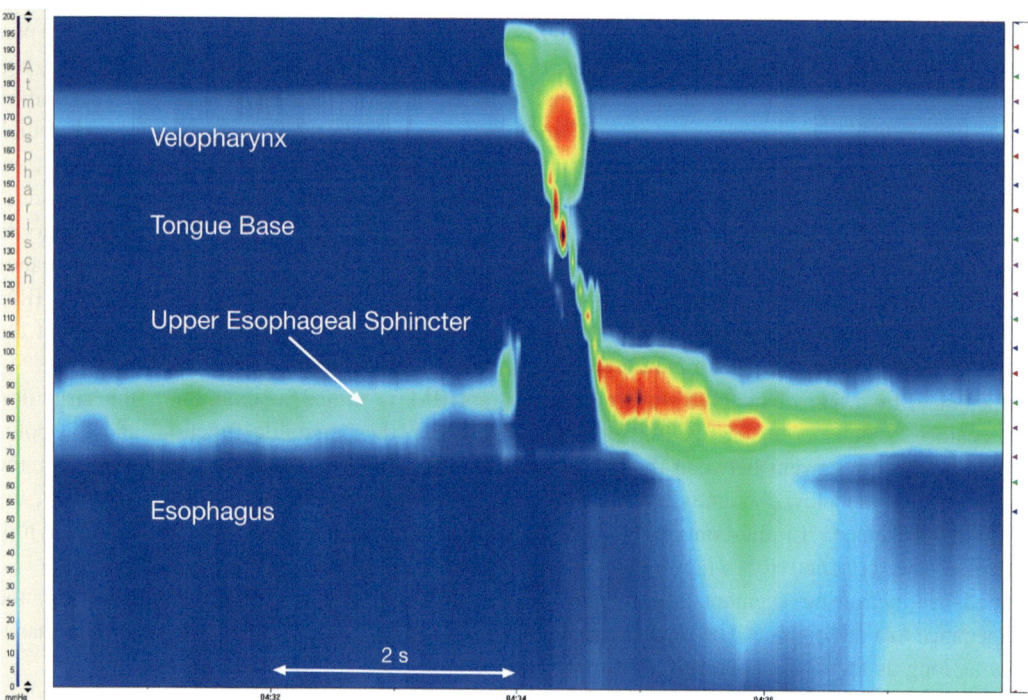

**Fig. 28.27** Pharyngeal high-resolution manometry: spatiotemporal-pressure plot of a 2 mL water bolus swallow. Abscissa: time, ordinate: probe position, colouring on scale left: actual pressure (mmHg). The regions of interest (velopharynx, tongue base, upper oesophageal sphincter, and oesophagus) are indicated. (Figure by Michael Jungheim with kind permission of Laborie, Mississauga, Canada)

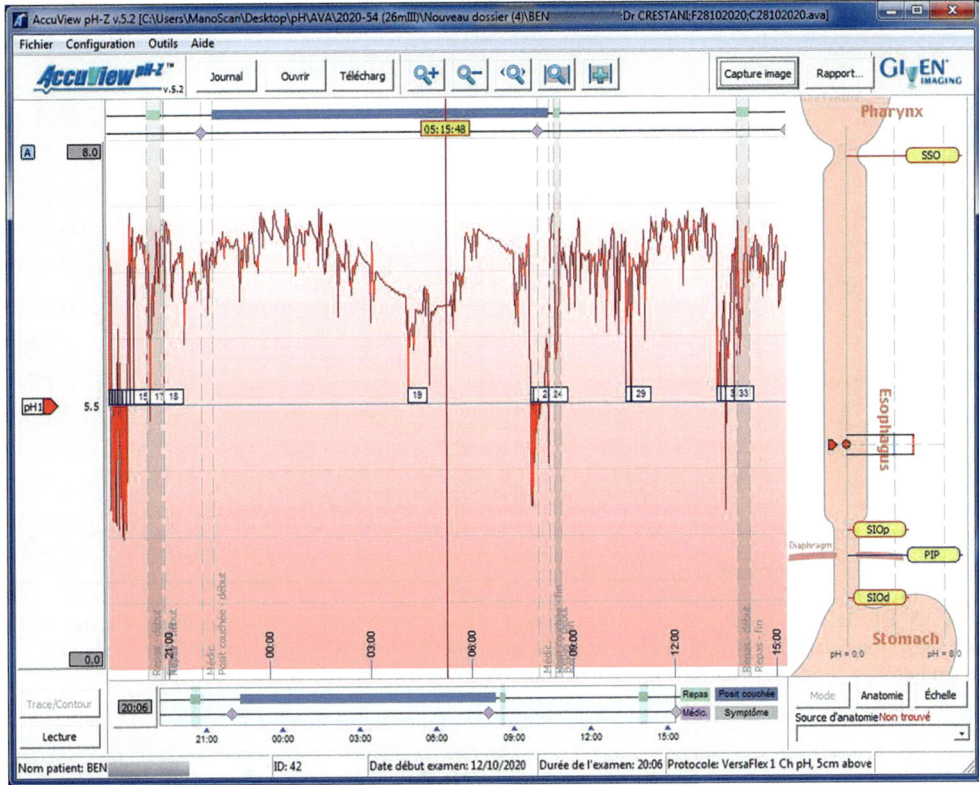

**Fig. 28.28** GERD on therapy with PPI (HR-manometry: low UES and LES pressures, ineffective oesophageal motility). (Figure by Marie-Françoise Napoleon, Clinique Rive Gauche, Toulouse, France with kind permission of Medtronic France, Paris)

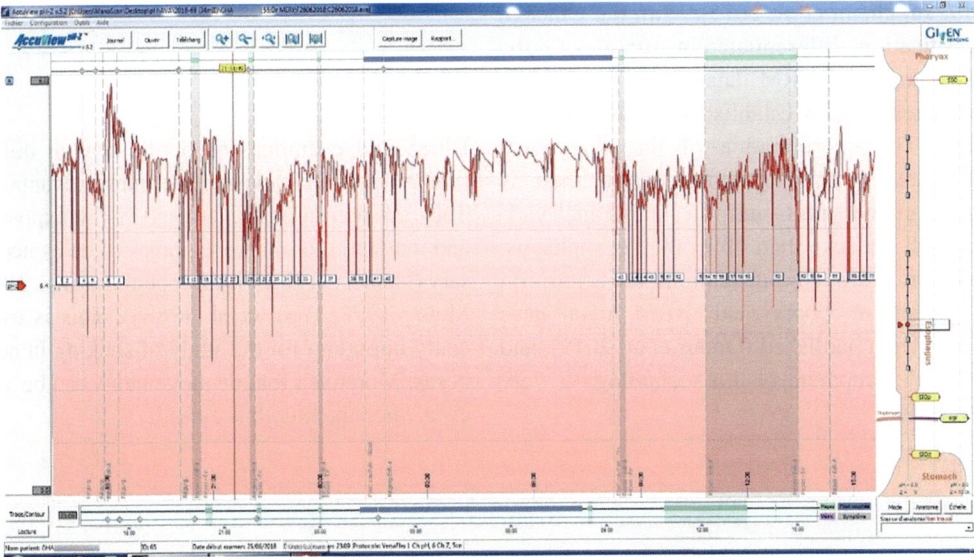

**Fig. 28.29** Correlation with weak acid reflux (HR-manometry: ineffective oesophageal motility, lack of upper airway protection). (Figure by Marie-Françoise Napoleon, Clinique Rive Gauche, Toulouse, France with kind permission of Medtronic France, Paris)

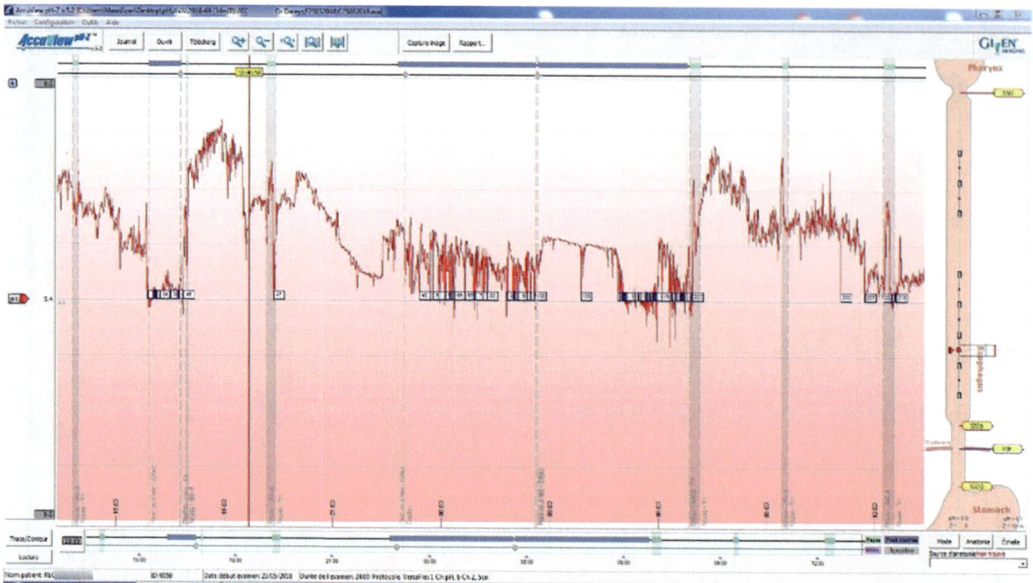

**Fig. 28.30** GERD with probable dysfunction of lower oesophageal sphincter (LES) (HR-manometry: absent contractility, low LES pressure). (Figure by Marie-Françoise Napoleon, Clinique Rive Gauche, Toulouse, France with kind permission of Medtronic France, Paris)

of different parameters have been proposed for evaluating the motor function. Accurate interpretation of parameters requires normative data, which are available for both the oesophagus and the pharynx (Kahrilas et al. 2015; Omari et al. 2019; Jungheim et al. 2015). With the Chicago Classification, differentiated instructions for the interpretation of HRM data of the oesophagus have already been established (Kahrilas et al. 2015). The interpretation of the pharyngeal HRM data is more difficult because there is often a greater intra- and inter-individual variance of values than for the oesophagus. However, first recommendations for a uniform evaluation of pharyngeal HRM data have already been published (Omari et al. 2019), and further development of this technology is very promising.

## 28.7 Sonography of the Tongue During Swallowing and Infant Sucking

Wolfgang Angerstein

### 28.7.1 Introduction

Ultrasound examinations of the tongue during swallowing and sucking have many advantages. They are non-invasive, have no X-ray-exposure, and may therefore be repeated as often as necessary (Fanucci et al. 1994; Koppenburg et al. 1988; Müßig 1992; Wein et al. 1988a). This is especially important for the study of sucking in newborns. Moreover, tongue movements can be seen even when the mouth is closed.

## 28.7.2 Examination Methods

The equipment[1] necessary for sonography of the tongue is described in Sect. 11.15 of Volume 1. A 5 or 7.5 MHz transducer with a 90° or 100° sector is needed (convex for adults, linear for babies), which is placed submentally lengthwise beneath the chin. The monitor should be split, showing the two-dimensional B-mode image on one side and the corresponding (T)M-mode image on the other side (Cheng et al. 2002; Kikyo et al. 1999; Peng et al. 1995, 2000, 2003; Watkin 1999). Usually, the transducer is handheld by the examiner. This might cause artefacts due to unvoluntary movements of the transducer or the head of the patient. In clinical routine, these blurring effects can be tolerated (Chi-Fishman 2005). For exact and reproducible scientific measurements, however, the transducer and the head of the patient should be fixed. Head and transducer stabilisation are important to eliminate motion artefacts (Chi-Fishman 2005; Peng et al. 1995, 2000, 2007; Stone and Davis 1995). Adults are examined in a sitting position on a chair, babies lie comfortably and cozy in the arms of their mothers. Some researchers prefer an additional transbuccal scanning approach for newborns (Fanucci et al. 1994; Smith et al. 1985).

## 28.7.3 Normal Tongue Motions During Swallowing

The physiological tongue movements during swallowing can be subdivided into a sequence of different phases running consecutively one after the other. Most researchers divide these subsequent tongue movements during a normal swallow into four phases (Böckler et al. 1989; Fuhrmann and Diedrich 1992, 1993; Ohtsuka et al. 1998; Peng et al. 2003; Shawker et al. 1984; Wein et al. 1988a, 1991, 1993a).

Initially, the tongue dorsum is in close contact with the hard and soft palate (see Fig. 28.31, 1).

When a bolus enters the mouth, the tip of the tongue is lowered to collect the bolus (collection phase) (see Fig. 28.31, 2–4). Afterwards the tip of the tongue is elevated to the hard palate, hereby the bolus is loaded and shovelled into a groove in the middle of the tongue (see Fig. 28.31, 5–7). The posterior third of the tongue is still elevated and has loose contact with the hard palate (loading phase or shovelling phase or preparation phase, since the bolus is prepared for reaching the hypopharynx). Then the posterior third of the tongue is rapidly lowered, so that the bolus can flow down into the hypopharynx (transport phase or displacement phase, since the bolus is displaced into the hypopharynx). This very short and quick third phase is the genuine effective swallowing movement of the tongue (see Fig. 28.31, 8). Finally, the tongue returns to its initial resting position (final or resting phase) (see Fig. 28.31, 9–10).

During these swallowing phases, the tongue dorsum movements can be seen in real-time midsagittal ultrasound B-mode sectional images. Corresponding simultaneous (T)M-mode scans show the typical pattern of sequential downward and upward movements of the tongue dorsum on a timeline (see Fig. 28.32a–f) (Cheng et al. 2002; Kikyo et al. 1999; Peng et al. 2007).

These (T)M-mode scans may also detect double or triple swallows and incomplete swallowing attempts (see Fig. 28.33a–c). ©Angerstein2021.

## 28.7.4 Normal Tongue Motions During Infant Sucking

Tongue motions during sucking of babies (either at their mother's breasts or during bottle feeding) can also be easily and reproducible examined by ultrasound.

Initially, the anterior third of the baby's tongue slides under its mother's nipple or the pacifier. Optimally, the tip of the nipple/pacifier should be placed close to the hard-soft palate junction of the baby (Geddes et al. 2008, 2017; Sakalidis et al. 2012). The tongue squeezes the nipple/pacifier from underneath, while the tip of the nipple/pacifier is in close contact with the hard-soft palate

---

[1] My special thanks go to Dipl.-Ing. Ursula Willems (Canon Medical Systems, Neuss/Germany) for providing us with the equipment and technical support free of charge.

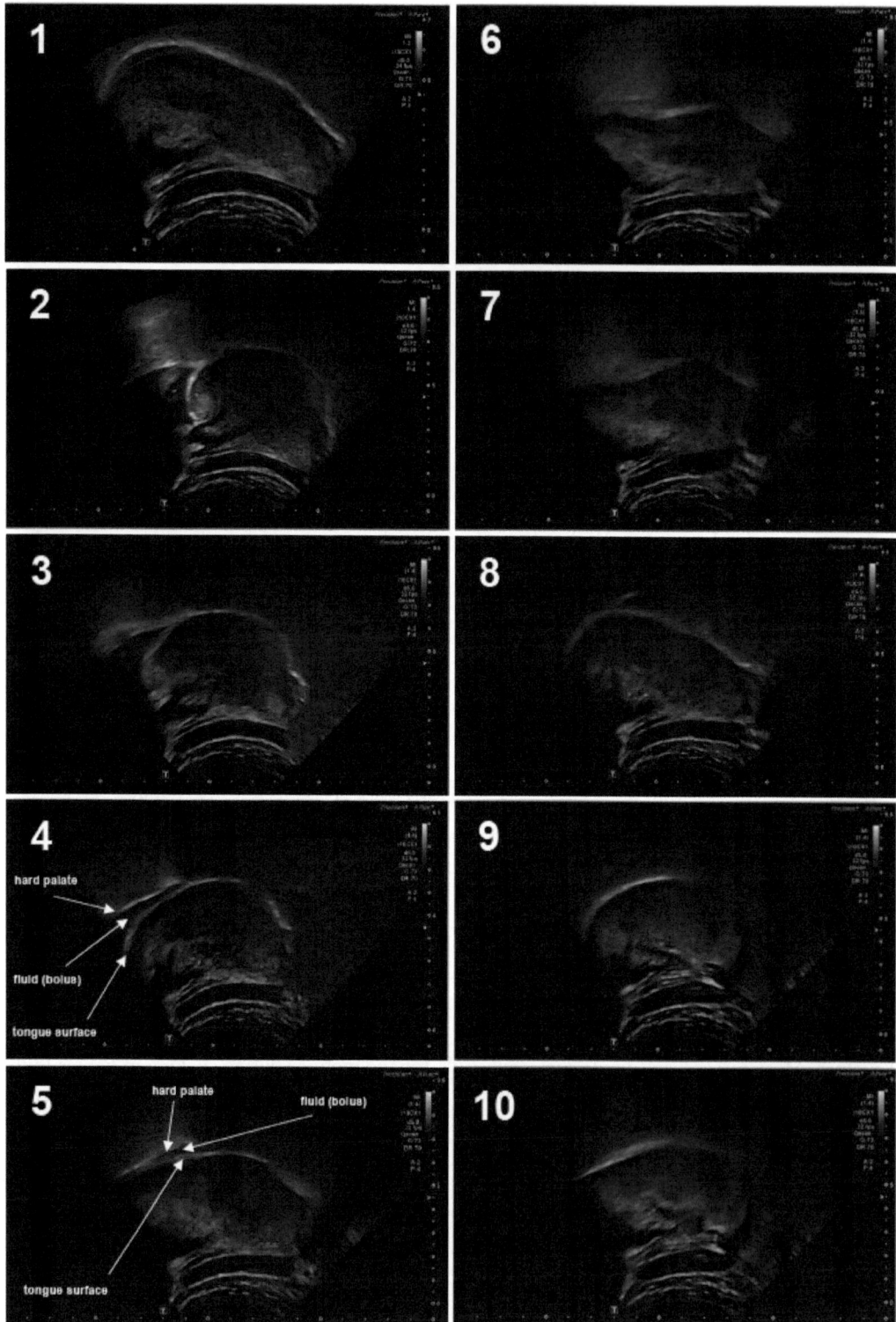

**Fig. 28.31** (1–10) Physiological tongue movements during swallowing (midsagittal B-mode scans). (©Angerstein2021)

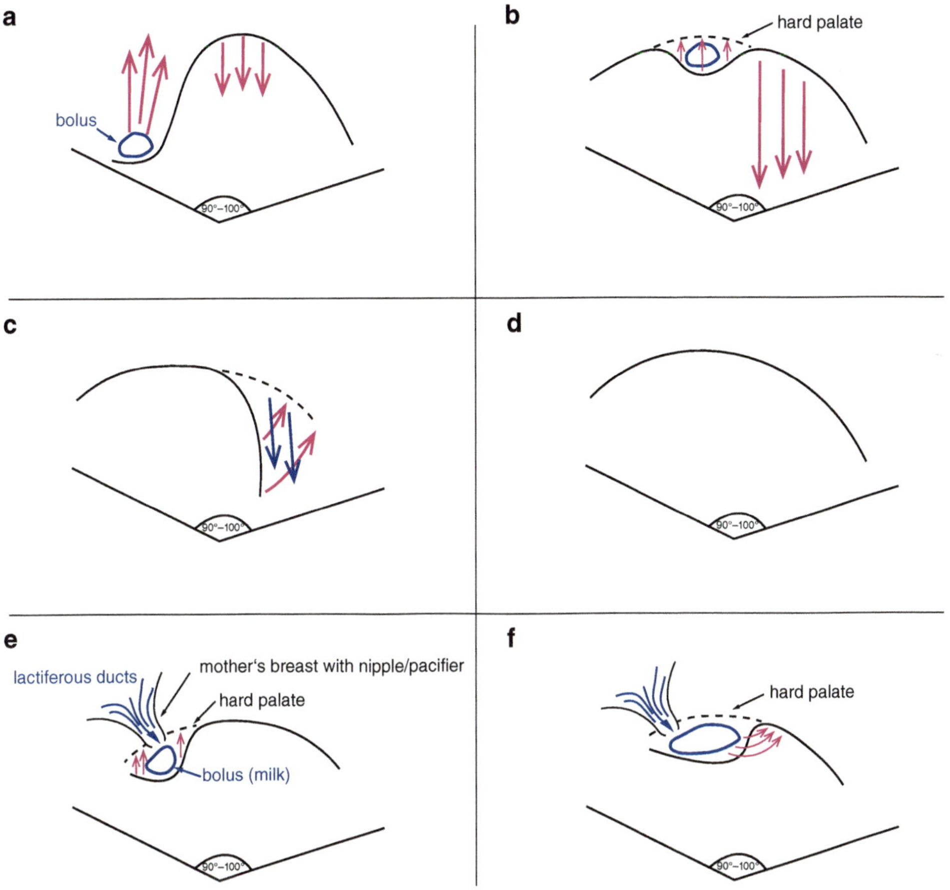

**Fig. 28.32** (a–f) Schematic midsagittal B-mode scans of the tongue dorsum during physiological swallowing and infant sucking. (a) Top left collection phase, (b) top right loading/shovelling/preparation phase, (c) middle left transport/displacement phase, (d) middle right final/rest- ing phase, (e) bottom left milking phase (overpressure), (f) bottom right suction phase (negative pressure/vacuum) (red arrows = tongue dorsum movements/blue = liquid bolus). (©Angerstein2021)

junction that lies above. Thus, the tip of the nipple/pacifier is compressed between the baby's tongue (from below) and the palate (from above). The milk is driven out by the resulting overpressure (the so-called milking phase). Afterwards, the whole tongue retracts backwards (in a dorso-cranial direction), resulting in a negative pressure (vacuum) within the anterior oral cavity. In this way, the rest of the milk is sucked out of the mother's lactiferous ducts (the so-called suction phase). Subsequently, the milk is swallowed according to the multiphase tongue movements described above. Thus, infantile sucking is a combination of alternating overpressure (milking) and negative pressure/vacuum (suction) within the baby's mouth. In older publications, squeezing of the

nipple/pacifier (resulting in overpressure) was regarded as the main reason for milk flow (Bosma et al. 1990; Fanucci et al. 1994; Hayashi et al. 1997; Weber et al. 1986). Recent literature, how-ever, considers the vacuum (negative pressure) as much more important for removal of milk from the breast/bottle, whereas peristaltic compression of the nipple/pacifier seems to be much less crucial (Geddes et al. 2008, 2012, 2017; Wein et al. 1993a). Therefore, the larger amount of milk reaches the baby's mouth during the suction phase. During the milking phase, milk flow is consider-ably smaller. Sucking and swallowing movements of the neonatal tongue are sometimes so fast that slow motion sequences are needed for detailed evaluation.

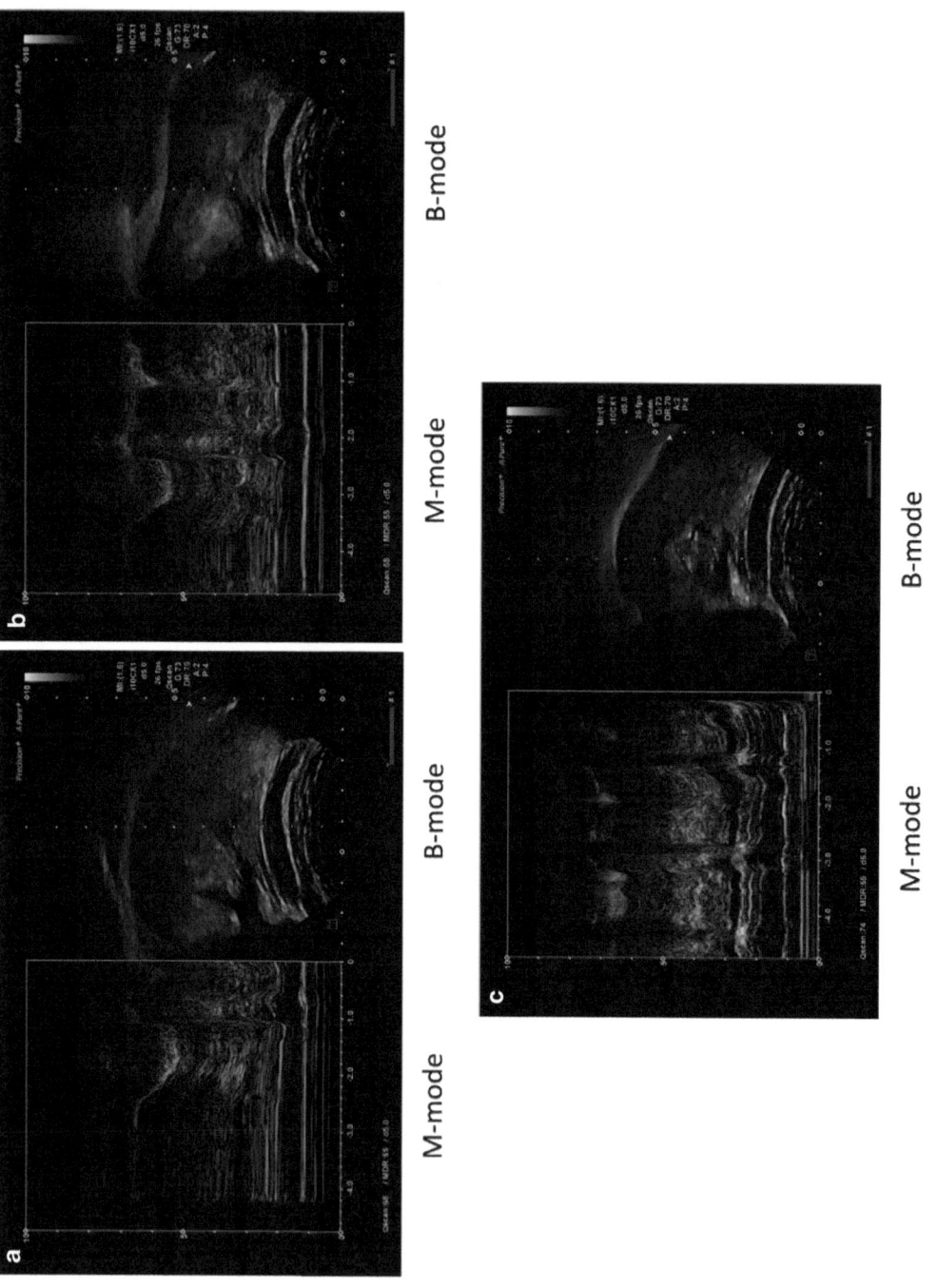

**Fig. 28.33** (**a**) M- and B-mode ultrasound scans of normal swallowing. (©Angerstein2021). (**b**) M- and B-mode ultrasound scans of normal swallowing with a subsequent incomplete post-deglutitive swallowing attempt. (©Angerstein2021). (**c**) M- and B-mode ultrasound scans of a triple swallow. (©Angerstein2021)

When the milking-suction cycle is insufficient (e.g. in cases of neonatal drinking weakness due to orofacial muscular hypotonia of the baby), the newborns suffer from impaired nutrition, and breast milk partly remains within the mother's lactiferous ducts where it may cause mastitis. Therefore, sonographic examination of infantile sucking and swallowing is clinically important in cases of neonatal drinking/feeding problems.

## 28.7.5 Possible Diagnostic Applications of Ultrasound of Tongue Movements

Other medical indications for ultrasound (B-mode, (T)M-mode) investigations of disturbed tongue movements during swallowing may be:

- Tongue thrust during visceral swallowing (often seen in combination with malocclusion of the front teeth/frontal open bite) (Kikyo et al. 1999; Peng et al. 2003, 2004).
- Cleft lip and palate (Koppenburg et al. 1988).
- Neurological disorders (e.g. Parkinson's disease, amyotrophic lateral sclerosis (ALS), stroke) (Wein et al. 1988a, 1991, 1998).
- Malignomas of the oral cavity (especially cancer of the tongue or the floor of the mouth) (Wein et al. 1991).

## 28.7.6 Digital Developments and Advances

During the last 35 years, multiple software algorithms for automated digital contour tracking and extraction of the tongue dorsum shape from ultrasound images were developed. Here is a short overview of the progress:

- Initially, 2D (a single plane or a single cross section, e.g. sagittal or coronal) B-mode images were used to visualise the tongue dorsum (Chi-Fishman 2005).
- When these 2D images are lined up on a time scale, temporal representations of the tongue

dorsum movements result (Böckler et al. 1989; Kikyo et al. 1999; Miller and Kang 2007; Wein et al. 1988a, b, 1991, 1993a, b, 1998). Such time-dependent image sequences are called pseudo-3D reconstructions.

- Real spatial 3D recordings of the tongue require algorithms for processing volume data (Chi-Fishman 2005; Watkin 1999).
- If the 3D images are moving, they are called 4D (Chi-Fishman 2005). Thus, 4D recordings are real-time "live" 3D recordings or live streamings of 3D images ("live 3D in motion").
- Finally, enhanced 4D (also called high resolution 4D, high definition (HD) 4D, or HD live) images were recently introduced by several commercial producers. Those moving 3D pictures with detailed surface profiles and realistic colours are advertised as 5D.

This rapid development highlights the digital progress in sonographic visualisation of tongue motions. And some ultrasound companies already philosophise about 6D.

## 28.8 Health-Related Quality-of-Life (HRQoL) Questionnaires for Swallowing Disorders

Devora Kiagiadaki, Mieke Moerman, and Christina Pflug

## 28.8.1 Dysphagia and Health-Related Quality of Life

Dysphagia has implications for morbidity, mortality, and health-related quality of life (HRQoL) (Logeman 1998). In congruence with the World Health Organization (WHO) definition of "health" (Centers for Disease Control and Prevention 1948), HRQoL is the physical and mental health, and social well-being, of a person or a group over time (Centers for Disease Control and Prevention 2014). The "Functional Health Status" (FHS) refers more precisely to the functioning in variable domains (physical, social, psychological) and how that ability is lost or limited owing to a disease or its treatment (Speyer et al. 2014). In 2001, WHO established the "International Classification of Functioning, Disability and Health" (ICF) (WHO 2001), which allows comparison of all conditions of health and disability with regard to their impact on the functioning of the individual.

There is a variety of self-administered instruments for evaluation of HRQoL—even disease-specific for dysphagic patients. Most dysphagia-specific questionnaires also have a component of specific functional health status, but of low methodological quality (Speyer et al. 2014).

For routine use in clinical practice, HRQoL questionnaires should fulfil a number of characteristics and objectives. They should:

- Be self-administered, easy, and time-saving.
- Evaluate the natural course of disease and the effects of treatment, facilitate clinical decisions, and improve the quality of care.
- Identify and prioritise restrictions.
- Facilitate communication.
- Screen for hidden or overlooked problems (Higginson and Carr 2001).

## 28.8.2 Generic QoL Instruments

An example of a validated and broadly used generic instrument is the "Short Form Health Survey" (SF-36), which is a multi-item scale, measuring vitality, physical functioning, bodily pain, general health perceptions, physical role functioning, social role functioning, emotional role functioning, and mental health (Ware and Sherbourne 1992).

## 28.8.3 Dysphagia-Specific QoL Questionnaires

In accordance with the objectives and recommendations of the "Union of the European Phoniatricians" (UEP), four dysphagia-specific questionnaires are reviewed, which fulfil the criteria of adequate psychometric quality and interpretability. They all have been developed and validated in adult populations with oropharyngeal dysphagia of multiple aetiology (swallowing quality-of-life questionnaire (SWAL-QoL), Deglutition Handicap Index (DHI), Dysphagia Handicap Index (D'HI)) and specific aetiology M.D. Anderson Dysphagia Inventory (MDADI) for head and neck cancer (Higginson and Carr 2001).

### 28.8.3.1 Swallowing Quality-of-Life Questionnaire (SWAL-QoL)

The SWAL-QoL was established by using data from adult patients with structural or neurological oropharyngeal dysphagia. In the final phase (III) of validation (McHorney et al. 2002), a questionnaire with 44 items divided into 10 scales was presented, relating to various aspects of the impact of dysphagia on everyday life (Table 28.8).

This questionnaire allows a differentiation between normal adults and patients and an assessment of the different degrees of dysphagia. The SWAL-QoL is characterised by a convergent validity that is shown in a positive correlation with the generic SF-36 (McHorney et al. 2002).

In addition, the SWAL-CARE, a 15-item questionnaire to assess quality of care and patient satisfaction, was simultaneously developed and validated.

### 28.8.3.2 M.D. Anderson Dysphagia Inventory (MDADI)

The MDADI was developed to study the effects of dysphagia on quality of life in patients with head and neck cancer (Chen et al. 2001). It consists of four subscales (global, emotional, functional, physical) with five to eight items. The MDADI has been used in follow-up studies regarding the evaluation of swallowing outcomes after surgery, e.g. for glottal cancer (Peretti et al. 2013) or cerebellopontine angle surgery (Starmer et al. 2014).

Convergent validity was verified by positive correlations of MDADI subscales and domains of the SF-36 (vitality, social functioning, role-emotional domain). It has been translated and validated in several languages, e.g. Swedish (Carlsson et al. 2012), Italian (Schindler et al. 2008), Brazilian (Guedes et al. 2013) Korean (Kwon et al. 2013) and Dutch (Samuels et al. 2021).

**Table 28.8** Dysphagia-specific quality-of-life questionnaires © J.C. Nienstedt 2018

| Dysphagia-specific QoL questionnaires | Swallowing quality-of-life questionnaire (SWAL-QoL) | M.D. Anderson Dysphagia Inventory (MDADI) | Deglutition Handicap Index (DHI) | Dysphagia Handicap Index (D'HI) | Feeding/Swallowing Impact Survey (FS-IS) |
|---|---|---|---|---|---|
| **Structure** | *A total of 44 items divided into 10 scales* | *A total of 20 items divided into 4 scales* | *A total of 30 items divided into 3 scales (10 per scale)* | *A total of 25 items divided into 3 scales and one question for self-perceived dysphagia severity on a 7-point equal-appearing interval scale* | *A total of 18 items divided into 3 scales* |
| **Validated for** | *Adults* | *Adults* | *Adults* | *Adults* | *Children (median age: 14 months; IQR 7, 35)* |
| *– With aetiology of dysphagia* | *Any* | *Specific: head and neck cancer patients* | *Any* | *Any* | *Any* |
| **(Sub-) Scales** | *– Burden (2)*<br>*– Eating duration (2)*<br>*– Eating desire (3)*<br>*– Food selection (2)*<br>*– Communication (2)*<br>*– Fear (4)*<br>*– Mental health (5)*<br>*– Social functioning (5)*<br>*– Fatigue (3)*<br>*– Sleep (2)* | *– Global (1)*<br>*– Emotional (6)*<br>*– Functional (5)*<br>*– Physical (8)* | *– Physical (10)*<br>*– Functional (10)*<br>*– Emotional (10)* | *– Physical (9)*<br>*– Functional (9)*<br>*– Emotional (7)*<br>*– Self-perceived severity (1)* | *– Daily activities (5)*<br>*– Worry (7)*<br>*– Feeding difficulties (6)* |
| **Patient's agreement** | *++/+/0/–/–* | *++/+/0/–/–* | | | |
| **Duration** | *++/+/0/–/–* | | | | |
| Frequency | *++/+/0/–/–* | | *++/+/0/–/–* | *++/0/–* | *++/+/0/–/–* |
| **Scoring** | *Range 0–100 (most-least favourable state)* | *Range 20–100 (extremely low-high functioning) global subscale is scored individually, all other are summed, and the mean score multiplied by 20* | *Range from 0 to 120 (least-most disabled)* | *Range from 0 to 100 (no-extremely severe impairment).*<br>*++/0/– scored: 4/2/0* | *All items summed, divided, and average score calculated* |

*++/+/0/–/–:* **Patient's agreement** (strongly, agree, uncertain, disagree, strongly disagree), **Duration** (all of the time, most of the time, some of the time, a little of the time, none of the time), **Frequency** ((almost) always, often, sometimes, hardly ever, never) of the stated condition; *IQR Interquartile Range Calculator*

### 28.8.3.3 Deglutition Handicap Index (DHI)

The DHI was designed on the model of the "Voice Handicap Index" by Woisard et al. (2006), Woisard and Lepage (2010), and Crestani et al. (2011) and validated for patients with dysphagia of any aetiology. It is a 3-scale model (physical, functional, emotional) with 30 items and available in French and English.

### 28.8.3.4 Dysphagia Handicap Index (D'HI)

The D'HI was developed by Silbergleit et al. (2012) to assess the disabling effect of dysphagia of different aetiology (neurological, oesophageal, reflux-related, postoperative, unknown). It has a 3-scale construct (physical, functional, emotional) with 25 items and one question for global dysphagia, rated on a visual analogue scale (VAS 0–7). The D'HI is easy to understand and may therefore be used in individuals with lower literacy levels. Initially developed in English, the D'HI has been validated in recent years in various languages including Iranian (Asadollahpour et al. 2015), Arabic (Farahat et al. 2014), and Japanese (Oda et al. 2017).

### 28.8.4 Paediatric Dysphagia-Related HRQoL Measures

To date, there are no universally validated HRQoL measures available for clinical use that focus on paediatric dysphagia. The Feeding/Swallowing Impact Survey (FS-IS) (Lefton-Greif et al. 2014) was designed to measure and improve understanding of the issues of caregivers for children with deglutition disorders. In an observational cross-sectional study, children with a median age of 14 months and their parents were included. All children had different diagnoses, all of which led to feeding/swallowing problems or restrictions in the parents' daily lives. The FS-IS has a 3-scale structure (daily activities, worry, feeding difficulties) and 18 items. Although FS-IS is well orientated and potentially useful, it lacks quality in terms of internal validity (use of a control group) and reproducibility and has yet to be validated in an extended population.

### 28.8.5 HRQoL in the Elderly with Dysphagia

Swallowing difficulties are common in the elderly, owing to normal ageing or comorbidities (e.g. neurological, neurodegenerative) or both.

Although there have been no questionnaires especially designed for dysphagia in geriatric populations, dysphagia impact QoL can be assessed by any of the validated, fore-mentioned instruments for adults (Chen et al. 2009).

### 28.8.6 Questionnaires for Primary Diseases That Often Result in Oropharyngeal Dysphagia

Timmerman et al. (2014) reviewed a number of questionnaires for other primary diseases that combine the "Functional Health Status" and the HRQoL: the European Dysphagia Group Questionnaire (EDGQ), and three modules for specific patient populations used as a supplement to the European Organisation for Research and Treatment of Cancer Quality of Life Questionnaire (QLQ-C30), the gastric cancer module (EORTC QLQ-STO22), the oesophageal, oesophagogastric junction, or gastric cancer module (EORTC QLQ-OG25), and the head and neck cancer module (EORTC QLQ-H&N35). However, they contain only a limited number of items or subscales for dysphagia and therefore cannot be considered dysphagia-specific.

Moreover, Speyer et al. (2014) include the DYMUS (dysphagia in multiple sclerosis questionnaire) in the list of oropharyngeal dysphagia-related "functional health status" questionnaires. DYMUS is useful for assessing dysphagia symptoms in patients with multiple sclerosis and thus can be considered more a screening tool rather than a HRQoL questionnaire (Bergamaschi et al. 2009).

### 28.8.7 Summary

From the questionnaires described above, the clinician/phoniatrician has a choice of four validated dysphagia-specific HRQoL instruments that fulfil the necessary quality requirements: the SWAL-QoL, the MDADI, the DHI, and the D'HI. The SWAL-QoL is the longer and the more detailed one and is of high psychometric quality, assessing dysphagia under the International

Classification of Functioning, Disability and Health (ICF) concept as well. The DHI is shorter and available in French and English. The D'HI is the shortest questionnaire, requiring possibly less effort by the patient. Finally, the MDADI is useful for oncological patients and is also available in four languages other than English.

In the future, further efforts should be made to validate these questionnaires in larger and multicentre studies involving paediatric populations. In addition, follow-up studies are needed to develop validated treatment recommendations for better improved quality of health care.

## 28.9 Automatic Digital Recording of Swallowing

Frank Müller and Christina Pflug

### 28.9.1 Introduction

The aim of swallowing diagnostics is to assess the patient's act of swallowing and to detect the pathophysiology. It assesses motor and sensory functions, such as pharyngeal residues, decreased swallowing frequency, or penetration/aspiration. Only an accurate diagnosis allows a targeted therapy and the evaluation of the patient's individual aspiration risk. An experienced clinician will follow an examination protocol and use diagnostic equipment. For many years, the gold standard of a detailed examination was videofluoroscopy with its disadvantage of X-irradiation, among others. With improved image quality in recent years, endoscopy has become a good alternative approach with lack of radiation exposure and some other advantages (Langmore 2003).

One question in clinical swallowing diagnostics is the relevance of findings for the everyday situation during food intake, drinking, or unconscious saliva transport. Recordings of these events would give the clinician valuable supplemental information. The basis of such recordings is a mobile recording system with an automatic detection of the swallowing process. With this information, the recorded data may be reduced to short samples or contain markers in a continuous recording.

### 28.9.2 Detection of Swallowing Events

An established screening test for the detection of aspiration and laryngeal penetration is cervical auscultation. A stethoscope is placed on the neck and a trained examiner listens to the sounds during swallowing. Leslie et al. (2007) questioned the evidence of the procedure, but the non-invasive approach and the sound processing on computers are reasons for research teams to follow this direction. Dudik et al. (2015) have provided an overview on various approaches to analysing this signal.

For simple swallowing events in a quiet situation, the listening-based detection of swallowing sounds works as reliably as multichannel physiological recordings (Crary et al. 2013) and has been used to analyse swallowing frequency. Golabbakhsh et al. (2014) used a skin-mounted microphone to detect spontaneous swallowing and reached a sensitivity of 87% (specificity: 78%). The challenge in the processing of microphone signals is to separate breathing, coughs, speech, and room sounds from the swallowing sound.

With a separate nostril microphone (Fig. 28.34), Fukuike et al. (2015) could detect breathing sounds and exclude those events from those of the swallows. With the help of a foot pedal (Fig. 28.35), the test persons marked the swallowing events and a sensitivity of the algorithm of 97% was determined (specificity: 95%). During the recording, no examiner is necessary but the sound analysis afterwards requires an expert.

At least the influence of room sounds can be reduced by using contact microphones or accelerometers on the skin instead of airborne microphones. Damouras et al. (2010) glued an accelerometer on the skin outside the larynx and reached a precision of 93% in healthy subjects and 40% in dysphagic patients. Lee et al. (2011) assumed that the recording of the nasal airflow

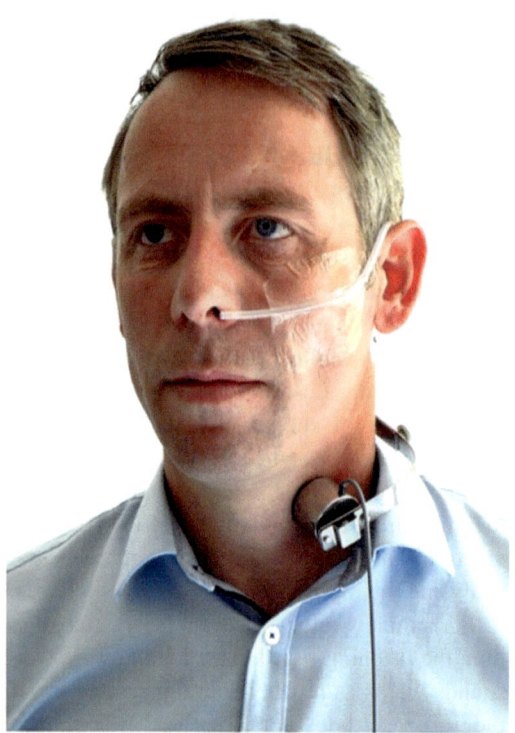

**Fig. 28.34** Typical placement of nostril microphone and contact microphone for a swallowing sound recording

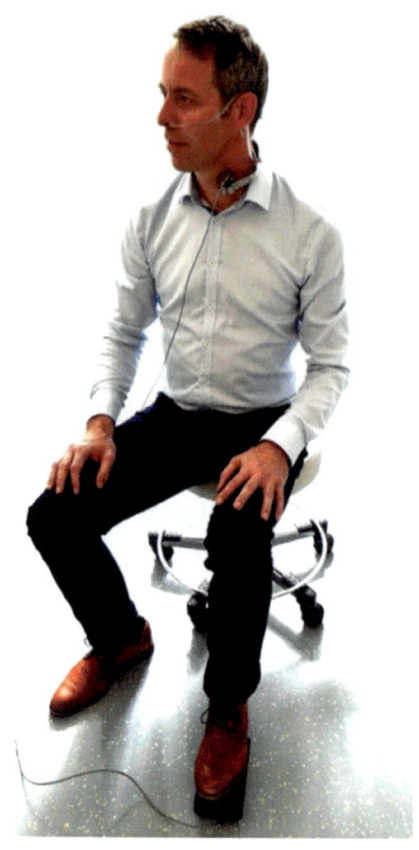

**Fig. 28.35** Setup with foot pedal. Here, the test subject marks the swallowing events during data recording. This information can be used to analyse the swallowing signals at those times or to provide a gold standard for evaluation of automatic swallowing detection

signal would improve the data analysis. During physiological swallowing, the airway closes (swallow apnoea). The team did not intend to detect swallowing events automatically, but to gain information on supraglottal and laryngeal closure. This approach was abandoned when the team found swallowing apnoea in patients with total laryngectomy, obviously without closure of laryngeal structures.

Alternative signals for swallowing detection come from the muscle activity (EMG) and the change of bio-impedance due to closing of the airway during each swallow. Schultheiss et al. (2014) used this signal combination and reached a sensitivity of 96% (specificity: 97%). This requires a laboratory setup but is independent of room noise or speech production. Lee et al. (2009) tried the combination of four signals (two-dimensional accelerometry, nasal airflow, mechanomyogram—MMG) and concluded that more signals led to a better swallowing detec-

tion accuracy (sensitivity 98%, specificity 95%, accuracy 94%) A non-contact approach for swallowing detection is the use of depth cameras in combination with artificial intelligence (AI). Lai et al. (2023) presented the stereo video sequences to several AI networks and reached a predictive performance (adjusted F1) of 0.885 when trying to classify swallowing and non-swallowing events.

A side branch of swallowing detection is the detection of drinking. Kobayashi and Mineno (2014) used a throat contact microphone to estimate daily water intake. They found a detection accuracy for drinking of 95% in relation to other events such as eating, breathing, and talking.

### 28.9.3 Diagnostics of Swallowing Events

Besides the mere detection of swallowing events, there is current research on categorising the quality of swallowing into diagnostic groups. Lim et al. (2001) used a pulse oximeter to detect aspiration in stroke patients. The group reported a sensitivity of 77% and a specificity of 83%, using flexible endoscopic evaluation of swallowing (FEES) as reference. Nikjoo (2011) used an accelerometer signal from the neck surface to distinguish between safe and unsafe swallows, i.e. swallows in which the bolus enters the airway. The sensitivity achieved was 97%, the specificity 64% (accuracy 80%). Lee et al. (2006) tested the separation of normal swallows and aspirations by means of an accelerometer signal with an accuracy of 80%. A mobile "aspirometre" prototype for paediatric surveillance has been developed (Lee et al. 2006). Later this group tried to distinguish between "depth-of-airway invasion", "bolus clearance from the valleculae", and "bolus clearance from the pyriform sinuses" (Lee et al. 2011). The team reported accuracy values of 75%, 84%, and 84%, respectively. Dudik et al. (2018) tried the combination of a two-dimensional accelerometer signal on the skin outside the larynx with a nearby contact microphone. From the additional information from the microphone, the algorithm could find statistically significant differences of thin versus viscous boluses. Miyagi et al. (2020) used a single neck-mounted microphone in combination with artificial intelligence of support vector machines (SVMs) to separate the recordings of swallow events in normal and abnormal regarding the VE swallowing test. The maximum accuracy with optimised parameters was 78%. Recently, Frakking (2022) used a contact microphone on the neck in combination with speech recognition technology to distinguish between normal and aspirating swallows. The demonstrated sensitivity of 89% and specificity of 100% (accuracy 98%) for the detection of aspiration was superior to the results described above.

### 28.9.4 Mobile Devices

Pehlivan et al. (1996) tested a mobile device termed a "digital phagometer", which records the vertical movement of the larynx with a piezoelectric sensor on the skin. The agreement of detected swallows and visual control was reported to be in "perfect agreement". The device was used to determine the swallowing rate of normal subjects and patients with Parkinson disease. The mean swallowing rate of the patient group was significantly lower ($p < 0.05$, normal subjects: 1.18 swallows per minute, patients: 0.80).

Lee et al. (2006) proposed a mobile device called an "aspirometer" for paediatric surveillance. The group provided an algorithm to differentiate between normal swallowing and aspiration, but each swallowing event had to be selected by an expert.

Afkari (2007) reported on a multi-sensory non-invasive portable system that records and analyses electromyogram, accelerometer, and microphone signals for the detection of swallows. Ninety-four percent of dry swallows were correctly detected. A swallow rate of 1.32 spontaneous swallows per minute was reported.

A prospective multicentre study reported in Steele et al. (2019) used the self-developed device "dysphagia detection system (DDS)" described in Steele et al. (2013) for an analysis of swallowing safety and efficiency in dysphagic patients. The device consists of a two-dimensional accelerometer on the skin above the larynx that is connected to a data recording PC-system. The swallowing events are selected manually in agreement with videofluoroscopy. The accelerometer signal of each swallow is categorised into safe/unsafe swallows (sensitivity 89%, specificity 60%, accuracy 80%) and efficient/inefficient swallows (sensitivity 79%, specificity 59%, accuracy 72%).

The group of O'Brien (2021) tested a combination of mechano-acoustic sensors on throat and chest in combination with a smartphone for data recording. The swallow tasks included several consistencies and instructions of intake. Machine learning approaches classified the severity of each swallow event according to the Mann Assessment of Swallowing Ability (MASA). Consistency puree gave the biggest contrast in the comparison of normal and impaired swallows.

In summary, it has to be stated that there is no device available that is established in clinical routine as a mobile data recorder for swallowing detection (So 2023). The main problem seems to be swallowing detection in a real-life environment with multiple noise sources and movement artefacts. Although Pehlivan et al. (1996) reported "perfect agreement" between automatic swallowing detection and visual verification, no other group has followed the use of piezoelectric sensors on the skin of the neck. Instead, research focuses on the detection of aspiration in stationary devices that need an expert to select the actual swallowing events.

# References

Afkari S (2007) Measuring frequency of spontaneous swallowing. Australas Phys Eng Sci Med 30(4):313–317

Allen JE, White CJ, Leonard RJ et al (2010) Prevalence of penetration and aspiration on videofluoroscopy in normal individuals without dysphagia. Otolaryngol Head Neck Surg 142(2):208–213

Arens C, Herrmann IF, Rohrbach S et al (2015) Position paper of the German Society of Oto-Rhino-Laryngology, Head and Neck Surgery and the German Society of Phoniatrics and Pediatric Audiology—current state of clinical and endoscopic diagnostics, evaluation, and therapy of swallowing disorders in children. GMS Curr Top Otorhinolaryngol Head Neck Surg 14:Doc02. https://doi.org/10.3205/cto000117

Arens C, Betz C, Kraft M et al (2016) "Narrow band imaging" zur Früherkennung epithelialer Dysplasien und mikroinvasiver Karzinome im oberen Luft-Speise-Weg (Narrow band imaging for early diagnosis of epithelial dysplasias and microinvasive tumors in the upper aerodigestive tract). HNO 64(1):19–26

Asadollahpour F, Baghban K, Asadi M (2015) Validity and reliability of the Persian version of the Dysphagia Handicap Index (DHI). Iran J Otorhinolaryngol 27(80):185–191

Ashraf HH, Palmer J, Dalton HR et al (2017) Can patients determine the level of their dysphagia? World J Gastroenterol 23(6):1038–1043

Audag N, Goubau C, Toussaint M et al (2019) Screening and evaluation tools of dysphagia in adults with neuromuscular diseases: a systematic review. Ther Adv Chronic Dis 10:2040622318821622. https://doi.org/10.1177/2040622318821622

Aviv JE, Martin JG, Sacco RL et al (1996) Supraglottic and pharyngeal sensory abnormalities in stroke patients with dysphagia. Ann Orol Rhinol Laryngol 105(2):92–97

Aviv JE, Kim T, Sacco RL et al (1998) FEESST: a new bedside endoscopic test of the motor and sensory components of swallowing. Ann Otol Rhinol Laryngol 107(5–1):378–387

Ayazi S, Lipham JC, Hagen JA et al (2009) A new technique for measurement of pharyngeal pH: normal values and discriminating pH threshold. J Gastrointest Surg 13(8):1422–1429

Baijens LW, Speyer R, Passos VL et al (2011) Swallowing in Parkinson patients versus healthy controls: reliability of measurements in videofluoroscopy. Gastroenterol Res Pract 2011:380682. https://doi.org/10.1155/2011/380682

Baijens LW, Speyer R, Pilz W et al (2014) FEES protocol derived estimates of sensitivity: aspiration in dysphagic patients. Dysphagia 29(5):583–590

Bartolome G, Schröter-Morasch H (2018) Schluckstörungen Interdisziplinäre Diagnostik und Rehabilitation (Interdisciplinary dysphagia diagnosis and rehabilitation). Elsevier, Urban & Fischer, Munich

Bastian RW (1991) Videoendoscopic evaluation of patients with dysphagia: an adjunct to the modified barium swallow. Otolaryngol Head Neck Surg 104(3):339–349

Battel I, Calvo I, Walshe M (2018) Cross-cultural validation of the Italian version of the Functional Oral Intake Scale. Folia Phoniatr Logop 70(3–4):117–123

Belafsky PC, Rees CJ, Allen J et al (2010) Pharyngeal dilation in cricopharyngeus muscle dysfunction and Zenker diverticulum. Laryngoscope 120(5):889–894

Bergamaschi R, Rezzani C, Minguzzi S et al (2009) Validation of the DYMUS questionnaire for the assessment of dysphagia in multiple sclerosis. Funct Neurol 24(3):159–162

Böckler R, Wein B, Klajman S (1989) Ultraschalluntersuchung der aktiven und passiven eweglichkeit der Zunge (Ultrasound examination of the active and passive mobility of the tongue). Folia Phoniatr 41(6):277–282

Bohr C, Dollinger M, Kniesburges S et al (2016) 3D-Visualisierung und Analyse von Stimmlippenschwingungen (3D visualisation and analysis of vocal fold vibrations). HNO 64(4):254–261

Boland K, Abdul-Hussein M, Tutuian R et al (2016) Characteristics of consecutive esophageal motility diagnoses after a decade of change. J Clin Gastroenterol 50:301–306

Bonilha HS, Blair J, Carnes B et al (2013) Preliminary investigation of the effect of pulse rate on judgments of swallowing impairment and treatment recommendations. Dysphagia 28(4):528–538

Bonilha HS, Reedy EL, Wilmskoetter J et al (2024) Impact of reducing fluoroscopy pulse rate on adult modified barium swallow studies. Dysphagia 39(4):632–641

Bosma JF, Hepburn LG, Josell SD et al (1990) Ultrasound demonstration of tongue motions during suckle feeding. Dev Med Child Neurol 32(3):223–229

Bours GJ, Speyer R, Lemmens J et al (2009) Bedside screening tests vs. videofluoroscopy or fibreoptic endoscopic evaluation of swallowing to detect dysphagia in patients with neurological disorders: systematic review. J Adv Nurs 65(3):477–493

Brady SL, Hildner CD, Hutchins BF (1999) Simultaneous videofluoroscopic swallow study and modified Evans blue dye procedure: an evaluation of blue dye visualization in cases of known aspiration. Dysphagia 14(3):146–149

Brodsky MB, Suiter DM, Gonzalez-Fernandez M et al (2016) Screening accuracy for aspiration using bedside water swallow tests: a systematic review and meta-analysis. Chest 150(1):148–163

Buhmann C, Bihler M, Emich K et al (2019) Pill swallowing in Parkinson's disease: a prospective study based on flexible endoscopic evaluation of swallowing. Parkinsonism Relat Disord 62:51–56

Butler SG, Markley L, Sanders B et al (2015) Reliability of the penetration aspiration scale with flexible endoscopic evaluation of swallowing. Ann Otol Rhinol Laryngol 124(6):480–483

Carlsson S, Rydén A, Rudberg I et al (2012) Validation of the Swedish M.D. Anderson Dysphagia Inventory (MDADI) in patients with head and neck cancer and neurologic swallowing disturbances. Dysphagia 27(3):361–369

Carnaby GD, Crary MA (2014) Development and validation of a cancer-specific swallowing assessment tool: MASA-C. Support Care Cancer 22(3):595–602

Centers for Disease Control and Prevention (1948) Preamble to the Constitution of the World Health Organization as adopted by the International Health Conference, New York, 19–22 June, 1946; signed on 22 July 1946 by the representatives of 61 States (Official Records of the World Health Organization, no. 2, p. 100) and entered into force on 7 April 1948

Centers for Disease Control and Prevention (2014). http://www.cdc.gov/chronicdisease/stats/index.htm. Accessed 11 Feb 2022

Chen AY, Frankowski R, Bishop-Leone J et al (2001) The development and validation of a dysphagia specific quality-of-life questionnaire for patients with head and neck cancer. Arch Otolaryngol Head Neck Surg 127(7):870–876

Chen PH, Golub JS, Hapner ER et al (2009) Prevalence of perceived dysphagia and quality-of-life impairment in a geriatric population. Dysphagia 24(1):1–6

Chen PC, Chuang CH, Leong CP et al (2016) Systematic review and meta-analysis of the diagnostic accuracy of the water swallow test for screening aspiration in stroke patients. J Adv Nurs 72(11):2575–2586

Cheng CF, Peng CL, Chiou HY et al (2002) Dentofacial morphology and tongue function during swallowing. Am J Orthod Dentofacial Orthop 122(5):491–499

Chi-Fishman G (2005) Quantitative lingual, pharyngeal and laryngeal ultrasonography in swallowing research: a technical review. Clin Linguist Phon 19(6–7):589–604

Cichero JA, Lam P, Steele CM et al (2017) Development of international terminology and definitions for texture-modified foods and thickened fluids used in dysphagia management: the IDDSI framework. Dysphagia 32(2):293–314. https://doi.org/10.1007/s00455-016-9758-y. Epub 2016 Dec 2. PMID: 27913916; PMCID: PMC5380696

Clouse RE, Staiano A (1993) Topography of normal and high-amplitude esophageal peristalsis. Am J Phys 265:G1098–G1107

Colodny N (2002) Interjudge and intrajudge reliabilities in fiberoptic endoscopic evaluation of swallowing (FEES) using the penetration-aspiration scale: a replication study. Dysphagia 17(4):308–315

Crary MA, Mann GD, Groher ME (2005) Initial psychometric assessment of a functional oral intake scale for dysphagia in stroke patients. Arch Phys Med Rehabil 86(8):1516–1520

Crary MA, Sura L, Carnaby G (2013) Validation and demonstration of an isolated acoustic recording technique to estimate spontaneous swallow frequency. Dysphagia 28(1):86–94

Crestani S, Moerman M, Woisard V (2011) The "Deglutition Handicap Index" a self-adminitrated [sic] dysphagia-specific quality of life questionnaire: sensibility to change. Rev Laryngol Otol Rhinol (Bord) 132(1):3–7

Damouras S, Sejdic E, Steele CM et al (2010) An online swallow detection algorithm based on the quadratic variation of dual-axis accelerometry. IEEE Trans Signal Process 58(6):3352–3359

Daniels SK, Anderson JA, Willson PC (2012) Valid items for screening dysphagia risk in patients with stroke: a systematic review. Stroke 43(3):892–897

Davies NJ (1973) A new fiberoptic laryngoscope for nasal intubation. Anesth Analg 52:807–808

DePippo KL, Holas MA, Reding MJ (1992) Validation of the 3-oz water swallow test for aspiration following stroke. Arch Neurol 49(12):1259–1261

Deutschmann MW, McDonough A, Dort JC et al (2013) Fiber-optic endoscopic evaluation of swallowing (FEES): predictor of swallowing-related complications in the head and neck cancer population. Head Neck 35(7):974–979

Doggett DL, Turkelson CM, Coates V (2002) Recent developments in diagnosis and intervention for aspiration and dysphagia in stroke and other neuromuscular disorders. Curr Atheroscler Rep 4(4):311–318

Donovan NJ, Daniels SK, Edmiaston J et al (2013) Dysphagia screening: state of the art: invitational conference proceeding from the State-of-the-Art Nursing Symposium, International Stroke Conference 2012. Stroke 44(4):e24–e31

Dudik JM, Coyle JL, Sejdić E (2015) Dysphagia screening: contributions of cervical auscultation signals and modern signal-processing techniques. IEEE Trans Hum Mach Syst 45(4):465–477

Dudik JM, Kurosu A, Coyle JL et al (2018) Dysphagia and its effects on swallowing sounds and vibrations in adults. Biomed Eng Online 17(1):69. https://doi.org/10.1186/s12938-018-0501-9

Dyer JC, Leslie P, Drinnan MJ (2008) Objective computer-based assessment of valleculae residue—is it useful? Dysphagia 23(1):7–15

Dziewas R, Warnecke T, Olenberg S et al (2008) Towards a basic endoscopic assessment of swallowing in acute stroke—development and evaluation of a simple dysphagia score. Cerebrovasc Dis 26(1):41–47

Eisenhuber E, Schima W, Schober E et al (2002) Videofluoroscopic assessment of patients with dysphagia: pharyngeal retention is a predictive factor for aspiration. AJR Am J Roentgenol 178(2):393–398

Ekberg O, Pokieser P (1997) Radiologic evaluation of the dysphagic patient. Eur Radiol 7(8):1285–1295

Eller R, Ginsburg M, Lurie D et al (2008) Flexible laryngoscopy: a comparison of fiber optic and distal chip technologies. Part 1: vocal fold masses. J Voice 22(6):746–750

Fanucci A, Cerro P, Ietto F et al (1994) Physiology of oral swallowing studied by ultrasonography. Dentomaxillofac Radiol 23(4):221–225

Farahat M, Malki KH, Mesallam TA et al (2014) Development of the Arabic version of Dysphagia Handicap Index (DHI). Dysphagia 29(4):459–467

Farneti D (2008) Pooling score: an endoscopic model for evaluating severity of dysphagia. Acta Otorhinolaryngol Ital 28(3):135–140

Farneti D (2012) Voice and dysphagia. In: Ekberg O (ed) Dysphagia: diagnosis and treatment. Springer, Heidelberg

Farneti D (2014) The instrumental gold standard: FEES. J Gastroenterol Hepatol 3(10):1055–1060

Farneti D, Favero E (2010) Valutazione videoendoscopica infantile, adulta e senile (Infant, adult and senile videoendoscopic evaluation). In: Schindler O, Ruoppolo G, Schindler A (eds) Deglutologia. II edizione (Swallowing), 2nd edn. Omega, Torino, pp 167–179

Farneti D, Fattori B, Nacci A et al (2014) The Pooling-score (P-score): inter- and intra-rater reliability in endoscopic assessment of the severity of dysphagia. Acta Otorhinolaryngol Ital 34(2):105–110

Fife TA, Butler SG, Langmore SE et al (2015) Use of topical nasal anesthesia during flexible endoscopic evaluation of swallowing in dysphagic patients. Ann Otol Rhinol Laryngol 124(3):206–211

Fox MR, Bredenoord AJ (2008) Oesophageal high-resolution manometry: moving from research into clinical practice. Gut 57(3):405–423. https://doi.org/10.1136/gut.2007.127993. Epub 2007 Sep 25. PMID: 17895358

Frakking TT et al (2022) Using an automated speech recognition approach to differentiate between normal and aspirating swallowing sounds recorded from digital cervical auscultation in children. Dysphagia 37:1482. https://doi.org/10.1007/s00455-022-10410-y

Fuhrmann R, Diedrich P (1992) Einsatzmöglichkeiten der dynamischen Sonographie bei der Diagnostik von Zungenfunktionsstörungen (Possible applications of dynamic sonography in the diagnosis of tongue dysfunction). Dtsch Zahnärztl Z 47(9):586–590

Fuhrmann R, Diedrich P (1993) Videogestützte dynamische B-Mode-Sonographie der Zungenfunktion während des Schluckens (Video-based dynamic B-mode sonography of tongue function during swallowing). Fortschr Kieferorthop 54(1):17–26

Fukuike C, Kodama N, Manda Y et al (2015) A novel automated detection system for swallowing sounds during eating and speech under everyday conditions. J Oral Rehabil 42(5):340–347

Garon BR, Sierzant T, Ormiston C (2009) Silent aspiration: results of 2,000 video fluoroscopic evaluations. J Neurosci Nurs 41(4):178–185, 186–187

Geddes DT, Kent JC, Mitoulas LR et al (2008) Tongue movement and intra-oral vacuum in breastfeeding infants. Early Hum Dev 84(7):417–477

Geddes DT, Sakalidis VS, Hepworth AR et al (2012) Tongue movement and intra-oral vacuum of term infants during breastfeeding and feeding from an experimental teat that released milk under vacuum only. Early Hum Dev 88(6):443–449

Geddes DT, Chooi K, Nancarrow K et al (2017) Characterisation of sucking dynamics of breastfeeding preterm infants: a cross sectional study. BMC Pregnancy Childbirth 17(1):386–397

Gerschke M, Schöttker-Königer T, Förster A et al (2019) Validation of the German version of the Yale Pharyngeal Residue Severity Rating Scale. Dysphagia 34(3):308–314. https://doi.org/10.1007/s00455-018-9935-2. Epub 2018 Aug 16. PMID: 30116884

Golabbakhsh M, Rajaei A, Derakhshan M et al (2014) Automated acoustic analysis in detection of spontaneous swallows in Parkinson's disease. Dysphagia 29(5):572–577

Graf S, Keilmann A, Dazert S et al (2019) Ausbildungscurriculum für das Zertifikat "Diagnostik und Therapie der oropharyngealen Dysphagie, einschließlich FEES" der Deutschen Gesellschaft für Phoniatrie und Pedaudiologie und der Deutschen Gesellschaft für Hals-Nasen-Ohrenheilkunde, Kopf- und Halschirurgie (Training curriculum for the certificate "Diagnostics and therapy of oropharyngeal dysphagia, including FEES", of the German Society for Phoniatrics and Pedaudiology and the German Society for Otolaryngology, Head and Neck Surgery). Laryngorhinootologie 98:695–700

Guedes RL, Angelis EC, Chen AY et al (2013) Validation and application of the M.D. Anderson Dysphagia Inventory in patients treated for head and neck cancer in Brazil. Dysphagia 28(1):24–32

Hayashi Y, Hoashi E, Nara T (1997) Ultrasonographic analysis of sucking behavior of newborn infants: the driving force of sucking pressure. Early Hum Dev 49(1):33–38

Hey C, Pluschinski P, Stanschus S et al (2011) A documentation system to save time and ensure proper application of the fiberoptic endoscopic evaluation of swallowing (FEES®). Folia Phoniatr Logop 63(4):201–208

Hey C, Lange BP, Eberle S et al (2013) Water swallow screening test for patients after surgery for head and neck cancer: early identification of dysphagia, aspiration and limitations of oral intake. Anticancer Res 33(9):4017–4021

Hey C, Pluschinski P, Zaretsky Y et al (2014) Penetrations-aspirations-Skala nach Rosenbek. Validierung der deutschen Version für die endoskopische Dysphagiediagnostik (Penetration-aspiration scale according to Rosenbek. Validation of the German version for endoscopic dysphagia diagnostics). HNO 62(4):276–281

Hey C, Pluschinski P, Pajunk R et al (2015) Penetration-aspiration: is their detection in FEES® reliable without video recording? Dysphagia 30(4):418–422

Higginson IJ, Carr AJ (2001) Using quality of life measures in the clinical setting. BMJ 322:1297–1300

Hinchey JA, Shephard T, Furie K et al (2005) Formal dysphagia screening protocols prevent pneumonia. Stroke 36(9):1972–1976

Huggins PS, Tuomi SK, Young C (1999) Effects of nasogastric tubes on the young, normal swallowing mechanism. Dysphagia 14(3):157–161

Jamieson JR, Stein HJ, DeMeester TR et al (1992) Ambulatory 24-h esophageal pH monitoring: normal values, optimal thresholds, specificity, sensitivity, and reproducibility. Am J Gastroenterol 87:1102–1111

Johnson LF, Demeester TR (1974) Twenty-four-hour pH monitoring of the distal esophagus. A quantitative measure of gastroesophageal reflux. Am J Gastroenterol 62:325–332

Jones B, Donner MW (1989) How I do it: examination of the patient with dysphagia. Dysphagia 4(3):162–172

Jungheim M, Ptok M (2011) Extraesophageal reflux. Overview and discussion of a new method for pH monitoring. HNO 59:893–899

Jungheim M, Miller S, Ptok M (2013) Methodologische Aspekte zur Hochauflösungsmanometrie des Pharynx und des oberen Ösophagussphinkters (Methodological aspects of high-resolution manometry of the pharynx and the upper oesophageal sphincter). Laryngorhinootologie 92:158–164

Jungheim M, Schubert C, Miller S et al (2015) Normative data of pharyngeal and upper esophageal sphincter high resolution manometry. Laryngorhinootologie 94:601–608

Kahrilas PJ, Shaheen NJ, Vaezi MF et al (2008) American Gastroenterological Association Medical Position Statement on the management of gastroesophageal reflux disease. Gastroenterology 135:1383–1391

Kahrilas PJ, Bredenoord AJ, Fox M et al (2015) International High Resolution Manometry Working Group. The Chicago Classification of esophageal motility disorders, v3.0. Neurogastroenterol Motil 27:160–174

Kaneoka AS, Langmore SE, Krisciunas GP et al (2013) The Boston Residue and Clearance Scale: preliminary reliability and validity testing. Folia Phoniatr Logop 65(6):312–317

Kikyo T, Saito M, Ishikawa M (1999) A study comparing ultrasound images of tongue movements between open bite children and normal children in the early mixed dentition period. J Med Dent Sci 46(3):127–137

Kobayashi Y, Mineno H (2014) Fluid intake recognition for nursing care support by leveraging swallowing sound. In: IEEE 3rd global conference on consumer electronics (GCCE), pp 620–621. https://doi.org/10.1109/GCCE.2014.7031280

Koppenburg P, Leidig E, Bacher M et al (1988) Die Darstellung von Lage und Beweglichkeit der Zunge bei Neugeborenen mit oralen Spaltfehlbildungen durch transorale Ultraschallsonographie (The visualisation of tongue position and mobility in newborns with oral cleft deformities by transoral ultrasonography). Dtsch Zahnaerztl Z 43(7):806–809

Koufman J, Aviv J, Casiano R et al (2002) Laryngopharyngeal reflux: position statement of the committee on speech, voice and swallowing disorders of the American Academy of Otolaryngology-Head and Neck Surgery. Otolaryngol Head Neck Surg 127:32–35

Kumar AR, Katz PO (2013) Functional esophageal disorders: a review of diagnosis and management. Expert Rev Gastroenterol Hepatol 7:453–461

Kwon CH, Kim YH, Park JH et al (2013) Validity and reliability of the Korean version of the MD Anderson Dysphagia inventory for head and neck cancer patients. Ann Rehabil Med 37(4):479–487

Lai DKH (2023) Transformer models and convolutional networks with different activation functions for swallow classification using depth video data. Mathematics 11(14):3081. https://doi.org/10.3390/math11143081

Lakshminarayan K, Tsai AW, Tong X et al (2010) Utility of dysphagia screening results in predicting poststroke pneumonia. Stroke 41(12):2849–2854

Langmore SE (2000) Endoscopic evaluation and treatment of swallowing disorders, 2nd edn. Thieme Verlag, New York

Langmore SE (2001) Endoscopic evaluation and treatment of swallowing disorders. Thieme, New York

Langmore SE (2003) Evaluation of oropharyngeal dysphagia: which diagnostic tool is superior? Curr Opin Otolaryngol Head Neck Surg 11(6):485–489

Langmore SE (2017) History of fiberoptic endoscopic evaluation of swallowing for evaluation and management of pharyngeal dysphagia: changes over the years. Dysphagia 32(1):27–38

Langmore SE, Schatz K, Olsen N (1988) Fiberoptic endoscopic examination of swallowing safety: a new procedure. Dysphagia 2(4):216–219

Langmore SE, Schatz K, Olson N (1991) Endoscopic and videofluoroscopic evaluations of swallowing and aspiration. Ann Otol Rhinol Laryngol 100:678–681

Langmore SE, Olney RK, Lomen-Hoerth C et al (2007) Dysphagia in patients with frontotemporal lobar dementia. Arch Neurol 64:58–62

Leder SB, Suiter DM, Green BG (2011) Silent aspiration risk is volume-dependent. Dysphagia 26(3):304–309

Lee J, Blain S, Casas M et al (2006) A radial basis classifier for the automatic detection of aspiration in children with dysphagia. J Neuroeng Rehabil 3:14. https://doi.org/10.1186/1743-0003-3-14

Lee J, Steele CM, Chau T (2009) Swallow segmentation with artificial neural networks and multi-sensor fusion. Med Eng Phys 31(9):1049–1055

Lee J, Steele CM, Chau T (2011) Classification of healthy and abnormal swallows based on accelerometry and nasal airflow signals. Artif Intell Med 52(1):17–25

Lefton-Greif MA, Okelo SO, Wright JM et al (2014) Impact of children's feeding/swallowing problems: validation of a new caregiver instrument. Dysphagia 29(6):671–677

Leonard R, Kendall K, McKenzie S (2004) UES opening and cricopharyngeal bar in nondysphagic elderly and nonelderly adults. Dysphagia 19(3):182–191

Leslie P, Drinnan MJ, Zammit-Maempel I et al (2007) Cervical auscultation synchronized with images from endoscopy swallow evaluations. Dysphagia 22(4):290–298

Levine MS, Carucci LR, DiSantis DJ, Einstein DM, Hawn MT, Martin-Harris B, Katzka DA, Morgan DE, Rubesin SE, Scholz FJ, Turner MA, Wolf EL, Canon CL (2016) Consensus Statement of Society of abdominal radiology disease-focused panel on barium esophagography in gastroesophageal reflux disease. AJR Am J Roentgenol 207(5):1009–1015. https://doi.org/10.2214/AJR.16.16323

Lim SH, Lieu PK, Phua SY et al (2001) Accuracy of bedside clinical methods compared with fiberoptic endoscopic examination of swallowing (FEES) in determining the risk of aspiration in acute stroke patients. Dysphagia 16(1):1–6

Logeman JA (1997) Therapy for oropharyngeal swallowing disorders. In: Perlman AL, Schulze-Delrieu K (eds) Deglutition and its disorders. Singular Publishing Group, San Diego, pp 449–461

Logeman JA (1998) Evaluation and treatment of swallowing disorders, vol 6, 2nd edn. PRO-ED, Austin, p 395

Logemann JA (2006) Medical and rehabilitative therapy of oral, pharyngeal motor disorders. PART 1: oral cavity, pharynx and esophagus. GI Motility online. https://doi.org/10.1038/gimo50

Logemann JA, Pauloski BR, Colangelo L et al (1995) Effects of sour bolus on oropharyngeal swallowing measures in patients with neurogenic dysphagia. J Speech Hear Res 38(3):556–563

Logemann JA, Veis S, Colangelo L (1999) A screening procedure for oropharyngeal dysphagia. Dysphagia 14(1):44–51

Martin-Harris B, Brodsky MB, Michel Y et al (2007) Delayed initiation of the pharyngeal swallow: normal variability in adult swallows. J Speech Lang Hear Res 50(3):585–594

Massey BT (2013) Manometry of the UES including high-resolution manometry. In: Shaker R, Easterling C, Belafsky PC et al (eds) Manual of diagnostic and therapeutic techniques for disorders of deglutition. Springer, New York, pp 129–149

McHorney CA, Robbins J, Lomax K et al (2002) The SWAL-QOL and SWAL-CARE outcomes tool for oropharyngeal dysphagia in adults: III documentation of reliability and validity. Dysphagia 17(2):97–111

Mercado-Deane MG, Burton EM, Harlow SA et al (2001) Swallowing dysfunction in infants less than 1 year of age. Pediatr Radiol 31(6):423–428

Meyer S, Jungheim M, Ptok M (2012) Ultra-Hochauflösungsmanometrie des oberen Ösophagussphinkters (Ultra-high-resolution manometry of the upper esophageal sphincter). HNO 60:318–326

Miller JL, Kang SM (2007) Preliminary ultrasound observation of lingual movement patterns during nutritive versus non-nutritive sucking in a premature infant. Dysphagia 22(2):150–160

Miller CK, Willging JP (2020) Fiberoptic endoscopic evaluation of swallowing in infants and children: protocol, safety, and clinical efficacy: 25 years of experience. Ann Otol Rhinol Laryngol 129(5):469–481

Miller CK, Schroeder JW, Langmore SE (2020) Fiberoptic endoscopic evaluation of swallowing across the age spectrum. Am J Speech Lang Pathol 29(2S):967–978

Miyagi S et al (2020) Classifying dysphagic swallowing sounds with support vector machines. Healthcare (Basel) 8:E103

Moreno I, Sun CC (2008) Modeling the radiation pattern of LEDs. Opt Exp 16(3):1808–1819

Morishima Y, Chida K, Watanabe H (2016) Estimation of the dose of radiation received by patient and physician during a videofluoroscopic swallowing study. Dysphagia 31(4):574–578

Murray J, Langmore SE, Ginsberg S et al (1996) The significance of accumulated oropharyngeal secretions and swallowing frequency in predicting aspiration. Dysphagia 11(2):99–103

Müßig D (1992) Die Sonographie—ein diagnostisches Mittel zur dynamischen Funktionsanalyse der Zunge (Sonography—a diagnostic tool for dynamic functional analysis of the tongue). Fortschr Kieferorthop 53(6):338–343

Muto M, Nakane M, Katada C et al (2004) Squamous cell carcinoma in situ at oropharyngeal and hypopharyngeal mucosal sites. Cancer 101(6):1375–1381

Nacci A, Simoni F, Pagani R et al (2022) Complications during Fiberoptic Endoscopic Evaluation of Swallowing (FEES) in 5680 examinations. Folia Phoniatr Logop 74:352. https://doi.org/10.1159/000521145

Nascimento A, Carvalho M, Nogueira J et al (2018) Complications associated with nasogastric tube placement in the acute phase of stroke: a systematic review. J Neurosci Nurs 50(4):193–198

Nativ-Zeltzer N, Kahrilas PJ, Logemann JA (2012) Manofluorography in the evaluation of oropharyngeal dysphagia. Dysphagia 27(2):151–161

Nativ-Zeltzer N, Rameau A, Kuhn MA et al (2018) The relationship between hiatal hernia and cricopharyngeus muscle dysfunction. Dysphagia 34:391. https://doi.org/10.1007/s00455-018-9950-3

Neubauer PD, Rademaker AW, Leder SB (2015) The Yale Pharyngeal Residue Severity Rating Scale: an anatomically defined and image-based tool. Dysphagia 30(5):521–528

Nienstedt JC, Müller F, Nießen A et al (2017) Narrow band imaging enhances the detection rate of penetration and aspiration in FEES. Dysphagia 32(3):443–448

Nienstedt JC, Pflug C, Fluegel T (2018a) Dysphagie - Effiziente Schluckdiagnostik in der Praxis (Dysphagia—efficient swallowing diagnostics in practice). HNO Nachrichten Ausgabe. https://doi.org/10.1007/s00060-018-5674-0. Accessed 22 Feb 2022

Nienstedt JC, Bihler M, Niessen A et al (2018b) Predictive clinical factors for penetration and aspiration in Parkinson's disease. Neurogastroenterol Motil 31(4):13524. https://doi.org/10.1111/nmo.13524

Niessen A, Nienstedt JC, Flügel T et al (2023) Narrow band imaging in flexible endoscopic evaluation of swallowing—how does it work? J Speech Lang Hear Res 66(6):2035–2046. https://doi.org/10.1044/2023_JSLHR-22-00579. Epub 2023 Jun 6. PMID: 37279337

Nikjoo MS, Steele CM, Sejdić E et al (2011) Automatic discrimination between safe and unsafe swallowing using a reputation-based classifier. Biomed Eng Online 10:100. https://doi.org/10.1186/1475-925X-10-100

O'Brien MK et al (2021) Advanced machine learning tools to monitor biomarkers of dysphagia: a wearable sensor proof-of-concept study. Digit Biomark 5:167–175

O'Dea MB, Langmore SE, Krisciunas GP et al (2015) Effect of lidocaine on swallowing during FEES in patients with dysphagia. Ann Otol Rhinol Laryngol 124(7):537–544

O'Horo JC, Rogus-Pulia N, Garcia-Arguello L et al (2015) Bedside diagnosis of dysphagia: a systematic review. J Hosp Med 10(4):256–265

Oda C, Yamamoto T, Fukumoto Y et al (2017) Validation of the Japanese translation of the Dysphagia Handicap Index. Patient Prefer Adherence 11:193–198

Odderson IR, Keaton JC, McKenna BS (1995) Swallow management in patients on an acute stroke pathway: quality is cost effective. Arch Phys Med Rehabil 76(12):1130–1133

Ohtsuka Y, Watanabe S, Ishida R et al (1998) Developmental changes of tongue movement during swallowing in infants (in Japanese). Jpn J Pediatr Dent 36(5):867–876

Omari TI, Ciucci M, Gozdzikowska K et al (2019) High-resolution pharyngeal manometry and impedance: protocols and metrics-recommendations of a high-resolution pharyngeal manometry International Working Group. Dysphagia 35:281–295

Palmer J, Rudin N, Lara G et al (1992) Coordination of mastication and swallowing. Dysphagia 7(4):187–200

Pandolfino JE, Kwiatek MA (2008) Use and utility of the Bravo pH capsule. J Clin Gastroenterol 42:571–578

Pandolfino JE, Richter JE, Ours T et al (2003) Ambulatory esophageal pH monitoring using a wireless system. Am J Gastroenterol 98:740–749

Pearson WG, Molfenter SM, Smith ZM et al (2013) Image-based measurement of post-swallow residue: the normalized residue ratio scale. Dysphagia 28(2):167–177

Pearson WG, Taylor BK, Blair J et al (2016) Computational analysis of swallowing mechanics underlying impaired epiglottic inversion. Laryngoscope 126(8):1854–1858

Pehlivan M, Yüceyar N, Ertekin C et al (1996) An electronic device measuring the frequency of spontaneous swallowing; digital phagometer. Dysphagia 11(4):259–264

Peng CL, Jost-Brinkmann PG, Lin CT (1995) Einteilung und Interpretation der oralen Schluckphase mittels B + M-Mode-Sonographie (Classification and interpretation of the oral swallowing phase using B+M mode ultrasound). Radiologe 35(10):747–752

Peng CL, Jost-Brinkmann PG, Miethke RR et al (2000) Ultrasonographic measurement of tongue movement during swallowing. J Ultrasound Med 19(1):15–20

Peng CL, Jost-Brinkmann PG, Yoshida N et al (2003) Differential diagnosis between infantile and mature swallowing with ultrasonography. Eur J Orthod 25(5):451–456

Peng CL, Jost-Brinkmann PG, Yoshida N et al (2004) Comparison of tongue functions between mature and tongue-thrust swallowing—an ultrasound investigation. Am J Orthod Dentofacial Orthop 125(5):562–570

Peng CL, Miethke RR, Pong SJ et al (2007) Investigation of tongue movements during swallowing with M-mode ultrasonography. J Orofac Orthop 68(1):17–25

Peretti G, Piazza C, Del Bon F et al (2013) Function preservation using transoral laser surgery for T2-T3 glottic cancer: oncologic, vocal, and swallowing outcomes. Eur Arch Otorrinolaringol 270(8):2275–2281

Perry L (2001a) Screening swallowing function of patients with acute stroke. Part one: identification, implementation and initial evaluation of a screening tool for use by nurses. J Clin Nurs 10(4):463–473

Perry L (2001b) Screening swallowing function of patients with acute stroke. Part two: detailed evaluation of the tool used by nurses. J Clin Nurs 10(4):474–481

Piazza C, Dessouky O, Peretti G et al (2008) Narrow-band imaging: a new tool for evaluation of head and neck squamous cell carcinomas. Review of the literature. Acta Otorhinolaryngol Ital 28(2):49–54

Pisegna JM, Kaneoka A, Leonard R et al (2018) Rethinking residue: determining the perceptual continuum of residue on FEES to enable better measurement. Dysphagia 33(1):100–108

Pisegna JM, Murray J (2018) Clinical application of flexible endoscopic evaluation of swallowing in stroke. Semin Speech Lang 39(1):3–14. https://doi.org/10.1055/s-0037-1608855. Epub 2018 Jan 22. PMID: 29359301

Plaat BE, van der Laan BF, Wedman J et al (2014) Distal chip versus fiberoptic flexible laryngoscopy using endoscopic sheaths: diagnostic accuracy and image quality. Eur Arch Otorrinolaringol 271(8):2227–2232

Pluschinski P, Zaretsky Y, Stover T et al (2015) Qualitätssicherung der endoskopischen Schluckdiagnostik (FEES) (Quality assurance in the endoscopic evaluation of swallowing (FEES)). Laryngorhinootologie 94(8):505–508

Pluschinski P, Zaretsky E, Stover T et al (2016) Validation of the secretion severity rating scale. Eur Arch Otorrinolaringol 273(10):3215–3218

Prosiegel M, Weber S (2010) Dysphagie (Dysphagia). Springer, Heidelberg

Ricci Maccarini A, Stacchini M, Salsi D et al (2007) Trans-tracheostomic endoscopy of the larynx in the evaluation of dysphagia. Acta Otorhinolaryngol Ital 27(6):290–293

Rodriguez KH, Roth CR, Rees CJ et al (2007) Reliability of the pharyngeal squeeze maneuver. Ann Otol Rhinol Laryngol 116(6):399–401

Rommel N, Borgers C, Van Beckevoort D et al (2015) Bolus Residue Scale: an easy-to-use and reliable videofluoroscopic analysis tool to score bolus residue in patients with dysphagia. Int J Otolaryngol 2015:780197. https://doi.org/10.1155/2015/780197

Rosen CA, Amin MR, Sulica L et al (2009) Advances in office-based diagnosis and treatment in laryngology. Laryngoscope 119(Suppl 2):S185–S212

Rosenbek JC, Robbins JA, Roecker EB et al (1996) A penetration-aspiration scale. Dysphagia 11(2):93–98

Rubesin SE, Levine MS (2018) Pharyngeal manifestations of gastroesophageal reflux disease. Abdom Radiol (NY) 43(6):1294–1305

Sakalidis VS, Williams TM, Garbin CP et al (2012) Ultrasound imaging of infant sucking dynamics during the establishment of lactation. J Hum Lact 29(2):205–213

Samuels EE, van Hooren M, Baijens LWJ et al (2021) Validation of the Dutch version of the M.D. Anderson Dysphagia Inventory for neurogenic patients. Folia Phoniatr Logop 73(1):42–49

Sawashima HD, Hirose H (1963) New laryngoscopic technique by use of fiberoptics. J Acoust Soc Am 43:168–169

Scharitzer M, Pokieser P, Schober E et al (2002) Morphological findings in dynamic swallowing studies of symptomatic patients. Eur Radiol 12(5):1139–1144

Scharitzer M, Pokieser P, Wagner-Menghin M et al (2017a) Taking the history in patients with swallowing disorders: an international multidisciplinary survey. Abdom Radiol (NY) 42(3):786–793

Scharitzer M, Lenglinger J, Schima W et al (2017b) Comparison of videofluoroscopy and impedance planimetry for the evaluation of oesophageal stenosis: a retrospective study. Eur Radiol 27(4):1760–1767

Scharitzer M, Pokieser P, Ekberg O (2024) Oesophageal fluoroscopy in adults—when and why? Br J Radiol 97(1159):1222–1233

Schepp SK, Tirschwell DL, Miller RM et al (2012) Swallowing screens after acute stroke: a systematic review. Stroke 43(3):869–871

Schindler A, Spadola Bisetti M, Favero E et al (2005) Role of videoendoscopy in phoniatrics: data from three years of daily practice. Acta Otorhinolaryngol Ital 25(1):43–49

Schindler A, Borghi E, Tiddia C et al (2008) Adaptation and validation of the Italian MD Anderson Dysphagia Inventory (MDADI). Rev Laryngol Otol Rhinol (Bord) 129(2):97–100

Schindler A, Biondi S, Farneti D et al (2009) La valutazione fibroendoscopica della deglutizione. Position statement del GISD (Gruppo Italiano Studio Disfagia) (The fibroendoscopic evaluation of swallowing. Position statement of the GISD (Italian Dysphagia Study Group)). Argomenti di ACTA Otorhinolaryngol Ital 3:6–9

Schindler A, Baijens LWJ, Geneid A et al (2021) Phoniatricians and otorhinolaryngologists approaching oropharyngeal dysphagia: an update on FEES. Eur Arch Otorrinolaringol 279:2727. https://doi.org/10.1007/s00405-021-07161-1

Schultheiss C, Schauer T, Nahrstaedt H et al (2014) Automated detection and evaluation of swallowing using a combined EMG/bio-impedance measurement system. Sci World J 2014:405471. https://www.hindawi.com/journals/tswj/2014/405471

Shawker TH, Sonies BC, Stone M (1984) Sonography of speech and swallowing. In: Sanders RC, Hill MC (eds) Ultrasound annual 1984. Raven Press, New York, pp 237–260

Sifrim D, Castell D, Dent J et al (2004) Gastroesophageal reflux monitoring: review and consensus report on detection and definitions of acid, non-acid, and gas reflux. Gut 53:1024–1031

Silbergleit AK, Schultz L, Jacobson BH et al (2012) The dysphagia handicap index: development and validation. Dysphagia 27(1):46–52

Silny J (1991) Intraluminal multiple electric impedance procedure for measurement of gastrointestinal motility. J Gastrointest Motil 3:151–162

Smith WL, Erenberg A, Nowak A et al (1985) Physiology of sucking in the normal term infant using real-time US. Radiology 156(2):379–381

So BPH (2023) Swallow detection with acoustics and accelerometric-based wearable technology: a scoping review. Int J Environ Res Public Health 20(1):170. https://doi.org/10.3390/ijerph20010170

Speyer R, Cordier R, Kertscher B et al (2014) Psychometric properties of questionnaires on functional health status in oropharyngeal dysphagia: a systematic literature review. Biomed Res Int 2014:458678. https://doi.org/10.1155/2014/458678

Starmer HM, Ward BK, Best SR et al (2014) Patient-perceived long-term communication and swallow function following cerebellopontine angle surgery. Laryngoscope 124(2):476–480

Steele CM, Cichero JA (2014) Physiological factors related to aspiration risk: a systematic review. Dysphagia 29(3):295–304

Steele CM, Sejdic E, Chau T (2013) Noninvasive detection of thin-liquid aspiration using dual-axis swallowing accelerometry. Dysphagia 28(1):105–112

Steele CM, Mukherjee R, Kortelainen JM et al (2019) Development of a non-invasive device for swallow screening in patients at risk of oropharyngeal dysphagia: results from a prospective exploratory study. Dysphagia 34(5):698–707

Steiger S, Veprek RG, Witzigmann B (2009) tdkp/AQUA: unified modelling of electroluminescence in nanostructures. In: 9th international conference on numerical simulation of optoelectronic devices, pp 73–74. https://doi.org/10.1109/NUSOD.2009.5297218

Stein J, Wehrmann T (2006) Funktionsdiagnostik in der Gastroenterologie (Functional diagnostics in gastroenterology). Springer, Heidelberg

Stone M, Davis EP (1995) A head and transducer support system for making ultrasound images of tongue/jaw movement. J Acoust Soc Am 98(6):3107–3112

Streets CG, DeMeester TR, Peter JH et al (2001) Clinical evaluation of the Bravo probe: a catheter-free ambulatory esophageal pH monitoring system. Gastroenterology 120:A35

Suiter DM, Leder SB (2008) Clinical utility of the 3-ounce water swallow test. Dysphagia 23(3):244–250

Swan K, Cordier R, Brown T et al (2019) Psychometric properties of visuoperceptual measures of video-fluoroscopic and fibre-endoscopic evaluations of swallowing: a systematic review. Dysphagia 34(1):2–33

Timmerman AA, Speyer R, Heijnen BJ et al (2014) Psychometric characteristics of health-related quality-of-life questionnaires in oropharyngeal dysphagia. Dysphagia 29(2):183–198

Trapl M, Enderle P, Nowotny M et al (2007) Dysphagia bedside screening for acute-stroke patients: the Gugging Swallowing Screen. Stroke 38(11):2948–2952

Tsunoda A, Hatanaka A, Tsunoda R et al (2008) A full digital, high definition video system (1080i) for laryngoscopy and stroboscopy. J Laryngol Otol 122(1):78–81

Tutuian R, Vela MF, Shay SS et al (2001) Multichannel intraluminal impedance in esophageal function testing and gastroesophageal reflux monitoring. J Clin Gastroenterol 37:206–215

Ward EM, Devault KR, Bouras EP et al (2004) Successful oesophageal pH monitoring with a catheter-free system. Aliment Pharmacol Ther 19:449–454

Ware JE, Sherbourne CD (1992) The MOS 36-item short-form health survey (SF-36). Conceptual framework and item selection. Med Care 30(6):473–483

Warnecke T, Ritter MA, Kroger B et al (2009a) Fiberoptic endoscopic dysphagia severity scale predicts outcome after acute stroke. Cerebrovasc Dis 28(3):283–289

Warnecke T, Teismann I, Oelenberg S et al (2009b) Towards a basic endoscopic evaluation of swallowing in acute stroke—identification of salient findings by the inexperienced examiner. BMC Med Educ 9:13. https://doi.org/10.1186/1472-6920-9-13

Warnecke T, Oelenberg S, Teismann I et al (2010) Endoscopic characteristics and levodopa responsiveness of swallowing function in progressive supranuclear palsy. Mov Disord 25(9):1239–1245

Warnecke T, Hamacher C, Oelenberg S et al (2014) Off and on state assessment of swallowing function in Parkinson's disease. Parkinsonism Relat Disord 20(9):1033–1034

Warnecke T, Im S, Kaiser C et al (2017) Aspiration and dysphagia screening in acute stroke—the Gugging Swallowing Screen revisited. Eur J Neurol 24(4):594–601

Watkin KL (1999) Ultrasound and swallowing. Folia Phoniatr Logop 51(4–5):183–198

Weber F, Woolridge MW, Baum JM (1986) An ultrasonographic study of the organisation of sucking and swallowing by newborn infants. Dev Med Child Neurol 28(1):19–24

Wein B, Klajman S, Huber W et al (1988a) Ultraschalluntersuchung von Koordinationsstörungen der Zungenbewegung beim Schlucken (Ultrasound examination of coordination disorders of tongue movement when swallowing). Nervenarzt 59(3):154–158

Wein B, Alzen G, Tolxdorff T et al (1988b) Computersonographische Darstellung der Zungenmotilität mittels Pseudo-3D-Rekonstruktion (Computerised sonographic imaging of tongue motility using pseudo-3 dimensional reconstruction). Ultraschall Med 9(2):95–97

Wein B, Böckler R, Klajman S (1991) Temporal reconstruction of sonographic imaging of disturbed tongue movements. Dysphagia 6(3):135–139

Wein B, Angerstein W, Klajman S et al (1993a) Zungensonographie und Druckmessungen beim Säuglingssaugen (Tongue sonography and pressure measurements during infant sucking). Klin Pädiatr 205(2):103–106

Wein B, Angerstein W, Klajman S (1993b) Darstellung der Bewegungsfolgen des Schluckvorganges mittels Sonographie und Röntgenvideofluoroskopie (Representation of the movement sequences of the swallowing process by means of sonography and X-ray video fluoroscopy). Sprache-Stimme-Gehör 17(2):65–67

Wein B, Neuschaefer-Rube C, Fischer-Wein G et al (1998) Analyse der Ultraschallbildsequenzen von Zungenbewegungen peripher und zentral verursachter Schluckstörungen (Analysis of ultrasound image sequences of tongue movements of peripheral and centrally caused swallowing disorders). Otorhinolaryngol Nova 8:82–87

WHO (World Health Organization) (2001) International classification of functioning, disability and health (ICF). World Health Organization, Geneva

Woisard V, Lepage B (2010) The "Deglutition Handicap Index" a self-administrated [sic] dysphagia-specific quality of life questionnaire: temporal reliability. Rev Laryngol Otol Rhinol (Bord) 131(1):19–22

Woisard V, Andrieux MP, Puech M (2006) Validation d'un questionnaire d'auto-évaluation du handicap pour les troubles de la déglutition oropharyngée (Deglutition Handicap Index) (Validation of a self-assessment questionnaire for swallowing disorders (deglutition handicap index)). Rev Laryngol Otol Rhinol 127(5):315–325

Woo P (2016) 4K video-laryngoscopy and video-stroboscopy: preliminary findings. Ann Otol Rhinol Laryngol 125(1):77–81

Zhou H, Zhu Y, Zhang X (2017) Validation of the Chinese Version of the Functional Oral Intake Scale (FOIS) score in the assessment of acute stroke patients with dysphagia. Stud Health Technol Inform 245:1195–1199

# Prevention of Dysphagia

**29**

Carl-Albert Bader

## 29.1 Prevention of Oropharyngeal Dysphagia

Carl-Albert Bader

### 29.1.1 Introduction

Oropharyngeal dysphagia has a symptomatic characteristic and is typically caused by structural lesions of the oral cavity, the pharynx or the larynx or by impaired sensory-motor control of the swallowing process. Many cases of oropharyngeal dysphagia are unavoidable but have far-reaching consequences. Thus, the question arises whether there are measures that mitigate the expression of dysphagia or even counteract their formation.

The preventive aspect of oropharyngeal dysphagia will be discussed below with selected examples:

- Dysphagia prevention in patients with head and neck malignancy who have undergone primary radio(chemo)therapy.
- Dysphagia prevention in head and neck surgery.

C.-A. Bader (✉)
Department of Otorhinolaryngology, University Hospital Saarland Homburg, Homburg/Saar, Germany
e-mail: c-a.bader@web.de

- Dysphagia prevention in the elderly.
- Dysphagia prevention when administering drugs.

### 29.1.2 Dysphagia Prevention in Primary Radio(chemo) therapy-Treated Patients with a Head and Neck Malignancy

Despite its principle organ-preserving approach, radio(chemo)therapy does not necessarily lead to a good maintenance of swallowing function: even with a conservative estimate poor swallowing can be assumed in more than half of the primarily radiotherapy- or radio(chemo)therapy-treated head and neck tumour patients, in some cases occurring even after many years (Lazarus 2009; Patterson et al. 2016). It is considered the most common long-term side effect of the therapy.

Although dysphagia may initially be underestimated in its severity, duration, and relevance by the patient himself (Brockbank et al. 2015), it is associated with a potentially life-threatening respiratory distress (Xu et al. 2015), a significant effect on nutrition and, in particular, on the social activities of those affected. Furthermore, it is expected to lead to a significant reduction in quality of life (Paleri et al. 2014).

Radio(chemo)therapy causes early and acute problems such as mucositis, mucosal oedema, and xerostomia as well as pain in the radiation field. However, the long-term characteristics of the dysphagia are mainly determined by the later effects of radiation presenting as fibrosis, and an alteration of the muscles involved in the swallowing process. Disturbances in the act of swallowing because of reduced laryngeal elevation, weakened pharyngeal constriction, reduced tongue retraction, and impaired epiglottal movement have been described, and the latter two have been reported in more than 75% of irradiated patients (Wall et al. 2013).

With regard to the prevention, or the best possible limitation, of the adverse side effects of radio(chemo)therapy, various strategies can be followed for which relevant studies can be found (see overview in Paleri et al. 2014):

- The use of a prophylactic, pre-therapeutic swallowing therapy.
- The appropriate use of feeding tubes.
- Taking radiological measures to reduce the tissue strain.

In *prophylactic swallowing therapy,* exercises are either performed before the beginning of the radio(chemo)therapy or immediately after the beginning of its application, provided the patient's condition allows it. The treatment approaches sometimes include a single therapy, sometimes a combination of several, and contain, for example, the following measures (Ahlberg et al. 2011; Carroll et al. 2008; Carnaby-Mann and Crary 2012; Daniels K et al. 2024; Kotz et al. 2012; Kulbersh et al. 2006; van der Molen et al. 2011):

- Exercises for the organs involved in the swallowing act, such as retraction of the tongue, pharynx constriction, elevation of the larynx and movements of the temporo-mandibular joint.
- Physiotherapeutic exercises for the throat, neck, and shoulder area.
- Additional speech and voice exercises.

The acceptance and the consistent execution of the exercises by the patients are described quite differently. Limitations due to motivational, cognitive and other reasons are to be expected (Cnossen et al. 2014; Shinn et al. 2013; van der Molen et al. 2011). Competent counselling is essential to ensure the best possible compliance by the patient (Brockbank et al. 2015). In addition, it should be ensured that the measures are accompanied by sufficient anti-pain therapy, adequate mucosal care, and psycho-oncological measures (Patterson et al. 2016).

The mechanism of the therapeutic effect is apparently not yet fully understood. It is assumed that the movement exercises counteract muscular fibrosis and strengthen muscle structures.

Positive effects of prophylactic swallowing therapy have been shown, for example, by using videofluoroscopic examination for specific aspects of the physiology of swallowing, such as the extent of tongue retraction or hyoid movement (Carroll et al. 2008; Ohba et al. 2016) and by evaluating dietary aspects (Kotz et al. 2012). In addition, favourable effects of a prophylactic swallowing therapy on the volume and structure of muscles involved in the process of swallowing have been documented by magnetic resonance imaging (Carnaby-Mann and Crary 2012). So far, none of the therapeutic procedures has turned out to be superior.

Pettersson et al. (2024) who assessed the swallowing performance in patients with head and neck cancer using a FEES protocol specifically adapted to their situation (Starmer et al. 2021) did however not find significant differences between treated and non-treated patients. Although positive effects have been demonstrated in several studies there is a need for randomised trials with a sufficiently large number of patients and comparable study designs (Messing et al. 2017; Perry et al. 2016; Roe and Ashforth 2011).

In addition to prophylactic swallowing therapy, the second strategy for the prophylaxis of dysphagia emphasises adequate *feeding tube management.*

For enteral feeding tubes, the nasogastric tube and percutaneous endoscopic gastrostomy (PEG) are available. Both are associated with typical advantages and disadvantages (Bartholome and Schröter-Morasch 2022), whereby the practical advantages of PEG for the patient are above all that it is less visible and is less likely to be blocked. There are different and quite controversial points of view regarding the choice of the tube (see overview in Paleri and Patterson 2010; Paleri et al. 2014).

For the radio-chemotherapy patient, the attachment of a PEG is typically indicated when food intake, due to pain, xerostomia and swelling in the treatment area, is impaired or expected to be impaired over a period of several weeks or more, and especially, of course, if aspiration does not allow safe oral food intake.

Especially in patients at risk of aspiration and in patients who have already started radio-chemotherapy with a relevant pre-therapeutic dysphagia, renunciation of PEG will be risky or unreasonable.

In other cases, however, a critical examination of the medical need for PEG is advisable. The exemplary study by Hutcheson et al. (2013) with nearly 500 patients, the study by Barbon et al. (2022) with nearly 600 patients, and the study by Langmore et al. (2012), suggest that nutrition per os for as long as possible, avoiding prolonged periods of non oral feeding, and not performing prophylactic PEG will lead to a better swallowing competence, more frequent oral food intake after treatment, and a higher tolerance of food of different consistencies.

The positive effects of this strategy are attributed to the prevention of disuse of swallowing muscles and thus to the inhibition of fibrous and atrophic processes of the oropharyngeal swallowing muscle (Hutcheson et al. 2013). They are probably based on similar mechanisms as assumed in prophylactic exercise therapy.

A third relevant aspect in the prophylaxis of radio(chemo)therapy-associated dysphagia concerns *radiological measures*.

As expected, the radiological literature describes close correlations between the dose applied in the neck area and the extent of damage to the pharyngeal, laryngeal and oesophageal muscles involved in the process of swallowing (Servagi-Vernat et al. 2015). For example, if the radiation dose of 50 Gy is exceeded, increasing damage to the pharyngeal constrictors is likely to happen. Therefore, requirements of therapeutic effectiveness need to take account the least possible muscle damage.

The most commonly reported side-effect of radio(chemo)therapy is xerostomia, which is experienced as very stressful by the patients. By using IMRT (Intensity-Modulated Radiation Therapy) while sparing parotid glands from radiation, Xerostomia can be effectively reduced (Nutting et al. 2011).

A surgical transfer of the submandibular gland from the irradiation field to the contralateral side can reduce radiogenic xerostomia as well (Sood et al. 2014).

### 29.1.3 Dysphagia Prevention in Surgical Procedures in the Head and Neck Area

In *oncological patients* who have undergone surgical therapy, the surgery-associated swallowing disorder is determined by the extent and in particular the functional relevance of the resected structures as well as the type of reconstructive measures (Mittal et al. 2003). Previously existing disorders of the swallowing process play an additional role (Manikantan et al. 2009).

Compared with primarily radio(chemo)-treated patients, there is only sparse knowledge on the effects of prophylactic exercises to prevent swallowing disorders in surgically treated oncological patients.

In cases of partial laryngeal resections, prophylactic preoperative exercises have pointed to a more rapid restoration of the swallowing process (Cavalot et al. 2009) but the data are considered insufficient for general recommendations (Lips et al. 2015).

In *spinal surgery* factors have been identified that can counteract postoperative dysphagia such as preoperative practice, specific surgical techniques, measures of anaesthesia, and drug application (Joaquim et al. 2014; Siribumrungwong et al. 2022; Yu et al. 2024).

### 29.1.4 Dysphagia Prevention in the Elderly

In old age, the increased incidence of dysphagia-triggering diseases and the purely age-related changes in the swallowing process itself as well as polypharmacy lead to an increase in oropharyngeal dysphagia (Jungheim et al. 2014; Wolf et al. 2021).

Above all, the best way of prevention is to preserve the *masticatory function*. Repair of existing tooth damage, avoidance of tooth loss as well as the best possible tooth replacement allowing regular mastication are regarded as crucial factors preventing swallowing disturbances. This also applies to acute diseases such as stroke events, which by themselves are associated with a high risk of dysphagia (Mituuti et al. 2015).

### 29.1.5 Dysphagia Prevention during the Administration of Drugs

Unwanted side effects on swallowing ability are caused by a number of drugs. The site of the drug action may be central (and usually sedating), central with peripheral effect (e.g., with reduction of salivation), neuromuscular, local-mucosal or may be unknown (see detailed overview in Schwemmle et al. 2015). Because of the specific pharmacodynamics and pharmacokinetics of these drugs in the elderly and in children special caution in required in these patient groups.

Table 29.1 illustrates a selection of drug groups with potential effects on the swallowing

**Table 29.1** Selection of drug groups that can trigger or enhance oropharyngeal dysphagia (Cichero and Murdoch 2006; Edholm 2010; Polmann et al. 2023)

| Drugs with central nervous, sedating side effects | Tranquilizers/ Benzodiazepines Barbiturates Antipsychotics/ Neuroleptics Central-acting Analgesics |
| --- | --- |
| Drugs with special extra-pyramidal side effects | Antipsychotics/ Neuroleptics Metoclopramide |
| Drugs with effects on the mucous membrane texture (xerostomia) | Anticholinergics Antihypertensives Diuretics Opiates Antidepressants Muscle relaxants Antihistamines |
| Drugs that affect the muscular parts of the swallowing apparatus | Statins |

ability. Indication and individual dosage must be carefully assessed.

### 29.1.6 Summary

- Prophylactic measures to reduce oropharyngeal dysphagia have been reported to be effective in primary radio(chemo)-treated oncological patients.
- These treatment approaches include, above all, movement exercises for the structures involved in the process of swallowing, adequate nutrition management, and technical measures of radiotherapy.
- Outside of the oncological field, preventive measures are particularly relevant for the elderly.

## References

Ahlberg A, Engström T, Nikolaidis P et al (2011) Early self-care rehabilitation of head and neck cancer patients. Acta Otolaryngol 131(5):552–561

Barbon CEA, Peterson CB, Moreno AC et al (2022) Adhering to eat and exercise status during radiotherapy for oropharyngeal cancer for prevention and mitigation of radiotherapy-associated dysphagia. JAMA Otolaryngol Head Neck Surg 148(10):956–964

Bartholome G, Schröter-Morasch H (eds) (2022) Schluckstörungen. Interdisziplinäre Diagnostik und Rehabilitation, 7th edn. Elsevier, Munich

Brockbank S, Miller N, Owen S et al (2015) Pretreatment Information of dysphagia: exploring the views of head and neck cancer patients. J Pain Symptom Manage 49(1):89–97

Carnaby-Mann G, Crary MA (2012) "Pharyngocise": randomized controlled trial of preventative exercises to maintain muscle structure and swallowing function during head-and-neck chemoradiotherapy. Int J Radiat Oncol Biol Phys 83(1):210–219

Carroll WR, Locher JL, Canon CL et al (2008) Pretreatment swallowing exercises improve swallow function after chemoradiation. Laryngoscope 118(1):39–43

Cavalot AL, Ricci E, Schindler A et al (2009) The importance of preoperative swallowing therapy in subtotal laryngectomies. Otolaryngol Head Neck Surg 140(6):822–825

Cichero JA, Murdoch BE (eds) (2006) Dysphagia. Foundation, theory, and practice. Wiley, Chichester

Cnossen IC, van Uden-Kraan CF, Rinkel RN et al (2014) Multimodal guided self-help exercise program to prevent speech, swallowing, and shoulder problems among head and neck cancer patients: a feasibility study. J Med Internet Res 16(3):e74. https://doi.org/10.2196/jmir.2990

Daniels K, Chanda A, Berry L et al (2024) A survey of manual therapy techniques and protocols used to prevent or treat dysphagia in head and neck cancer patients during and after radiation therapy. Glob Adv Integr Med Health 13:1–11

Edholm B (2010) Statin-induced dysphagia. Ugeskr Laeger 172(7):544–545

Hutcheson KA, Bhayani MK, Beadle BM et al (2013) Eat and exercise during radiotherapy or chemoradiotherapy for pharyngeal cancers: use it or lose it. JAMA Otolaryngol Head Neck Surg 139(11):1127–1134

Joaquim AF, Murar J, Savage JW et al (2014) Dysphagia after anterior cervical spine surgery: a systematic review of potential preventative measures. Spine J 14(9):2246–2260

Jungheim M, Schwemmle C, Miller S et al (2014) Schlucken und Schluckstörungen im Alter (Swallowing and dysphagia in the elderly). HNO 62(9):644–651

Kotz T, Federman AD, Kao J et al (2012) Prophylactic swallowing exercises in patients with head and neck cancer undergoing chemoradiation: a randomized trial. Arch Otolaryngol Head Neck Surg 138(4):376–382

Kulbersh BD, Rosenthal EL, McGrew BM et al (2006) Pretreatment, preoperative swallowing exercises may improve dysphagia quality of life. Laryngoscope 116(6):883–886

Langmore S, Krisciunas GP, Miloro KV et al (2012) Does PEG use cause dysphagia in head and neck cancer patients? Dysphagia 27(2):251–259

Lazarus CL (2009) Effects of chemoradiotherapy on voice and swallowing. Curr Opin Otolaryngol Head Neck Surg 17(3):172–178

Lips M, Speyer R, Zumach A et al (2015) Supracricoid laryngectomy and dysphagia: a systematic literature review. Laryngoscope 125(9):2143–2156

Manikantan K, Khode S, Sayed SI et al (2009) Dysphagia in head and neck cancer. Cancer Treat Rev 35(8):724–732

Messing BP, Ward EC, Lazarus CL et al (2017) Prophylactic swallow therapy for patients with head and neck cancer undergoing chemoradiotherapy: a randomized trial. Dysphagia 32(4):487–500

Mittal BB, Pauloski BR, Haraf DJ et al (2003) Swallowing dysfunction—preventative and rehabilitation strategies in patients with head-and-neck cancer treated with surgery, radiotherapy, and chemotherapy: a critical review. Int J Radiat Oncol Biol Phys 57(5):1219–1230

Mituuti CT, Bianco VC, Bentim CG et al (2015) Influence of oral health condition on swallowing and oral intake level for patients affected by chronic stroke. Clin Interv Aging 10:29–35

Nutting CM, Morden JP, Harrington KJ et al (2011) Parotid-sparing intensity modulated versus conventional radiotherapy in head and neck cancer (PARSPORT): a phase 3 multicentre randomised controlled trial. Lancet Oncol 12(2):127–136

Ohba S, Yokohama J, Kojima M et al (2016) Significant preservation of swallowing function in chemoradiotherapy for advanced head and neck cancer by prophylactic swallowing exercise. Head Neck 38(4):517–521

Paleri V, Patterson J (2010) Use of gastrostomy in head and neck cancer: a systematic review to identify areas for future research. Clin Otolaryngol 35(3):177–189

Paleri V, Roe JWG, Strojan P et al (2014) Strategies to reduce long-term postchemoradiation dysphagia in patients with head and neck cancer: an evidence-based review. Head Neck 36(3):431–443

Patterson JM, Brady GC, Roe JWG (2016) Research into prevention and rehabilitation of dysphagia in head and neck cancer: a UK perspective. Curr Opin Otolaryngol Head Neck Surg 24(3):208–214

Perry A, Lee SH, Cotton S et al (2016) Therapeutic exercises for affecting post-treatment swallowing in people treated for advanced-stage head and neck cancers (review). Cochrane Database Syst Rev 8:CD011112

Pettersson K, Finizia C, Pauli N et al (2024) Preventing radiation-induced dysphagia and trismus in head and neck cancer—a randomized controlled trial. Head Neck. Online ahead of print

Polmann MB, Suarez RI, Saad A et al (2023) A case report of an atypical presentation of statin-induced necrotizing myositis. Cureus 15(8):e43587

Roe JWG, Ashforth KM (2011) Prophylactic swallowing exercises for patients receiving radiotherapy for head and neck cancer. Curr Opin Otolaryngol Head Neck Surg 19(3):144–149

Schwemmle C, Jungheim M, Miller S et al (2015) Medikamenteninduzierte Dysphagien. Ein Überblick (Medication-induced dysphagia. An overview). HNO 63(7):504–510

Servagi-Vernat S, Ali D, Roubieu C et al (2015) Dysphagia after radiotherapy: state of the art and prevention. Eur Ann Otorhinolaryngol Head Neck Dis 132(1):25–29

Shinn EH, Basen-Engquist K, Baum G et al (2013) Adherence to preventive exercises and self-reported swallowing outcomes in post-radiation head and neck cancer patients. Head Neck 35(12):1707–1712

Siribumrungwong K, Kanjanapirom P, Dhanachanvisith N et al (2022) Effect of single-dose preemptive systemic dexamethasone on postoperative dysphagia and odynophagia following anterior cervical spine surgery: a double-blinded, prospective, randomized controlled trial. Clin Orthop Surg 14(2):253–262

Sood AJ, Fox NF, O'Connell BP et al (2014) Salivary gland transfer to prevent radiation-induced xerostomia: a systematic review and meta-analysis. Oral Oncol 50(2):77–83

Starmer HM, Arrese L, Langmore S et al (2021) Adaptation and validation of the dynamic imaging grade of swallowing toxicity for flexible endoscopic evaluation of swallowing: DIGEST-FEES. J Speech Lang Hear Res 64(6):1802–1810

van der Molen L, van Rossum MA, Burkhead LM et al
(2011) A randomized preventive rehabilitation trial
in advanced head and neck cancer patients treated
with chemoradiotherapy: feasibility, compliance, and
short-term effects. Dysphagia 26(2):155–170

Wall LR, Ward EC, Cartmill B et al (2013) Physiological
changes to the swallowing mechanism following
(chemo)radiotherapy for head and neck cancer: a systematic review. Dysphagia 28(4):481–493

Wolf U, Eckert S, Walter G et al (2021) Prevalence of
oropharyngeal dysphagia in geriatric patients and

real-life associations with diseases and drugs. Sci Rep
11(1):21955. www.nature.com/scientificreports

Xu B, Boero IJ, Hwang L et al (2015) Aspiration pneumonia after concurrent chemoradiotherapy for head and
neck cancer. Cancer 121(8):1303–1311

Yu C, Chunmei L, Qin L et al (2024) Application of intra-
operative neurophysiological monitoring (IONM) for
preventing dysphagia after anterior cervical surgery:
a prospective study. World Neurosurg 184:e390–e396

# Rehabilitation and Prognosis of Dysphagia

**30**

Tamer Abou-Elsaad, Carmelo Perez Alvarez, Carl-Albert Bader, Florence Baert, Jörg Edgar Bohlender, Doris-Maria Denk-Linnert, Mohamed Farahat, Žofia Korim, Peter Kummer, Tamer Mesallam, Tadeus Nawka, Renée Speyer, Miroslav Tedla, Geertrui Vlaemynck, and Patrick G. Zorowka

**Supplementary Information** The online version contains supplementary material available at https://doi.org/10.1007/978-3-031-48091-1_15.

T. Abou-Elsaad (✉)
Phoniatrics Unit, ORL Department, Mansoura University, Faculty of Medicine, Mansoura, Egypt
e-mail: taboelsaad@mans.edu.eg

C. P. Alvarez
Department of Otorhinolaryngology, University Hospital Regensburg, Regensburg, Germany
e-mail: carmelo.alvarez@klink.uni-regensburg.de

C.-A. Bader
Department of Otorhinolaryngology, University Hospital Saarland Homburg, Homburg/Saar, Germany
e-mail: c-a.bader@web.de

F. Baert
Vitaflow Company, Antwerpen, Belgium
e-mail: florence.baert@vitaflo.co.uk

J. E. Bohlender
Department of Phoniatrics and Speech Pathology, University Hospital Zurich (USZ), Zurich, Switzerland
e-mail: joerg.bohlender@usz.ch

D.-M. Denk-Linnert
Division of Phoniatrics and Speech Language Therapy, Department of Otorhinolaryngology, Medical University of Vienna, Vienna, Austria
e-mail: doris-maria.denk-linnert@meduni.wien.ac.at

M. Farahat
Department of Otolaryngology, Communication and Swallowing Disorders Unit, King Saud University, College of Medicine, ENT Department, Riyadh, Saudi Arabia
e-mail: mfarahat@ksu.edu.sa

Ž. Korim · M. Tedla
Department of Otolaryngology, Head and Neck Surgery, Faculty of Medicine, Comenius University, University Hospital Bratislava, Bratislava, Slovakia
e-mail: korim7@uniba.sk; miroslav.tedla@unb.sk

P. Kummer
Department of Phoniatrics and Pediatric Audiology, ENT-Clinic, University Hospital Regensburg, Regensburg, Germany
e-mail: peter.kummer@ukr.de

T. Mesallam
Otolaryngology Department, King Saud University College of Medicinde, Riyadh, Saudi Arabia
e-mail: t.mesallam@ksu.edu.sa

T. Nawka
Department of Audiology and Phoniatrics, Charité - Universitätsmedizin Berlin, Berlin, Germany
e-mail: tadeus.nawka@charite.de

R. Speyer
Discipline of Speech and Language Therapy, School of Health Sciences, College of Medicine, Nursing & Health Sciences, University of Galway, Galway, Ireland

School of Occupational Therapy, Social Work and Speech Pathology, Curtin University, Faculty of Health Sciences, Perth, WA, Australia
e-mail: renee.speyer@universityofgalway.ie

G. Vlaemynck
Technology and Food Science Unit, Flanders Research Institute for Agriculture, Fisheries and Food (ILVO), Flanders, Melle, Belgium
e-mail: geertrui.vlaemynck@ilvo.vlaanderen.be

## 30.1 Concepts of Swallowing Therapy

Jörg Edgar Bohlender

### 30.1.1 Introduction

The careful decision-making on which kind of dysphagia rehabilitation programme is appropriate requires a thorough personal history and clinical examination. Additionally, the clinical examination should include an accurate instrumental assessment that defines the type and nature of the specific swallowing disorder, and the underlying cause and conditions such as stroke (Daniels and Huckabee 2014; Johnson et al. 2014; Vose et al. 2014) and head and neck cancer (Kraaijenga et al. 2014). Instrumental evaluation plays a crucial role in dysphagia management and is the essential tool that guides the course of treatment and assesses the benefit or failure of dysphagia therapy. The evaluation and treatment of patients with swallowing disorders is generally a comprehensive, multidisciplinary approach with a team of phoniatricians and speech language pathologists, otolaryngologists, neurologists, gastroenterologists, radiologists, nurses and dieticians. A range of different direct and indirect treatment interventions exists for swallowing problems: swallowing therapy (Hegland and Murry 2013), dietary modifications, pharmacological treatment and surgery. Major goals of swallowing therapy are generally restoration and maintenance of the ability to swallow safely and effectively without aspiration.

### 30.1.2 Compensatory Strategies

Compensatory manoeuvres are designed to direct bolus flow and to alter the flow velocity of the bolus for safe and efficient oral intake. These techniques are usually used to compensate for structural deficits and physiological insufficiencies. Compensatory strategies focus on safe swallowing by alterations in diet consistency, changes in the patient's posture and in the mechanism of swallowing. The outcome of these manoeuvres is temporary and depends on the appropriate conditions. The purpose is a short-term adjustment to facilitate swallowing function, but it does not involve a direct treatment of the impaired physiology.

Compensatory strategies include:

- Texture-modified diet (TMD).
- Sensory-based enhancement.
- Changing posture/position.
- Volitional control of swallowing.
- Volitional breath-hold manoeuvres:
- Supraglottic swallowing.
- Super-supraglottic swallowing.
- Mendelsohn manoeuvre.

#### 30.1.2.1 Texture Modified Diet (TMD)

Besides specific rehabilitative approaches and surgical options, the clinician should advise the safest food and fluid texture for the patient to swallow. In addition to volume and rate delivery, the provision of texture-modified food and thickened fluids is an important and routine part of dysphagia therapy to maintain the individual nutritional needs, to support the quality of life (for instance, disengagement from tube feeding) and to prevent more weight loss. Modifying the viscosity of fluids or food texture enhances safer eating and drinking. Altering the volume of food and food consistency is based on a range of different assessment methods designed to recommend whether an individual can take food or drink orally. The appropriate texture should be drawn from medical history, clinical swallowing examination (CSE), instrumental assessment: a videofluoroscopic swallowing study (VFSS) or flexible endoscopic evaluation of swallowing (FEES).

In response to patient safety in dysphagia, the following questions on diet modification should be answered:

P. G. Zorowka
Department for Hearing, Voice and Speech Disorders,
Medical University Innsbruck,
Innsbruck, Austria
e-mail: patrick.zorowka@i-med.ac.at

- Can be food taken orally?
- Is no or insufficient oral food intake possible?
- Is nutritional supplement with a texture-modified diet necessary?
- Is complete tube feeding necessary?

**Oral Care**

The highly vulnerable group of elderly patients with poorly fitted dentures and missing teeth shows a predisposition to aspiration with chewing and swallowing. Poor oral and dental hygiene frequently occurs with a significant pathogenic colonisation of the mouth, leading to an increasing risk of aspiration pneumonia. As part of responsible care, routine regular daily oral and dental care, also including those patients on feeding tubes, is effective in improving the quality of life by preventing aspiration pneumonia. The maintenance of oral care hygiene by thorough oral care and quality oral care equipment is a crucial factor in the therapeutic management of dysphagia, by reducing the negative side effects associated with poor oral hygiene. A comprehensive oral rehabilitation programme includes both oral hygiene and indirect oral training of mastication and swallowing.

### 30.1.2.2 Sensory Based Enhancement

Bolus modification means not only varying the texture, consistency and viscosity of food and liquids. By taking into account the decrease in sensory awareness in dysphagic elderly and neurogenic dysphagia patients, the sensory strategy pursues the goal of improving sensory deficits by altering *temperature*, *carbonation* and *taste*. Sensory-based enhancement techniques are judged automatically with a positive impact but should be handled with care and linked to known evidence-based strategies.

### 30.1.2.3 Changing in Posture/Position

Postural techniques are a part of compensatory strategies to prevent aspiration and minimise residues. They are targeted at modification of oral and pharyngeal physiology. Usually these postures and postural combinations have specific effects on the flow of the bolus.

These facilitatory postures include:

- Chin tuck.
- Chin elevation.
- Head rotation.
- Head tilt.
- Side-lying.
- Combinations of different positions.

**Chin Tuck**

The chin-tuck technique (Fig. 30.1) is often equated with swallowing safety. The anticipated efficacy of this popular method still remains unclear. In particular cases, patients without residue in the pyriform sinuses benefit by merely tucking the chin towards the neck to prevent aspiration from the vallecular regions. The indication of postural techniques should always be confirmed critically and evaluated by instrumental assessment (FEES/VFSS).

### 30.1.2.4 Volitional Control of Swallowing

Volitional control of swallowing includes established methods with promising results in clinical practice. The patients are previously advised to delay volitionally the beginning of the oral transfer. The *three-second preparation* occurs over a silent counting of 1, 2 and 3 before the oral transfer is executed.

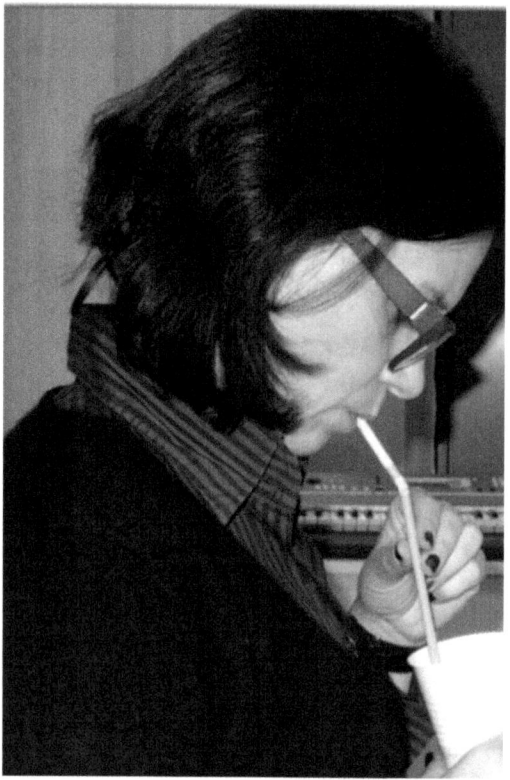

**Fig. 30.1** The chin-tuck technique prevents aspiration form the vallecular regions. With kind permission of the test person

### 30.1.2.5 Volitional Breath-Hold Manoeuvres

This group of swallowing manoeuvres includes also the so-called breath-holding techniques, which are excellent methods to eliminate penetration and aspiration. These specific strategies are primarily developed for postsurgical head and neck cancer patients and also used now for other patient groups. A successful teaching and realisation of both exercises requires a minimum of comprehension and memory to compensate a swallowing problem.

The *supraglottal swallow manoeuvre* protects the airway from aspiration at the vocal fold level. This technique includes simultaneous breath-holding and swallowing, which is immediately followed by a cough after swallowing before the next inhalation starts.

The *super-supraglottal manoeuvre* protects the airway from penetration and aspiration primarily at the level of the laryngeal vestibule. This exercise is similar to the supraglottal swallow manoeuvre; following the supraglottal exercise the patient has to hold his breath again while bearing down before the next inhalation starts. The additional bearing-down-technique increases the duration of pressure of the base of the tongue on the posterior pharyngeal wall and also of the muscular effort at the false and true vocal fold level.

The *Mendelsohn manoeuvre* is a special form of breath-holding exercise. It combines compensatory and strengthening exercise strategies in dysphagia management. Initially the Mendelsohn technique was developed to increase hyolaryngeal motion and to support a prolonged opening and width of the upper oesophageal segment (UES) during swallowing. The patient is instructed to keep the larynx elevated and hold it in the middle of the swallow for 2–3 s, when the larynx is felt to elevate, and then relax. The effort of holding the larynx up is an exhausting swallowing exercise and in some cases challenging to use consistently owing to the effects of fatigue. In conclusion the Mendelsohn manoeuvre is helpful in selected patient groups by decreasing aspiration and pyriform sinus residuals (McCullough and Kim 2013).

### 30.1.3 Oral Motor Exercises

Rehabilitation manoeuvres include the so-called oral motor exercises. The rehabilitative concept of performing oropharyngeal strengthening therapy is an important component in swallowing therapy. These specific exercises permit modification of the force, length and range of motion of oropharyngeal and also laryngeal structures occurring during swallowing. Oral motor exercises include generally:

• Lingual resistance exercises.
• Effortful swallowing.
• Masako Manoeuvre.
• Shaker Exercise.

### 30.1.3.1 Strengthening Tongue Muscles by Lingual Resistance Exercises

Numerous devices and tools are provided for lingual strengthening exercises: tongue depressors, Iowa Oral Performance Instrument (IOPI®), SwallowSTRONG®, Madison Oral Strengthening Therapeutic (MOST®). *Isometric lingual resistance* exercises require a patient-specific training regimen that is mainly based on specificity, repetition, intensity and time. The principles of training and overload are represented in isometric progressive oropharyngeal (I-PRO) therapy programmes, using for instance the IOPI® (with both anterior and posterior lingual pressure bulbs) or SwallowSTRONG® device. The promising results for patients with dysphagia due to oropharyngeal weakness show an improvement not only in isometric and swallowing pressures and tongue mass, but also in speed of oral transit time and quality of life measures, and in a significant decrease in airway invasion (Chua et al. 2024).

### 30.1.3.2 Effortful Swallowing

Effortful swallowing as an established and well-used rehabilitation technique containing elements of compensatory as well as strengthening exercises. The trained method 'to swallow hard' influences to an increasing degree the pharyngeal pressure and duration of orolingual pressure. Furthermore, the effects of effortful swallowing result in an improvement of hyo-laryngeal movement, protection of the deeper airways and UES opening. The application of effortful swallowing is useful in oral pharyngeal impairment and improves the base of tongue retraction and decreases vallecular residue. Clinicians should bear in mind that the recommended technique has also adverse effects on hyo-laryngeal excursion and nasal backflow.

### 30.1.3.3 Masako Manoeuvre

The *Masako* or *tongue-hold manoeuvre* describes solely a focused strengthening technique. The patient is instructed to protrude the anterior part of the tongue between the front teeth (edentulous patients place it between the lips) and maintain this posture while swallowing saliva. In the first instance the Masako manoeuvre is considered to strengthen the pharyngeal constrictor muscles and supports the reduction of vallecular residues. The application of this encouraging technique in clinical routine remains rare.

### 30.1.3.4 Shaker Exercise

The *Shaker exercise* (Fig. 30.2) is an isometric and isokinetic exercise designed to increase the antero-posterior deglutitive opening of the UES by strengthening the suprahyoid muscles (Shaker et al. 2013). The patient is instructed to lie flat on the back and keep the shoulders on the base and raise the head to look at the toes.

The goal of this simple but demanding exercise is initially to maintain raising the head position for 1 min (isometric strengthening part). The patient has to repeat the head lift three times. Subsequently the patient has to perform a repetitive head-lift manoeuvre 30 times with a 1 min rest between (isokinetic strengthening part). The Shaker exercise is usually performed three times a day for 6–8 weeks.

The exercise should be not recommended for patients with neck immobility, heart problems and stroke, or patients with a tracheal cannula.

**Fig. 30.2** The Shaker exercise. With kind permission of the test person

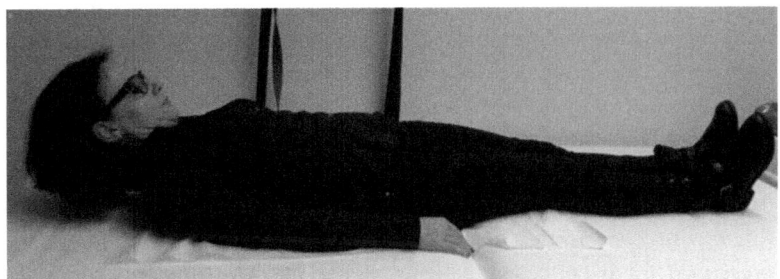

## 30.1.4 Rehabilitation Adjuncts

*Neuromuscular electrical stimulation* (NMES) (e.g., Suntrup et al. 2015) is an increasingly popular but still controversially discussed therapeutic strategy in dysphagia management. The effectiveness and efficacy of electrical stimulation as a new treatment modality of individuals with dysphagia still remains vague. In healthy subjects intra-pharyngeal electrical stimulation demonstrates temporary changes in cortical swallowing processing. Nevertheless, first studies show the equivocal potential of NMES compared with traditional swallowing rehabilitation regimens.

For instance, active *pharyngeal electrical stimulation* (PES) compared with sham PES contributes evidence that the swallowing disability, the feeding status and the duration of hospitalisation in patients after a brain lesion are effectively modulated. In summary NMES is a promising tool for future dysphagia therapy.

The application of the non-invasive *repetitive transcranial magnetic stimulation* (rTMS) as a therapeutic tool in swallowing disorders is currently under investigation. This promising treatment needs further trials with larger sample sizes to clarify the long-term functional outcome in dysphagic patients.

## 30.1.5 Medical and Surgical Intervention

In addition to the traditional treatments for dysphagia, many pharmacological agents have been studied for possible beneficial effects on dysphagia patients. But there is only a small number of possible medications that can facilitate swallowing problems. Beside phosphodiesterase inhibitors, amantadine, dopamine and capsaicin, angiotensin converting enzyme (ACE) inhibitors play a crucial part by the sensitising effects on the cough and swallowing reflexes.

### 30.1.5.1 Medical Interventions
*Angiotensin converting enzyme* (ACE) *inhibitors* prescribed for hypertensive patients reduce the risk of aspiration pneumonia. Studies in hypertensive patients with dysphagia and stroke have confirmed that ACE inhibitors induce the cough reflex and decrease the delay of the swallowing reflex and reduce silent aspirations. This positive and important protective impact on the ability to swallow is related to the elevation of substance P (SP). The increased serum level of neurotransmitter SP due to the medical intervention by ACE inhibitors confirms a strong link to the improvement of swallowing functions.

*Botulinum toxin* (BTX) is a potent neurotoxin acting by inhibiting acetylcholine release at the neuromuscular junction. The therapeutic achieved effect of decreased muscle activity and motor control is used for instance as a common treatment in dystonia, spasticity disorders and muscular atrophy.

In dysphagia, BTX injections are also recommended in particular cases to relieve spasm in patients with oesophageal achalasia, characterised by incomplete lower oesophageal sphincter (LES) relaxation, diffuse oesophageal spasms or failed cricopharyngeal relaxation. Furthermore, BTX is provided as a beneficial treatment in unintentional loss of saliva from the mouth (drooling) and excessive salivation, which interferes with severe swallowing problems. BTX minimises salivary secretions by blocking cholinergic autonomic parasympathetic and postganglionic sympathetic acetylcholine release at the endings in the salivary glands. The injection of BTX into salivary glands helps to reduce sialorrhoea and shows therapeutic effects in dysphagia patients. BTX injection should always be considered before performing an invasive surgical procedure, usage of anticholinergic medication or radiation therapy.

In conclusion BTX injections are generally a reasonable approach to diminish the specific symptoms of dysphagia. At least patients should be informed that repeated injections are necessary for continued relief.

### 30.1.5.2 Surgical Options
Surgical procedures are a part of the treatment options in dysphagia and should be always considered as a choice of procedure depending upon the specific cause of dysphagia. The choice of surgery depends on accurately identifying the cause of swallowing problems. In particular, Zenker's diverticulum surgery, including open

and endoscopic approaches, is an effective method and improves patients' quality of life.

Treatment of chronic intractable aspiration should initially include all conservative options: aggressive pulmonary hygiene to clear mucus and secretions from the airways, suitable antibiotics, oral hygiene and continued nutritional and fluid supplementation by enteral (nasogastric tube, cervical oesophagotomy, gastrostomy and jejunostomy) or parenteral route (see Table 30.1).

**Preventive Dysphagia Therapy**

Acute and long-term swallowing side effects due to radiochemotherapy for advanced head and neck cancer is a leading functional complication for many patients during non-operative treatments. A crucial component of modern, multidisciplinary head and neck care involves swallowing exercises before, during and after the course of radiotherapy, and additionally provides the maintenance of oral intake with specific dietary modifications. The initiation of swallowing therapy requires initially an extensive functional and instrumental assessment to develop an individual rehabilitation plan before the therapy starts. This derived proactive pre-, per- and post-treatment strategy pursues the goal to reduce radiation-associated dysphagia risks following the 'Use it or lose it' paradigm. Recent encouraging studies support the positive impact of prophylactic intervention for head and neck cancer patients on several levels after radiation:

Risk reduction for loss of functional swallowing ability.

More normal oral diet levels.

Less weight loss.

Improvement of swallowing-related quality of life.

Shorter duration of feeding tube dependence.

Significant preservation of muscle mass due to swallowing-related musculature.

Better base of tongue and epiglottal movement.

**Table 30.1** Surgical procedures in dysphagia

| Problem | Surgical procedure |
| --- | --- |
| Chronic intractable aspiration | Tracheostomy (reversible, phonation possible) |
| | Laryngectomy (irreversible, no phonation) |
| | Tracheo-oesophageal diversion (reversible, no phonation) |
| | Laryngotracheal separation (reversible, no phonation) |
| | Glottal closure (irreversible, no phonation) |
| | Laryngeal suspension (reversible, phonation possible) |
| | Total and partial cricoid resection |
| Hypertonic cricopharyngeus muscle | Cricopharyngealmyotomy (endoscopic or external approach) |
| Zenker's diverticulum | Endoscopic or open transcervical approach |
| Oesophageal strictures due to malignant or benign stenotic lesions | Endoscopic dilation |
| Unilateral paralysis of the vocal folds with inefficient cough and aspiration | Vocal fold medialisation Thyroplasty Arytenoid adduction |

## 30.2 Planning and Supervision of Dysphagia Interventions by Therapists

Renée Speyer

### 30.2.1 Introduction

Oropharyngeal dysphagia has many aetiologies and can affect a person of any age. Paediatric dysphagia is mainly associated with neurodevelopmental delay. Dysphagia in middle age frequently has gastro-oesophageal and immunological causes. In people older than 60 years it is mostly associated with oncological and neurological pathologies. In the elderly it is related to stroke, neurodegenerative disease and dementia (Roden and Altman 2013). Prevalence data (Takizawa et al. 2016) vary widely, depending on the characteristics of the study population, the way dysphagia is defined, and the choice of screening or assessment tools and outcome variables. Dysphagia may lead to complications such as dehydration, malnutrition, aspiration pneumonia and even death. In addition, it has a major impact on a patient's psychosocial and emotional well-being (Timmerman et al. 2014; Jones et al. 2018).

Best clinical practice for oropharyngeal dysphagia usually entails a multidisciplinary approach to the care and management of dysphagia and calls for early detection and assessment of swallowing problems. Then, in light of an individual's needs, the assessment will be followed by medical, surgical or behavioural treatment. Behavioural intervention strategies are generally implemented by allied health professionals, usually speech and language therapists (SLPs). Next, the evaluation of intervention outcomes is an essential part of the overall treatment and management of oropharyngeal dysphagia.

## 30.2.2  Multidisciplinary Team

Both the diagnosis and the planning of treatment are generally done by a multidisciplinary team that includes medical specialists such as a phoniatrician, oto-rhino-laryngologist, neurologist or oncologist. The team may also include allied health professionals—a nurse, SLP, physiotherapist, occupational therapist, social worker or dietician. But other disciplines such as psychology or dentistry may be involved as well. The role of each team member may overlap disciplines or differ by country. Mostly, SLPs play a dominant role in the supervision and planning of behavioural intervention techniques. In some countries, Denmark for example, behavioural swallowing treatment may be the responsibility of an occupational therapist instead.

Even though behavioural interventions are usually carried out by SLPs, other health-care providers may also be responsible for some parts, reflecting regional and cultural differences. To capture that diversity, the term *dysphagia therapist* is introduced in this section. The term denotes any of the professionals involved in planning,

performing and evaluating behavioural treatment for patients with oropharyngeal dysphagia.

Countries may organise the care for dysphagia differently. The ratio of therapists to patients treated may differ considerably, as may education and training. The European Society for Swallowing Disorders (ESSD) is one of the stakeholders in education, offering and formulating new proposals for international education in oropharyngeal dysphagia at postgraduate and master levels. Such initiatives could standardise the learning outcomes and thereby ensure comparable levels of education among health-care providers. Recently, professional and patient organisations have shown interest in developing national and international guidelines on dysphagia. These efforts have generated evidence-based reviews of assessment and treatment outcomes for various patient populations. Altogether, the initiatives in education, guideline development and awareness-raising should lead to optimisation of the care for patients with dysphagia.

## 30.2.3  Screening and Assessment

The first step in the management of the population at risk for oropharyngeal dysphagia is screening. The aim is early detection of patients at risk for dysphagia and unsafe swallowing. Screening should meet certain clinical criteria: administration should be easy, not time-consuming and preferably non-invasive, to minimise patient distress. But the procedure should also meet certain psychometric criteria on diagnostic performance. Bours et al. (2009) and Kertscher et al. (2014) published detailed overviews of screening methods with sufficiently high sensitivity ($\geq 70\%$) and moderate specificity ($\geq 60\%$). In clinical practice, too many false positives will increase the number of referrals for further assessment, with the attendant bottlenecks: insufficient workforce capacity and limited access to assessment tools. On the other hand, too many false negatives may lead to an underestimation of the actual number of patients suffering from dysphagia. A list of screening methods meeting both clinical and psychometric criteria is provided in Table 30.2.

Nurses generally conduct the screening, but other allied healthcare providers may be involved as well, particularly SLPs. Decisions on the type of screening tool are usually made by the SLPs, who are also responsible for training and education on screening within the workplace.

When a subject fails the initial screening, further assessment is usually required. Two 'gold standards' for this purpose are described in the literature: videofluoroscopy of swallowing (VFS) and flexible endoscopic evaluation of swallowing (FEES). Both VFS and FEES are aimed at detailed detection and quantification of abnormalities in swallowing function, physiology and anatomical structures. Depending on the clinical setting, these assessments will be performed by medical specialists or dysphagia therapists. However, access to either of these 'gold standard' tools may differ greatly between settings and no international consensus exists regarding which visuoperceptual or software-based measures to use for interpretation and assessment of these video recordings (Speyer et al. 2021). Therefore,

dysphagia therapists generally use other assessment tools as well (Table 30.2).

There is a wide range of clinical assessment methods in daily practice: from taking the patient's history to the evaluation of anatomy, physiology and function of the oral cavity, larynx and pharynx. For instance, particular methods may cover oral intake evaluation and mealtime observation, the assessment of communication and cognition, or the evaluation of trial interventions (to determine effects of bolus modification, postural adjustments and swallowing manoeuvres). To assess Functional Health Status (FHS) and Health-Related Quality of Life (HRQoL), the dysphagia therapist will use patient self-administered questionnaires. The literature offers detailed information on the reliability and validity of FHS and HRQoL questionnaires in oropharyngeal dysphagia (respectively, Speyer et al. 2014 and Timmerman et al. 2014). Sometimes additional assessments will be required, namely, video-manometry, oesophageal pH monitoring, EMG or cervical auscultation. Depending on the supplementary method selected, the clinical assessment will call upon certain disciplines.

**Table 30.2** Screening and multidisciplinary assessment in oropharyngeal dysphagia (data from Bours et al. 2009; Kertscher et al. 2014; Speyer 2013)

| Method | Description | Main purpose |
|---|---|---|
| Screening | → trial swallow with water, different viscosities, water in combination with oxygen desaturation, or different viscosities in combination with oxygen desaturation<br>→ oxygen desaturation<br>→ clinical features<br>→standardised form with clinical features | Detection of patients at risk for oropharyngeal dysphagia |
| Assessment | 'Gold standard'<br>→ VFS (Videofluoroscopy of swallowing)<br>→ FEES (Flexible endoscopic evaluation of swallowing) | Detection and quantification of abnormalities in swallowing function/ physiology or anatomical structures |
| | Clinical assessment<br>→ e.g. patient/medical history, Assessment of cognition, assessment of communication, mealtime observation, trial intervention, functional/anatomical/physiological evaluation of oral cavity/larynx/pharynx | Detection and quantification of abnormalities in swallowing function/ physiology or anatomical structures |
| | Patient self-evaluation<br>→ functional health status questionnaire<br>→ health-related quality of life questionnaire | Description of functional health status or impact of oropharyngeal dysphagia on quality of life as experienced by the patient |
| | Supplementary methods<br>→ e.g. Videomanometry, Oesophageal pH monitoring, EMG, cervical auscultation | (additional information depending on supplementary method) |

In general, the dysphagia therapist is responsible for choices in assessment and for the planning of future assessment of therapy outcomes. However, the use of an instrument can only be justified if it has sufficient reliability and validity and is deemed appropriate in light of the discriminative and evaluative purposes of the assessment (Speyer 2013, 2021).

### 30.2.4  Behavioural Treatment

Behavioural interventions have shown promising effects in people with oropharyngeal dysphagia as reported in a recent systematic review and meta-analysis of randomised controlled trials (Speyer et al. 2022). Behavioural treatment may be recommended on the basis of an assessment outcome. There are various techniques to choose from, depending on the therapist's professional expertise and a patient's particular swallowing problems. Swallowing manoeuvres, for instance,

may require relatively high cognitive functioning and active patient participation, unlike interventions such as bolus modification or postural adjustments. Table 30.3 provides an overview of the most commonly used behavioural techniques in oropharyngeal dysphagia implemented by therapists (Speyer et al. 2010; Speyer 2018).

In the management of dysphagia, a balance must be kept between aspiration risk and safe swallowing, which might require a compromise between pursuing treatment goals and making urgent changes in the feeding route. In making that trade-off, the estimated risks of oral intake and aspiration pneumonia, malnutrition or dehydration need to be taken into account. It may be necessary to give additional tube-feeding combined with nutritional supplements. Obviously, the multidisciplinary team will play an important role in the decision-making. While dysphagia management relies, among other things, on collaboration between the dietician and dysphagia therapist, the key to its success lies also in edu-

**Table 30.3**  Behavioural interventions in oropharyngeal dysphagia. Based on Speyer (2018)

| Method | Main Purpose |
|---|---|
| Bolus modification and management → Bolus consistency/viscosity, size/volume, temperature, taste | Reduction of risk of penetration/aspiration and residue by deceleration of bolus transport into pharynx Improved bolus-forming Reduced need for chewing/effort |
| Postural adjustment → Body posture (e.g., lying down, lying on the side) → Head posture (e.g., head extension, flexion, rotation, tilt) | Reduction or elimination of aspiration risk by changing oropharyngeal dimensions Redirection and facilitation of bolus flow, improvement of oral and pharyngeal transit times, and decrease in amount of residue after swallowing |
| Motor behavioural techniques → Muscle strength, range of movement, muscle tone, steadiness, accuracy and coordination | Increased awareness of the bolus, control and its passage direction, and maximised driving and propulsive force of the bolus in transit to the oropharynx |
| Swallowing manoeuvres → e.g., Supraglottal swallowing, super supraglottal swallowing, Mendelsohn manoeuvre, effortful swallow, Masako manoeuvre, Shaker exercise | Physiological modification of the swallowing mechanism by gaining an improved and voluntary control of the swallowing process, including bolus propulsion and airway protection |
| Sensory and neurophysiological interventions → Chemical stimulation (e.g., acid, menthol, carbonation, pungency) → Physical stimulation (e.g., tactile-thermal stimulation of faucial pillars, bolus temperature) → Neuromuscular electrical stimulation (e.g., intrapharyngeal or trancutaneous) | Increased sensitivity of the oropharynx by providing stimuli before a swallowing attempt, alerting or triggering the nervous system and preparing the swallowing mechanism for the subsequent swallow |
| Adjunctive biofeedback → e.g., surface electromyographic feedback, flexible video-endoscopic or videofluoroscopic biofeedback | Facilitating processes of complex motor learning and enhancing the rate of motor learning |

cating other healthcare providers, especially nurses, who implement the nutritional and therapy recommendations in daily care. Accordingly, the dysphagia therapist sets the goals for behavioural treatment and should take the lead in supervising the health care providers and patients to ensure their compliance with the recommendations made within the multidisciplinary team.

When the team discusses the behavioural treatment options, a minimal treatment protocol is usually considered an adequate first step. That protocol consists of bolus modification in combination with postural adjustments. Bolus modification amounts to adjusting food viscosity, bolus volume, temperature, acidity or taste. Postural adjustments entail whole-body positioning or head positioning strategies such as chin tuck or head flexion. The aim of the protocol is to lower or eliminate the risk of aspiration and reduce the amount of residue. By changing the oropharyngeal dimensions, the bolus flow will be redirected and facilitated, thus improving oral and pharyngeal transit times (Speyer et al. 2010; Speyer 2018).

Other behavioural options involve various motor techniques, swallowing manoeuvres, sensory and neurophysiological interventions and adjunctive biofeedback.

The *motor techniques* address particular features of motor function: muscle strength, range of movement, muscle tone, steadiness, accuracy and coordination. The main goals of oral motor exercises are to increase awareness of the bolus, to improve control and the direction of passage and to maximise the driving and propulsive force of the bolus in transit to the oropharynx.

*Swallowing manoeuvres* allow a patient to gain more voluntary control of the swallowing process, particularly the aspects of bolus propulsion and airway protection. The literature describes a wide variety of manoeuvres, most of which require active patient participation and intensive practice before leading to positive therapy outcomes.

*Sensory and neurophysiological interventions* include chemical, physical and neuromuscular stimulation. The interventions may prompt increased sensitivity of the oropharynx by providing stimuli before a swallowing attempt. By triggering or alerting the nervous system, these stimuli help prepare the swallowing mechanism for the subsequent swallow.

Finally, the application of *biofeedback* as an adjunct to dysphagia therapy can facilitate the process of complex motor learning and enhance the rate of learning (Speyer et al. 2010; Speyer 2018). While these are the most common behavioural treatment techniques, new ones are constantly being developed. More detailed information can be found in textbooks such as Ekberg (2018), Leonard and Kendall (2014) and Shaker et al. (2013).

The success of behavioural treatment depends on the compliance of patients, healthcare providers, treatment assistants and spouses or relatives. It is essential to provide these parties with information, emphasising the rationale for compliance with the dysphagia recommendations made by the multidisciplinary team. That essential task, which is mainly the responsibility of the dysphagia therapist, includes instructing the parties in how to implement the behavioural techniques. But it also includes supervising all those involved in the daily care of dysphagic patients. There is no such thing as a single treatment for all patients with oropharyngeal dysphagia. A treatment plan must be tailor-made for each individual, specifying the supervision and management goals for his or her swallowing problems. Both the treatment and the goals may have to be adjusted in the course of the intervention, not only in keeping with a patient's preferences but also depending on the effectiveness of the treatment.

### 30.2.5 Evaluation and Reporting

After initial screening and assessment, the next step is to specify the therapy outcomes in objective terms. Several systematic reviews have been published on the evidence-based effects of behavioural treatment (e.g., Ashford et al. 2009; McCabe et al. 2009; Speyer et al. 2010, 2022). They underscore the importance of using valid and reliable tools when comparing pre- and post-treatment outcomes which is in line with the recommendations on screening and non-instrumental assessment for dysphagia in adults as reported by the European Society for Swallowing Disorders (Speyer et al. 2021). The issue is that therapeutic effects measured with different assessment tools are not necessarily correlated with each other; measurements based on visuoperceptual assessment of VFS or FEES, may not always show similar trends in therapy effects when compared with other changes, for example, functional health status or health-related quality of life as reported by the patient. It is therefore recommended to use tools covering distinct aspects of oropharyngeal dysphagia (Speyer 2018).

The literature gives little information on the long-term effects of treatment in oropharyngeal dysphagia. Therefore, to generate benchmarks, changes in swallowing capacity can be evaluated after a period of no treatment as part of the overall planning of the patient's care. The dysphagia therapist has a major role in planning the follow-up assessment and in counselling health-care providers and relatives when necessary. Notably for patients with degenerative disorders or in palliative care, ethical concerns need to be discussed within a multidisciplinary setting. Especially in the palliative or dying phase, information from the dysphagia therapist on the care and management of swallowing problems can be useful to both relatives and health-care providers (Bogaardt et al. 2015).

To facilitate the supervision and management of swallowing disorders by a dysphagia therapist, all members of the multidisciplinary team should report adequately on aspects within their realm of expertise. Healthcare providers need to be trained in concise and objective reporting and the use of professional jargon when participating in multidisciplinary care for patients with oropharyngeal dysphagia.

## 30.2.6 Conclusions

In most countries, an SLP will play a dominant role in the supervision and planning of behav-

ioural intervention techniques in oropharyngeal dysphagia. Depending on the cultural setting, though, members of other disciplines could also perform this role. Dysphagia therapists are usually responsible for decisions on the type of screening tools, for providing training and education on screening, and for its implementation within the workplace setting. The therapist selects evidence-based assessment tools with robust psychometric properties and plans future assessment of therapy outcomes. Providing information and motivation for compliance with multidisciplinary dysphagia recommendations is essential for a successful intervention. The dysphagia therapist will assist in instructing other caregivers on how to apply behavioural techniques and supervising those involved in the daily care of patients suffering from swallowing problems. Still, the care for patients with oropharyngeal dysphagia is not the responsibility of a single dysphagia therapist. Rather, it is a group effort that is highly dependent on the contribution of individual members of the multidisciplinary team.

## 30.3 Phoniatric Aspects of Functional (Behavioural) Swallowing Therapy

Doris-Maria Denk-Linnert

### 30.3.1 Introduction

In the management of the dysphagic patient, the phoniatrician and the speech-language pathologist (SLP) play a vital role within the multidisciplinary and multi-professional dysphagia team. A holistic approach is necessary to manage the dysphagic patient appropriately. The patient's cognitive status and motivation has to be taken into account. Owing to the problem of silent aspiration, dynamic instrumental swallowing examinations are necessary and cannot be replaced by any clinical (bedside) observations or screening protocols. In recent decades, the fibreoptic endoscopic evaluation of swallowing has become an indispensable tool in clinical routine for revealing the aetiology and pathophysiology of dysphagia, for testing compensatory and adaptive treatment techniques, and for recommending further diagnostic and therapeutic approaches. Owing to the implementation of chip-on-the tip flexible endoscopes (i.e., video endoscopes), the terminology of FEES has been updated. Instead of 'fibreoptic', the term 'flexible' is used.

Video-endoscopic and videofluoroscopic findings are comparable with respect to the identification of aspiration, penetration and retention (Schima and Denk 1998; Aviv 2000; Langmore 2000, 2003; Schröter-Morasch and Graf 2014), each having its advantages and limitations (Pisegna and Langmore 2016), and proven to be complementary dynamic instrumental diagnostic methods. Simultaneous use of FEES and videofluoroscopy [simultaneous radiological and fibre-endoscopic (flexible) evaluation of swallowing SIRFES] provides different benefits from the two methods and provides additional information, especially in complex cases (Scharitzer et al. 2019).

## 30.3.2 The Phoniatrician and FEES

In the phoniatric endoscopic workup of dysphagic patients, morphological as well as functional aspects have to be examined. The FEES procedure offers a close view of the upper aerodigestive tract and the pharyngeal stage of swallowing. Especially during swallowing rehabilitation of head and neck cancer patients, oncological aspects (tumour recurrence!) also have to be considered.

During FEES follow-up examination, compensatory and adaptive treatment techniques are tested (see Sects. 28.2–28.4) to determine how the treatment programme must be adapted to the patient's current needs, and if further conservative or surgical interventions are indicated. Therefore, the phoniatrician has to be familiar with the causal, compensatory and adaptive methods of functional dysphagia therapy. Digital recording of video-endoscopic findings is of great clinical value and a matter of quality

assurance (Pluschinski et al. 2015; Hey et al. 2015). It enables discussion of the findings not only within the rehabilitation team, but also with the patient and his family. This helps the patient to understand his swallowing problems better and increases his motivation and cooperation during therapy. Furthermore, FEES can be used as a biofeedback tool in swallowing treatment (Denk and Kaider 1997): in patients after head and neck surgery the use of FEES significantly increases the therapeutic success by shortening the period of functional rehabilitation and non-oral feeding.

In many European countries, such as Austria, Germany, Italy and France, FEES is a phoniatric/otorhinolaryngological task (Langmore 2017). This is due, inter alia, to the historical development of the medical discipline of phoniatrics as well as to the necessary medical expertise, e.g., to exclude/recognise endangering malignant diseases of the upper aerodigestive tract (Fig. 30.3 shows a supraglottal tumour in a patient with Parkinson's disease, diagnosed in the phoniatric exam, including FEES) and to manage possible complications of endoscopy (e.g., laryngospasm, epistaxis).

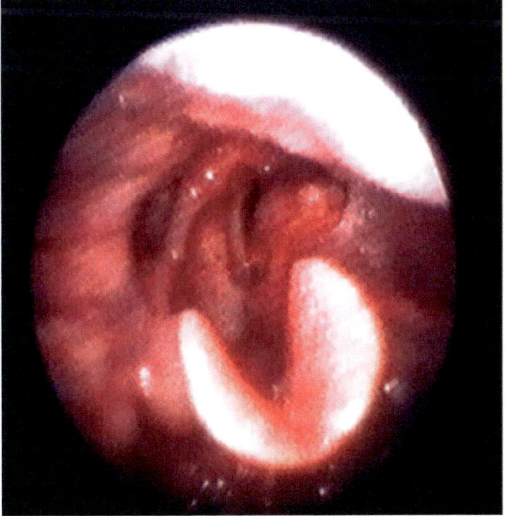

**Fig. 30.3** Supraglottal tumour in a patient with Parkinson's disease—the patient was referred for behavioural (functional) dysphagia therapy. ©Denk-Linnert 2019

However, in the USA the situation is different: FEES has been carried out by speech language therapists (SLTs) since its inception and description by Susan E. Langmore in 1988. In any case, a medical doctor must be within easy access (i.e., in the same building) to provide emergency medical backup should a complication arise (Kelly et al. 2007). In 1992, the American Speech-Language-Hearing Association published a written position paper stating that the practice of endoscopy to evaluate swallowing function was within the scope of practice of speech-language pathologists (ASHA 1992). Nowadays, the growing demand and interest in FEES has attracted the interest of, in addition to ENT specialists/phoniatricians, other medical specialties and speech therapists around the world, who are also seeking FEES training to practice FEES (Dziewas et al. 2014, 2017). Nevertheless, only the ENT specialist/phoniatrician has the endoscopic expertise to diagnose and treat pathologies of the upper aerodigestive tract (Denk-Linnert et al. 2023).

### 30.3.3 Patient-Specific Aspects of Dysphagia Management

#### 30.3.3.1 Geriatric Patients

The epidemiological development resulting in a much older population, often presenting with the problem of dementia, has brought about an urgent increase in dysphagia management. 27–91% of the population of 70 years or older is affected by oropharyngeal dysphagia (Ortega et al. 2017). The FEES procedure will help to manage patients, including those in nursing homes, adequately. Figure 30.4 is taken from a FEES procedure of a patient with Alzheimer's disease: silently aspirated liquid material is seen below the glottis, and a lot of saliva and jelly retention in the valleculae and the hypopharynx indicates a risk of aspiration after the swallow. The patient was then given liquids only thickened, and he and his caregiver were instructed to perform repetitive and effortful swallows during the meals and to clear his throat after each swallow.

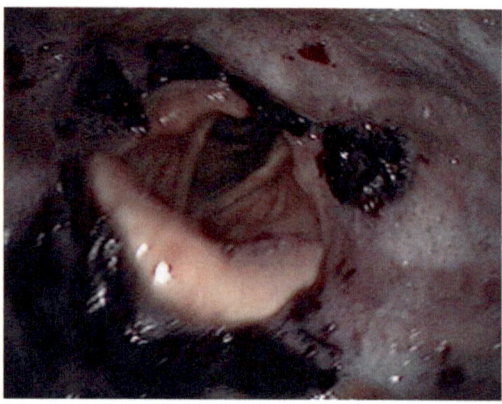

**Fig. 30.4** Aspiration of liquid, retentions of saliva and jelly with a high risk of aspiration after the swallow in a patient with Alzheimer's disease. ©Denk-Linnert 2019

#### 30.3.3.2 Paediatric Patients

FEES is also a safe and effective tool for evaluating dysphagia in the paediatric population (Dodrill and Gosa 2015) and in the neonatal intensive care unit (Suterwala et al. 2017). It can even be performed on breast-feeding infants (Willette et al. 2016). In recent years, the survival rate of preterm infants has significantly increased. This patient group, often suffering from severe comorbidities, syndromes or airway issues, has become a challenge for the dysphagia team, especially for the phoniatrician performing FEES.

#### 30.3.3.3 Intensive Care Unit (ICU) Patients

Dysphagia and aspiration occur in a high number of patients after prolonged intubation, with varying incidence given in the literature (56% aspiration, 25% silent (Ajemian et al. 2001), 35.9% aspiration (de Oliveira et al. 2018)). Dysphagia and aspiration are associated with a prolonged length of stay in hospital, high mortality and poor outcome (Macht et al. 2011, 2013a, b). Pathological laryngeal findings as well as post-extubation and ICU-related dysphagia was also observed in patients after COVID-19 (Frajkova et al. 2020; Lagier et al. 2021; Piazza et al. 2021; Svennerholm et al. 2021), for whom detection of aspiration/dysphagia is of great prognostic relevance.

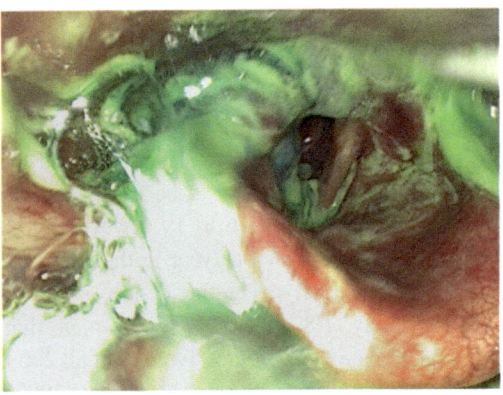

**Fig. 30.5** Silent aspiration—aspirated material below the vocal folds, no sign of cough reflex. ©Denk-Linnert 2019

In ICU patients whose general condition often does not allow a transfer to the radiological department, FEES can be performed as a bedside exam, and its findings are the basis for further management (Hafner et al. 2008, Dziewas et al. 2019). It helps to detect silent aspiration (Fig. 30.5) and therefore to prevent aspiration pneumonia.

### 30.3.3.4 Patients with Tracheostomy

In tracheostomised patients, the precondition for functional swallowing therapy is adequate tracheal cannula management. The phoniatrician recommends the apt tracheal cannula: as early as possible an uncuffed fenestrated tracheal cannula with speaking valve is used to enable laryngeal airflow, phonation and coughing, as preconditions for the improvement of laryngeal sensibility, throat clearing and swallow manoeuvres (Denk-Linnert 2018). The so-called multifunctional tracheal cannulae can be used as speaking cannulae during speech-language therapy and, if necessary, be cuffed if the patient has to be ventilated for some time. Furthermore, the swallowing exam can be performed with or without a cannula. In many cases, the removal of the tracheostomy tube makes no difference to the incidence of aspiration or laryngeal penetration (Donzelli et al. 2005).

Swallowing also plays a determining role in the process of decannulation. The following criteria have to be taken into account when planning the decannulation:

- Patient awake.
- No need for ventilation.
- Patent airway (no glottal or tracheal stenosis).
- Coughing is possible to clean the airway from tracheal secretions.
- Adequate secretion management.
- Swallowing without aspiration or, in case of minor aspiration, the capability of clearing the airway (cough reflex or voluntary coughing).
- Step-by-step procedure under in-patient conditions: downsizing the tracheal cannula, occlusion—first during the day with close monitoring, then, if without problems, for 1–2 days.

### 30.3.3.5 Head and Neck Cancer Patients

Swallowing rehabilitation is an essential issue in head and neck cancer patients and their rehabilitation—not only as a vital need but also to improve the quality of life. Organ-preserving treatment regimens do not enable the preservation of functions. The patients have to be treated in close cooperation with head and neck oncological surgeons, oncologists and radiotherapists (Denk-Linnert 2019). In many cases, voice rehabilitation also has to be carried out. Maintaining an oral diet and performing prophylactic swallowing exercises are regarded to be the most evidence-based strategies for dysphagia prevention in these patients (Starmer 2014). Helpful to maintain swallowing ability and to avoid/reduce aspiration are exercises to strengthen the strap muscles in the neck (e.g., the Shaker Exercise (Shaker et al. 1997), Mendelsohn Manoeuvre) or the base of the tongue (e.g., Masako Exercise) or airway protection exercises (e.g., supraglottal swallow). Knowing that aspiration cannot be avoided entirely in some cases, expiratory muscle strength training and voluntary coughing (Hutcheson et al. 2018) and respiratory-swallow training (Martin-Harris et al. 2015) help to compensate and clear the subglottal airway.

## 30.4 Basic Principles of Drug Treatment in Dysphagia

Tamer Abou-Elsaad

### 30.4.1 Introduction

Currently, no medications have been identified as beneficial in non-specific oropharyngeal swallowing dysfunction. Medical intervention in treating dysphagia has been based on recognition of the disorder underlying the swallowing dysfunction, since improvement of dysphagia may occur when the underlying pathology is treated. Unfortunately many neurological and myopathic causes of dysphagia, such as multiple sclerosis or muscular dystrophy, have no substantiated medical treatment (Ergun and Kahrilas 2003). This discussion will be divided into two parts. The first part will be limited to those diseases that are more common or have better recognised therapeutic options. The second part provides an overview of the medications that potentially affect the swallowing function.

### 30.4.2 Pharmacological Intervention for Swallowing Problems in Degenerative Neurological Diseases

A variety of pharmacological agents may be employed to target the symptoms in degenerative neurological diseases. This type of intervention is not directed at a cure of the underlying disease; rather it is aimed at reducing the level of functional limitation.

**Parkinson's Disease** Parkinson's disease (PD) is the second-most common neurodegenerative disorder after Alzheimer's disease (de Lau and Breteler 2006). It is a slowly progressive disorder of the basal ganglia that is manifested by motor as well as non-motor symptoms. These symptoms are due to a gradual loss of dopaminergic neurons located in the substantia nigra (Chaudhuri et al. 2006) in addition to autonomic dysfunction (Chaudhuri et al. 2006; Wood

et al. 2010; Yoritaka et al. 2013). Dysphagia in PD appears to be related to changes in both striated musculature under dopaminergic control and smooth musculature under autonomic control (Morrell 1992). The overall incidence of the disease has been estimated to be from 12 to 15 (Hirtz et al. 2007) and 16 to 19 (Twelves et al. 2003) per 100,000 persons/year in the USA and Europe, respectively. The incidence of PD is approximately 1.8 times higher in men than women (Mayeux et al. 1995; Twelves et al. 2003; Van Den Eeden et al. 2003; Hirtz et al. 2007). Age is the greatest risk factor for PD with the number of world-wide cases increasing from an estimated 4.1 million in 2005 to nearly 8.7 million by 2030 (Dorsey et al. 2007). Oropharyngeal dysphagia (OD) is prevalent in at least a third of PD patients (Kalf et al. 2012).

Although anticholinergic agents are almost universally helpful in the initial control of muscular tremors and skeletal muscle rigidity, the symptoms of bradykinesia and OD may or may not be improved with anticholinergics (Hughes et al. 1993). In fact, the oral and pharyngeal phase defects may even be exaggerated by drug use. For example, impaired bolus containment and poor propulsion due to muscular rigidity may be aggravated by xerostomia induced by the anticholinergics used to treat the disorder. The mainstays of long-term therapy of PD are predominantly dopamine precursors. However, the OD in idiopathic PD appears to be resistant to drug treatment. Some researchers have already examined the deglutition process in a group of patients in different periods (at one time under dopaminergic influence; at another without the use of dopaminergic drugs) and discovered that the abnormalities generally persist after administration of drugs, despite an increase in dose (Gross et al. 2008), or demonstrate only a low improvement in dysphagia in a group of participants, with decline of function in other (Lim et al. 2008).

On the other hand, the natural tendency to swallow slows down in many Parkinson patients so that they do not swallow as often as they used to, and as a consequence they tend to drool. The treatment of drooling in PD has been attempted with anticholinergic drugs, which reduce drooling by restricting saliva production (National Parkinson Foundation 2013). Some researchers have proposed botulinum toxin injections as a better alternative option for saliva reduction in Parkinson patients (Ellies et al. 2003; Lagalla et al. 2009; Kalf 2013). Botulinum toxin is injected directly into the submandibular and parotid salivary glands bilaterally under ultrasound guidance or blindly. The injected botulinum toxin is bound to the cholinergic nerve terminal, absorbed into the cytoplasm of the nerve terminal, and blocks acetylcholine release.

**Multiple Sclerosis** Multiple sclerosis (MS) is a chronic inflammatory disease of the central nervous system that typically presents in the third or fourth decade of life. It is estimated that more than two million people have MS worldwide and the disease is among the more common causes of neurological disability in young adults (Atlas: multiple sclerosis resources in the world 2008). Estimated annual incidence rates for populations in Europe range widely from <1/100,000 (Becuş and Popoviciu 1994; Dean et al. 2002) to >10/100,000 (Rothwell and Charlton 1998; Sumelahti et al. 2000; Nicoletti et al. 2001). Swallowing disorders are commonly observed in MS patients. About one-third of MS patients suffer from dysphagia (Poorjavad et al. 2010). Several potential factors, such as involvement of the corticobulbar tracts, cerebellar and brainstem dysfunction, lower cranial nerve paresis and cognitive impairment, can cause dysphagia in MS patients (Calcagno et al. 2002). The complications of dysphagia are common causes of morbidity and death in late stages of MS (Marchese-Ragona et al. 2006). Other authors have proposed anticholinergics and botulinum toxins for hypersalivation, N-acetylcysteine for thick secretions and botulinium toxin for upper oesophageal sphincter dysfunction in MS. On the other hand, patients with MS are likely to be on a large number of medications, many of which have the potential to cause or exacerbate dysphagia (Balzer and Pharm 2000). For example, anticholinergics and antimuscarinics may impair the function and coordination of the oesophageal smooth muscles and may also decrease salivation

and hence impair bolus preparation (Schechter 1998). Anti-epileptics, benzodiazepines and skeletal muscle relaxants may decrease awareness and control of voluntary muscle leading to difficulty in initiating a swallow (Feinberg 1994). Antipsychotics block dopaminergic transmission, which can result in an extrapyramidal syndrome similar to PD (Stoschus and Allescher 1993). Over time the resultant dopaminergic super-sensitivity may lead to an irreversible syndrome known as tardive dyskinesia (Sliwa and Lis 1993). Prolonged use of immunosuppressants predisposes the patient to viral and fungal infections of the oesophagus (Schechter 1998).

**Amyotrophic Lateral Sclerosis** Amyotrophic lateral sclerosis (ALS) is a neurodegenerative disorder characterised by progressive loss of upper and lower motor neurons in the motor cortex, brainstem and spinal cord (Wijesekera and Leigh 2009; Roche et al. 2012). Homogeneous incidence rates have been reported in populations from Europe, Northern America and New Zealand (1.81/100,000 person/year) (Marin et al. 2017). The mean age of onset for sporadic ALS is about 60 years, with a slight prevalence among men (male:female ratio approximately 1.5:1). OD is very frequent serious consequence during the course of ALS, especially in its bulbar form, and is caused by the degeneration of bulbar motor neurons. It manifests with functional impairments in both swallowing safety and efficiency (Ruoppolo et al. 2013; Tabor et al. 2017; Waito et al. 2017).

The changes in the oral phase of swallowing are late manifestations but often they are the first to be noticed by the patient when the pharyngeal phase is compromised (Watts and Vanryckeghem 2001; Goeleven et al. 2006). Transdermal patches that dispense scopolamine (hyoscinehydrobromide) over a period of 72 h to reduce salivary flow and control the drooling problems in ALS patients have been proposed. Atropine or drugs with anticholinergic effects, such as tricyclic antidepressants (amitriptyline or doxepin), can also be used for the same purpose (Heffernan et al. 2004). Botulinum toxin injection into the parotid glands has been shown to be an efficient and cost-effective alternative to these approaches.

Furthermore, botulinum toxin injection into the upper oesophageal sphincter (UES) has been found to reduce significantly the score of the penetration aspiration scale (PAS). This significant improvement has been observed in patients who suffered from UES dysfunction with no signs of lower motor neuron impairment (Restivo et al. 2014). Thick mucus secretions are frequently reported by patients with ALS and could be a sign of dehydration. Liquefaction of thick mucus secretions by use of N-acetylcysteine might also be helpful (Simmons 2006).

**Huntington's Disease** Huntington's disease (HD) is a neurodegenerative autosomal dominant disease involving progressive, selective loss of neurons primarily in the striatum and cortexVenuto et al. 2012). It is characterised by motor disturbance, behaviour and cognitive decline. The motor disturbances are both choreiform and hypokinetic. The combination of these signs can result in dysphagia in many patients with HD (Cardoso et al. 2006). The incidence of HD is 0.38 per 100,000 persons/year. The worldwide prevalence of HD is 2.71 per 100,000 (Pringsheim et al. 2012).

At this time, there is no cure for HD, and medical treatment is symptomatic. There are some potential therapies that have been described in animal models and in small open-label human studies; however, definitive results from large randomised placebo controlled trials are not yet available. Most studies have been insufficient in duration and underpowered to provide clear evidence of disease modificationVenuto et al. 2012). Unfortunately, pharmacological treatment of one symptom may aggravate others. For example, tricyclic antidepressants (amitriptyline) can alleviate depression but aggravate dysphagia by causing dry mouth and a sour or metallic taste (Hunt and Walker 1991). In addition, the empirical use of neuroleptics such as phenothiazines to treat associated choreas has not been effective in ameliorating the oro-pharyngeal symptoms (Leopold and Kagel 1985). Moreover, bolus formation, swallow initiation and transfer may even be adversely affected, owing to the associated xerostomia from the anticholinergic effect (Ergun

and Kahrilas 2003). Nash et al. (2004) have proposed Botulinum toxin for management of jaw clenching in HD.

**Myasthenia Gravis** Myasthenia gravis (MG) is a chronic autoimmune neuromuscular disease characterised by fluctuating weakness of the skeletal muscles. Patients with MG have acetylcholine receptor antibodies, which block acetylcholine from binding to muscle cell receptors. The impulse transmission is therefore impaired and muscle fibres are incapable of contracting (Juel and Massey 2007). The incidence for populations in Europe from 1970 to 2000 varied from 4.1 (Somnier and Engel 2002) to 30/1,000,000/ year (MacDonald et al. 2000). Approximately 20% of patients with MG will present with OD (Kaminsky 2002). Improvement of dysphagia in response to medical therapy for MG is variable and often less satisfactory than the response of other manifestations (Cook and Kahrilas 1999). Oral anticholinesterase inhibitors are the first-line treatment for MG. It improves the neuromuscular transmission by prolonging the availability of acetylcholine at neuromuscular junction (Skeie et al. 2010). Steroid (prednisone) and immunosuppressants (Azathioprine) are usually used on a chronic therapeutic regimen (Mantegazza et al. 2011). The Myasthenia Gravis Foundation of America, Inc. (2013) recommends to time meals around the peak of MG medication, i.e., eating about an hour after taking medication, for instance, intended to improve muscle function.

### 30.4.3 Medications that Potentially Affect Swallowing Function

The effect of medications on swallowing function is poorly recognised. Some medications have been proposed as having harmful actions on swallowing function, whereas others have been found to have promising positive effects (Loeb et al. 2003). The following lists the classes of drugs and the mechanisms by which they may affect swallowing function.

**Antibiotics** Broad-spectrum antibiotics may eliminate the competing bacteria and disrupt the normally balanced ecology of oral micro-organisms causing secondary mucosal infection from yeast overgrowth (Neville et al. 2002).

**Antipsychotic Medications** Antipsychotic medications (also known as neuroleptics) have been found to be associated with OD. Patients on antipsychotic treatment present double the risk of suffering OD than those that are not taking these drugs (Miarons et al. 2016). The use of loxapine (Sokoloff and Pavlakovic 1997), fluphenazine (Stewart 2001), risperidone (Stewart 2003), trifluoperazine (Bashford and Bradd 1996) and haloperidol (Gonzalez 2008) has been reported to have detrimental effects on swallowing function when administered to older patients. Adverse effects of antipsychotics, such as extrapyramidal symptoms (more common in older patients) and tardive dyskinesia, could be the cause of OD in the reported cases.

**Antidepressants** It has been suggested that some antidepressants with anticholinergic actions, such as tricyclic antidepressants, can produce xerostomia, leading to impaired oropharyngeal bolus transport (Brandt 1999). Miarons et al. (2016) have found that there is no significant association between OD and the use of antidepressants.

**Drugs decreasing Arousal and directly suppressing Brainstem Function** These include some sedatives, e.g., benzodiazepines (BZs). The exact relationship between BZs and swallowing function remains unknown owing to conflicting research results. The association between BZs and OD has been reported through some case studies. BZs could affect the swallowing function through their depressive action on the central nervous system (Dantas and Souza 1997). However, Miarons et al. (2016) have stated that there is no association between BZs and OD. Moreover, it has been suggested that BZs could exert a protective effect in community-acquired pneumonia (CAP), commonly associated with OD in older people. It was thought that BZs could inhibit the rapid eye movement (REM) phase of sleep, and thus prevent bronchial micro-aspirations associated with this phase of sleep (Gaillard 1989; Almirall et al. 2008, 2013). Anti-emetic drugs that have anticholinergic effects, e.g., chlorpromazine, and antiepileptic medications may decrease awareness and voluntary muscle control with difficulty in initiating a swallow. They may also cause dryness of the mucosa (Feinberg 1994).

**Medications resulting in Myopathy** Corticosteroids may result in myopathy, either through a direct catabolic effect on skeletal muscle, via effects on intermediary metabolism that provide amino acids as a substrate for gluconeogenesis (Sun et al. 2008), or by interfering with insulin-like growth factor-I (IGF-I) leading to increased myocyte apoptosis (Singleton et al. 2000). Colchicine may result in myopathy as a result of its effect on cellular mitosis after long-term use at normal doses or as a result of toxicity secondary to organ failure (Saleh and Seidman 2003). Lipid-lowering agents, e.g., HMG-CoA reductase inhibitors, may disrupt muscle energy production by reducing ubiquinone (coenzyme Q10) production (Ghirlanda et al. 1993). Other lipid-lowering agents, such as fibric acid derivatives (clofibrate, gemfibrozil) and niacin, also have low myotoxic potential (Chucrallah et al. 1992).

**Medications Compromising Neuromuscular Transmission** These include aminoglygoside antibiotics, e.g., gentamicin (Paradelis et al. 1980), and local injection of botulinum toxin type A into neck muscles (Bakheit 2001). These drugs have been found to cause harmful effects on swallowing function.

**Topical Anaesthetics** Benzocaine, as an example, causes loss of sensory afferent input, which results in a feeling of impaired or uncontrolled swallowing and suppresses the laryngeal cough reflex and thus may promote silent aspiration (Schechter 1998).

**Drug-related Movement Disorders** Dopamine antagonists, including neuroleptics, e.g., chlorpromazine, block dopaminergic transmission, which can result in an extrapyramidal syndrome similar to PD (Stoschus and Allescher 1993). Over time, the resultant dopaminergic super-sensitivity may lead to an irreversible syndrome known as tardive dyskinesia (Sliwa and Lis 1993).

**Anticholinergic Medications** These include atropine, opiates and some anti-arrhythmic (e.g., disopyramide) and anti-hypertensive (e.g., mecamylamine) drugs. These medications decrease salivation and thus impair bolus preparation (Brandt 1999). They may also impair oesophageal motility (Schechter 1998).

**Drugs that increase Salivation** Clonazepam (Lacy 2002), clozapine (Syed et al. 2008) and anticholinesterases (Pappano 2012) can result in difficulty in managing secretions in neurogenic OD.

**Corrosive Drugs** Some drugs in high concentration with little fluid intake, especially when oesophageal motility does not clear the material, can result in pill oesophagitis and painful swallowing (odynophagia) owing to disruption of the mucosal integrity (Boyce 1998). These include antibiotics (especially tetracycline), non-steroidal anti-inflammatory drugs (acetylsalicylic acid (ASA), indomethacin, ibuprofen, etc.) and iron preparations.

**Chemotherapeutic Drugs** These directly injure the oesophageal mucosa owing to their cytotoxic effects (Stoschus and Allescher 1993; Schechter 1998). 40% of chemotherapy patients present with mucositis, which manifests as odynophagia during mastication (stomatitis), oral bleeding and dysphagia (Oral Cancer Foundation 2014).

**Prolonged Use of Immunosuppressants** This predisposes the patient to viral and fungal infections of the oesophagus (Stoschus and Allescher 1993; Schechter 1998).

**Acetylcholine** This is a central and peripherally acting neurotransmitter that is responsible for excitation at the neuromuscular junction. The cholinergic medication can be effective in improving swallowing function in selected patients with OD (Sukys-Claudino et al. 2012).

**Anticholinergic drugs** These can be used to reduce drooling in PD (National Parkinson Foundation 2013), MS (Prosiegel et al. 2004) and ALS (Hefferman et al. 2004) by restricting saliva production.

**Botulinum Toxin Type A** This is used to treat oro-mandibular dystonia, torticollis and spasmodic dysphonia and may result in short-term dysphagia and even short-term aspiration of fluids (Deron 1994; Palmer et al. 1995). Some research-

ers have proposed botulinum toxin injections as a better alternative option for saliva reduction in Parkinson patients (Ellies et al. 2003; Lagalla et al. 2009; Kalf 2013), MS (Prosiegel et al. 2004) and ALS (Verma and Steele 2006). Furthermore, botulinum toxin can be used for the management of UES dysfunction in MS (Prosiegel et al. 2004), ALS (Restivo et al. 2014). Nash et al. (2004) have proposed botulinum toxin for management of jaw clenching in HD. The injected botulinum toxin is bound to the cholinergic nerve terminal, absorbed into the cytoplasm of the nerve terminal and blocks acetylcholine release.

**Antagonists of Angiotensin** These are likely to protect against OD (Miarons et al. 2016). This could be explained by the ability of the antagonists to improve muscle remodelling and protect against disuse atrophy (sarcopenia) in old patients. This improvement in muscle function could be responsible for the facilitation of swallowing function in these patients (Burks et al. 2011).

**Beta-blocker Agents** It has been reported that fast skeletal muscle beta-adrenergic receptors are up-regulated in response to chronic $\beta2$-adrenergic blockade and that this up-regulation increases isometric contractile forces in muscles (Murphy et al. 1997). This beneficial effect on pharyngeal muscles is responsible for the lower rates of OD in older patients chronically taking beta-blocker agents (Miarons et al. 2016). Moreover, beta-adrenergic stimulation increases the production of protein and mucus-rich secretions, which may thicken saliva and make it especially difficult for patients to manage. Administration of beta-blocker agents reduces the thickness of oral, nasal and pulmonary secretions, which would also improve the swallowing function of older patients (Bradley et al. 2000).

**Angiotensin Converting Enzyme (ACE) Inhibitors** Some studies, most of them performed on Japanese populations and on post-stroke patients, have reported that treatment with ACE inhibitors significantly reduces the risk of pneumonia among Asian participants but not non-Asians. The mechanism by which ACE inhibitors affect the swallowing function is thought to be through elevation of substance P, a neurotransmitter for primary sensory afferent nerves that is normally degraded by ACE. Elevated levels of substance P have been associated with an enhanced swallowing reflex. It has been reported that Asian and European populations differ in the distribution of a particular polymorphism in the ACE gene, affecting its activity and substance P levels (Arai et al. 1998; Nakayama et al. 1998; Perez et al. 1998; Ohkubo et al. 2004; Shimizu et al. 2008). On the other hand, Miarons et al. (2016) stated that there is no favourable effect of ACE inhibitors on swallowing function. The genetic characteristics, together with the fact that their patients were not limited to post-stroke patients, could explain the differences between the results of the previous studies and their study.

**Acknowledgement** I should like to thank Mrs. Aliaa Sabry, MSc assistant lecturer of phoniatrics, Mansoura Faculty of Medicine, Egypt, for her valuable assistance in collecting the references for this section, and my appreciation also goes to Prof. Mohamed Hisham Daba and Prof. Hussein El-Beltagi, professors of clinical pharmacology, Mansoura Faculty of Medicine, Egypt, for their valuable scientific comments.

## 30.5 Botulinum Toxin Treatment of Sphincter Diseases

Tamer Mesallam

### 30.5.1 Dysfunction of the Pharyngo-Oesophageal Segment

Dysphagia due to cricopharyngeal muscle (CPM) dysfunction can have a significant impact on patients' quality of life (Kelly et al. 2013). The cricopharyngeus muscle is located in a region referred to as the pharyngo-oesophageal segment (PES), comprising the main part of the upper oesophageal sphincter (UES) (Kuhn and Belafsky 2013). The CPM contains two types of muscle fibre; mostly slow type I muscle fibres and also some fast type II muscle fibres, providing a balancing action between rapid reflexive reactions and maintaining baseline tonicity (Kuhn and Belafsky 2013). The muscle receives dual innervation from the recurrent laryngeal nerve and the ipsilateral pharyngeal plexus, whereas the sensory signals are carried through the glossopharyngeal nerve and cervical sympathetics (Schulze et al. 2002). Uncoordinated peristalsis of the PES could be the result of cricopharyngeus muscle dysfunction and can present as dysphagia (Allen et al. 2010). Cricopharyngeus muscle dysfunction can result from a variety of causes including cerebrovascular accidents, pharyngeal diverticula, surgical skull base lesions, laryngectomy and oculopharyngeal muscular dystrophy (Kuhn and Belafsky 2013). Accurate diagnosis of cricopharyngeal dysfunction (CPD) is challenging and needs comprehensive evaluation. It can be reached through a detailed history, bedside assessment tests and instrumental assessment, whether flexible endoscopic evaluation of swallowing (FEES) (Fig. 30.6) or videofluoroscopic swallowing studies (Fig. 30.7). Furthermore, oesophageal manometric techniques can provide additional information (see Chap. 28).

### 30.5.2 Botulinum Toxin as a Therapeutic Option

Given the variable aetiology of CPD, treatment options vary accordingly. Current surgical interventions for this problem are also variable and include mechanical dilation, CPM myotomy and pharyngeal plexus neurectomy. However, there are not enough data supporting the greater effectiveness of one intervention over another (Kelly et al. 2013; Ross et al. 1982; McKenna and Dedo 1992).

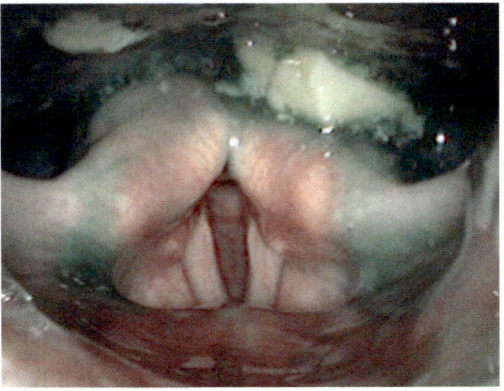

**Fig. 30.6** Flexible endoscopic evaluation of swallowing (FEES) for a patient with CPD showing a bolus residue over the UES and on both pyriform sinuses despite intact pharyngeal peristalsis. Mesallam©2019

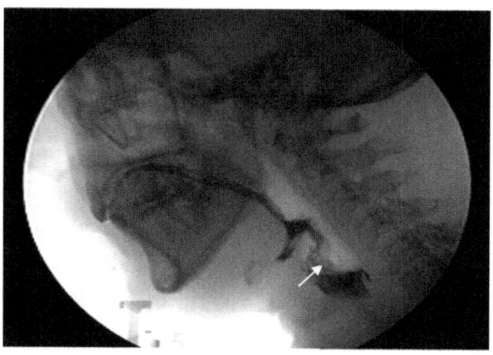

**Fig. 30.7** Videofluoroscopic swallowing study (VFSS) of a patient with CPD showing narrowing of the UES segment because of cricopharyngeus spasm (indicated by the arrow). Mesallam©2019

Before 1994, the main treatment of UES dysfunction was surgical, either through myotomy, dilation or neurectomy of the pharyngeal plexus (Woodson 1997; Singer et al. 1986). Since its first introduction in 1994, Botulinum Toxin (BTX) injection has been used for treatment of CPM dysfunction by many clinicians (Schneider et al. 1994). The potential role of BTX as an alternative to surgery is appealing: it is used in a variety of hypertonic muscular disorders with minimal or no side effects (Zaninotto et al. 2004); it is a virtually non-invasive procedure, relatively simple to implement, and certainly less costly than surgery. The main drawback of the therapeutic use of BTX is that its effect is relatively short-lived, but it can be useful in identifying patients who would benefit from definitive surgical treatment: it has been suggested that if the toxin fails to improve CP disorders, then myotomy is also unlikely to be helpful (Blitzer and Brin 1997).

Seven BTX serotypes have been isolated, with serotypes A and B commercially available for clinical use, most commonly by neurologists, ophthalmologists, otolaryngologists and plastic surgeons, among others, for a variety of conditions (Kuhn and Belafsky 2013). There are different types of Botulinum Toxin type A that can be used in CPM dysfunction; Dysport® (Ipsen, Paris, France) and Botox® (Al-lergan, Irvine California, USA). The dose of Botulinum Toxin administered to the CPM varies according to the type

used. In the case of Botox the dose ranges from 4 to 120 units, whereas for Dysport the range is from 60 to 180 units. There are different techniques for administering BTX into the CPM including endoscopic injection under general anaesthesia or mask ventilation, percutaneous injection with or without electromyographic guidance, and injection via flexible endoscopy (Kelly et al. 2013). Office-based BTX injection of CPM can be performed whether fluoroscopically or electromyogram guided. The injection approach should be done while the patient is awake through a flexible endoscope, or transcervically (Murry et al. 2005; Parameswaran and Soliman 2002). CMP BTX injection under general anaesthesia can also be done through rigid laryngoscopy or oesophagoscopy with direct visualisation of the CPM, allowing a more controlled BTX injection and concurrent UES dilation (Kuhn and Belafsky 2013). The effect of BTX injection is expected within a few weeks of injection and usually lasts up to 5–6 months, although some individuals might experience longer durations of improvement (Chiu et al. 2004).

In general, there are few reported complications following CPM BTX injection, including transient vocal fold paresis, temporary worsening of dysphagia, neck cellulitis and aspiration pneumonia. There are no reported deaths in the literature that are directly related to CP injection of BTX (Kelly et al. 2013).

### 30.5.3 Summary

Botulinum Toxin injection is commonly used for treating isolated cricopharyngeal dysfunction or upper oesophageal sphincter spasm, and it strongly competes with the traditional surgical interventions. The technique is relatively simple and can be conducted in an office-based setup or under general anaesthesia. Although the effect of injection lasts for 5–6 months, longer duration of improvement can be expected. It appears to be a safe and effective treatment with a very few complications compared with the success of the outcomes.

## 30.6 Oral, Enteral and Parenteral Nutrition Management in Dysphagic Patients and Refeeding Syndrome— An Overview

Mohamed Farahat

### 30.6.1 Introduction

The aim of managing patients with oropharyngeal dysphagia is to put the patient in a state of safe and sufficient nutritional intake. So it is important to prevent any incidence of aspiration pneumonia, to maintain adequate food and fluid intake, and to correct nutritional deficiencies. Because oral feeding has a great impact on the social and psychological aspects of the patients and their families, it should be continued whenever possible and safe.

The management of oropharyngeal dysphagia includes behavioural management, medical treatment, intra-oral prosthetics, surgical intervention, and in some cases the patient may need artificial nutrition (enteral or parenteral nutrition) (Abou-Elsaad and Kotby 2002). Some of these modalities will be discussed in this section (for further information see Sect. 30.7).

### 30.6.2 Behavioural Management

Behavioural management of oropharyngeal dysphagia starts immediately after assessing the patients, and may also be conducted during the Modified Barium Swallow (MBS) or Flexible Endoscopic Evaluation of Swallowing (FEES), after defining the patient's anatomical or physiological disorder (Logemann 1993; Logemann et al. 1998, 1999). Behavioural management includes (1) compensatory treatment, which redirects or improves the food flow and (2) therapy procedures that change swallowing physiology (Logemann 1999). Compensatory treatment includes: postural techniques (chin tuck, head back, head rotation, lying down and head tilt), sensory enhancement before swallowing (ther-

mal stimulation and sour bolus), changing diet volumes and viscosities, and introduction of intra-oral prosthetics (Logemann 1999). Therapy procedures include: exercises (resistance, range of motion and bolus control exercises) to improve the range of movement of oral and pharyngeal structures, and swallow manoeuvres (effortful swallow, supraglottal swallow, super supraglottal swallow, Mendhelson's manoeuvre), which voluntarily change pharyngeal physiology (Logemann 1999).

### 30.6.3 Medical Treatment

There is no medication that is specific for targeting certain aspects of oropharyngeal swallowing. However, in some neurological disorders, such as Parkinson's disease and myasthenia gravis, the patient's problem in oropharyngeal swallowing physiology can be improved with the general improvement of the original neurological condition if he or she is compliant to the medications (Logemann 1999).

### 30.6.4 Alternative Routes of Alimentation

Enteral nutrition represents the direct delivery of nutrients into the stomach (or into the jejunum) via a feeding tube, which is frequently used as the sole method of nutritional support of severely dysphagic patients who are at risk of aspiration pneumonia if fed orally. However, in some cases, for example, when easy fatigability makes swallowing unsafe, or if there is a certain food consistency that puts the patient at risk of developing aspiration pneumonia, tube feeding can be used to supplement the daily oral intake. The patients will then be able to take their favourite foods orally and the rest of the caloric requirements or the unsafe consistency will be given through the tube.

Feeding via percutaneous gastrostomy (PEG) should be considered when dysphagia is likely to be progressive or to persist for long periods of time. For example, most clinicians would consider gastrostomy tube feeding in stroke patients if there are no signs of recovery of swallowing after the first week (Bakheit 2001).

Parenteral nutrition (PN) represents delivery of all nutrients in special solutions to a person intravenously, bypassing the usual process of eating and digestion. The person receives nutritional formulae that contain nutrients such as glucose, salts, amino acids, lipids and added vitamins and oligo-elements and minerals. This is called total parenteral nutrition (TPN) or total nutrient admixture (TNA) when no significant nutrition is obtained by other routes, and partial parenteral nutrition (PPN) when nutrition is also partially enteric. It may also be called peripheral parenteral nutrition (PPN) when administered through veins accessible in a limb rather than through a central vein as in central venous nutrition (CVN).

Total parenteral nutrition (TPN) is provided when the gastrointestinal tract is non-functional because of an interruption in its continuity (it is blocked or has a leak or fistula) or because its absorptive capacity is impaired (Kozier et al. 2004). It has been used for comatose patients, although here enteral feeding is usually preferable, and less prone to complications. Parenteral nutrition is used to prevent malnutrition in patients who are unable to obtain adequate nutrients by oral or enteral routes (AGA 2007).

Solutions for total parenteral nutrition may be customised to individual patient requirements, or standardised ('all in one' three-chamber bag) solutions may be used. The use of standardised parenteral nutrition solutions is cost-effective and provides good control of serum electrolytes (Schnitker et al. 1951). Ideally, each patient is assessed individually before commencing parenteral nutrition, and a team consisting of specialised physicians, nurses, clinical pharmacists and registered dietitians evaluate the patient's individual data and decide which PN formula to use and at what infusion rate.

## 30.6.5 Refeeding Syndrome

Refeeding syndrome was first described in Far East prisoners of war after the Second World War (Schnitker et al. 1951). Starting to eat again after a period of prolonged starvation seemed to precipitate cardiac failure. The pathophysiology of refeeding syndrome has now been elucidated (Crook et al. 2001). In starvation, the secretion of insulin is decreased in response to a reduced intake of carbohydrates. Fat and protein stores, instead of carbohydrates, are catabolised to produce energy. This results in an intracellular loss of electrolytes, in particular phosphate. Malnourished patients' intracellular phosphate stores can be depleted despite normal serum phosphate concentrations. When they start to feed, a sudden shift from fat to carbohydrate metabolism occurs and secretion of insulin increases. This stimulates cellular uptake of phosphate, which can lead to profound hypophosphataemia (Crook and Swaminathan 1996). This phenomenon usually occurs within 3–4 days of starting to feed again.

Refeeding syndrome can occur with either enteral or parenteral nutrition. Understanding of refeeding syndrome and its treatment is limited among general physicians and surgeons. Many patients at risk of refeeding syndrome are not treated at specialist nutrition units. Serum phosphate may not be measured in patients at risk, and when it is the importance of grossly abnormal results may not be appreciated.

Treatment of refeeding syndrome can be helped by the input from hospitals' nutrition teams. Dietitians and nutrition nurses can help in identifying malnourished patients at risk of developing refeeding syndrome. When these patients require artificial feeding (enteral or parenteral), this should be started at a reduced caloric rate (25–50% of estimated requirements) to reduce the risk of developing refeeding syndrome. Serum phosphate, magnesium, calcium, potassium, urea and creatinine concentrations should be measured before feeding, and repeated daily for at least 4 days after feeding is started (Hearing 2004).

## 30.6.6 Summary

There are many choices for tackling the problem of patients with dysphagia. Each patient should have a regimen for treatment that is carefully tailored to bypass his disability.

## 30.7 Challenges in the Production of Texture-Modified Food in Oropharyngeal Dysphagia

Florence Baert and Geertrui Vlaemynck

### 30.7.1 Introduction

Besides surgical or medicinal treatment and rehabilitation strategies, nutritional management forms an integral part of the management of oropharyngeal dysphagia (OD). And as mentioned in Sect. 30.6 by Mohamed Farahat, it is important that oral feeding be continued whenever possible and safe. There is a strong correlation between malnutrition and OD, which confirms the clear need for nutritional guidance in this population (Clavé et al. 2006; Raheem et al. 2021). As malnutrition and dehydration are highly prevalent complications in OD, both the nutritional and the hydration status of OD persons should be assessed regularly. One of the cornerstones of nutritional management in OD is the modification of food texture (Hansen et al. 2022). The goal of food texture modification is to improve both the safety and the efficacy of the swallowing process.

### 30.7.2 Texture-Modified Food (TMF)

#### 30.7.2.1 Liquids

Food texture modification or bolus modification typically consists of thickening liquids and softening solid foods, although there is still discussion about it (Swan et al. 2015). Thickened liquids are recommended in OD to prevent aspiration during the swallowing process and to avoid dehydration. The strategy behind thickening fluids is to change the flow properties of the fluid by increasing the bolus viscosity. These changes in flow properties result in a prolonged time for the airway to close during swallowing and thus reducing the risk of aspiration (Steele et al. 2015).

There are different methods to increase the viscosity of liquids, but most often starch- or gum-based thickening agents are used. It is also possible to use naturally thicker (more viscous) beverages or foods, e.g., smoothies or custards, yoghurt drinks, depending on the patient's needs. In the last example thickeners (polysaccharides) are produced in situ during the fermentation process. Traditionally, starch-based thickening agents were used to increase the bolus viscosity of liquids. Different starches can be used, including corn starch, potato starch, tapioca starch, etc., however, it is important to realise that different starches have different thickening or swelling characteristics (Dewar and Malcolm 2006). Although starch-based thickeners are often used in dysphagia management, an increased risk of post-swallow aspiration, due to increased post-swallow oropharyngeal residue, has been reported, depending on the administered thickness of the liquid (Vilardell et al. 2016). Furthermore, starches often add a grainy texture to the beverages and can be broken down by the amylase enzyme (Matta et al. 2006).

Therefore, another generation of thickening agents based on different gums, such as xanthan gum, guar gum and Arabic gum, was developed to both improve the therapeutic effect and the palatability of thickened liquids (Rofes et al. 2014). Gum-based thickeners mainly maintain the clarity of beverages, are amylase-resistant and are mostly stable at different temperature ranges, in contrast to starch-based thickeners (Rofes et al. 2014). Besides starch- and gum-based thickeners, which can be added by the consumer, there also different pre-thickened beverages on the market.

Although there is evidence for the therapeutic effect of thickening liquids in OD, there are also various disadvantages of this strategy (Newman et al. 2016). The non-compliance rates vary from 40 to 80%, mostly owing to the patient's dislike of the thickened liquids (McCurtin et al. 2018). The mouth feel caused by the rheological structure of the thickened beverage is also often disliked. Thickening agents have a negative effect on the sensory qualities of beverages (Matta et al. 2006). Different studies have demonstrated that thickeners reduce the perceived taste intensity and sometimes even impart off-flavours (Matta et al. 2006; Cassani et al. 2017; Baert et al. 2021; Hollowood et al. 2002).

Of course, the organo-leptic characteristics of thickened liquids, including taste, aroma and texture, determine the palatability and finally the acceptability of the product. Horwarth et al. (2005) therefore investigated in healthy adults whether a natural thickener was preferred over commercial thickening agents. Their results demonstrated that the acceptance of the thickened liquid not only depends on the thickening agent, but also on the temperature of the liquid. Their results also demonstrated a taste difference in thickened hot chocolate, where both the natural thickener as SimplyThick (a gum-based thickener) was preferred over the other commercial thickener, Thick It; however, no significant taste difference was found in thickened fruit juice (Horwarth et al. 2005). Further research is needed to develop new thickening agents with fewer effects on organoleptic properties of beverages to increase the compliance rates of thickened liquids.

Although one of the objectives of thickened liquids is to avoid dehydration, some studies have suggested that thickeners reduce the bioavailability of water. Hill et al. (2010), however, have shown that water bioavailability is unaffected by thickeners, independent of the used thickness (Hill et al. 2010; Cichero 2013). Potentially, the non-compliance due to the dislike of the thickened liquids results in reduced fluid intake and therefore increases the risk of dehydration (Gallegos et al. 2017). As well as this, thickened beverages often lead to a sticky feeling in the mouth, rather than quenching thirst (Cichero 2013). Another disadvantage of thickened liquids is their effect on the bioavailability of some drugs. For instance, the intake of guar gum-thickened water combined with the intake of penicillin reduces absorption of penicillin (Cichero 2013).

### 30.7.2.2 Solid Foods

A texture-modified diet also includes texture-modified solid foods, often recommended for people with mastication and swallowing dysfunction. Solid foods are softened or reduced in particle size through mincing, pureeing or liquidising (Aguilera and Park 2016). A bolus that is 'safe to swallow' should be soft, cohesive, homogeneous in texture and slide easily into the throat.

Hard, dry, fibrous or adhesive (sticky) food textures should be avoided, since they are more difficult to process (Cichero 2016).

However, this texture modification often results in blended meals with an unappetising appearance, wherein the ingredients are difficult to recognise (Nakatsu et al. 2014). Currently, already known food technologies are evaluated to create TMF that maintain their flavour and appearance combined with a softer texture (Van den Steen et al. 2024). These methods include freeze-thawing infusion, enzymatic treatments, sonication and high-pressure treatment (Aguilera and Park 2016).

### 30.7.3 Challenges Concerning an Unambiguous Description of the Desired Food Texture

One of the main challenges in TMF is the lack of a universal language to describe the various consistencies of thickened liquids and softened, moisturised solid foods. Different studies have demonstrated that the terminology used to describe different consistency levels varies greatly, even within countries (Atherton et al. 2007; Felt 1999; Cichero et al. 2017). Even greater differences in terminology exist between countries, owing to cultural differences. There have been efforts in different countries to create a national standardised dysphagia diet (Atherton et al. 2007; Felt 1999; Watanabe et al. 2018; IASLT and INDI 2009; National Patient Safety Agency 2011; Beck et al. 2018). For example, the National Dysphagia Diet Task Force determined four texture levels for solid food and four consistency levels for liquids: NDD Level 1: Dysphagia-Pureed (homogeneous, very cohesive, pudding-like, requiring very little chewing ability); NDD Level 2: Dysphagia-Mechanical Altered (cohesive, moist, semi-solid foods, requiring some chewing); NDD Level 3: Dysphagia-Advanced (soft foods that require more chewing ability) and Regular food and four consistency levels for liquids (thin <50 mPa; Nectar-like 51–350 mPa; Honey-like 351–1750 mPa; Spoon-thick >1750 mPa with shear viscosities measured at 25 °C and a shear rate of 50 s$^{-1}$) (McCullough et al. 2003;

Zwiefelhofer 2012). In other countries, including Australia, Ireland, the UK, Denmark and Japan, national standardised viscosity levels and descriptors have been accepted (Atherton et al. 2007; Felt 1999; Watanabe et al. 2018; IASLT and INDI 2009; National Patient Safety Agency 2011; Beck et al. 2018).

Currently no international guidelines concerning the dysphagia diet are globally used. However, in 2013, the International Dysphagia Diet Standardization Initiative (IDDSI) was established with the aim of developing global descriptors and definitions for TMF (Cichero et al. 2017). In 2017 it published a framework consisting of a continuum of eight levels for both solid foods and liquids. In this framework they combine descriptors with colours and numbers to label the different consistency levels.

Independent of the descriptor used, each patient should be prescribed the appropriate consistency in line with his needs. The appropriate texture should be determined from the medical history, clinical swallowing examination and the instrumental assessment of the swallowing process: videofluoroscopic swallowing study (VFSS) or flexible endoscopic evaluation of swallowing (FEES). However, the current practice of connecting the clinical measurements with the appropriate texture relies often on subjective assessment of the viscosity, using relatively vague descriptors such as 'syrup-thickness'. This subjective assessment results in poor repeatability for a safe dysphagia treatment (Gallegos et al. 2017). The consistency of a thickened liquid is influenced by various factors, including temperature, type of thickener used and storage time.

### 30.7.4 Challenges Concerning the Analysis of the Texture of Texture-Modified Foods

IDDSI is working on measuring techniques and also provides testing methods for the different viscosity levels (Cichero et al. 2017). These were designed so that they can be easily carried out in different settings, including nursing homes, hospitals etc. Currently, it is working on the implementation of this framework step by step, all over the world. Although IDDSI provides various testing methods for assessing the consistency both of liquids and solid foods, they are influenced by the executer, and the assignment after a spoon test or fork test at a certain level is not always easy, as the differences in results by performing a fork or spoon test within a certain level can be quite large and are not yet fully standardised. Therefore, they are a useful option in a care facility but should be documented and underpinned with results of objective measurements of consistency.

The consistency of liquids can be determined by viscosity measurements, but also by determination of the visco-elastic profile of the liquids. Currently, however, there is no consensus on the appropriate measurement method for thickened liquids used for dysphagia. Often shear viscosity of thickened liquids is measured, but there is no general consensus yet on which shear rate, or rather range of shear rates, is most representative of the physiological shear rates occurring during the whole swallowing process. A shear rate of $50 \text{ s}^{-1}$ is often used as representative, but some studies report varying shear rates from 1 to $1000 \text{ s}^{-1}$ for swallowing (Popa Nita et al. 2013; Gallegos et al. 2012). Furthermore, different types of rheological measurement apparatus are used in various scientific papers, which complicates the comparison of their results. Similarly, there is no global agreement on the textural measurement of solid and semisolid foods (Gallegos et al. 2017). Different food texture characteristics can be used to describe the (modified) texture of solids or semi-solid foods, including cohesiveness, adhesiveness, hardness, firmness, fracturability and springiness (Felt 1999; Hadde and Chen 2021).

In conclusion, a lack of both standardised measurement methods, accompanied by a lack of global consistency standards, undermine the efficiency of the dysphagia diet.

### 30.7.5 Oral, Enteral, Parenteral or Mixed Feeding?

Some patients, depending on the aetiology and the severity of their OD, will not be able to take any food orally, even when the texture is modified. According to the European Society for Clinical Nutrition and Metabolism (ESPEN) guidelines, enteral nutrition is recommended for these patients, including those with very severe neurological dysphagia (Volkert et al. 2006; Burgos et al. 2018). There are different enteral nutrition routes, including naso-gastric tubes, naso-jejunal tubes and percutaneous endoscopic gastrostomy, and the appropriate route is determined according to the anticipated duration and the type of nutritional support needed, as described in detail in Sect. 30.6.

## 30.8 Indication for Surgical Procedures in Dysphagia

Tadeus Nawka

### 30.8.1 Introduction

In cases of dysphagia with chronic aspiration and even recurrent aspiration pneumonia the severity of the risk depends on the quantity of aspiration. . A tracheostomy is the acute life-saving intervention to protect the airway; a nasogastric tube or percutaneous endoscopic gastrostomy (PEG) ensures nutrition.

The following disorders are a reason for surgical intervention:

1. Acute diseases of the motor system for reparative surgery.
2. Neurodegenerative diseases, as long as they are slowly progredient and thus a realistic chance exists for a lifetime with fewer complaints after surgery.
3. Diseases associated with sensitivity disorders or loss.
4. Dysphagia as sequel of therapeutic measures for tumour disease.

The most important rule for surgery of dysphagia is to preserve existing functions and residual functions of swallowing comparable to their natural state. High diagnostic precision is required regarding the high number of involved muscles and brain nerves. The decision for surgical measures is made on an interdisciplinary

scale in cases of neurologically based disease; it has to be discussed intensively with the patient and individually adapted. In the following, the surgical therapy steps with dysphagia relevant techniques are summarised.

### 30.8.2 Surgical Therapy of Specific Organ Structures

#### 30.8.2.1 Positioning of the Laryngohyoid Unit

Aspiration may be reduced by displacement of the larynx and hyoid from the oesophagus in a ventral direction to protect the laryngeal entrance by the base of tongue.

Different laryngeal suspension techniques have been described (Calcaterra 1971) in order to minimise the aspiration problem after tumour surgery. The authors used suture techniques to displace the thyroid cartilage in an anterior direction and approach it to the mandible.

Hillel and Goode (1983) suspended the larynx laterally with sutures to solve the problem of aspiration after resection of the base of the tongue. Herrmann (1992); Herrmann and Arce-Recio 1998) described a suspension technique in severe neurological swallowing disorders, using fascia lata for laryngo-hyoidopexy to the chin and myotomy of the upper oesophageal sphincter. This technique respects the correct position of the laryngohyoid unit in the pharynx and considers the function of the suprahyoid muscles and the elevation of the epiglottis in order to protect the laryngeal entrance.

**Technique of Laryngo-hyoidopexy** At the beginning of the intervention, PEG is applied in order to immobilise postoperatively the surgical site and to secure nutrition. The existing tracheostoma is circumcised and a cranially pedicled flap is prepared. If no tracheostoma is present, this is the first surgical step. The thyroid gland is identified, the isthmus is transected and the trachea is exposed. Trachea and pharynx are disconnected from the thyroid and mobilised. The recurrent nerves are protected.

Afterwards the following steps are performed:

1. Myotomy of the cricopharyngeal muscle.
2. Transection of the infrahyoid muscles: in order to get the functionally impaired larynx out of the swallowing pathway and to protect it by the tongue base, the infrahyoid muscles except the thyrohyoid muscle are transected (Herrmann 1992). The unit of larynx and hyoid can now be placed in the desired position.
3. Laryngo-hyoidopexy and suspension of the laryngo-hyoid unit at the chin: with two strong sutures (non-absorbable) the thyroid cartilage is fixed at the hyoid in such a way that the hyoid is positioned behind the anterior edge of the thyroid cartilage (Fig. 30.8) (Mahieu et al. 1999). The threads connect the thyroid cartilage to the hyoid (Herrmann 1998).
4. In order to avoid overcorrection, i.e., closure of the laryngeal entrance, the sutures for suspension are placed under endoscopic control.
5. Since the laryngohyoid unit is displaced in cranial and ventral directions the tracheostoma has to be made at a lower position.
6. PEG nutrition and a blocked cannula are generally maintained for about 10 days.

### 30.8.2.2  Protection of the Laryngeal Entrance (Lowering of the Epiglottis)

The slightly inclined position of the epiglottis results from the pre-epiglottal fatty tissue and the suspension by the thyro-epiglottal ligament, the glosso-epiglottal fold, and both pharyngo-epiglottal folds.

The epiglottis can be lowered in a dorsal direction to protect the laryngeal entrance by applying an endoscopic technique described by Laurian et al. (1986), or in a modified manner by bilaterally transecting the plicae pharyngo-epiglotticae and disconnecting the plica glosso-epiglottica from the tongue (Herrmann and Arce-Recio 1999).

### 30.8.2.3  Insufficiency of the Glottal Closure and Dysphagia

Insufficiencies of glottal closure at the membranous or cartilaginous part of the glottis caused by unilateral paresis and defects are permanent or transitory, partial or total (Voigt-Zimmermann and

Arens 2013). They may not only impair the voice (see Sect. 5.7) but also lead to penetration and aspiration. To improve swallowing, different therapeutic measures are applied (modified according to Giraldez-Rodriguez and Johns (2013)):

- Training of swallowing.
- Injection and implantation augmentation.
- Thyroplasty with or without arytenoid adduction.
- Partial unilateral pharyngeal resection.
- Myotomy of the cricopharyngeal muscle.

Injection and implantation augmentations can be performed transorally and transcervically; they are mainly applied in the treatment of low-to-moderate glottic insufficiencies. These methods are still most frequently used in total and also partial vocal fold paresis; however, they are also useful for the treatment of vocal fold atrophies, e.g., in cases of presbylarynx, as well as scarring of the vocal folds. Increasingly often they successfully accompany interventions of the laryngeal framework.

The aim is the medialisation of the vocal folds by augmentation of the insufficient vocal fold, e.g., in paresis, defects and scarring of the vocal folds. In this context, injection or implantation is performed laterally into the lateral part of the vocalis muscle or deeper between the thyroid cartilage and the vocalis muscle. As material for augmentation, usually fat, fascia, cartilage, hyaluronic acid, hydroxyapatite and silicone are used (Voigt-Zimmermann and Arens 2013). However, there is limited evidence that injection augmentation and medialization thyroplasty improve swallowing function and/or safety (Dhar SI et al. 2022).

**Thyroplasty** Isshiki (2000) made medialisation thyroplasty internationally known as type I thyroplasty. It is predominantly applied in paresis and atrophies of the vocal folds, but also in dysphagia. The complex structure of the parts of the vocal folds that are relevant for the quality of the voice are not destroyed.

After previous creation of a defined thyroid cartilage window, a displacement of the lateral vocal fold in direction of the midline is achieved by inserting, and if needed fixing, autologous or allogeneic material. These materials are for example autologous cartilage (septum or thyroid cartilage), Gore-Tex, titanium clips or silicone blocs (Voigt-Zimmermann and Arens 2013).

**Arytenoid Adduction** In 1978, Isshiki (2000) was the first to describe arytenoid adduction as a surgical technique for correction of glottal insufficiency. It is mostly combined with thyroplasty. In the context of this intervention, first the posterior edge of the thyroid cartilage of the affected side is identified and after creation of a cartilaginous window according to Maragos, the muscular process of the arytenoid cartilage is exposed (Nawka and Hosemann 2005). A Vicryl thread (4 × 0) is then pulled through the muscular process and fixed ventrally at the inferior edge of the thyroplasty cartilage window. By rotating the arytenoid cartilage, an improved glottal closure in the posterior part of the vocal folds is achieved and thus the voice and swallowing function are optimised.

### 30.8.2.4 Myotomy of the Upper Oesophageal Sphincter

Myotomy is indicated when the upper oesophageal sphincter does not, or does not sufficiently, relax during the swallowing act (Herrmann 1986, 1987; Kocdor et al. 2016). The causative diseases may lie in the central nervous system (cerebellar infarct, brain stem infarct, Parkinsonism, amyotrophic lateral sclerosis, base of skull neoplasm), the peripheral nervous system (peripheral neuropathy, diabetic neuropathy, bulbar poliomyelitis, myasthenia gravis, neoplasm), the cricopharyngeal muscle (polymyositis, oculopharyngeal muscular dystrophy, hyperthyroidism, hypothyroidism), cricopharyngeal disruption (laryngectomy, supraglottal laryngectomy, radical oropharyngeal resections, pulmonary resections) and cricopharyngeal spasm (hiatal hernia, gastro-oesophageal reflux, idiopathic cricopharyngeal achalasia).

For diagnosis the most important component is a thorough history. Further diagnostic procedures are videofluoroscopic swallowing studies, manometry, manofluoroscopy, a combination of both methods, and electromyography. These not only demonstrate the dysfunctional UES, but also demonstrate laryngeal elevation, the strength of the pharyngeal muscles, and laryngeal penetration or aspiration. Although some authors find

manometry cumbersome and of limited value, others strongly advocate its use, especially if coupled with fluoroscopy. The latter allows assessment of pressures at known sensor locations during swallowing. However, it is still not available and not a part of the workup in many institutions. The disadvantage of lateral myotomy is that the neural supply of the constrictor muscle is partly destroyed on the side of the myotomy.

Before the intervention, a nasogastric tube is inserted into the hypopharynx and upper oesophagus. The incision is performed at the anterior edge of the sternocleidomastoid muscle and in a skin line at the level of the cricoid cartilage. The prevertebral space is reached between the neurovascular cord of the carotid artery, jugular vein and vagus nerve and the hypopharynx. The external branch of the superior laryngeal nerve must be preserved.

In order not to jeopardise the neural supply of the pharynx and oesophagus, the preferred localisation of the myotomy is dorso-medial (Fig. 30.8a, b) over the venous plexus and the mucosa under the muscles extending to the upper oesophagus and thyropharyngeal muscle. The possibility that the muscle stubs merge again is excluded by suturing them on the constrictor or longus colli muscle of the same side (Herrmann and Arce-Recio 1998).

In the case of single spasm of the cricopharyngeal muscle with formation of Zenker's diverticulum, an endosopic approach and dissection of the muscle is possible. This can be done via flexible endoscopy or micro-laryngo-hypopharyngoscopy with a laser (Krespi et al. 2002) or stapler (Lang et al. 2007).

The success rate of myotomy is significantly higher than the success rate of botulinum toxin injections in cricopharyngeal dysfunction (see also Sect. 30.5). Moreover, endoscopic myotomy compared with open myotomy was found to have a higher success rate in one review (Kocdor et al. 2016) and a lower success but also lower complication rate in another (Verdonck and Morton 2015). Systematic reviews revealed insufficient evidence for guiding clinical practice (Knigge and Thibeault 2018). Reliable and valid evidence on the following is required to support increasing clinical usage of endoscopic cricopharyngeal

a

b

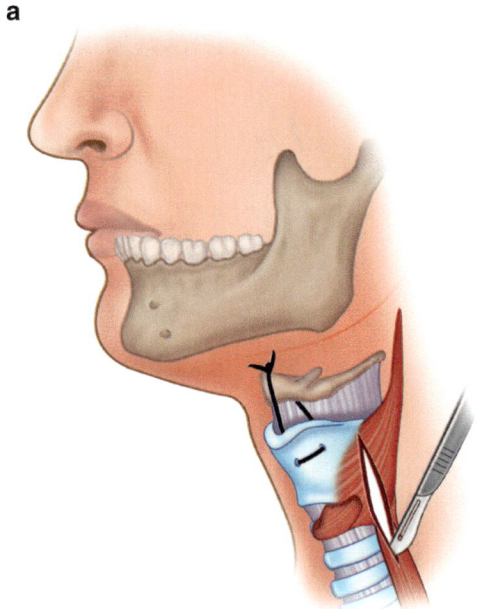
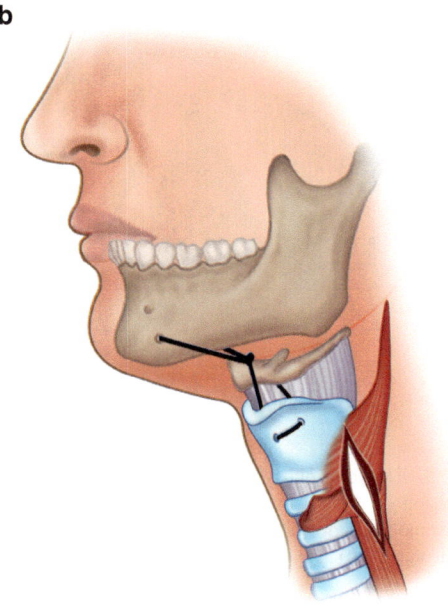

**Fig. 30.8** (**a, b**) Schematic presentation of upper oesophageal sphincter (UES) myotomy and laryngeal suspension procedure. (**a**) UES myotomy performed; thyrohyoid approximation by non-absorbable 0-suture tied as mattress suture over Gore-tex bolsters on the thyroid cartilage and around the body of the hyoid bone. (**b**) Thyrohyoid complex suspended from the mandible by non-absorbable 0-sutures, which have been passed around the body of thy hyoid bone and through holes drilled in the mandible. (Figure reprinted from Mahieu et al. (1999) with permission from Elsevier)

myotomy: optimal candidacy selection; standardised post-operative management protocol; complications; and endoscopic cricopharyngeal myotomy effects on aspiration of food and laryngeal penetration, mean upper oesophageal sphincter resting pressure and quality of life (Gilheaney et al. 2016).

### 30.8.2.5 Elevation Plasty of the Interarytenoid Region

In cases of slight interarytenoid aspiration where no or only a slow progression of the disease is observed, an endoscopic, plastic-surgical intervention may reduce the existing problem. Saliva or liquids flow over the lowest point, i.e., the interarytenoid region, into the larynx. A postcricoid transposition flap that is also applied in small laryngeal gaps (grade 1) can lead to raising the interarytenoid region (Fig. 30.9).

Age-related swallowing disorders or beginning neurodegenerative diseases (Parkinson) more often reveal this type of dysphagia. Patients complain about a desire to clear their throats and coughing, especially when eating or drinking. In cases of sensitivity disorders, the complaints even occur in rest. The indication is made based on interdisciplinary cooperation, after functional endoscopy and videofluoroscopy. The cricopharyngeal dysfunction or a tumour disease must be excluded.

After tracheostomy, the surgical intervention is performed. The distending laryngoscope is applied and the interarytenoid region is exposed. For treatment of aspiration, a mucosal flap of the postcricoid region is circumcised (Herrmann and Arce-Recio 1998; Herrmann 1992). Only the mucosal incision is performed with the $CO_2$ laser after identification of the arytenoid cartilage. The mucosa of the inter-arytenoid region is prepared to the side. The flap is freely prepared in a postcricoid direction. It is generously dimensioned as a transposition flap and turned into the prepared bed of the inter-arytenoid region, fixed with sutures, and sealed at the wound edges with tissue glue (Fig. 30.9).

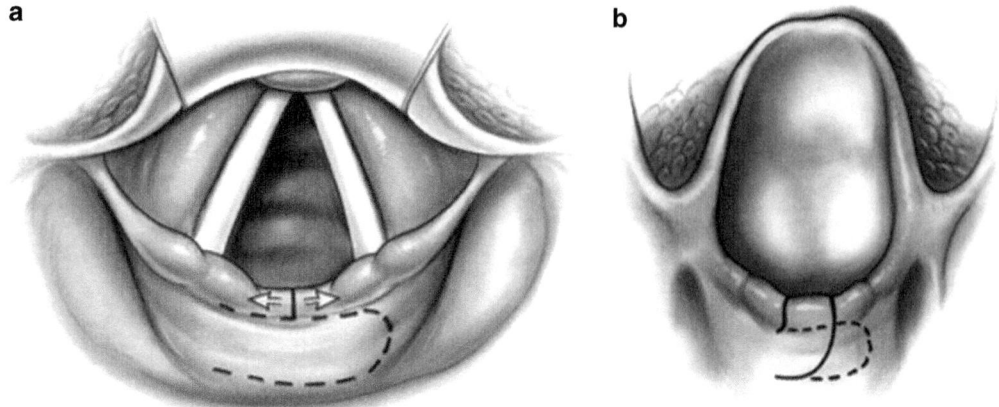

**Fig. 30.9** Elevation plasty of the interarytenoid region. (**a**) Incision of the mucosa in the interarytenoid region, which is mobilised towards the arytenoids. A postcricoid flap is isolated. (**b**) The postcricoid flap is mobilised and transferred to the interarytenoid region with the goal of elevating this area. (Figure reprinted from (Herrmann and Arce-Recio 1999) with permission from Elsevier)

### 30.8.2.6 Transsection of Velar Formations

Velar or tissue formations occur as a sequel to inflammations in the hypopharynx, upper oesophageal entrance and upper oesophagus. These scars can be transected with the laser and dissolved.

### 30.8.3 Special Surgery for Severe Aspiration

Silent aspiration often occurs in combination with motor disorders and is characterised by reduced sensitivity. The extent of sensitivity loss can be slight to severe. The progressive course of the disease should be considered in the therapeutic concept. The airway has to be protected against aspiration.

The following findings may be revealed during functional endoscopy:

- Overflow into the larynx without coughing.
- Foamy or thick, sticky saliva diffusely spread in the oro- and hypopharynx, no inflammation.
- Reduced bolus control.
- Food residues in the pharynx.
- Increased reflux.

Anamnestic data give important hints:

- Transient ischaemic attack or stroke.
- Tumours or sequelae of surgery in the posterior cranial fossa or the bulb area.
- Neurodegenerative diseases.
- Head injury.
- Sequelae of surgery—scars, defects, etc.
- Late consequences of radiochemotherapy, etc.
- Fractures, strictures and stenoses, etc.

A tracheostomy secures respiration. Nutrition is secured via PEG. Silent aspiration must be stopped. Communication should be possible.

The following questions should be answered:

- Is breathing regular?
- Is voice production possible?
- How is the muscular function of the oral cavity, the pharynx, larynx and the trachea?
- Which innervation is disturbed?
- What is the general condition of the patient?
- What is the prognosis?

Depending on the answers to these questions, the decision of surgical intervention is made on an interdisciplinary basis. The head and neck surgeon has to choose the procedure adapted to the patient's individual situation. If the disease allows phonation on the glottal level, the according techniques have to be preferred (Herrmann and Arce-Recio 1998). If the structures relevant for articulation are damaged in such a way that the patient can no longer speak, surgical procedures with this regard are not indicated. In certain cases, the reversibility of this surgery is an important factor. On the basis of the results with reversible techniques, the former technique of total laryngectomy with surgical voice rehabilitation is indicated only in very rare cases. Aspiration prevention surgeries prevent aspiration and increase oral intake in 50-80% of patients (Ueha et al. 2023).

### 30.8.3.1 Laryngo-Tracheal Separation

Laryngo-tracheal separation is a surgical treatment of silent or severe aspiration without preservation of the individual voice, in order to achieve complete separation of the airway and the swallowing tract (Fig. 30.10, Eisele et al. 1989).

Whether to proceed with this separation is ethically a very difficult decision for every surgeon because normal laryngeal or tracheal tissue is surgically altered and the procedure has a high complication rate of 58% and an inefficiency of 27% (Zocratto et al. 2006). By contrast, Hara et al. (2014) reported successful laryngo-tracheal separation in two thirds of their neurologically impaired paediatric patients. Laryngo-tracheal separation is a reversible procedure.

### 30.8.3.2 Supraglottal Closure of the Larynx

Supraglottal separation can be performed by means of transoral endoscopy. The epiglottis is mobilised ventral and laterally and the cartilage is incised and reduced to diminish the tension. Afterwards, partial de-epithelialisation of the aryepiglottic folds is performed. The epiglottal flap is turned in a dorsal direction and sutured over the laryngeal entrance with the aryepiglottal folds. After closure, phonation is no longer possible; however, the procedure is reversible.

### 30.8.3.3 Plastic Closure of the Airway Between Larynx and Trachea with Preservation of the Individual Voice and the Continuity of the Membranous Wall of the Trachea

The aim of the reversible tracheal closure by means of laryngo-hyoidopexy (LHP), suspension to the chin, and subsequent restitution of the individual voice, is for the patient to be able to speak after the intervention with his own voice without aspiration (Herrmann 1987). LHP with suspension is necessary to control the quantity of aspiration below the vocal folds and above the closure because otherwise the quality of the voice may be impaired.

Via a median incision from the thyroid cartilage into the jugular fossa, the trachea is exposed after transection of the thyroid isthmus. The anterior tracheal wall is split at the level of the first to fourth tracheal ring in the median line or opened in form of a swing door. A small tube is inserted at the level of the fourth tracheal ring for ventilation. A cranially pedicled mucosal flap of the membranous wall is circumcised, shifted upwards, and sutured in such a way that is closes

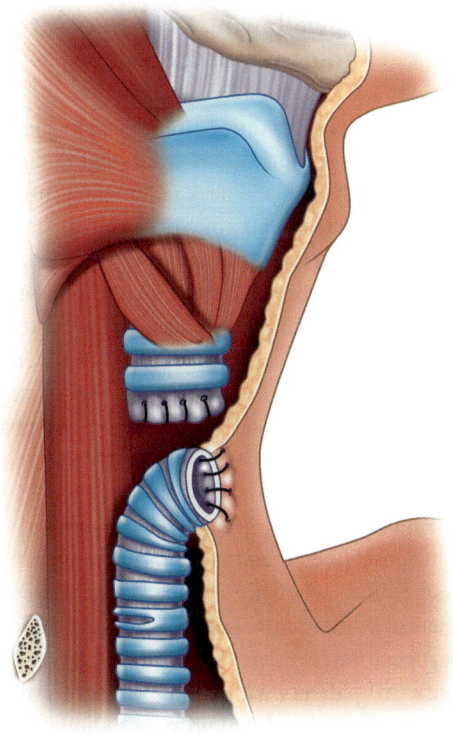

**Fig. 30.10** Laryngo-tracheal separation. Lateral view. (Figure reprinted from Eisele et al. (1989) with permission from Elsevier)

the trachea at the level of the first or second tracheal ring with the mucosa without tension. The caudal covering of the closure is performed with a skin-platysma, fascia graft.

After planning of the flap, the hatched area of the pedicle is de-epithelialised so that it may heal under the skin. The pedicle should be sufficiently large to secure good vascular supply to the graft. The graft is dimensioned to the extent that it covers the inferior surface of the cranially pedicled mucosal flap, and the donor defect at the posterior tracheal wall, both without tension. Both flaps are fixed together with fibrin glue. In order to avoid pressure on the pedicle, the anterior part of the second tracheal ring is resected. A slight tamponade stabilises the position of the graft. It is recommended to create a bigger tracheostoma and to suture the skin with the skin-platysma fascia graft with tension at the superior circumference of the tracheostoma. The same applies for the suture of the other parts of the tracheostoma between skin and tracheal mucosa. Generally, the insertion of a cannula after extubation is not necessary.

Two months after intervention, the secondary restitution of the voice is performed by puncture through the tracheostoma closure with insertion of a voice prosthesis. Speech therapy starts 1 week after insertion of the shunt valve.

Another technique has been described to avoid laryngectomy; this allows phonation via a voice prosthesis inserted into a shunt from the trachea at the posterior wall of the tracheal stoma to the superior laryngotracheal segment. Via this tracheo-tracheolaryngeal shunt (TTLS) the patient brings the air from the lungs to the larynx when closing the tracheal stoma during expiration similar to the routine tracheo-oesophageal puncture after laryngectomy. But in this case the air drives the vocal folds of the structurally intact larynx to produce voice (Ford et al. 1999).

### 30.8.3.4 Laryngectomy

Dysphagia and laryngectomy may interrelate in different ways. The laryngo-tracheal separation or laryngectomy are applied therapeutically for irreversible, neurological or oncological diseases with severe aspiration. Laryngectomy is the most radical method to prevent aspiration.

Laryngectomy with partial resection of the hypopharynx leads to swallowing disorders.

Severe dysphagia is often the result of therapy of advanced laryngeal and hypopharyngeal carcinomas. In this context, patients have the poorest result of their swallowing function after radiochemotherapy or laryngectomy (Burnip et al. 2013). Stenosis in the neopharynx can be avoided by primary application of a radial flap. Bougienage of the stenosis may improve the patient's situation. Sweeny et al. (2012) evaluated stenoses of the neopharynx or the pharyngo-oesophageal transition after laryngectomy. Hereby, stenoses occurred in 19% of laryngectomised patients. 82% of these stenoses became apparent within the first postoperative year. There was no difference between primary or salvage laryngectomy. Patients who underwent dilatation only once had a better prognosis regarding dysphagia than laryngectomised patients after several dilatation procedures.

### 30.8.4 Surgical Therapy of Swallowing Disorders After Radiochemotherapy

By means of modified fluoroscopic barium-swallowing examination and endoscopy in patients with head and neck carcinomas after primary radiochemotherapy, or surgical therapy combined with radiochemotherapy, Nguyen et al. (2008) could show stenoses in the pharynx or oesophagus in 11% of the cases that led to persisting dysphagia after therapy. Those stenoses were treated with dilatation. In 50% dilatation performed once was sufficient for dysphagia treatment. In 21% of the patients, dilatation was needed at least 4 times.

Hutcheson et al. (2012) analysed 23 recurrence-free patients with laryngo-pharyngeal dysfunction who had to be laryngectomised because of tumour therapy. These were 6% of all laryngectomies in an evaluation interval of 6 years. All patients with laryngo-pharyngeal dysfunction had to undergo primary radiotherapy or radiochemotherapy because of a carcinoma of the head and neck.

### 30.8.5 Percutaneous Endoscopic Gastrostomy

Percutaneous endoscopic gastrostomy (PEG) is an established endoscopic surgical procedure for patients suffering from dysphagia who are not able, for a determined time or even permanently, to care for the necessary daily intake of liquid or calories (see also Sect. 30.9). In this context, the nutrition via PEG tube secures the energy supply. Indications for PEG are obstructive or neurogenic dysphagia with reversible and irreversible swallowing disorders as well as aspiration (Kurien et al. 2010). Depending on their abilities, the patients may still pursue oral food intake. Currently, the method of pulling a thread according to the Seldinger technique, and direct puncture are established procedures, but the method of pulling through a thread is considered a safe and simple method that is most frequently applied. A description of the procedure is described in Kurien et al. (2010). In prospective clinical studies, it has been confirmed that nutrition via PEG is well accepted and tolerated. Mays et al. (2014) developed predictors for the application of PEG tubes in order to secure enteral nutrition in the context of therapies. Influencing factors are preoperative irradiation, supraglottal partial resection of the larynx, tracheostomy, clinical status of the cervical lymph nodes (N0 vs. N2, N1 vs. N2), preoperative weight loss, dysphagia, type of reconstruction and the tumour stage. Mays prefers the early application of PEG so that complications in the context of postoperative wound healing can be avoided in high-risk patients and the prognosis and quality of life may be improved.

### 30.8.6 Radiologically Inserted Gastrostomy

Radiologically Inserted Gastrostomy (RIG) is a technique of creating a percutaneous gastrostomy while using radiological guidance to create the gastrostomy. The indications are similar to those described above for a PEG. The procedure is done under sedation and local anaesthesia by a skilled radiologist. A nasogastric tube is inserted to place air within the stomach in order to oppose the stomach wall to the anterior abdominal wall. Following initial gastric puncture, often with a specialised gastropexy device, contrast is inserted to confirm the gastric lumen. The gastric wall is anchored to the abdominal wall while a guidewire is placed into the lumen of the stomach. A series of dilators are passed over the guidewire until the gastrostomy tube can be inserted over the guidewire. The gastrostomy tube is then fixed by sutures. Feeding should not commence for at least 12 h (Behrbohm et al. 2022).

**Remark** This section is an excerpt from Arens C, Herrmann IF, Rohrbach S, Schwemmle C, Nawka T (2015) For more detailed information, see this source https://doi.org/10.1055/s-0035-1545298 (Arens et al. 2015)

## 30.9 Percutaneous Endoscopic Gastrostomy (PEG): Indications and Ethical Issues

Patrick G. Zorowka

### 30.9.1 Introduction

Since its introduction in 1980 (Gauderer et al. 1980), Percutaneous Endoscopic Gastrostomy (PEG) has become the method of choice for provision of nutritional support in patients who require long-term enteral nutrition. PEG is safe and effective (Gomes et al. 2012); it is minimally invasive and usually does not require general anaesthesia during tube insertion (Ho et al. 1988). These factors facilitate its use in a wide range of patients, including the very old, frail and debilitated. PEG placement is the preferred method of enteral nutrition in patients with a functional gastrointestinal tract and with a long-lasting incapability of orally ingesting food. In patients with a short-time need for artificial nutrition (< 30 days), nasogastric tube feeding may be the more appropriate treatment method.

Nevertheless, after decades of PEG insertions it is time to consider PEG placement in a more precise way. First, it must be recognised that the mortality rate in PEG patients may be raised: a recent study recorded 18% deaths within 2 months after PEG insertion (Blomberg et al. 2024). The surgical risks of PEG placement are now well known from the literature and daily practice. Among them peritonitis, perforation and abdominal bleeding may be the more serious ones and seem to occur in 1–4% of cases. Buried bumper syndrome (BBS) may also occur as a rare, but potentially fatal complication of PEG placement (Cyrany et al. 2016). Peristomal infection, abdominal pain, diarrhea, granulation tissue, leakage and tube dislocation are the most frequent complications occurring in 10 to 40% of PEG patients (Blomberg et al. 2024; Orlandoni and Peladic 2024). Given the fact that most of the patients selected for PEG placement suffer from chronic disease, impairment of wound healing and poor immune function have to be considered as additional complications. As a consequence some patients may be predisposed for pneumonia and surgical complications. Therefore the indication should be made on an individual basis, taking into account several factors including nutritional status, comorbidity, prognosis, the anticipated quality of life improvement and last, but not least, the wishes of the patient.

## 30.9.2 Indications for PEG

The main indication for PEG is a long-lasting incapability of oral food intake, which puts the patient at risk of malnourishment. As malnutrition syndromes such as cachexia and sarcopenia are difficult to reverse when fully established, the indication of nutritional support should not be delayed. Indication for nutritional therapy and PEG placement should be based on identifying nutritional risk. For this purpose in daily practice, validated screening instruments such as the Nutrition Risk Screening 2002 (Kondrup et al. 2003) or the Mini Nutritional Assessment (MNA) (Guigoz et al. 1994) for geriatric patients should be applied. Meanwhile some instruments have been validated for the differentiated indication of

PEG placement in certain patient groups (e.g., Alshekhlee et al. 2010; Chung et al. 2024). Brown et al. (2014) integrated the underlying extent of disease, nutritional status and the therapy planned in an instrument made to identify patients with head and neck cancer who are in need for early PEG placement.

Among the conditions typically associated with this incapability, are:

- Dysphagia due to an advanced neurological disease (e.g., amyotrophic lateral sclerosis, cerebrovascular disease, dementia, Huntington's disease, Multiple sclerosis, Parkinson's disease, status after stroke).
- Dysphagia due to mechanical obstruction (e.g., oropharyngeal or oesophageal cancer).
- Dysphagia due to anatomical anomalies (e.g., trachea-oesophageal fistula).
- Dysphagia due to functional impairment of the oropharyngeal tract (e.g., traumatic lesions, recent surgery, cystic fibrosis).
- Inability to eat effectively owing to reduced level of consciousness or cognitive functioning (e.g., advanced dementia, coma, head trauma).
- Psychiatric conditions (e.g., anorexia).

Another group of indications for PEG tubes refers to gut decompression. This may be needed in patients with abdominal malignancies, with bowel obstruction or with ileus. This group is not considered here.

In some of the conditions listed above it is questionable whether the patients really do benefit from PEG tubes. For instance, evidence suggests that survival rates in patients with advanced dementia are not improved through PEG feeding (Candy et al. 2009; van Bruchem-Visser et al. 2019). Also uncertain is the effect of PEG tubes on survival rates of patients with amyotrophic lateral sclerosis (Katzberg and Benatar 2011; Cui et al. 2018). These findings are considered as questioning the appropriateness of PEG tubes, when it is unclear wherein their benefit lies. At this point, medical indications alone fail to give a well-justified decision for a PEG. In addition, ethical aspects have to be considered. I shall refer to this point below.

### 30.9.3  Contra-Indications to PEG

Contra-indications are traditionally divided into the absolute and relative. Absolute contra-indications are any conditions where a treatment (a) causes more harm than benefit to the patient, or (b) involves side effects that are by no means acceptable (but likely to occur). Relative contra-indications are any conditions where a treatment involves side effects that are normally unacceptable but—in particular cases or in the light of specific considerations—may appear acceptable. Whether or not such specific considerations apply depends essentially on the patient's condition. Hence, relative contra-indications require individualised risk assessment and the results may differ between patients.

Regarding PEG there is little agreement in the literature as to which conditions constitute absolute contra-indications and which constitute relative ones. Among those frequently listed as absolute are:

- Uncorrected bleeding disorders: coagulopathy or thrombocytopenia (platelets $<50 \times 10^9/l$) (Kurien et al. 2010).
- Severe intra-abdominal afflictions: active peritonitis, massive ascites, perforation, acute infections.
- Gastric anomalies: gastric outlet obstruction, gastroparesis, varices, history of gastrectomy.
- Severe systemic diseases: e.g., haemodynamic instability, sepsis, recent myocardial infarction.
- Any contra-indication to endoscopy: e.g., oropharyngeal or oesophageal obstruction.

Relative contra-indications include conditions such as:

- Abdominal wall abnormalities (e.g., open wounds, ventral hernia, recent abdominal surgery).
- Intra-abdominal pathologies (e.g., portal hypertension, hepatomegaly, splenomegaly).
- Neoplastic or metastatic infiltration of abdominal structures.
- Morbid obesity.
- Cachexia.

Oropharyngeal and oesophageal cancer are also considered relative contra-indications, because of the potential spread of cancer cells into the gastrointestinal tract (Pickhardt et al. 2002). In this case, alternative methods such as radiographically placed percutaneous gastrostomy or surgical gastrostomy tube may be chosen. It has also long been questionable whether ventriculoperitoneal shunt (VPS) insertion is a contra-indication to PEG, but recent literature suggests that the combination of the two may have a tolerable complication risk (Oterdoom et al. 2017).

Finally, evidence indicates that a few conditions exist that are risk factors for poorer outcome and increased mortality after PEG placement. These conditions, too, must be seen as relative contra-indications. Among them are hypo-albuminaemia, elevated CRP, diabetes mellitus, high age and low BMI (Tominaga et al. 2010).

### 30.9.4  Ethical Issues

It is widely recognised today that the decision for PEG-feeding requires both a medical indication and an ethical justification (Loeser 2013). While the medical indication warrants the safety and effectiveness of the treatment, ethical reflections determine in what way and to what degree the patient will benefit from PEG.

As frequently found with medical treatments, their benefit is not fully assessed by applying a single measure (e.g., prolonged life expectancy). Rather, benefit assessment requires consideration of various aspects that, in one way or another, contribute to the patient's condition. Among the most important aspects to consider in the case of PEG tube feeding, are:

- Maintenance of the patient's life.
- Avoiding malnutrition.
- Avoiding other complications of his or her condition.
- Improving (or maintaining) quality of life.
- Respecting the patient's personal wishes regarding the way of being nourished.

Careful assessment of these aspects (and probably additional ones) will result in a highly individualised decision whether or not PEG is appropriate. The decision cannot be based on one person's view but requires consultation with the members of the healthcare team, including representatives from subspecialties (e.g., oncology, geriatrics, neurology). Ideally, the final decision is made by the whole healthcare team.

There is broad agreement that PEG tubes are no alternative to oral food intake as long as it is possible. For instance, in patients with advanced dementia or with an advanced neurodegenerative disorder, eating and drinking become difficult but not impossible. In such patients dietary modifications can help reduce the swallowing difficulties (e.g., altering the consistency of foods and liquids, or adding tasty ingredients). Additionally, assisted feeding through trained staff (logopaedics, nurses) can enable the patient to experience successful swallowing again and to diminish the fears and aversions associated with oral food intake.

If, despite the above measures, the nutritional status of the patient cannot be maintained by oral feeding, a PEG tube is indicated: not as an alternative to oral feeding, but as a supportive means. Oral ingestion should continue (as long as possible), and supplemental nutrition is provided through the PEG tube to prevent malnutrition. It is only after the risks associated with dysphagia (e.g., aspiration) become uncontrollable that the nutrition is provided only via the PEG tube.

Another group of patients for which the use of PEG tubes has fuelled discussion is that of the terminally ill (Dev et al. 2012). These patients typically reduce food and fluid intake, which results in weight loss and cachexia. Their family members often misperceive the physical changes as a sign of starvation due to ineffective eating and drinking—and demand that the patient receive artificial nutrition as a life-sustaining treatment. However, terminally ill people do not die owing to not eating and drinking but the converse; they do not eat or drink owing to dying. As their metabolic functions decrease, they experience less thirst and hunger, and have little desire for eating and drinking. Supplying them with a PEG tube will neither provide them more comfort nor stop their physical decline. In addition, PEG tubes also do not improve functional, nutritional or subjective outcomes of the health status of older adults (Callahan et al. 2000).

An important aspect to consider is the patient's personal wish regarding artificial nutrition. It seems that agreement to tube feeding is sparse. A survey (O'Brien et al. 1997) among residents of nursing homes found that only 33% of them favoured tube feeding in the case they would be no longer able to eat, while 62% opposed it. Of those who initially favoured it, 20% changed their mind after they received additional information about the possible need of being physically restrained in order to facilitate tube feeding. This finding suggests that only a small percentage of patients would finally consent to tube feeding when they receive full information about this procedure.

PEG tubes may also have a psychological impact on the patients. Some patients may miss the pleasure of tasting and eating together with others. In younger people, e.g., in patients with cystic fibrosis, tube feeding may have a negative effect on self-esteem and body image (Morton and Wolfe 2015).

It is the clinician's ethical responsibility to provide all relevant information to the patient before asking him or her whether he or she has a preference for a PEG tube. If the patient is incapable of comprehending the information and making the decision, his or her surrogate caregiver must be consulted. In addition, the clinician must determine whether the patient has already executed an advance directive whose provisions could apply to the PEG tube decision. Only with the patient's informed consent to PEG is the health care team authorised to continue the decision-making process. In full length, this process consists of three steps:

- First step: Medical indication.
  - Not given: no PEG.
  - Given: proceed to second step.
- Second step: Patient's (or surrogate caregiver's) informed consent.
  - Not given: no PEG.

- Given: proceed to third step.
- Third step: Ethical justification (assessment of pros and cons).
  - Ethically not justified: no PEG.
  - Ethically justified: decision to PEG.

### 30.9.5 Conclusion

Given the potential benefits and risks of PEG placement, the indication should be made on an individual basis. Especially in situations where the indication for long-term enteral nutrition is not obvious, caution is needed. Over- and undertreatment should be avoided. In general a compromised nutritional status has negative effects on clinical outcome and predisposes the patient to surgical and non-surgical complications. Therefore, validated screening tools should be applied to identify patients being nutritionally at risk. For some patient groups special validated instruments are available and should be used in clinical practice. Besides this, ethical considerations are of utmost importance and need to be considered when indicating a PEG tube.

---

## 30.10  Tracheal Tube Management

Peter Kummer and Carmelo Perez Alvarez

### 30.10.1 Introduction

The management of the tracheal cannula is often one of the key components during rehabilitation in dysphagia (Dziewas and Pflug 2020). Early and ongoing swallowing diagnostics should aim at determining adequate tracheal tube management, matching the requirements of the individual patient, which may change during the rehabilitation process. On the one hand, secure protection against aspiration is essential, regularly combined with limited oral food intake. Rehabilitation, on the other hand, requires permanent searching for options that enable early verbal communication, support adequate nutrition and improve the quality of life, finally aim-

ing at decannulation. A thorough knowledge of different tracheostomy tubes and their individual advantages is therefore mandatory.

### 30.10.2  Cuffed Tracheal Tubes

Cuffed tracheal tubes are necessary for mechanical ventilation, depending on the pulmonary situation and whether there is a need to protect the lower airways from aspiration of saliva and food, even during tube feeding (see Fig. 30.11a, b). This is especially true in cases of recurrent aspiration pneumonia; mostly, but not only, in severe neurological dysphagia. Cuffed tracheal tubes also allow the suctioning of secretions and food through the cannula and the evacuation of aspirated foreign bodies after cannula removal.

To prevent ulcerations and the formation of tracheo-oesophageal fistulas, the use of low-pressure-high-volume cuffs and the measurement of the cuff pressure are mandatory. The ideal pressure ranges from 15 to 25 mmHg in order to ensure sufficient tracheal sealing. Pressures below 15 mmHg promote the risk of aspiration, although a cuffed tracheal tube cannot prevent aspiration with 100% certainty. In no case does a cuffed tracheal tube sufficiently prevent aspiration following oral food intake (Winklmaier et al. 2005; Dullenkopf et al. 2003; Oikkonen and Aromaa 1997).

On the other hand, for rehabilitation purposes, which aim to restore swallowing, breathing and phonation, the question is regularly raised of whether inflation of the cuff and protection against aspiration is (still) necessary or whether this rather impedes the next rehabilitation steps, especially when considering that the severity of the dysphagia may have decreased owing to recovery from the underlying disease. Eventually, the cannula and inflation of the cuff itself result in severe restraints on respiration, voice generation and swallowing.

Although often primarily indicated for reasons of airway protection, tracheostomy and cuffed tracheal cannulae differentially impede physiological respiration. Both impair heating, moisturisation and particle filtration of the

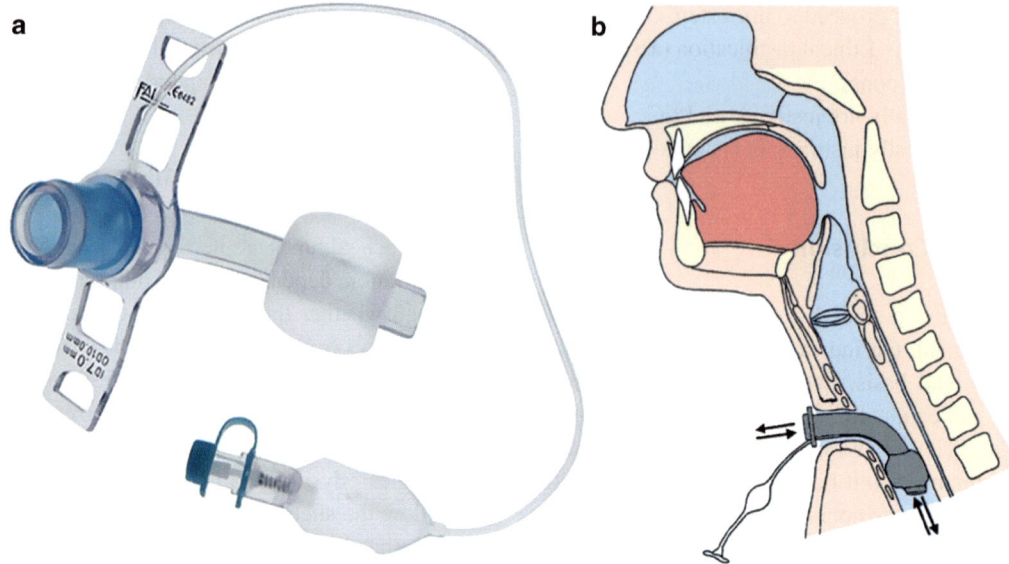

**Fig. 30.11** (**a**) Cuffed tracheal tube, for mechanical ventilation and airway protection. With kind permission from Andreas Fahl Medizintechnik-Vertrieb GmbH. (**b**) Arrows indicate that both inhaled and exhaled air bypasses the trachea, larynx and pharynx. (Reprinted from Schröter-Morasch 2022 in Bartolome G, Schröter-Morasch H: Swallowing Disorders, sixth Edition 2018 © Elsevier GmbH, Urban & Fischer, Munic. With kind permission from Elsevier)

inhaled air, leading to inflammation, desiccation and increased mucus secretion of the airways. The pulmonary clearance is also impaired, since subglottal pressure build-up and coughing up are not possible. The respiration is regularly flattened and does not reach the deeper airways. Similarly, voice production is not possible, as the exhaled air does not pass through the larynx. In addition to communication limitations, psychosocial isolation and anxiety may result. The vocal folds may suffer from atrophy leading to voice fatigue (Schwegler et al. 2021).

Tracheostomy and cuffed tracheal cannulae, however, may also differentially contribute to the maintenance as well as the formation of dysphagia. The mucosa of the trachea, larynx and pharynx are left unstimulated, when exhaled air is bypassed through the cannula (see Fig. 30.11b). It is also impossible to cough up saliva and secretions that are not swallowed. First pooling in the pharynx, secretions penetrate into the larynx, are aspirated through the glottis, pooled in the subglottal spaces, and accumulate above the cuff, potentially leaking from the tracheostoma (see Fig. 30.12). Both the absence of physiological

stimulation through the respiratory air flow and the pooling of secretions reduce mucosal sensitivity, which finally impairs such mechanisms as the cough and swallowing reflexes (Frank et al. 2007, 2021; Tolep et al. 1996). Both oral and pharyngeal stages of swallowing are involved, i.e. in terms of prolonged triggering of swallowing, reduced tongue functioning and strength, laryngeal closure and impaired relaxation of the upper oesophageal sphincter, leading to aspiration (Seo et al. 2017). The tracheal tube and cuff, however, also mechanically impede the swallowing process, by inhibiting laryngeal elevation and promoting laryngeal fixation (Ding and Logemann 2005; Feldman et al. 1966; Jung et al. 2012).

### 30.10.3 Stepwise Approach to Rehabilitation of Voice and Swallowing

A heat and moisture exchanger (HME) fitted onto the end of the tracheal tube not only provides filtering of small particles entering the tube and

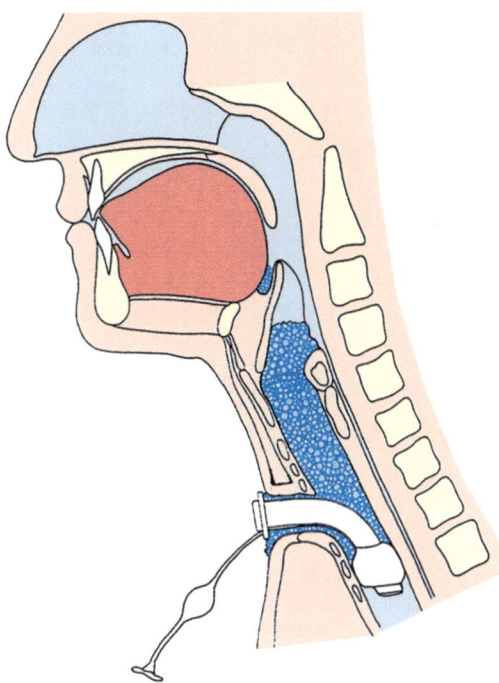

**Fig. 30.12** Cuffed tracheal cannula. Pooling of aspirated secretions in the trachea that accumulate above the cuff and leak from the tracheostoma. (Reprinted from Schröter-Morasch (2022) in Bartolome G, Schröter-Morasch H: Swallowing Disorders, 7th Edition 2022 © Elsevier GmbH, Urban & Fischer, Munic. With kind permission from Elsevier)

humidification to keep secretions thin and to avoid mucus plugs, but also improves pulmonary rehabilitation, as part of respiratory therapy. Tracheal cannulae with a subglottal suctioning tube may allow removal of mucus above the cuff and therefore facilitate coughing up after deflating the cuff. Infectious complications may be reduced and monitoring subglottal saliva may indicate proper timing of decuffing. With the cuff deflated, even cuffed tracheal tubes allow speaking and coughing, as long as the tracheal cannula size is small enough and the air can move around the tube upwards. More easily applicable and therapeutically flexible in this sense are cuffed and fenestrated tubes with both fenestrated and unfenestrated inner cannulae. Mechanical ventilation and protection against aspiration are possible by using an unfenestrated inner cannula that blocks the fenestrations of the cuffed outer can-

nula. If mechanical ventilation is interrupted for spontaneous ventilation, respiratory and swallowing therapy, the cuff is deflated and the fenestrated inner cannula is inserted, such that the patient is able to breathe spontaneously, to generate voice and cough up secretions. It has to be confirmed that the fenestration is at the correct site and endoscopic examination has to check if granulation tissue forms there.

A speaking valve, i.e., a one-way valve attached to the outside opening of the tracheostomy tube, is usually required to build-up subglottal pressure and air flow (see Fig. 30.13a, b). Exhaled air thus is no longer bypassed but passed through the trachea, larynx and pharynx, not only for phonation and coughing but also for restoring normal mucosal sensitivity, as a basis of swallowing and coughing reflex sensory input (Suiter et al., 2003). A speaking valve may be crucial when compensatory manoeuvres, e.g. the supraglottal manoeuvre, are necessary for swallowing rehabilitation. Lack of tolerance of a speaking valve may require testing a smaller diameter tracheal tube and clarifying tracheal or laryngeal stenosis. It is imperative that the speaking valve not be set on the cannula when the cuff is inflated, as this would trap the air in the lungs. Personnel must be instructed to observe this rule strictly.

Cuffless cannulae are used when no protection against aspiration is needed in patients with upper airway obstructions. Even this type of tracheal tube, however, mechanically impedes laryngeal elevation and promotes laryngeal fixation and silent aspiration (Oikkonen and Aromaa 1997).

When the indication for the insertion of a tracheostomy tube has been resolved, the decannulation, i.e., the permanent removal of the tracheal tube, can be performed. Criteria for decannulation include that the patient is alert, orientated and responsive to commands; that he no longer depends on a ventilator for assisted breathing; that he requires tracheal suctioning less than once a day, manages oral secretions without the risk of aspiration, coughs and cleans tracheal secretions, and tolerates tube occlusion with no evidence of respiratory difficulty or requiring suctioning of the tracheal tube (Bianchi et al. 2012; Warnecke et al. 2013).

a

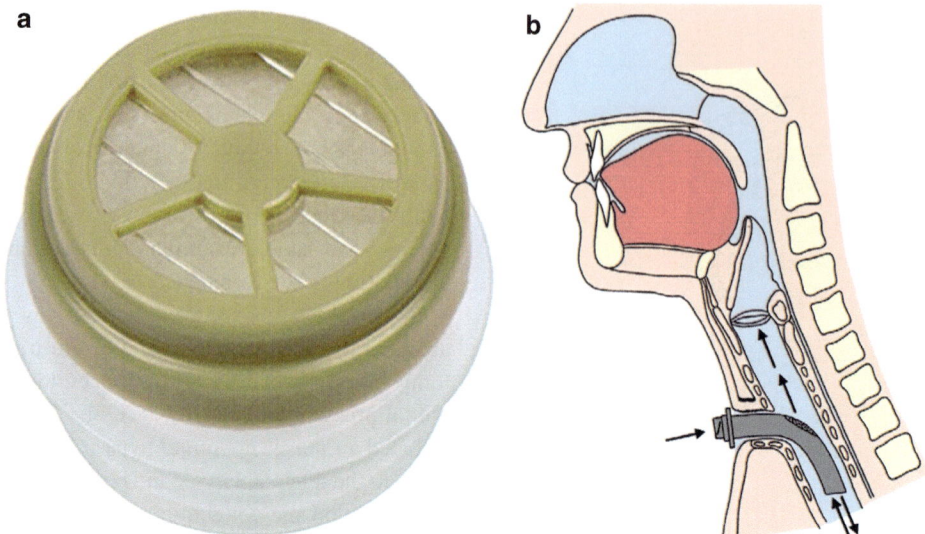

b

**Fig. 30.13** (**a**) Fahl speaking valve: Speaking valve that can be mounted to a decuffed tracheostomy tube. (With kind permission from Andreas Fahl Medizintechnik-Vertrieb GmbH). (**b**) Fenestrated tracheal tube with a speaking valve. Arrows indicate air flow that allows build-ing up subglottal air pressure and air flow during exhala-tion. (Reprinted from Schröter-Morasch (2022) in Bartolome G, Schröter-Morasch H: Swallowing Disorders, 7th Edition 2022 © Elsevier GmbH, Urban & Fischer, Munic. With kind permission from Elsevier)

In summary, the following steps are advised in tracheal tube management (Schröter-Morasch (2022)):

1. Mounting an HME to the cuffed cannula.
2. Deflating the cuff.
3. Attaching a speaking valve to the tracheal tube, and increasing time with the speaking valve mounted until cuffing is needed no more.
4. Inserting a cuffless cannula with a speaking valve.
5. Using a tracheal place holder instead of the tracheal tube (see Fig. 30.14).
6. Decannulation.

### 30.10.4 Complications of Tracheal Cannula Usage

Complications resulting from tracheal cannula usage may first appear as signs of respiratory dis-tress or bleeding. Dyspnoea most often arises from dry mucus in the cannula and may require

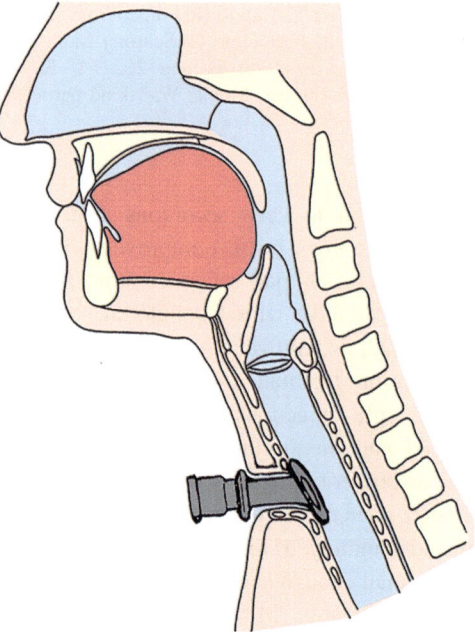

**Fig. 30.14** Montgomery tube (place holder) inserted into the tracheostoma. (Reprinted from Schröter-Morasch (2022) in Bartolome G, Schröter-Morasch H: Swallowing Disorders, 7th Edition 2022 © Elsevier GmbH, Urban & Fischer, Munic. With kind permission from Elsevier)

emergency measures, i.e., following initial removal of the cannula, instrumental removal of dry mucus from the trachea and cleaning or replacing of the cannula. Moisturisation of inhaled air via HMEs is critical and can be combined with inhalation and antibiotic therapy if necessary. Dyspnoea may also occur during dislocation of the cannula (via falsa), something especially dangerous in cases of non-epithelialised tracheostomy where endoscopically guided reintubation may be required. Granulation tissue at the distal cannula end, erosion and bleeding may be prevented by regular endoscopy and monitoring of cannula position and the tracheal wall, both with and without the cannula. By utilising tubes of various lengths, ulcerations of the tracheal wall may be treated or even prevented. Granulation tissue forms when cannulae are not changed for more than 2–4 weeks. In these instances, secretions cause maceration of the stoma canal tissue. Granulations may protrude not only externally, but also internally, blocking the cannula lumen during its change.

In addition to airway protection and respiration, ease of phonation should also be emphasised when selecting the proper cannula diameter and length. Phonation should not be hampered by overly large cannula diameters when non-fenestrated tubes are used. On the other hand, cannulae should be large enough to seal the stoma sufficiently. In cases of severe insufficiency, additional measures may be required for sealing. Moreover, phonation may also interfere with protrusion of the anterior tracheal wall or subglottal stenosis. In these cases, surgical revision or stabilisation via Montgomery t-tube stents or trachea placeholders (trachea-safe) may be required.

Severe bleeding occurs most commonly as an early complication following epithelialised tracheostomy. Surgical revision will be required. In case of emergency, cuffing of the cannula protects the airways until surgical revision can be performed. A speculum, a cuffing syringe, a cannula with a cuff, as well as a suction apparatus, should therefore always be within the immediate vicinity of a tracheostomised patient. Moderate bleeding may arise from granulation tissue formation at the stoma and requires only local measures, e.g., ablation or cauterisation. Bleeding granulations may stress the patient when replacement of the cannula is necessary, especially when the patient is anxious and coughs. Periodic replacement of the cannula, keeping the stoma clean and dry, and use of cortisol-containing unguents may prevent formation of granulation tissue.

## 30.11 Dysphagia in Non-surgically Treated Patients with Head and Neck Cancer

Žofia Korim and Miroslav Tedla

### 30.11.1 Introduction

The causes of dysphagia in patients with head and neck cancer (HNC) can be multifactorial. At the time of HNC diagnosis, two-thirds of patients have a swallowing disorder (van der Molen et al. 2009). According to Pauloski et al. (2000), 28.2% of patients with stage T2 or more oral cancer, 50.9% of patients with pharyngeal cancer, and 28.6% of patients with laryngeal cancer have dysphagia at the time of diagnosis of HNC. Tumours in the laryngeal sphincters that spread to the suprahyoid muscles, pre-epiglottal space and prevertebral fascia may restrict movement of the hyolaryngeal complex during swallowing, and cause pain (odynophagia) (Russi et al. 2012). In the non-surgical oncological treatment of head and neck cancer (radiotherapy and chemotherapy), the incidence of dysphagia is 2.5 times higher than in patients undergoing surgical treatment. Ten percent of these patients will experience aspiration pneumonia within 3 years of starting treatment (Francis et al. 2010).

During non-surgical treatment, almost all patients require nutritional support. Some patients may avoid the need for enteral nutrition if they undergo ingestion therapy at the beginning of treatment, with optimal pain relief and increased nutritional support (Paleri et al. 2014).

## 30.11.2 Toxicity of Radiotherapy

Dysphagia develops in two phases in patients with HNC undergoing non-surgical treatment. Acute difficulties occur during or shortly after treatment. There is radiation-induced dermatitis or mucositis, appetite disorder, salivary gland damage, lymphoedema and swallowing pain (Barbon et al. 2017; Ihara et al. 2018). These difficulties worsen food intake, which can lead to reduced food intake or the need for enteral nutrition. By limiting oral intake, less swallowing occurs, which accelerates the atrophy of unused tissues and exacerbates post-radiation oedema and fibrosis (Hutcheson et al. 2013). Mucosal damage is associated with cell death and the subsequent inflammatory process. Other tissue responses are associated with damage to mucosal vascularisation and adjacent connective tissue (King et al. 2016). Acute symptoms are alleviated within three to 6 months of stopping treatment.

However, continued hypoxia can damage exposed tissues, and dysphagia may develop years after the end of HNC treatment (Raber-Durlacher et al. 2012; Jeans et al. 2019). Patients who have not experienced acute difficulty swallowing during treatment may still have problems in the late post-treatment phase (Chelakkot 2018). A specific complication after radiotherapy is mandibular osteoradionecrosis. After irradiation, the salivary glands are permanently damaged (xerostomia). Tissue fibrosis is a major cause of long-term dysphagia after non-surgical HNC treatment. The difference between normal wound healing and the treatment of radiation damage is that during radiation the tissue damage repeats at regular intervals. Therefore, healing cannot be continuous and is disrupted by other radiation doses (Chelakkot 2018).

Several inflammatory and cellular signalling mediators are activated during wound healing. One of the mediators, Transforming Growth Factor-Beta (TGF-β), signals to cells in the wound-healing process to repair damaged tissue. These cells form new tissue, and the process stops when the tissue heals. Radiation-induced fibrosis does not undergo a normal wound healing process. Some TGF-β is formed, leading to the activation of another mediator, CTGF (Connective Tissue Growth Factor) (Okunieff et al. 2008). CTGF is inhibited during standard wound healing, but in the case of its wound reproduction, the process cannot be stopped. CTGF and TGF-β can activate other cells and spread fibrosis within the anatomical structure. The process of fibrosis is triggered by a critical amount of TGF-β.

Patients who have fibrosis are expected to reach this threshold soon after radiotherapy. However, it is not known what influences the onset and course of fibrotisation in HNC patients (Langmore and Krisciunas 2010). Fibrous tissue envelops muscle fibres and makes them ineffective. As a result of not using muscle fibres, they weaken and the swallowing act worsens. After radiotherapy, the organisation of muscle fibrils changes, their course is less organised and they lose their linear structure (Tedla et al. 2012). Biological processes under the influence of radiotherapy alter the cellular, molecular pathways of oxidative stress and signal transduction (King et al. 2016). Fibrosis leads to muscle atrophy, fasciculation, vocal fold weakness, incompetence of the velopharyngeal mechanism, and weakening of the pharyngeal constrictors may occur (Chelakkot 2018). Fibrosis can cause trismus. In addition to tissue changes, radiotherapy causes thermal and mechanical damage that triggers inflammatory mediators such as cytokines, neuropeptides and glutamate receptors (King et al. 2016). The most common deficits in the swallowing act are tongue root dysfunction, decreased pharyngeal contraction, impaired movement of the epiglottis and hyolaryngeal complex, delayed transit through the pharyngeal phase, impaired swallowing muscle coordination (Logemann et al. 2008).

## 30.11.3 Causes and Predictors of Dysphagia

Dysphagia before non-surgical treatment can be caused by:

- Tumour mass, infiltrating or ulcerating lesion of swallow structures or cranial nerves involved in swallowing.

- Tumour damage of the laryngeal and oesophageal sphincters.
- Pain (Russi et al. 2012).

Treatment intensity, younger age and lower scores in the subjective swallow assessment predict long-term dysphagia (Wilson et al. 2011). Swallowing difficulties are exacerbated by the addition of concomitant chemotherapy and by increasing the radiation dose to the swallowing structures. Acute xerostomia and dysphagia during radiotherapy are strong prognostic factors for late dysphagia (van der Laan et al. 2015a, b). The risk of developing dysphagia after curative (chemo) radiotherapy can be identified from the Total Dysphagia Risk Score (TDRS) (Langendijk et al. 2009; Nevens et al. 2016). This score identifies patients who could benefit from a preventive intervention before swallowing difficulties arise. Unfavourable prognostic factors for dysphagia are: T3-T4 tumour, bilateral neck radiotherapy, weight loss before radiotherapy, oropharyngeal and nasopharyngeal tumour, accelerated and concomitant chemoradiotherapy.

Three risk groups have been identified: a low-risk group, a medium-risk group and a high-risk dysphagia group (Langendijk et al. 2009). Grouping expresses the risk of acute dysphagia (Koiwai et al. 2010) and late dysphagia 12, 18 and 24 months after treatment. It may also be beneficial in identifying patients requiring intensity-modulated radiation therapy (IMRT) aimed at preserving the anatomical structures involved in swallowing (Langendijk et al. 2009). The Italian Association of Radiation Oncology recommends the use of TDRS to assess the risk of ingestion dysfunction. With TDRS greater than 9 points, the patient should be advised to prevent swallowing strategies (Russi et al. 2012). However, TDRS is not screening for dysphagia and the score does not correlate with objective swallowing examinations (Nevens et al. 2018).

## 30.11.4 Incidence of Aspiration and Aspiration Pneumonia

The incidence of aspiration in patients with HNC before treatment is 11–53% (Rosen et al. 2001;

Graner et al. 2003; Nguyen et al. 2006; Langerman et al. 2007; Feng et al. 2010); silent aspiration occurs in 14–18% of these patients (Stenson et al. 2000; Rosen et al. 2001). Dysphagia reported by patients is a predictor of aspiration pneumonia. Dysphagia reported by healthcare professionals has not been identified as a significant predictor of aspiration pneumonia (Hunter et al. 2014). This suggests that swallowing dysfunction alone is not the only cause of aspiration pneumonia. The development of aspiration pneumonia is conditioned by inhalation of colonised oropharyngeal contents (Marik 2001). If the protective mechanisms are intact and the amount of aspirated bolus is small, aspiration pneumonia usually does not develop (Tedlová and Mucska 2018). A meta-analysis of 30,962 patients found that risk factors for pneumonia in HNC patients were: male sex, regular alcohol consumption, poor oral hygiene before treatment, dysphagia before treatment, hypopharyngeal and nasopharyngeal tumour, (chemo)radiotherapy versus surgical treatment itself, the addition of chemotherapy to radiotherapy, recurrent radiotherapy, neck dissection, longer duration of tracheostomy, use of sleep medication (Reddy et al. 2020).

## 30.11.5 Dysphagia Stages According to Swallowing Phases

### 30.11.5.1 Oral Phase

Tumours of the tongue or mouth act as an obstruction, causing pain or restricting the movement of the structures of the mouth. Impairment of the lingual nerve causes changes in sensitivity (Murphy and Gilbert 2009). Injury of the hypoglossal nerve causes dysfunction of the tongue. These deficits disrupt the oral preparation and transport phase of the swallowing act. Loss of soft palate function causes nasal regurgitation or premature bolus leakage into the pharynx. Xerostomia causes difficulties in the oral preparation phase and in shifting the bolus through the pharyngeal swallowing phase (Simental and Carrau 2004). Reduced salivation leads to insufficient protection of soft and hard tissues, which increases the number of cariogenic bacteria.

Calcium deficiency can cause structural damage to teeth (Epstein and Barasch 2018).

### 30.11.5.2 Pharyngeal Phase

The pharyngeal phase of swallowing can be disordered by the tumour itself, fixation of the swallowing muscles, fibrosis of the pharyngeal and laryngeal structures. Tumours in the suprahyoid muscle, pre-epiglottal space and prevertebral fascia limit elevation and protrusion of the hyolaryngeal complex. Radiotherapy in this area causes cranial nerve neuropathy, exacerbating swallowing deficits (Simental and Carrau 2004). Research has shown a significant reduction in laryngeal nerve perineurium thickness after radiotherapy (Tedla et al. 2012). Changes in the perineurium of the laryngeal nerve may affect swallowing. In patients with HNC, complete loss of function of swallowing structures may occur as a result of cancer destruction or cancer treatment (Denaro et al. 2013). Pharyngeal residues are a significant problem in dysphagic patients with HNC (Langmore et al. 2016; Pisegna et al. 2020). Bolus aspiration occurs mainly after ingestion, which is associated with pharyngeal residues (Denaro et al. 2013; Servagi-Vernat et al. 2015; Langmore et al. 2016).

Aspiration after swallowing is the result of:

- Decreased pharyngeal peristalsis (Servagi-Vernat et al. 2015).
- Limited elevation of the hyolaryngeal complex.
- Laryngeal sphincter insufficiency at the level of arytenoid cartilages and epiglottis.
- Upper oesophageal sphincter dysfunction (Denaro et al. 2013; Langmore et al. 2016; Pisegna et al. 2020).

Penetration and aspiration are debilitating for the patient and worsen the quality of life (Meyer et al. 2017). Therefore, they should be identified and managed in a timely manner.

### 30.11.5.3 Oesophageal Phase

Narrowing or complete stricture of the oesophagus is a possible form of damage after non-surgical treatment of HNC. A so-called corkscrew

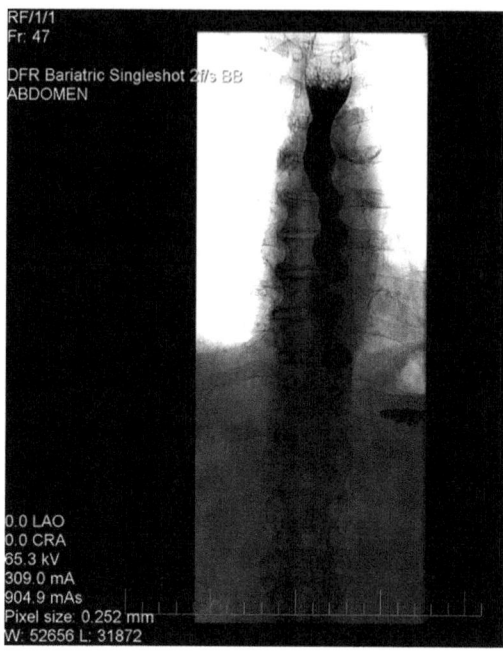

**Fig. 30.15** Corkscrew oesophagus

oesophagus is shown in Fig. 30.15. It occurs in 8–24% of patients after chemoradiotherapy and affects swallowing by blocking the passage of the bolus into the stomach (Pauloski 2008). In terms of pathophysiology, stricture formation begins with ulceration after severe mucositis. At the same time, the limited mobility of the larynx with radiation-induced fibrosis also has an adverse effect. Gastrostomy may also contribute to the development of fibrosis, as the risk of non-use and inactivity of the upper oesophageal sphincter increases (Mekhail et al. 2001).

## 30.11.6 Multidisciplinary Management of Swallowing Before Non-surgical Treatment of HNC

According to multidisciplinary guidelines of head and neck oncology, speech and swallowing intervention is part of the care of patients with HNC (Clarke et al. 2016; NICE (2004); Paleri and Roland 2016). Every patient should undergo a clinical swallowing evaluation before HNC treatment (Clarke et al. 2016).

The aim of the evaluation is:

- Identification of abnormalities in the swallowing act.
- Recommendations for further evaluations to assess the risk of aspiration.
- Developing an appropriate treatment plan for the impaired swallowing act (Schindler et al. 2015).

Head and neck cancer patients should be managed by a multidisciplinary team (MDT) focusing on head and neck cancer. MDT integrates experts from several fields (Kuhn et al., 2023). The goal of MDT is to increase the effectiveness of treatment, shorten the hospital stay, improve the oncological outcome of treatment and the patient's quality of life. MDT includes ENT and maxillofacial surgeons, phoniatricians, clinical and radiation oncologists, diagnostic radiographers, histopathologists, speech-language therapists and nutritionists (Cohen et al. 2016). The surgeon and oncologist lead the MDT and plan a treatment strategy. The role of the speech-language therapist/phoniatrician in the team is to ensure an adequate and safe way of swallowing (Ackerman et al. 2018). The speech-language therapist/phoniatrician applies measures to prevent swallowing difficulties, participates in the diagnostic process in HNC patients, and determines the treatment options for dysphagia according to the nature and severity of the deficits (Cohen et al. 2016).

Maintaining partial safe oral intake during radiotherapy and chemotherapy is the main goal of proactive intervention in the patient's HNC. Swallowing assessment should include a quality of life measurement that helps explain the difficulties from the patient's perspective and determines the balance between the optimal effect of cancer treatment and an acceptable quality of life (Heutte et al. 2014). Early care of swallowing and nutrition leads to shorter duration of enteral feeding, lower weight loss, and earlier return to oral intake. Therefore, this should be an integral part of standard processes in the care of patients with HNC (Messing et al. 2019). Three main strategies for reducing long-term dysphagia after non-surgical treatment HNC treatment are pre-ventive exercises to preserve oral and pharyngeal structures, providing enteral nutrition during CHRT, reduction of the radiation dose to the structures involved in swallowing (Paleri et al. 2014). However, a unified approach to dysphagia in HNC patients does not yet exist (Krisciunas et al. 2012).

### 30.11.6.1  Oral Versus Enteral Nutrition

There is no consensus on the optimal timing of enteral nutrition in HNC patients undergoing non-surgical cancer treatment (Nugent et al. 2010; Langmore et al. 2012; Shaw et al. 2015). The nasogastric tube (NGS) in non-surgically treated patients with HNC causes discomfort and increases the risk of extra-oesophageal reflux (Denaro et al. 2013). Therefore, this method of nutrition is used the least. However, there is also an opinion that NGS promotes more frequent swallowing, which reduces the risk of muscle fibrosis and improves swallowing results. In addition, NGS serves as a stent, reducing the risk of severe swallowing stricture (Dutta and Thankappan 2018).

Some patients with HNC are malnourished before treatment, and tumour localisation and toxicity of planned therapy may increase the need for nutritional intake. Therefore, percutaneous endoscopic gastrostomy (PEG) before treatment provides patients with adequate nutrition during therapy and helps them recover more rapidly (Pfister et al. 2020). However, it is not recommended to introduce PEG or NGS prophylactically in patients without significant weight loss, airway obstruction and severe dysphagia. These patients should be monitored and weight changes should be recorded. They may require enteral nutrition during treatment.

Prophylactic introduction of PEG is strongly recommended if the patient:

- Severe weight loss before treatment, 5% weight over the last month or 10% weight over the last 6 months.
- Dehydration or dysphagia, anorexia or pain preventing adequate oral intake.
- Severe aspiration or mild aspiration in elderly patients or patients with impaired cardiopulmonary function;

- Presumed prolonged dysphagia, including patients undergoing prolonged radiotherapy in other areas. Other risk factors for swallowing failure should be considered when considering (Pfister et al. 2020).

In contrast to prophylactic PEG placement, enteral nutrition is thought to adversely affect the ability to swallow. If PEG is placed before the start of non-surgical treatment, the patient's nutrition depends on enteral intake. Changes in taste, dry mucosa and anorexia are associated with this, which reduces or interrupts oral food and fluid intake. It is thought that reducing the frequency of swallowing may lead to muscle atrophy and worsen the severity of radiation-induced neck fibrosis. According to the results of the Langmore et al. study, a significant difference in weight loss was not confirmed in patients with prophylactic PEG and patients without PEG/with therapeutic PEG (Langmore et al. 2012). Other studies suggest that prophylactic PEG placement helps maintain the nutritional status of HNC patients, prevents weight loss during non-surgical treatment, and reduces the number of treatment interruptions (Beer et al. 2005; Mercuri et al. 2009). According to a recent systematic review, prophylactic gastrostomy is one of the prognostic factors for enteral nutrition dependence ≥6 months (Wopken et al. 2018). The prophylactic placement of PEG is associated with long-term dependence on enteral nutrition compared to the reactive introduction of PEG (McClelland et al. 2018).

### 30.11.6.2 Oral Nutrition and Exercise as Preventive Measures for Dysphagia

Radiotherapy has the effect of limiting the range of motion of important pharyngeal and laryngeal muscles, thereby disrupting the shift of the bolus when swallowing and thus reducing lower respiratory protection. Long-term dietary restrictions are necessary in patients with severe dysphagia, and dependence on enteral nutrition may persist for the rest of their lives (Goldsmith and Jacobson 2018). Reducing oral intake lowers the use of swallowing muscles and accelerates their atrophy

when underloaded. Failure to use aerodigestive tract muscles is likely to exacerbate oedema and radiation-induced fibrosis (Hutcheson et al. 2013). Restriction of oral nutrition longer than 14 days is significantly associated with prolonged post-treatment dysphagia and reduced quality of life (Gillespie et al. 2004). Patients whose PEG was not prevented and those with partially preserved oral intake during non-surgical treatment had significantly better preserved oral intake 3, 6 and 12 months after treatment (Langmore et al. 2012).

Patients who maintained partial oral intake during non-surgical HNC treatment and at the same time proactively exercised had the highest return to normal oral intake and the shortest time of dependence on enteral nutrition (Hutcheson et al. 2013). Such an approach appears to reduce the risk of treatment complications and is a key component in improving the patient's quality of life (Carnaby and Crary 2014). In addition to providing information to the patient, there may be a positive effect of preventive exercises aimed at swallowing. This type of intervention is also referred to in the literature as proactive or prophylactic and should be part of the care of HNC patients (Carnaby and Madhavan 2013; Govender et al. 2017).

Preventive swallowing exercises serve to increase the strength and range of movement of the muscles involved in swallowing, can prevent muscle atrophy, and reduce or delay the risk of radiation fibrosis (van der Molen et al. 2009). The studies performed so far are highly variable in the inclusion criteria, the exercises performed, their intensity and frequency (Carroll et al. 2008; Wall et al. 2013; Paleri et al. 2014, Dotevall et al., 2022). Dynamic and clinically achievable goals need to be formulated when planning therapy (Cheville 2005). Rehabilitation approaches constantly change the physiology of swallowing. They can be aimed at gaining skill or muscle strength. The design of the study in swallow therapy should include components of frequency, duration, repetition and intensity so that the results are measurable, repeatable, comparable (Krekeler et al. 2020).

## 30.12 Prognosis of Oropharyngeal Dysphagia

Carl-Albert Bader

### 30.12.1 Introduction

The course and prognosis of oropharyngeal dysphagia are determined by many factors. One is the disease underlying the swallowing disorder. Another is the individual ability for compensation, which depends, for example, on the general condition, the age and the cognitive conditions of the patient. Finally, the course of the dysphagia will be affected by a conservative swallowing therapy (see overview in Speyer et al. 2010). The complex interactions of these factors suggests that reliable prognostic statements may be difficult.

### 30.12.2 Oropharyngeal Dysphagia in Neurological Disorders

For oropharyngeal dysphagia of neurological cause, data are available primarily for patients with *stroke* (Table 30.4).

However, it should be noted that the statements from the studies were made only partially on the basis of imaging procedures, and otherwise based on clinical examinations only, some of them just with screening characteristic.

By using endoscopic or radiological techniques in the acute phase of an apoplectic insult, a dysphagia prevalence of 50-60 % is realistic (Broadley et al. 2003, 2005; Mann et al. 1999; Smithard et al. 1997). Apparently, in the first few days after the insult a significant regression of the swallowing disorder occurs (i.e., in about 30–50% of the dysphagic patients) (Broadley et al. 2003, 2005). However, studies involving periods beyond the acute phase show that after 6 months and more, aspirations may still be detectable in imaging in up to 40% of dysphagic patients, even though some studies have been done

in selected patients (Terré and Mearin 2009). Similarly, the need for tube feeding amounts to up to 60% after one year (Oto et al. 2009).

Different relevant factors are mentioned for the prognosis of the progression: age, cognition and mobility play an important role, as well as initial findings in imaging, as far as available, and above all an initially existing aspiration. Overall, consistent profiles of prognostic factors do not exist.

Chronic progressive disorders of the nervous system such as Parkinson's disease or disseminated encephalitis are also associated with oropharyngeal dysphagia (Alali et al. 2016; Calcagno et al. 2002; van Hooren et al. 2014), which may worsen the prognosis of the underlying disease. Significant predictors of the course of dysphagia itself could not be identified from the available data.

### 30.12.3 Oropharyngeal Dysphagia after Therapy of ENT Malignancies

Oropharyngeal dysphagia with structural causes is typically found after treatment of malignancies in the ENT area. It occurs both because of surgery itself and as a result of radio(chemo) therapy, and is based on disorders of the motor function, sensitivity and salivation. Experience has shown that, in principle, all phases of the swallowing process may be affected, with defects, scars and paralyses having an effect on the oral and pharyngeal phases. The adverse effects of a radio(chemo)therapy on swallowing function are generally more pronounced than those on vocal function (Lewin 2007). The supposedly beneficial organ preservation in radio(chemo)therapy does not necessarily mean the simultaneous maintenance of functionality (Lewin 2007). Local tissue changes (such as oedema, fibrosis or necrosis) and systemic effects of radio(chemo)therapy (such as neutropenia, general physical weakness and nausea) lead to dysphagia in the acute treatment phase (Lewin 2007). But even years after radiation

**Table 30.4** Neurogenic oropharyngeal dysphagia

| Reference | Number of patients | Determination of dysphagia extent | Recorded period post-onset | Prognostic statements | Course | Remarks |
|---|---|---|---|---|---|---|
| Broadley et al. (2003) | 149 | Clinical | $r$ = 0–97 d $m$ = 18 d | Dysphagia of >14 days to be expected from 1 Conspicuous water swallow test plus 2 Presence of two of the four factors: (a) Barthel index <20 (b) Paramatta score < 70 (c) Dysphasia (d) Lesion in the frontal or insular cortex | 74/149 (50%) initially dysphagic, Normalised at >50% within the first 5 days; At discharge ($n$ = 123): – 80% fully oralised – 14% oral with diet – 6% non-oral | Patients with acute stroke; 26 died during the course. |
| Broadley et al. (2005) | 104 | Clinical | $r$ = 16–40 d $m$ = 31 d | 'Positive RAPIDS' (corresponds to the negative prognosis factors, see Broadley et al. 2003) significantly influences the prognosis. | 55/104 (53%) initially dysphagic. 34% complete recovery within 14 days; 19% >14 days dysphagic; 4% fed non-oral at discharge. | Patients with acute stroke; 9 patients died during the course. Validation study for 'RAPIDS' (Royal Adelaide Prognostic Index for Dysphagic stroke). |
| Han et al. (2008) | 83 | Videofluoroscopy (VFSS) | 6 mon | Prognostically significantly unfavourable VFSS findings, e.g.: – Vallecular and sinusoidal residuals – Prolonged pharyngeal transit time – Initial aspiration – Symptoms of apractic dysphagia | 11 out of 83 (13%) patients with persistent aspiration >6 Mon | VFSS was carried out 40 days after stroke on average |
| Ikenaga et al. (2017) | 72 | FEES or VFSS | $r$ = 22–54 d | Prognostically relevant factors for achieving a completely oral diet were: – Initial nutritional status – Cognitive requirements – Initial severity of dysphagia | Of 72 initially dysphagic patients 38 could be completely fed orally and 34 partially orally fed at discharge | Patients in a rehabilitation clinic with an acute stroke. |
| Kojima et al. (2014) | 123 | Clinical + FEES, partly VFSS | Max. 1 y | Significant factors for a lack of improvement in terms of prognosis: - Presence of dementia - Immobility | Initially in 85/123 patients no oral nutrition possible; After 2–4 weeks no change in 39/85 patients, in 24/85 partial and in 22/85 complete oralisation possible | Group with high proportion of stroke patients (>50%). All patients received swallowing therapy. |

| | | | | | | |
|---|---|---|---|---|---|---|
| Kumar et al. (2014) | 323 | Clinical; Partly + VFSS | 10 ± 7 d | Significantly unfavourable factors in terms of prognosis:<br>– Initial positive proof of aspiration<br>– Bi-hemispheric infarction<br>– Condition after intubation<br>– NIHSS score ≤ 12 | Initial dysphagia signs in all 323 patients and proof of aspiration in 211/323 (65%) patients;<br>At discharge:<br>– 30% oral nutrition<br>– 70% no full or largely oral tasting<br>– 28% supplied with PEG | Patients with acute stroke. |
| Maeshima et al. (2013) | 334 | Clinical | r = 7–317 d<br>x = 100 d | Unfavourable forecast:<br>– Age > 70 years<br>– Extent of motor and cognitive impairments (according to FIM® score) | 334 patients initially fed by tube;<br>After rehab:<br>– in 291/334 oral nutrition<br>– in 43/334 tube feeding | Patients in a rehabilitation clinic with an acute stroke. |
| Mann et al. (1999) | 128 | Clinical + VFSS | 6 mon | Unfavourable forecast:<br>– Age > 70 years<br>– Male sex<br>– At initial VFSS: Delayed pharyngeal transit time and laryngeal penetration | Initial clinical suspicion of dysphagia in 65/128 (51%) patients;<br>VFSS abnormalities in 82/128 (64%) and evidence of aspiration in 28/128 (22%);<br>After 6 months:<br>– in 56/112 (50%) clinical dysphagia signs<br>– Evidence of aspiration in 17/67 (25%) patients examined with VFSS | Patients with acute stroke; 5 patients died, 11 'lost to follow-up'. |
| McMicken and Muzzy (2009) | 100 | Clinical | r = 1–48 d<br>x = 20 d | Prognostically significant factors for improvement in ingestion of food:<br>– Cognition<br>– Ingestion of food at admission<br>– Duration of the stay<br>– Number of therapy units | Initially no oral food intake possible in 26/100 patients;<br>at discharge in 4/100 patients no food intake per os | Patients with acute stroke; all patients received swallowing therapy. Study focuses on changes in food ingestion. |
| Neumann et al. (1995) | 58 | Clinical + VFSS | r = 3–156 w<br>m = 10 w | Same success rates of therapy for prolonged (≥25 w) and shorter (≤25 w) past acute injury.<br>None of the pre-therapeutic variables age, lesion site, time interval between onset of lesion and initiation of therapy, cognition, type, and extent of aspiration were significantly predictive. | Initially 86% exclusively or 14% partly fed by tube;<br>VFSS detection of laryngeal penetration or aspiration in 79%;<br>at discharge only oral nutrition in 67% | Patients of a rehabilitation facility with various underlying neurological diseases; all patients received therapy; outcome clinically recorded only. |

(continued)

| Reference | Number of patients | Determination of dysphagia extent | Recorded period post-onset | Prognostic statements | Course | Remarks |
|---|---|---|---|---|---|---|
| Oto et al. (2009) | 30 | Clinical | r = 109–262 d, m = 158 d | – Age > 70 years<br>– Extent of motor and cognitive limitations (according to FIM® score) | Initially all patients fed by tube; at discharge<br>– 12 patients orally fed<br>– 18 patients fed with tube | Patients of a rehabilitation facility with stroke. |
| Prosiegel et al. (2002) | 208 | Clinical + VFSS ± FEES | r = 2–322 d, m = 66 d | Prognostically relevant factors for outcome:<br>– Extent of dysphagia at baseline<br>– Endoscopically determined degree of aspiration<br>– Barthel index<br>– Duration of the disease | Initially tube feeding in 75% (n = 157); after therapy oral food intake in 55 % possible | 48 % patients with stroke. All patients received swallowing therapy |
| Smithard et al. (1997) | 121 | Clinical; Partly + VFSS | Max. 180 d | No prognostically significant influence of age, sex, lesion site, Barthel index, and presence of neglect | After clinical evaluation dysphagia signs<br>– initially in 51%<br>– after 7 days in 27%<br>– after 4 weeks in 17%<br>– after 6 months in 11%<br>VFSS evidence of aspiration<br>– initially 22%<br>– after 4 weeks 15% | Patients with acute stroke; 73/121 patients were followed up to 6 months. Partially newly occurring dysphagia observed in the course. |
| Terré and Mearin (2009) | 20 | VFSS | 12 mon | Prognostically significant factors, e.g.:<br>1 lesion district ('posterior stromal path')<br>2 VFSS findings at baseline:<br>- prolonged pharyngeal transit time<br>- delayed triggering of swallow reflex | VFSS detection of aspiration in 100% (35% silent), decreased to 40% after 1 year (silent aspiration to 0%) | Patients with acute stroke. |

Abbreviations: r range, x average, m median, d days, w weeks, max maximum, mon months, y years, VFSS Video Fluoroscopic Swallowing Study, FEES Flexible Endoscopic Evaluation of Swallowing, FIM Functional Independence Measure, NIHSS National Institutes of Health Stroke Score, RAPIDS Royal Adelaide Prognostic Index for Dysphagic Stroke therapy, existing dysphagia symptoms may worsen or may appear as late effects for the first time (Denaro et al. 2014).

### 30.12.4 Radio(Chemo)-Treated Patients with Head and Neck Malignancies

The negative effects of radio(chemo)therapy on the physiology of swallowing that can be detected by imaging are summed up in the review article by Wall et al. (2013). The authors report not only on the frequency of individual functional deficits, but also on their time course. Thus, for the prevalence of aspiration, a bell-shaped curve is described with an initial frequency immediately after the end of radio(chemo)therapy of almost 10%, an increase in prevalence to around 50% 3 months after the end of therapy, and a subsequent drop to approximately 10% 12 months after the end of therapy. A similar curve is given for the deficit in larynx elevation (initially up to 20%, 3 months after the end of therapy to almost 70%, and 12 months after the end of treatment about 35%). The initially frequent restrictions of tongue retraction (prevalence approx. 50–80%), however, persist at a high level (>80%) and are thus prognostically unfavourable.

As with neurogenic dysphagia, prognostic statements are limited because data derive mainly from clinical findings or questionnaires rather than from imaging examinations. There are reasonable doubts as to whether the former methods are suitable for adequately depicting the actual functional conditions (Lewin 2007). In addition, clinical data and questionnaire results highlight different aspects of a disease course (Pedersen et al. 2016).

From a particularly large number of patients (over 1400), Mortensen et al. (2013) collected data on the dysphagia progress after primary radiotherapy by using a clinical scoring system. It was found that the incidence of severe dysphagia, in which patients could only ingest liquid or no food per os, increased within the first 3 months after initiation of therapy. The tumour locations of the oral cavity and pharynx were especially affected (frequency of severe dysphagia around 50–60%). After 6 months, the frequency decreased significantly to about 30%. Over a period of 5 years, the incidence of severe dysphagia in the tumour locations of the oral cavity, pharynx and supraglottis was 30%, significantly higher than in glottal malignancy (3%). In addition to the primary tumour location and the local and regional extent, the presence of early (acute) dysphagia was considered as a prognostically relevant factor. Similarly, van der Laan et al. (2015a, b) rated an early dysphagia appearing within first 3-6 weeks as prognostically unfavourable.

From a questionnaire study, Szczesniak et al. (2014) examined a period of up to 8 years in primary radiotherapy for 83 head and neck cancer patients and reported a dysphagia rate of 59% at the end of the follow-up. However, they were unable to identify any statistically significant predictors (such as age, tumour location, or stage).

Tulunay-Ugur et al. (2013) analysed dysphagia progression in their study based on the presence of percutaneous endoscopic gastronomy (PEG). They showed that initial PEG was required in 144 out of 320 (59%) primary radiochemotherapy-treated patients with a head and neck malignancy but only 53 patients (37%) needed a PEG after a 1-year follow-up. Two-thirds of PEG-requiring patients had T3 and T4 tumours.

### 30.12.5 Primarily Surgically Treated Patients with Head and Neck Malignancies

#### 30.12.5.1 Various Tumour Locations

Denk et al. (1997) used imaging techniques to examine 32 patients with head and neck malignancies who received functional dysphagia therapy. They saw in 75% a complete recovery of oral food ingestion. The extent of resection defects and the severity of dysphagia before the start of swallowing therapy were identified as prognostically relevant factors. Dejonckere and Hordijk (1998) regarded the existence of aspiration before the beginning of rehabilitation as prognostically unfavourable in the 82 patients they examined, whereas the sole evidence of a transport disorder apparently led to a better outcome.

### 30.12.5.2 Special Tumour Locations

A selection of dysphagia studies relating to oropharyngeal malignancies is given in Table 30.5.

A review by Mahalingam et al. (2016) refers to studies from the years 1970–2014, which were done on patients with hypopharyngeal carcinomas and primary laryngectomy or pharyngolaryngectomy. Eleven studies including almost 900 patients were identified, which rated the short-term prognosis of postoperative dysphagia favourably and described a return to oral food ingestion after an average of 14 days. Eight studies including around 600 patients provided long-term prognostic statements: for predominantly multi-year observation periods, a frequency of 6.5% for the necessity of long-term tube-feeding was reported.

For laryngeal malignomas treated by partial laryngectomy, there is also a review: Lips et al.

(2015) report on the prognosis of 'supracricoid laryngectomy' on the basis of 31 articles with an overall inhomogeneous patient group. Several authors report a complete restoration of swallowing function after 3 months in 75% of patients after an initially 100% dysphagia incidence in the first postoperative days. Prognostically relevant factors could not be derived from the surgical method or from the extent of resection in the arytenoid region or from the patient's age.

### 30.12.6 Other Disorders with Oropharyngeal Dysphagia

For intensive care there are data on progression and prognoses, for example in patients with injuries to the cervical spinal cord (Brady et al. 2004), in patients with traumatic brain injury (Ward et al. 2007), and in burn patients (Ward et al. 2001). As prognostically adverse factors for the remission of dysphagia, the age of the patient, the presence of a tracheostoma as well as the underlying disease are

**Table 30.5** Oropharyngeal dysphagia after surgical or combined therapy of oropharyngeal malignancies

| References | Number of patients | Therapy | Period of follow-up | Proportion of patients receiving tube-feeding in the acute phase (≤3 mon) | Proportion of patients with tube feeding during the follow-up | Prognostic factors |
|---|---|---|---|---|---|---|
| Dale et al. (2015) | 72 | OP±RCT | r = 53–165 mon; m = 93 mon | 22% | After 1 year, no patient with PEG-obligation anymore. | Adverse effect owing to higher age and local extent of tumour |
| Rich et al. (2009) | 84 | OP±RCT | x = 53 mon | 33% | 1 y 19% 2 y 9% 3 y 3% 4 y 5% 5 y 4% | Adverse effect on the course by adjuvant RCT |
| Skoner et al. (2003) | 20 | OP+RT | r = 4.5–78 mon | | After 4 months 4/20 patients completely fed via PEG, 6/20 patients partially fed via PEG. | Tendency for more favourable outcomes in patients <60 y and for location in tonsil/soft palate |
| Zafereo et al. (2010) | 65 | OP±RT | r = 1.3–144.2 mon; x = 36 mon | 100% | 65% of patients were fed by tube at the end of follow-up. | Preoperative swallowing ability and extent of tongue resection |

Abbreviations: *r* range, *x* average, *m* median, *mon* months, *y* years, *OP* Operative therapy, *RCT* Radiochemotherapy, *RT* Radiotherapy mentioned. In prolonged intubated patients, the progression appears to be mainly determined by the severity of the initial dysphagia within the first 48 hours (Moraes et al. 2013).

## 30.12.7 Summary

The prognosis of oropharyngeal dysphagia is generally difficult to make, as its progress is determined by a complex interaction of various factors. In addition, prognostic statements can only partially be based on studies that use accurate diagnostic imaging for the detection of dysphagia.

For neurogenic dysphagia associated with acute stroke, the prognosis in the acute phase is favourable and a remission of dysphagia symptoms is expected in up to 50% of the patients. In up to 40% of patients after more than 6 months aspiration is present. Prognostic factors are likely to be the patient's age, general physical and cognitive status, and the initial diagnostic findings of dysphagia in imaging.

The prognosis of oropharyngeal dysphagia after treatment of malignancies in the ENT area is, above all, unfavourable in patients who received radio(chemo) therapy or had large tumours in the pharyngeal area, even if the data here are inconsistent.

Overall, there is a further need for studies that monitor the progress of oropharyngeal dysphagia over long-term periods, particularly with meaningful imaging techniques.

## References

Abou-Elsaad T, Kotby MN (2002) Efficacy of behavior readjustment therapy for oro-pharyngeal dysphagia. Paper presented at the 17th world congress of the IFOS, 28th sept–3rd Oct., Cairo, Egypt

Ackerman D, Laszlo M, Provisor A et al (2018) Nutrition management for the head and neck cancer patient. Cancer Treat Res 174:187–208

AGA (American Gastroenterological Association) (2007) AGA medical position statement: parenteral nutrition. Archived from the original on 2007-07-30. Accessed 5 Jan 2008

Aguilera JM, Park DJ (2016) Texture-modified foods for the elderly: status, technology and opportunities. Trends Food Sci Technol 57:156–164

Ajemian MS, Nirmul GB, Anderson MT et al (2001) Routine fiberoptic endoscopic evaluation of swallowing following prolonged intubation: implications for management. Arch Surg 136(4):434–437

Alali D, Ballard K, Bogaardt H et al (2016) Treatment effects for dysphagia in adults with multiple sclerosis: a systematic review. Dysphagia 31(5):610–618

Allen J, White CJ, Leonard R et al (2010) Effect of cricopharyngeus muscle surgery on the pharynx. Laryngoscope 120(8):1498–1503

Almirall J, Bolíbar I, Serra-Prat M et al (2008) New evidence of risk factors for community-acquired pneumonia: a population-based study. Eur Respir J 31:1274–1284

Almirall J, Serra-Prat M, Baron F et al (2013) The use of benzodiazepines could be a protective factor for community-acquired pneumonia in <60-year-old subjects. Thorax 68(10):965–966

Alshekhlee A, Ranawat N, Syed TU et al (2010) National Institutes of Health stroke scale assists in predicting the need for percutaneous endoscopic gastrostomy tube placement in acute ischemic stroke. J Stroke Cerebrovasc Dis 19(5):347–352. https://doi.org/10.1016/j.jstrokecerebrovasdis.2009.07.014

Arai T, Yasuda Y, Toshima S et al (1998) ACE inhibitors and pneumonia in elderly people. Lancet 352(9144):1937–1938

Arens C, Herrmann IF, Rohrbach S et al (2015) Position paper of the German Society of Oto-Rhino-Laryngology, head and neck surgery and the German Society of Phoniatrics and Pediatric Audiology — current state of clinical and endoscopic diagnostics, evaluation, and therapy of swallowing disorders in children. Laryngo-Rhino-Otol 94:S306–S354

ASHA (American Speech-Language-Hearing Association) (1992) Instrumental diagnostic procedures for swallowing. ASHA 34(7):25–33

Ashford J, McCabe D, Wheeler-Hegland K et al (2009) Evidence-based systematic review: oropharyngeal dysphagia behavioural treatments. Part III—impact of dysphagia treatments on populations with neurological disorders. J Rehabil Res Dev 46(2):195–204

Atherton M, Bellis-Smith N, Cichero JAY et al (2007) Texture-modified foods and thickened fluids as used for individuals with dysphagia: Australian standardised labels and definitions. Nutr Diet 64(2):53–76

Atlas: multiple sclerosis resources in the world (2008) Atlas: multiple sclerosis resources in the world. World Health Organization, Geneva

Aviv JE (2000) Prospective, randomized outcome study of endoscopy versus modified barium swallow in patients with dysphagia. Laryngoscope 110(4):563–574

Baert F, Vlaemynck G, Beeckman AS et al (2021) Dysphagia management in Parkinson's disease: comparison of the effect of thickening agents on taste, aroma and texture. J Food Sci 86(3):1039–1047

Bakheit AM (2001) Management of neurogenic dysphagia. Postgrad Med J 77(913):694–699

Balzer KM, Pharm D (2000) Drug-induced dysphagia. Int J MS Care 2(1):40–50

Barbon C, Hope A, Steele CM (2017) Radiation 101: A Guide for Speech-Language Pathologists. Perspect ASHA Spec Interest Groups 13:63–72

Bashford G, Bradd P (1996) Drug-induced parkinsonism associated with dysphagia and aspiration: a brief report. J Geriatr Psychiatry Neurol 9(3):133–135

Beck AM, Kjaersgaard J, Hansen T et al (2018) Systematic review and evidence-based recommendations on texture modified foods and thickened liquids for adults (above 17 years) with oropharyngeal dysphagia—an updated clinical guideline. Clin Nutr 37(6A):1980–1991

Becuş T, Popoviciu L (1994) Epidemiologic survey of multiple sclerosis in Mureş County, Romania. Rom J Neurol Psychiat 32(2):115–122

Beer KT, Krause KB, Zuercher T et al (2005) Early percutaneous endoscopic gastrostomy insertion maintains nutritional state in patients with aerodigestive tract cancer. Nutr Cancer 52:29–34

Behrbohm H, Nawka T, Kaschke O et al (2022) Ear, nose, and throat diseases with head and neck surgery, 4th edn. Thieme, London. ISBN 978-3-13-671204-7

Bianchi C, Baiardi P, Khirani S et al (2012) Cough peak flow as a predictor of pulmonary morbidity in patients with dysphagia. Am J Phys Med Rehabil 91(9):783–788

Blitzer A, Brin MF (1997) Use of botulinum toxin for diagnosis and management of cricopharyngeal achalasia. Otolaryngol Head Neck Surg 116(3):328–330

Blomberg J, Lagergren J, Mattsson F et al (2024) Complications after percutaneous endoscopic gastrostomy in a prospective study. Scand J Gastroenterol 47(6):737–742

Bogaardt HCA, Veerbeek L, van der Heide A et al (2015) Swallowing problems at the end of the palliative phase: incidence and severity in 164 unsedated patients. Dysphagia 30(2):145–151

Bours GJJW, Speyer R, de Wit R et al (2009) Bedside screening methods for dysphagia in neurologic patients: a systematic review. J Adv Nurs 65(3):477–493

Boyce HW (1998) Drug-induced esophageal damage: diseases of medical progress. Gastrointest Endosc 47(6):547–550

Bradley W, Daroff R, Fenichel G et al (2000) Neurology in clinical practice, the neurological disorders, 3rd edn. Butterworth, Woburn, MA

Brady S, Miserendino R, Statkus D et al (2004) Predictors to dysphagia and recovery after cervical spine cord injury during acute rehabilitation. J Appl Res 4(1):1–11

Brandt N (1999) Medications and dysphagia: how do they impact each other? Nutr Clin Pract 14(5S):S27–S30

Broadley S, Croser D, Cottrell J et al (2003) Predictors of prolonged dysphagia following acute stroke. J Clin Neurosci 10(3):300–305

Broadley S, Cheek A, Salonikis S et al (2005) Predicting prolonged dysphagia in acute stroke: the Royal Adelaide Prognostic Index for Dysphagic stroke (RAPIDS). Dysphagia 20(4):303–310

Brown T, Banks M, Hughes B et al (2014) Protocol for a randomized controlled trial of early prophylactic feeding via gastrostomy versus standard care in high risk patients with head and neck cancer. BMC Nurs 13:17. https://doi.org/10.1186/1472-6955-13-17

Burgos R, Bretón I, Cereda E et al (2018) ESPEN guideline clinical nutrition in neurology. Clin Nutr 37(1):354–396

Burks TN, Andres-Mateos E, Marx R et al (2011) Losartan restores skeletal muscle remodeling and protects against disuse atrophy in sarcopenia. Sci Transl Med 3(82):82ra37. https://doi.org/10.1126/scitranslmed.3002227

Burnip E, Owen SJ, Barker S et al (2013) Swallowing outcomes following surgical and non-surgical treatment for advanced laryngeal cancer. J Laryngol Otol 127(11):1116–1121

Calcagno P, Ruoppolo G, Grasso MG et al (2002) Dysphagia in multiple sclerosis—prevalence and prognostic factors. Acta Neurol Scand 105(1):40–43

Calcaterra TC (1971) Laryngeal suspension after supraglottic laryngectomy. Arch Otolaryngol 94(4):306–309

Callahan CM, Haag KM, Weinberger M et al (2000) Outcomes of percutaneous endoscopic gastrostomy among older adults in a community setting. J Am Geriatr Soc 48(9):1048–1054

Candy B, Sampson EL, Jones L (2009, 2009) Enteral tube feeding for older people with advanced dementia. Cochrane Database Syst Rev:CD007209

Cardoso F, Seppi K, Mair KJ et al (2006) Seminar on choreas. Lancet Neurol 5:589–602

Carnaby GD, Crary MA (2014) Development and validation of a cancer-specific swallowing assessment tool: MASA-C. Support Care Cancer 22:595–602

Carnaby G, Madhavan A (2013) A systematic review of randomized controlled trials in the field of dysphagia rehabilitation. Curr Phys Med Rehabil Rep 1:197–215

Carroll WR, Locher JL, Canon CL et al (2008) Pretreatment swallowing exercises improve swallow function after chemoradiation. Laryngoscope 118:39–43

Cassani E, Barichella M, Ferri V et al (2017) Dietary habits in Parkinson's disease: adherence to Mediterranean diet. Parkinsonism Relat Disord 42:40–46

Chaudhuri KR, Healy DG, Schapira AH (2006) Non-motor symptoms of Parkinson's disease: diagnosis and management. Lancet Neurol 5(3):235–245

Chelakkot P (2018) Swallowing dysfunction after radiotherapy and chemotherapy. In: Thankappan K, Iyer S, Menon JR (eds) Dysphagia management in head and neck cancers: a manual and atlas. Springer, Singapore, pp 305–320

Cheville AL (2005) Cancer rehabilitation. Semin Oncol 32:219–224

Chiu MJ, Chang YC, Hsiao TY (2004) Prolonged effect of botulinum toxin injection in the treatment of cricopharyngeal dysphagia: case report and literature review. Dysphagia 19(1):52–57

Chua DMN, Choi YY, Chan KM (2024) Effects of oropharyngeal exercises on the swallowing mechanism of older adults: a systematic review. Int J Speech Lang Pathol 26(5):696–713

Chucrallah A, De Girolami U, Freeman R et al (1992) Lovastain/gemfibrozil myopathy: a clinical, histochemical, and ultrastructural study. Eur Neurol 32(5):293–296

Chung HT, Lee JY, Joo MK et al (2024) Clinical practice guideline for percutaneous endoscopic gastrostomy. Gut Liver 18(1):10–26

Cichero JAY (2013) Thickening agents used for dysphagia management: effect on bioavailability of water, medication and feelings of satiety. Nutrition J 12(1):54–54

Cichero JAY (2016) Adjustment of food textural properties for elderly patients. J Texture Stud 47(4):277–283

Cichero JAY, Lam P, Steele CM et al (2017) Development of international terminology and definitions for texture-modified foods and thickened fluids used in dysphagia management: the IDDSI framework. Dysphagia 32(2):293–314

Clarke P, Radford K, Coffey M et al (2016) Speech and swallow rehabilitation in head and neck cancer: United Kingdom National Multidisciplinary Guidelines. J Laryngol Otol 130:S176–S180

Clavé P, De Kraa M, Arreola V et al (2006) The effect of bolus viscosity on swallowing function in neurogenic dysphagia. Aliment Pharmacol Ther 24:1385–1394

Cohen EEW, LaMonte SJ, Erb NL et al (2016) American Cancer Society head and neck cancer survivorship care guideline. CA Cancer J Clin 66:203–239

Cook IJ, Kahrilas PJ (1999) AGA technical review on management of oropharyngeal dysphagia. Gastroenterology 116(2):455–478

Crook M, Swaminathan R (1996) Disorders of plasma phosphate and indications for its measurement. Ann Clin Biochem 33(5):376–396

Crook MA, Hally V, Panteli JV (2001) The importance of the refeeding syndrome. Nutrition 17(7–8):632–637

Cui F, Sun L, Xiong J, Li J et al (2018) Therapeutic effects of percutaneous endoscopic gastrostomy on survival in patients with amyotrophic lateral sclerosis: a meta-analysis. PLoS One 13(2):e0192243. https://doi.org/10.1371/journal.pone.0192243

Cyrany J, Rejchrt S, Kopacova M et al (2016) Buried bumper syndrome: a complication of percutaneous endoscopic gastrostomy. World J Gastroenterol 22(2):618–627. https://doi.org/10.3748/wjg.v22.i2.618

Dale OT, Han C, Burgess CA et al (2015) Long-term functional outcomes in surgically treated patients with oropharyngeal cancer. Laryngoscope 125(7):1637–1643

Daniels SK, Huckabee ML (2014) Dysphagia following stroke, 2nd edn. Plural Publishing Inc., San Diego, CA

Dantas R, Souza R (1997) Dysphagia induced by chronic ingestion of benzodiazepine. Am J Gastroenterol 92(7):1194–1196

De Lau LML, Breteler MMB (2006) Epidemiology of Parkinson's disease. Lancet Neurol 5(6):525–535

de Oliveira ACM, Friche AAL, Salomão MS et al (2018) Predictive factors for oropharyngeal dysphagia after prolonged orotracheal intubation. Braz J Otorhinolaryngol 84(6):722–728

Dean G, Elian M, Galea de Bono A et al (2002) Multiple sclerosis in Malta in 1999: an update. J Neurol Neurosurg Psychiatry 73(3):256–260

Dejonckere PH, Hordijk GJ (1998) Prognostic factors for swallowing after treatment of head and neck cancer. Clin Otolaryngol Allied Sci 23(3):218–223

Denaro N, Merlano MC, Russi EG (2013) Dysphagia in head and neck cancer patients: pretreatment evaluation, predictive factors, and assessment during radio-chemotherapy, recommendations. Clin Exp Otorhinolaryngol 6:117–126

Denaro N, Russi EG, Lefebvre JL et al (2014) A systematic review of current and emerging approaches in the field of larynx preservation. Radiother Oncol 110(1):16–24

Denk D-M, Kaider A (1997) Videoendoscopic biofeedback: a simple method to improve the efficacy of swallowing rehabilitation of patients after head and neck surgery. ORL J Otorhinolaryngol Relat Spec 59(2):100–105

Denk DM, Swoboda H, Schima W et al (1997) Prognostic factors for swallowing rehabilitation following head and neck cancer surgery. Acta Otolaryngol 117(5):769–774

Denk-Linnert D-M (2018) Schlucken nach Tracheostomie (swallowing after tracheostomy). In: Schneider-Stickler B, Kress P (eds) Tracheotomie und Tracheostomaversorgung (tracheotomy and tracheostomy care). Springer, Vienna, pp 303–319

Denk-Linnert D-M (2019) Schluck—und Stimmstörungen in der onkologischen rehabilitation (dysphagia and voice disorders in the oncological rehabilitation). In: Crevenna R (ed) Onkologische Rehabilitation (oncological rehabilitation). Springer, Berlin, pp 203–225

Denk-Linnert DM, Farneti D, Nawka T et al (2023) Position statement of the Union of European Phoniatricians (UEP): fees and phoniatricians' role in multidisciplinary and multiprofessional dysphagia management team. Dysphagia 38(2):711–718

Deron PH (1994) Dysphagia with systemic diseases. Acta Otorhinolaryngol Bel 48(2):191–200

Dev R, Dalal S, Bruera E (2012) Is there a role of parenteral nutrition or hydration at the end of life? Curr Opin Support Palliat Care 6(3):365–370

Dewar RJ, Malcolm JJ (2006) Time-dependent rheology of starch thickeners and the clinical implications for dysphagia therapy. Dysphagia 21:264–269

Dhar SI, Ryan MA, Davis AC et al (2022) Does medialization improve swallowing function in patients with unilateral vocal fold paralysis? A systematic review. Dysphagia 37(6):1769–1776. https://doi.org/10.1007/s00455-022-10441-5. Epub 2022 Apr 12. PMID: 35412149

Ding R, Logemann JA (2005) Swallow physiology in patients with trach cuff inflated or deflated: a retrospective study. Head Neck 27(9):809–813

Dodrill P, Gosa MM (2015) Pediatric dysphagia: physiology, assessment, and management. Ann Nutr Metab 66(5):24–31

Donzelli J, Brady S, Wesling M et al (2005) Effects of the removal of the tracheotomy tube on swallowing during the fiberoptic endoscopic exam of the swallow (FEES). Dysphagia 20(4):283–289

Dorsey ER, Constantinescu R, Thompson JP et al (2007) Projected number of people with Parkinson disease in the most populous nations, 2005 through 2030. Neurology 68(5):384–386

Dotevall H, Tuomi L, Petersson K et al (2022) Treatment with head-lift exercise in head and neck cancer patients with dysphagia: results from a randomized, controlled trial with flexible endoscopic evaluation of swallowing (FEES). Support Care Cancer 31(1):56. https://doi.org/10.1007/s00520-022-07462-z. PMID: 36526734; PMCID: PMC9758100

Dullenkopf A, Gerber A, Weiss M (2003) Fluid leakage past tracheal tube cuffs: evaluation of the new microcuff endotracheal tube. Intensive Care Med 29(10):1849–1853

Dutta D, Thankappan K (2018) Preventive strategies in radiation-associated dysphagia. In: Thankappan K, Iyer S, Menon JR (eds) Dysphagia management in head and neck cancers: a manual and atlas. Springer, Singapore, pp 321–331

Dziewas R, Warnecke T (2019) ICU-related dysphagia. In: Ekberg O (ed) Dysphagia. Medical radiology. Springer, Berlin, pp 157–164

Dziewas R, Pflug C (2020) Neurogene Dysphagie (Neurogenic Dysphagia) Leitlinien für Diagnostik und Therapie in der Neurologie (Guidelines for Diagnostics and Therapy in Neurology) Arbeitsgemeinschaft der Wissenschaftlichen Medizinischen Fachgesellschaften) (Association of the Scientific Medical Societies in Germany) AWMF online 030/111. https://www.awmf.org/uploads/tx_szleitlinien/030-111l_Neurogene-Dysphagie_2020-05.pdf. Accessed 17 Feb 2022

Dziewas R, Glahn J, Helfer C et al (2014) FEES für neurogene Dysphagien. Ausbildungscurriculum der Deutschen Gesellschaft für Neurologie und Deutschen Schlaganfall-Gesellschaft (FEES for neurogenic dysphagia: training curriculum of the German Society of Neurology and the German Stroke Society). Nervenarzt 85(8):1006–1015

Dziewas R, Baijens L, Schindler A et al (2017) European Society for Swallowing Disorders FEES accreditation program for neurogenic and geriatric oropharyngeal dysphagia. Dysphagia 32(6):725–733

Eisele DW, Yarington CT, Lindeman RC et al (1989) The tracheoesophageal diversion and laryngotracheal separation procedures for treatment of intractable aspiration. Am J Surg 157(2):230–236

Ekberg O (2018) Dysphagia: diagnosis and treatment. In: Medical radiology: diagnostic imaging, 2nd edn. Springer, Berlin

Ellies M, Laskawi R, Rohrbach-Volland S et al (2003) Up-to-date report of botulinum toxin therapy in patients with drooling caused by different etiologies. J Oral Maxillofac Surg 61(4):454–457

Epstein JB, Barasch A (2018) Oral and dental health in head and neck cancer patients. In: Maghami E, Ho AS (eds) Multidisciplinary care of the head and neck cancer patient. Springer International Publishing, Cham, pp 43–57

Ergun GA, Kahrilas PJ (2003) Medical and surgical treatment interventions in deglutitive dysfunction. In: Perlman A, Schultze-Delrieu K (eds) Deglutition and its disorders: anatomy, physiology, clinical diagnosis and management. Singular Publishing Inc., San Diego, CA, pp 363–490

Feinberg M (1994) The effects of medication on swallowing. In: Sonies BC (ed) Dysphagia-a continuum of care. Aspen Publishing, New York, NY

Feldman SA, Deal CW, Urquhart W (1966) Disturbance of swallowing after tracheostomy. Lancet 1(7444):954–955

Felt P (1999) The National Dysphagia Diet Project: the science and practice. Nutr Clin Pract 14(5S):S60–S65

Feng FY, Kim HM, Lyden TH et al (2010) Intensity-modulated chemoradiotherapy aiming to reduce dysphagia in patients with oropharyngeal cancer: clinical and functional results. J Clin Oncol 28:2732–2738

Ford CN, Samlan R, Robbins J (1999) Voice restoration by tracheo-tracheolaryngeal shunt after laryngotracheal diversion for chronic aspiration. Oper Tech Otolaryngol Head Neck Sur 10(4):303–304

Frajkova Z, Tedla M, Tedlova E, Suchankova M, Geneid A (2020) Postintubation dysphagia during COVID-19 outbreak-contemporary review. Dysphagia 35(4):549–557

Francis DO, Weymuller EA, Parvathaneni U et al (2010) Dysphagia, stricture, and pneumonia in head and neck cancer patients: does treatment modality matter? Ann Otol Rhinol Laryngol 119:391–397

Frank U, Mäder M, Sticher H (2007) Dysphagic patients with tracheotomies: a multidisciplinary approach to treatment and decannulation management. Dysphagia 22(1):20–29

Frank U, Pluschinski P, Hofmaier A et al (2021) FAQ Dysphagie (question answer format dysphagia). Urban & Fischer in Elsevier Publisher, Munich

Gaillard JM (1989) Benzodiazepines and GABA-ergic transmision. In: Kryger MH, Roth T, Dement WC (eds) Principles and practice of sleep medicine. WB Saunders, Philadelphia, PA, pp 213–218

Gallegos C, Quinchia L, Ascanio G et al (2012) Rheology and dysphagia: an overview. Ann Trans Nordic Rheol Soc 20:3–10

Gallegos C, Brito-de La Fuente E, Clavé P et al (2017) Nutritional aspects of dysphagia management. Adv Food Nutr Res 81:271–318

Gauderer MW, Ponsky JL, Izant RJ (1980) Gastrostomy without laparotomy: a percutaneous endoscopic technique. J Pediatr Surg 15(6):872–875

Ghirlanda G, Oradei A, Manto A (1993) Evidence of plasma CoQ10-lowering effect by HMG-CoA reductase inhibitors: a double-blind, placebo-controlled study. J Clin Pharmacol 33(3):226–229

Gilheaney Ó, Kerr P, Béchet S et al (2016) Effectiveness of endoscopic cricopharyngeal myotomy in adults with neurological disease: systematic review. J Laryngol Otol 130(12):1077–1085. https://doi.org/10.1017/S0022215116008975. PMID: 27938463

Gillespie MB, Brodsky MB, Day TA et al (2004) Swallowing-related quality of life after head and neck cancer treatment. Laryngoscope 114:1362–1367

Giraldez-Rodriguez LA, Johns M (2013) Glottal insufficiency with aspiration risk in dysphagia. Otolaryngol Clin N Am 46(6):1113–1121

Goeleven E, De Raedt R, Baert S et al (2006) Deficient inhibition of emotional information in depression. J Affect Disord 93(1–3):149–157

Goldsmith T, Jacobson MC (2018) Managing the late effects of chemoradiation on swallowing: bolstering the beginning, minding the middle, and cocreating the end. Curr Opin Otolaryngol Head Neck Surg 26:180–187

Gomes CAR, Lustosa SAS, Matos D et al (2012) Percutaneous endoscopic gastrostomy versus nasogastric tube feeding for adults with swallowing disturbances. Cochrane Database of Syst Rev Art 2012:CD008096

Gonzalez F (2008) Extrapyramidal syndrome presenting as dysphagia: a case report. Am J Hosp Palliat Care 25(5):398–400

Govender R, Smith CH, Taylor SA et al (2017) Swallowing interventions for the treatment of dysphagia after head and neck cancer: a systematic review of behavioural strategies used to promote patient adherence to swallowing exercises. BMC Cancer 17:43. https://doi.org/10.1186/s12885-016-2990-x

Graner DE, Foote RL, Kasperbauer JL et al (2003) Swallow function in patients before and after intra-arterial chemoradiation. Laryngoscope 113:573–579

Gross RD, Atwood CW, Ross SB et al (2008) The coordination of breathing and swallowing in Parkinson's disease. Dysphagia 23(2):136–145

Guigoz Y, Vellas BJ, Garry PJ (1994) Mini nutritional assessment: a practical assessment tool for grading the nutritional state of elderly patients. Facts and research in gerontology. Nutr Aging 1997(Suppl (2)):15–59

Hafner G, Neuhuber A, Hirtenfelder S et al (2008) Fiberoptic endoscopic evaluation of swallowing in intensive care unit patients. Eur Arch Otorrinolaringol 265(4):441–446

Hadde EK, Chen J (2021) Texture and texture assessment of thickened fluids and texture modified food for dysphagia management. J Texture Stud 52(1):4–15

Han TR, Paik NJ, Park JW et al (2008) The prediction of persistent dysphagia beyond six months after stroke. Dysphagia 23(1):59–64

Hansen T, Beck AM, Kjaersgaard A et al (2022) Second update of a systematic review and evidence-based recommendations on texture modified foods and thickened liquids for adults (above 17 years) with oropharyngeal dysphagia. Clin Nutr Espen 49:551–555

Hara H, Hori T, Sugahara K et al (2014) Effectiveness of laryngotracheal separation in neurologically impaired pediatric patients. Acta Otolaryngol 134(6):626–630

Hearing SD (2004) Refeeding syndrome. BMJ 328(7445):908–909

Heffernan C, Jenkinson C, Holmes T et al (2004) Nutritional management in MND/ALS patients: an evidence based review. Amyotroph Lateral Scler Other Motor Neuron Disord 5(2):72–83

Hegland KW, Murry T (2013) Nonsurgical treatment: swallowing rehabilitation. Otolaryngol Clin N Am 46(6):1073–1085

Herrmann IF (1986) Glottoplasty with functional pharynx surgery and tracheostomaplasty. In: Herrmann IF (ed) Speech restoration via voice prosthesis. Springer, Stuttgart, pp 116–124

Herrmann IF (1987) Die sekundäre chirurgische Stimmrehabilitation (secondary surgical voice rehabilitation). HNO 35(8):351–354

Herrmann IF (1992) Surgical solutions for aspiration problems. J JPN Bronchoesophagol Soc 43(2):72–79

Herrmann IF, Arce-Recio S (1998) Special techniques for resolving aspiration problems. Oper Tech Otolaryngol Head Neck Surg 9(4):180–191

Herrmann IF, Arce-Recio S (1999) Special techniques for resolving aspiration problems. Oper Tech Otolaryngol Head Neck Surg 10(4):244–252

Heutte N, Plisson L, Lange M et al (2014) Quality of life tools in head and neck oncology. Eur Ann Otorhinolaryngol Head Neck Dis 131:33–47

Hey C, Pluschinski P, Pajunk R et al (2015) Penetration-aspiration: is their detection in FEES® reliable without video recording? Dysphagia 30(4):418–422

Hill R, Dodrill P, Bluck L et al (2010) A novel stable isotope approach for determining the impact of thickening agents on water absorption. Dysphagia 25:1–5

Hillel AD, Goode RL (1983) Lateral laryngeal suspension: a new procedure to minimize swallowing disorders following tongue base resection. Laryngoscope 93(1):26–31

Hirtz D, Thurman DJ, Gwinn-Hardy K et al (2007) How common are the "common" neurologic disorders? Neurology 68(5):326–337

Ho CS, Yee AC, McPherson R (1988) Complications of surgical and percutaneous nonendoscopic gastrostomy: review of 233 patients. Gastroenterology 95(5):1206–1210

Hollowood TA, Linforth RS, Taylor AJ (2002) The effect of viscosity on the perception of flavour. Chem Senses 27:583–591

Horwarth M, Ball A, Smith R (2005) Taste preference and rating of commercial and natural thickeners. Rehabil Nurs 30:239–246

Hughes JA, Daniel SE, Blankson S et al (1993) A clinicophathologic study of 100 cases of Parkinson's disease. Arch Neurol 50(2):140–148

Hunt V, Walker FO (1991) Learning to live at risk for Huntington's disease. J Neurosci Nurs 23(3):179–182

Hunter KU, Lee OE, Lyden TH et al (2014) Aspiration pneumonia after chemo–intensity-modulated radiation therapy of oropharyngeal carcinoma and its clinical and dysphagia-related predictors. Head Neck 36:120–125

Hutcheson KA, Alvarez CP, Barringer DA et al (2012) Outcomes of elective total laryngectomy for laryngopharyngeal dysfunction in disease-free head and neck cancer survivors. Otolaryngol Head Neck Surg 146(4):585–590

Hutcheson KA, Bhayani MK, Beadle BM et al (2013) Eat and exercise during radiotherapy or chemoradiotherapy for pharyngeal cancers: use it or lose it. JAMA Otolaryngol Head Neck Surg 139:1127–1134

Hutcheson KA, Barrow MP, Warneke CL et al (2018) Cough strength and expiratory force in aspirating and nonaspirating postradiation head and neck cancer survivors. Laryngoscope 128(7):1615–1621

IASLT (Irish Association of Speech and Language Therapists), INDI (Irish nutrition and dietetic institute) (2009) Irish consistency descriptors for modified fluids and food. INDI, Ashgrove house, kill avenue, dun Laoghaire, Dublin

Ihara Y, Crary MA, Madhavan A et al (2018) Dysphagia and oral morbidities in chemoradiation-treated head and neck cancer patients. Dysphagia 33:739–748

Ikenaga Y, Nakayama S, Taniguchi H et al (2017) Factors predicting recovery of oral intake in stroke survivors with dysphagia in a convalescent rehabilitation ward. J Stroke Cerebrovasc Dis 26(5):1013–1019

Isshiki N (2000) Progress in laryngeal framework surgery. Acta Otolaryngol 120(2):120–127

Jeans C, Ward EC, Cartmill B et al (2019) Patient perceptions of living with head and neck lymphoedema and the impacts to swallowing, voice and speech function. Eur J Cancer Care (Engl) 28:e12894. https://doi.org/10.1111/ecc.12894

Johnson DN, Herring HJ, Daniels SK (2014) Dysphagia management in stroke rehabilitation. Curr Phys Med Rehabil Rep 2(4):207–218

Jones E, Speyer R, Kertscher B et al (2018) Health-related quality of life in oropharyngeal dysphagia. Dysphagia 33(2):141–172

Juel VC, Massey JM (2007) Myasthenia gravis. Orphanet J Rare Dis 2:44. https://doi.org/10.1186/1750-1172-2-44. Accessed 14 Feb 2022

Jung SJ, Kim DY, Kim YW et al (2012) Effect of decannulation on pharyngeal and laryngeal movement in post-stroke tracheostomized patients. Ann Rehabil Med 36(3):356–364

Kalf JG (2013) Review. Management of dysphagia and drooling in patients with Parkinson's disease. Neurodegen Dis Manag 3(1):71–79

Kalf JG, de Swart BJ, Bloem BR et al (2012) Prevalence of oropharyngeal dysphagia in Parkinson's disease: a meta-analysis. Parkinsonism Relat Disord 18(4):311–315

Kaminsky H (2002) Myasthenia gravis. In: Katirji B, Kaminsky H, Preston D (eds) Neuromuscular disorders in clinical practice. Butterworth-Heinemann, Boston, MA, pp 916–930

Katzberg HD, Benatar M (2011) Enteral tube feeding for amyotrophic lateral sclerosis/motor neuron disease. Cochrane Database Syst Rev 2011:CD004030

Kelly AM, Hydes K, McLaughlin C et al (2007) Fiberoptic endoscopic evaluation of swallowing (FEES): the role of speech and language therapy. RCSLT policy statement 2007. http://www.sld.cu/galerias/pdf/sitios/rehabilitacion-logo/evaluacion_endoscopica_de_la_deglucion.pdf. Accessed 14 Feb 2022

Kelly EA, Koszewski IJ, Jaradeh SS et al (2013) Botulinum toxin injection for the treatment of upper esophageal sphincter dysfunction. Ann Otol Rhinol Laryngol 122(2):100–108

Kertscher B, Speyer R, Palmieri M et al (2014) Bedside screening methods for oropharyngeal dysphagia: an updated systematic review. Dysphagia 30(2):114–120

King SN, Dunlap NE, Tennant PA et al (2016) Pathophysiology of radiation-induced dysphagia in head and neck cancer. Dysphagia 31:339–351

Knigge MA, Thibeault SL (2018) Swallowing outcomes after cricopharyngeal myotomy: a systematic review. Head Neck 40(1):203–212. https://doi.org/10.1002/hed.24977. Epub 2017 Oct 30. PMID: 29083513

Kocdor P, Siegel ER, Tulunay-Ugur OE (2016) Cricopharyngeal dysfunction: a systematic review comparing outcomes of dilatation, botulinum toxin injection, and myotomy. Laryngoscope 126(1):135–141

Koiwai K, Shikama N, Sasaki S et al (2010) Validation of the Total dysphagia risk score (TDRS) as a predictive measure for acute swallowing dysfunction induced by chemoradiotherapy for head and neck cancers. Radiother Oncol 97:132–135

Kojima A, Imoto Y, Osawa Y et al (2014) Predictor of rehabilitation outcome for dysphagia. Auris Nasus Larynx 41(3):294–298

Kondrup J, Allison SP, Elia M et al (2003) ESPEN guidelines for nutrition screening 2002. Clin Nutr 22(4):415–421

Kozier B, Erb G, Berman AJ et al (2004) Fundamentals of nursing: the nature of nursing practice in Canada. Canadian Edition. Prentice Hall Health, Toronto

Kraaijenga SA, van der Molen L, van den Brekel MW et al (2014) Current assessment and treatment strategies of dysphagia in head and neck cancer patients: a systematic review of the 2012/13 literature. Curr Opin Support Palliat Care 8(2):152–163

Krekeler BN, Rowe LM, Connor NP (2020) Dose in exercise-based dysphagia therapies: a scoping review. Dysphagia 36:1. https://doi.org/10.1007/s00455-020-10104-3

Krespi Y, Kacker A, Remacle M (2002) Endoscopic treatment of Zenker's diverticulum using $CO_2$ laser. Otolaryngol Head Neck Surg 127(4):309–314

Krisciunas GP, Sokoloff W, Stepas K et al (2012) Survey of usual practice: dysphagia therapy in head and neck cancer patients. Dysphagia 27:538–549

Kuhn MA, Belafsky PC (2013) Management of cricopharyngeus muscle dysfunction. Otolaryngol Clin N Am 46(6):1087–1099

Kuhn MA, Gillespie MB, Ishman SL et al (2023) Expert consensus statement: management of dysphagia in head and neck cancer patients. Otolaryngol Head Neck Surg 168(4):571–592. https://doi.org/10.1002/ohn.302. PMID: 36965195

Kumar S, Doughty C, Doros G et al (2014) Recovery of swallowing after dysphagic stroke: an analysis of prognostic factors. J Stroke Cerebrovasc Dis 23(1):56–62

Kurien M, McAlindon ME, Westaby D et al (2010) Percutaneous endoscopic gastrostomy (PEG) feeding. BMJ 340:c2414. https://doi.org/10.1136/bmj.c2414

Lacy CF (2002) Drug information handbook, 10th edn. Lexi-Comp Inc., Hudson, OH

Lagalla G, Millevolte M, Capecci M et al (2009) Long-lasting benefits of botulinum toxin type B in Parkinson's disease-related drooling. J Neurol 256(4):563–567

Lagier A, Melotte E, Poncelet M et al (2021) Swallowing function after severe COVID-19: early videofluoroscopic findings. Eur Arch Otorrinolaringol 278(8):3119–3123

Lang RA, Spelsberg FW, Winter H et al (2007) Transoral diverticulostomy with a modified Endo-Gia stapler: results after 4 years of experience. Surg Endosc 21(4):532–536

Langendijk JA, Doornaert P, Rietveld DHF et al (2009) A predictive model for swallowing dysfunction after curative radiotherapy in head and neck cancer. Radiother Oncol 90:189–195

Langerman A, MacCracken E, Kasza K et al (2007) Aspiration in chemoradiated patients with head and neck cancer. Arch Otolaryngol Head Neck Surg 133:1289–1295

Langmore SE (2000) Evaluation and treatment of swallowing disorders. Thieme, New York, NY

Langmore SE (2003) Evaluation of oropharyngeal dysphagia: which diagnostic tool is superior? Curr Opin Otolaryngol Head Neck Surg 11(6):485–489

Langmore SE (2017) History of fiberoptic endoscopic evaluation of swallowing for evaluation and management of pharyngeal dysphagia: changes over the years. Dysphagia 32:27–38

Langmore SE, Krisciunas GP (2010) Dysphagia after radiotherapy for head and neck cancer: etiology, clinical presentation, and efficacy of current treatments. Perspect Swall Swallow Disord (Dysphagia) 19:32–38

Langmore S, Krisciunas GP, Miloro KV et al (2012) Does PEG use cause dysphagia in head and neck cancer patients? Dysphagia 27:251–259

Langmore SE, Pisegna JM, Krisciunas GP et al (2016) A closer look at residue in the post-radiated HNC population. In: Conference of the dysphagia society, Tucson, AZ

Laurian N, Shvili Y, Zohar Y (1986) Epiglotto-aryepiglottopexy: a surgical procedure for severe aspiration. Laryngoscope 96(1):78–81

Leonard R, Kendall K (2014) Dysphagia assessment and treatment planning: a team approach, 3rd edn. Plural Publishing, San Diego, CA

Leopold NA, Kagel MC (1985) Dysphagia in Huntington's disease. Arch Neurol 42(1):57–60

Lewin JS (2007) Dysphagia after chemoradiation: prevention and treatment. Int J Radiat Oncol Biol Phys 69(Suppl 2):S86–S87

Lim A, Leow L, Huckabee ML et al (2008) A pilot study of respiration and swallowing integration in Parkinson's disease: "on" and "off" levodopa. Dysphagia 23(1):76–81

Lips M, Speyer R, Zumach A et al (2015) Supracricoid laryngectomy and dysphagia: a systematic literature review. Laryngoscope 125(9):143–156

Loeb M, Becker M, Eady A et al (2003) Interventions to prevent aspiration pneumonia in older adults: a systematic review. J Am Geriatr Soc 51(7):1018–1022

Loeser C (2013) Das PEG-dilemma—Plädoyer für ein ethisch verantwortungsbewusstes ärztliches Handeln (the PEG-dilemma—pleading for an ethically responsible medical treatment). Z Gastroenterol 51(5):444–449

Logemann J (1993) A manual for videofluoroscopic evaluation of swallowing, 2nd edn. Pro-Ed, Austin

Logemann JA (1999) Behavioral management for oropharyngeal dysphagia. Folia Phoniatr Logop 51(4–5):199–212

Logemann JA, Rademaker AW, Pauloski BR et al (1998) Normal swallowing physiology as viewed by videofluoroscopy and videoendoscopy. Folia Phoniatr Logop 50(6):311–319

Logemann JA, Rademaker AW, Pauloski BR et al (1999) Interobserver agreement on normal swallowing physiology as viewed by videoendoscopy. Folia Phoniatr Logop 51(3):91–98

Logemann JA, Pauloski BR, Rademaker AW et al (2008) Swallowing disorders in the first year after radiation and chemoradiation. Head Neck 30:148–158

MacDonald BK, Cockerell OC, Sander JW et al (2000) The incidence and lifetime prevalence of neurological disorders in a prospective community-based study in the UK. Brain 123(4):665–676

Macht M, Wimbish T, Clark BJ et al (2011) Postextubation dysphagia is persistent and associated with poor outcomes in survivors of critical illness. Crit Care 15(5):R231. https://doi.org/10.1186/cc10472

Macht M, Wimbish T, Bodine C et al (2013a) ICU-acquired swallowing disorders. Crit Care Med 41(10):2396–2405

Macht M, King CJ, Wimbish T et al (2013b) Postextubation dysphagia is associated with longer hospitalization in survivors of critical illness with neurologic impairment. Crit Care 17(3):R119. https://doi.org/10.1186/cc12791

Maeshima S, Osawa A, Hayashi T et al (2013) Factors associated with prognosis of eating and swallowing disability after stroke: a study from a community-based stroke care system. J Stroke Cerebrovasc Dis 22(7):926–930

Mahalingam S, Srinivasan R, Spielmann P et al (2016) Quality-of-life and functional outcome following pharyngolaryngectomy: a systematic review of literature. Clin Otolaryngol 41(1):25–43

Mahieu HF, de Bree R, Westerveld GJ et al (1999) Laryngeal suspension and upper esophageal sphincter myotomy as a surgical option for treatment of severe aspiration. Oper Tech Otolaryngol Head Neck Surg 10(4):305–310

Mann G, Hankey GJ, Cameron D (1999) Swallowing function after stroke. Prognosis and prognostic factors at 6 months. Stroke 30(4):744–748

Mantegazza R, Bonanno S, Camera G et al (2011) Current and emerging therapies for the treatment of myasthenia gravis. Neuropsychiatr Dis Treat 7:151–160

Marchese-Ragona R, Restivo DA, Marioni G et al (2006) Evaluation of swallowing disorders in multiple sclerosis. Neurol Sci 27(Suppl 4):335–337

Marik PE (2001) Aspiration pneumonitis and aspiration pneumonia. N Engl J Med 344:665–671

Marin B, Boumediene F, Logroscino G et al (2017) Variation in worldwide incidence of amyotrophic lateral sclerosis: a meta-analysis. Int J Epidemiol 46(1):57–74

Martin-Harris B, McFarland D, Hill EG et al (2015) Respiratory-swallow training in patients with head and neck cancer. Arch Phys Med Rehabil 96(5):885–893

Matta Z, Chambers E, Mertz Garcia J et al (2006) Sensory characteristics of beverages prepared with commercial thickeners used for dysphagia diets. J Am Diet Assoc 106:1049–1054

Mayeux R, Marder K, Cote LJ et al (1995) The frequency of idiopathic Parkinson's disease by age, ethnic group, and sex in northern Manhattan, 1988–1993. Am J Epidemiol 142(8):820–827

Mays AC, Moustafa F, Worley M et al (2014) A model for predicting gastrostomy tube placement in patients undergoing surgery for upper aerodigestive tract lesions. JAMA Otolaryngol Head Neck Surg 140(12):1198–1206

McCabe D, Ashford J, Wheeler-Hegland K et al (2009) Evidence-based systematic review: oropharyngeal dysphagia behavioural treatments. Part IV—impact of dysphagia treatment on individuals' postcancer treatments. J Rehabil Res Dev 46(2):205–214

McClelland S, Andrews JZ, Chaudhry H et al (2018) Prophylactic versus reactive gastrostomy tube placement in advanced head and neck cancer treated with definitive chemoradiotherapy: a systematic review. Oral Oncol 87:77–81

McCullough GH, Kim Y (2013) Effects of the Mendelsohn maneuver on extent of hyoid movement and UES opening post-stroke. Dysphagia 28(4):511–519

McCullough G, Pelletier C, Steele C (2003) National Dysphagia Diet: what to swallow? The ASHA leader. https://leader.pubs.asha.org/doi/10.1044/leader.FTR3.08202003.16. Accessed 16 Feb 2022

McCurtin A, Healy C, Kelly L et al (2018) Plugging the patient evidence gap: what patients with swallowing disorders post-stroke say about thickened liquids. Int J Lang Commun Disord 53(1):30–39

McKenna JA, Dedo HH (1992) Cricopharyngeal myotomy: indications and technique. Ann Otol Rhinol Laryngol 101(3):216–221

McMicken BL, Muzzy CL (2009) Prognostic indicators of functional outcomes in first time documented acute stroke patients following standard dysphagia treatment. Disabil Rehabil 31(26):2196–2203

Mekhail TM, Adelstein DJ, Rybicki LA et al (2001) Enteral nutrition during the treatment of head and neck carcinoma: is a percutaneous endoscopic gastrostomy tube preferable to a nasogastric tube? Cancer 91:1785–1790

Mercuri A, Lim Joon D, Wada M et al (2009) The effect of an intensive nutritional program on daily set-up variations and radiotherapy planning margins of head and neck cancer patients. J Med Imaging Radiat Oncol 53:500–505

Messing BP, Ward EC, Lazarus C et al (2019) Establishing a multidisciplinary head and neck clinical pathway: an implementation evaluation and audit of dysphagia-related services and outcomes. Dysphagia 34:89–104

Meyer TK, Pisegna J, Krisciunas GP et al (2017) Residue influences QoL independently of penetration and aspiration in H&N cancer survivors. Laryngoscope 127:1615–1621

Miarons M, Campins L, Palomera E et al (2016) Drugs related to oropharyngeal dysphagia in older people. Dysphagia 31(5):697–705

Moraes DP, Sassi FC, Mangilli LD et al (2013) Clinical prognostic indicators of dysphagia following prolonged orotracheal intubation in ICU patients. Crit Care 17(5):R243. https://doi.org/10.1186/cc13069

Morrell RM (1992) Neurologic disorders of swallowing. In: Groher ME (ed) Dysphagia, diagnosis and management. Butterworth, Stoneham, MA, pp 37–60

Mortensen HR, Overgaard J, Jensen K et al (2013) Factors associated with acute and late dysphagia in the DAHANCA 6 & 7 randomized trial with accelerated radiotherapy for head and neck cancer. Acta Oncol 52(7):1535–1542

Morton A, Wolfe S (2015) Enteral tube feeding for cystic fibrosis. Cochrane Database Systematic Reviews Art 2015:CD001198

Murphy BA, Gilbert J (2009) Dysphagia in head and neck cancer patients treated with radiation: assessment, sequelae, and rehabilitation. Semin Radiat Oncol 19:35–42

Murphy R, Gardiner P, Rousseau G et al (1997) Chronic β-blockade increases skeletal muscle β-adrenergic receptor density and enhances contractile force. J Appl Physiol 83(2):459–465

Murry T, Wasserman T, Carrau RL et al (2005) Injection of botulinum toxin a for the treatment of dysfunction of the upper esophageal sphincter. Am J Otolaryngol 26(3):157–162

Myasthenia Gravis Foundation of America, Inc (2013) Effects of myasthenia gravis on voice, speech, and swallowing. https://myasthenia.org/MG-Education/Learn-More-About-MG-Treatments/MG-Brochures/effects-of-mg-on-voice-speech-and-swallowing. Accessed 14 Feb 2022

Nakatsu S, Shimoda M, Shibata K et al (2014) Effect of citrate ions on the softening of root crops prepared with freeze-thaw impregnation of macerating enzymes. J Food Sci 79(3):E333–E334

Nakayama K, Sekizawa K, Sasaki H (1998) ACE inhibitor and swallowing reflex. Chest 113(5):1425. https://doi.org/10.1378/chest.113.5.1425

Nash MC, Ferrell RB, Lombardo MA et al (2004) Treatment of bruxism in Huntington's disease with botulinum toxin. J Neuropsychiatry Clin Neurosci 16(3):381–382

National Parkinson Foundation (2013) Difficulty swallowing can be fatal for people with Parkinson's. http://www.parkinson.org. Accessed 14 Feb 2022

National Patient Safety Agency (2011) Royal College of Speech and Language Therapists, British Dietetic Association, National Nurses Nutrition Group, Hospital Caterers Association Dysphagia diet food texture descriptions. https://www.independentliving.co.uk/Dysphagia-food-texture-descriptors.pdf. Accessed 16 Feb 2022

Nawka T, Hosemann W (2005) Surgical procedures for voice restoration. GMS Curr Top Otorhinolaryngol Head Neck Surg 4:Doc14

Neumann S, Bartolome G, Buchholz D et al (1995) Swallowing therapy of neurologic patients: correlation with pretreatment variables and therapeutic methods. Dysphagia 10(1):1–5

Nevens D, Deschuymer S, Langendijk JA et al (2016) Validation of the total dysphagia risk score (TDRS) in head and neck cancer patients in a conventional and a partially accelerated radiotherapy scheme. Radiother Oncol 118:293–297

Nevens D, Goeleven A, Duprez F et al (2018) Does the total dysphagia risk score correlate with swallowing function examined by videofluoroscopy? Br J Radiol 91:20170714. https://doi.org/10.1259/bjr.20170714

Neville BW, Damm DD, Bouquot JE et al (2002) Fungal and protozoal diseases. In: Neville BW (ed) Oral & maxillofacial pathology. WB Saunders, Philadelphia, PA, pp 189–197

Newman R, Vilardell N, Clavé P et al (2016) Effect of bolus viscosity on the safety and efficacy of swallowing and the kinematics of the swallow response in patients with oropharyngeal dysphagia: White paper by the European Society for Swallowing Disorders (ESSD). Dysphagia 31:232–249

Nguyen NP, Frank C, Moltz CC et al (2006) Aspiration rate following chemoradiation for head and neck cancer: an underreported occurrence. Radiother Oncol 80:302–306

Nguyen NP, Smith HJ, Moltz CC et al (2008) Prevalence of pharyngeal and esophageal stenosis following radiation for head and neck cancer. J Otolaryngol Head Neck Surg 37(2):219–224

NICE (National Institute for Clinical Excellence) (2004) Improving outcomes in head and neck cancers—The Manual. NICE, London. https://www.nice.org.uk/guidance/csg6/resources/improving-outcomes-in-head-and-neck-cancers-update-pdf-773377597. Accessed 9 Dec 2021

Nicoletti A, Lo Bartolo ML, Lo Fermo S et al (2001) Prevalence and incidence of multiple sclerosis in Catania. Sicily Neurol 56(1):62–66

Nugent B, Lewis S, O'Sullivan JM (2010) Enteral feeding methods for nutritional management in patients with head and neck cancers being treated with radiotherapy and/or chemotherapy. Cochrane Database Syst Rev 2013:1. https://doi.org/10.1002/14651858.CD007904.pub2

O'Brien LA, Siegert EA, Grisso JA et al (1997) Tube feeding preferences among nursing home residents. J Ger Intern Med 12(6):364–371

Ohkubo T, Chapman N, Neal B et al (2004) Effects of an angiotensin-converting enzyme inhibitor-based regimen on pneumonia risk. Am J Respir Crit Care Med 169(9):1041–1045

Oikkonen M, Aromaa U (1997) Leakage of fluid around low-pressure tracheal tube cuffs. Anaesthesia 52(6):567–569

Okunieff P, Chen Y, Maguire DJ et al (2008) Molecular markers of radiation-related normal tissue toxicity. Cancer Metastasis Rev 27:363–374

Oral Cancer Foundation (2014) Evaluation and Management of Oropharyngeal Dysphagia in Head and Neck Cancer. http://www.oralcancerfoundation.org/complications/dysphagia. Accessed 14 Feb 2022

Orlandoni P, Peladic NJ (2024) Safety and effectiveness of percutaneous endoscopic gastrostomy may be improved by proper pre- and post-positioning management of elderly patients with multimorbidity. Nutrients 16(17):2893

Ortega O, Martín A, Clavé P (2017) Diagnosis and management of oropharyngeal dysphagia among older persons, state of the art. J Am Med Dir Assoc 18(7):576–582

Oterdoom LH, Marinus Oterdoom DL et al (2017) Systematic review of ventricular peritoneal shunt and percutaneous endoscopic gastrostomy: a safe combination. J Neurosurg 127(4):899–904. https://doi.org/10.3171/2016.8.JNS152701

Oto T, Kandori Y, Ohta T et al (2009) Predicting the chance of weaning dysphagic stroke patients from enteral nutrition: a multivariate logistic modelling study. Eur J Phys Rehabil Med 45(3):355–362

Paleri V, Roland N (2016) Introduction to the United Kingdom National Multidisciplinary Guidelines for head and neck cancer. J Laryngol Otol 130:S3–S4

Paleri V, Roe JWG, Strojan P et al (2014) Strategies to reduce long-term postchemoradiation dysphagia in patients with head and neck cancer: an evidence-based review. Head Neck 36:431–443

Palmer PM, McCulloch TM, Lemke JH et al (1995) Analysis of magnitude and duration of swallowing disorders following treatment with botulinum toxin in patients with spasmodic dysphonia. Abstracts of scientific papers presented at the third annual dysphagia research society meeting McLean, Virginia, October 14–16, 1994. Dysphagia 10(2):135–141

Pappano AJ (2012) Cholinoceptor-activating & cholinesterase-inhibiting drugs. In: Katzung BG, Masters SB, Trevor AJ (eds) Basic & clinical pharmacology. McGraw-Hill-Lange, New York, NY

Paradelis AG, Triantaphyllidis C, Giala MM (1980) Neuromuscular blocking activity of aminoglycoside antibiotics. Methods Find Exp Clin Pharmacol 2(1):45–51

Parameswaran MS, Soliman AM (2002) Endoscopic botulinum toxin injection for cricopharyngeal dysphagia. Ann Otol Rhinol Laryngol 111(10):871–874

Pauloski BR (2008) Rehabilitation of dysphagia following head and neck cancer. Phys Med Rehabil Clin N Am 19:889–928

Pauloski BR, Rademaker AW, Logemann JA et al (2000) Pretreatment swallowing function in patients with head and neck cancer. Head Neck 22:474–482

Pedersen A, Wilson J, McColl E et al (2016) Swallowing outcome measures in head and neck cancer—how do they compare? Oral Oncol 52:104–108

Perez I, Smithard DG, Davies H et al (1998) Pharmacological treatment of dysphagia in stroke. Dysphagia 13(1):12–16

Pfister DG, Spencer S, Adelstein D et al (2020) Head and neck cancers NCCN clinical practice guidelines in oncology, version 2.2020. J Natl Compr Cancer Netw 18(7):873–898

Piazza C, Filauro M, Dikkers FG et al (2021) Long-term intubation and high rate of tracheostomy in COVID-19 patients might determine an unprecedented increase of airway stenoses: a call to action from the European laryngological society. Eur Arch Otorrinolaringol 278(1):1–7

Pickhardt PJ, Rohrmann CA, Cossentino MJ (2002) Stomal metastases complicating percutaneous endoscopic gastrostomy: CT findings and the argument for radiologic tube placement. Am J Roentgenol 179(3):735–739

Pisegna JM, Langmore SE (2016) Parameters of instrumental swallowing evaluations: describing a diagnostic dilemma. Dysphagia 31(3):462–472

Pisegna JM, Langmore SE, Meyer TK et al (2020) Swallowing patterns in the HNC population: timing of penetration-aspiration events and residue. Otolaryngol Head Neck Surg 163(6):1232–1239

Pluschinski P, Zaretsky Y, Stöver T et al (2015) Qualitätssicherung der endoskopischen Schluckdiagnostik (FEES) (quality assurance in the endoscopic evaluation of swallowing (FEES)). Laryngorhinootologie 94(8):505–508

Poorjavad M, Derakhshandeh F, Etemadifar M et al (2010) Oropharyngeal dysphagia in multiple sclerosis. Mult Scler 16(3):362–365

Popa Nita S, Murith M, Chisholm H et al (2013) Matching the rheological properties of videofluoroscopic contrast agents and thickened liquid prescriptions. Dysphagia 28:245–252

Pringsheim T, Wiltshire K, Day L et al (2012) The incidence and prevalence of Huntington's disease: a systematic review and meta-analysis. Mov Disord 27(9):1083–1091

Prosiegel M, Heintze M, Wagner-Sonntag E et al (2002) Schluckstörungen bei neurologischen Patienten (Dysphagia in neurologicalpatients.). Nervenarzt 73(4):364–370

Prosiegel M, Schelling A, Wagner-Sonntag E (2004) Dysphagia and multiple sclerosis. Int MS J 11(1):22–31

Raber-Durlacher JE, Brennan MT, Verdonck-de Leeuw IM et al (2012) Swallowing dysfunction in cancer patients. Support Care Cancer 20:433–443

Raheem D, Carrascosa C, Ramos F et al (2021) Texture-modified food for dysphagic patients; a comprehensive review. Int J Environ Res Public Health 18(10):5125

Reddy PD, Yan F, Nguyen SA et al (2020) Factors influencing the development of pneumonia in patients with head and neck cancer: a meta-analysis. Otolaryngol Head Neck Surg 164(2):234–243

Restivo D, Casabona A, Alfonsi E et al (2014) P921: ALS dysphagia: different BoNT/a response for different pathophysiology. Clin Neurophysiol 125(Suppl 1):S291

Rich JT, Milov S, Lewis JS et al (2009) Transoral laser microsurgery (TLM) +/− adjuvant therapy for advanced stage oropharyngeal cancer: outcomes and prognostic factors. Laryngoscope 119(9):1709–1719

Roche JC, Rojas-Garcia R, Scott KM et al (2012) A proposed staging system for amyotrophic lateral sclerosis. Brain 135(3):847–852

Roden DF, Altman W (2013) Causes of dysphagia among different age groups: a systematic review of the literature. Otolaryngol Clin North Am 46(6):965–987

Rofes L, Arreola V, Mukherjee R et al (2014) The effects of a xanthan gum-based thickener on the swallowing function of patients with dysphagia. Aliment Pharmacol Ther 39:1169–1179

Rosen A, Rhee TH, Kaufman R (2001) Prediction of aspiration in patients with newly diagnosed untreated advanced head and neck cancer. Arch Otolaryngol Head Neck Surg 127:975–979

Ross ER, Green R, Auslander MO et al (1982) Cricopharyngeal myotomy: management of cervical dysphagia. Otolaryngol Head Neck Surg 90(4):434–441

Rothwell PM, Charlton D (1998) High incidence and prevalence of multiple sclerosis in south East Scotland: evidence of a genetic predisposition. J Neurol Neurosurg Psychiatry 64(6):730–735

Ruoppolo G, Schettino I, Frasca V et al (2013) Dysphagia in amyotrophic lateral sclerosis: prevalence and clinical findings. Acta Neurol Scand 128(6):397–401

Russi EG, Corvò R, Merlotti A et al (2012) Swallowing dysfunction in head and neck cancer patients treated by radiotherapy: review and recommendations of the supportive task group of the Italian Association of Radiation Oncology. Cancer Treat Rev 38:1033–1049

Saleh FG, Seidman RJ (2003) Drug-induced myopathy and neuropathy. J Clin Neuromuscul Disord 5(2):81–92

Scharitzer M, Roesner I, Pokieser P et al (2019) Simultaneous radiological and fiberendoscopic evaluation of swallowing ("SIRFES") in patients after surgery of oropharyngeal/laryngeal cancer and postoperative dysphagia. Dysphagia 34:852. https://doi.org/10.1007/s00455-019-09979-8

Schechter GL (1998) Systemic causes of dysphagia in adults. Otolaryngol Clin N Am 31(3):525–535

Schima W, Denk D-M (1998) Videofluoroscopic and videoendoscopic studies: complementary methods for assessment of dysphagia. In: Proceedings European Study Group for *Dysphagia* and Globus. EGDG, Vienna

Schindler A, Denaro N, Russi EG et al (2015) Dysphagia in head and neck cancer patients treated with radiotherapy and systemic therapies: literature review and consensus. Crit Rev Oncol Hematol 96:372–384

Schneider I, Thumfart WF, Pototschnig C et al (1994) Treatment of dysfunction of the cricopharyngeal muscle with botulinum a toxin: introduction of a new, noninvasive method. Ann Otol Rhinol Laryngol 103(1):31–35

Schnitker MA, Mattman PE, Bliss TL (1951) A clinical study of malnutrition in Japanese prisoners of war. Ann Intern Med 35(1):69–96

Schröter-Morasch H (2022) Medizinische Basisversorgung von Patienten mit Schluckstörung—Trachealkanülen—Sondenernährung (basic medical care for patients with dysphagia—tracheostomy tubes—tube feeding). In: Bartolome G, Schröter-Morasch H (eds) Schluckstörungen. Interdisziplinäre Diagnostik und rehabilitation (dysphagia. Interdisciplinary diagnostics and rehabilitation), 7th edn. Elsevier GmbH, Urban & Fischer, Munich

Schröter-Morasch H, Graf S (2014) Dysphagiediagnostik durch den HNO-Arzt (swallowing examination for ENT specialists). HNO 62(5):324–334

Schulze SL, Rhee JS, Kulpa JI et al (2002) Morphology of the cricopharyngeal muscle in Zenker and control specimens. Ann Otol Rhinol Laryngol 111(7–1):573–578

Schwegler H, Peter S, Frank U (2021) Tracheal cannula management. In: Frank U, Pluschinski P, Hofmaier A et al (eds) FAQ Dysphagie (question answer format dysphagia). Kapitel 5 Trachealkanülen-Management. Urban and Fischer in Elsevier Publisher, Munic

Seo HG, Kim JG, Nam HS et al (2017) Swallowing function and kinematics in stroke patients with tracheostomies. Dysphagia 32(3):393–400

Servagi-Vernat S, Ali D, Roubieu C et al (2015) Dysphagia after radiotherapy: state of the art and prevention. Eur Ann Otorhinolaryngol Head Neck Dis 132:25–29

Shaker R, Kern M, Bardan E et al (1997) Augmentation of deglutitive upper esophageal sphincter opening in the elderly by exercise. Am J Phys 272(6–1):G1518–G1522

Shaker R, Belafsky PC, Postma GN et al (eds) (2013) Principles of deglutition. A multidisciplinary text for swallowing and its disorders. Springer, New York NY

Shaw SM, Flowers H, O'Sullivan B et al (2015) The effect of prophylactic percutaneous endoscopic gastrostomy (PEG) tube placement on swallowing and swallow-related outcomes in patients undergoing radiotherapy for head and neck cancer: a systematic review. Dysphagia 30:152–175

Shimizu T, Fujioka S, Otonashi H et al (2008) ACE inhibitor and swallowing difficulties in stroke. A preliminary study. J Neurol 255(2):288–289

Simental AA, Carrau RL (2004) Assessment of swallowing function in patients with head and neck cancer. Curr Oncol Rep 6:162–165

Simmons Z (2006) Management strategies for patients with amyotrophic lateral sclerosis from diagnosis through death. Neurologist 11(5):257–270

Singer MI, Blom ED, Hamaker RC (1986) Pharyngeal plexus neurectomy for a laryngeal speech rehabilitation. Laryngoscope 96(1):50–54

Singleton JR, Baker BL, Thorburn A (2000) Dexamethasone inhibits insulin-like growth factor signaling and potentiates myoblast apoptosis. Endocrinology 141(8):2945–2950

Skeie GO, Apostolski S, Evoli A et al (2010) Guidelines for the treatment of autoimmune neuromuscular transmission disorders. Eur J Neurol 17(7):893–902

Skoner JM, Andersen PE, Cohen JI et al (2003) Swallowing function and tracheotomy dependence after combined-modality treatment including free tissue transfer for advanced-stage oropharyngeal cancer. Laryngoscope 113(8):1294–1298

Sliwa JA, Lis S (1993) Drug-induced dysphagia. Arch Phys Med Rehabil 74(4):445–447

Smithard DG, O'Neill PA, England RE et al (1997) The natural history of dysphagia following a stroke. Dysphagia 12(4):188–193

Sokoloff LG, Pavlakovic R (1997) Neuroleptic-induced dysphagia. Dysphagia 12(4):177–179

Somnier FE, Engel PJH (2002) The occurrence of antititin antibodies and thymomas: a population survey of myasthenia gravis, 1970–1999. Neurology 59(1):92–98

Speyer R (2013) Oropharyngeal dysphagia: screening and assessment. Otolaryngol Clin North Am 46(6):989–1008

Speyer R (2018) Behavioural treatment of oropharyngeal dysphagia. In: Ekberg O (ed) Dysphagia: diagnosis and treatment, 2nd edn). Medical Radiology: Diagnostic Imaging. Springer, Berlin

Speyer R, Baijens LW, Heijnen MAM et al (2010) The effects of therapy in oropharyngeal dysphagia by speech therapists: a systematic review. Dysphagia 25(1):40–65

Speyer R, Cordier R, Kertscher B et al (2014) Psychometric properties of questionnaires on functional health status in oropharyngeal dysphagia: a systematic literature review. Bio Med Res Int 458678:1–11

Speyer R, Cordier R, Farneti F et al (2021) White paper by the European society for swallowing disorders: screening and non-instrumental assessment for dysphagia in adults. Dysphagia 37:333. https://doi.org/10.1007/s00455-021-10283-7

Speyer R, Cordier R, Sutt A-L et al (2022) Behavioural interventions in people with oropharyngeal dysphagia: a systematic review and meta-analysis of randomised clinical trials. J Clin Med 11(3):685. https://doi.org/10.3390/jcm11030685

Starmer HM (2014) Dysphagia in head and neck cancer: prevention and treatment. Curr Opin Otolaryngol Head Neck Surg 22(3):195–200

Steele C, Alsanei WA, Ayanikalath S et al (2015) The influence of food texture and liquid consistency modification on swallowing physiology and function: a systematic review. Dysphagia 30:2–26

Stenson KM, MacCracken E, List M et al (2000) Swallowing function in patients with head and neck cancer prior to treatment. Arch Otolaryngol Head Neck Surg 126:371–377

Stewart JT (2001) Reversible dysphagia associated with neuroleptic treatment. J Am Geriatr Soc 49(9):1260–1261

Stewart JT (2003) Dysphagia associated with risperidone therapy. Dysphagia 18(4):274–275

Stoschus B, Allescher HD (1993) Drug-induced dysphagia. Dysphagia 8(2):154–159

Sukys-Claudino L, Moraes W, Guilleminault C et al (2012) Beneficial effect of donepezil on obstructive sleep apnea: a double-blind, placebo-controlled clinical trial. Sleep Med 13(3):290–296

Suiter DM, McCullough GH, Powell PW (2003) Effects of cuff deflation and one-way tracheostomy speaking valve placement on swallow physiology. Dysphagia 18(4):284–292. https://doi.org/10.1007/s00455-003-0022-x. PMID: 14571334

Sumelahti ML, Tienari PJ, Wikström J et al (2000) Regional and temporal variation in the incidence of multiple sclerosis in Finland 1979–1993. Neuroepidemiology 19(2):67–75

Sun L, Trausch-Azar JS, Muglia LJ et al (2008) Glucocorticoids differentially regulate degradation of MyoD and Id1 by N-terminal ubiquitination to promote muscle protein catabolism. Proc Natl Acad Sci USA 105(9):3339–3344

Suntrup S, Teismann I, Wollbrink A et al (2015) Pharyngeal electrical stimulation can modulate swallowing in cortical processing and behavior—magnetoencephalographic evidence. NeuroImage 104:117–124

Suterwala MS, Reynolds J, Carroll S et al (2017) Using fiberoptic endoscopic evaluation of swallowing to detect laryngeal penetration and aspiration in infants in the neonatal intensive care unit. J Perinatol 37(4):404–408

Svennerholm K, Doteval H, Svennerholme K et al (2021) Characterization of dysphagia and laryn-geal findings in COVID-19 patients treated in the ICU-an observational clinical study. PLoS One 16(6):e0252347

Swan K, Speyer R, Heijnen BJ et al (2015) Living with oropharyngeal dysphagia: effects of bolus modification on health-related quality of life—a systematic review. Qual Life Res 24:2447–2456

Sweeny L, Golden JB, White HN et al (2012) Incidence and outcomes of stricture formation postlaryngectomy. Otolaryngol Head Neck Surg 146(3):395–402

Syed R, Au K, Cahill C et al (2008) Pharmacologic interventions for clozapine-induced hypersalivation (review). Cochrane Database Syst Rev 3:CD005579. https://doi.org/10.1002/14651858.CD005579.pub2

Szczesniak MM, Maclean J, Zhang T et al (2014) Persistent dysphagia after head and neck radiotherapy: a common and under-reported complication with significant effect on non-cancer-related mortality. Clin Oncol 26(11):697–703

Tabor LC, Plowman EK, Romero-Clark C et al (2017) Oropharyngeal dysphagia in oculopharyngeal muscular dystrophy. Neurogastroenterol Motil 30(4):e13251

Takizawa C, Speyer R, Gemmell E et al (2016) A systematic literature review of oropharyngeal dysphagia in stroke, Parkinson's disease, head injury, community acquired pneumonia, and Alzheimer's disease. Dysphagia 31(3):434–441

Tedla M, Valach M, Carrau RL et al (2012) Impact of radiotherapy on laryngeal intrinsic muscles. Eur Arch Otorrinolaringol 269:953–958

Tedlová E, Mucska I (2018) Aspiračná pneumónia a aspiračná pneumonitída. Poruchy polykání, II, Tobiáš, pp 148–152

Terré R, Mearin F (2009) Resolution of tracheal aspiration after the acute phase of stroke-related oropharyngeal dysphagia. Am J Gastroenterol 104(4):923–932

Timmerman A, Speyer R, Heijnen BJ et al (2014) Psychometric characteristics of quality of life questionnaires in oropharyngeal dysphagia. Dysphagia 29(2):183–198

Tolep K, Getch CL, Criner GJ (1996) Swallowing dysfunction in patients receiving prolonged mechanical ventilation. Chest 109(1):167–172

Tominaga N, Shimoda R, Iwakiri R et al (2010) Low serum albumin level is a risk factor for patients with percutaneous endoscopic gastrostomy. Intern Med 49(21):2283–2288

Tulunay-Ugur OE, McClinton C, Young Z et al (2013) Functional outcomes of chemoradiation in patients with head and neck cancer. Otolaryngol Head Neck Surg 148(1):64–68

Twelves D, Perkins KS, Counsell C (2003) Systematic review of incidence studies of Parkinson's disease. Mov Disord 18(1):19–31

Ueha R, Magdayao RB, Koyama M et al (2023) Aspiration prevention surgeries: a review. Respir Res 24(1):43. https://doi.org/10.1186/s12931-023-02354-0. Erratum in: Respir Res. 2023 May 3;24(1):123. https://doi.

org/10.1186/s12931-023-02398-2. PMID: 36747240; PMCID: PMC9901145

van Bruchem-Visser RL, Mattace-Raso FUS, de Beaufort ID et al (2019) Percutaneous endoscopic gastrostomy in older patients with and without dementia: survival and ethical considerations. J Gastroenterol Hepatol 34(4):736–741. https://doi.org/10.1111/jgh.14573

Van Den Eeden SK, Tanner CM, Bernstein AL et al (2003) Incidence of Parkinson's disease: variation by age, gender, and race/ethnicity. Am J Epidemiol 157(11):1015–1022

van der Laan HP, Bijl HP, Steenbakkers RJ et al (2015a) Acute symptoms during the course of head and neck radiotherapy or chemoradiation are strong predictors of late dysphagia. Radiother Oncol 115(1):56–62

van der Laan HP, Bijl HP, Steenbakkers RJHM et al (2015b) Acute symptoms during the course of head and neck radiotherapy or chemoradiation are strong predictors of late dysphagia. Radiother Oncol 115:56–62

van der Molen L, van Rossum MA, Ackerstaff AH et al (2009) Pretreatment organ function in patients with advanced head and neck cancer: clinical outcome measures and patients' views. BMC Ear Nose Throat Disord 9:10. https://doi.org/10.1186/1472-6815-9-10

van Hooren MR, Baijens LW, Voskuilen S et al (2014) Treatment effects for dysphagia in Parkinson's disease: a systematic review. Parkinsonism Relat Disord 20(8):800–807

Van den Steen L, Goossens E, Van Gemst M et al (2024) The effects of adding particles in texture modified food on tongue strength and swallowing function in patients with oropharyngeal dysphagia: a proof of concept study. Dysphagia

Venuto C, McGarry A, Ma Q et al (2012) Pharmacologic approaches to the treatment of Huntington's disease. Mov Disord 27(1):31–41

Verdonck J, Morton RP (2015) Systematic review on treatment of Zenker's diverticulum. Eur Arch Otorrinolaringol 272(11):3095–3107

Verma A, Steele J (2006) Botulinum toxin improves sialorrhea and quality of living in bulbar amyotrophic lateral sclerosis. Muscle Nerve 34(2):235–237

Vilardell N, Rofes L, Arreola V et al (2016) A comparative study between modified starch and xanthan gum thickeners in post-stroke oropharyngeal dysphagia. Dysphagia 31:169–179

Voigt-Zimmermann S, Arens C (2013) Behandlung von Glottisschlussinsuffizienzen (Treatment of glottal gap). HNO 61(2):117–134

Volkert D, Berner YN, Berry E et al (2006) ESPEN guidelines on enteral nutrition: geriatrics. Clin Nutr 25:330–360

Vose A, Nonnenmacher J, Singer ML et al (2014) Dysphagia management in acute and sub-acute stroke. Curr Phys Med Rehabil Rep 2(4):197–206

Waito AA, Valenzano TJ, Peladeau-Pigeon M et al (2017) Trends in research literature describing dysphagia in motor neuron diseases (MND): a scoping review. Dysphagia 32(6):734–747

Wall LR, Ward EC, Cartmill B et al (2013) Physiological changes to the swallowing mechanism following (chemo)radiotherapy for head and neck cancer: a systematic review. Dysphagia 28(4):481–493

Ward EC, Uriarte M, Sppath B et al (2001) Duration of dysphagic symptoms and swallowing outcomes after thermal burn injury. J Burn Care Rehabil 22(6):441–453

Ward EC, Green K, Morton AL et al (2007) Patterns and predictors of swallowing resolution following adult traumatic brain injury. J Head Trauma Rehabil 22(3):184–191

Warnecke T, Suntrup S, Teismann IK et al (2013) Standardized endoscopic swallowing evaluation for tracheostomy decannulation in critically ill neurologic patients. Crit Care Med 41(7):1728–1732

Watanabe E, Yamagata Y, Fujitani J et al (2018) The criteria of thickened liquid for dysphagia management in Japan. Dysphagia 33:26–32

Watts CR, Vanryckeghem M (2001) Laryngeal dysfunction in amyotrophic lateral sclerosis: a review and case report. BMC Ear Nose Throat Disord 1(1):1. https://doi.org/10.1186/1472-6815-1-1

Wijesekera LC, Leigh PN (2009) Amyotrophic lateral sclerosis. Orphanet J Rare Dis 4:3. https://doi.org/10.1186/1750-1172-4-3

Willette S, Molinaro LH, Thompson DM et al (2016) Fiberoptic examination of swallowing in the breast-feeding infant. Laryngoscope 126(7):1681–1686

Wilson JA, Carding PN, Patterson JM (2011) Dysphagia after nonsurgical head and neck cancer treatment: patients' perspectives. Otolaryngol Head Neck Surg 145:767–771

Winklmaier U, Wüst K, Wallner F (2005) Evaluation des Aspirationsschutzes blockbarer Trachealkanülen (evaluation of the aspiration protection of blockable tracheostomy tubes). HNO 53(12):1057–1062

Wood AM, Froh JJ, Geraghty AWA (2010) Gratitude and Well-being: a review and theoretical integration. Clin Psychol Rev 30(7):890–905

Woodson G (1997) Cricopharyngeal myotomy and arytenoid adduction in the management of combined laryngeal and pharyngeal paralysis. Otolaryngol Head Neck Surg 116(3):339–343

Wopken K, Bijl HP, Langendijk JA (2018) Prognostic factors for tube feeding dependence after curative (chemo-) radiation in head and neck cancer:

a systematic review of literature. Radiother Oncol 126:56–67

Yoritaka A, Shimo Y, Takanashi M et al (2013) Motor and non-motor symptoms of 1453 patients with Parkinson's disease: prevalence and risks. Parkinsonism Relat Disord 19(8):725–731

Zafereo ME, Weber RS, Lewin JS et al (2010) Complications and functional outcomes following complex oropharyngeal reconstruction. Head Neck 32(8):1003–1011

Zaninotto G, Marchese Ragona R et al (2004) The role of botulinum toxin injection and upper esophageal sphincter myotomy in treating oropharyngeal dysphagia. J Gastrointest Surg 8(8):997–1006

Zocratto OB, Savassi-Rocha PR, Paixao RM et al (2006) Laryngotracheal separation surgery: outcome in 60 patients. Otolaryngol Head Neck Surg 135(4):571–575

Zwiefelhofer D (2012) Making dysphagia easier to swallow. Nutrition and Foodservice Edge Magazine 21:16–20

# Part VII

# Phoniatrics and COVID-19

Editor: Antoinette am Zehnhoff-Dinnesen
Lectors: no further lector

# Telepractice

# 31

Mirela Duranović

## 31.1 Telepractice in Speech-Language Pathology

Mirela Duranović

### 31.1.1 Introduction

Investigation of the usefulness of telepractice, the use of communication technology in speech-language pathology (SLP) practice, has been conducted since the 1970s (see Vaughn 1976; Wertz et al. 1992). It is not a new field of research because the rapid growth of information technology has long influenced the emergence of a broad professional interest in this model of service delivery. Accordingly, different professional associations have been initiated and developed guidelines for the use of telepractice in SLP.

The American Telemedicine Association defines telerehabilitation as

> the delivery of rehabilitation services through information and communications technology (ICT)—Brennan et al. (2010)

It refers to a new and innovative approach involving rehabilitation at home with the goal of improving the patient's motor, cognitive or psychological disorders. Different types of interven-

tion can be included, such as physiotherapy, speech, cognitive, and behavioural therapy, occupational therapy, telemonitoring, and teleconsultation (Piron et al. 2004).

The American Speech-Language-Hearing Association (ASHA), the professional and scientific association that comprises 218,000 members who are audiologists, speech-language pathologists, speech, language and hearing scientists, audiology and speech-language pathology-support personnel, and students from the USA, is one of the associations that support the use of telepractice in work with clients who have speech, language, and hearing disorders. ASHA defines telepractice as

> the application of telecommunications technology to the delivery of SLP and audiology professional services at a distance by linking clinician to client, or clinician to clinician, for assessment, intervention, and/or consultation—ASHA (2021)

Different terms are in use for "telepractice" such as: telehealth, telerehabilitation, telespeech, and teleSLP. The first intention was to use telepractice with the aim of overcoming such barriers as distance from the place of residence to the place of treatment, problems with patient transport, a discrepancy in the work schedule of the patient or family member, and an insufficient number of experts in certain areas (ASHA, cited in Tucker 2012, p. 47); later it provided continuity of treatment upon return from the hospital (Turolla et al. 2013) for which the costs were sig-

M. Duranović (✉)
Department of Speech and Language Pathology,
University of Tuzla, Tuzla, Bosnia and Herzegovina
e-mail: mirela.duranovic@bih.net.ba

© The Author(s), under exclusive license to Springer Nature Switzerland AG 2025
A. am Zehnhoff-Dinnesen et al. (eds.), *Phoniatrics III*, European Manual of Medicine,
https://doi.org/10.1007/978-3-031-48091-1_16

nificantly lower (Mutingi and Mbohwa 2015). Telepractice can

> extend clinical services to remote, rural, and underserved populations, and to culturally and linguistically diverse populations—Tucker (2012, p. 47)

In 2020, the virus causing coronavirus disease 2019 (COVID-19) had become pandemic and spread around the world, leading to demands for social distancing, and a restructured social life and people's working activities. Since then telepractice has become even more important for SLP services and has found its place in reducing the transmission risk of COVID-19. Telepractice has provided admission to SLP and learning services during the COVID-19 pandemic, and will be important after the pandemic when social relations return to normal (Sarti et al. 2020).

## 31.1.2 Types of Telepractice Models

Telepractice may include individual and group sessions, specialist clinical consultation, and clinical training/supervision (Speech Pathology Association of Australia Limited 2014). It includes:

- Synchronous (client interactive) models—services are provided through interactive audio and video connections in real time and the experience is in-person, approximately the same as in traditional treatment. Synchronous services may include the work of a client or group of clients with a clinician, or the consultation of clinicians and specialist.
- Asynchronous (store-and-forward) models—images or data are recorded (i.e., stored) and transmitted (i.e., forwarded) for review or interpretation by experts.
- Hybrid models—combinations of synchronous, asynchronous, and in-person services (ASHA 2021).

Synchronous services have been used to provide speech, language, cognitive communication, voice, and swallowing services and have been found to correspond with those provided in person (see Duffy et al. 1997; Hill et al. 2006;

Theodoros et al. 2006; Waite et al. 2006; Grogan-Johnson et al. 2010; Kully 2002; Mashima et al. 2003; Perlman and Witthawaskul 2002). Asynchronous services have been provided in person or to review and validate data observed and recorded during synchronous teleservices (see Hill et al. 2006, 2009; O'Brian et al. 2010; Onslow et al. 2003; Theodoros et al. 2006, 2008; Waite et al. 2006; Ward et al. 2007, 2009; Wilson et al. 2004; Constantinescu et al. 2010).

## 31.1.3 SLP Telepractice Research

It is very important to have enough information on the outcomes and satisfaction levels of SLP services delivered through telepractice (Mashima and Doarn 2008) and on results of research that have analysed whether service delivery via telepractice is comparable with traditional, face-to-face, speech, and language therapy. Telepractice in speech-language therapy for assessment and intervention purposes should be documented.

The use of telepractice is being analysed for different speech and language disorders. It has been investigated through analysis assessment and treatment services in an online and face-to-face environment. Results have been obtained for a wide range of speech and language disorders:

- Aphasia
  - Theodoros et al. (2008) assessed aphasia with the short forms of the Boston Diagnostic Aphasia Examination (BDAE-3) (Goodglass et al. 2001) and the Boston Naming Test (BNT, second edition) (Kaplan et al. 2001) via an internet-based videoconferencing system. Results confirmed the validity and reliability of standardised assessments of aphasia online.
  - Macoir et al. (2017) used a telerehabilitation platform and software based on the Promoting Aphasics' Communicative Effectiveness (PACE) approach (see Davis and Wilcox 1985). Patients with chronic post-stroke aphasia were included in nine speech therapy sessions over a 3-week period. Positive effects of language therapy

on functional communication in chronic aphasia delivered through synchronous telerehabilitation were noted.

- Articulation disorders
  - Cole et al. (1986) noted overall positive results for providing SLP services through an audio teleconferencing system. Only the lack of video was a problem for the articulation assessment as the clinician could not perceive an interdental lisp because the child's tongue placement was unable to viewed. The results were only preliminary.
  - Grogan-Johnson et al. (2013) analysed the success of using traditional and telepractice intervention for school-age children with speech sound impairments. Children in both delivery services made progress in their speech sound production.
  - Waite et al. (2006) investigated the feasibility of assessing childhood speech disorders via an Internet-based telehealth system (eREHAB) (see Hill et al. 2006), with scoring for in-person and online services. High levels of agreement between the two scoring environments were found for single-word articulation, speech intelligibility and oro-motor tasks.
- Language disorders
  - Cole et al. (1986) investigated the telepractice assessment of speech and language in school-age children by using an audio teleconferencing system with a microphone and loudspeaker that operated via a telephone landline. No differences were found between the two SLPs' ratings on the language test, showing the acceptability of an audio-only system for this assessment of expressive language.
  - Waite et al. (2010a) assessed the core language subtests online and face to face. No significant difference was found between the scores for each subtest for either delivery service.
- Motor speech disorders
  - Hill et al. (2006) investigated the efficacy of an internet-based application for the assessment of motor speech disorders in

adults with acquired neurological impairment. A battery of perceptual tests was used for the assessment of patients with dysarthria. Most measurements were found to be within the clinically acceptable criteria, while several ratings were not comparable between two environments.
  - Hill et al. (2009) explored assessment of apraxia via telepractice and found that using the Apraxia Battery for Adults-2 over the internet is possible. Participant satisfaction was at an acceptable level. However, comments from the SLPs indicated that participants exhibiting severe apraxia of speech might be better suited to face-to-face assessment.
  - Constantinescu et al. (2010) investigated a telerehabilitation application for assessing the speech and voice disorder associated with Parkinson's disease with hypokinetic dysarthria, in an online and face-to-face environment. The assessment protocol included perceptual measures of voice and oro-motor function, articulatory precision, speech intelligibility, and acoustic measures of vocal sound pressure levels, phonation time, and pitch range. For the majority of measures, comparable levels of agreement were reached between the two service models.
- Autism
  - Gibson et al. (2010) assessed the impact of functional communication training via videoconference in preschool students with autism. The results showed that the teaching staff were able to intervene successfully by using this type of service and that unsupervised departing the healthcare system in children was significantly reduced.
  - Iacono et al. (2016) explored the use of technology by parent and practitioner, and their views about telehealth service delivery for early autism intervention. Mothers were interested in applying telehealth, and practitioners would like to apply it for consulting with other professionals and their professional development. They detected problems in telehealth application, such as

limited experience, practitioners not knowing what a telehealth service might look like, poor access to reliable and fast internet, lack of skills and technical support, and practitioners believing that families preferred face-to-face services.

– Parmanto et al. (2013) developed an intuitive software platform for autism assessment, as close to face-to-face assessment as possible, integrating video-conferencing, stimuli presentation, recording, image and video presentation, and electronic assessment scoring. The results showed that the system was easy to use and provided high-quality interaction.

– Boisvert et al. (2010) and Sutherland et al. (2018) reviewed studies including the use of telepractice in the delivery of services to individuals with autism spectrum disorders (ASD). Outcomes were largely positive, indicating that services delivered via telehealth were comparable to services delivered face to face, and suggesting that telepractice is a promising service delivery approach in the treatment of individuals with ASD.

– Sutherland et al. (2019) investigated the validity and reliability of telehealth during language assessments for children with autism and found strong inter-rater reliability between the telehealth and face-to-face environments. Positive feedback was noted from parents.

• Specific learning disorders
– Waite et al. (2010b) investigated the validity and reliability of the use of videoconferencing in assessing children's literacy by standardised assessments. Problems with audio latency, break-up, and echo were reported. Nevertheless, overall positive results of this research were obtained.

– Hodge et al. (2019a) studied the feasibility and reliability of telepractice literacy assessments in children with reading difficulties. Strong agreement between telepractice and face-to-face-rated scores were found.

– Hodge et al. (2019b) assessed cognitive function in children with learning difficulties

by using telehealth. High associations were found between two testing methodologies.

• Fluency disorders
– Kully (2002) showed that interactive video conferencing can be a useful format for providing services to some patients who stutter.

– Wilson et al. (2004) and Lewis et al. (2008) analysed the outcomes of a telehealth adaptation of the Lidcombe Program of Early Stuttering Intervention for children with early stuttering (see Onslow et al. 2003). The results showed that telehealth delivery of the programme was effective and could give the desired results.

– The viability of telehealth delivery of the Camperdown Program (see O'Brian et al. 2010) was investigated for stuttering adults (O'Brian et al. 2008) and adolescents (Carey et al. 2012). The results showed that the service delivery model was efficacious and efficient. Carey et al. (2014) conducted a phase II trial of the same programme, with adolescents who stutter, delivered over the internet. The results showed a positive effect for the adolescents as a group, who significantly reduced their stuttering frequency and severity.

• Swallowing disorders
– Ward et al. (2007, 2009) investigated laryngectomy patients with a multimedia video conferencing system. The remote clinician and the face-to-face assessors of swallowing, stoma, and communication status agreed in the assessment. The image quality determined through the use of a stand-alone camera was rated slightly lower than direct observation, but still sufficient to assess the stoma and status of the voice prosthesis.

– Cassel (2016) analysed the possibility of realising the goals typically targeted in the in-person setting when using tele-dysphagia therapeutic intervention, and found that it could be used as a successful delivery method.

– Malandraki et al. (2011) assessed a real-time internet-based protocol for remote, telefluoroscopic evaluation of oropharyngeal swallowing and found an acceptable level of agreement with evaluations performed in the fluoroscopy suite by traditional videofluoroscopic methodology.

- Perlman and Witthawaskul (2002) tested an internet system for real-time, interactive evaluation of oral/pharyngeal swallowing function, and noted that it can be easily integrated into commercially available fluoroscopic equipment.

- Voice disorders
  - Mashima et al. (2003) evaluated treatment outcomes for vocal rehabilitation delivered to patients with voice disorders. No differences were found between the conventional and the remote video teleconference group for outcome measures including perceptual judgments of voice quality, acoustic analyses of voice, patient satisfaction ratings, and fibre-optic laryngoscopy.
  - Theodoros et al. (2006), Tindall et al. (2008), and Halpern et al. (2012) investigated the usefulness of an internet-based telerehabilitation application for the delivery of the Lee Silverman Voice Treatment (LSVT®) developed by Ramig et al. (1994), to persons with Parkinson's disease (PD). In all studies there were significant improvements in many outcome measures and all of them supported the use of the telerehabilitation in treatment of dysarthria in individuals with PD.
  - Towey (2012) retrospectively reviewed patients with vocal fold dysfunction referred to speech therapy at Waldo County General Hospital (WCGH) and noted that the use of telepractice might result in significant cost-savings for patients insurers and society.

### 31.1.4 Telepractice in SLP during COVID-19 Pandemic

A newly discovered virus that causes an infectious disease called COVID-19 has spread around the world. The disease endangers human lives, causes mortality, and brings various problems such as quarantine, social exclusion, and the obligation to use protective tools, which negatively influence different jobs and services, including rehabilitation services. The disease has also hampered the provision and services of SLP. Therefore, described here are the quality of SLP service delivery during the COVID-19 pandemic and the negative effects of the disease on SLP service delivery.

The proclamation of a pandemic due to the spread of Coronavirus 2019 (COVID-19) affected a change in service delivery by health professionals, who had to adapt to the changes and provide their services via telepractice during the pandemic. The use of telepractice is accepted as the most sustainable alternative to face-to-face assessment, as it allows the provision of basic health care without compromising the safety of the patient or clinician. SLPs also had to adopt new approaches to their professional activities, such as telepractice.

The use of telepractice among SLPs during the COVID-19 pandemic has been studied in different countries (in India: Aggarwal et al. 2020; in Hong Kong: Fong et al. 2021; Lam et al. 2021; in Croatia: Kuvač Kraljević et al. 2020; in the United States: Sylvan et al. 2020). SLPs redirected their services to telepractice during the COVID-19 pandemic with a generally positive attitude towards its use. The most commonly used platform was the WhatsApp video calling feature, although more than one platform was used. The biggest challenges were dealing with network problems and the child's lack of cooperation (Aggarwal et al. 2020). Reasons for a client's refusal of therapy delivered via telepractice include the lack of equipment, insufficient independence, and doubts on the effectiveness of telepractice (Kuvač Kraljević et al. 2020). Face-to-face service is preferred by parents and SLPs (Fong et al. 2021; Lam et al. 2021). Most SLPs had no previous experience with telepractice (Sylvan et al. 2020) or training with it (Fong et al. 2021). It is very important for SLPs to be trained to provide telepractice services, with the aim of increasing the quality of these services (Tohidast et al. 2020), reducing their low self-confidence and their workload, which is present in SLPs as result of the use of a new model of work (Sylvan et al. 2020).

## 31.1.5 Conclusion

Telepractice can alleviate the shortage of SLPs, especially in rural and under-served areas, reduce costs, allow wider connectivity, reducing the inaccessible environment and may also be a suitable means of SLP service during pandemics and social exclusion conditions. In addition, telepractice allows patients to access services in their natural environment, increases the participation of family members in this process, and enhances the efficiency of service delivery (Brady 2007). Crutchley and Campbell (2010) found that parents/carers, teachers, and administrators consider telepractice to be a satisfactory service delivery model.

Telepractice can be an effective way to provide SLP intervention to people with speech and language impairments as shown by numerous studies. However, the provision of reliable SLP-standardised assessments and interventions through telepractice, monitoring progress, client and parent satisfaction, and also the SLPs' satisfaction with the provision of telepractice services need further research. In previous studies, SLPs have positively assessed the potential of telepractice but have also noted barriers such as cost, lack of professional standards, and lack of data on its effectiveness and cost-effectiveness (Mashima and Doarn 2008).

Telepractice can provide great access to SLP services for children with speech and language disorders in a variety of situations and challenges. Further consideration and rationale for this delivery model is needed to make it an accepted alternative delivery model that could remove many obstacles and shortcomings and be a useful alternative tool for providing services in SLP.

## References

Aggarwal K, Patel R, Ravi R et al (2020) Uptake of telepractice among speech-language therapists following COVID-19 pandemic in India. Speech Lang Hear 2(1):118–124

ASHA (American Speech-Language-Hearing Association) (2021) Telepractice. https://www.asha.org/practice-portal/professional-issues/telepractice/#collapse_3. Accessed Feb 2021

Boisvert M, Lang R, Andrianopoulos M et al (2010) Telepractice in the assessment and treatment of individuals with autism spectrum disorders: a systematic review. Dev Neurorehabil 13(6):423–432

Brady A (2007) Moving toward the future: providing speech-language pathology services via telehealth. Home Healthcare Nurse 25:240–244

Brennan D, Tindall L, Theodoros D et al (2010) A blueprint for telerehabilitation guidelines. Int J Telerehabil 2(2):31–34

Carey B, O'Brian S, Onslow M et al (2012) Webcam delivery of the Camperdown Program for adolescents who stutter: a phase I trial. Lang Speech Hear Serv Sch 43(3):370–380

Carey B, O'Brian S, Lowe R et al (2014) Webcam delivery of the Camperdown Program for adolescents who stutter: a phase II trial. Lang Speech Hear Serv Sch 45(4):314–324

Cassel S (2016) Case reports: trial dysphagia interventions conducted via telehealth. Int J Telerehabil 8(2):71–76

Cole C, Martin V, Moody J et al (1986) Speech pathology at a distance. Aust Commun Q 2:17–19

Constantinescu G, Theodoros D, Russell T et al (2010) Assessing disordered speech and voice in Parkinson's disease: a telerehabilitation application. Int J Lang Commun Disord 45(6):630–644

Crutchley S, Campbell M (2010) TeleSpeech therapy pilot project: stakeholder satisfaction. Int J Telerehabil 2(1):23–30

Davis GA, Wilcox MJ (1985) Adult aphasia rehabilitation: applied pragmatics. College-Hill Press, San Diego, CA

Duffy JR, Werven GW, Aronson AE (1997) Telemedicine and the diagnosis of speech and language disorders. Mayo Clin Proc 72(12):1116–1122

Fong R, Tsai CF, Yiu OY (2021) The implementation of telepractice in speech language pathology in Hong Kong during the COVID-19 pandemic. Telemed J E Health 27(1):30–38

Gibson JL, Pennington RC, Stenhoff DM et al (2010) Using desktop videoconferencing to deliver interventions to a preschool student with autism. Topics Early Child Spec Educ 29(4):214–225

Goodglass H, Kaplan E, Barresi B (2001) Boston diagnostic aphasia examination, 3rd edn. Lippincott Williams & Wilkin, Baltimore, MD

Grogan-Johnson S, Alvares RL, Rowan L et al (2010) A pilot study comparing the effectiveness of speech-language therapy provided by telepractice. J Telem Telecare 16(3):134–139

Grogan-Johnson S, Schmidt AM, Schenker J et al (2013) A comparison of speech sound intervention delivered by telepractice and side-by-side service delivery models. Commun Disord Q 34(4):210–220

Halpern AE, Ramig LO, Matos CEC et al (2012) Innovative technology for the assisted delivery of intensive voice treatment (LSVT®LOUD) for Parkinson disease. Am J Speech Lang Pathol 21(4):354–367

Hill AJ, Theodoros DG, Russell TG et al (2006) An internet-based telerehabilitation system for the assessment of motor speech disorders: a pilot study. Am J Speech Lang Pathol 15(1):45–56

Hill AJ, Theodoros D, Russell T et al (2009) Using telerehabilitation to assess apraxia of speech in adults. Int J Lang Commun Disord 44(5):731–747

Hodge MA, Sutherland R, Jeng K et al (2019a) Literacy assessment via telepractice is comparable to face-to-face assessment in children with reading difficulties living in rural Australia. Telemed J E Health 25(4):279–287

Hodge MA, Sutherland R, Jeng K et al (2019b) Agreement between telehealth and face-to-face assessment of intellectual ability in children with specific learning disorder. J Telemed Telecare 25(7):431–437

Iacono T, Dissanayake C, Trembath D et al (2016) Family and practitioner perspectives on telehealth for services to young children with autism. Stud Health Technol Inform 231:63–73

Kaplan E, Goodglass H, Weintraub S (2001) Boston Naming Test, 2nd edn. Lippincott Williams & Wilkin, Baltimore, MD

Kully D (2002) Telehealth in speech-language pathology: applications to the treatment of stuttering. J Telemed Telecare 6(2):39–41

Kuvač Kraljević J, Matić A, Pavičić Dokoza K (2020) Telepractice as a reaction to the COVID-19 crisis: insights from Croatian SLP Settings. Int J Telerehabil 12(2):93–104

Lam J, Lee S, Tong X (2021) Parents' and students' perceptions of telepractice services for speech-language therapy during the COVID-19 pandemic: survey study. JMIR Pediatr Parent 4(1):e25675. https://doi.org/10.2196/25675

Lewis C, Packman A, Onslow M et al (2008) A phase II trial of telehealth delivery of the Lidcombe Program of Early Stuttering Intervention. Am J Speech Lang Pathol 17(2):139–149

Macoir J, Martel Sauvageau V, Boissy P et al (2017) In-home synchronous telespeech therapy to improve functional communication in chronic poststroke aphasia: results from a quasi-experimental study. Telemed J E Health 23(8):630–639

Malandraki GA, McCullough G, He X et al (2011) Teledynamic evaluation of oropharyngeal swallowing. J Speech Lang Hear Res 54(6):1497–1505

Mashima PA, Doarn CR (2008) Overview of telehealth activities in speech-language pathology. Telemed J E Health 14(10):1101–1117

Mashima PA, Birkmire-Peters DP, Syms MJ et al (2003) Telehealth: voice therapy using telecommunications technology. Am J Speech Lang Pathol 12(4):432–439

Mutingi M, Mbohwa C (2015) Developing multi-agent systems for mHealth drug delivery. Mobile Health 1:671–683

O'Brian S, Packman A, Onslow M (2008) Telehealth delivery of the Camperdown Program for adults who stutter: a phase I trial. J Speech Lang Hear Res 51(1):184–195

O'Brian S, Carey B, Onslow M et al (2010) The Camperdown Program of Stuttering: treatment manual. https://www.yumpu.com/en/document/read/10974808/camperdown-treatment-manual-the-university-of-sydney. Accessed 7 Apr 2021

Onslow M, Packman A, Harrison E (2003) The Lidcombe Program of Early Stuttering Intervention: a clinician's guide. Pro-Ed, Austin, TX

Parmanto B, Pulantara W, Schutte J et al (2013) An integrated telehealth system for remote administration of an adult autism assessment. Telemed J E Health 19:88–94

Perlman AL, Witthawaskul W (2002) Real-time remote telefluoroscopic assessment of patients with dysphagia. Dysphagia 17(2):162–167

Piron L, Tonin P, Trivello E et al (2004) Motor tele-rehabilitation in post-stroke patients. Med Inform Internet Med 29(2):119–125

Ramig LO, Bonitati C, Lemke J et al (1994) Voice treatment for patients with Parkinson disease: development of an approach and preliminary efficacy data. J Med Speech-Language Pathol 2:191–209

Sarti D, De Salvatore M, Gazzola S et al (2020) So far so close: an insight into smart working and telehealth reorganization of a language and learning disorders service in Milan during COVID-19 pandemic. Neurol Sci 41(7):1659–1662

Speech Pathology Association of Australia Limited (2014) Telepractice in speech pathology. https://www.telemedecine-360.com/wp-content/uploads/2019/02/2015-SPA-0113_Position_Statement_Telepractice_in_Speech.pdf. Accessed Feb 2021

Sutherland R, Trembath D, Roberts J (2018) Telehealth and autism: a systematic search and review of the literature. Int J Speech Lang Pathol 20(3):324–336

Sutherland R, Trembath D, Hodge MA et al (2019) Telehealth and autism: are telehealth language assessments reliable and feasible for children with autism? Int J Lang Commun Disord 54(2):281–291

Sylvan L, Goldstein E, Crandall M (2020) Capturing a moment in time: a survey of school-based speech-language pathologists' experiences in the immediate aftermath of the COVID-19 public health emergency. Perspect ASHA Spec Interest Groups 5:1735–1749

Theodoros DG, Constantinescu AG, Russell TG et al (2006) Treating the speech disorder in Parkinson's disease online. J Telemed Telecare 12(3):88–91

Theodoros D, Hill A, Russell T et al (2008) Assessing acquired language disorders in adults via the Internet. Telemed J E Health 14(6):552–559

Tindall LR, Huebner RA, Stemple JC et al (2008) Videophone-delivered voice therapy: a comparative analysis of outcomes to traditional delivery for adults with Parkinson's disease. Telemedic J E Health 14(10):1070–1077

Tohidast SA, Mansuri B, Bagheri R et al (2020) Provision of speech-language pathology services for the treatment of speech and language disorders in children during the COVID-19 pandemic: problems, concerns, and solutions. Int J Pediatr Otorhinolaryngol 138:110262. https://doi.org/10.1016/j.ijporl.2020.110262

Towey M (2012) Speech therapy telepractice for vocal cord dysfunction (VCD): MaineCare (Medicaid) cost savings. Int J Telerehabil 4(1):34–36

Tucker JK (2012) Perspectives of speech-language pathologists on the use of telepractice in schools: the qualitative view. Int J Telerehabil 4(2):47–59

Turolla A, Dam M, Ventura L et al (2013) Virtual reality for the rehabilitation of the upper limb motor function after stroke: a prospective controlled trial. J Neuroeng Rehabil 10:85. https://doi.org/10.1186/1743-0003-10-85

Vaughn GR (1976) Tele-communicology: health-care delivery system for persons with communication disorders. ASHA 18(1):13–17

Waite MC, Cahill LM, Theodoras DG et al (2006) A pilot study of online assessment of childhood speech disorders. J Telemed Telecare 12(3):92–94

Waite MC, Theodoros D, Russell TG et al (2010a) Internet-based telehealth assessment of language using the CELF-4. Lang Speech Hear Serv Sch 41(4):445–448

Waite MC, Theodoros DG, Russell TG et al (2010b) Assessment of children's literacy via an Internet-based telehealth system. Telemed J E Health 16(5):564–575

Ward L, White J, Russell T et al (2007) Assessment of communication and swallowing function post laryngectomy: a telerehabilitation trial. J Telemed Telecare 13(Suppl 3):88–91

Ward E, Crombie J, Trickey M et al (2009) Assessment of communication and swallowing post-laryngectomy: a telerehabilitation trial. J Telemed Telecare 15(5):232–237

Wertz RT, Dronkers NF, Bernstein-Ellis E et al (1992) Potential of telephonic and television technology for appraising and diagnosing neurogenic communication disorders in remote settings. Aphasiology 6(2):195–202

Wilson L, Onslow M, Lincoln M (2004) Telehealth adaptation of the Lidcombe Program of early stuttering intervention: five case studies. Am J Speech Lang Pathol 13(1):81–93

# Aerosol Particle Emissions During Voice Production/Playing Wind Instruments

# 32

Wolfgang Angerstein, Mario Fleischer,
and Dirk Mürbe

## 32.1 Aerosol Particle Emissions During Speaking, Singing, and Shouting

Dirk Mürbe and Mario Fleischer

### 32.1.1 Aerosols and Voice Production

The respiratory system is the main transmission route for airborne viruses, which might be carried by aerosols and droplets. Whereas aerosol particles (smaller than 100 µm in diameter) remain airborne for a long-time, larger particles (denoted as droplets) fall rapidly to the ground after emission. The problem of particle generation within the respiratory system has initiated immense research activities during the *SARS-CoV-2* pandemic because of life-threatening COVID-19 disease (Prather et al. 2020).

The respiratory tract has a dual function: it is not only the main tool for ventilation, but also the source of voice and spoken language production.

Particle formation occurs in the pulmonary alveoli (Johnson and Morawska 2009), but also by means of flow effects of the vibrating vocal folds, and adjustments of the articulation instruments during speaking and singing (Johnson et al. 2011). When aerosol particles are exhaled, the fluid component of the virus-containing particles evaporates. They become lighter, can float in the air for long periods (Stadnytskyi et al. 2020), and spread in enclosed rooms by airflow and turbulent diffusion (Gao and Niu 2007).

Activities such as speaking and singing are regarded as being linked to increased aerosol particle emission from the respiratory system, dependent on the used vocal intensity (Asadi et al. 2020). With higher emission rates, the risk of transmission increases within the near- and far-field of an infectious person in enclosed spaces, through the increased concentrations of virus-carrying aerosol particles.

To contribute to the risk management of airborne virus transmission a series of studies with a Laser-Particle-Counter under cleanroom conditions was carried out to measure particle emission rates of aerosols during speaking, singing, and shouting. The investigations were to assess differences of aerosol emission rates between different age groups, namely children, adolescents, and adults. Furthermore, the measurements addressed previously described effects of vocal loudness (Asadi et al. 2020). From a phoniatricians point of view it is a particular motiva-

---

tion to assess aerosol emission rates of voice and spoken language production because singing activities in enclosed spaces has been strictly regulated since the outbreak of the COVID-19 pandemic owing to the risk of infection from the *SARS-CoV-2* virus, transmitted by virus-carrying aerosols. These constraints have strongly influenced cultural and public life throughout society. Especially for children and young people this was associated with far-reaching consequences for music education in schools and such extra-curricular activities as ensemble and choir singing.

### 32.1.2 Experimental Set-Up Under Cleanroom Conditions

To determine the number of aerosol particles emitted during a variety of phonatory activities of different age groups (denoted as particle emission rate $P_M$), we used a Laser-Particle-Counter (LPC) under cleanroom conditions in cooperation with the Technische Universität Berlin. The measured particles were assigned to six size classes from 0.3 μm to 25 μm diameter. To avoid any disturbances and artifacts in the data caused by abrasion of clothing and hair, all participants wore cleanroom clothing and headgear (see Mürbe et al. 2021a, b).

We investigated different phonatory test conditions in three age groups. Firstly, 15 pre-adolescent children (8–10 years old) with singing experience of 1.5–4.5 years were asked to breathe at rest, read a text ("Seefahrt nach Rio"), sing a song (Ludwig van Beethoven, Ode to Joy, ninth Symphony in D Minor op. 125), and shout as enthusiastically as possible for about 10–30 s (Fleischer et al. 2022). Secondly, eight adolescents (13–15 years old) were also asked to read a text ("Der Nordwind und die Sonne"), sing a song (Swedish folk song "Vem kan segla" in G Major), and cheer as loudly as possible (Mürbe et al. 2021a). Thirdly, an adult group ($N = 15$, 23–64 years old) was also asked for breathing at rest, speaking a text ("Der Nordwind und die Sonne"), singing a song (Ludwig van Beethoven,

Ode to Joy, ninth Symphony in D Minor op. 125), and shout as loudly as possible.

### 32.1.3 Aerosol Emission Rates for Children, Adolescents, and Adults

Similar size distributions of $P_M$ were observed for children, adolescents, and adults. Moreover, the shape of the size distributions was nearly independent of the different phonatory conditions and skewed to the small values. Within the measuring range between 0.3 μm and 25 μm, most of the measured particles for all conditions were smaller than 3 μm (Fig. 32.1).

For all age groups investigated the aerosol emission rates $P_M$ for speaking were clearly lower than for singing. Furthermore, children and adolescents showed even higher emission rates for shouting than singing. In detail, for the children the group median $P_M$ was 8 P/s for breathing at rest. For the different conditions speaking, singing, and shouting, the group medians $P_M$ were 24 P/s, 118 P/s, and 1083 P/s, respectively. The measurements of the adolescents showed group median values $P_M$ of 75 P/s for speaking and 490 P/s for singing. For shouting, the group median of $P_M$ was still higher (2472 P/s). Within the adult group, the group median of the cumulative $P_M$ for breathing at rest was 20 P/s. For the different conditions speaking, singing, and shouting, the group medians $P_M$ were 204 P/s, 1640 P/s, and 1295 P/s, respectively (Fig. 32.2).

Because previous measurements described a strong effect of vocal loudness on aerosol emission rates (Mürbe et al. 2021b; Asadi et al. 2020) the contribution of this effect was assessed by means of the measured maximum sound pressure level $L_{AFmax}$. While $P_M$ decreased from adults to children for speaking and singing by factors of 8.7 and 13.9, respectively, $L_{AFmax}$ values decreased from adults to children for speaking and singing by factors of 1.3 and 2.9, respectively. Thus, the differences between the aerosol emission rates are only partly due to different vocal loudness

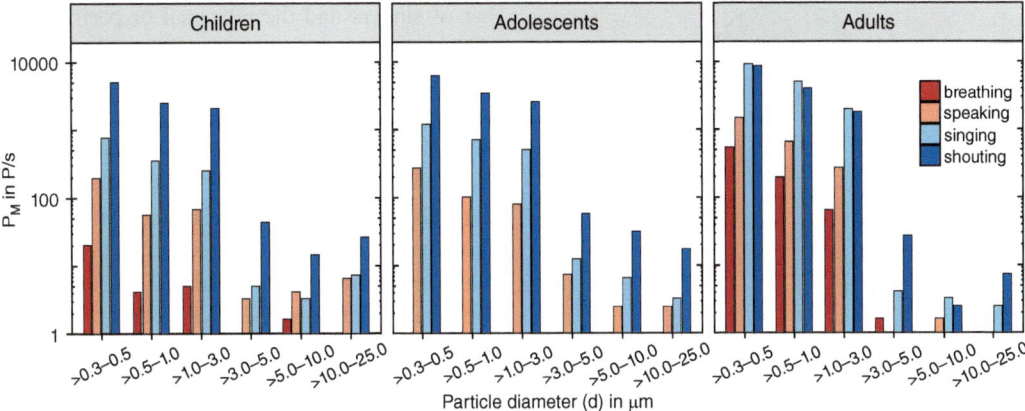

**Fig. 32.1** Aerosol particle distributions in P/s (Particles/second) for different size classes up to 25 μm normalised to the number of participants in each age group (children, adolescents, and adults). (Modified from Fleischer et al. (2022). Pre-adolescent children exhibit lower aerosol par-ticle volume emissions than adults for breathing, speaking, singing, and shouting. J R Soc Interface 19:20210833.20210833 and from Mürbe et al. (2021a) Aerosol emission of adolescents voices during speaking, singing, and shouting. PLoS ONE 16(2): e0246819)

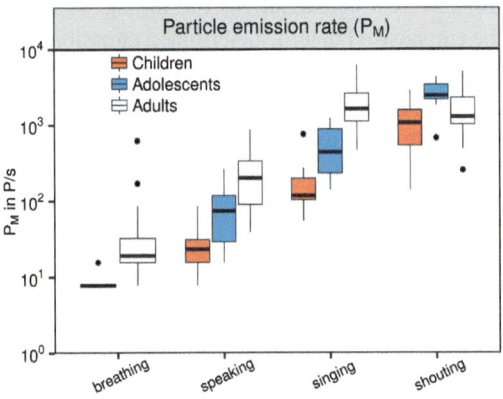

**Fig. 32.2** Comparison of particle emission rate $P_M$ in particle per second for the conditions breathing, speaking, singing, and shouting comparing children, adolescents, and adults. (Modified from Fleischer et al. (2022). Pre-adolescent children exhibit lower aerosol particle volume emissions than adults for breathing, speaking, singing, and shouting. J R Soc Interface 19:20210833.20210833 and from Mürbe et al. (2021a) Aerosol emission of adolescents voices during speaking, singing, and shouting. PLoS ONE 16(2): e0246819. The box-and-whisker plots show the inter-quartile range (box), median (line in box), and maximum and minimum values (whiskers extending from box))

levels. For adolescents, $L_{AFmax}$ was in between that of children and adults for the different conditions.

## 32.1.4 Relevance for Singing and Speaking Activities

The present studies confirm the dependence of aerosol emission rates on different phonatory tasks. Considerably more aerosol particles were emitted during speaking than breathing at rest. Even higher particle emission rates have been recorded for singing than speaking (Mürbe et al. 2021b; Asadi et al. 2019; Alsved et al. 2020; Gregson et al. 2021), both of which are surpassed by emission rates observed during shouting (Mürbe et al. 2021a). Furthermore, the rate of emission depends substantially on the loudness of the vocalisation (Fig. 32.3).

Similar to the previous studies of particle emissions during speaking and singing, a large inter-subject variability was observed in all measurements. Thus, the aspect of high-emitters or super-emitters might need to be considered (Asadi et al. 2019).

Compared with adults', children's aerosol emission rates were substantially reduced for breathing at rest, speaking and singing conditions. More precisely, children emitted $P_M$ during speaking of the same order of magnitude as adults during breathing, and while singing, they emitted similar $P_M$ to the adults while speaking.

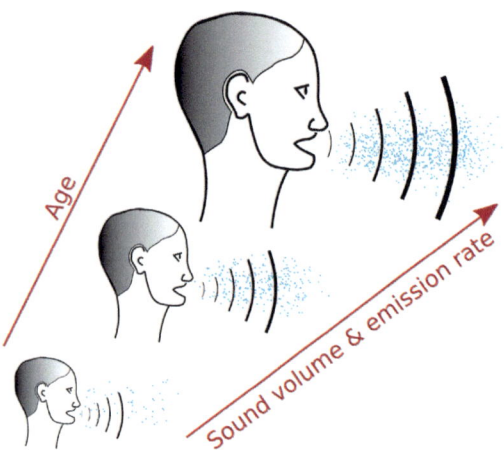

**Fig. 32.3** Dependence of aerosol emission rates during speaking and singing on vocal loudness and age. ©Mürbe and Fleischer 2022

Adolescents' emission rates were between the emission rates of adults and children. There might be different reasons for the low emission rates for child voices in comparison with that of adults. Before puberty voice changes, there are considerable differences in the vibration characteristics of the vocal folds from those of adults. Typical features of a child's vocal register in singing include differences in subglottal pressure and in contact time and contact area of the vocal folds during each vibration cycle. Furthermore, there are smaller anatomical proportions of the child's airways and vocal folds are shorter before pubertal voice changes. The lower sound intensity of the child group only partially explains the observed difference in these measures.

Owing to the increased risk of transmission of *SARS-CoV-2* viruses during singing and the described accumulation of these infections during choir rehearsals, the survey of particle emissions and the assessment of aerosols in rooms are key elements in the risk management of ensemble and choir singing in enclosed rooms (Hamner et al. 2020; Charlotte 2020; Miller et al. 2021). Since aerosols emitted during breathing, speaking, and singing are mainly <3 μm diameter, it cannot be assumed that they sink quickly to the ground, so the retention time might be in the range of minutes to hours.

Activities to reduce the aerosol input in closed rooms during singing include limiting the number of singers and the rehearsal or performance time, which contributes to a lower cumulative aerosol concentration. Apart from these issues, the individual emission rates of the singers determine the aerosol input into closed rooms. Other than emission rates, the risk of transmission depends on several further factors, including a prolonged stay of the infected person(s), insufficient ventilation (Shao et al. 2020), and small dimensions of the venue. As the basis of an aerogenic virus transmission, the spatial distribution of aerosols is dependent on several factors of the surrounding air, such as temperature and humidity (Morawska 2006).

The low aerosol emissions for children's voices during singing in comparison with those of adult singers could contribute to the development of more specific risk management strategies for different constellations of singing. It should be emphasised that the determined emission rates do not provide information about possible concentrations of *SARS-CoV-2* viruses yet. However, there are reasons to assume that an increasing amount of viral RNA will be emitted when the aerosol emission rate is increased. The number of aerosol particles likely to stay airborne because of their size is highly relevant for airborne transmission studies and estimating the infection risk. In contrast to particle concentrations, emission rates as determined within these studies can directly be applied in infection risk models for airborne viral transmission.

## 32.2 Flow Visualisation of Droplets and Aerosols During Singing and Playing Wind Instruments

Wolfgang Angerstein

### 32.2.1 Introduction

In March/April and July 2020 multiple outbreaks of COVID-19 were noticed in several choirs and during church singing (Charlotte 2020; Hamner et al. 2020; Katelaris et al. 2021; van der Lint 2020; Miller et al. 2021). It became clear pretty soon that the reason for these superspreading events was the transmission of SARS-CoV-2 by inhalation of aerosols with high viral loads. Thus, airborne transmission of the virus is nowadays considered to be the main mode of infection with COVID-19 (Abraham et al. 2021; Brockmann et al. 2021; Buonanno et al. 2020; Hartmann et al. 2020a, b; Lange et al. 2020; Morawska and Milton 2020; Morawska et al. 2020; Naunheim et al. 2021; Setti et al. 2020; Stadnytskyi et al. 2020; Sun et al. 2021; Tan et al. 2021; Zhang et al. 2020).

Consequently, the question came up, how airflow and the spreading of exhaled aerosols during musical performance (singing, playing wind instruments) can be visualised in order to protect the artists. This review is based on a study of roughly 250 literature sources. The survey is focused on:

- Explaining different flow visualisation methods and their historical development.
- Assessing the risk for Corona virus infections during singing and playing different wind instruments.
- Identifying possible prophylactic measures to prevent those infections.

The visualisation of flow started with the pioneering experiments of Leonardo da Vinci around 1500 (Cheng 1997). Today, flow visualisation is a world-wide recognised special field of physics that was scientifically established roughly during the last 50 years (Cheng 1997; Merzkirch 1987; Smits and Lim 2012). The rapid spread of this speciality was promoted by the progress in microelectronics and computational research.

## 32.2.2 Techniques for Visualisation of Aerosols in Exhaled Air Besides Schlieren Techniques

Due to vibrations of the vocal folds (in singers), of the lips (in brass players) or of the reed (in woodwind players), droplets are generated, swirled, and propelled into the exhaled air. Since the beginning of the Corona pandemic in early 2020, several techniques have been applied to visualise those exhaled air clouds during singing and playing wind instruments. These techniques represent fascinating interfaces somewhere between physics (flow dynamics), medicine (phoniatrics), and performing arts (music). They may be divided into direct and indirect examination methods.

### 32.2.2.1 Direct Methods for Visualising Exhaled Air Clouds

These either track and count the exhaled aerosol particles or visualise their clouds. Already in 1942 droplets were being visualised during articulation of consonants and vowels by stroboscopic illumination and high-speed photography (Jennison 1942). For particle tracking, nowadays light (laser, LED, halogen) beams are used. The exhaled aerosol particles are spotted with light.

"Due to refraction and reflection, the incident light ray is split into several rays" Chao et al. (2009)

and the deflection or scattering of the beam is registered by high-speed digital cameras. Thus, "light scattered by the droplets/particles" (Abraham et al. 2021; Bahl et al. 2021; Cheng et al. 2000; Brandt 2020; Merghani et al. 2021; Stadnytskyi et al. 2020) is recorded. Exactly the same principle was applied by Jennison in 1942 with stroboscopic light (Jennison 1942).

To perform particle tracking (Bahl et al. 2020, 2021; Dunker et al. 2020a, b), the background noise has to be subtracted and thus eliminated from the raw images. Within these background-subtracted frames, the facial contour of the examined person is detected in order to generate a mask for removing erroneous data spots. Finally, each particle is tracked and counted individually (see Figs. 32.4 and 32.5).

All these imaging steps (background noise subtraction, discarding data outside the area of interest by means of a facial contour mask, particle tracking and counting) are realised with computer-aided digital processing algorithms. For particle image velocimetry (PIV), the particles are illuminated with pulsed laser light (Chao et al. 2009; Cheng et al. 2000; Raffel et al. 2018; Zhu et al. 2006). A digital

**Fig. 32.4** Visualisation of an extreme (not representative) event of exhaled particles during singing (image composed of ten consecutive frames with an exposure time of 0.01 s each; image dimensions approximately 20 cm by 20 cm). (With kind permission of T. Dunker, J. Tschudi and M. O'Farrell (Dunker et al. 2020a))

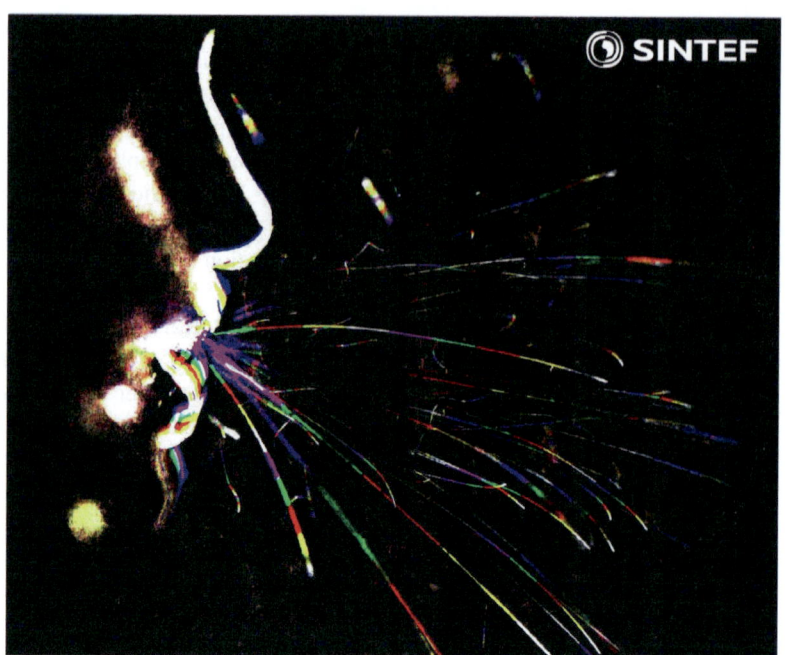

**Fig. 32.5** Droplets ejected from a horizontally held tuba's mouthpiece, its opening partially blocked by a finger (image composed of ten consecutive frames with an exposure time of 0.01 s each; image dimensions approximately 20 cm by 20 cm). (With kind permission of T. Dunker, J. Tschudi and M. O'Farrell (Dunker et al. 2020a))

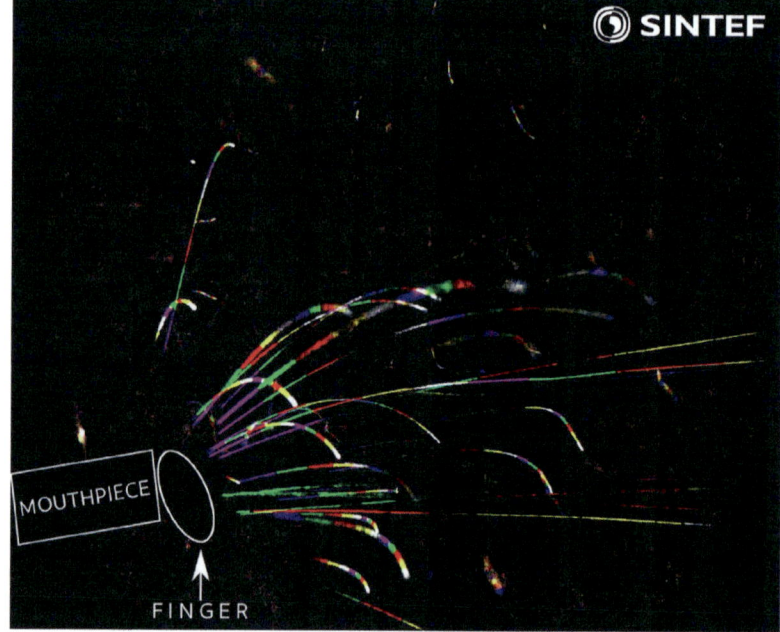

"camera acquires two single exposed images taken shortly one after another. By comparing these two sequential pictures, the travelled distance of individual particles can be determined" Kähler and Hain (2020); Merghani et al. (2021)

"The motion of small seeding particles is evaluated from a single frame recorded with double exposure or from two frames recorded in a suitable interval" Meier (2002)

Thus, the pathways of the particles can be tracked (Kwon et al. 2012).

For volumetric 3D representations, at least three synchronised high-resolution cameras are necessary. Thus, indoor flow fields (e.g., human thermal plumes or flows generated by breathing and speaking) may be studied with PIV (Cao et al. 2014). - Moreover, there are direct methods for visualising the spread of exhaled aerosol clouds. To detect the expansion of those clouds, illuminated smoke (e.g., that produced by e-cigarettes), illuminated artificial saline mist (theatrical/stage fog either from commercially available spray cans or generated by nebulisers) and schlieren may be used (Abkarian and Stone 2020; Echternach et al. 2020, 2021a; Gantner et al. 2021; Hermann et al. 2021; Ho et al. 2021a, b; Kniesburges et al. 2021; Lange et al. 2020; Merghani et al. 2021; Sterz 2020a, b; Stockman et al. 2021). The schlieren techniques will be explained later.

Flour (either in the mouth or in the palm of a hand during coughing, speaking, singing or in the bell of a brass instrument while playing) can also serve as a tracer to visualise the spreading of air (Bertsch 2020; Lau 2020; Zhu et al. 2006). Finally, chalk dust impregnated with fluorescent dye (strontium aluminate crystals) may be used to study the spreading of the dust cloud when the fluorescent chalk is placed within the bell of a brass instrument and illuminated by ultraviolet light (Moore and Cannaday 2020).

#### 32.2.2.2  Indirect Methods for Examining the Flow of Exhaled Aerosols

These measure the velocity of the air flow/particle stream (anemometry) (Richter et al. 2021; Spahn et al. 2021), the temperature changes caused by exhaled air jets (thermography with thermal imaging cameras) (Izdebski et al. 2017) or the room concentration of carbon dioxide ($CO_2$-monitors/visual displays with red/yellow/green "ventilation traffic lights") (Hartmann et al. 2020a, b).

$CO_2$ monitoring is used to indicate indoor air quality (Hartmann et al. 2020a, b; Nusseck et al. 2020; Umweltbundesamt 2008): the $CO_2$ concentration in rooms should not exceed 1000 ppm, and 800 ppm is

"the threshold at which ventilation especially during musical activities should take place" Nusseck et al. (2020)

$CO_2$ monitoring can also

"work as an indirect marker estimating the COVID-19-infection risk" Schade et al. (2021)

Monitoring the local $CO_2$ distribution in a room is an indirect measure of aerosol dispersion; the $CO_2$ concentration allows conclusions to be drawn about the concentration of infectious aerosols (Hartmann et al. 2020a, b; Nusseck et al. 2020; Schade et al. 2021). Lowering the $CO_2$ concentration by frequent ventilation reduces the aerosol concentration and thus the risk of infection (Hartmann et al. 2020a, b). Indoor $CO_2$ measurements may serve as a risk-reducing measure to prevent Coronavirus infections (Hartmann et al. 2020a, b; Nusseck et al. 2020; Schade et al. 2021). $CO_2$ monitoring is important for assessing the potential hazard of viral contamination.

Another indirect method for visualising the spread of exhaled aerosol clouds is the use of candles or tea lights lined up every 50 cm in a row (Bertsch 2020; Lau 2020): The emitted airflow during singing or playing a wind instrument makes the candles/tea lights flicker or even blows them out when they form a straight line.

### 32.2.3  Schlieren Techniques

The German word "Schlieren "means "streaks", "striae", "striations" or "cords" (though the German noun is always capitalised, in customary English usage the capitalisation is dropped) (Rienitz 1997; Settles 2001).

The German word "Schliere" designates a local optical inhomogeneity in a transparent medium. Raffel et al. (2018).

Schliere

"describe disturbances in inhomogeneous transparent media" Becher et al. (2020a, c)

with streak-like flow. They arise from light refractions due to density variations in the atmosphere, in liquids (Settles 2001) or in glass lenses and mirrors. Schlieren represent local differences or inequalities of light refraction (Rienitz 1997).

Density gradients in transparent media (gases and vapours, fluids, glasses, and mirrors) generating unequal optical densities cause unequal light refraction (Merghani et al. 2021; Rienitz 1975) due to different indices of refraction.

> "If light reaches a medium with different density, light rays will change their speed and therefore become deflected to the extent defined by the density gradient. The result is discontinuous movement which occurs as a schliere" Becher et al. (2020a, c)

These density gradients or changes in refractive index are based on differences in temperature or pressure (Abraham et al. 2021; Becher et al. 2021; Gena et al. 2020; Raffel 2015), they allow visualisation of local optical inhomogeneities in transparent media as bright and dark areas in schlieren pictures (Krehl and Engemann 1995). The differences in brightness correspond to the differences in density (Becher et al. 2020a). Thus,

non-invasive real-time observations of liquid and gaseous flow are possible.

It was the German physicist and chemist August Töpler (1836–1912) who introduced the name "schlieren". He made the technique popular and widely known among scientists. In 1864 and 1867 he published an experimental set-up for visualising schlieren (Krehl and Engemann 1995; Raffel 2015; Töpler 1864, 1867). His apparatus with a telescope is shown in Fig. 32.6.

He demonstrated it at the World Fair in Paris. The physicist Ernst Abbe was one of the early scientists who designed handier and more practical advancements of Töpler's schlieren apparatus (Czapski 1885). But only Töpler re-invented and further developed the schlieren method. Its first known description dates back to Robert Hooke (1635–1703): in 1672 he introduced his schlieren experiments to the Royal Society of London (Mazumdar 2013; Rienitz 1975, 1997; Settles

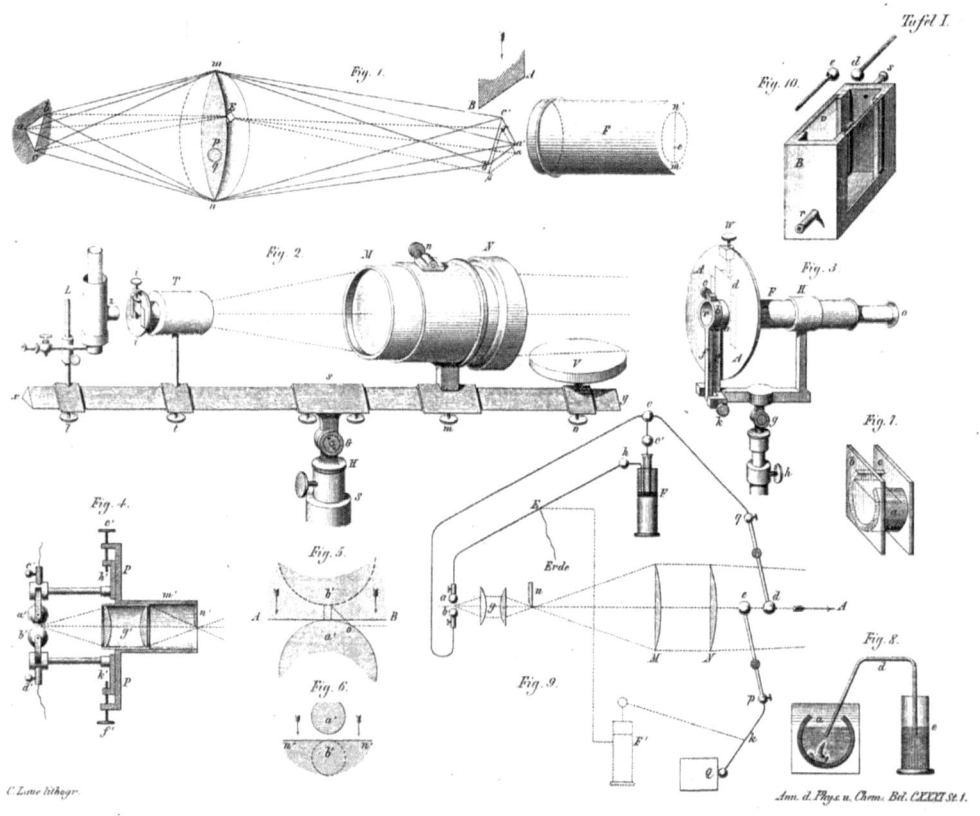

**Fig. 32.6** Schlieren observation apparatus with a telescope for optical studies (Töpler 1867)

2001). In his book "Micrographia" (published in 1665) he even explained the "heat haze" (mirage, fata morgana) as a schlieren phenomenon: this optical illusion is due to density and temperature variations in the atmosphere with thermal air disturbances (warm air is less dense than the ambient) causing unequal refractions of the sunlight (Settles 2001). Thus, air ascending from dry, hot earth makes objects appear "to be undulated or shaken", and

> "you shall find a tremulation and wavering of the remote object"   Hooke cited by Rienitz (1997), Settles (2001)

So

> "the principle of schlieren is similar to the observation of heat shimmer or fata morganas when density changes between the human eye and a distant object lead to distortion or even reflections"   Becher et al. (2020c)

like a mirror (Raffel 2015). Later on, the schlieren technique was described and applied by the well-known scientists Christiaan Huygens in 1685 and Léon Foucault in 1859 (Mazumdar 2013; Rienitz 1975, 1997; Settles 2001). In 1780, the French revolutionary Jean Paul Marat was the first medical doctor who mentioned schlieren, when he published pictures of thermal plumes of candles and heated metal objects (Rienitz 1997; Settles 2001).

By using his schlieren method, Töpler was the first to visualise the propagation and reflection of shock waves (Krehl and Engemann 1995). Shock waves are supersonic phenomena with abrupt, almost instantaneous pressure changes. The wave front is a region of propagating disturbance with sudden and violent changes in pressure, density and temperature of the medium in which shock waves travel (e.g. air). Thus, shock waves are characterised by a very short but extremely strong impulse of air, they are "sharp pressure waves" (Krehl and Engemann 1995) with steep high amplitudes. August Töpler was the first to visualise shock waves (Krehl and Engemann 1995), the physicist Ernst Mach (1838–1916) was the first to publish photos of shock waves in 1886 and 1887 (Cheng 1997; Dvořák 1990). His son Ludwig

Mach (1868–1951), a medical doctor, continued his father's schlieren research with shock waves. In 1896 he published a paper "On the visualisation of air streamlines" ("Ueber die Sichtbarmachung von Luftstromlinien") in the "Journal of Airship Travel and Physics of the Atmosphere" ("Zeitschrift für Luftschiffahrt und Physik der Atmosphäre") (Mach 1896).

Thus, at least two medical doctors (Jean Paul Marat and Ludwig Mach) participated in establishing and applying the schlieren method. But what does schlieren imaging have to do with musical performance (singing, playing on wind instruments)?

- Schlieren techniques have been used to visualise shock waves radiating from the open end of brass wind instruments (trombones: Hirschberg et al. 1996; Zielinski 2011; trumpets: López-Carromero et al. 2017; Pandya et al. 2003; Rendón et al. 2018; didjeridu: Tarnopolsky and Fletcher 2004; Tarnopolsky et al. 2006).
- "Shock waves represent a stark and sudden change in refractive index" of the air, therefore "they show up clearly in schlieren photographs" Zielinsky (2011)
- Schlieren techniques allow the documentation and examination of indoor air flows (Becher et al. 2020c; Settles and Via 1987). They are also useful for studying the human thermal plume (Gena et al. 2020; Settles 1985; Settles and Kuhns 1984). Exhaled human airflows during such respiratory activities as breathing, coughing, laughing, sneezing, speaking or whistling may also be observed with the schlieren technique (Settles and Kuhns 1984; Stockman et al. 2021; Tang et al. 2011). Finally, the spread of exhaled air from wind instruments and singers may be visualised by schlieren (Becher et al. 2020a, b, 2021).

The air emerging from the human body (e.g., during expiratory activities like speaking, singing or playing a wind instrument)

> "has a higher temperature or humidity (or both) than the surrounding air" Becher et al. (2020a)

Thus,

"a density gradient is induced by the temperature difference between the (colder) ambient air and the (warmer) exhaled air" Abraham et al. (2021); Merghani et al. (2021)

This allows visualising the air escaping from the mouth or from wind instruments.

Owing to the immense progress in computational imaging and the rapid development of high-speed digital cameras with ultrafast framing rates, the "Background-Orientated Schlieren" (BOS) method was established by 1999 (Becher et al. 2020a, c; Gardner et al. 2020; Hargather and Settles 2012; Mazumdar 2013; Meier 2002; Raffel 2015; Settles and Hargather 2017). Nowadays, high-speed schlieren systems with digital image processing are "state of the art". "Background-orientated" describes the fact that the focus and the reference of this technique is the illuminated background and the object behind the flow (Elsinga et al. 2004; Meier 2002; Raffel 2015). This irregular background of the test volume is a random dot pattern (randomised grid of tiny black pixels on a white surface) (Elsinga et al. 2004; Gardner et al. 2020; Goldhahn and Seume 2007; Hargather and Settles 2012; Meier 2002; Raffel 2015). The background is visualised once without flow (reference image, no deflection, no distortion) and once with flow (measurement image, deflected by schlieren object, distortions due to refraction) (Elsinga et al. 2004; Hargather and Settles 2012; Richard and Raffel 2001; Settles and Hargather 2017). Thus, both the undisturbed background structure ("flowoff") and the density gradient in front of the background ("flow-on") are recorded by cameras.

"Due to the refractive index, each light ray passing through the measuring field is refracted, so that a pixel on the flow-on image appears at a different position compared to the reference (flow-off) image. Using computer-aided algorithms, it is then possible to determine the image shift of each individual pixel and thus, to visualise the density gradient" Becher et al. (2020a)

So,

"BOS systems detect refractive-index deflections by comparing an image of an undistorted background with a schlieren distorted background

obstructed by refracting flow" Mazumdar (2013); Meier (2002)

The virtual displacement or movement of the background patterns can be calculated by numerical comparison with image correlation algorithms (Hargather and Settles 2012; Meier 2002; Richard and Raffel 2001; Settles and Hargather 2017), it is related to and contains information about the refractive index of the test volume. For even more precise studies, light rays coming from the schlieren probe may be optically encoded with colour and intensity variations (Mazumdar 2013; Settles 1985, 2001; Settles and Hargather 2017). By using several synchronised digital cameras at different viewing angles, the flow field can be reconstructed stereoscopically, i.e., three-dimensionally (Goldhahn and Seume 2007; Meier 2002). Thus, owing to a large number of synchronised images from different observation points, a visualisation of three-dimensional flow fields of schlieren objects is possible (Becher et al. 2020c; Mazumdar 2013; Meier 2002). Schlieren and BOS imaging of thermal plumes is nowadays even possible on smartphones (Miller and Loebner 2016; Settles 2018). The BOS method has been applied to study airflows during singing and playing different wind instruments (Becher et al. 2020a, 2021).

### 32.2.4  Results of Visualisation of Droplets and Aerosols

Droplets are not only expelled during coughing (Jennison 1942; Lange et al. 2020; Tan et al. 2021; Xie et al. 2009; Zhu et al. 2006) and sneezing (Bahl et al. 2020; Jennison 1942), but also during speaking (Anfinrud et al. 2020; Lange et al. 2020; Jennison 1942; Xie et al. 2009) and singing (Bahl et al. 2021; Lange et al. 2020). These droplets

"do not settle rapidly and may follow the ambient airflow pattern" Bahl et al. (2021)

Therefore, it is possible

"that small particles containing the SARS-CoV-2 virus may diffuse in indoor environments covering distances up to 10 m from the emission sources" Setti et al. (2020)

thus representing airborne transmission of virus-laden aerosols.

"These particles are too small to settle because of gravity, but they are carried by air currents and dispersed by diffusion and air turbulence" Meselson (2020)

The aerosol particles

"continue to linger in the air and disperse" due to "convection by ambient air currents" or due to "turbulent eddy-driven diffusion" Tan et al. (2021)

For hitherto unknown reasons,

certain persons called "super spreaders" produce many more aerosol particles than other persons   Gregson et al. (2021); Meselson (2020)

These

"individuals emit particles at a rate more than an order of magnitude larger than their peers, they behave as speech super-emitters. … Speech super-emitters might contribute to the phenomenon of "superspreading", in which relative few contagious individuals infect a … large number of secondary cases" Asadi et al. (2019)

"Super-emitters produce an unusually large number of droplets during speech, and super-shedders have large viral titers in their mucus and saliva, and the combination has been suggested to be a defining characteristic of superspreaders" Abkarian and Stone (2020)

### 32.2.4.1  Results of Visualisation of Droplets and Aerosols in Speaking and Singing

There is

"a strong correlation between the amplitude of human speech and the emission rate of … aerosol particles"  Asadi et al. (2020)

The louder the vocalisation, the more particles are emitted (Alsved et al. 2020; Anfinrud et al. 2020; Archer et al. 2022; Asadi et al. 2019; Gregson et al. 2021; Jennison 1942; McCarthy et al. 2021; Mürbe et al. 2021a, b; Stadnytskyi et al. 2020). This is true for both speaking and singing (e.g. increasing loudness from piano to forte). Singing generates many more aerosol particles than speaking (Alsved et al. 2020; Archer

et al. 2022; Dunker et al. 2020a, b; Gregson et al. 2021; Hartmann et al. 2020c, d; Mürbe et al. 2021a, b, c; Nusseck et al. 2020):

"Compared to breathing through the nose, an average increase of about factor 10 was described for speaking, and for singing an average increase of about factor 30 was described compared to speaking" Hartmann et al. (2020c, d)

Archer et al. found even greater differences between breathing and speaking (Archer et al. 2022). For children and adolescents, lower aerosol emission rates during singing were measured than for adult singers (Mürbe et al. 2021b, c). But another study showed that

"children and adults generate similar aerosol concentrations when performing the same activity" (speaking, singing) Archer et al. (2022)

There is still another study with different results: here,

"singing a note produced the most droplets (more droplets over a longer period), whereas singing Happy Birthday produced a similar number to speaking". There was "no consistency between participants as to which task (speaking, singing) generated the most droplets…", and "no clear hierarchy between vocal tasks" could be observed, since "wide variation existed for droplet production" Ho et al. (2021a, b)

In adult singers, voices with higher pitches tend to higher particle emission rates compared with lower pitched voices (Mürbe et al. 2021a).

According to a Japanese study (Ono 2020), a bass singer produced more aerosol particles than a soprano singer and also more aerosol particles than wind instrument players. Songs with "many bursts on the consonants" created particularly many aerosol particles. When the singer

"stood 0.65 m from the measuring instrument, it clearly registered the aerosol. When he stood 1.8 m away from it, the reading was much smaller" Ono (2020)

"A warm-up exercise where one lets the lips vibrate during exhalation (without activating the vocal cords) generated immense amounts of droplets" Alsved et al. (2020)

This exercise is very popular among singers and wind instrument players. The voiceless plosive or stop consonant /t/ seems to have a high airflow rate. This is the only consistent result of almost all studies dealing with the exhalation of droplets during articulation of different vowels, consonants, and syllables (Abkarian and Stone 2020; Alsved et al. 2020; Jennison 1942; Lau 2020; Tan et al. 2021). Compared with vowels,

> "consonants … largely enhance the distance reached by the impulse dispersion" of aerosols. "Consonants are associated with greater dispersions than vowels," Westphalen et al. (2021)

they

> "generate the largest number of droplets, … much greater than those for vowels". Abkarian and Stone (2020)

Within a glycerine-propylene glycol cloud (e-cigarettes)

> "vowels … in loud and whispered voices" show higher airflow velocities "than in normal voice". There is a "great variability in the expired air velocities", but the "velocities … during vocal exercises" are generally "slower than in long exhalation" Giovanni et al. (2021)

Speaking made a candle flicker at a distance of 1 m and blew the candle out at a distance of 0.4 m (Bertsch 2020).

The length of a propylene cloud (e-cigarettes) during sustained phonation of the vowel /a/ was 0.45 m (Giovanni et al. 2021). Another group of researchers conducted several studies (Echternach et al. 2020, 2021a; Hermann et al. 2021; Kniesburges et al. 2021) with the vapour of e-cigarettes (glycerine and propylene glycol) to evaluate the dimensions of aerosol clouds during singing: the maximum expansion in sagittal direction (front−back) was 1.96 m, in horizontal direction (left side−right side) 1.98 m and in vertical direction (upwards−downwards resp. top-bottom) 1.38 m. Thus, the biggest aerosol clouds were a little less than 2 m long and wide and less than 1.5 m high. Amateur singers showed

> "larger distances for all spatial directions in comparison to professional singers", probably due to "less efficient breath control and smaller mouth openings" of the amateurs. Hermann et al. (2021)

Increasing mouth opening decreases the airflow velocity during singing (Kähler and Hain 2020). In a study with air velocity sensors (anemometers) and artificial mist (commercially available stage fog consisting of water droplets), no airflows during singing were measurable beyond a distance of 1.5 m (Richter et al. 2021). These results did "not depend on volume, pitch or the style of singing." Singing reached higher air velocities than woodwind playing and about the same air velocities as speaking. Significant airflows during singing were measured only at a distance of 1 m from the singers' mouths. Two other studies (Kähler and Hain 2020; Sterz 2020b) had similar results: droplets and air clouds produced by singers were illuminated with a laser (Kähler and Hain 2020) or with powerful spotlights (Sterz 2020b).

> "The experiments clearly showed that air was only set in motion in the immediate vicinity of the mouth when singing. … At a distance of around 0.5 m almost no air movement could be detected" Kähler and Hain (2020)

regardless of volume, pitch or whether the singer was a professional or an amateur. The second study (Sterz 2020b) demonstrated that during singing the "extension of the aerosol cloud, particularly in frontal direction", reached a maximum of 0.9 m. "Strong expiration" (especially of the bass singer) resulted in an extension of 1.5 m, and normal breathing showed a maximum extension of 0.5 m. When tracked by stroboscopic light and high-speed photography,

> "in speaking the majority of droplets was not expelled farther than about one foot" Jennison (1942)

The maximum droplet penetration distance during "loud" vocalisation was about 1.3 m and about 0.6 m during "normal" vocalisation (Tan et al. 2021), when measured by particle image velocimetry (PIV).

### 32.2.4.2 Results of Visualisation of Droplets and Aerosols in Playing Wind Instruments

Compared with breathing, aerosol emission rates while playing wind instruments seem to be lower (Parker and Crookston 2020) or at least similar

(McCarthy et al. 2021). Compared with speaking and singing at high volume, aerosol emission rates while playing wind instruments were lower (McCarthy et al. 2021; Ono 2020; Parker and Crookston 2020). In one Japanese study (Ono 2020), the aerosol production of wind instrument players

> "was less than that of a male singer (bass). The wind instrument tests showed that players make less spray during a concert than they do in daily conversations" Ono (2020)

But another

> "study showed that performing with musical instruments produced a greater number of airborne particles compared to normal speaking levels and comparable levels to singing and theater performances" Stockman et al. (2021)

When measuring the dimensions of aerosol clouds produced by the vapour of e-cigarettes (glycerine and propylene glycol), speaking showed "much lower" expansions in the frontal direction than playing wind instruments (Gantner et al. 2021), while von Zadow et al. (2021) measured higher aerosol emission rates for playing flutes, oboes, trumpets or clarinets than during speaking. Compared with singing, aerosol emission rates in this study (von Zadow et al. 2021) were lower for playing flutes or oboes and similar to the aerosol emission rates of trumpets or clarinets. Parker and Crookston (2020) found more large droplets by playing brass instruments than during breathing.

Many wind instruments have been examined for particle emission (see Table 32.1).

Their aerosol generation and concentration depends on several factors concerning the musician and his environment, the instrument, and the piece of music played (see Table 32.2). In brass instruments (trumpet, bass trombone, French horn, tuba), for example, the total tube length is inversely correlated with the aerosol concentration at the outlet (He et al. 2021). – A Japanese study revealed "much less... aerosol from wind instruments compared with... European Orchestras.... This might relate to the difference in humidity of the air in Japan – the air in Europe is much drier than in Japan" Ono (2020)

Regarding the amount of expelled droplets and aerosols, high risk and low risk instruments can be identified:

> "Plastic blowing horns (vuvuzelas)" emit "extremely large numbers of aerosols", namely "approximately 4 million particles per second" Lai et al. (2011)

> "Straight, long instruments with conically increasing diameter like vuvuzelas have the capacity to propel very large numbers of aerosols into the air" Gantner et al. (2021)

The vuvuzela can therefore be regarded as a "super spreader".–In classical orchestras, transverse flutes distribute aerosols up to 2 m in enclosed rooms (Tur et al. 2021). Transverse flutes are mentioned most often as high or the highest risk instruments (Becher et al. 2020a, b, 2021; Brandt 2020; Gantner et al. 2021; Kähler and Hain 2020; Lau 2020; Sterz 2020a; Tur et al. 2021), followed by the oboe (Becher et al. 2020a, 2021; Brandt 2020; He et al. 2021; Kähler and Hain 2020; Spahn et al. 2021) and

**Table 32.1** Wind instruments examined for particle emissions or exhaled air clouds (Abraham et al. 2021; Becher et al. 2020a, b, 2021; Bertsch 2020; Brandt 2020; Dunker et al. 2020a, b; Eiche 2020; Gantner et al. 2021; He et al. 2021; Kähler and Hain 2020; Lai et al. 2011; Lau 2020; McCarthy et al. 2021; Moore and Cannaday 2020; Nusseck et al. 2020; Parker and Crookston 2020; Spahn et al. 2021; Sterz 2020a; Stockman et al. 2021; Tur et al. 2021; von Zadow et al. 2021)

| Brass instruments | Cornet, trumpet, French horn, tenor horn, baritone (horn), tenor trombone, bass trombone, tuba, euphonium, vuvuzela |
|---|---|
| Single reed woodwind instruments | Clarinet, bass clarinet, basset horn, Alto saxophone, tenor saxophone |
| Double reed woodwind instruments | Bassoon, contrabassoon, oboe, oboe d'amore, English horn/cor anglais |
| Flutes/recorders/ Air jet instruments | Piccolo flute, soprano flute, alto flute, Grand/traverse/transverse/cross flute |

**Table 32.2** Factors affecting aerosol generation and concentration of wind instruments (Abraham et al. 2021; Becher et al. 2020a, b, 2021; Gantner et al. 2021; He et al. 2021; Kähler and Hain 2020; Ono 2020; Spahn et al. 2021)

- Pitch, dynamic level (loudness/musical amplitude), and note/phrase duration
- Articulation (smooth, slurred and connected = legato vs. short, impulsive and separated = staccato)
- Lung volumes, breathing patterns, respiratory pressure, intermittent exhalation between phrases
- Movements of musicians and instruments (e.g., trombone slide)
- Angle at which the instrument is held and at which the air escapes
- Individual playing styles/blowing techniques (e.g., such tongue and lip motions as tongue ram, fluttering tongue, jet whistle)
- Dampers and stopping mutes
- Design of instrument (coiling, tube length, tube diameter, tube straight or bent/tortuous, bell size/diameter = width of outlet, bore size, inlet, inner walls, bifurcations, mouthpiece)
- Air leakage (at labium, mouth plate with blow hole, near mouthpiece or at tone holes = key holes), air flow (laminar, turbulent), and air velocity
- REED selection (width of opening, hardness/stiffness)
- Air humidity and temperature

bassoon (Abraham et al. 2021; Becher et al. 2020a, 2021; Brandt 2020; Kähler and Hain 2020), trumpets (Abraham et al. 2021; He et al. 2021; von Zadow et al. 2021) and clarinets (Abraham et al. 2021; Becher et al. 2020a, 2021; Kähler and Hain 2020; Tur et al. 2021; von Zadow et al. 2021). On the other hand, tubas are usually considered as low risk instruments (Abraham et al. 2021; Becher et al. 2020a, 2021; Brandt 2020; Dunker et al. 2020a, b). Only two studies (McCarthy et al. 2021; Parker and Crookston 2020) found no significant differences in particle emission between the various wind instruments:

"No single instrument consistently emits significantly more or fewer particles than any other instrument" McCarthy et al. (2021)

"The variation in particle release between different instruments appeared to be less significant than ... between individual players ... as no discernible pattern related to either instrument size or design could be established" Parker and Crookston (2020)

In a study with air velocity sensors (anemometers) and artificial mist (commercially available stage fog consisting of water droplets),

"no airflows escaping from any of the 14 wind instruments ... were measurable beyond a distance of 1.5 m, regardless of volume, pitch or what was played" Spahn et al. (2021)

Closer than 1.5 m, oboes produced the highest air velocities in the frontal direction.

"Most wind instruments did not have any visual or measurable influence on the movement of compartment air" in the concert hall. Spahn et al. (2021)

Two other studies (Kähler and Hain 2020; Sterz 2020a) had similar results: droplets and air clouds produced by wind instrument players were illuminated with a laser (Kähler and Hain 2020) or with powerful spotlights (Sterz 2020a).

"The moving air area in front of the brass instruments ... was smaller than 0.5 m. ... With a clarinet, an oboe and a bassoon, especially low and long-lasting tones could lead to larger flow movements (in the range around 1 m for the clarinet and oboe and above 1 m for the bassoon). ... An even greater range could be achieved with a transverse flute for long, low notes. ... The risk of infection emanating from this instrument is much greater than from any other instrument examined. ... The large brass instruments (trombone, euphonium) were not able to influence the flow over a large area" Kähler and Hain (2020)

The second study (Sterz 2020a) demonstrated that during wind instrument play the exhaled air clouds had a maximum extension of 0.5 m. The only exception was the transverse flute with a dissemination up to 0.75 m. The exhaled air originated almost entirely from the players' mouths and noses, the openings of the instruments showed hardly any outflow. The maximum range of air jets generated by playing wind instruments was about 2 m when measured with the illuminated vapour of e-cigarettes (glycerine and propylene glycol) (Echternach et al. 2020, 2021a; Hermann et al. 2021; Kniesburges et al. 2021; Tur et al. 2021), usually the spreading distance of the exhaled air jets was less than 1.2 m (Becher et al. 2020a, b, 2021). This holds true for all the above-mentioned studies. Wind instruments (both brass and woodwinds) had the highest $CO_2$ emissions of all instruments tested, whereas

> "singers showed low $CO_2$ emission rates comparable to the control group which only spoke and listened" Nusseck et al. (2020)

### 32.2.4.3  Summary of the Distance Measurements

Summing up the results of all the above-mentioned studies that measured the extension of aerosol clouds during singing or playing wind instruments, the maximum extension for singing was 1.96 m in the frontal direction, 1.98 m in the horizontal, and 1.38 m in the vertical direction. For playing wind instruments, the maximum frontal extension of air jets was 2 m. Therefore, a distance of 2.5 m between singers or wind instrumentalists should be fairly safe regarding airborne virus transmission.

### 32.2.5  Discussion and Conclusions

When evaluating the risk of airborne infections, droplets (larger particles) and aerosols (smaller particles) must be distinguished: droplets have spit-like ballistic trajectories (see Figs. 32.4 and 32.5) and fall to the ground within less than 2 m from their origin (mostly less than 1.2 m) (Dunker et al. 2020a, b; Kähler and Hain 2020). Aerosols spread because of air movements which are often induced by human thermal plumes (Craven and Settles 2006; Salmanzadeh et al. 2012; Sun et al. 2021) and convection flows (Kriegel and Hartmann 2020a, b). The aerosols may easily be transported for several metres by such air streams (Jennison 1942).

> "Large particles (droplets) quickly settle to the ground, while small particles (aerosols) are entrained with the air flow" Hedworth et al. (2021)

Thus, long distance infections by aerosols are much more important than short distance infections by droplets when considering the risk of airborne virus dissemination.

### 32.2.5.1  Mitigation Strategies

> "While virus transmission via droplets can be mainly handled by distance and hygiene rules, the risk management of transmission through virus carrying aerosols has to be addressed with further strategies" Mürbe et al. (2021b)

These mitigation strategies include the rearranging of musicians within their orchestras (e.g., staggered positioning, placing wind instrumentalists with high emission rates in the front row or near the doors), altering the airflow (e.g., by opening doors or windows, introducing air conditioning and air filtration systems) and thereby improving ventilation and cleaning, limiting the numbers of singers or wind instrumentalists according to the size of the room or stage, or limiting the rehearsal or performance time (Abraham et al. 2021; Hartmann et al. 2020c, d; Hedworth et al. 2021; Kähler and Hain 2020; Mürbe et al. 2021b).

The air cleaning and ventilation measures should take advantage of the upward motion of the human thermal plume (Craven and Settles 2006; Gena et al. 2020; Salmanzadeh et al. 2012). Thus, air cleaning systems are most effective when they are positioned above the musicians close to the ceiling.

> "The thermal plume is generated by the temperature difference between the human body and the surroundings. This plume can be strengthened by increasing the temperature difference, i.e., reducing the ambient temperature" Abraham et al. (2021)

By lowering the temperature on stage (e.g., from 25 °C to 20 °C), the upward motion of the thermal plume becomes stronger, thereby driving more aerosols vertically upwards into the air cleaners. Thus, the air "filtration efficiency increases considerably" (Abraham et al. 2021).

Beside these strategies for minimising the risk of aerosol accumulation and spread, ultraviolet (UV) light may be used to inactivate airborne human corona viruses (Buonanno et al. 2020; Reed 2010; Schuit et al. 2020). It seems quite conceivable to install UV light barriers or UV light "showers" on stages (Wieser et al. 2021).

### 32.2.5.2 Limitations

The above-mentioned examination techniques have certain limitations:

- Schlieren, smoke from e-cigarettes, artificial fog, flour, chalk dust, the flickering of candles/tea lights and thermography only show the spreading and extent of exhaled air clouds and
- "can be used to determine the direction of the expelled particles" Becher et al. (2021)
- But they do not give any information regarding the number or concentration of aerosols within those clouds.

"The actual dispersion of aerosols is not recorded. Therefore, the evaluations can only be used to determine how far and to which extent the exhaled air is transported directly into the room" Becher et al. (2020a)

"The actual spread of infectious particles cannot be estimated" Becher et al. (2021)

- Particle tracking devices with light beams are able to count the number of emitted aerosols, but they do not show their clouds. They

"deliver the particle count and size only at a specific point in the room and thus are not applicable to acquire the spatial and temporal dynamics of an aerosol cloud" Kniesburges et al. (2021)

Thus, a combination of these complementary examination methods would be optimal. But for economical reasons, such a combination can hardly ever be realised.

None of the above-mentioned techniques allow any statement as to whether the exhaled particles contain viruses or not: they

"do not provide quantification of viral load" Archer et al. (2022)

which depends, among other factors, on air temperature and humidity. It is also unclear how many virus particles are necessary for an infection (Echternach et al. 2021b).

- Schlieren techniques including BOS (background-orientated schlieren)

"only visualize refractive index gradients that occur due to density gradients in transparent media", thus they "only detect flows based on a density gradient". "If the density gradients (i.e., differences in temperature or pressure) become too small, neither the schlieren imaging nor the BOS method can visualize these gradients" Becher et al. (2021)

- "Longer instruments with wide bores can cool the breathing air to the extent that it cannot be visualized using the schlieren method (e.g. F tuba)" Becher et al. (2020a)

- Another problem may occur with trombones and French horns:

"The musician's hand in or near the bell interferes with … flow measurements using schlieren data" Abraham et al. (2021)

- And finally, sometimes

"the air stream is transported further into the room than the schlieren mirror can detect" Becher et al. (2020a)

This happens when the diameter of the mirror is smaller than the length of the exhaled cloud. Then the air stream extends beyond the margin of the schlieren mirror. – But even when all these limitations are taken into account, computer-assisted flow visualisation techniques nowadays permit accurate measurements of exhaled particles during singing and playing wind instruments. Thus, these techniques contribute significantly to reduce the risk of airborne virus infections.

**Research is a virus that will never stop infecting.**

## References

Abkarian M, Stone HA (2020) Stretching and break-up of saliva filaments during speech: a route for pathogen aerosolization and its potential mitigation. Phys Rev Fluids 5(10):102301. https://doi.org/10.1103/PhysRevFluids.5.102301

Abkarian M, Mendez S, Xue N, Yang F, Stone HA (2020) Speech can produce jet-like transport relevant to asymptomatic spreading of virus. Proc Natl Acad Sci USA 117(41):25237–25245

Abraham A, He R, Shao S et al (2021) Risk assessment and mitigation of airborne disease transmission in orchestral wind instrument performance. J Aerosol Sci 157:105797. https://doi.org/10.1101/2020.12.23.20248652

Alsved M, Matamis A, Bohlin R et al (2020) Exhaled respiratory particles during singing and talking. Aerosol Sci Technol 54(11):1245–1248

Anfinrud P, Stadnytskyi V, Bax CE et al (2020) Visualizing speech-generated oral fluid droplets with laser light scattering. N Engl J Med 382(21):2061–2063

Archer J, McCarthy LP, Symons HE et al (2022) Comparing aerosol number and mass exhalation rates from children and adults during breathing, speaking and singing. Interface Focus 12(2):20210078. https://doi.org/10.1098/rsfs.2021.0078

Asadi S, Wexler AS, Cappa CD et al (2019) Aerosol emission and superemission during human speech increase with voice loudness. Sci Rep 9(1):2348. https://doi.org/10.1038/s41598-019-38808-z

Asadi S, Wexler AS, Cappa CD et al (2020) Effect of voicing and articulation manner on aerosol particle emission during human speech. PLoS One 15(1):e0227699. https://doi.org/10.1371/journal.pone.0227699

Bahl P, de Silva CM, Chughtai AA et al (2020) An experimental framework to capture the flow dynamics of droplets expelled by a sneeze. Exp Fluids 61(8):176. https://doi.org/10.1007/s00348-020-03008-3

Bahl P, de Silva CM, Bhattacharjee S et al (2021) Droplets and aerosols generated by singing and the risk of coronavirus disease 2019 for choirs. Clin Infect Dis 72(10):e639–e641

Becher L, Gena AW, Voelker C et al (2020a) Risk assessment of the spread of breathing air from wind instruments and singers during the COVID-19 pandemic. Bauhaus-Universität, Weimar. https://www.uni-weimar.de/fileadmin/user/fak/bauing/professuren_institute/Bauphysik/00_Aktuelles/Risk_assessment_of_the_spread_of_breathing_air_from_wind_instruments_and_singers_during_the_COVID-19_pandemic_01.pdf. https://doi.org/10.13140/RG.2.2.18313.67683/1

Becher L, Mühlenberend A, Gena AW et al (2020b) Einsatz von Filtern zur Reduktion der Ausbreitung der Atemluft beim Spielen von Blasinstrumenten und beim Singen während der COVID-19 Pandemie. (use of filters to reduce the spread of breathing air when playing wind instruments and singing during the COVID-19 pandemic). Musik Musik 27(3):97–102

Becher L, Voelker C, Rodehorst V et al (2020c) Background-oriented Schlieren technique for two-dimensional visualization of convective indoor air flows. Opt Lasers Eng 134:106282. https://doi.org/10.1016/j.optlaseng.2020.106282

Becher L, Gena AW, Alsaad H et al (2021) The spread of breathing air from wind instruments and singers using Schlieren techniques. Indoor Air 31(6):1798–1814

Bertsch M (2020) Sind Blasinstrumente Virenschleudern? Experimente und Erklärungen mit Trompete und Posaune (Are wind instruments virus slingshots? Experiments and explanations with trumpet and trombone). https://www.mdw.ac.at/mrm/iasbs/virenschleuder-blasinstrumente/. Accessed 23 Jun 2022

Brandt L (2020) Measurement of aerosol from brass and woodwind instruments playing 5 minutes in distances from 0.5 to 4 meter. Center for Performing Arts Medicine, Odense University Hospital, University of Southern Denmark. https://www.makingmusic.org.uk/sites/makingmusic.org.uk/files/Measurement%20of%20aerosol%20from%20brass%20and%20woodwind%20instruments%20.pdf. Accessed 23 Jun 2022

Brockmann S, Dittler A, Grün G et al (2021) Stellungnahme des "Expertenkreises Aerosole": aerosole und SARS-CoV-2—Entstehung, Infektiosität, Ausbreitung und Minderung luftgetragener, virenhaltiger Teilchen in der Atemluft (statement of the "expert group aerosols": aerosols and SARS-CoV-2—formation, infectivity, spread and reduction of airborne, virus-containing particles in the air we breathe). Gesundheitswesen 83(3):231–234

Buonanno M, Welch D, Shuryak I, Brenner DJ (2020) Far-UVC light (222 nm) efficiently and safely inactivates airborne human coronaviruses. Sci Rep 10(1):10285. https://doi.org/10.1038/s41598-020-67211-2

Cao X, Liu J, Jiang N et al (2014) Particle image velocimetry measurement of indoor airflow field: a review of the technologies and applications. Energ Buildings 69:367–380

Chao CYH, Wan MP, Morawska L et al (2009) Characterization of expiration air jets and droplet size distributions immediately at the mouth opening. J Aerosol Sci 40(2):122–133

Charlotte N (2020) High rate of SARS-CoV-2 transmission due to choir practice in France at the beginning of the COVID-19 pandemic. J Voice S0892-1997(20):30452–30455

Cheng KC (1997) A history of flow visualization: chronology. J Flow Vis Image Proc 4(1):9–27

Cheng CY, Atkinson JF, van Benschoten JE et al (2000) Image-based system for particle counting and sizing. J Environ Eng 126(3):258–266

Craven BA, Settles GS (2006) A computational and experimental investigation of the human thermal plume. J Fluids Eng 128(6):1251–1258

Czapski S (1885) Einige neue optische Apparate von prof. Abbe. Instrument für die Aufsuchung von Schlieren (some new optical apparatuses by prof. Abbe. Instrument for the search of streaks). Zeitschrift für Instrumentenkunde 5:117–121

Dunker T, Tschudi J, O'Farrell M (2020a) Measurements of droplets from singing, laughing, reciting poetry, and playing wind instruments. Preprint arXiv 2203:04763. https://doi.org/10.48550/arxiv.2203.04763

Dunker T, Tschudi J, O'Farrell M (2020b) Project Memo: measurements of droplets from singing and some other activities. https://www.sintef.no/contentassets/c443f8aad9324279a2c8734674dde6e9/memo_measurement_of_droplets_signed.pdf. Accessed 23 Jun 2022

Dvořák R (1990) Prague's contribution to the science of flow visualization. In: Řezníček R (ed) Flow visualization V. Proceedings of The fifth international symposium on flow visualization, august 21–25, 1989,

Prague, Czechoslovakia. Hemisphere, New York, NY, pp 4–8

Echternach M, Gantner S, Peters G et al (2020) Impulse dispersion of aerosols during singing and speaking: a potential COVID-19 transmission pathway. Am J Respir Crit Care Med 202(11):1584–1587

Echternach M, Herrmann L, Gantner S et al (2021a) The effect of singers' masks on the impulse dispersion of aerosols during singing. J Voice 38:247.e1. https://doi.org/10.1016/j.jvoice.2021.08.011

Echternach M, Westphalen C, Köberlein MC et al (2021b) Reply to Philip et al.: aerosol transmission of SARS-CoV-2: inhalation as well as exhalation matters for COVID-19. Am J Respir Crit Care Med 203(8):1042–1043

Eiche T (2020) Schutzkonzept im Rahmen der schritt- weisen Lockerung der BAG-Massnahmen zum Schutz der Bevölkerung vor dem Coronavirus (COVID-19). Version 2.2, S. 8, Kap. 1.11: Untersuchung über Aerosole und Tröpfchen (Protection concept as part of the gradual relaxation of the FOPH measures to pro- tect the population from the coronavirus (COVID-19). Version 2.2, p. 8, chap. 1.11: Investigation of aero- sols and droplets). https://www.theaterschweiz.ch/ wp-content/uploads/2020/05/200508-Schutzkonzept_ COVID-19_Theater_Konzert_Veranstaltung_V2_1. pdf. Accessed 23 Jun 2022

Elsinga GE, van Oudheusden BW, Scarano F et al (2004) Assessment and application of quantitative Schlieren methods: calibrated color Schlieren and background oriented Schlieren. Exp Fluids 36(2):309–325

Fleischer M, Schumann L, Hartmann A et al (2022) Pre-adolescent children exhibit lower aerosol par- ticle volume emissions than adults for breathing, speaking, singing and shouting. J R Soc Interface 19(187):20210833. https://doi.org/10.1098/ rsif.2021.0833

Gantner S, Echternach M, Veltrup R et al (2021) Impulse dispersion of aerosols during playing wind instru- ments. PLoS One 17(3):e0262994. https://doi. org/10.1371/journal.pone.0262994

Gao N, Niu J (2007) Modeling particle dispersion and deposition in indoor environments. Atmos Environ 41(18):3862–3876

Gardner AD, Raffel M, Schwarz C et al (2020) Reference- free digital shadowgraphy using a moving BOS back- ground. Exp Fluids 61(2):1. https://doi.org/10.1007/ s00348-019-2865-4

Gena AW, Voelker C, Settles GS (2020) Qualitative and quantitative Schlieren optical measurement of the human thermal plume. Indoor Air 30(4):757–766

Giovanni A, Radulesco T, Bouchet G et al (2021) Transmission of droplet-conveyed infectious agents such as SARS-CoV-2 by speech and vocal exercises during speech therapy: preliminary experiment con- cerning airflow velocity. Eur Arch Otorrinolaringol 278(5):1687–1692

Goldhahn E, Seume J (2007) The background oriented Schlieren technique: sensitivity, accuracy, resolution

and application to a three-dimensional density field. Exp Fluids 43(2–3):241–249

Gregson FKA, Watson NA, Orton CM et al (2021) Comparing aerosol concentrations and particle size distributions generated by singing, speaking and breathing. Aerosol Sci Technol 55(6):681–691

Hamner L, Dubbel P, Capron I et al (2020) High SARS- CoV-2 attack rate following exposure at a choir prac- tice—Skagit County, Washington. Morb Mortal Wkly Rep 69(19):606–610

Hargather MJ, Settles GS (2012) A comparison of three quantitative Schlieren techniques. Opt Lasers Eng 50(1):8–17

Hartmann A, Lange J, Rotheudt H et al (2020a) Emission rate and particle size of bioaerosols during breathing, speaking and coughing. Technical University of Berlin, Berlin. https://doi.org/10.14279/depositonce-10331

Hartmann A, Lange J, Rotheudt H et al (2020b) Emissionsrate und Partikelgröße von Bioaerosolen beim Atmen, Sprechen und Husten. Technische Universität Berlin, Berlin. https://doi.org/10.14279/ depositonce-10332

Hartmann A, Mürbe D, Kriegel M et al (2020c) Risikobewertung von Probenräumen für Chöre hin- sichtlich virenbeladenen Aerosolen. Technische Universität Berlin, Berlin. https://doi.org/10.14279/ depositonce-10372

Hartmann A, Mürbe D, Kriegel M et al (2020d) Risk assessment of rehearsal rooms for choir singing regarding aerosols loaded with virus. Technical University of Berlin, Berlin. https://doi.org/10.14279/ depositonce-10388

He R, Gao L, Trifonov M et al (2021) Aerosol gen- eration from different wind instruments. J Aerosol Sci 151:105669. https://doi.org/10.1016/j. jaerosci.2020.105669

Hedworth HA, Karam M, McConnell J et al (2021) Mitigation strategies for airborne disease transmission in orchestras using computational fluid dynamics. Sci Adv 7(26):eabg4511. https://doi.org/10.1126/sciadv. abg4511

Hermann LA, Tur B, Köberlein MC et al (2021) Aerosol dispersion during different phonatory tasks in ama- teur singers. J Voice. https://doi.org/10.1016/j. jvoice.2021.11.005

Hirschberg A, Gilbert J, Msallam R et al (1996) Shock waves in trombones. J Acoust Soc Am 99(3):1754–1758

Ho KMA, Davies H, Epstein R et al (2021a) Spatiotemporal droplet dispersion measurements demonstrate face masks reduce risks from singing. Sci Rep 11(1):24183. https://doi.org/10.1038/s41598-021-03519-x

Ho KMA, Davies H, Epstein R et al (2021b) Spatiotemporal droplet dispersion measurements dem- onstrate face masks reduce risks from singing: results from the COvid aNd FacEmaSkS Study (CONFESS) https://doi.org/10.1101/2021.07.09.21260247

Izdebski K, Jarosz P, Usydus I (2017) Thermographic imaging of facial and ventilatory activity during vocalization, speech and expiration (conference presentation). Proc SPIE vol 10039. In: BJF W, Ilgner JF, Izdebski K (eds) Optical imaging, therapeutics, and advanced technology in head and neck surgery and otolaryngology, p 1003908. https://doi.org/10.1117/12.2256474

Jennison MW (1942) Atomizing of mouth and nose secretions into the air as revealed by high-speed photography. In: Moulton FR (ed) Aerobiology. American Association for the Advancement of Science, Washington, DC, pp 106–128

Johnson GR, Morawska L (2009) The mechanism of breath aerosol formation. J Aerosol Med Pulm Drug Deliv 22(3):229–237

Johnson GR, Morawska L, Ristovski ZD et al (2011) Modality of human expired aerosol size distributions. J Aerosol Sci 42(12):839–851

Kähler CJ, Hain R (2020) Singing in choirs and making music with wind instruments. Is that safe during the SARS-CoV-2 pandemic? https://doi.org/10.13140/RG.2.2.36405.29926

Katelaris AL, Wells J, Norton S et al (2021) Epidemiologic evidence for airborne transmission of SARS-CoV-2 during church singing, Australia. Emerg Infect Dis 27(6):1677–1680

Kniesburges S, Schlegel P, Peters G et al (2021) Effects of surgical masks on aerosol dispersion in professional singing. J Expo Sci Environ Epidemiol 32:727. https://doi.org/10.1038/s41370-021-00385-7

Krehl P, Engemann S (1995) August Toepler—the first who visualized shock waves. Shock Waves 5(1–2):1–18

Kriegel M, Hartmann A (2020a) Ausbreitungsdistanz und -dynamik von Aerosolen in Innenräumen durch Konvektionsströme. Technische Universität Berlin, Berlin. https://doi.org/10.14279/depositonce-10391

Kriegel M, Hartmann A (2020b) Spreading distance and dynamic of aerosols in internal spaces by convection flows. Technical University of Berlin, Berlin. https://doi.org/10.14279/depositonce-10392

Kwon S-B, Park J, Jang J et al (2012) Study on the initial velocity distribution of exhaled air from coughing and speaking. Chemosphere 87(11):1260–1264

Lai K-M, Bottomley C, McNerney R (2011) Propagation of respiratory aerosols by the vuvuzela. PLoS One 6(5):e20086. https://doi.org/10.1371/journal.pone.0020086

Lange J, Schumann L, Hartmann A et al (2020) SARS-CoV-2 und Aerosole (1): was wir bis heute Wissen (SARS-CoV-2 and aerosols (1): what we know to this day). Dtsch Ärztebl Online 2:12–14. https://doi.org/10.3238/PersPneumo.2020.12.11.03

Lau J (2020) Sind Blasinstrumente Virenschleudern? (Are wind instruments virus slingshots?). https://www.derstandard.de/story/2000118106449/sind-blasinstrumente-virenschleudern. Acccessed 23 Jun 2022

López-Carromero A, Campbell DM, Rendón PL et al (2017) Validation of brass wind instrument radiation models in relation to their physical accuracy using an optical Schlieren imaging setup. Proc Mtgs Acoustic 28(1):35003. https://doi.org/10.1121/2.0000386

Mach L (1896) Ueber die Sichtbarmachung von Luftstromlinien (on the visualization of air streamlines). Zeitschrift für Luftschiffahrt und Physik der Atmosphäre 15(6):129–139

Mazumdar A (2013) Principles and techniques of Schlieren imaging systems. Columbia University Computer Science Technical Reports, New York. https://doi.org/10.7916/D8TX3PWV

McCarthy LP, Orton CM, Watson NA et al (2021) Aerosol and droplet generation from performing with woodwind and brass instruments. Aerosol Sci Technol 55(11):1277–1287

Meier G (2002) Computerized background-oriented Schlieren. Exp Fluids 33(1):181–187

Merghani K, Sagot B, Gehin E et al (2021) A review on the applied techniques of exhaled airflow and droplets characterization. Indoor Air 31(1):7–25

Merzkirch W (1987) Flow visualization, 2nd edn. Academic Press, New York, NY

Meselson M (2020) Droplets and aerosols in the transmission of SARS-CoV-2. N Engl J Med 382(21):2063. https://doi.org/10.1056/NEJMc2009324

Miller VA, Loebner KT (2016) Smartphone schlieren. arXiv https://doi.org/10.48550/arXiv.1609.04298

Miller SL, Nazaroff WW, Jimenez JL et al (2021) Transmission of SARS-CoV-2 by inhalation of respiratory aerosol in the Skagit Valley chorale superspreading event. Indoor Air 31(2):314–323

Moore TR, Cannaday AE (2020) Do "brassy" sounding musical instruments need increased safe distancing requirements to minimize the spread of COVID-19? J Acoust Soc Am 148(4):2096. https://doi.org/10.1121/10.0002182

Morawska L (2006) Droplet fate in indoor environments, or can we prevent the spread of infection? Indoor Air 16(5):335–347

Morawska L, Milton DK (2020) It is time to address airborne transmission of coronavirus disease 2019 (COVID-19). Clin Infect Dis 71(9):2311–2313

Morawska L, Johnson GR, Ristovski ZD et al (2006) Size distribution and sites of origin of droplets expelled from the human respiratory tract during expiratory activities. J Aerosol Sci 40(3):256–269

Morawska L, Tang JW, Bahnfleth W et al (2020) How can airborne transmission of COVID-19 indoors be minimised? Environ Int 142:105832. https://doi.org/10.1016/j.envint.2020.105832

Mürbe D, Kriegel M, Lange J et al (2021b) Aerosol emission in professional singing of classical music. Sci Rep 11(1):14861. https://doi.org/10.1038/s41598-021-93281-x

Mürbe D, Kriegel M, Lange J et al (2021a) Aerosol emission of adolescents voices during speaking, singing and shouting. PLoS One 16(2):e0246819. https://doi.org/10.1371/journal.pone.0246819

Mürbe D, Schumann L, von Zadow D et al (2021c) Aerosolpartikelemissionen von Kindern, Jugendlichen und Erwachsenen beim Sprechen, Singen und Rufen (aerosol particle emissions from children, adolescents and adults when speaking, singing and shouting). German medical science GMS publishing house. In: Caffier PP, Echternach M (eds) Aktuelle phoniatrisch-pädaudiologische Aspekte (current phoniatric-paediatric audiological aspects), vol 28, pp 117–118

Naunheim MR, Bock J, Doucette PA et al (2021) Safer singing during the SARS-CoV-2 pandemic: what we know and what we don't. J Voice 35(5):765–771

Nusseck M, Richter B, Holtmeier L et al (2020) $CO_2$ measurements in instrumental and vocal closed room settings as a risk reducing measure for a coronavirus infection. https://doi.org/10.1101/2020.10.26.20218354

Ono K (2020) Reshaping the concert stage. https://maestroarts.com/articles/reshaping-the-concert-stage. Accessed 23 Jun 2022

Pandya BH, Settles GS, Miller JD (2003) Schlieren imaging of shock waves from a trumpet. J Acoust Soc Am 114(6):3363–3367

Parker AS, Crookston K (2020) Investigation into the release of respiratory aerosols by brass instruments and mitigation measures with respect to Covid-19. https://doi.org/10.1101/2020.07.31.20165837

Prather KA, Ma LC, Schooley RT et al (2020) Airborne transmission of SARS-CoV-2. Science 370(6514):303–304

Raffel M (2015) Background-oriented Schlieren (BOS) techniques. Exp Fluids 56(3):60. https://doi.org/10.1007/s00348-015-1927-5

Raffel M, Willert CE, Scarano F et al (2018) Particle image velocimetry. A practical guide, 3rd edn. Springer, Cham. https://doi.org/10.1007/978-3-319-68852-7

Reed NG (2010) The history of ultraviolet germicidal irradiation for air disinfection. Public Health Rep 125(1):15–27

Rendón PL, Velasco-Segura R, Echeverría C et al (2018) Using Schlieren imaging to estimate the geometry of a shock wave radiated by a trumpet bell. J Acoust Soc Am 144(4):EL310. https://doi.org/10.1121/1.5063810

Richard H, Raffel M (2001) Principle and applications of the background oriented Schlieren (BOS) method. Meas Sci Technol 12(9):1576–1585

Richter B, Hipp A, Schubert B et al (2021) From classic to rap: airborne transmission of different singing styles, with respect to risk assessment of a SARS-CoV-2 infection. doi:https://doi.org/10.1101/2021.03.25.21253694

Rienitz J (1975) Schlieren experiment 300 years ago. Nature 254(5498):293–295

Rienitz J (1997) Optical inhomogeneities: Schlieren and shadowgraph methods in the seventeenth and eighteenth centuries. Endeavour 21(2):77–81

Salmanzadeh M, Zahedi G, Ahmadi G et al (2012) Computational modeling of effects of thermal plume adjacent to the body on the indoor airflow and particle transport. J Aerosol Sci 53:29–39

Schade W, Reimer V, Seipenbusch M et al (2021) Experimental investigation of aerosol and $CO_2$ dispersion for evaluation of COVID-19 infection risk in a concert hall. Int J Environ Res Public Health 18(6):3037. https://doi.org/10.3390/ijerph18063037

Schuit M, Ratnesar-Shumate S, Yolitz J et al (2020) Airborne SARS-CoV-2 is rapidly inactivated by simulated sunlight. J Infect Dis 222(4):564–571

Setti L, Passarini F, de Gennaro G et al (2020) Airborne transmission route of COVID-19: why 2 meters/6 feet of inter-personal distance could not be enough. Int J Environ Res Public Health 17(8):2932. https://doi.org/10.3390/ijerph17082932

Settles GS (1985) Colour-coding Schlieren techniques for the optical study of heat and fluid flow. Int J Heat Fluid Flow 6(1):3–15

Settles GS (2001) Schlieren and shadowgraph techniques. Visualizing phenomena in transparent media. Experimental fluid mechanics. Springer, Berlin, pp 1–15, 122–129

Settles GS (2018) Smartphone Schlieren and shadowgraph imaging. Opt Lasers Eng 104:9–21

Settles GS, Hargather MJ (2017) A review of recent developments in Schlieren and shadowgraph techniques. Meas Sci Technol 28(4):42001. https://doi.org/10.1088/1361-6501/aa5748

Settles GS, Kuhns JW (1984) Visualization of airflow and convection phenomena about the human body. Bull Am Phys Soc 29(9):1515

Settles GS, Via GG (1986) A portable schlieren optical system for clean room applications. Proceedings of the 8th International Symposium on Contamination Control: 381–392

Settles GS, Via GG (1987) A portable Schlieren optical system for clean-room airflow analysis. J Environ Sci 30(5):17–21

Shao S, Zhou D, He R et al (2020) Risk assessment of airborne transmission of COVID-19 by asymptomatic individuals under different practical settings. J Aerosol Sci 151:105661. https://doi.org/10.1016/j.jaerosci.2020.105661

Smits AJ, Lim TT (eds) (2012) Flow visualization. Techniques and examples, 2nd edn. Imperial College Press, London

Spahn C, Hipp AM, Schubert B et al (2021) Airflow and air velocity measurements while playing wind instruments, with respect to risk assessment of a SARS-CoV-2 infection. Int J Environ Res 18(10):5413. https://doi.org/10.3390/ijerph18105413

Stadnytskyi V, Bax CE, Bax A et al (2020) The airborne lifetime of small speech droplets and their potential importance in SARS-CoV-2 transmission. Proc Natl Acad Sci USA 117(22):11875–11877

Sterz F (2020a) Philharmoniker zeigen geringe Infektionsgefahr auf (Philharmonic orchestras show low risk of infection). https://wien.orf.at/stories/3049099/. Accessed 23 Jun 2022

Sterz F (2020b) Untersuchung und fotografische Dokumentation von aerosol-und Kondenswasseremission bei Chor Mitgliedern. Medizinische Universität Wien (investigation and photographic documentation of aerosol and condensation water emissions in choir members. Medical University of Vienna). https://www.meduniwien.ac.at/hp/fileadmin/notfallmedizin/pamuv/2020_05_26_SterzF_protokoll_aerosolchor_002.pdf. Accessed 23 Jun 2022

Stockman T, Zhu S, Kumar A et al (2021) Measurements and simulations of aerosol released while singing and playing wind instruments. ACS Environ Au 1(1):71–84

Sun S, Li J, Han J (2021) How human thermal plume influences near-human transport of respiratory droplets and airborne particles: a review. Environ Chem Lett 19(3):1973–1982

Tan ZP, Silwal L, Bhatt SP et al (2021) Experimental characterization of speech aerosol dispersion dynamics. Sci Rep 11(1):3953. https://doi.org/10.1038/s41598-021-83298-7

Tang JW, Nicolle ADG, Pantelic J et al (2011) Qualitative real-time Schlieren and shadowgraph imaging of human exhaled airflows: an aid to aerosol infection control. PLoS One 6(6):1–6

Tarnopolsky AZ, Fletcher NH (2004) Schlieren flow visualisation technique: applications to musical wind instruments, especially the didjeridu. Proc 18th international congress on acoustics (ICA), Kyoto/Japan: II 955- II 958 (paper no. Tu2.C1.4)

Tarnopolsky AZ, Fletcher NH, Hollenberg LCL et al (2006) Vocal tract resonances and the sound of the Australian didjeridu (yidaki) I. Experiment. J Acoust Soc Am 119(2):1194–1204

Töpler A (1864) Beobachtungen nach einer neuen optischen Methode. Ein Beitrag zur Experimentalphysik (observations from a new optical method. A contribution to experimental physics). Cohen, Bonn

Töpler A (1867) II. Optische Studien nach der Methode der Schlierenbeobachtung (optical studies from the method of streak observation). I. Verbesserter Beobachtungsapparat.; II. Einige Versuche über die Empfindlichkeit der Beobachtungsmethode. (I. Improved observation apparatus.; II. Some experiments on the sensitivity of the observation method). Pogg Ann Phys Chem 131(5):33–55

Tur B, Veltrup R, Hermann L et al (2021) Projekt zur Untersuchung der Aerosoldynamik beim Singen und Spielen von Blasinstrumenten während der Covid-19-Pandemie (project to investigate aerosol dynamics when singing and playing wind instruments during the Covid-19 pandemic). German medical science GMS publishing house. In: Caffier PP, Echternach M (eds) Aktuelle phoniatrisch-pädaudiologische Aspekte (current phoniatric-paediatric audiological aspects), vol 28, pp 114–116

Umweltbundesamt (2008) Gesundheitliche Bewertung von Kohlendioxid in der Innenraumluft. Mitteilungen der Ad-hoc-Arbeitsgruppe Innenraumrichtwerte der Innenraumlufthygiene-Kommission des Umweltbundesamtes und der Obersten Landesgesundheitsbehörden (Health assessment of carbon dioxide in indoor air. Announcements of the Ad Hoc Working Group on Interior Guideline Values of the Indoor Air Hygiene Commission of the Federal Environment Agency and the Supreme State Health Authorities). Bundesgesundheitsblatt Gesundheitsforschung Gesundheitsschutz (Federal Health Gazette Health Research Health Protection) 51(11):1358–1369

van der Lint P (2020) Die ene passion die wel doorging, met rampzalige gevolgen. (the passion that proceeded with disastrous consequences). Trouw. https://www.trouw.nl/verdieping/die-ene-passion-die-weldoorging-met-rampzalige-gevolgen~b4ced33e/?referrer=https%3A%2F%2Fwww.google.com%2F. Accessed 23 Jun 2022

von Zadow D, Schumann L, Ifrim L et al (2021) Aerosolpartikelemissionen beim Spielen verschiedener Blasinstrumente im Vergleich zum Atmen, Sprechen und Singen (aerosol particle emissions when playing different wind instruments compared with breathing, speaking and singing). German medical science GMS publishing house. In: Caffier PP, Echternach M (eds) Aktuelle phoniatrisch-pädaudiologische Aspekte (current phoniatric-paediatric audiological aspects), vol 28, pp 119–121

Westphalen C, Kniesburges S, Veltrup R et al (2021) Sources of aerosol dispersion during singing and potential safety procedures for singers. J Voice 37:504. https://doi.org/10.1016/j.jvoice.2021.03.013

Wieser A, Beyerl J, Brunn A Von et al (2021) Aerosol decontamination and spatial separation using a free-space LED-based UV-C light curtain. https://doi.org/10.1101/2021.12.16.21267937

Xie X, Li Y, Sun H et al (2009) Exhaled droplets due to talking and coughing. J R Soc Interface 6(6):S703–S714

Zhang R, Li Y, Zhang AL et al (2020) Identifying airborne transmission as the dominant route for the spread of COVID-19. Proc Natl Acad Sci USA 117(26):14857–14863

Zhu S, Kato S, Yang JH (2006) Study on transport characteristics of saliva droplets produced by coughing in a calm indoor environment. Build Environ 41(12):16971702. https://doi.org/10.1016/j.buildenv.2005.06.024

Zielinski S (2011) Watch a trombone's shock wave. Scientists have generated the first video of a shock wave from a trombone. Smithsonian Magazine. https://www.smithsonianmag.com/science-nature/watch-a-trombones-shock-wave-180274743/. Accessed 23 Jun 2022

# Correction to: Phoniatrics III

Antoinette am Zehnhoff-Dinnesen,
Antonio Schindler, and Patrick G. Zorowka

## Correction to:
## Chapters 20 and 27 in: A. am Zehnhoff-Dinnesen et al. (eds.), *Phoniatrics III*, European Manual of Medicine, https://doi.org/10.1007/978-3-031-48091-1

The original version of this book was inadvertently published with the below errors and was corrected as given in the below corrections:

Chapter 20, Sect. 20.10: The name of the section author "Dr. Michelangelo Dini" was inadvertently deleted from the section opening page and instead "Dr. Angelica De Sandi" was inserted by oversight. This has now been corrected.

Chapter 27, Sect. 27.7: By oversight, the incorrect affiliation of author Dr Dirk Vanneste was published. This has now been corrected as Privatpraxis for speech and voice therapy, Kooigem (Kortrijk), Belgium.

---

The updated version of these chapters can be found at:
https://doi.org/10.1007/978-3-031-48091-1_5
https://doi.org/10.1007/978-3-031-48091-1_12

# Description of Videos and Audios Plus Still Images of Videos for the European Manual of Medicine Phoniatrics III

Katrin Neumann, Corinna Gietmann,
and Antoinette am Zehnhoff-Dinnesen

**V. Woisard**
Voice and Deglutition Unit, Department of Otorhinolaryngology and Head and Neck Surgery, Larrey Hospital, University Hospital of Toulouse, Toulouse, France
e-mail: woisard.virginie@iuct-incopole.fr

**School of Logopedics**
University Hospital Münster, Münster, Germany
e-mail: logoschule@ukmuenster.de

**M. Boentert**
Department of Neurology, University Hospital, Münster, University Münster, Germany
e-mail: Matthias.boentert@ukmuenster.de

**R. Shprintzen**
Connecticut Children's (WDG), Farmington; and The Virtual Center for Velo-Cardio-Facial Syndrome (RJS), Manlius, NY, USA
e-mail: robert.shprintzen@vcfscenter.org

**M. Tedla** and **Z. Korim**
Department of ENT and HNS, Faculty of Medicine, University Hospital Bratislava, Comenius University, Bratislava, Slovakia
e-mail: miro.tedla@gmail.com; korim7@uniba.sk

**M. Farahat**
Department of Otolaryngology, Research Chair of Voice, Swallowing, and Communication Disorders, Head and Neck Surgery, College of Medicine, King Saud University, Riyadh, Saudi Arabia
e-mail: mfarahat@KSU.EDU.SA

**K. Neumann**
*Department of Phoniatrics and Pedaudiology, University Hospital Münster, University Münster, Germany
e-mail: Katrin.neumann@uni-muenster.de
**formerly: Division of Phoniatrics and Pediatric Audiology, Department of Otorhinolaryngology, Head and Neck Surgery, St. Elisabeth Hospital, Ruhr University Bochum, Bochum, Germany

K. Neumann · C. Gietmann
A. am Zehnhoff-Dinnesen
Department of Phoniatrics and Pedaudiology,
University Hospital Münster,
Münster, Germany

**Case Study Audio 16.1a–c**: Ataxic dysarthria in a French-speaking women with cerebellar syndrome (dysfunction of the cerebellum, including afferent and efferent cerebellar pathways): alternating pressed, creaky, and sometimes breathy; instable voice quality; mild fluctuations in voice pitch and volume, occasionally "voice tremor"; sometimes slurred articulation, but sometimes also "explosive", i.e. overly clear articulation; predominantly monotone, slowed, and scanding (syllabic) speech with unnatural prosody, occasionally mild hypernasality.

1. **Case Study Audio 16.1a**: Spontaneous speech
2. **Case Study Audio 16.1b**: Reading
3. **Case Study Audio 16.1c**: Dialogue
   **Source audios 16.1a–c: V. Woisard**
4. **Case Study Audio 16.2**: Moderate to severe, mixed, predominantly flaccid dysarthria with peripheral paretic (hypotonic; lesion of the second motoneuron or the neuromuscular junction) and central paretic (spastic; lesion of the second motoneuron) components in a German-speaking woman 9 years after a severe traumatic brain injury with cerebral contusions, traumatic subarachnoid haemorrhage with ventricular haemorrhage, skull base, and midface fracture. In addition, mild oropharyngeal dysphagia. Velopharyngoplasty 7 years ago. The patient's speech is characterised by disturbed speech breathing with shortened expiratory duration, a somewhat pressed and breathy voice quality, a reduced voice volume, a strongly blurred articulation, mild hypernasality (rhinophonia aperta), and a disturbed prosody with slowed and monotonous speech.
   **Source: School of Logopedics, University Hospital Münster**
5. **Case Study Video 16.1**: Male patient, 73 years, with amyotrophic lateral sclerosis (ALS) of upper motor neuron predominant phenotype and pseudobulbar dysarthria and dysphagia. Symptom onset 14 years ago, slow disease progression, paraplegia, bilateral arm weakness, chronic hypercapnic respiratory failure, non-invasive home ventilation 20 h a day, moderate dysphagia with

impaired oral and pharyngeal phase on flexible endoscopic evaluation of swallowing (FEES), no tube feeding. Speech characteristics: slow, "spastic" phonation (resulting from bilateral damage to the upper motor neuron), moderate impairment of articulation, still understandable, speech dyspnea (loss of breath when speaking). Tongue without atrophy or fibrillations. Note hypomimic facial movements.

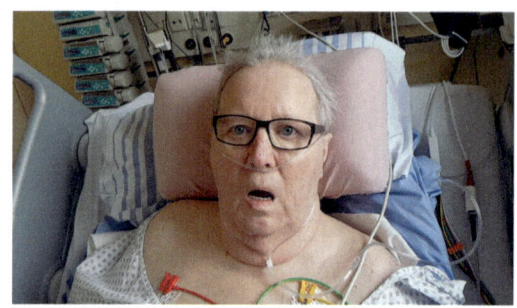

6. **Case Study Video 16.2**: Male patient, 80 years, ALS, bulbar phenotype, symptom onset 1.5 years ago. Tongue atrophy, weakness, and fibrillations. Severe dysphagia with aspiration and weight loss, enterostomy tube feeding. No weakness of arms and legs, but ubiquitous fasciculations of limb and trunk muscles during the last few months. No sleep-disordered breathing. Severe weakness of cough due to incomplete closure of the glottis. Speech characteristics: bulbar dysarthria, slurred, paretic, slow, severe impairment of articulation, very hard to understand.

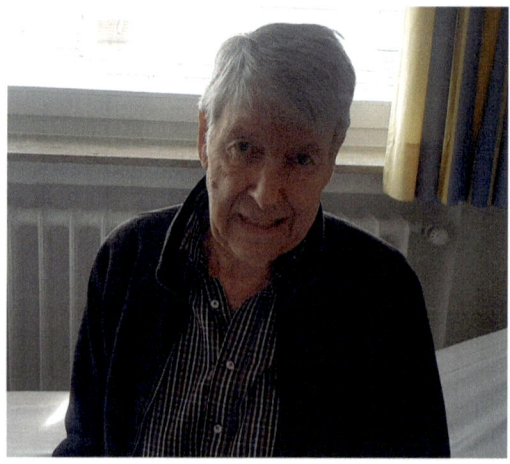

7. **Case Study Video 16.3**: Male patient, 63 years, ALS, upper motor neuron predominant phenotype, but evolving bulbar weakness (lower motor neuron), disease onset 3 years ago, spastic gait, bilateral foot drop, atrophy of intrinsic hand muscles (dorsal interosseous). Mild dysphagia, no tube feeding, no sleep-disordered breathing. Speech characteristics: bulbar and pseudobulbar dysarthria with slow, "spastic" speech and moderately impaired, slurred, articulation.

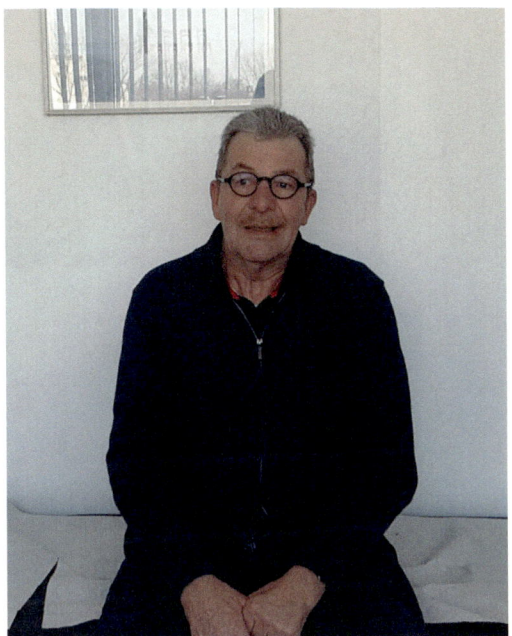

8. **Case Study Video 16.4**: Female patient, 62 years, ALS of upper motor neuron predominant phenotype, symptom onset 2 years ago, slow disease progression, spastic gait, no arm weakness, no dysphagia, no sleep-disordered breathing. Speech characteristics: bulbar and pseudobulbar dysarthria, slow, "spastic" phonation, mild impairment of articulation. Tongue without atrophy or fibrillations. Weakness of the soft palate with resulting "hypernasality" (rhinolalia aperta).

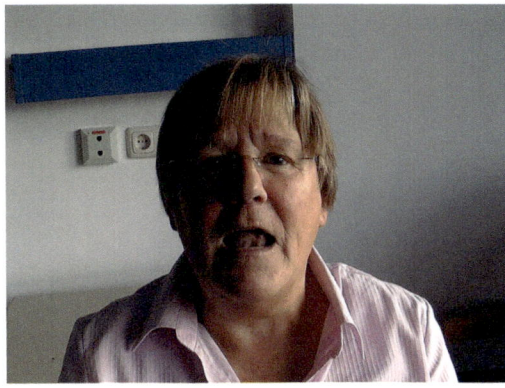

Source videos 16.1–16.4: M. Boentert

9. **Case Study Video 16.5**: Young German-speaking man who had experienced a severe diffuse axonal traumatic brain injury (shearing injury due to acceleration or deceleration movements with a simultaneous rotatory component) 14 years ago. He suffers from spastic tetraparesis and moderate central paretic (spastic) dysarthria. This video shows him during speaking spontaneously, and Video 20.1 shows him in a therapy situation applying learned speech techniques during reading.

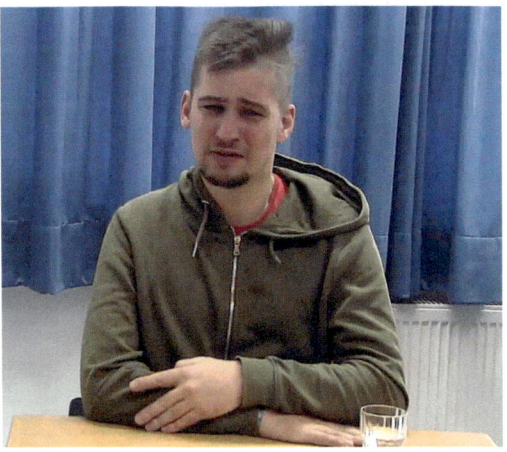

**Source videos 16.5 and 20.1: School of Logopedics, University Hospital Münster**

10. **Case Study Video 16.6**: Man with ataxic dysarthria

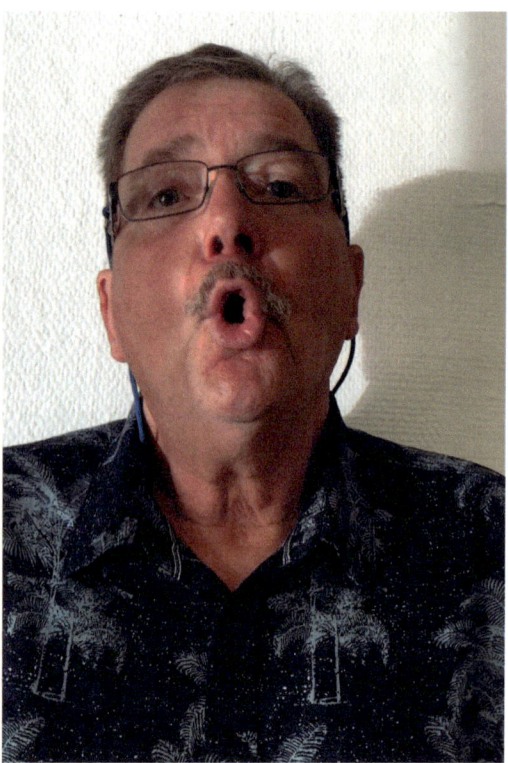

Source: **School of Logopedics, University Hospital Münster**

11. **Case Study Video 16.7**: Woman with spastic dysarthria and dysphagia after stroke

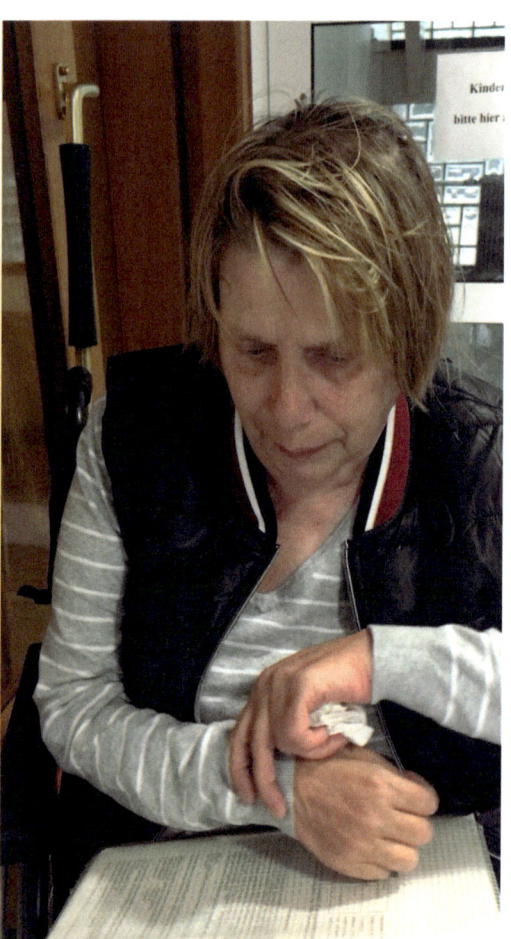

12. **Case Study Video 16.8**: Woman with beginning ALS and mixed flaccid (hypotonic) and ataxic dysarthria

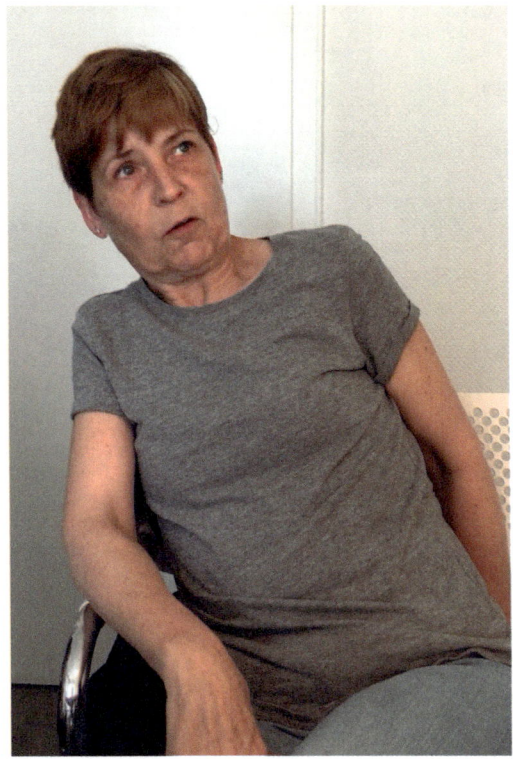

**Source: \*\*K. Neumann**

13. **Case Study Video 20.1**: Young German-speaking man, the same as in Video 16.5, who had a severe diffuse axonal traumatic brain injury 14 years ago. He suffers from spastic tetraparesis and moderate central paretic (spastic) dysarthria. This video shows him in a therapy situation using learned speech techniques while reading, such as conscious control of body tension, breath control, pauses, and control of voice pitch.

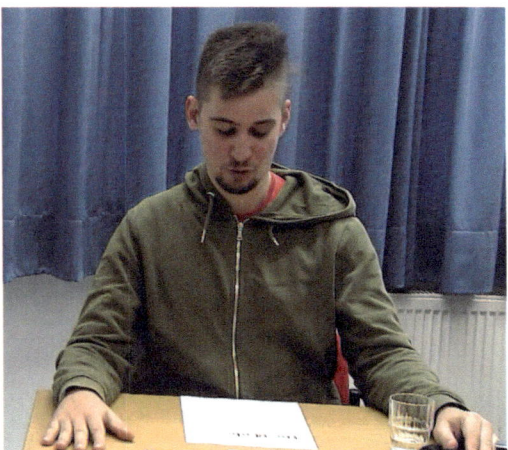

**Source videos 16.5 and 20.1: School of Logopedics, University Hospital Münster**

**Case Study Videos 23.1a–e**: Assessment of language abilities in a German-speaking patient with mild to moderate Broca's aphasia by the Aachen Aphasia Test. The aphasia together with a meanwhile mild apraxia of speech occurred after a left medial infarction 6 years ago with haemorrhage of cardiogenic-embolic origin in the context of a paradoxical embolism with atrial septal defect. It is characterised by word-finding difficulties, many semantic paraphasias, sentence breaks, and missing or false inflections in the context of agrammatism.

14. **Case Study Video 23.1a**: Aachen Aphasia Test, subtest *Naming objects* (nouns and composites): Patient laboriously searches for words, especially compound ones; tries to paraphrase them, helped by gestures: „Das ist eine Staub – Staub-sauger (*correct:* „ein Staubsauger")." – „Das ist eine (*correct:* „ein") Kühlschrank." – „Ähm Schraub- nee Hubschrauber" – "Steck-nadel" (*correct* "Sicherheitsnadel" - semantic paraphasia) – „Das ist ähm (*obligatory article* „eine" *is lacking*) Schreibmaschine." - „Doden - Dosen öffnen, öffner" (*correct:* „Dosenöffner") – "Lampe" (*correct:* "Taschenlampe") – "Schraubenzicher" – "Schuh-öffel, nee Schuh -öff, nein Schuhlöffel" – "Das ist (*obligatory article* „ein" *is lacking*) Rollschuh."

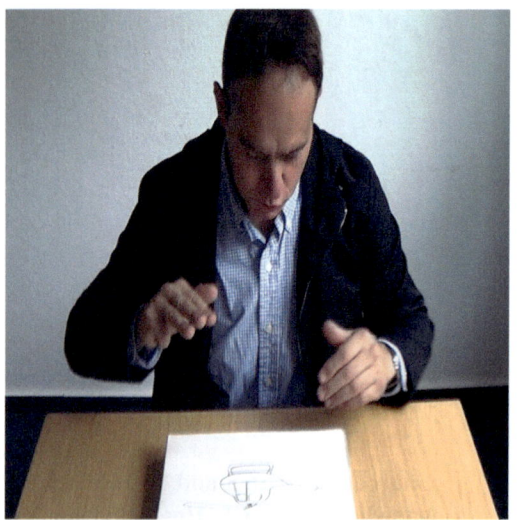

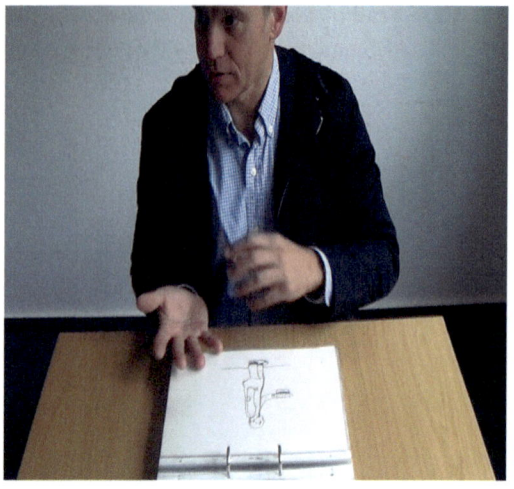

16. **Case Study Video 23.1c**: Aachen Aphasia Test, subtest *Repeating loan and foreign words*

15. **Case Study Video 23.1b**: Aachen Aphasia Test, subtest *Describing situations and actions:*

„Der Bettler…hat einen Hut…danach für eine Gabe." (*correct:* „Der Bettler bittet mit seinem Hut um Geld.") – „Die Frau, die Frau…den….Tanne (*correction*) nee Ka-Kanne…Kaffeekanne putzt." (*correct:* „Die Frau trocknet die Kaffeekanne ab.") – Die… (*correction*) der…ähm der….der Junge… gibt einen…einen Ding für Hund." (*correct:* „Der Junge gibt dem Hund etwas.") – „Der Junge hat verbrochen… (*correction* phonematic paraphasia) äf...zerbrochen plötzlich." (*correct*: „Dem Jungen ist die Tasse herunter-gefallen.") – "Der…die die Lehrerin, ähm, malt…malt, ähm, gegenüber…gegenüber ihrer Schülerin." (*correct:* „Die Lehrerin schreibt ihrer Schülerin etwas an die Tafel.")

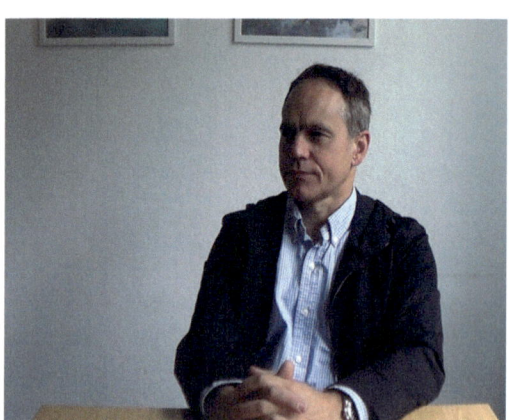

17. **Case Study Video 23.1d**: Aachen Aphasia Test, subtest *Repeating sentences*

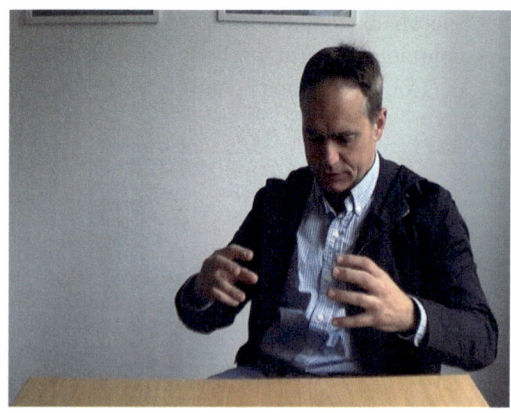

18. **Case Study Video 23.1e**: Aachen Aphasia Test, subtest *Repeating compound words*

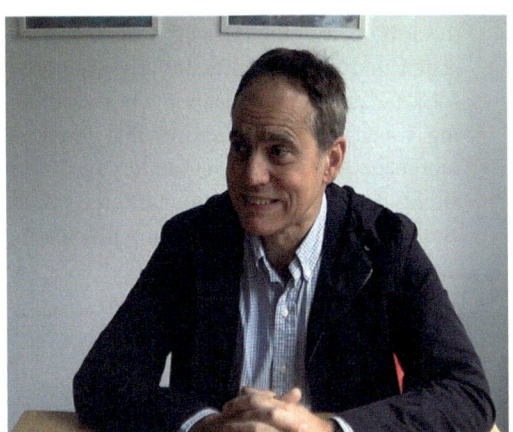

**Source videos 23.1a–e: School of Logopedics, University Hospital Münster**

19. **Case Study Video 26.1**: Globus pharyngis and dysphagia in a 16-year-old adolescent due to hypertrophic lingual tonsils leading to obstruction of the valleculae, as demonstrated by flexible endoscopic evaluation of swallowing (FEES).

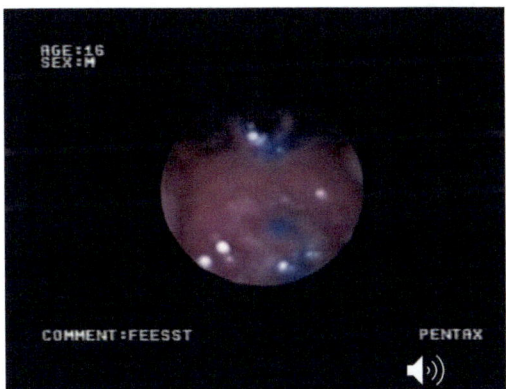

**Source: R. Shprintzen**

20. **Case Study Video 26.2**: A 76-year-old man after non-surgical treatment of squamous cell carcinoma of the hypopharynx (piriform sinus, T2N1M0) by chemoradiotherapy and subsequent neck dissection due to persistence of a nodular lesion. Dysphagia developed after surgery and a nasogastric tube had to be placed. The video shows salivary pooling in the vallecular space, bilaterally in the piriform sinus and penetration through the posterior glottic chink and via the left aryepiglottic fold. During FEES, there was delayed opening of the upper oesophageal sphincter and aspiration after swallowing with residue in the glottis area (green colour).

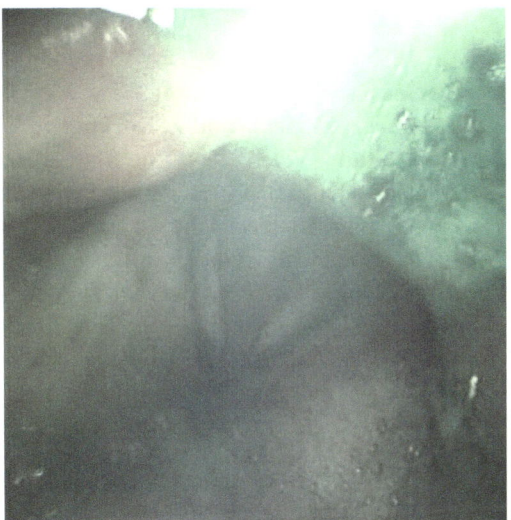

**Source: M. Tedla and Z. Korim**

21. **Case Study Video 26.3**: A 52-year-old patient with laryngeal cancer (T2N0M0) who had undergone one cycle of chemotherapy after radiotherapy. He did not tolerate another and refused further tumour treatment. The video shows thick, sticky secretions pooling mainly in the pharynx and laryngeal vestibule as well as decreased laryngeal sensitivity, with salivary aspiration. The supraglottis was inflamed as a result of the chemoradiotherapy, a condition that worsened oral intake and caused odynophagia.

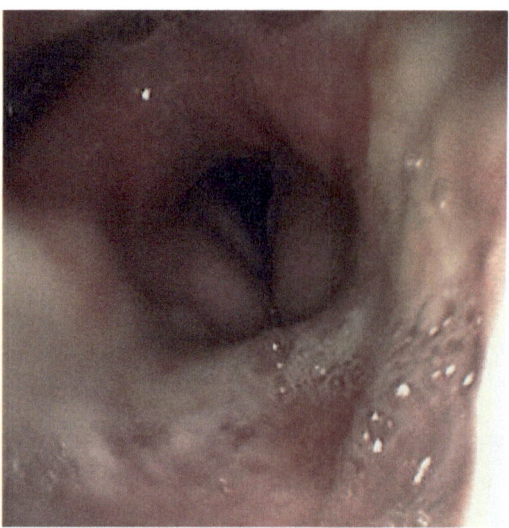

**Source: M. Tedla and Z. Korim**

22. **Case Study Video 26.4**: An 87-year-old woman with presbyphagia and no significant comorbidities. Subjectively, she reported difficulty swallowing, food jams in her throat, and prolonged eating. The video shows ineffective swallowing of puree, weakened pharyngeal constriction, and pressure of the tongue on the posterior pharyngeal wall. Multiple swallows and after-drinking after meals are required.

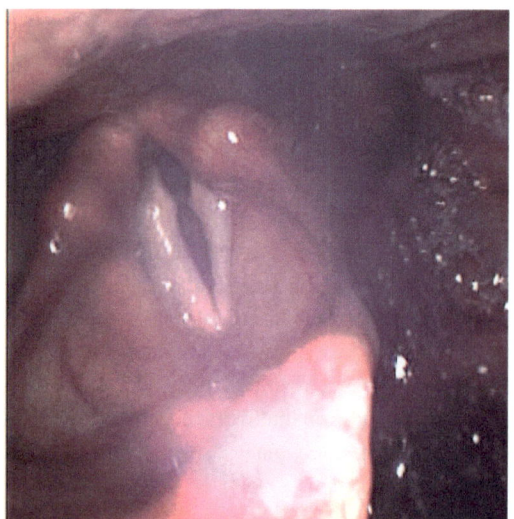

**Source: M. Tedla and Z. Korim**

23. **Case Study Video 26.5**: Neurogenic dysphagia in a woman with motor neuron disease and bulbar symptoms of progressive bulbar dysarthria, dysphonia, and dysphagia. She stated that she had difficulty chewing solid food and a choking sensation when swallowing water. The video shows that impaired motor function and decreased laryngeal sensitivity led to aspiration of an offered biscuit and a subsequent reflex cough with clearing of the lower respiratory tract.

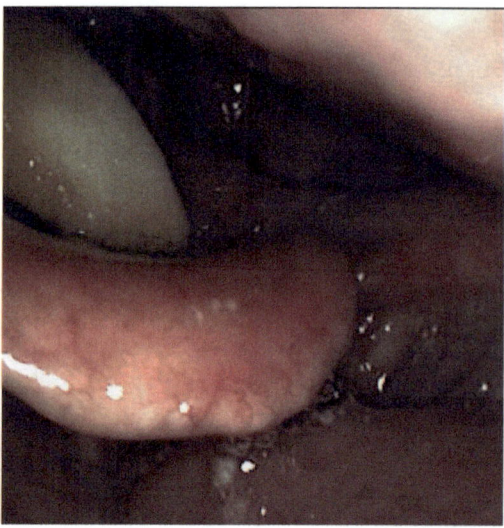

**Source: M. Tedla and Z. Korim**

24. **Case Study Video 26.6**: Neurogenic dysphagia in a 71-year-old man who had been diagnosed with Parkinson's disease 12 years earlier and was therefore treated with medication. He had been suffering for one and a half years from the feeling that food was stuck in his throat and had a thicker consistency. The video shows piecemeal swallowing and a pooling of puree in the valleculae and piriform sinuses, but these residues were largely eliminated by repeated dry swallowing (not shown in the video).

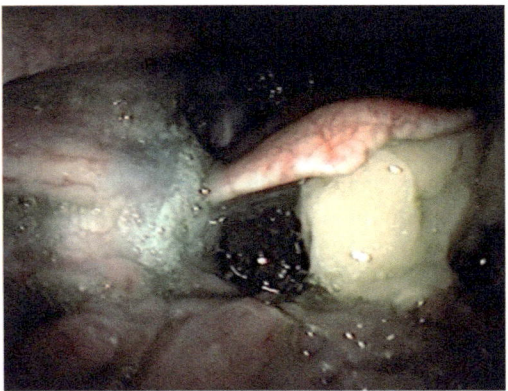

**Source: M. Farahat**

25. **Case Study Video 26.7**: Neurogenic dysphagia in a 58-year-old teacher one month after an ischaemic stroke. With intact consciousness and good cognitive abilities, he coughed when drinking. The video shows delayed triggering of the swallowing reflex for liquids. When the patient swallows, he aspirates with reflexive coughing to clear the trachea of the aspiration bolus.

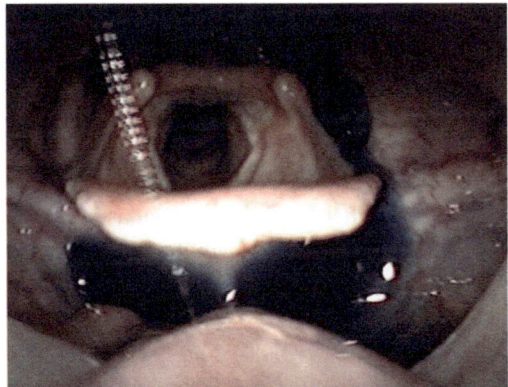

**Source: M. Farahat**

26. **Case Study Video 26.8**: Neurogenic dysphagia in a 44-year-old man who had undergone open-heart surgery one year earlier and had postoperative paralysis of the left recurrent laryngeal nerve. He noticed a change in his voice afterwards and recurrent coughing when drinking water. The video shows the right vocal fold that is free to move and the left vocal fold that is immobile and excavated. When the patient swallows liquids, aspiration occurs

with the cough reflex intact so that the aspirated bolus can be removed from the laryngeal vestibule.

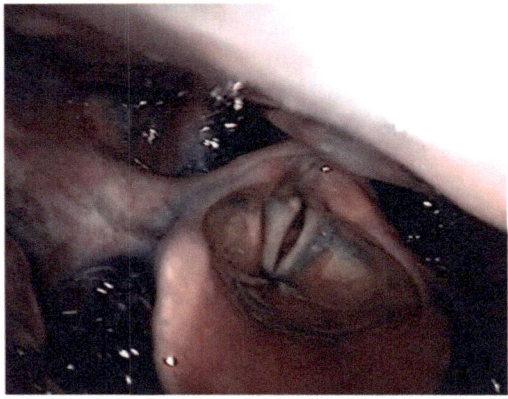

**Source: M. Farahat**

27. **Case Study Video 26.9**: Neurogenic dysphagia in a 66-year-old woman after an ischaemic stroke 7 months ago. She was fed with a nasogastric tube (NGT) for 3 weeks, then the NGT was weaned. She complained of coughing during meals thereafter. The video shows swallowing thin liquids, with the patient safely swallowing the first part of the bolus presented. However, the remaining part of the bolus is shown to run down into the valleculae without triggering the swallowing reflex, indicating impaired sensation in the oral cavity and oropharynx, putting the patient at risk of penetration and/or aspiration before swallowing.

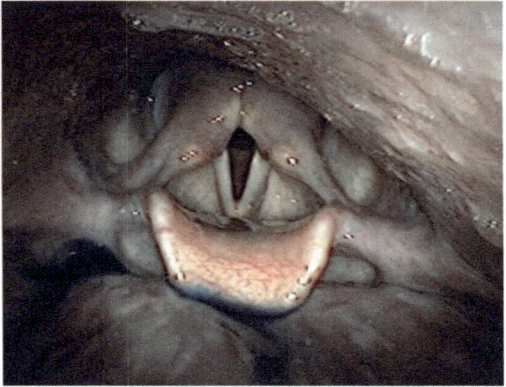

**Source: M. Farahat**

28. **Case Study Video 26.10**: Neurogenic dysphagia of a 64-year-old male patient who is recovering from haemorrhagic stroke that he had 8 weeks ago. FEES was performed 2 weeks post-insult and did not find any safe volumes or consistencies to be presented orally with high risk of developing aspiration pneumonia. The patient was NPO (*nil per os*) and put on nasogastric tube feeding for 8 weeks after which a second FEES was performed. The video shows this second FEES and a safe swallow of puree with an accumulation of residue in the valleculae and right piriform sinus. The patient was then switched to pureed and liquid food and over time learned to clear the residue with controlled bolus volumes and multiple dry swallows (not shown in the video).

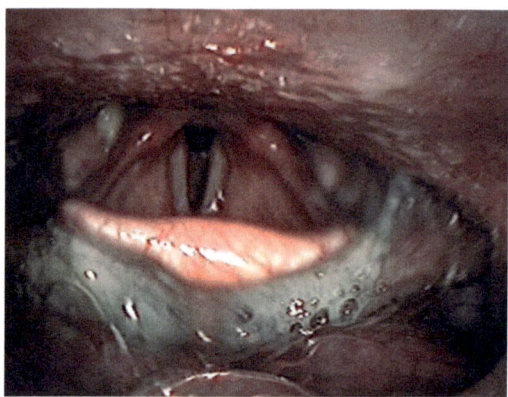

**Source: M. Farahat**

29. **Case Study Video 26.11**: Neurogenic dysphagia in a 69-year-old man who had undergone surgery to remove a tumour from the left cerebello-pontine angle 6 weeks previously and suffered from cranial nerve injury (pharyngeal plexus). Postoperatively, he started regurgitating food in the left side of the mouth, nasal tone, gurgling voice quality, and coughing with all types of food and drinks. The patient was fed via an NGT but developed aspiration pneumonia, following which a percutaneous endoscopic gastrostomy (PEG) tube was placed. The relatives insisted that nothing was fed to him by mouth, including fluids, but the nurse in charge noted

that the patient had poor oral hygiene. The short video shows an accumulation of foamy secretions in both valleculae, on the left pharyngeal wall and in the left piriform fossa, and that the patient was unable to control his own secretions. This case shows the importance of proper oral hygiene even in patients who are NPO (*nil per os*) to prevent the occurrence of aspiration pneumonia due to bacterial colonisation of the mouth that could be aspirated into the lungs.

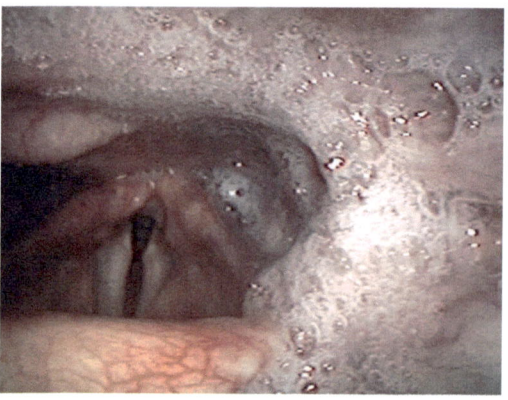

**Source: M. Farahat**

30. **Case Study Video 26.12**: Neurogenic dysphagia in a 52-year-old engineer who suffered an ischaemic stroke one month ago. He was properly treated and discharged from hospital after 2 weeks on regular oral diet. He suffered from an inability to manage soft mechanical consistencies (feeling like something was stuck at the back of his tongue and he had to wash it down with water if he could not swallow it). The video shows the swallowed small piece of bread on the right vallecula, and despite several attempts at dry swallowing, the patient was unable to remove it. The other thinner consistencies were unobjectionable. So the patient was instructed to take small bolus amounts of soft food to be chewed thoroughly and swallowed several times, and sips of thick liquids were allowed during meals to wash down any residues. In addition, the Masako manoeuvre was explained to the patient to practice at home.

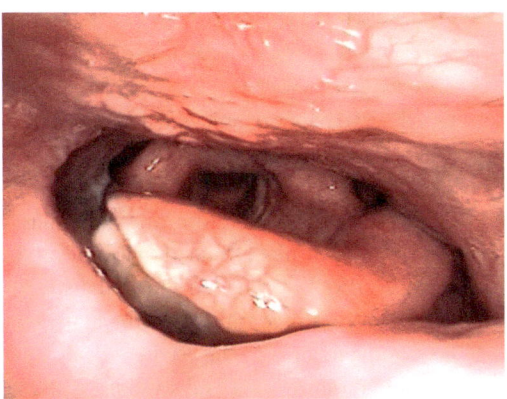

**Source: M. Farahat**

31. **Case Study Video 26.13**: Neurogenic dysphagia in a 56-year-old woman who had a traffic accident two months earlier. She was admitted to the intensive care unit and was intubated for 4 weeks. After extubation, she developed low saturation and a tracheostomy tube had to be inserted. She was fitted with a tracheal mask for 2 weeks and then gradually weaned off the tracheal tube within 2 weeks. She wore an NGT tube for 4 weeks and was then switched to a normal oral diet, but the primary team noted that she had an unclear chest with a low fever and referred her to the swallow team for assessment. The video shows a silent aspiration with thin fluid content. This demonstrates the impact of tracheostomy, endotracheal and NGT tubes on pharyngeal and laryngeal sensitivity. Thus, silent aspiration must always be watched for, even if caregivers or nursing staff claim that a patient is being fed without signs of choking.

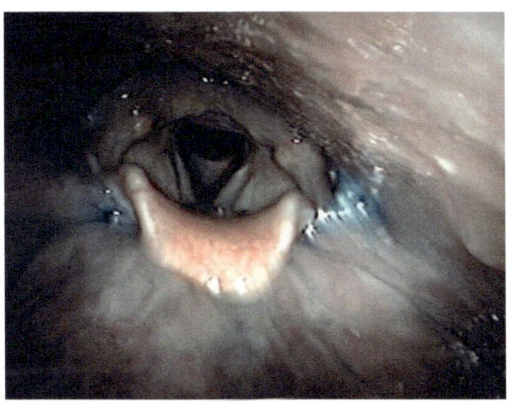

**Source: M. Farahat**

32. **Case Study Video 26.14**: A man with hypoxic brain injury after resuscitation for catecholaminergic polymorphic ventricular tachycardia (CPVT) due to a near drowning accident 2 years ago, treated with an implantable cardioverter defibrillator (ICD). The patient suffers from moderate mixed dysarthria with central paretic (spastic) and ataxic components and uses a compensatory ventricular fold voice. Initial dysphagia was treated with a percutaneous endoscopic gastrostomy tube for 3 months and gradually improved. The patient can now swallow food in all consistencies but needs time to do so. The video (without sound) shows his vocal fold use during phonation. Furthermore, it shows in the FEES prolonged transport times for liquid, puree, and solid food, an elongated swallowing reflex and temporary residuals in the valleculae (for liquids), the piriform sinuses and the retrocricoidal region as well as at the posterior pharyngeal wall for puree and solid consistencies. However, the patient always manages to clear completely in between and there is no penetration into the larynx and no aspiration.

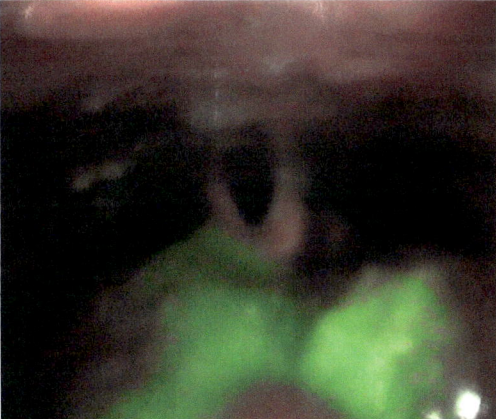

**Source: **Katrin Neumann**

33. **Case Study Video 28.1**: FEES of a women with normal swallowing conditions: The video shows nasal passage through the left side of the nasal cavity. The function of the velopharyngeal sphincter, tested during phonation and swallowing, is normal. There are

no structural abnormalities in the oropharynx, hypopharynx, and larynx. The women was asked to stick out the tongue to have a better view of the laryngeal cavity. Then she was asked to phonate /i:/ and count to five. Three consistencies were then tested. When swallowing a thickened liquid (white colour), four swallows were taken with no penetration, aspiration, or residue in the hypopharynx. The video then shows four swallows of liquid (green coloured water), then chewing and swallowing a cookie. At the end of the video, the backward passage from the hypopharyngeal and laryngeal view through the oropharynx and nasopharynx to the nasal cavity is shown.

34. **Case Study Video 30.1**: FEES of a 29-year-old woman after right-sided vestibular schwannoma surgery and postoperative facial nerve palsy, dysphagia, and dysphonia. She stated that she was not able to swallow after the surgery; she was coughing while drinking liquids. Therefore, she had a nasogastric tube in place. Functional oral intake scale (FOIS) 2. The video shows the stagnation of saliva in the right piriform sinus, limited movement of the right vocal fold, inefficient shift, and subsequent multiple swallowing of the concentrated fluid. By compensating the manoeuvre by tilting the head to the side of the paresis, the stagnation of the bolus and saliva is cleared.

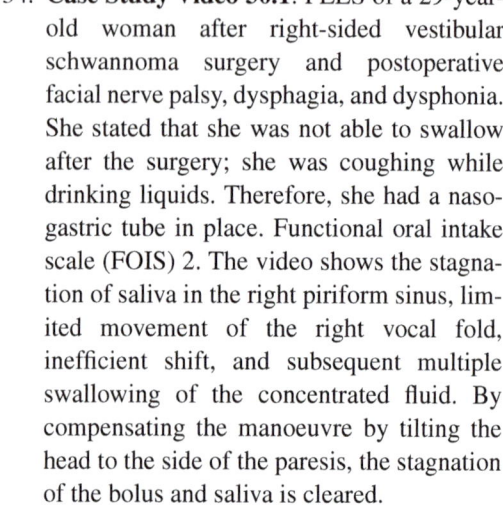

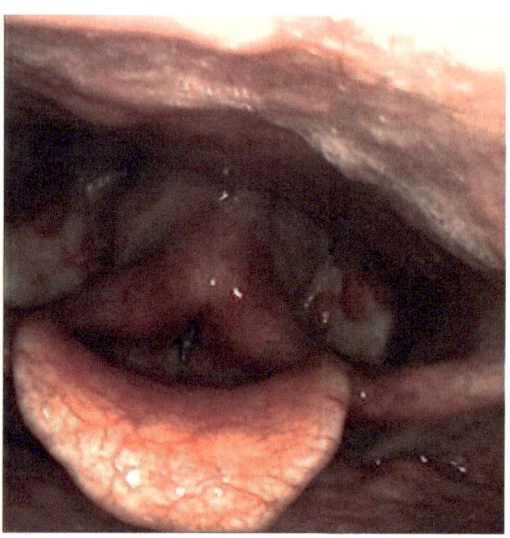

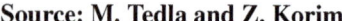

**Source: M. Tedla and Z. Korim**

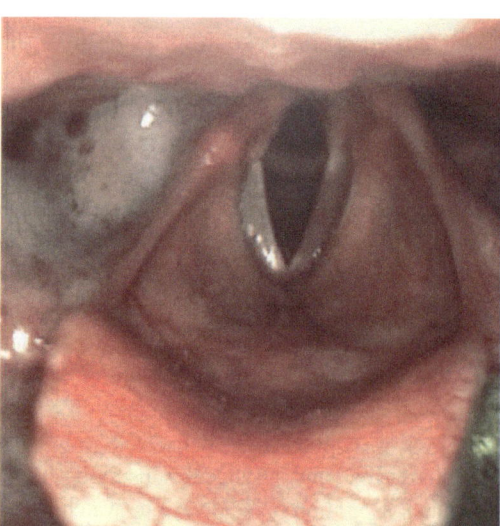

**Source: M. Tedla and Z. Korim**

# Index

A. am Zehnhoff-Dinnesen et al. (eds.), *Phoniatrics III*, European Manual of Medicine, https://doi.org/10.1007/978-3-031-48091-1